Interesting Facts and Quotes

"SEVENTY-FOUR per cent of the U.S. population 25 or older are overweight, up from 71 per cent just a year ago, 69 per cent in 1994, 66 per cent in 1992 and only 59 per cent 10 years ago, Louis Harris and Associates reported."
—*Associated Press*, Feb. 1996

BETTY Rollin of *NBC News* recently reported that baby boomers weigh more than their parents weighed at the same age.

"MEASURING changes in one's body composition . . . is very valuable. You can then alter your training and diet program accordingly."
—Arnold Schwarzenegger, *Encyclopedia of Modern Bodybuilding*

"IN THE next few years calorie charts will become available telling you how many calories you can eat based on your pounds of lean body mass."
—Covert Bailey, *The New Fit or Fat*, 1991

"AFTER THEY failed to achieve permanent weight control with conventional diets, I realized my clients needed what Covert Bailey predicted: up-to-date calorie charts to help them analyze their energy balance. Also, as Arnold suggested, they needed an easy way to measure their body composition. Having no other book to recommend, I wrote *The Body Fat Guide: The Easy Way to Analyze Your Body Composition and Energy Balance*."
—Ron Brown, Certified Fitness Trainer

Weight Lbs.	Waist % Fat %	Fat Lbs.	LBM Lbs.	BMR Cal.
100	10.49	10.49	89.51	1738
100.5	10.40	10.45	90.05	1245
101	10.30	10.41	90.59	1251
101.5	10.21	10.37	91.13	1350
108	10.12	10.33	91.67	1288
102.5	10.03	10.29	90.22	1275
109	9.95	10.24	92.76	1283
103.5	9.88	10.20	88.30	1290

Weight Lbs.	Waist % Fat %	Fat Lbs.	LBM Lbs.	BMR Cal.
100	10.49	10.49	89.51	1738
100.5	10.40	10.45	90.05	1245
101	10.30	10.41	90.59	1251
101.5	10.21	10.37	91.13	1350
108	10.12	10.33	91.67	1288
102.5	10.03	10.29	90.22	1275
109	9.95	10.24	92.76	1283
103.5	9.88	10.20	88.30	1290

THE BODY FAT GUIDE

THE BODY FAT GUIDE

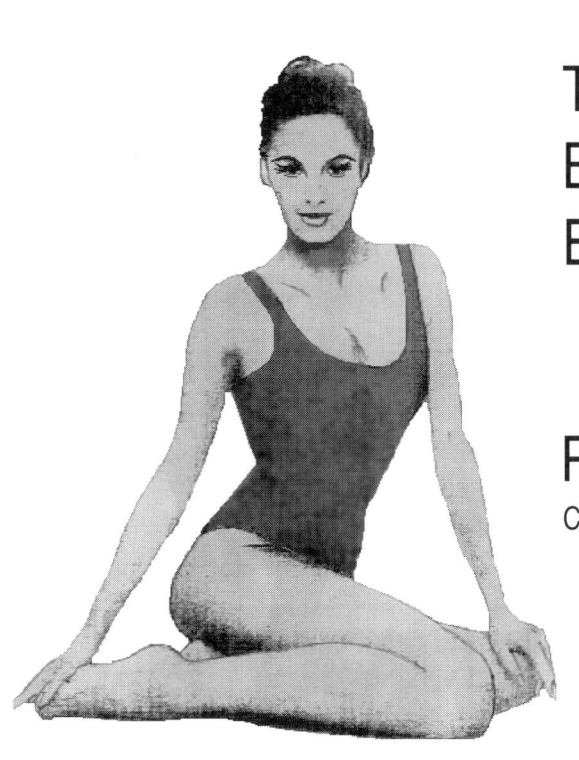

The Easy Way to Analyze Your
Body Composition and
Energy Balance

RON BROWN
CERTIFIED FITNESS TRAINER, NASM

HEALTH*STYLE*

Canadian Cataloguing in Publication Data

Brown, Ron, 1950–
    The body fat guide: the easy way to analyze your
body composition and energy balance

Includes bibliographical references and index.
ISBN 0–9681910–0–2

    1. Weight loss. 2. Health. 3. Physical fitness.
4. Nutrition. I. Title.

RA776.5B77 1997   613   C97–900270–2

Cover

Model: Nikki Novak

Makeup and Wardrobe: The Plutino Group

Photographers: David Benchitrit, Keith Penner (rear black and white)

Design: Scott Richardson

Prepress: Alko Graphics

Interior

Models: Lisa Maslanka, Helen Daniel, Sherry Parsons, Yovanca Summers

Photographers: Gee Wong, PKG Photography, Ron Brown

Copy Editor: Mary Pequegnat

Art Work, Page Layout and Index: Ron Brown

Printed in Canada

Distributed by BookWorld

1933 Whitfield Park Loop
Sarasota, FL 34243 USA
Orders: Tel: 800/444-2524, Fax: 800/777-2525
e-mail: sales@bookworld, www.bookworld.com

A 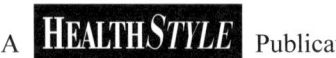 Publication

HEALTHSTYLE
250 Frederick Street, #805
Kitchener, Ontario, Canada N2H 2N1
Tel. & Fax: 519/578-2094

e-mail: healthst@home.com
Visit www.bodyfatguide.com

Table Of Contents

(Continued on next page)

Acknowledgments

Dedicated to my Father, who always kept me surrounded with books.

THANKS TO THE following people for their guidance, support and assistance during the preparation of this book:
Helen Daniel, Mary Pequegnat, Sherry Parsons, Lisa Maslanka, Roxolana Sawka, Marianne Wiens, Nikki Novak, The Plutino Group, Elmer Olsen and Elite Modeling Agency, David Benchitrit, Alko Graphics, Scott Richardson, Best Book Manufacturers, Ralph Schmidt and A Bit Better Computers, PKG Photography and Gee Wong.

Thanks to my family and to all my fitness clients who were the inspiration for this book. Also thanks to all the authors, doctors, health care professionals, athletes, journalists and scientists listed in the Bibliography who provided the valuable information that formed the basis for this book.

Finally, I would like to acknowledge the assistance of the numerous reference materials and desktop publishing tools that gave me the confidence and skill to write and publish this book. Particularly valuable were Microsoft Office (besides writing the text on Microsoft Word, the Body Composition Tables in this book were generated on Excel spreadsheets), Adobe PageMaker, and the works of Dan Poynter and Avery Cardoza.

Author's Note

WARNING: THE information in this book is not intended to be used as a substitute for therapeutic care. The author and publisher assume no responsibility for any adverse effect on your health that may result from the application of the information in this book, and shall not be held responsible for any claims attributable to errors, omissions, or inaccuracies.

The Body Composition Tables in this book are not intended for children and should not be used by pregnant women. Children and pregnant women should never be placed on a weight-loss diet unless under the care of a physician.

Consult your physician before attempting the diet and exercise program outlined in this book.

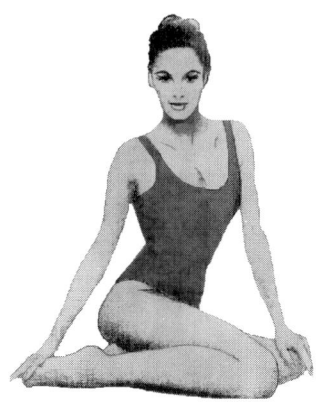

"Like having a personal trainer at your fingertips!"

Introduction

What This Book Can Do for You

- How much of your body is muscle?
- How much of your body is fat?
- How much weight do you need to lose?
- How much should you eat?
- How much should you exercise?

FOR THE first time, the answers to all these questions are contained in one book. *The Body Fat Guide* is the world's first book to analyze your body weight to the nearest $1/100^{th}$ of a pound of fat and muscle. As well, it analyzes your daily energy requirement to the nearest calorie. And it only takes seconds to look it up! There are no confusing calculations. What's more, it provides information that is more accurate than Body Mass Index tables.

You don't need to fuss with skin-fold calipers, electrical gadgets or expensive laboratory equipment. All that is required is a tape measure and a bathroom scale. Everything else you need to get started is in this book.

The Body Fat Guide explains how you can reshape your body by changing the ratio of your body fat to muscle. Did you know you could become leaner by gaining the right kind of weight? Or fatter by losing the wrong kind of weight? *The Body Fat Guide* will make it all clear to you. It's like having a personal trainer at your finger tips!

The information in this book is based on sound scientific principles of nutrition, anatomy, kinesiology and physiology. Much of this information is not new—it has been known by the experts for a long time. Unfortunately, few of these experts have had their findings successfully conveyed into an applicable program for the general public— until now!

In addition to a program that is simple, safe and effective, the public requires the hands-on guidance of a personal trainer who is comfortable working with people. Being pleasant, entertaining, sympathetic and encouraging to people, however, is only part of the requirements of a trainer. A motivating personal trainer or self-proclaimed fitness expert who lacks a scientific background is as compromised as an academic expert who lacks empathy for people and their problems.

The mission of this book is to combine the best of both scientific knowledge and friendly, practical training advice into one system.

Getting and staying in shape is rewarding and fun when done properly, but if it isn't a pleasurable experience, you won't stick with it. Following a program like the one offered in this book will make achieving permanent weight control a pleasurable challenge and a rewarding experience.

Weight Loss and Health

ACCORDING TO Dr. Philip James, chair of a World Health Organization task force on obesity:

> "We have a huge epidemic and a disaster on our hands . . . Obesity is doubling every five years."

Being overweight contributes to much physical and mental suffering in our society. A study by the U. S. Centers for Disease Control and Prevention, released in 1997, indicates that 34.9% of U.S. adults are dangerously overweight. Former U.S. Surgeon General C. Everett Coop claims that obesity causes the loss of 300,000 U. S. lives every year. He states that obesity is the second leading preventable cause of death in the U.S., just behind cigarette smoking.

Adult-onset diabetes, heart disease, hypertension, back problems, lower limb osteoarthritis and other types of arthritis are some of the physical conditions caused or exacerbated by being overweight.

The primary and preferred medical treatment for these conditions, before drugs and surgery, is weight loss and life-style modification of diet and activity. By providing you with an easy way to analyze your body weight, and by showing you the proper way to monitor and adjust your diet and activity, this book can point you toward improved health.

"For temporary weight loss, just run your body on less food.
But for permanent weight control, learn how your body runs on food."

Don't expect to have an attractive, trim, fit and healthy body without putting in the time or effort to get it. The proper way to permanently control your weight requires work, not quick fixes. It takes more than just *running* your body on less food. You need to learn how your body *runs* on food.

The Body Fat Guide will help you. It will teach you how to balance your body's flow of energy and improve your body composition, regardless of whether you want to lose, gain or just maintain your weight. There's also a section on how to tone, shape and strengthen your body—without using any special exercise equipment!

At last, you have a dependable guide through the maze of dieting misinformation, guesswork and quick fix rip-offs. No longer will you have to settle for the disappointment of temporary weight loss. *The Body Fat Guide* shows you the one proper way to permanently control your weight. From an elite athlete to a couch potato, everyone will benefit from this book. As indispensable as a dictionary and a bathroom scale, every home needs a copy of *The Body Fat Guide*.

PART ONE: DIET and EXERCISE GUIDE

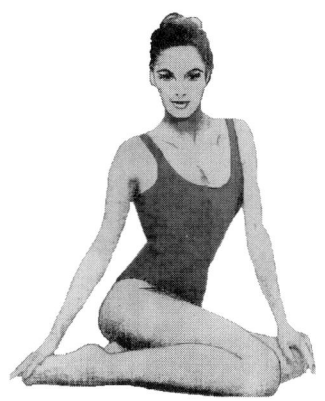

"Take a few seconds to look up your body fat level."

Chapter 1

Quick Checkup

How Fat Are You?

"How fat am I? I don't want to know!"

IF YOU ARE thinking something similar to the above statement, and you are feeling anxious and intimidated, don't worry. You will probably be interested in skipping ahead to the next chapter, *Pounds Don't Count*. It will encourage you with a fresh point of view. Otherwise, if you have the stomach for it (yes, that was intended to be a pun), read on.

This book contains Body Composition Tables that allow you to instantly and accurately analyze your level of muscle and body fat to the nearest ¹/₁₀₀th of a pound. If you wish, you can quickly check your body fat level now by using the following directions:

In the Table of Contents, find the section in Part Two of this book that lists your sex and weight class. Turn to that section and proceed to the page that lists your waist size across the top of the page. Waist sizes are listed in numerical order in differences of ¹/₄ of an inch. If your weight or waist size is not listed, turn to the section titled *Special Weight Class— Male and Female*, page 294.

On the page with your waist size, find your weight in the column on the left. Move to the right in the row with your weight until you are in the box under your waist size. The number in the first of the four columns of that box is your percentage body fat. Healthy adult males should have no higher than approximately 15% body fat and healthy adult females should have no higher than approximately 22% body fat.

Weight Lbs.	Waist 99 inches			
	Fat %	Fat Lbs.	LBM Lbs.	BMR Cal.
100	10.49	10.49	89.51	1236
100.5	10.40	10.45	90.05	1245
101	10.30	10.41	90.59	1253
101.5	10.21	10.37	91.13	1250
102	10.12	10.33	91.67	1268
102.5	10.03	10.29	92.22	1274
103	9.95	10.24	92.76	1283
103.5	9.88	10.20	93.30	1290

Weight Lbs.	Waist 99 inches			
	Fat %	Fat Lbs.	LBM Lbs.	BMR Cal.
100	10.49	10.49	89.51	1236
100.5	10.40	10.45	90.05	1245
101	10.30	10.41	90.59	1253
101.5	10.21	10.37	91.13	1250
102	10.12	10.33	91.67	1268
102.5	10.03	10.29	92.22	1274
103	9.95	10.24	92.76	1283
103.5	9.88	10.20	93.30	1290

What Do You Do Now?

YOU HAVE two choices:

1. Put this book on the shelf to collect dust and pull it out every now and then to check your percentage body fat.

2. Plan a course of action to make some changes.

But before you consider doing anything drastic, continue reading through Part One of this book. Part One consists of a Diet and Exercise Guide. It will give you a better understanding of how your percentage body fat affects your health and appearance, and it will show you what you can do about it. You will learn the secrets of permanent weight control, and you will learn how to change your body by altering your body fat and muscle levels. As you make specific diet and activity adjustments, the Body Composition Tables analyze the effect of your adjustments. This is the most effective way to work toward your body weight goals.

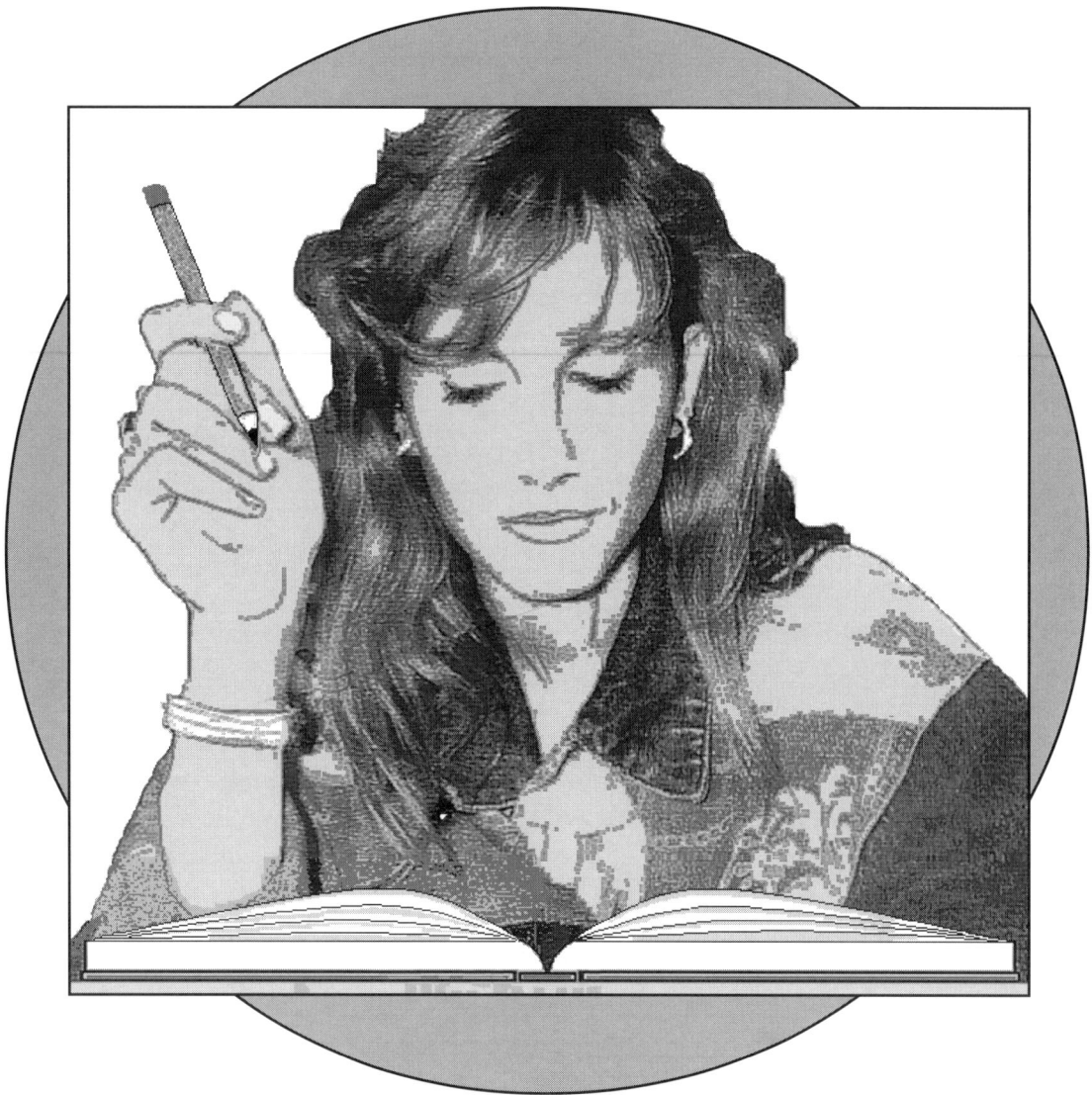

The Body Fat Guide is a quick, easy and inexpensive way to look up your body composition and energy requirements.

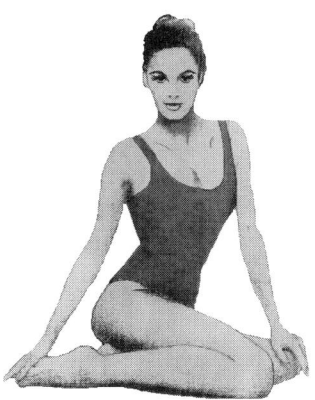

"You could be large and lean or thin and flabby!"

Chapter 2

Pounds Don't Count

A New Way to Watch Your Weight

- Are you thinking of taking off a few pounds?
- Did you know you could become leaner by *gaining* weight?
- Would you like to be thin?
- Did you know becoming thinner could make you *fatter*?
- Do you weigh the same as you weighed when you were younger?
- Did you know you may have *gained* body fat even though the scale says you haven't?

IF YOU are surprised by any of these statements, you, and millions of others like you, are being tricked and misled by counting pounds. That's right, watching your weight by counting pounds is preventing you from achieving your optimum body weight. There's a new and better way to watch your weight.

A Pound Is a Pound

WHICH WEIGHS more, a pound of gold coins or a pound of feathers? Since a pound is a pound, it doesn't matter whether you are comparing gold, feathers or whatever, a pound of something always weighs as much as a pound of something else. It just takes a greater volume of feathers than gold coins to add up to a pound. On a pound for pound basis, a small stack of gold coins and a large bundle of feathers are equal, even though gold is essentially different from feathers.

The same is true of your body fat and muscle. Even though they weigh the same, a pound of body fat looks and functions differently than a pound of muscle. A pound of body fat is less dense than a pound of muscle, so it takes up more space on your figure than a pound of muscle.

15

All Pounds Are Not Created Equal

WHAT GOOD is knowing how many total pounds you weigh if you don't know how many of those pounds are body fat and how many of them are muscle? What good is taking off a few pounds if it is mostly valuable muscle? What good is fighting a weight gain if it is useful lean tissue? How can you tell the difference between pounds of muscle and pounds of body fat? A pound of muscle may weigh the same as a pound of body fat, but, like comparing a pound of gold to a pound of feathers, they have little else in common. Measuring your weight in pounds simply does not give you the kind of information you need to effectively guide you in determining your proper weight.

Thin Isn't the Same As Lean

SIZE ALONE doesn't give you the true inside story either. You could be large and lean or thin and flabby—heavy and firm or light and fat. This book offers you a way to separate the lean from the fat, regardless of what shape you are in and regardless of whether you want to lose body fat, gain muscle, or do both. You will learn a new way to watch your weight. So forget about pounds. From now on *pounds don't count!*

Percentage Body Fat—The Inside Story

YOUR BODY is composed of two main ingredients: body fat, and everything else. A term used to describe the part of your body that isn't body fat is *lean body mass* or *LBM*. While LBM includes bone, blood and internal organs, lean body mass gains and losses mentioned in this book usually refer only to skeletal muscle (muscle attached to

bone). The combined amount of your body fat and LBM makes up your *body composition.*

Your *percentage body fat* is the percent of your body composition that is fat—the amount of body fat you have in relation to your total body weight. The more you increase your weight by adding body fat, the more your percentage body fat increases. The more you decrease your weight by reducing body fat, the more your percentage body fat decreases.

However, if your weight goes *up* because you are gaining muscle instead of body fat, your percentage body fat goes *down.* That's how gaining weight can make you leaner. If your weight goes *down,* and you are losing more muscle than body fat, as often happens on a quick fix, crash diet, your percentage body fat goes *up.* That's how getting thin can actually make you fatter. Even if your weight stays the same, you could be exchanging muscle for body fat and thus changing your percentage body fat either *up* or *down.* Sound confusing?

The following example illustrates how changes in your percentage body fat occur, and it explains how these changes affect your body's appearance.

The Painted Balloon

IMAGINE YOUR body is an air-filled painted balloon. The amount of air inside represents your LBM, or your lean body mass, and the paint covering the balloon represents your layer of subcutaneous body fat, which lies under your skin and over your muscles. As you increase the air inside the balloon, the layer of paint stretches out over a greater area and appears thinner. This thinning effect is what happens to your subcutaneous body fat when you gain LBM as muscle. Your

The Painted Balloon

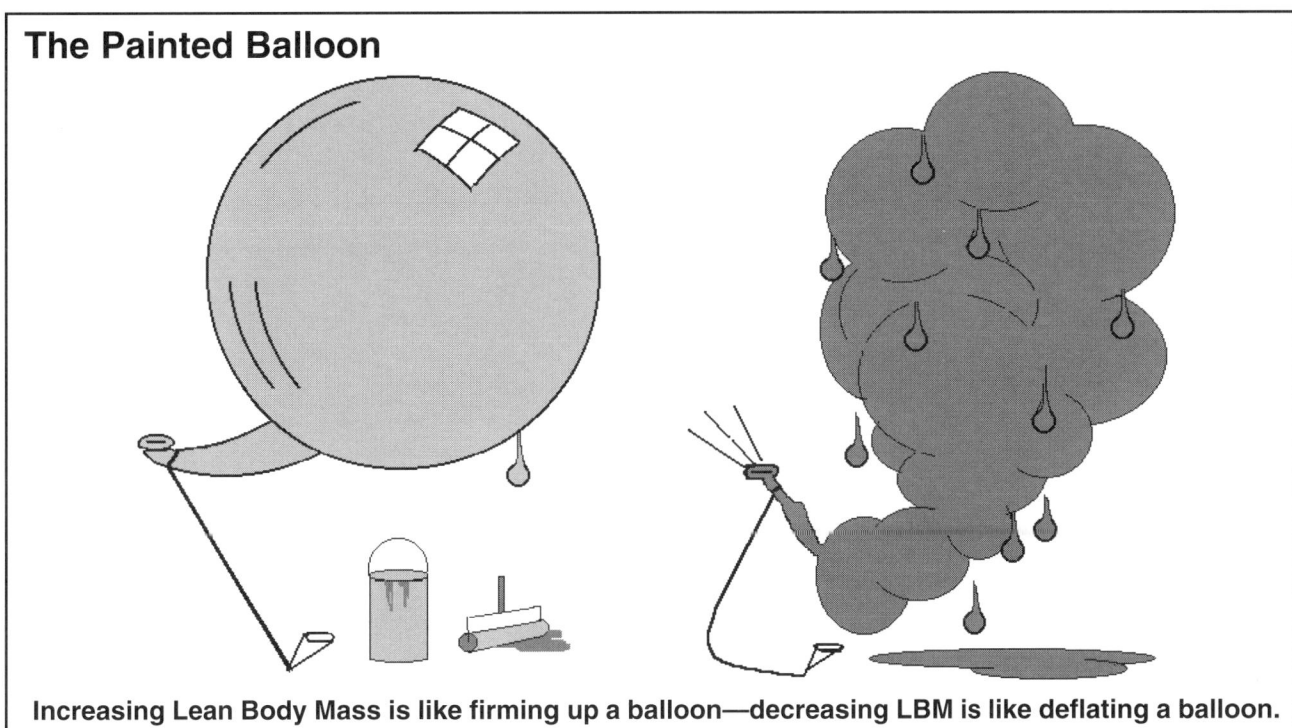

Increasing Lean Body Mass is like firming up a balloon—decreasing LBM is like deflating a balloon.

percentage body fat decreases and you look leaner and firmer—*toned.*

Whether you realize it or not, whenever you refer to "toning" your body, you are really referring to the process of maintaining or increasing your LBM with muscle-building exercise—exactly like a bodybuilder, although perhaps not to the same degree. This book will show you how to do that.

What happens when you let air out of the painted balloon? It sags and the paint looks thicker. This is the same effect that occurs to your body when you lose more muscle than body fat—for example, while crash dieting. Your body sags and your body fat looks thicker. The lean appearance of your body is diminished—you have increased your percentage body fat. Often, people misinterpret this change in body appearance as a failure to burn body fat. They may stubbornly continue on with even more crash dieting, which makes matters worse.

What people need is an easy way to analyze their body composition so they can estimate their percentage body fat. Then, as they attempt to lose body fat, tone, strengthen muscle and shape their bodies, they can make accurate adjustments in their diet and activity level. This will allow them to progress towards their goals faster and easier. By getting you to focus on your percentage body fat, this book will teach you a new, more accurate way to watch your weight. You will achieve your body weight goals faster and easier than you ever thought possible.

Quick, Easy and Accurate

THERE ARE many scientific methods available to the public that are good indicators of one's body composition and percentage body fat. Some methods are more accurate than others, but few are completely error-free. Besides being expensive and time consuming, many methods require special equipment as well as the assistance of another person to measure you. Such methods, although usually very accurate, may not serve you well in the long-run if you can't afford them or you don't have instant access to them on a regular basis.

Finding a method you can use consistently and easily to quickly note changes in your body composition is just as important as finding one that is accurate. Such a method is presented in this book. Noting *changes* in body fat and muscle levels is often more important than estimating the precise amount of your body fat and muscle. Noting changes is a reliable indictor of the effectiveness of your diet and exercise program, or lack of one, and can guide you in making adjustments.

No Calipers, Electrodes or Water Tanks

THIS BOOK does not require you to fuss with skin-fold calipers; a device that pinches a fold of your skin to measure the thickness of your subcutaneous body fat (**A**). No one likes to get pinched, anyway! Besides, it is very easy to misuse skin-fold calipers and get readings that are not consistent or accurate.

(A) **Calipers**

(B) **Bioelectrical Impedance**

(C) **Hydrostatic Weighing**

You also do not need to hook electrodes to your body, as in bioelectrical impedance testing (**B**), or dunk your body into a tank of water, as in hydrostatic weighing (**C**).

Body Composition Tables provided in this book allow you to instantly look up your percentage body fat and other body composition information. You need not do complicated calculations to figure out your percentage body fat. You can complete your measurements by yourself and look up your body composition information quickly, conveniently and inexpensively.

Body Mass Index

IN THE PAST, many people relied upon Body Mass Index tables to determine their proper weight. Based simply on weight and height (weight/height^2), while ignoring individual differences in body fat percentages, Body Mass Index tables alone are too general to help you determine your ideal body weight. Similarly, Metropolitan Life Insurance tables, which average together weight, height and mortality, are also limited.

This book gives you more specific information about your weight by allowing you to zero-in on changes in your body composition to the nearest $^1/_{100}$th of a pound of body fat and muscle. So, if you choose to describe your weight by pounds instead of by body fat percentage, you will be able to specify the type of pounds you are describing: pounds of body fat or pounds of muscle.

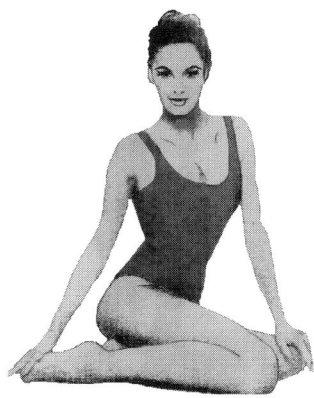

"Few people can guess their way to permanent weight control."

Chapter 3

How to Use This Book

The Energy Balance Chart

THE BALANCE between your energy output and your calorie intake is called your *energy balance*. An Energy Balance Chart is provided on page 295. You have permission to make photocopies of this chart if you need them. Page 297 shows you how to create an Electronic Energy Balance Chart that automatically calculates your body composition and energy balance information for you. This chapter explains how to use the Energy Balance Chart. A sample of the chart, reduced in size, is illustrated here:

Energy Balance Chart										
MEASUREMENTS			BODY COMPOSITION			ENERGY OUTPUT				CALORIE INTAKE	
Date	Weight	Waist	Fat	Fat	LBM	RMR	+ Activity Calories		= Total	Diet	Net
Month/Day	Lb.	Inches	%	Lb.	Lb.	Calories	Aerobic	Anaerobic	Calories	Calories	+/-

On your chart, you will record your daily:
• *measurements*
• *body composition*
• *energy output*
• *calorie intake*

Continue using the Energy Balance Chart until you have learned to control your energy balance and body composition with proper eating and activity habits. How long will that take? A few days, a few weeks, several months—it doesn't matter. It will take as long as it takes.

Measurements

THE FIRST heading on the Energy Balance Chart is **MEASUREMENTS**. Begin by filling in the date under this heading. The next column to the right of the date is where you record your weight. Yes, you will have to weigh yourself, but do not despair. Hopefully, you have gotten the message by now that your pounds of body weight is meaningless by itself.

MEASUREMENTS		
Date	Weight	Waist
Month/Day	Lb.	Inches
1/7	154.5	

If possible, record your weight to the nearest half-pound. Many newer scales today display body weight, digitally, in half-pounds. If you

19

can, obtain a strain-gage scale to weigh yourself. They are more accurate.

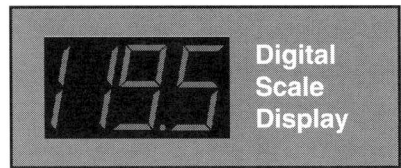

**Digital
Scale
Display**

At first, you will be weighing and recording your measurements every day.

Important—*Do not go into a panic over small daily fluctuations in your measurements. Pay more attention to changes that last over several days.*

This does not mean, however, that you should ignore taking your daily measurements. You need to learn to distinguish daily fluctuations from real body fat gains. To do that, you have to begin with daily monitoring. Remember, it only takes one day of overeating to produce body fat. Why wait several days to check it?

In the past, you may have been encouraged not to weigh yourself more than once a week when following a weight-loss diet. That may work for temporary weight-loss purposes. However, the purpose of this book is to teach you permanent weight control. You will create your own custom-designed diet and exercise program that is based on your total daily energy requirements. This goes far beyond a simple weight-loss plan. Once you have set up your program and have successfully changed your living habits to achieve and maintain your ideal body weight, you may only occasionally need to check your body weight and body composition information.

Since your weight will normally fluctuate throughout the day, try to schedule your daily weigh-in to a consistent time of the day. Most people weigh themselves first thing in the morning.

Your Waistline

NEXT TO your weight, under the **MEASUREMENTS** heading on the Energy Balance Chart, record your waist size to the nearest quarter of an inch. Obtain an accurate tape measure (surprisingly, they do

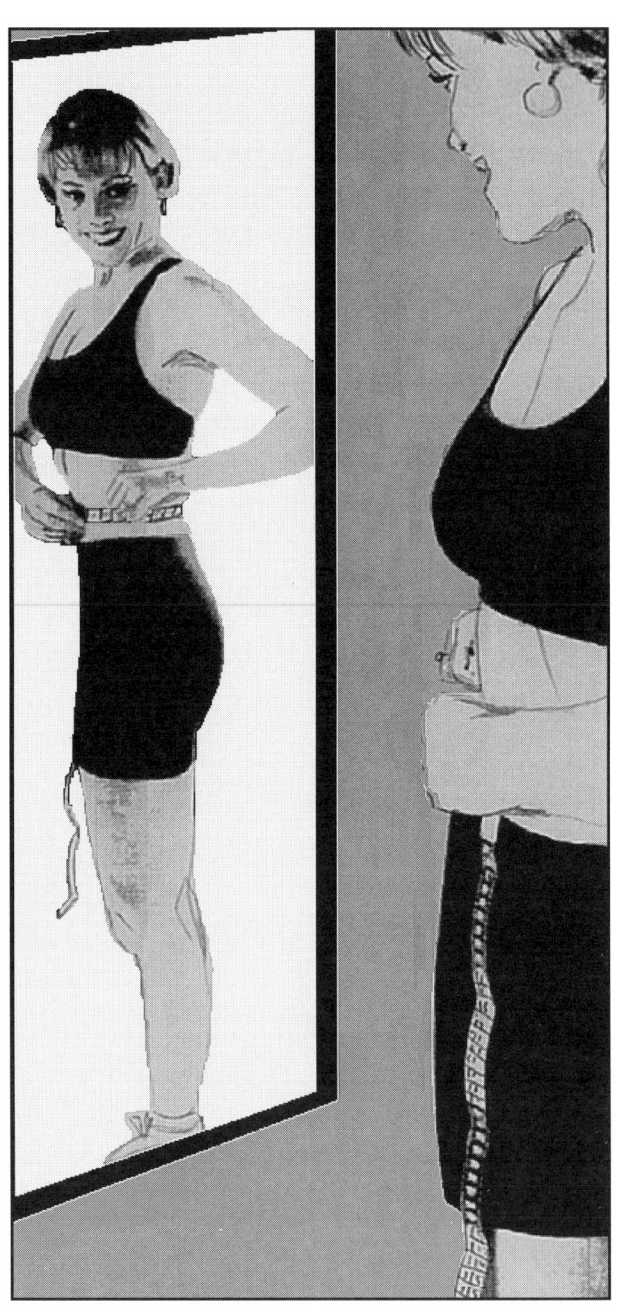

Check your waist measurement by standing sideways in front of a mirror. Make sure the tape is level from front to back.

not all measure the same!) and *measure your waistline at the level of your navel.*

MEASUREMENTS		
Date	Weight	Waist
Month/Day	Lb.	Inches
1/7	154.5	29.25

(Note: See page 302 for metric conversion.)

Many people are tempted to place the measuring tape several inches higher than their waistline, at the narrower portion of their torso known as the *midriff.* No, no! Ideally, your waistline should be the narrowest portion of your torso (figure below, left). However, as you gain body fat, your waist expands faster than your midriff, so your midriff becomes the narrowest portion of your torso (figure below, right). But just because you buckle your belt there, that doesn't mean it is your real waistline. Eventually, if you lower your percentage body fat enough, your true navel-level

waistline will become narrower than your midriff, like on a clothes-store mannequin.

Do not suck in your stomach or pull the measuring tape too tight when measuring your waist. Stand up straight and tall. When released, the tape should gently fall away from your body without springing out across the room. Regardless of the accuracy of your waist-measuring technique, it is important not to vary the way you take your waist measurements from day to day. Consistency in your waist-measuring technique will give you readings that are a reliable indication of any *changes* in your waist size.

Day to day changes in your waist size may indicate a change in your body composition. Even if your waistline is not your problem area, measuring changes in the size of your

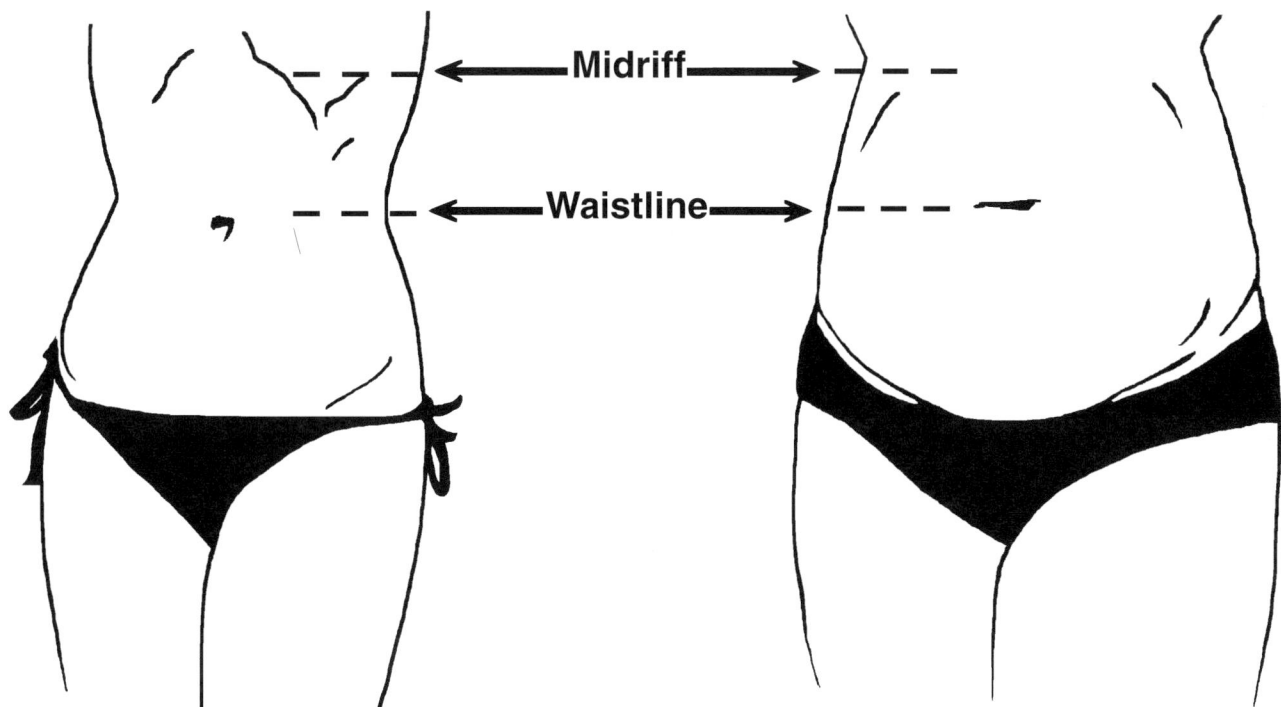

As your body fat increases, your waistline expands and your midriff gradually becomes the narrowest portion of your torso—but that doesn't mean you should measure your waist at your midriff.

waist will indicate relative body fat changes throughout the rest of your body.

Since there is little bone in the area of your waist (just your spinal column), your general bone size—their thickness and length—hardly affects your waistline. So do not blame your large girth on your "heavy bones." Methods of body composition analysis that use hip size can be misleading. You can not distinguish how much of your hip measurement is due to bone size and how much is due to body fat.

Being tall or having a large frame does not entitle you to carry a higher percentage body fat. Although you may weigh more and carry more pounds of body fat than a shorter or smaller framed person, your percentage body fat should be no higher.

Generally, *a gain or loss of one pound of body fat will change your waist size by about ¼ of an inch.* It takes a gain or loss of 12 pounds of muscle to change your waist size by an equal amount. Like your weight, your waist size varies throughout the day, so measure it at the same time of each day—at your designated weigh-in, preferably in the morning.

There may be times when your waist size will be larger or smaller than expected at your weigh-in simply because of changes in your eating schedule. Changing the normal timing of a meal can result in a greater or lesser amount of food lying in your gastrointestinal tract at weigh-in, even if your overall daily amount of food remains the same. This can temporarily throw off your waist measurement. For example, if you eat your normal dinner several hours later than usual, you may wake up the next morning with a slightly larger waistline, even though you haven't eaten more than your usual amount of food for the day.

Levels of gastrointestinal contents can also be affected by constipation, gas, the quantity of fiber in your diet, diarrhea, dehydration—all this may temporarily alter your waist size.

Fluid Retention

AS YOU LEARN to interpret how your energy balance affects your body composition, you may discover that changes in your weight and waist size are not always due to changes in your body fat or muscle, nor to changes in gastrointestinal contents. Body weight changes may be due to temporary bloating from fluid retention. This often results from eating foods containing added sodium chloride—common table salt.

When you eat salt, your body retains excess water to dilute it, thus lessening salt's harmful effect on your tissues. Salt diluted with water creates a brine that is stored throughout your body. This brine remains in your system until your kidneys and other excretory organs can eliminate it. An ounce of salt requires about 96 times its own weight in water to be held in solution in your body. The average person eating the conventional diet of modern western society may have 3–4 ounces of sodium chloride in their body. This means the average person may be retaining as much as 16–24 pounds of excess water (2–3 gallons)! People who remove sodium chloride from their diet rapidly lose much of this weight.

Fluid retention may occur as part of a woman's menstrual cycle—bloating associated with premenstrual syndrome or PMS. Indirectly, this bloating may be due more to temporary changes in a woman's eating habits than to direct hormonal changes. There may be cravings for stimulating foods, including foods processed with salt. Many women have reduced or eliminated monthly bloating by following a program that includes exercise and a low-salt diet of natural, unrefined foods.

Steroids: Growth or Bloat?

FLUID RETENTION may also result from drug use. For example, consider this hypothesis explaining how synthetic steroids affect your body: Steroids produce intramuscular bloating by absorbing into the muscle cell membrane and blocking the muscle cell's ability to excrete liquid cellular waste. The resulting increase in muscle size would be due to bloating from the retention of this liquid waste, not from genuine biosynthesis of new tissue. Although these drugs are used medically to help patients gain weight, the extra weight gained may not be real muscle growth. Bloat is not the same as growth.

Muscle bloating from using steroids would affect the muscle cells in your face and abdomen and would give you a puffy face while altering your natural waist size. Bodybuilders who alter their physiques in this way are destroying the natural aesthetic appeal of having a trim waist in proportion to the rest of their physique. In addition, here are some other adverse effects of steroid use:

1. Cardiovascular disease.
2. Liver disease.
3. Reproductive disease.
4. Impaired immune response.
5. Behavioral changes.

Is it Body Fat, Muscle, Food or Fluid?

WHEN ESTIMATING your body composition, always consider which of the following factors are affecting your daily weight and waistline measurements:

1. Changes in body fat and muscle levels.
2. Changes in gastrointestinal contents.
3. Fluid retention from salt and drugs.

Oh yes, there could be one more reason why your waist size and weight are increasing:

Important—*If you are pregnant, or if you think you are pregnant, do not use your weight and waist measurements to analyze your body composition as described in this book.*

Body Composition—The Tables

THE NEXT section on the Energy Balance Chart is titled **BODY COMPOSITION**. You will record your body composition information under this heading after referring to the Body Composition Tables in Part Two of this book. Check the Table of Contents to locate the table in your body weight class.

BODY COMPOSITION		
Fat	Fat	LBM
%	Lb.	Lb.

The science of measuring the human body is known as *anthropometry*. The Body Composition Tables in this book are based on accurate anthropometric formulas developed by the research of two scientists, J. H. Wilmore and A. T. Benke.* These Body Composition Tables were specially prepared by the author and are appearing in this book for the first time anywhere. It is important to note that they are intended for normal adults only and *are not applicable to children. Neither are they intended for pregnant females.* If you are an adult, are not pregnant, and your weight or waist size is not listed in the Body Composition Tables, turn to the section titled *Special Weight Class—Male and Female*, page 294, and follow the directions there.

*Source: Myers, C. and Sinning, W. E. *Y's Way to Physical Fitness: The Complete Guide to Fitness Testing and Instruction.* 3rd Edition. 1989.

The figure below illustrates a sample from the Body Composition Tables for Males.

Body Composition MALE 152–183.5 Lb.

Weight: Lb.	Waist: 29 inches				29.25 inches			
	Fat: %	Fat: Lb.	LBM: Lb.	RMR: Cal.	Fat: %	Fat: Lb.	LBM: Lb.	RMR: Cal.
152	6.23	9.47	142.53	1971	6.91	10.50	141.50	1957
152.5	6.18	9.42	143.08	1979	6.86	10.46	142.04	1964
153	6.13	9.38	143.62	1986	6.81	10.42	142.58	1972
153.5	6.09	9.34	144.16	1994	6.76	10.38	143.12	1979
154	6.04	9.30	144.70	2001	6.71	10.34	143.66	1987
154.5	5.99	9.26	145.24	2009	6.67	10.30	144.20	1994
155	5.95	9.22	145.78	2016	6.62	10.26	144.74	2002

Notice, each waist size sits on top of a box that contains headings to four vertical columns. Before describing what these headings mean, notice the separate column on the left side of the table. This column lists your weight by half-pounds. In this column, find the row with your weight and move directly to the right in that row until you come to the box under your waist size. Note the four numbers in that box. The first three of these numbers are transferred to the Energy Balance Chart. Enter them into their respective places, as

BODY COMPOSITION		
Fat	Fat	LBM
%	Lb.	Lb.
6.67	10.30	144.20

shown in the figure above, under the heading: **BODY COMPOSITION**.

The number in the first column of the box from the Body Composition Table is under the column heading:

Fat: %

This is your percentage body fat. It tells you what percentage of your total body weight is fat. This number is useful for setting and maintaining health and

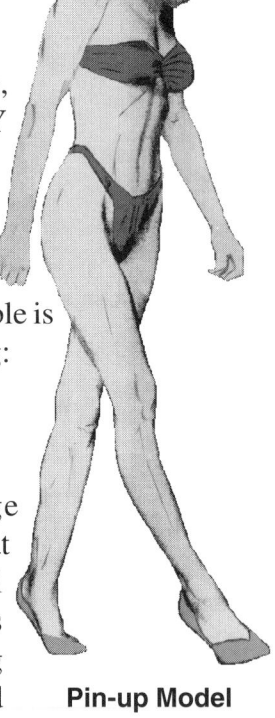

Pin-up Model

Body Fat Percentages of Models

FEMALE PIN-UP models, and "glamour" stars who are known for their figures, tend to have body fat percentages at the lower end of normal. In her early career, Marilyn Monroe's waist measured 23½ inches and her weight was 118 pounds, putting her at just under 10% body fat.

The average weight of all the women who have posed for *Playboy* centerfolds since Marilyn Monroe, who appeared as the first centerfold, is 115 pounds. Their average waist size is 23 inches—average height, 5 foot 6 inches. Similar to Marilyn Monroe, the centerfolds also averaged around 10% body fat. The illustration above shows a woman at 10% body fat.

Measuring 3 inches taller, at a basic minimum height of 5 foot 9 inches, today's female fashion model averages 110 pounds. Claudia Schiffer represents the ideal *healthy* model (not emaciated). Weighing 126 pounds, with a 24 inch waist, she is taller than Marilyn Monroe and most *Playboy* centerfolds, but still maintains 10% body fat.

Athletes, like the one illustrated on the next page, often have low body fat percentages, bottoming out as low as 3% or less for males and 6% for females. Arnold Schwarzenegger competed as a world-class champion bodybuilder with a body fat percentage between 3–4%.

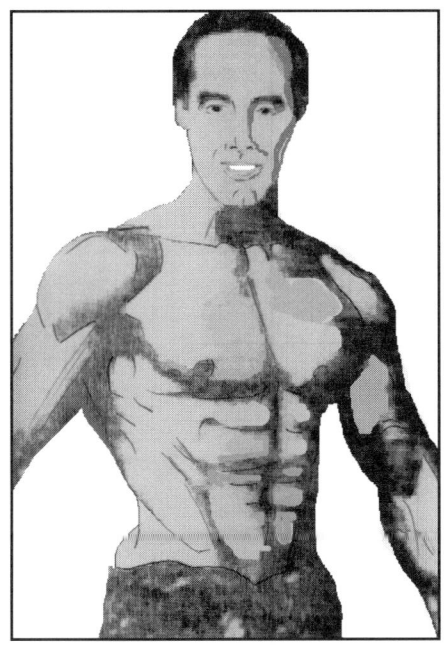

Athlete

fitness goals. For example, physiologists have determined that normal body fat percentages are no higher than approximately 15% for males, and 22% for females. Averages are unfortunately higher than that at 23% for males and 32% for females. *Obesity* is defined as 20% over "ideal" body weight. Taking 15% and 22% body fat as ideals, obesity starts at 29% body fat for males and 35% for females.

There are conflicting views on how low a percentage body fat one may safely attain. Apparently, the manner in which one reduces and maintains a low percentage body fat plays a large part in this. Dieting on coffee, cigarettes and diet pills is not recommended.

Physiologists estimate the human body's reserve of *essential body fat* to be around 3% of total body weight. Essential body fat is found around your internal organs, as part of your nervous system and within all your body's cell membranes. Unlike subcutaneous body fat under your skin, essential body fat is hardly reduced, even in death by starvation.

The number in the second column of the box from the Body Composition Table is under the column heading:

Fat: Lb.

This is your amount of body fat listed by pounds. This specifically indicates changes in only your body fat level. Your body fat cells may change in size and increase in number, but they can't decrease in number (except by surgery) or change into muscle cells.

The number in the third column of the box is under the column heading:

LBM: Lb.

This is the amount of your lean body mass listed by pounds. Changes in this number are usually due to gains and losses in skeletal muscle. Note that changes in your overall percentage body fat may occur from various combinations of gains and losses in your pounds of body fat *combined* with changes in your pounds of LBM.

Energy Output

THE NEXT section on the Energy Balance Chart is titled **ENERGY OUTPUT**. Here, there is a column with the heading:

RMR: Cal.

As shown below, you will enter the number you found in the *fourth* column of the box from the Body Composition Table. This is the number of calories (units of heat used to measure energy)

ENERGY OUTPUT			
RMR	+ Activity Calories		= Total
Calories	Aerobic	Anaerobic	Calories
1994			

that comprise your *Resting Metabolic Rate* or your *RMR*.

Your RMR is how many calories you burn at rest. Muscle burns calories at rest—body fat hardly burns any calories at rest. The more muscle you have, the more calories you require to maintain your weight. If you didn't get out of bed all day, your RMR is the approximate number of calories you would need to eat to maintain your body weight.

RMR is determined by your lean body mass;[*] *not* by your body weight. Two people may differ widely in total body weight, but if they have identical amounts of LBM, they would also have identical RMRs. So, though one carries more body fat and is heavier than the other, if the calorie output of their activities is similar, their total daily energy requirements would be similar also. That's why your skinny friend, who is all muscle and no fat, can eat as much as you and not gain weight.

In 1991, health expert Covert Bailey predicted there would soon be a chart to tell you how much to eat based upon your LBM. The Energy Balance Chart is such a chart! Calculate your total daily energy output by adding your RMR to the caloric output of your other activities.

Analyzing Your Activities

NEXT ON the Energy Balance Chart, you will record the number of calories you burn while performing your daily activities. Many people cannot accurately guess the number of calories they burn throughout the day. The following guide will help you estimate the calorie output of your activities. Do not be overly concerned about the accuracy of

[*] Source: Schwarzenegger, Arnold. *Encyclopedia Of Modern Bodybuilding.* Simon And Schuster. 1985, p.677.

your calorie estimates at this point. You will have a chance to correct them later.

Each activity, and its corresponding calorie output, is classified according to intensity. Start by making an estimate of 200–300 calories per day. This estimate represents the total of all your daily *sedentary* and *light* activities. This includes activities such as eating, dressing, washing, desk-work, automobile driving—all the little activities that are too difficult to keep track of individually.

Adjust this number up or down by 100 calories or so if you are generally more active on some days—burning off a lot of energy—or less active—conserving energy. Also consider the current climate. Regular exposure to very cold climatic conditions can increase your estimate. Regular exposure to very hot climatic conditions can decrease it. If you do a few extra hours of automobile driving, increase your estimate by an additional 140 calories for each extra hour of driving.

Add 200–300 calories to your estimate for each hour of *moderate* activities. This level of intensity includes activities such as slow walking, shopping, and performing activities with your arms while standing—for example, doing light house work, playing a musical instrument, or giving someone a haircut. By the way, women burn off an average of 4.5 calories per minute during sex, or 270 calories per hour. This places female sexual activity within the moderate activity level.

Men burn off more calories during sex—6 calories per minute, or 360 calories per hour. Three hundred to 400 calories per hour falls within the *vigorous* intensity level. This level includes brisk walking at 3.5 mph (depending on your weight—see *Weight and Intensity*, page 60).

As you can see, the intensity level of love-making for most people is not much greater than going shopping or taking a walk around the block!

Activities at the *strenuous* intensity level burn calories at a rate of 7–8+ calories per minute, or about 400–500+ calories per hour. Fast running and other very intense activities burn calories at a rate of 600–1000+ calories per hour and are classified as *very strenuous*.

All of the above calorie estimates are combined into one estimate and recorded in the Aerobic column on the Energy Balance Chart. Don't forget to include 200–300 calories or so for your daily sedentary and light activities.

ENERGY OUTPUT		
RMR	+ Activity Calories	= Total
Calories	Aerobic	Anaerobic	Calories
1994	550	100	

Aerobic activities use oxygen to burn fat as fuel for energy. Strenuous activities can be aerobic, but some strenuous activities, such as weight lifting, are listed in the Anaerobic column. For fuel, anaerobic activities require no oxygen as they burn a starch, *glycogen*, stored in your muscles.

It's easy to distinguish anaerobic activity from aerobic activity. Whether you are performing abdominal crunches or running a marathon, whenever you feel your muscles burning you are performing anaerobic activity—you are burning glycogen for fuel, *not* fat. You can't feel fat burning in your muscles. Since glycogen is part of muscle, it is correct to say that anaerobic activities burn LBM as fuel for energy.

Record any anaerobic activity in the Anaerobic column on the Energy Balance Chart. The intensity level of many sporting activities may fall somewhere between vigorous and strenuous and may be a mixture of aerobic and anaerobic activity.

Check the Activity Calorie Table in Appendix D, page 301. It lists the calorie output of various activities. Learn to identify the intensity level of your activities by "feel"—your perceived rate of exertion. Determine the feel of an activity by noting your breath rate when performing that activity. Activities at the vigorous level should allow you to carry on a steady conversation, haltingly between breathes—a good indication you are working within your aerobic fat-burning zone.

Check your perceived rate of exertion at different intensity levels. As your fitness level changes, the efficiency of your breathing, heart rate, and oxygen uptake change. If this improves, you'll feel like you're doing less work than before. Adjust your perceived rate of exertion to match changes in your intensity level.

Summing up, classify your activities according to the following intensity levels:

Activity Intensity Levels

- **sedentary plus light :**
  200–300 calories *per day.*
- **moderate :** 200–300 calories *per hour.*
- **vigorous :** 300–400 calories *per hour.*
- **strenuous :** 7–8+ calories *per minute* or 400–500+ calories *per hour.*
- **very strenuous:** 10+ calories *per minute* or 600–1000+ calories *per hour.*

Once you take the time to figure out the calorie output of your most common daily activities, like house chores, shopping, exercise and working at your occupation, store your information so it can be easily recalled when you need it. The use of an electronic organizer is recommended for this purpose. Add up your activities as you go through the day and it won't be long before you can quickly perform all your daily aerobic and anaerobic calorie estimates in your head.

ENERGY OUTPUT			
RMR	+ Activity Calories		= Total
Calories	Aerobic	Anaerobic	Calories
1994	550	100	2649

Under the **ENERGY OUTPUT** heading, on the Energy Balance Chart, add together your RMR plus the calorie output of your daily aerobic and anaerobic activities. As shown above, enter this sum in the Total column. This is the caloric value of your total day's energy output.

Diet—Your Calorie Intake

YOUR DIET provides energy to your body in the form of calories. Your calorie intake counterbalances your energy output. Many people are poor at estimating the number of calories in their food. A study at St. Luke's Roosevelt Hospital in New York shows that some people's estimates are off by about 100%.

People often complain that no matter how little food they eat, they can't control their weight. They blame their problem on their glands, genes, or "slow metabolism." These people need to add up their calories to see how much they are actually eating and burning-off. Few people can correctly guess their way to permanent weight control. *Until you gain some proficiency at estimating your daily calorie intake, you will continue to have difficulty controlling your weight.*

Quick fix diet plans may encourage you to ignore calories while you follow some

unbalanced diet or while you temporarily restrict yourself to certain foods. You will never receive more than temporary results this way. There are so-called negative-calorie foods, high-protein diets, fat-free diets, mono-diets, water-diets, juice-diets, restrictive food combinations—some of these plans have value when used for other purposes. Unfortunately, many of these plans are *misused* as gimmicks to trick you into temporarily getting by on fewer calories. When considering such a plan for permanent weight control, stop and ask yourself, "Is this really teaching me to eat properly?"

There are 1001 ways you can eliminate or burn-off calories by abusing your body with unhealthy and unbalanced diets, with drugs, or with excessive energy-wasting activities. But there is only one proper way to plan your eating. *A proper plan of eating includes being calorie conscious.* If you cannot accurately estimate your daily calorie intake, you are not planning your eating properly.

Calories are no less important than any other part of your diet. You may choose to ignore your intake of calories, but calories will never ignore you—they will continue to affect your body composition. If you can remember your birthday, your telephone number, your shoe size, your mortgage payment and the price of gas, surely you can remember the number of calories you had for lunch. The following advice will help you become more calorie conscious.

Begin by analyzing the amount of calories in your diet. Look up the caloric value of everything you normally eat. A Food Calorie Table is included in Appendix C of this book to get you started, but eventually you may want to get a larger calorie reference book. Make sure you get one that includes *everything* you eat—

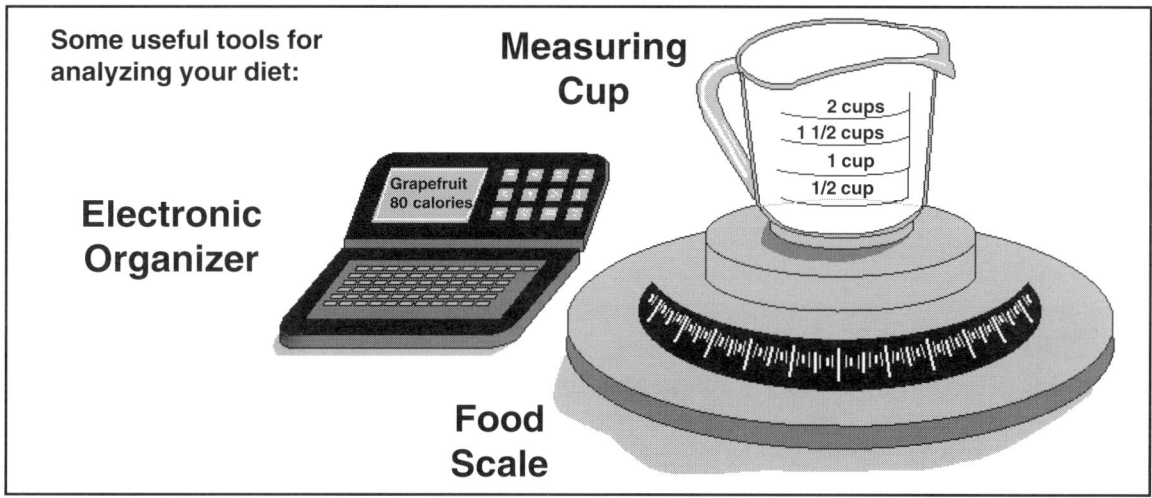

Some useful tools for analyzing your diet:

Electronic Organizer

Grapefruit 80 calories

Measuring Cup

2 cups
1 1/2 cups
1 cup
1/2 cup

Food Scale

brand names, special recipes, etc. Figure out the calories in each food you eat, in the portions you eat them. Include each ingredient.

Many people relate to their own custom-sized portions better than to "standardized" servings. Measure your portions in whichever way you wish—by weight (grams, ounces), by volume (cups, milliliters), or by plate size. Consult the Standard Measurement Table in Appendix E. Get to know what a measured cup of something looks like. Purchase a good quality food scale and learn what 4 ounces or 100 grams of something looks like.

Dietitians teach people to compare portion sizes to common objects; e.g., $3^1/2$ ounces of meat is the size of a deck of playing cards, 1 ounce of cheese is 4 dice, $^1/2$ cup of ice cream is a tennis ball.

Eventually you will combine typical portions of your favorite and most commonly eaten foods into meals—meals can be combined into personalized daily menus—all figured out by calories in predetermined amounts. Record and store this information where you can easily refer to it—you don't want to figure out everything all over again. A pocket-sized electronic organizer is perfect for keeping

track of this information. Use it to total your calorie intake and energy output throughout the day.

When dining out, base your calorie estimates on how you would prepare the same food at home. If you don't prepare your own meals, ask the person who prepares your meals for you if they would be kind enough to estimate the calories for you. If you are a regular customer in a restaurant, they would probably be happy to assist you this way. Otherwise, beware—a typical full-course feast served in a restaurant can total as much as 2000 calories! Remember, if you allow yourself to lose complete track of your calorie intake, it won't be long before it shows up as changes in your body composition—you'll get fat!

Keeping track of your calories takes the guesswork out of how much you are eating and eliminates the fear of unintentionally overeating. Once you learn how much to eat, you can relax, eat, and enjoy yourself— guilt-free. You won't feel the urge to run around the block 20 times every time you put something into your mouth!

Analyze the calories in all the foods in your diet at a pace that is comfortably manageable for you. Take as long as you need to calculate all your information. Do not think of counting calories as a dreary, lifelong task. Use it to temporarily analyze your eating while you form better eating habits. As better eating becomes a habit, your calories will automatically look after themselves.

When you have enough information, total up your daily calorie intake. As shown below, enter this amount in the Diet column, under the **CALORIE INTAKE** heading on the Energy Balance Chart. Don't worry if your calorie estimates are not accurate; just write something down. Later on, after analyzing changes in your body composition, you will be able to correct your estimates.

ENERGY OUTPUT				CALORIE INTAKE	
RMR	+ Activity Calories		= Total	Diet	Net
Calories	Aerobic	Anaerobic	Calories	Calories	+/-
1994	550	100	2649	2949	300

2949 – 2649 = 300

output from your calorie intake, as shown above.

CALORIE INTAKE	
Diet	Net
Calories	+/-
2949	

Net Calorie Intake

THE NUMBER you record in the Net column, on the Energy Balance Chart, represents how much your daily calorie intake is more or less equal to your daily energy output. This number will indicate whether you are likely to gain or lose body fat or muscle. Subtract the calories you recorded in the Total column, under the **ENERGY OUTPUT** heading, from the calories you recorded in the Diet column, under the **CALORIE INTAKE** heading. In other words, subtract your energy

"No matter how little fat you eat or how much you exercise, you will never lose body fat unless you are in negative calorie balance."

If the difference is a positive number, your calorie intake is greater than your energy output. You are likely storing calories as body fat and/or muscle. This is *positive calorie balance.*

A negative number means your energy output is greater than your calorie intake. You are burning-off stored calories from body fat and/or muscle. This is *negative calorie balance.*

If the number in the Net column calculates to zero, your calorie intake and energy output cancel each other out—you have no net storage or net loss of calories from body fat or muscle. This is *neutral calorie balance.*

Important—*Even if you are eating a low-fat diet and taking regular aerobic classes, you will never reduce your body fat level unless you are in negative calorie balance (see Chapter 8). Likewise, you will never gain muscle unless you are in positive calorie balance, no matter how much muscle-building protein food and muscle-building exercise you include in your program (see Chapter 9).*

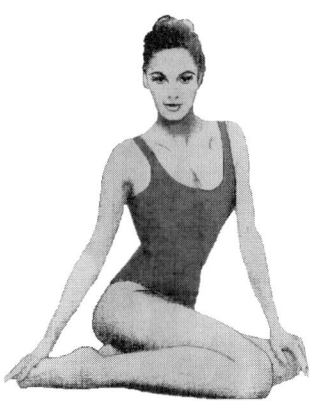

"Learn to eat properly before you reduce your body fat."

Chapter 4

Starting Your Program

Your First Goal

THIS CHAPTER will guide you through the first steps in creating a customized diet and exercise program that you can use to build strength, reshape your body, reduce body fat and permanently control your weight. Your body composition information will allow you to analyze and adjust the effectiveness of your program.

Your first goal will be to record, on the Energy Balance Chart, your normal eating and activity routine for one week. Do not alter your activity and eating habits during this period. Instead, concentrate on forming estimates of your normal calorie intake and energy output—how many calories you are consuming and how many you are burning.

Review Chapter 3 on how to use the Energy Balance Chart. Also review Chapter 3 on how to form your calorie intake estimates and energy output estimates.

Correct Your Estimates

USE YOUR body composition information to guide you in forming more accurate calorie intake and energy output estimates. If there are no changes in your body composition after a week, and your Net column is consistently showing zero (neutral calorie balance), then your calorie intake and output estimates are perfect. Congratulations! However, if your calorie intake and energy output estimates don't cancel out, or if they don't agree with changes in your body composition, you need to correct them.

The following troubleshooting list gives examples of discrepancies between your Net calorie calculations and your body composition information. These examples indicate when you need to correct your calorie intake and energy output estimates:

1. If you *gain* body fat and/or LBM over several days, but your Net indicates consistent *neutral* or *negative* calorie balance . . .

2. If you *lose* body fat and/or LBM over several days, but your Net indicates consistent *neutral* or *positive* calorie balance . . .

3. If there's no change in your body composition over several days but your Net indicates consistently large *negative* or *positive* calorie balances . . .

. . . then your calorie intake and/or energy output estimates are off and must be corrected to be consistent with any changes in your body fat and muscle. Did you underestimate the size of your food portions? Perhaps you overestimated the intensity level of some of your activities. Make small, gradual corrections until you have estimates that consistently agree with your body composition information.

Once you correct your estimates in the proper general direction, you can fine tune them even more. Compare any positive and negative numbers in your Net column with the theoretical calorie values of body fat and muscle.

For example: Suppose your body fat level changes. Theoretically, it takes an excess of 3500 calories to store one pound of body fat. If your calorie estimates are correct, you should see a *gain* of one pound of body fat in your body composition as your numbers under the Net column add up to 3500 calories (assuming you are not gaining any muscle).

If the figures under the Net column add up to *minus* 3500 calories, you should see a *loss* of one pound of body fat in your body composition (assuming you are not losing any muscle).

Suppose you gain or lose muscle. Some health authorities suggest it takes an excess of 600 calories to grow one pound of muscle. Six hundred calories is higher than the actual amount of calories stored in one pound of lean, fat-free muscle (one pound of muscle has 90 grams of protein, or 360 calories), but extra calories are probably required for the biosynthesis of that muscle. In addition, there are extra calories stored in a pound of muscle as glycogen. See *Chapter 9* to determine how many calories you require to gain muscle.

If your estimates are correct, and you are on a muscle-building program that includes an anaerobic exercise routine (see *Chapter 9*), your Net column should show a fairly consistent calorie surplus per pound of LBM growth.

The table below sums up the theoretical calorie values of body fat and, according to some health authorities, of muscle.

1 pound of body fat	3500 calories
$1/2$ pound of body fat	1500 calories
$1/4$ pound of body fat	750 calories
1 pound of muscle	600 calories
$1/2$ pound of muscle	300 calories
$1/4$ pound of muscle	150 calories

Compare these calorie values for body fat and muscle with your Net calorie calculations on the Energy Balance Chart. If you lose a quarter of a pound of body fat, your Net column should show an accumulated deficit of 750 calories; a gain of half a pound of muscle might show a surplus of around 300 calories in your Net column, etc.

Results Are Your Guide

REMEMBER, the calorie values of a pound of fat (3500 calories) and a pound of muscle (600 calories) are theoretical and should be considered *general guidelines* for most people. If, based on your corrected estimates, it consistently takes you more or less than 3500 calories to achieve a loss of one pound of body fat, or if it consistently takes you more or less than 600 calories to grow one pound of muscle, what does it matter? People are different at using calories. You may or may not burn up calories more efficiently than someone else. Some people may or may not assimilate calories from food more efficiently than others.

One's age and state of health play a large part in modifying one's ability to use calories. But regardless of age or other factors, it is best to let your body composition be your specific guide when assessing the state of your energy balance.

Important—*When determining the calorie value of changes in your body fat and muscle, if a particular number of calories per pound of body fat and per pound of muscle seems consistently right for you, that's the customized number with which you should work.*

After your personalized estimates are reasonably accurate and consistent, continue reading on in this book. You will learn how to make specific modifications in your energy balance to achieve your body composition goals. Use your body composition to check your energy balance modifications, readjust your modifications when necessary, and you'll never fail to achieve and maintain your body composition goals.

Rapid Weight Change

WEIGHT LOSS claims, such as: "I lost 20 pounds in two weeks," are achieved mainly from losing large amounts of fluid and muscle. Actual body fat losses in these claims are much smaller. If you add up the calories in 20 pounds of fat it comes to 70,000. You begin

to realize that, even if a person is in negative calorie balance by 2000–2500 calories a day, a person could never achieve 20 pounds of weight loss from pure body fat in just two weeks.

If the Body Composition Tables indicate you *lost* one pound of body fat, but you know you have not accrued a deficit of 3500 calories in your Net column, then you probably lost fluid. Likewise, if the Body Composition Tables indicate a one pound fat *gain*, but you know your actual calorie intake doesn't total anywhere near a surplus of 3500 calories, you probably are retaining extra fluid. Subtract actual changes in your body fat and muscle (determined by your Net calorie intake) from changes in your total body weight—the difference indicates how many pounds of fluid you have gained or lost.

Maintain Your Percentage Body Fat

AFTER A WEEK or so, you should have completed gathering your body composition information and finished improving the accuracy and consistency of your calorie intake and energy output estimates. You will be ready for your next goal: mastering the art of stabilizing and maintaining your percentage body fat.

Using the Energy Balance Chart, begin gradually balancing your daily calorie intake and energy output toward neutral calorie balance —if they aren't already balanced—by making small changes in your diet and activity. Tighten up your diet, increase your activity— do anything you can comfortably manage in order to balance your calorie intake with your energy output. Ideally, your Net should be coming out to zero and you should see no changes in your body composition.

You must properly adjust your diet to match your changing activity level from day to day. The difference in energy output between your average active days and your less active days can be quite large. Football players may require 5000 calories a day when active, but what happens on their days off ? If they rest and continue eating 5000 calories, their body fat will increase.

If you don't make the necessary calorie intake adjustments on your less active days, you could find yourself gaining body fat. Remember, it only takes one day of overeating to gain body fat and one day of undereating to lose muscle. For this reason, diets that restrict you to the same exact amount of food every day, despite your body's changing daily calorie requirements, may have an undesirable effect on your body composition. If you are exceptionally active for a few days, but you do not increase your calorie intake accordingly, you could lose a substantial amount of muscle.

Considering how your energy requirements may vary from day to day, what chance do you have of feeding yourself properly if you fail to adjust your daily calorie intake to your energy output? Can you imagine attempting to manage your finances this way? Imagine never knowing what your earned income was or how much you spent. How could you balance your account? Yet, this is precisely how most people attempt to manage their weight. No wonder they resort to quick fix diets.

When you have succeeded in achieving neutral calorie balance over a sufficiently long period, and when your daily Net on the Energy Balance Chart is consistently coming out to zero, your body composition measurements are remaining stable, your level of food intake is satisfying, and your activity output is comfortable, you will have taught yourself one of the most important principles of permanent weight control:

Maintaining your weight and your percentage body fat with proper amounts of food and activity requires much more precision, knowledge, practice and patience than losing weight on a quick fix diet.

The following analogy illustrates the difference between quick fix dieting and proper weight maintenance.

The Frisbee and the Barn

QUICK FIX dieting is like hitting the side of a barn with a ball. If you keep throwing the ball in the right direction, sooner or later you're bound to hit your target, the barn. And so, with quick fix dieting, if you keep undereating, no matter by how much or for how long, sooner or later you're bound to hit your target weight.

When you are quick fix dieting, you may or may not be precisely aware of body weight changes from day to day. And you may or may not be aware of the precise amount of calories your body is absorbing and burning-off every day. It doesn't really matter. As long as you are correctly *guessing* that the amount of calories you are absorbing is less than the amount of calories your body is burning-off (negative calorie balance) you will probably succeed in reducing your weight.

As you are losing weight, you may notice your clothes are feeling looser around your waist, even though you may not have any idea what your actual waist measurement is. Of course, you have no idea how much of your weight loss is muscle and how much is body fat. On a quick fix diet, you may be blissfully ignorant

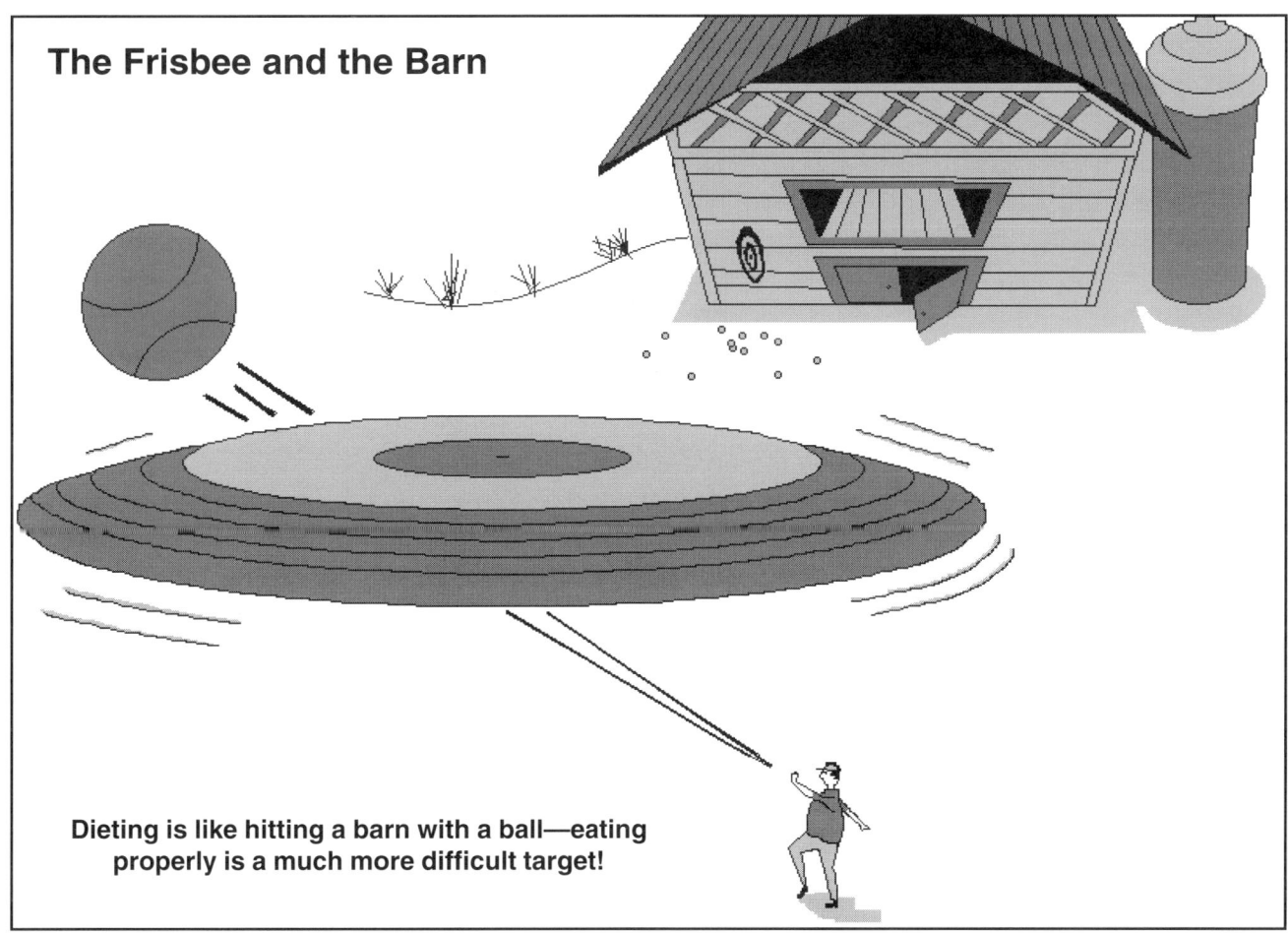

The Frisbee and the Barn

Dieting is like hitting a barn with a ball—eating properly is a much more difficult target!

of the precise measurable changes in all of these things, and still lose weight.

But when your goal is to maintain your weight and your percentage body fat, guessing isn't enough. As difficult as dieting may be, maintaining your proper weight is an altogether different and even tougher challenge. It is *essential* that you be aware of your daily weight, your daily waist measurement, your body composition and the daily caloric value of your food intake and activity output. You can't afford to undereat, you can't afford to overeat, and your daily calorie intake requirement varies with the changing level of your activity, the current amount of muscle on your body, the state of your digestion, your age, your sex, and even the weather!

So, if quick fix dieting is like hitting a barn with a ball, then maintaining your proper weight and body fat percentage is like hitting a Frisbee in flight with a ball. Not only is your target much smaller, but it's moving too.

A Diet Is the Last Thing You Need

DO NOT be in a hurry to start a diet until you have thoroughly learned to maintain your body composition by balancing your calorie intake with your energy output. Later in this book, you will learn the proper way to lower your body fat. In the meantime, you need to learn to eat properly before you reduce your body fat. After all, if you already knew how to maintain your weight and percentage body fat through proper eating, you wouldn't have body fat to lose now, would you?

If you simply yo-yo between improper eating, dieting, and improper eating again, what have you accomplished? Achieving weight loss through dieting only proves you have succeeded in temporarily underfeeding yourself. It doesn't prove you know how to feed yourself properly to prevent gaining body fat in the first place. It doesn't prove you know how to properly balance your calorie intake and energy output.

Before-and-after photos of people who have lost weight on diets can't reveal, by themselves, whether these people have learned to feed themselves properly to permanently maintain their weight.

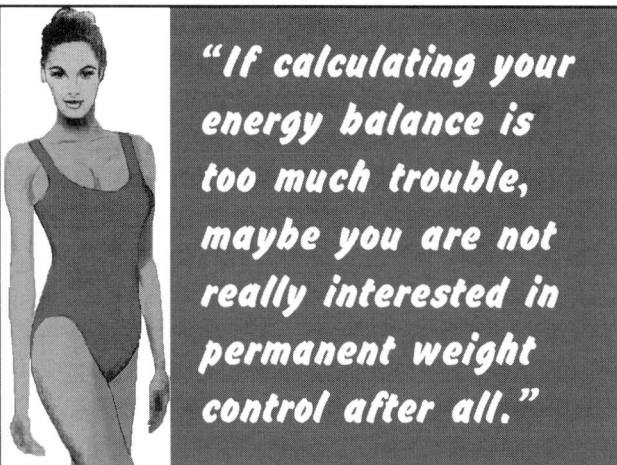

"If calculating your energy balance is too much trouble, maybe you are not really interested in permanent weight control after all."

Commercial weight-loss programs may claim to teach you the skills necessary to maintain your weight, but they still put the first and most important emphasis on immediate weight loss. This allows them to attract more customers because they know people want instant results. If these results are temporary, and if their repeat business is high, why should the people who earn money running weight-loss programs care? In the meantime, the general population continues to have a weight problem.

For most people, maintaining long-term weight loss after a diet is rare. The problem is not that diets don't work. Diets are meant to temporarily reduce your weight, nothing more. The problem is: *No one wants to take the time to learn to feed themselves properly.*

To repeat: Feeding yourself properly takes more skill, knowledge, practice and patience than following a crash diet. Feeding yourself properly means more than just memorizing calories. It means understanding, analyzing and adjusting your energy balance as described in this book.

There are many ways to temporarily reduce your weight, but there is only one way to permanently control it: by tracking and controlling your energy balance.

If you decide to continue quick fix dieting because it is easier than learning to eat properly—if attempting to become calorie conscious is a waste of your valuable time, then you have learned an important lesson. You have learned that you are not really interested in permanent weight control after all. Hopefully, at least you will no longer be tricked into thinking dieting alone can give you permanent results.

Once you get over the quick fix mentality, it probably won't be long before your thoughts turn toward doing something about your weight again. You can then decide if you want to continue trying to guess your way to permanent weight control (good luck), or if you want to try to tackle this problem the right way and solve it once and for all.

A man who jumps off a bridge doesn't defy the law of gravity—he demonstrates it! If you ignore balancing your calorie intake with your energy output, and you continue to have a weight problem, you won't be defying the law of energy balance—you'll be demonstrating it!

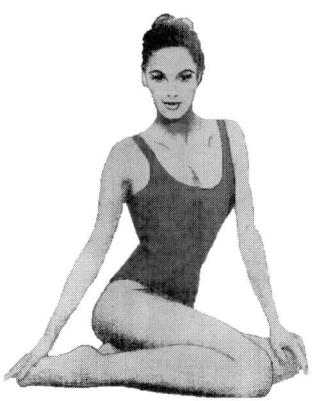

"Gaining and losing body fat is a matter of timing your food intake."

Chapter 5

Food, Nutrition and Health

Balance Your Nutrients

TO ENSURE that you make proper dietary adjustments when balancing your calorie intake and energy output, this chapter will present some fundamental basics about food, nutrition and health. You could visit a registered dietitian to have the nutrient content of your diet analyzed. Or you could get a nutrient guide, available in any bookstore, and take the time to analyze the nutrients in your diet yourself. A good plan these days is to use a personal-computer software program designed to analyze your diet for you. For more information, check the *Suggested Reading* section on page 307.

In calories, a generally balanced maintenance diet for an adult consists of approximately:

- 10–15% protein
- 20–30% fat
- 55–70% carbohydrates

Protein needs are slightly higher during periods of growth, while fats and carbohydrates should predominate during periods of vigorous physical activity. Adjust your diet accordingly. Adjust the overall amount of calories in your diet as well as the percentage of calories you derive from protein, carbohydrates and fat. (See chart on page 40.)

To help you determine the protein, fat and carbohydrate content of the foods you are eating, refer to the food classification chart below.

Food Classifications

- **Foods High in Protein:** meat, fish, poultry, eggs, dairy products, nuts, seeds, whole grains and legumes.

- **Foods High in Carbohydrates:** whole grains, legumes, tubers, starchy vegetables, sugars, syrups and fruit.

- **Foods High in Fat:** eggs, cheese, butter, cream, whole milk, fatty meats and fatty fish, oils, nuts, seeds and avocados.

Vitamins, minerals, enzymes and other micro-nutrients, although containing no caloric value, are critical for your health. Get them from fresh foods, especially from raw fruits and green vegetables. Fresh, whole, natural foods also contain necessary amounts of dietary fiber. Avoid empty-calorie foods that have had most of their micronutrients and fiber removed. This includes foods made from white sugar and white flour. In *The Hygienic System, Volume II, Orthotrophy*, Herbert Shelton points out that animals die quicker when fed a diet of empty-calorie foods than if given nothing but water.

Raw green vegetables, containing an abundance of vitamins, minerals and chlorophyll, are especially valuable for building your bones and your blood. A molecule of chlorophyll in green plants has a molecular structure that is almost identical to a molecule of hemoglobin in your blood. Raw, dark green leafy vegetables are an excellent food source to supply your body with the blood forming elements it needs.

Too many protein and energy-rich foods can clog your body and produce an abundance of metabolic acids that negatively affects your bone, blood, kidneys, and liver. Foods that contribute metabolic acids to your body include: grains, legumes (if not green), all animal foods (except breast milk for infants), most nuts and seeds, and any food that has had its nutrient content altered by cooking or processing. The metabolic acids resulting from the ingestion of large amounts of these foods must be promptly neutralized to preserve the proper pH balance (acid/alkaline balance) of your tissues. Any alteration in your body's pH could cause illness or death.

Fresh, raw fruits and vegetables, rich in vitamins and minerals, are considered alkaline foods because they counteract the pH-disturbing effect caused by metabolic acids. Raw, whole, natural fruits and green vegetables contribute elements that have an alkaline reaction in your blood and that neutralize metabolic acids. Even acidic fruits and vegetables, like tomatoes and citrus fruits, are alkaline in your blood once digested. They contribute minerals that bind with metabolic acids to neutralize or buffer these acids and prepare them for elimination by your kidneys.

If you don't supply enough alkaline foods in your diet, your body simply draws upon its reserve of alkaline elements stored in your bones, teeth, nerves, blood and other tissues to neutralize metabolic acids. Over time, this drain of alkaline minerals out of your body forms the basis for the development of many degenerative diseases ranging from dental caries and osteoporosis to anemia. As these alkaline reserves dwindle, un-neutralized metabolic acids accumulate and further poison your body. Illness, premature aging and death result.

Eat a balanced diet! Your diet should consist of 90% alkaline foods. Unlike the conventional diet that most people eat, a properly balanced diet should consist mainly of an abundance of fresh fruits and raw green vegetables.

In his book, *Health For The Millions*, Herbert Shelton says:

> *"If we do not cook and refine our foods, vitamin deficiency is practically impossible. . . If foods are eaten in their unprocessed, unrefined and uncooked state, there is no possibility of mineral deficiency. Our dietary deficiencies grow largely out of a refined and processed diet."*

Vitamin and Mineral Supplements

CONTRARY TO popular opinion, vitamin and mineral supplements cannot correct deficiencies caused by improper eating—or caused by eating empty-calorie foods, or foods whose nutrient content has been impaired by exposure to heat and air. Back in the early 1980's, The National Academy of Sciences in the U.S. declared it had not been scientifically proven that supplements are beneficial to your health. It *has* been proven many times that supplements are often toxic.

Will swallowing a vitamin and mineral pill teach you to eat properly? No, it does just the opposite by giving you a false sense of security and encouraging you to ignore proper eating. Only natural foods can deliver nutrients to your body that are usable and nontoxic.

Plants alone can take soil, water, sunlight and air and manufacture vitamins, minerals, amino acids (the building blocks of proteins) and other nutrients essential to your health. Vitamins and minerals extracted from food, exposed to heat and air, and packed into pills become as worthless as the soil from which they were originally derived. You can't eat soil. Only plants can provide nutrients in a usable form for humans and animals.

The threat of vitamin B_{12} deficiency is often used to scare vegetarians into taking supplements. Animal foods containing B_{12} come from animals who also eat no animal foods. They manufacture vitamin B_{12} themselves. If you are healthy, so do you. Vitamin B_{12} deficiency is said to cause pernicious anemia, but most people with pernicious anemia eat plenty of animal foods. Some experts point out that pernicious anemia is caused mainly by functional disturbances along the gastrointestinal tract, not by lack of vitamin B_{12}.

When humans rely on animal foods for nutrients, they are receiving them secondhand along with many undesirable by-products. Get your nutrients from whole, natural, unprocessed plant foods—mostly raw whenever possible.

No one ingredient in your diet is any more or less important than any other ingredient. It's the combination of all the ingredients working together in your diet that is important. A diet may be adequate in calories but lack essential nutrients such as adequate proteins, essential fat, vitamins and minerals. On the other hand, a diet that is adequate in nutrients, but not adequate in calories, may be just as harmful in the long run.

Food Guides

SHOULD YOU use government food guides to help you organize your diet? If you wish, but food guides only contain suggested foods that you may or may not wish to use. There are many other foods from which you can choose to properly balance your diet. Besides representing the welfare of the consumer, government food guides and food exchange programs, based on the old "four-basic-food-groups" idea, usually also represent the business interests of food manufacturers and food processors.

The Associated Press recently reported statements by Dr. Meir Stampfer, a Harvard Professor of Epidemiology and Nutrition, that indicates the government is subject to pressure from interest groups when making food recommendations. It is up to you to carefully assess the health and nutritional advice of any government or privately sponsored dietitian, nutritionist, physician or health expert.

There Are No Fattening Foods

DIETARY FAT contains essential nutrients and a concentrated source of calories (9 calories/gm) that supplies your body with slow-burning fuel. Polyunsaturated and monounsaturated fat, unhydrogenated with no trans—fatty-acids, occur naturally in plant foods and are better than saturated animal fat. An adequate supply of at least one fatty acid in dietary fat—linoleic acid—is essential to your health. The best sources of fat for adults and weaned children are in raw nuts, seeds, unheated vegetable oils, avocados and olives.

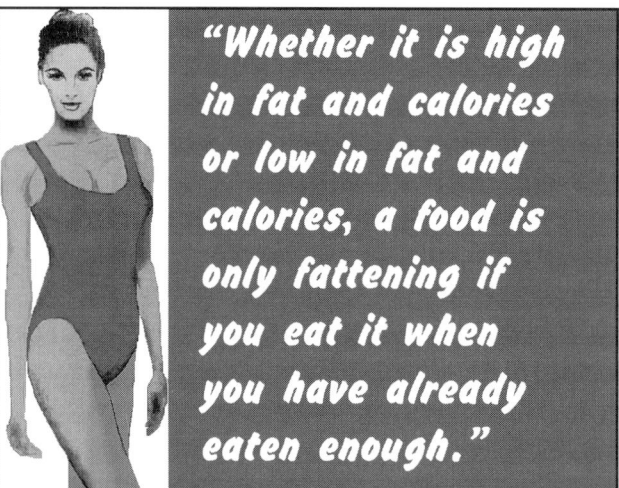

"Whether it is high in fat and calories or low in fat and calories, a food is only fattening if you eat it when you have already eaten enough."

Authorities warn that dietary fat should comprise no more than 30% of the calories in your diet—a percentage that is meaningless if you are not calorie conscious! You can figure your calorie and gram requirements for fat with the chart below; but why stop with fat? What

---

Calorie and Gram Requirements for
Fat (30%), Protein (15%), Carbohydrates (55%)

Calorie Requirement for:
Fat = total calorie intake x .3
Protein = total calorie intake x .15
Carbohydrates = total calorie intake x .55

Gram Requirement for:
Fat = calories from fat ·/. 9
Protein = calories from protein ·/. 4
Carbohydrates = calories from carbohydrates ·/. 4

---

about your calorie and gram requirements for protein (4 calories/gm) and carbohydrates (4 calories/gm.)? As you see, all these numbers can get overwhelming. *Is all this calculating really necessary?*

If your calorie intake is consistently meeting your energy requirements, you are probably eating close to a properly balanced diet, including proper amounts of fat. It is easier to eat proper amounts of food on a balanced diet. On the other hand, if you are consistently eating more or less calories than you need, check your diet's nutrient balance, especially of fat, since fat is more calorie-dense. It is easy to go over or under your calorie requirement on an unbalanced diet. Get on a balanced diet, pay close attention to your total calorie intake, and occasionally check your calorie and gram requirements for fat, protein and carbohydrates.

Cut down on your grams of fat if you are eating too much, but do not avoid fat. Restricting your *overall* diet to 30% fat does not mean eliminating *each* food whose calorie content is greater than 30% fat! Whether a food is high in dietary fat and calories or low in fat and calories, there are no fattening foods. It's the total amount of daily calories you consume, counterbalanced by your energy output, that can increase your body fat level.

Calorie-wise, it doesn't matter what time of day you eat your food. Eating late at night will no more cause an accumulation of body fat than eating at any other time of the day. People are more likely to associate nighttime eating with body fat gain because they are eating extra calories on top of what they have already consumed during the day. It's overeating at anytime, whether day or night, that puts you at risk for body fat gain. *A food, any food, only becomes fattening if you eat it when you have already eaten enough.*

Gaining and losing body fat is a matter of timing your intake of food. If you take three days to eat a normal two-day supply of food, you will lose body fat. But if you eat two-day's worth of food in *one* day, you will gain body fat. Think of body fat gain as an accumulation of surplus material you haven't gotten around to using for energy purposes yet. When cutting food intake to reduce body fat, you needn't feel deprived. You are just paying back the extra calories of energy you borrowed ahead of time, like paying back money borrowed from a bank.

You must get the proper balance of nutrients in your diet, including dietary fat, while controlling the overall amount of food you eat. Cutting dietary fat alone and overeating other foods will get you nowhere when trying to maintain your proper weight and percentage body fat. North Americans eat more low-fat food products than anyone else in the world. Yet, North Americans continue to have the most problems controlling their body fat. Is low-fat food being sold as the latest quick fix?

We live in a fat-phobic society. People equate the fat under their skin and the fat in their arteries with the fat in their food. But by making the generalization that all fat is bad, people are ignoring important distinctions. As you will see, the manner in which fat accumulates in your arteries as arterial plaque, in your food as dietary fat, and under your skin as subcutaneous fat, is very different.

Absorption of Food

YOUR SMALL intestine is where digested food absorbs into your blood and lymph and ultimately circulates to the rest of your body. The surface area of your small intestine is where contact and absorption of nutrients takes place. Your small intestine never quits absorbing as many nutrients as comes in contact with it. The size of your small intestine's surface area is the only factor that regulates its rate of nutrient absorption—an area equivalent to the size of a tennis court. If you can shovel the food in, digest it and give it time to reach your small intestine before it is voided out your colon as waste, it's going to be absorbed and become a part of you.

Dietary fat and sugar absorb more easily into your system and are converted to energy more easily than protein and starch. Through a more complicated process of digestion, protein provides a limited amount of calories to your body at a time. Protein must first be converted to amino acids. If there is not enough energy-supplying nutrients immediately available in your blood, these amino acids would be burned for energy. An adequate supply of carbohydrates has a *protein-sparing* effect in your body. It prevents amino acids from being used for fuel to supply energy, allowing them to be used for growth and repair instead.

Starch, although containing an abundant supply of concentrated energy, must be slowly converted by your digestive system into simple sugars called monosaccharides. However, since dietary fat and sugar require less complicated digestive processes, your small intestine can quickly and easily absorb an unlimited amount of calories directly from fat and sugar. Fat and sugar (galactose) are the two main nutrients in whole milk. The best sources of sugar (fructose, glucose) for adults and weaned children are in whole, unprocessed, uncooked, mineral-rich and vitamin-rich fruits and vegetables.

As stated previously, natural, unrefined fat and sugar foods are not more fattening. These foods just have a less complicated process of digestion and provide energy to your body more efficiently than other foods. Trying to control your weight by eating a greater proportion of foods that your body converts to energy less efficiently, like an excess of protein foods, puts a needless strain on your body. Eating large amounts of starch to replace a normal amount of fat in your diet also puts a needless strain on your body. This is not a substitute for eating a calorie-controlled, balanced diet containing proper amounts of fats, sugars, starches and proteins.

Many people who eat beyond their digestive capacity, especially of proteins and starches, pass a significant amount of undigested food past their small intestine and out their colon. This may result in undernourishment in some people. If these undernourished people were to eat a more properly balanced diet, replacing the amount of undigested protein and starch they are wasting with calorie equivalent amounts of natural, unrefined sugars and fats, they might find themselves absorbing more calories and gaining healthy weight.

Many overweight people also pass undigested food out their colon. If these people gradually cutback on their total food intake, they may not experience much weight loss at first. This is because the amount of digested food absorbed in their small intestine remains almost the same. They are simply wasting less of the food they are eating.

Sometimes, due to less strain on a person's digestive system, a reduction in food might improve a person's digestive ability, allowing greater intestinal absorption and producing a weight *gain*. This reduction in strain is easy to understand when you consider that, for most sedentary people, running a full day's supply of food through their gastrointestinal tract is the most energy consuming thing they do!

Specific dynamic effect is the term used to describe the amount of energy your body burns in the process of digesting food. Some foods, like green vegetables, actually cause your body to burn-off more calories during the process of digestion than they supply to your body. However, this does not mean that restricting yourself to a diet of so-called "negative-calorie foods" is a substitute for learning to eat properly.

Food swallowed, but not digested properly, provides no nourishment, no energy, and does more harm than good. *Calorie intake alone is no guarantee of energy*. Never eat when exhausted, ill or when hunger is lacking. To improve the efficiency of your digestion, consider exploring the subject of food combining. Check the *Suggested Reading* section. You will also find some valuable books listed there on vegetarianism, fasting, raw food and other health topics.

Diet and Heart Disease

THE FOLLOWING information is based on the research of one of the world's leading epidemiologists, T. Colin Campbell, Ph.D., of Cornell University. Dr. Campbell points out that dietary animal protein is more responsible for increased risk of heart and circulatory disease than dietary fat. An example of his findings is found in the effect of the Mediterranean diet. Moderately high in dietary fat, but low in animal protein, this diet causes significantly less heart disease than the typical western diet, which is high in dietary fat *and* animal protein.

Why would eating animal protein produce heart and circulatory disease? Scientists aren't sure, but apparently the human body is not designed to efficiently process this kind of nutritive material. Meat-eating plants and animals—carnivores—are better equipped anatomically to handle the ingestion of animal protein. The science of comparative anatomy has led some authorities to claim humans are fruit, nut and vegetable eaters—frugivores. These authorties say our health suffers when we stray from our true constitutional nature.

Cholesterol

CHOLESTEROL, a substance found in cell membranes, is a type of steroid lipid that helps form steroid hormones and bile. Your liver manufactures most of your body's cholesterol. Additional cholesterol is ingested from your diet, mainly from animal foods. There is *no* cholesterol in unprocessed foods that originate from plants, even in high-fat foods like nuts, seeds and avocados. Unlike dietary fat, cholesterol does not supply energy to your body.

There are two types of protein in your blood that transport cholesterol: high-density lipoproteins, HDLs, and low-density lipoproteins, LDLs. LDLs circulate and deposit cholesterol throughout your body and HDLs help remove cholesterol out of your body's circulation. Exercise increases HDL levels.

The theory that your arteries become blocked with fatty deposits because your body is clogged up with too much dietary fat and cholesterol may be too simplistic. It is not rare to find an overweight person with low serum cholesterol levels, or a lean person with high

levels. Salt and tobacco contribute to hardened and blocked arteries, but unlike animal foods, there is no fat or cholesterol in salt and tobacco. There must be another factor involved.

The latest research, reported by the Washington Post, April, 1997, proposes that blood vessels become hard and blocked due to inflammation. To illustrate: Exposing your skin to external irritants causes inflammation and results in a large and hard callus formation. Similarly, inflammation that leads to hardened and blocked arteries may be caused by exposing your arteries to irritating substances in your blood. One thing that salt, tobacco smoke and animal protein have in common is the irritation they can cause in your blood and blood vessels (*anaphylaxis* is the term used to describe an allergic hypersensitivity associated with foreign protein or drugs in the blood). This could be why they all contribute to hardened and blocked arteries (atherosclerosis and coronary occlusions) as well as to the cause of cancer, hypertension, arthritis and many more diseases.

Your serum cholesterol levels are a good indication of possible arterial plaque formation that could lead to a heart attack. People with cholesterol levels below 150 mg/dl (or about 4 mmol/L) rarely have heart attacks. According to Dr. William Castelli, the world renowned cardiac expert and director of the Framingham Heart Study in Massachusetts:

> *"We've never had a heart attack in 35 years in anyone who had a cholesterol level under 150."*

A balanced vegan or strict vegetarian diet of fruits, nuts, vegetables, legumes and grains, with no dairy, eggs or flesh (no fish, fowl or meat), along with other healthy life-style habits, will get most people's cholesterol levels down below 150 mg/dl—the level where heart attacks rarely occur. Epidemiological studies, such as Dr. Campbell's China study, *Diet, Life-style, and Mortality in China* (Oxford University Press, 1990), show striking evidence to support this claim.

Is Vegetarianism the Answer?

ARE YOU interested in ensuring a healthy life? Put the facts together:

1. Cardiovascular disease is the leading cause of death in our western culture.

2. Following a well-balanced vegan or strict vegetarian diet that totally eliminates animal foods, keeping sodium chloride intake low, eliminating smoking, and getting regular exercise will reduce your cholesterol down to a level that practically guarantees you will never have a heart attack.

This is true health *"ensurence"*—not health *insurance*, which pays you when you get sick. Surprisingly, the medical profession has known about the preventative effect of a vegetarian diet on strokes (thromboembolic disease) and blocked heart arteries (coronary occlusions) for some time. An article titled "Diet and Stress in Vascular Disease" appearing in the Journal of the American Medical Association, Vol. 176, No. 9, June 3, 1961, p.806 states:

> *"... a vegetarian diet can prevent 90 percent of our thromboembolic disease and 97 percent of our coronary occlusions."*

Recently, this statement has been verified by Dr. Dean Ornish, MD., who used a strict vegetarian diet to reverse heart disease in his patients. Unfortunately, a major criticism of Dr. Ornish's program is that his low-fat diet regime is too restrictive for most people to follow. The program developed by the late Nathan Pritikin, who also advocated a low-fat diet, received the same criticism.

It is true that arbitrarily restricting all forms of dietary fat, vegetable as well as animal fat, may make it difficult for you to comply with the type of diet advocated by Dr. Ornish and Nathan Pritikin. Dietary fat is an essential nutrient. The amount you need depends mainly on your body's daily energy requirement. Forcing your body to replace necessary amounts of dietary fat with large amounts of carbohydrates and proteins is not the correct way to balance your diet.

Considering Dr. Campbell's findings about animal protein and cardiovascular disease, the solution to complying with a healthy diet is clear. Put enough vegetable fat back in your diet, while excluding animal foods, and give yourself a chance to properly balance your diet. A small amount of dietary fat has a longer lasting effect on satisfying your hunger than other foods—satiety effect—and can actually help you feel satisfied on less food. The addition of fresh, raw, unsalted nuts, seeds, avocados, and unheated and unrefined vegetable oils are a delicious and nutritious way to help you balance your diet. If you are meeting your energy needs with a properly balanced diet, you will feel better and have a much better chance of long-term compliance with the diet.

Use this book to determine your daily calorie requirement. Restrict your dietary fat intake to no more than 30% of that requirement, investigate the vegetarian life-style in the *Suggested Reading* section of this book, and stay healthy while you permanently control your weight.

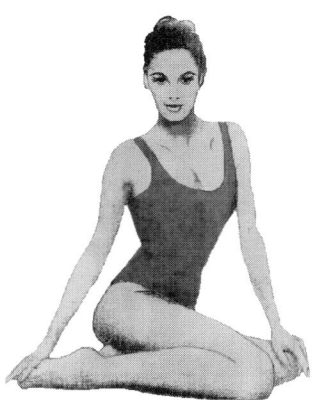

"Most people are days to months ahead in their feeding schedule!"

Chapter 6

The 4 Secrets of Weight Control

Quality, Quantity, Sensitivity and Satisfaction

YOU MAY learn to analyze your body composition and energy balance, and you may determine how much you *should* eat to control your weight, but if you attempt to follow a feeding program that does not satisfy you, you will never achieve lasting results. To be effective in the long run, changes in your living and eating habits must be based on pleasure—legitimate pleasure that is the result of wholesome living.

If you are having trouble controlling your calorie intake—the *quantity* of food you are eating—examine the *quality* of your food choices. Making changes in the direction of selecting more natural, unrefined, unprocessed and less seasoned foods will gradually allow your taste buds to restore their natural *sensitivity*. You will then derive more pleasure and *satisfaction* from eating normal amounts of nourishing food.

The 4 secrets of weight control are summed up as follows:

> ### The 4 Secrets of Weight Control:
>
> 1. Maintain control of the *quality* of food you eat to . . .
>
> 2. Maintain control of the *quantity* of food you eat by . . .
>
> 3. Restoring and maintaining the *sensitivity* of your taste buds, giving you . . .
>
> 4. Greater *satisfaction* as you enjoy normal amounts of wholesome food.

Restore Your Taste Buds

YOUR TASTE buds are nerve receptors located in your mouth. They sense information arriving from the external environment and activate signals along your sensory nerves to the taste center in your brain. Taste bud cells wear out and are replaced every ten days.

45

Overactivation of some nerve receptors can quickly tire them, causing them to lose their responsiveness. Overactivation of your taste buds occurs as you eat more stimulating foods. It then takes progressively stronger stimulation with stronger tasting foods in greater quantities to get your receptors working again. This can result in even more fatigue and reduced effectiveness of your taste buds. You are soon trapped in a vicious circle: overstimulation leading to fatigue and then back to more overstimulation. The more you overstimulate and fatigue your taste buds, the more you reduce their sensory effectiveness.

There is a way to break out of this vicious circle. Instead of developing a dependency on overstimulation to get your taste buds to function, why not give your taste buds a rest? Eat lighter for a while. This will allow your taste buds to restore their natural responsiveness. With a reestablished level of taste bud sensitivity, you will enjoy, and feel more satisfied, eating unrefined natural foods.

It has been shown that what you eat at one meal will influence what will satisfy you at your next meal. This illustrates the adaptation of your taste bud's response to the stimulation level of the food previously eaten. A meal of natural foods with their natural flavors intact will allow your taste buds to be satisfied with normal amounts of natural foods at subsequent meals. A meal of processed and overstimulating foods will drive your taste buds toward demanding larger amounts of overstimulating foods at subsequent meals.

Besides overstimulating your taste buds, refined foods, low in fiber, quickly slide down your throat with minimal chewing. You tend to swallow large amounts of this type of food before your gastrointestinal tract can signal your brain that you have eaten enough.

Because of their higher fiber and water content, eating natural foods gives your body time to feel satisfied before you have overeaten. Eating refined and processed foods that are low in nutrients can also cause your body to demand greater amounts of food because your body senses it isn't getting enough nutrients.

You may ask, "What harm is there in moderately indulging in unwholesome food?" The answer is that moderation only applies to the healthy things in life, as an excess of even wholesome things becomes a source of harm. Total abstinence from unwholesome things is the only way to preserve health. That's just the way things are.

If you occasionally eat highly processed food items, you may pay more than you bargained for by distorting the sensitivity of your taste buds. Your taste buds then become unreliable guardians of sane eating. You will have trouble feeling satisfied eating natural food. Distorting the natural sensitivity of your taste buds with processed foods and then trying to satisfy the cravings they cause is like trying to put out a fire with gasoline.

Controlling your eating by abstaining from processed foods altogether is far easier than attempting to control your eating while continually tempting your taste buds with overstimulating food.

Fun On a Bun

A PROPER plan of eating allows you to derive pleasure exclusively from simple meals of wholesome food with their natural flavors; not from fiery spices, or from refined sugar, salt, sauces, gravies, grease and stomach-irritating condiments added to improperly prepared, tasteless foods. Think of a young child's reaction of repulsion when they first taste these unwholesome things. The young and innocent need to be "educated" into enjoying spicey, refined foods.

Once you have acquired a taste for condiments and seasonings, their use may make tasteless foods more palatable, but not without blunting the natural sensitivity of your taste buds. It is difficult to control how much you eat when refined foods, spices and condiments are dominating your taste buds.

Consider the type of food served at your local *Fun On A Bun*. The "fun" is not in the unappealing taste of the bland food; it's in what's added to the food to cover it up and add zing to it! "Wake up your taste buds!" is the battle cry at *Fun On A Bun*. Salt, spices and condiments, sauces and gravies, pungent substances like strong onions and garlic—these may overexcite your worn out taste buds and add "taste" to overcooked and processed foods that you would normally not be interested in eating. But every time you resort to overexciting your taste buds this way, you leave them more desensitized. Revitalize your taste buds with rest, not with more stimulation.

It's bad enough that condiments and spices derange your taste sensibilities, but they do more harm than that. These substances irritate

your gastrointestinal system to such an extent that they impair digestion and cause irreparable injury to your digestive organs.

Why is so much fat added to "fun" food? Fat is not the tempting, irresistible taste treat most people think it is. Fat may absorb the flavors of other foods, but by itself, fat is tasteless or bland at most. If fat is such a treat, pour yourself a nice tall glass of oil (100% fat) and knock yourself out! Greasing food with fat simply allows the food to slide down easier. There are many foods you wouldn't even bother to eat if you didn't first grease them with fat.

Why not reject tasteless foods and their accompanying grease and seasonings? Give your body a chance to restore the natural sensitivity of your taste buds by returning to natural foods. Will you miss any pleasure? No, you won't miss any pleasure if you return to natural foods. You will gain more pleasure by rediscovering the abundant natural flavors of wholesome food, and you will have a much better chance of controlling your eating.

Damage Control

IT IS SOMETIMES difficult to retain control of your eating because of social

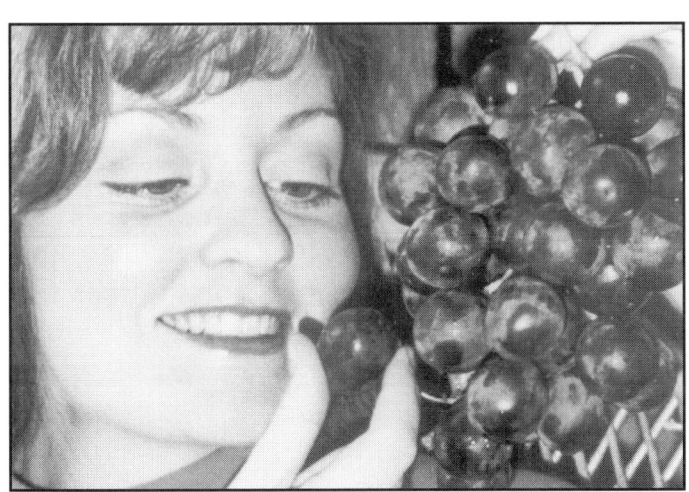

You will not miss any pleasure when you restore the sensitivity of your taste buds and rediscover the flavors of natural foods.

pressures. If you are at a dinner party, and you are hungry, and there isn't much to choose from as far as healthy food selections, what do you do? You could eat ahead of time and politely refuse the main course while nibbling on salad. You could call ahead and make arrangements for a special meal. You could even say to your host, "No thank you. If I eat that I will get sick right in front of you." Then you could sit there like an ascetic monk while everyone enjoys themselves. Use common sense. Often, it's best to politely accept what is offered and get back on track the next meal.

The best way to balance out a day that included one-too-many meals, or two- or three-too-many meals, is by having less meals the following day. If you go to bed stuffed the night before, it makes sense to miss next morning's breakfast to give your body more time to employ those extra calories. Whether or not you feel breakfast is important, in a sense, you already ate your morning breakfast the night before.

Use next morning's mealtime to work-off or walk-off the extra calories, or get extra rest by sleeping through breakfast. There's no need for concern about nutritional deficiencies when you're simply balancing out your extra calorie intake this way. Of course, this is assuming you are not stuffing yourself on empty-calorie food. Sadly, there is little you can do to correct the damage from eating empty-calorie food, no matter how much you try to balance it out with wholesome food. Get back to normal eating as soon as possible.

After you have given your taste buds time to rest and regain their sensitivity, and after you have used up the temporary food excess, it is important to give yourself a chance to feel

satisfied on natural foods again. When you resume eating, make sure your first meal consists of natural foods. This is a critical part of the process of regaining control of your eating. You are not out of the woods until you reestablish the enjoyment of eating natural foods again. If you don't, you run the risk of slipping back into more and more feeding indiscretions. Avoid this temptation, and by your second or third natural-food meal the thought of craving denatured food will be completely foreign to you.

Learn to balance out any eating indiscretions this way so you never get ahead of your feeding schedule. The amount of subcutaneous fat on your body is a good indicator of how many meals you are ahead in your feeding schedule. Most people are days, weeks, even months ahead in their feeding schedule. Take it one meal at a time. Decide now that if you get one single meal ahead of your normal feeding schedule, you will take measures to immediately get back on schedule. Remember, balancing out your eating to prevent body fat gain is a question of timing your food intake, not of deprivation.

Exercise Purging

DO NOT LET your damage-control strategy encourage you to blowout your diet on a regular basis. It makes no sense to deliberately stuff yourself with extra meals and force yourself to run a marathon the next day to balance out your extra calories. This becomes a form of *exercise purging*. Learning how to balance out temporary overeating with activity is not a substitute for learning how to eat properly. *Eating properly means never overeating in the first place!*

Overcoming Bad Habits

THOSE ACCUSTOMED to the conventional and haphazard way of life, which includes the consumption of caffeine, tobacco, alcohol, drugs and poor diets, often find it necessary to break bad habits in order to get back to a more natural way of living. Withdrawal pain and discomfort that accompanies the process of breaking away from bad habits occurs as your body remedies the aftereffects of your bad habits. This healing reaction should convince you once and for all of your bad habit's destructive nature.

If your body cannot *resist* and cast off the initial exposure to a harmful agent, it learns to accommodate or *tolerate* the damage done by that agent during subsequent exposures. By continuously weakening your body with harmful and poisonous substances, like drugs and bad food, you *suppress* your body's ability to resist and heal the effects of your bad habits. Thus, another cup of coffee or another cigarette suppresses and temporarily "relieves" the agitation caused by the caffeine in your previous cup of coffee or by the nicotine in your previous cigarette.

Consider this: Caffeine often causes headaches in coffee drinkers, but many headache remedies contain caffeine. How is that so? The inflammation of your headache is your body's way of eliminating caffeine and initializing healing. The temporary "relief" brought on by administering more caffeine is due to the overpowering, weakening and suppression of your body's remedial efforts to resist and overcome this toxic substance.

Just about any "treatment" or "remedy" that weakens your body will suppress symptoms. Toleration may be increased, but the damage to your body continues. Eventually this only further perpetuates weakness and pain. One becomes trapped in a cycle: pain, followed by relief that causes weakness, which leads back to more pain. The more you seek relief in this manner, the less likely you are to ever experience a return to genuine health, comfort and ease. How do you break this cycle?

Take a few days off, crawl into bed—cease weakening your body. Allow your natural resistance to do its job as it overcomes and casts off destructive agents. Check the *Suggested Reading* section of this book and investigate the benefits of fasting. Once you completely break away from bad habits, and the pain and discomfort have ceased, it is important to firmly establish new good habits in place of the former bad habits and start enjoying the pleasures and health benefits of wholesome living. All genuine health-building habits, including healthy eating habits, are pleasurable.

Caffeine

CAFFEINE, ONE of the most commonly used drugs in the world, stimulates your central nervous system. A similar drug is found in chocolate—theobromine—and in tea—theine. Besides causing headaches, as previously mentioned, caffeine also causes anxiety disorders, panic attacks, lowered potassium levels, heart palpitations and arrhythmias.

Because it mobilizes body fat from storage sites, caffeine is often contained in diet pills. However, if body fat that is mobilized by caffeine is not used for energy, it is deposited back into the body's adipose tissue where fat-storing cells lie.

To mobilize body fat, caffeine increases the activity of your adrenal glands, causing release of the fight-or-flight hormones, epinephrine and norepinephrine. Body fat is mobilized as these fight-or-flight hormones work in combination with another adrenal hormone, cortisol.

An increased level of cortisol can also mobilize body fat by itself. People with high levels of cortisol secretion, sometimes resulting from glucocorticoid therapy, may develop a condition known as Cushing's syndrome. Body fat is thinned out in their arms, legs and buttocks but extra body fat is deposited in their face—*moon face*—and in their abdomen, back and neck—*buffalo torso*. See the illustration below.

It is interesting to compare the effect of caffeine use with Cushing's syndrome. Common characteristics of both include:

1. Increased breakdown and redistribution of body fat.
2. Increased muscle breakdown.
3. Elevated blood glucose levels (hyperglycemia).
4. Elevated levels of fat-mobilizing adrenal hormones.
5. Insomnia.
6. Elevated blood pressure (hypertension).
7. Increased stomach acidity.

With so many similarities, one wonders if caffeine users, like people with Cushing's syndrome, redistribute their body fat into moon faces and buffalo torsos. Think about that over your next cup of coffee!

Food Addiction and Eating Disorders

DOES THIS sound like someone you know?

"My name is Amy, and I am a food addict. When I eat something, it never satisfies me for long. I'm constantly hungry, no matter how much I eat. I actually feel ill if I go without food. Eating food relieves my suffering, but I notice the more I eat, the more I suffer after. So I eat again to make the pain go away. I feel trapped, like I'm a slave to my desires. I can't control my actions no matter how hard I try. My pain is physical, mental and emotional."

The symptoms and behavior Amy describes above are strikingly similar to those seen in other addictions. Amy's addictive eating, sometimes referred to as *compulsive overeating*, is her attempt to suppress the pain and satisfy the cravings caused from eating improper foods.

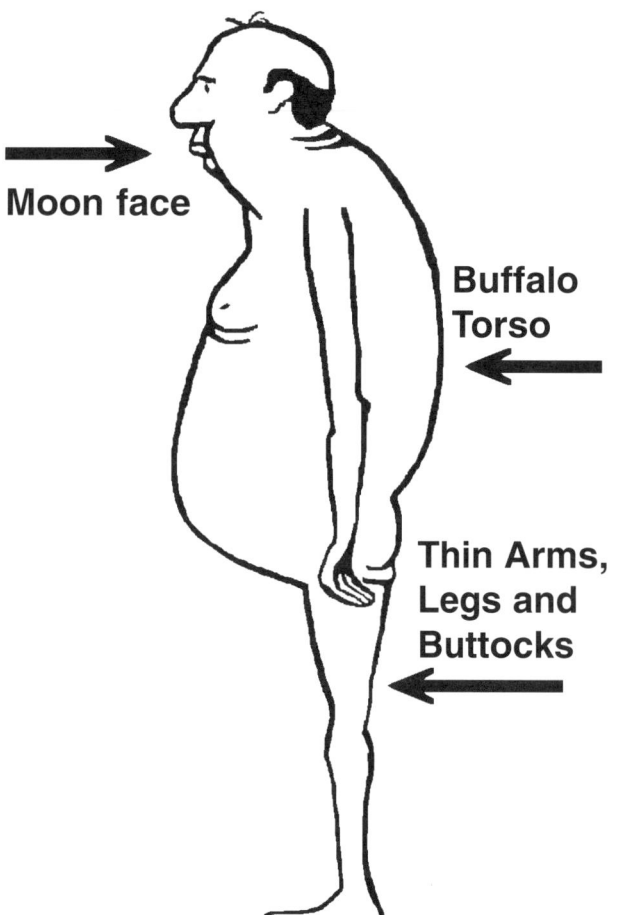

Moon face

Buffalo Torso

Thin Arms, Legs and Buttocks

People often suppress and "relieve" the gnawing, empty feeling in their stomach, an aftereffect of their previous bad eating habits, by quickly refilling their stomach with food again. Pain that accompanies your body's remedial efforts is an indication that you have been doing harm to yourself. A normal person with proper eating habits should experience no pain or discomfort if missing several meals.

Other than psychological factors, which may require separate attention, the quality of Amy's food choices and her lack of understanding about healthy eating is at the root of Amy's compulsive overeating. She needs education and living reform.

> *"You must learn to distinguish true hunger from cravings for relief and for overstimulation."*

Amy must learn to distinguish true hunger, which is a comfortable and pleasant sensation, from cravings for relief and for overstimulation. Wholesome eating is never dull when one is genuinely hungry. Cravings for unwholesome substances are never "natural" —they are deliberately cultivated.

It is possible to be a food addict and not have a weight problem. But if food addiction is leading to a weight problem, you should know it is almost *impossible* to become a food addict from eating natural foods. We just don't find overweight people who select natural, unrefined foods as the main part of their diet. It's actually difficult to eat enough unrefined food to produce a large amount of body fat.

To reform her life and bring about changes in her habits, Amy does not have to drop out of society and live in a grass hut for the rest of her life while eating sunflower seeds and lemons. How *far* she goes in reforming her living and eating habits will depend on what kind of weight control results will satisfy her. One thing is certain: As long as food addiction and other bad habits are causing Amy to eat greater than normal amounts of food, she will always have a weight control problem.

Most addictive behavior has a physical as well as a psychological component. A good therapy program deals with both. In normal eating, our relationship with food is very emotional— food naturally brings us pleasure and comfort. An insecure person who turns to food to provide extra amounts of comfort will obviously create an energy balance problem. But anyone can develop eating disorders and become obese by continually making the wrong food choices.

Eating disorders, such as anorexia nervosa and bulimia, often occur in achievement-oriented people. These disorders may sometimes be caused by a simple misunderstanding of what determines body composition. The problem may stem from confusing pounds of body weight with pounds of body fat. It is based on the mistaken assumption that dieting away body weight at all costs will improve body composition—that thin is the same as lean! Under this mistaken assumption, a person will always view their body image as too fat, even if they are already down to skin and bones.

These types of cases may not always be cries for help as some therapists claim. If a young person is successful at many extracurricular activities, why don't they ever chose something else to fail at as a cry for help? Perhaps they simply need better information about the proper way to achieve their body weight goals. A book like this can help these people achieve the outstanding figure they desire, not by trying to talk them out of it, but by showing them the proper way to achieve it!

The next chapter contains a table showing minimum lean body mass levels a person should maintain. If one follows these guidelines, there should never be concern about becoming anorexic.

For people with more severe psychological problems stemming from low self-confidence and low self-respect, resolving eating disorders and compulsive overeating often involves going beyond learning about proper

A Message to Therapists

This book offers an approach to permanent weight control and body shaping that the author believes to be intelligent, effective and safe. Therapists who deal with anorexic patients are no doubt well-intentioned when they try to convince young people to abandon their pursuit of conventional body ideals, e.g., looking like a swimsuit model. This alternative is certainly better than becoming anorexic, but is it the only alternative? Many people have attained splendid figures without becoming anorexic or appearing emaciated. How did they do it? Therapists interested in applying some of this book's ideas into their own practice are invited to contact the author through the publisher's address listed in this book.

food choices and body composition. Early experiences with sexual abuse, alcoholism, abandonment—these are issues that must be examined and resolved if a person is to break away from the habit of using food as an escape from reality or as a means of attempting to regain control of one's life.

In his book, *Love And Addiction*, Stanton Peele says:

> *"We have good grounds for tracing the addictive bent of many of today's young adults to their home environment and upbringing. But it doesn't make any more sense to shift the blame for our problems back one generation, onto people who themselves had to act to circumstances that they did not create, than it does to blame ourselves for not being able to break out of those problems all at once. A more constructive alternative is to accept that we are each given our own set of psychic and personal limitations to resolve."*

If the people who were responsible for raising you in a healthy manner didn't adequately fulfill their responsibilities, leaving you with damaged self-esteem and other psychological problems, you'll have to finish the job yourself. Again quoting Stanton Peele,

> *"Acceptance of personal responsibility is the first step toward freedom from addiction."*

There are many support groups and councilors available today offering worthwhile assistance in the areas of abuse, addiction, eating disorders and obesity. Check your local community services listings. Don't be afraid to ask for help.

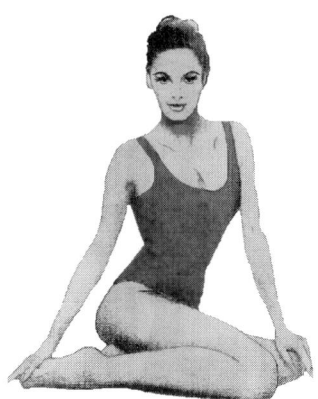

"You may need to gain muscle as well as lose body fat."

Chapter 7

Your Ideal Body

Selecting Your Goals

ONCE YOU have mastered the ability to properly stabilize and maintain your body composition, it's time to consider what changes you would like to make to achieve your ideal body. The two best approaches to take are:

1. Losing body fat while minimizing loss of muscle mass and tone.

2. Gaining and toning muscle while minimizing body fat gain.

Either of these two approaches will help you improve your percentage body fat while keeping your body firm and shapely. The next two chapters in this book will show you specifically how to reduce body fat and gain lean body mass. But first, an overview and a few general remarks about your program.

Losing body fat is a goal that requires negative calorie balance and aerobic activity. Gaining muscle is a goal that require positive calorie balance and anaerobic activity. Since it is impossible to have negative and positive calorie balance at the same time, you should not attempt to pursue both these goals at the same time. Performing excessive aerobic activity when attempting to gain muscle is counterproductive. Performing excessive anaerobic activity while dieting to lose body fat will make it difficult to prevent muscle loss.

Remember, for fuel, aerobic activities burn fat. Anaerobic activities burn glycogen for fuel, which is part of your lean body mass. As the intensity of an activity rises it gradually becomes less aerobic and more anaerobic. So, there are many activities that burn varying degrees of both fat and lean body mass. These activities, like running and sporting activities, are great for cardiovascular conditioning and other fitness goals, and the calories they burn helps prevent you from gaining additional body fat. But they pose a problem if your goal is to preserve muscle while lowering body fat.

Since, to lose body fat, you must stay in negative calorie balance on days you do these activities, you won't be able to eat enough food to fully replenish any LBM that is also being burned. For example, doing a lot of strenuous activity while on a continuous calorie-reduced diet might speed up body fat reduction, but it doesn't allow you enough calories to fully replace burned-off LBM. You are losing as much muscle as body fat—often, as the Body Composition Tables would reveal, you may lose *more* muscle than body fat. Our rule then for lowering body fat is:

To prevent LBM loss, avoid excessive anaerobic activity while on an extended low-calorie diet.

Stick with low-intensity aerobic activities when exercising to lower body fat. Keep your intensity well within your fat-burning zone.

To start your plan, it may be helpful to select your ideal body measurements and decide which specific goal to work towards first—body fat loss or muscle gain. You can then work out a specific timetable to achieve each separate goal at a pace that is comfortably manageable for you.

Select a program that allows you to strip off body fat on certain days you designate as "fat-burning days." On those days, stay in negative calorie balance, increase your low-intensity aerobics and keep your LBM losses to a minimum. Then, to add muscle without regaining any body fat, select other days designated as "muscle-building days." Perform anaerobic activity, such as resistance weight training or freehand exercises, and follow this up with appropriate rest. Stay in positive calorie balance by eating just enough of a nutrient-adequate diet to increase muscle growth.

If you do not want to increase the amount of muscle on your body, you can still maintain tone of your muscles by performing anaerobic exercise several times per week. On these days, do not eat extra calories. Eat only enough to keep you in neutral calorie balance.

To keep your muscles toned while dieting, take an occasional day off from dieting and increase your calorie intake back up to neutral calorie balance while you perform anaerobic exercise. Then, the following day, continue on with body fat reduction.

When you are happy with your body composition—your body fat and lean body mass levels—you can maintain your muscle tone by performing anaerobic activity 2–3 times a week. Keep your body fat level stable by including higher levels of aerobic activity if you wish, and eat enough to keep you in neutral calorie balance. That's it!

Does Height Count?

PREVIOUSLY, IT was mentioned that Body Mass Index tables, based on averages of weight and height, are not accurate in determining your proper body weight because they ignore body fat percentages. Nonetheless, height, as well as weight, are considerations when selecting your ideal body measurements.

The combination of your body fat percentage, your weight and your height should all be considered when selecting your ideal body measurements.

Body Mass Index tables, combined with body fat percentages, can be used as a starting point to determine your ideal body measurements. For example, the Body Mass Index table on the top of the next page suggests a person measuring 5' 10" should weigh no more than

Acceptable Body Mass Index Ranges*

4' 10" .... 96–119 lb.	5' 7" .... 127–159 lb.
4' 11" .... 99–124 lb.	5' 8" .... 131–164 lb.
5' 0" .... 102–128 lb.	5' 9" .... 135–169 lb.
5' 1" .... 106–132 lb.	5' 10" .. 139–174 lb.
5' 2" .... 109–136 lb.	5' 11" .. 143–179 lb.
5' 3" .... 113–141 lb.	6' 0" .... 147–184 lb.
5' 4" .... 116–145 lb.	6' 1" .... 151–189 lb.
5' 5" .... 120–150 lb.	6' 2" .... 155–194 lb.
5' 6" .... 124–155 lb.	6' 3" .... 160–200 lb.
	6' 4" .... 164–205 lb.

*Source: Grunwald, Lisa. *"Do I Look Fat To You?"* Life. February 1995, p.60.

174 pounds. How does this change when taking body fat percentages into consideration?

Let's assume a 174 pound, 5' 10" male has an acceptably healthy level of body fat—15%. What harm is there in this individual gaining muscular weight above 174 pounds, as long as he remains at 15% body fat or lower? Such a person could be carrying a lower percentage of body fat than a person considered normal on the Body Mass Index tables.

For example, during his competitive body-building years, Arnold Schwarzenegger's weight was above his Body Mass Index allowance. Weighing between 230–240 pounds and standing 6' 2", he was considered far too heavy for his height by Body Mass Index standards alone (155–194 lb.), even though he was in outstanding shape with 3–4% body fat.

Sometimes an individual may need to gain muscle as well as lose body fat to bring them around to normal levels. Even if one's body fat percentage is normal or lower, one's pounds of lean body mass—LBM— may be less than recommended when taking Body Mass Index standards into consideration.

The table below, based on Body Mass Index numbers and normal body fat percentages, was formulated by the author to show the *minimum* amount of LBM a male and female should carry. For example, a 5 foot 6 inch woman should carry no less than 96½ pounds of LBM, regardless how low her body fat percentage. So, if she weighs 110 pounds at 16% body fat, her LBM is only 92½ pounds. She should gain at least 4 pounds of muscle.

Minimum Lean Body Mass Levels

Females:

4' 10" .. 75.0 lb. LBM	5' 7" .... 99.0 lb. LBM		
4' 11" .. 77.0 lb. LBM	5' 8" ..... 102.0 lb. LBM		
5' 0" .... 79.5 lb. LBM	5' 9" ..... 105.5 lb. LBM		
5' 1" .... 82.5 lb. LBM	5' 10" ... 108.5 lb. LBM		
5' 2" .... 85.0 lb. LBM	5' 11" ... 111.5 lb. LBM		
5' 3" .... 88.0 lb. LBM	6' 0" ..... 114.5 lb. LBM		
5' 4" .... 90.5 lb. LBM	6' 1" ..... 118.0 lb. LBM		
5' 5" .... 93.5 lb. LBM	6' 2" ..... 121.0 lb. LBM		
5' 6" .... 96.5 lb. LBM	6' 3" ..... 125.0 lb. LBM		
	6' 4" ..... 128.0 lb. LBM		

Males:

4' 10" .. 81.5 lb. LBM	5' 7" ..... 108.0 lb. LBM
4' 11" .. 84.0 lb. LBM	5' 8" ..... 111.5 lb. LBM
5' 0" .... 86.0 lb. LBM	5' 9" ..... 115.0 lb. LBM
5' 1" .... 90.0 lb. LBM	5' 10" ... 118.0 lb. LBM
5' 2" .... 92.5 lb. LBM	5' 11" ... 121.5 lb. LBM
5' 3" .... 96.0 lb. LBM	6' 0" ..... 125.0 lb. LBM
5' 4" .... 98.5 lb. LBM	6' 1" ..... 128.5 lb. LBM
5' 5" .. 102.0 lb. LBM	6' 2" ..... 132.0 lb. LBM
5' 6" .. 105.5 lb. LBM	6' 3" ..... 136.0 lb. LBM
	6' 4" ..... 139.5 lb. LBM

As long as one's level of lean body mass is adequate, what harm is there in an individual weighing less than the recommended weight for their height on the Body Mass Index tables? Such a person could be carrying a greater amount of muscle than a person considered normal on the Body Mass Index tables.

For example, as an international model, Claudia Schiffer's weight is below her Body Mass Index allowance. Weighing 126 pounds and standing 5' 10", Claudia is considered too light for her height by Body Mass Index standards alone (139–174 lb.). However, even with a small 24 inch waist and only 10% body fat, Claudia still carries a healthy 113½ pounds of LBM—well above the minimum LBM recommendation for her height. This is why she appears healthy as well as light and lean. Because she has not sacrificed muscle for the sake of appearing thin, she does not appear emaciated.

Remember, of course, the average male with 23% body fat or average female with 32% body fat will need to lose body fat, regardless of their current weight and height.

Body Types

ONE'S SKELETAL frame—large, medium or small—is yet an additional consideration when choosing an ideal body weight. Obviously, larger-framed people can afford to carry slightly more total body weight than smaller-framed people. Some authorities classify people's overall body types as:

- **Ectomorphic:** lean, thin-muscled and narrow-boned.

- **Mesomorphic:** muscular, strong, large torso and large-boned.

- **Endomorphic:** soft, wide hips and more body fat.

Even though you cannot change your bone size, you can still dramatically alter your body type classification by adding muscle and/or lowering your percentage body fat.

Some health authorities evaluate general body proportions by using waist to hip ratio (WHR). Divide your hip size by your waist size. A quotient above .80—an apple-shaped body rather than a pear-shaped body—is considered an increasing risk for health problems.

Age Doesn't Count

GETTING FATTER with age may be a statistical reality, but there is no biological justification for it. Quoting Patricia A. Kreutler's textbook, *Nutrition In Perspective*:

> *"The customary assumption that weight gain with increasing age is normal and desirable is simply not so. This fallacious viewpoint grew from surveys of **actual**, rather than desirable, weights of typical men and women."*

Health authorities and the fitness and diet industries implore an aging population to eat less and exercise more to prevent weight gain—their advice has been largely ineffective. Why? No one denies the benefits of exercise and lighter eating. But the truth is, to maintain a desirable weight, it doesn't matter *how much* you eat or exercise— it's more important to know how to *balance* your energy output and your calorie intake.

By teaching you how to analyze and adjust your energy balance, *The Body Fat Guide* will help you achieve and maintain your ideal body weight for life!

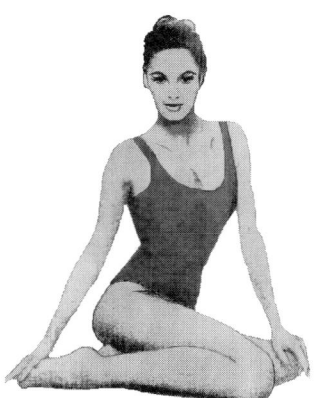

"Walking a mile burns as many calories as running a mile!"

Chapter 8

Reducing Body Fat

Proper Weight Loss

REDUCING BODY fat while avoiding a net loss of muscle is the proper way to lose weight. When losing weight, it is important to know if your body is burning calories from body fat or from muscle. Loss of lean body mass is easily checked by referring to changes in your body composition.

Muscle is 72% water, while body fat is only 20–25% water. A diet or exercise program that burns a large amount of muscle for energy (as when performing excessive anaerobic exercise while in negative calorie balance) will cause your weight to drop like a stone because of the large amount of water and glycogen lost from burned-off muscle.

In addition to losses from the elimination of fluid retention, most of the rapid weight loss seen in fasting and crash diets is due more to water lost from burned-off muscle rather than to calories lost from burned-off body fat. When returning to normal eating, much of this weight will be rapidly regained when muscle replenishes with glycogen and fluid. As muscle replenishes, it is not unusual for a person to regain muscular weight while eating an amount of food on which they would normally lose weight.

Note the difference between *weight* loss and *calorie* loss. In fasting, although most of the *weight* lost is from burned-off muscle (mostly glycogen and water with small amounts of protein), most of the *calories* lost are from burned-off body fat. Fasting is a subject that goes beyond the scope of this book. For more information on fasting, check the *Suggested Reading* section.

Dieting improves digestion and assimilation of calories from food. This is another reason why body weight is quickly and easily regained after a diet. Although dieting may increase levels of one's "fat-storing" enzymes, body fat can not be regained unless one absorbs excess calories.

It is practically impossible to avoid burning-off some muscle when in negative calorie balance. Through a process known as *gluconeogenesis*, your body draws upon all its tissues to release stored energy. The trick to preventing a *net* loss of muscle when attempting to reduce body fat is to periodically replenish your lost muscle mass. You can do this all at once following the end of a long period of continuous negative calorie balance —for example, following the breaking of a fast. Or you can do it intermittently by restricting negative calorie balance to short periods throughout the day, as occurs when following a moderate calorie-reduced diet. The best way to avoid losing muscle while burning body fat is to never accumulate the body fat in the first place!

Dieting At Last

A REDUCING diet is best composed of an abundance of fresh, raw, juicy fruit and succulent green vegetables with a minimum of concentrated starches, sugars and dietary fat. Drink all the pure water you desire, but do not force yourself to drink more than thirst calls for in an attempt to "flush" your body. Excess water will not speed up the ability of your kidneys to filter waste products from your blood—it may even slow it down.

The majority of foods in your diet should be naturally high in water content. Distilled or purified water, as pure as uncontaminated rain water, is the best to drink. Minerals dissolved in water are as unusable to your body as any

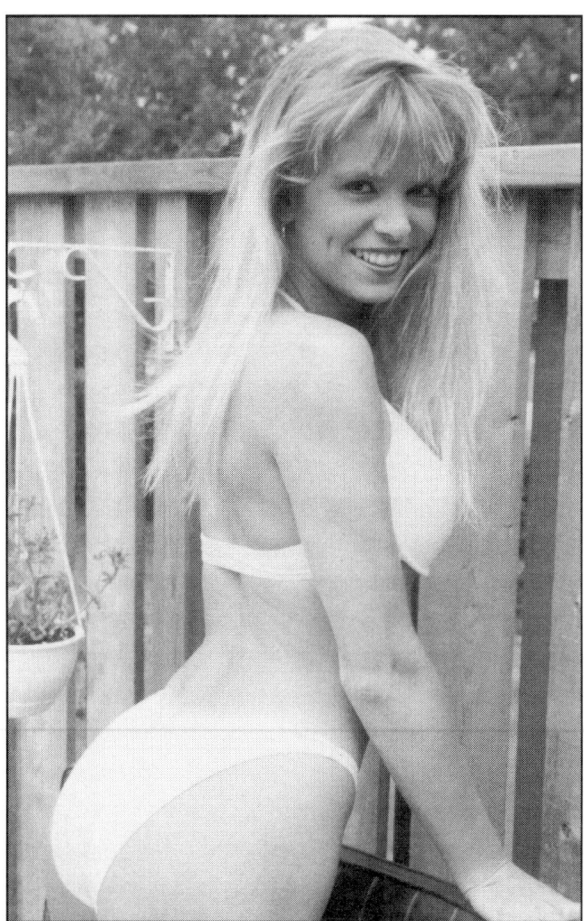

The results of a good diet and exercise program are worth the effort.

other dirt that comes direct from the ground. Only a properly balanced diet of fresh, natural, unrefined foods can provide you with minerals in a form your body can use.

Since a reducing diet is not a time for new growth, protein needs are reduced. Taking in extra protein while dieting in an attempt to build more muscle is ineffective because the extra protein will simply be burned for energy. Most adults only require about 25–30 grams of protein a day for maintenance. This is about half the usual daily recommended allowance of .8 grams of protein per kilogram (2.2 lbs.) of body weight. The recommended allowance for protein is doubled for growth purposes and does not take body composition into consideration.

The most difficult part of dieting is getting through the first day. When you cut back on supplying your body with energy from food, your system needs time to adjust to supplying extra energy from stored body fat to make up the difference. This will not occur until you withhold food.

As you begin to diet, your blood glucose may drop. This signals the part of your brain known as the *glucostat* to make you hungry. In addition, a healing crisis of symptoms resulting from previous bad eating habits may occur.

Once your body gets the message that you are no longer feeding it all it wants, it begins to change over to running on stored energy sources. As these new sources release their energy, they drive your blood glucose back to normal levels, which turns down your glucostat. The result: hunger is usually more manageable. Your vital tissues continue to be nourished with nutrients supplied from internal sources as well as external sources.

This physiological adaptation is even more pronounced while on an extended fast. On a fast with nothing but water, your body is running completely on internal sources. Since there is temporarily no need for any external sources of nourishment, hunger disappears altogether. Not until the fast is broken or your body's internal supply of stored energy runs out will hunger return. Absence of hunger on a severe diet is one of the reasons why people can easily get carried away and prolong their diet longer than necessary.

Calorie Deficit

HEALTH AUTHORITIES recommend losing no more than 2 pounds of body fat a week to prevent a net loss of muscle. To accomplish this in one week, you need to accumulate a deficit of −7000 calories, in the Net column on your Energy Balance Chart, at a suggested rate of −1000 calories per day. Cut back your daily calorie intake by 500 calories while simultaneously increasing your daily activity level by 500 calories, and you will come out right.

Any combination of cutting calorie intake and increasing activity that totals −1000 net calories a day will work just as well. For a slower

rate of weight loss, cut 250–500 calories a day to lose $1/2$–1 pound of body fat a week.

Combining some aerobic activity with reduced food intake is more beneficial than reducing food intake alone. However, do not expect that increased activity without dietary control will give you results. Trying to reduce body fat with more and more activity, while ignoring your food intake, is a losing battle. The relatively meager caloric expenditures of activity are no match for the ease with which those calories are almost instantly regained through eating.

Do not be concerned about "slowing down" your metabolism as you diet. Metabolism is the total of all the processes that build up your body and remove waste. While dieting, some parts of your metabolism may be temporarily slowed because your body is not working as hard to digest and burn food. However, the aftereffect of a proper diet or fast is to increase and improve your overall metabolism.

Exercise and Hunger

DOES EXERCISE decrease hunger? It's true, you may not feel like immediately sitting down to a large meal after running a marathon. Eventually though, after you have given your body time to rest, and after most of your blood is no longer concentrated within your exercising skeletal muscles, you would probably feel a stronger than usual urge to satisfy hunger.

Don't confuse the immediate short-term and long-term effects of exercise on hunger. Extra effort by your body uses up extra calories and usually creates extra hunger in the long run. The immediate effect of exercise may be to reduce hunger, but in the long run, exercise will increase your hunger.

Speed Doesn't Count

LOW-INTENSITY, long-duration aerobic activities, like walking, tend to burn calories from fat for fuel. High-intensity, short-duration anaerobic activities, like sprinting, tend to burn calories from muscle glycogen for fuel. Sprinters often have very well developed, muscular legs because of the muscle-building effect of the anaerobic exercise they perform. Slower-paced long-distance runners tend to have less developed muscle and less body fat.

On a calorie basis, walking a mile burns the same amount of calories as running a mile—it just takes longer to walk. But the sources of fuel for the calories burned during walking and running are different: fat as fuel for walking and glycogen as fuel for fast running. Since most people can walk farther than they can run, walking is a very potent fat-burning activity.

Here's a walking tip if you are climbing a steep hill. To maintain the same rate of exertion climbing the hill as you maintained on level ground, keep the pace of your stride the same (steps per minute), but shorten your stride's length. Use your perceived rate of exertion to determine if you are making the right adjustment as you ascend the hill.

If you want to perform aerobic exercise indoors, walking and running in place burns

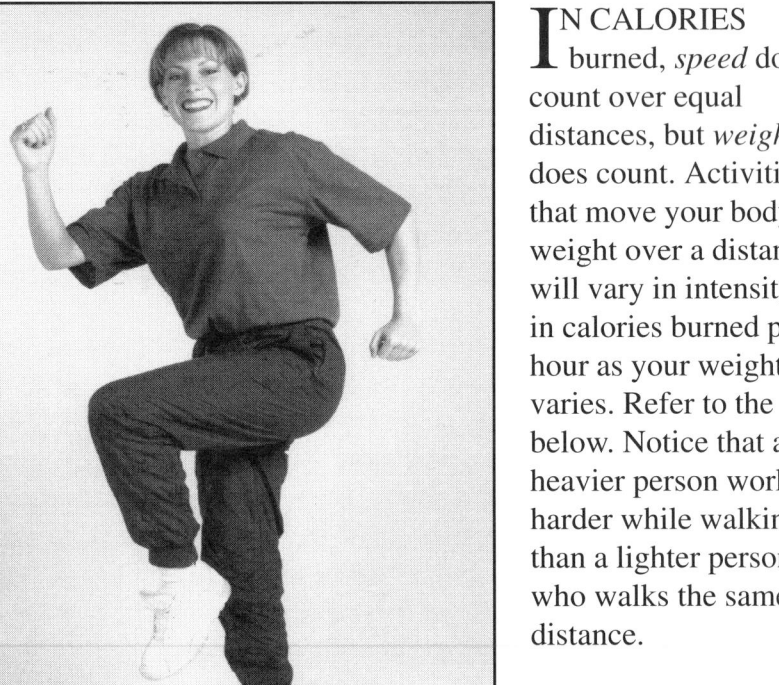

You don't need equipment—walk or run in place.

calories just as effectively as walking or running outside. And it's much cheaper than purchasing fancy aerobic-exercise equipment.

Weight and Intensity

IN CALORIES burned, *speed* doesn't count over equal distances, but *weight* does count. Activities that move your body weight over a distance will vary in intensity and in calories burned per hour as your weight varies. Refer to the chart below. Notice that a heavier person works harder while walking than a lighter person who walks the same distance.

For example, if you weigh 175 pounds, one hour of walking at 3.5 mph burns approximately 350 calories (100 calories per mile), mainly from fat. Weighing 115 pounds, you would burn 230 calories per hour (65.7 calories per mile)—within the *moderate* intensity level. But weighing 300 pounds, you would burn 600 calories per hour (171.4 calories per mile)—well past the *strenuous* level and burning more muscle.

Calories burned *per hour* at 3.5 mph (5.6 km/h) = 2 x body weight (including clothing).

Calories burned *per mile*, on foot (walking, running) = 2 x body weight ·/. 3.5

Calories burned *per kilometre*, on foot = 2 x body weight ·/. 5.6

Heavier people are better off doing aerobic activity that gets them off their feet, such as cycling or rowing. Nevertheless, exercise that requires you to stay on your feet generally allows you to burn more calories by increasing the total amount of muscle you are using. Cross country skiing burns more calories than most other activities because it uses the most muscle at the same time.

Heart Rate

IN ADDITION TO your perceived rate of exertion, many authorities recommend using your heart rate to gauge the intensity level and calorie output of your activities. Use gentle pressure with your fingertips to check your pulse at your carotid artery (beside your adam's apple) or radial artery (inner wrist, below your thumb). Your maximum heart rate (MHR), in beats per minute, is determined by subtracting your age from 220. Intensity levels are figured as percentages of your maximum heart rate; e.g., 65% of your MHR is considered your fat-burning zone. Note your heart rate during various activity intensity levels. If your cardiovascular fitness changes, you may find your heart rate has changed at different intensity levels.

Spot Reducing

AS YOU LOSE body fat, some body parts may thin out before others. Don't get discouraged. Body fat melts away from all areas evenly. Areas where body fat is piled up higher simply require more time to thin out.

Attempting to spot reduce body fat from problem areas with specific muscle-burning exercises is futile. When doing these exercises while dieting, you may temporarily reduce the size of your problem areas, but that is because you have reduced muscle, not body fat.

For example, losing two pounds of body fat in one week should reduce your waist size about $1/2$ inch. It is possible to temporarily decrease your waist size by more than this without losing any additional body fat. Performing excessive amounts of anaerobic abdominal exercise, while in negative calorie balance, would temporarily reduce the mass of your abdominal muscles. Your reduced calorie intake would temporarily prevent them from fully replenishing back to normal size.

Ironically, muscles in your abdomen, and in other problem areas that are exercised this way, would tighten up with more definition if allowed to fully replenish. They would look leaner and toned, as described in the example of the painted balloon. Of course, this assumes there is no excess body fat covering them in the first place. If you don't limit your calorie intake while attempting to spot reduce your problem areas with anaerobic exercise, you will actually build up the size of these areas, like a bodybuilder.

Cellulite and Liposuction

SOMETIMES FIBROUS compartments lying under the skin become overstuffed with fat, water and accumulated waste material. This can make tissue pucker out like an overstuffed quilt. People call this "orange peel" type of tissue *cellulite*. The fat stored in cellulite responds to the same reducing effect as any other type of surplus body fat. Additional steps must be taken to prevent the accumulation of waste material that produces the distinct appearance of cellulite.

An improved diet that includes an abundance of fresh, vitamin-mineral-rich, raw fruit and green vegetables will strengthen the walls of tiny blood vessels known as capillaries. Improved capillary strength reduces the seepage of waste material into the interstitial spaces between the subcutaneous cells where cellulite occurs. A diet low in sodium chloride will prevent the accumulation of excess salt water brine into these spaces as well.

Contraction of the muscles through regular exercise helps to drain off the waste deposits that lie trapped in the interstitial spaces between the subcutaneous cells. Regular exercise to promote overall circulation is all that is needed. Specific massage, lymph drainage, body wraps, skin creams and other treatments are not necessary. What good does it do to temporarily push this material out of local areas, as is claimed by people who employ these treatments, if it just gets backed up again in the general circulation?

In addition to reducing cellulite, a diet and exercise program that improves capillary strength, reduces salt, reduces abdominal fat, strengthens the abdominal muscles and promotes general circulation can help alleviate menstrual problems such as heavy bleeding, bloating and fatigue.

What about liposuction? According to an article, *"Lipo: Permanent Fat Loss or Quick Fix?"* by Nicole Garris Lorey. Vie. May 1996:

> *"While effective at removing fat, liposuction and liposculpture probably will not reduce the dimpled appearance of cellulite—a condition caused by the pulling of bands of fiber between the top of the skin and the deep layers of fat below."*

Diet Drugs

THE RECENT diet drug craze for those anxious to "look good naked" involved the fen/phen prescription. Fen/phen is a combination of drugs—one a stimulant, the other a depressant—that reduces appetite. Although resulting in miraculous weight loss, former U.S. Surgeon General C. Everett Coop reported that little weight loss is permanent when coming off drugs like fen/phen. The reason should be clear to you by now: Taking drugs does not teach you to eat properly. Eating properly is the only way to permanently control your weight.

Fen/phen works by upsetting the brain's normal balance of serotonin, a neurotransmitter. As with any new drug prescription that lacks long-term studies, there were suspected adverse effects when taking this prescription.

Many people had reported symptoms of insomnia, irritability, depression, amnesia, hallucinations and anxiety when taking these drugs. Fen/phen was implicated as a cause of primary pulmonary hypertension (PPH), a rare, but serious, disease. People taking this prescription were 25 times more likely to develop this disease than the regular population. Eventually, fen/phen was yanked off the market.

When fen/phen was legal, the "morbidly obese" were described as the only patients who should take this prescription. Yet, few people who took fen/phen would be characterized as morbidly obese. Considering the potential dangers and long-term ineffectiveness of most quick fix drug solutions for permanent weight control, why should *anyone*, including the morbidly obese, waste their time with these kinds of drugs?

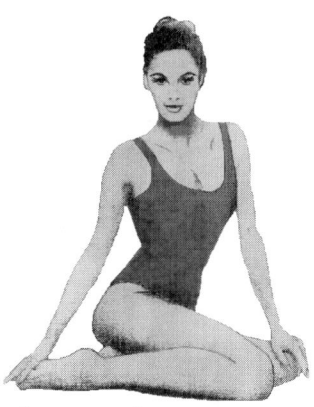

"Exercise tears down muscle. Recovery from exercise builds up muscle."

Chapter 9

Increasing Lean Body Mass

Proper Weight Gain

INCREASING LEAN body mass without gaining body fat is the proper way to build, tone and shape your physique. You must combine the right exercises, sufficient recovery time and adequate calorie intake to achieve your goal.

Although men naturally have more muscle mass than women, women should not underestimate their ability to gain useful, shapely muscle. Testosterone is the hormone responsible for the creation of extra muscle fiber in males as boys grow into adulthood. These muscle fibers are made of non-removable structural proteins. Once reaching adulthood, however, the effect of testosterone on the further development of muscle fiber is very limited.

In both male and female adults, muscle mass is generally increased by the addition of removable storage proteins, called *labile proteins*, rather than by the creation of new muscle fibers. Anaerobic exercise, rest and a well-balanced, calorie-sufficient diet are all that are needed to increase lean body mass in both males and females.

Calorie Surplus

SOME HEALTH authorities recommend gaining no more than $1/2$–1 pound of muscle per week to prevent a net gain of body fat. Other authorities suggest a 2–$2^{1}/_2$ pound per week limit. The total amount of muscle you can gain in a year is determined by how far away you are from your maximum potential. Theoretically, to gain 2 pounds of muscle in one week, at 600 calories per pound, you would need to perform anaerobic bodybuilding exercise and accumulate approximately 1200 surplus calories. Your Net column, on the Energy Balance Chart, would show an average daily surplus of 171 calories.

Creating a calorie surplus does not mean you have to stuff yourself with more food. *Getting more rest can be just as valuable in creating a calorie surplus as eating more food.* In nature, pregnant animals, who do not always have

63

access to additional food to support the growth of their offspring, create a calorie surplus by becoming less active.

For muscle growth, a number of health authorities recommend extra daily calories ranging from a minimum of approximately 200 extra calories a day, 300–500 (the most common recommendation), 700 and as high as 1000 extra calories. Incidently, 300 extra calories a day is recommended for pregnant women and 500 extra calories a day for lactating women.

Try experimenting for one week to see how many extra calories you should eat to add muscle without adding body fat. For example, you may wish to start at around 300 extra calories per day. Analyze your results with the Body Composition Tables and increase or decrease your calories as necessary. Soon you will be able to determine that *x* amount of extra calories allows you to grow *x* amount of muscle without adding body fat. Any extra protein required for muscle growth will be provided along with the extra calories you ingest, as long as you are eating a properly balanced diet.

Adding a small amount of body fat while gaining muscle is only permissible if your percentage body fat is not increasing. You can trim off any body fat accumulated this way later. However, adding large amounts of body fat along with muscle is not recommended.

Recovery

SINCE ANAEROBIC exercise burns glycogen for fuel, and since glycogen is part of your lean body mass, LBM is lost when performing anaerobic exercise. The recovery of burned-off LBM, through rest and diet, along with the addition of newly synthesized

LBM is what makes anaerobic activity a muscle-building and strength-building activity.

Notice, exercise alone does not build strength and muscle. Exercise temporarily depletes your energy and leaves you weaker. *Recovery* from exercise replenishes strength and muscle. *Overcompensation* of muscle reserves through replenishment builds additional strength and muscle.

To increase the mass of a muscle, you must force the muscle to contract against resistance and then allow 48–96 hours for that muscle to completely recover. If you are a beginner, you can ensure maximum growth of basic muscle mass by exercising your whole body in one session, performed 3 times per week. To bring out more shape and definition, you can work-out more often. Divide up your exercise routine, working some muscles on certain days while other muscles are recovering.

Eventually, as you gain muscle and strength, the intensity of your exercise routine will need to progress to a higher level if you want to continue developing muscle mass and strength. There are many fine books, videos, gyms and personal trainers available to assist you in planning a more advanced routine.

Freehand Exercises

THE FOLLOWING exercises require no equipment and are useful for any beginner interested in strengthening, shaping, toning and building muscle. All exercises should be performed starting with two sets of 15–20 repetitions or until fatigued. Concentrate on the feeling of the muscle being worked when performing the exercise.

There is no magic number of sets and repetitions per exercise that will guarantee results.

The most basic and important principle of muscle-building exercise is to achieve an increased flow of blood into the area being worked.

Work hard with as many sets and reps as it takes to achieve this blood flow—you'll know it when you feel it. Ideally, this flow should increase until tissue congestion prevents continuation of the exercise. When you can no longer increase the flow of blood into the muscle, you have finished working the muscle to its limit. Move on to the next exercise.

As a warm-up, the following exercise should be performed:

Warm-Up

Stand with your feet shoulder width apart. Bend over at the waist as you gently reach both hands towards the floor on the outside of your left foot. Keep your knees slightly bent. Do not force yourself downward. After reaching down, straighten half-way up and reach down with your hands again, this time between your feet. Come halfway up again and reach down towards the outside of your right foot. Now straighten all the way up and stretch your arms over your head as you gently bend backwards at the waist. Repeat this entire sequence 20 times. Perform the first ten sequences as described above and then reverse the order of the movements for the last ten sequences.

1. Push-Ups and Modified Push-Ups

Here's a classic upper body exercise for your chest, the back of your arms and the front of your shoulders. Lie face down (prone) on the floor with your hands under your shoulders, palms on the floor. Take a breath and exhale as you push your upper body away from the floor, keeping your entire body straight from toes to head. Breathe in as you dip your body back down so that only your chest touches the floor. *For all exercises in general, exhale on exertion and inhale on relaxation.* Repeat this movement. If this exercise is too strenuous, perform a modified version by keeping your knees on the floor throughout the exercise.

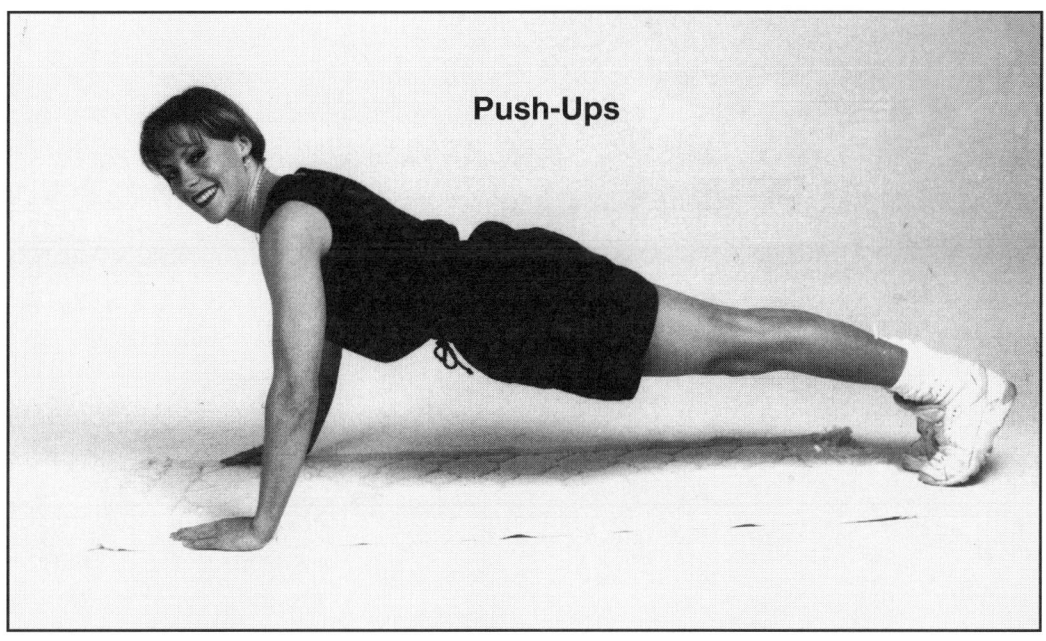

Push-Ups

2. Squats or Deep Knee-Bends

This exercise works the front and back of your thighs as well as your buttocks and lower back. It is also good for improving your breathing. Stand up straight with your feet about shoulder width apart and toes pointed out slightly. With hands on hips or holding on to a chair for balance, breathe in while you squat down, keeping your back straight and

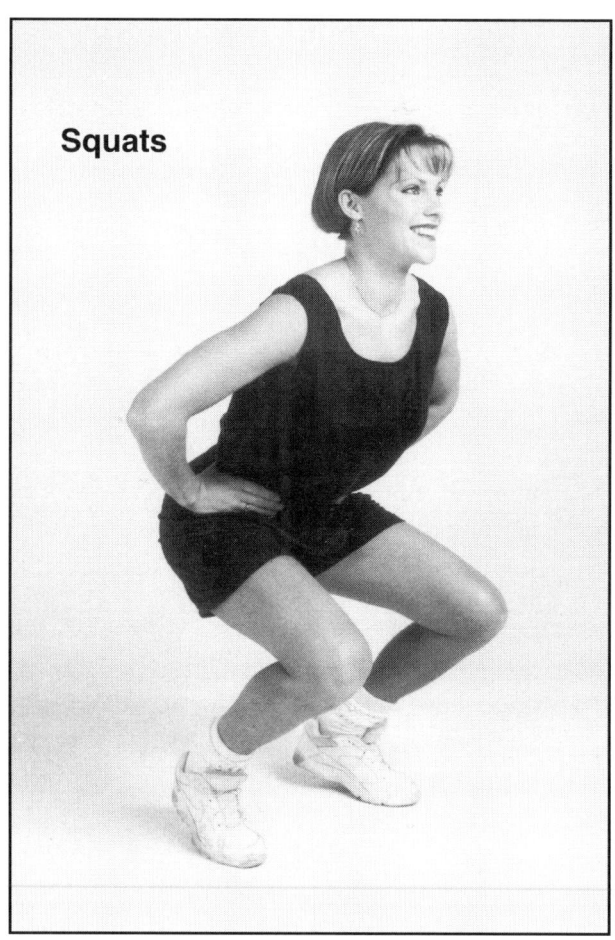

Squats

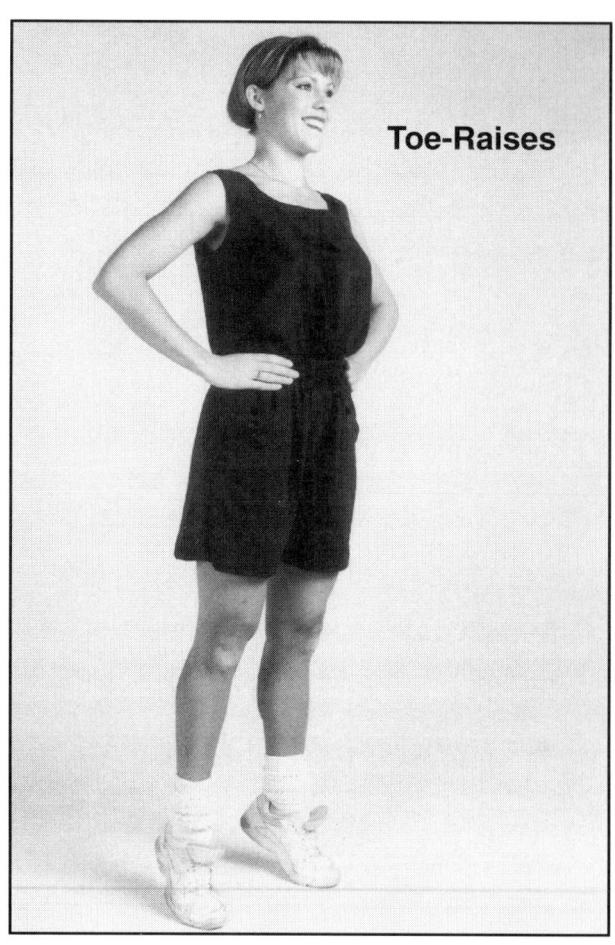

Toe-Raises

head up. Your knees should line up with the second toe of each foot. Squat down with your feet flat on the floor. Let your heels come off the floor if that feels more comfortable, or place a book under them. Squat down only until the tops of your thighs are parallel with the floor, no lower. Keep your back straight and head up at all times. Breathe out as you straighten your knees and return to an upright position. Repeat this movement.

3. One- and Two-Legged Toe-Raises or Calf-Raises

Stand up straight, rise up on the balls of your feet (the part of your sole at the base of your big toe) and slowly lower your heels back down to the floor. Repeat this movement. Stand with your toes on the edge of a step to lower your heels farther. Hold onto a chair and

make this exercise more difficult by rising up on one foot at a time. This exercise works the back of your lower leg, your calf.

4. Doorknob Rows

Here's one for your back and for the front of your arms. Face the narrow edge of an open door and grasp both doorknobs, one in each hand. Plant each foot firmly on the floor on opposite sides of the door and lean back until your arms are fully extended, your upper body straight. Pull your body toward the knobs while you tense your back muscles. Then lean back, straighten your arms and repeat.

5. Lying Hyper-Extensions

Lie prone on the floor (face down), your feet together and your arms under your body with your palms touching the front of your thighs.

Raise your upper body until your shoulders and chest do not touch the floor while simultaneously raising your legs until your thighs no longer touch your hands. Relax and repeat. This exercise requires very little movement, so do not strain. This is a powerful movement for your back and buttocks as well as for the back of your neck, shoulders and legs. Make this exercise more difficult by extending your arms out to the side and in front of you.

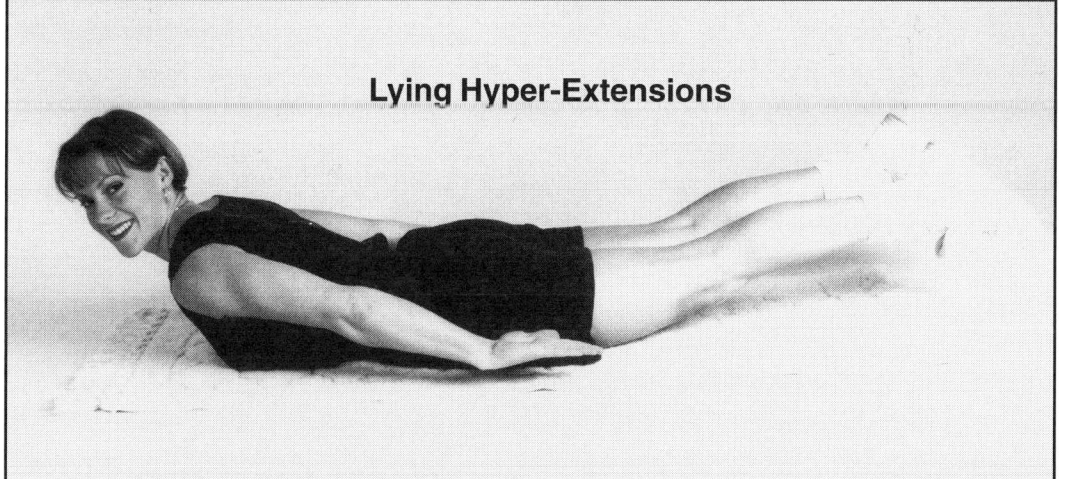

Lying Hyper-Extensions

your biceps, place your hands behind your neck and raise both elbows straight up. Then, turn your palms down and out, and point your thumbs straight up. Tense your biceps into tight balls of muscle and hold for several seconds. Relax and repeat.

For your triceps, extend your arms straight down by your sides. Rotate your arms inward so your thumbs move inward toward your body, and continue rotating your arms as far as they will go. Straighten your elbows and tense your triceps into hard knots. Hold a few seconds, relax and repeat. Try this exercise again with your arms fully rotated in the opposite direction— move your thumbs outward, away from your body. These are very powerful exercises—take care not to strain your muscles. Feeling a little stiff and sore the following day is normal, but don't overdo it.

6. Doorway Shoulder Isometrics

To exercise your shoulders, stand in a doorway and place the little-finger edge of each closed fist against opposite sides of the door frame, your arms straight and stiff. Take a breath and exhale as you vigorously push your fists into the frame. After several seconds, relax and repeat. Concentrate on keeping your arms straight throughout this exercise so you can feel the force being transferred throughout your arms into your shoulder muscles. This is an isometric exercise; it causes your muscles to contract without moving your limbs.

7. Triceps and Biceps Tensing

The back of your arm, your triceps, and the front of your arm, your biceps, can be exercised by placing your arm in various positions and vigorously tensing these muscles. For

8. Running in Place

Finish your routine with an exercise that promotes general circulation, clears waste products from your system, improves cardiovascular efficiency, and makes your skin glow. Raise your feet a few inches off the floor as you gently run in place for 5 minutes. Gradually build up your time to 20–30 minutes and eventually raise your feet and knees higher as you run at a faster pace. When you are finished, keep moving for several minutes as you allow your body to cool down.

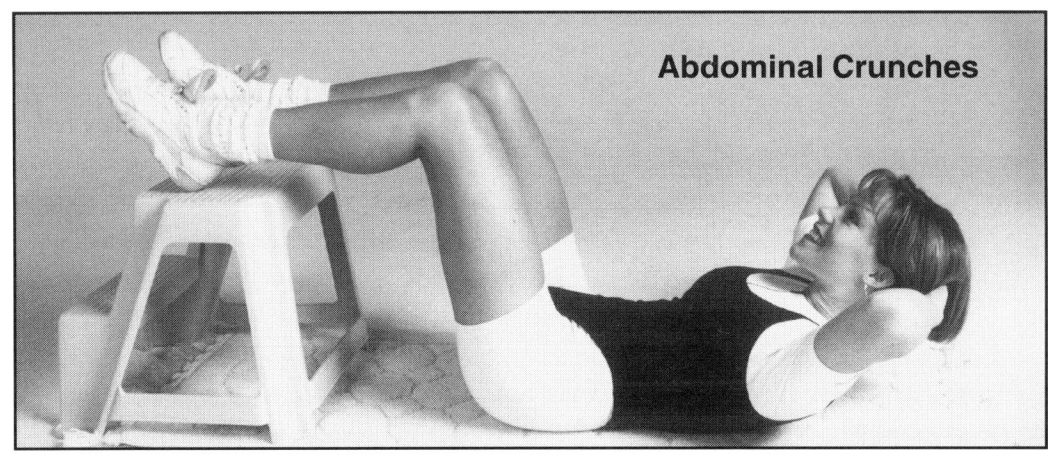

Abdominal Crunches

you do not pull on your neck to assist you in raising your torso. Keep your elbows spread out to the side and out of your line of vision. Slowly lower your torso and repeat.

Special Toning Exercises

THE FOLLOWING exercises can be added to your exercise routine to maintain the tone and shape of muscles in special areas like your waist, glutes (buttocks), thighs and lower back.

1. Abdominal Crunches and Reverse Crunches

Here's how to safely and effectively perform an abdominal crunch without purchasing any special exercise apparatus. Lie on your back with your feet resting on the seat of a chair and your knees bent. Raise only your upper torso by gently lifting and curling your chest bone toward your pelvis. You may place your hands behind your head for support as long as

Perform reverse crunches in this position by keeping your upper torso on the floor as you raise your pelvis up and away from the floor. Do not push your pelvis up with your legs. Let your lower abdominal muscles pull up your pelvis. Lower and repeat.

Simultaneously performing crunches and reverse crunches together in one movement is not as effective as performing them in separate movements. If you bring the chest-end and pelvis-end of your abdominal muscles closer together it tends to slacken your abdominal muscles, making them difficult to contract.

2. Lying Side Leg-Raises

This exercise is for the side of your waist, hips and thighs. Lie on your side, bend your bottom leg for a base of support, and raise your straight leg up and away from your body. Lower your leg slowly and repeat. When you are finished, lie on your opposite side and repeat.

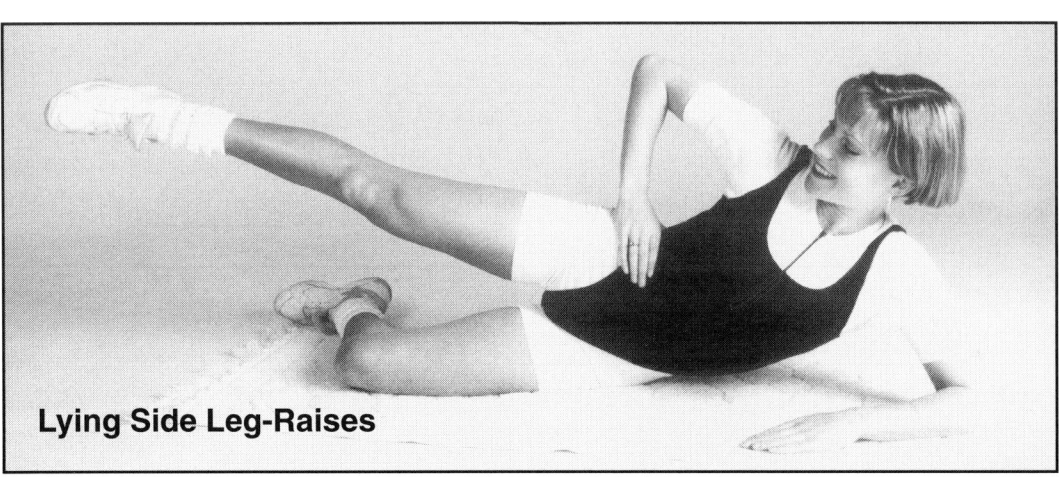

Lying Side Leg-Raises

3. Twisting Elbow-to-Opposite-Knee Sit-Ups

Lie on your back with your legs straight out and your hands behind your head. Sit up and twist to the left as you bring your left knee up to touch

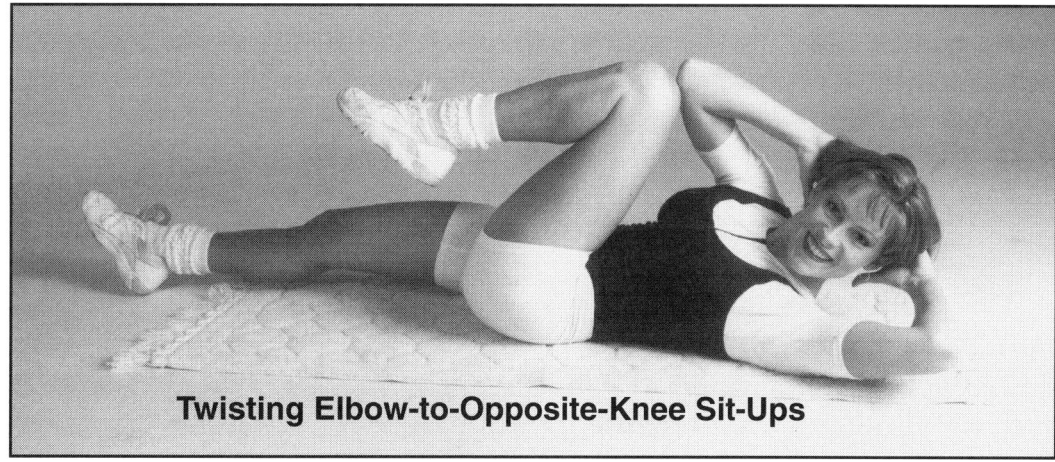

Twisting Elbow-to-Opposite-Knee Sit-Ups

your right elbow. Do not pull on your neck. Return to a lying position and repeat, this time sitting up and twisting to the right while bringing your right knee up to touch your left elbow. Continue alternating in this manner.

4. Side Sit-Ups

Lie on your back with your knees bent and your hands behind your head. Lower both knees to the left and turn your left hip into the floor while raising your upper body straight up. Do not pull on your neck. You should feel a contraction on the right side of your waist. Relax and repeat on the opposite side, lowering both knees to the right and turning your right hip into the floor while raising your upper body.

5. Seated Twists

Sit on a bench with both hands behind your head and your elbows pointing outward. Without bending over, turn your upper body to the right as you twist from your waist. Then turn to the

left as you twist in the opposite direction. Concentrate on pulling your abdominal muscles in tight while you continue twisting in alternate directions. (Photo on next page.)

6. Bent-Over Standing Twists

This one works your waist and lower back. Stand with your feet shoulder width apart and your hands behind your head. Unlock your knees as you bend your upper body forward from your hips until your upper body is parallel to the floor. Twist to the right from your waist until your right elbow is straight up. Then twist to the left in the same manner. Keep your abdominal muscles tight and continue alternating twists until tired. (Photo on next page.)

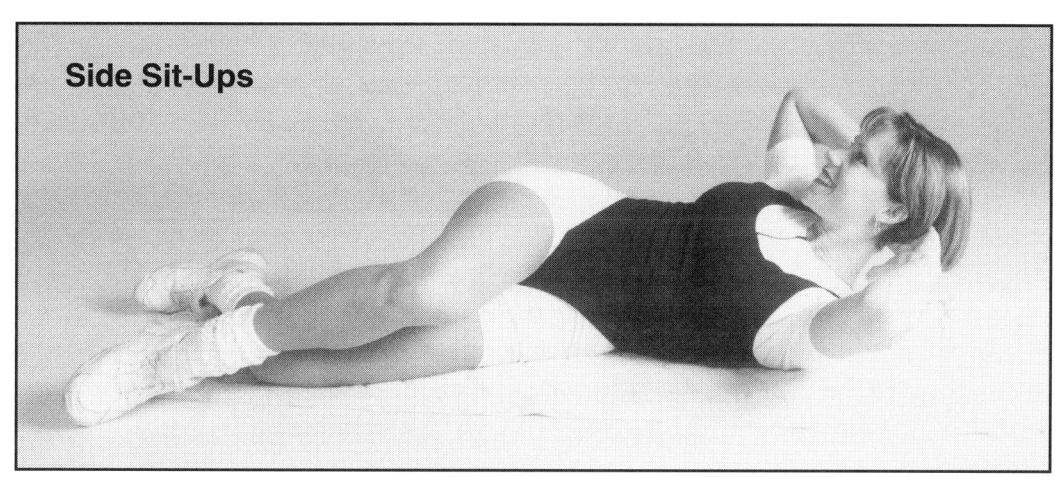

Side Sit-Ups

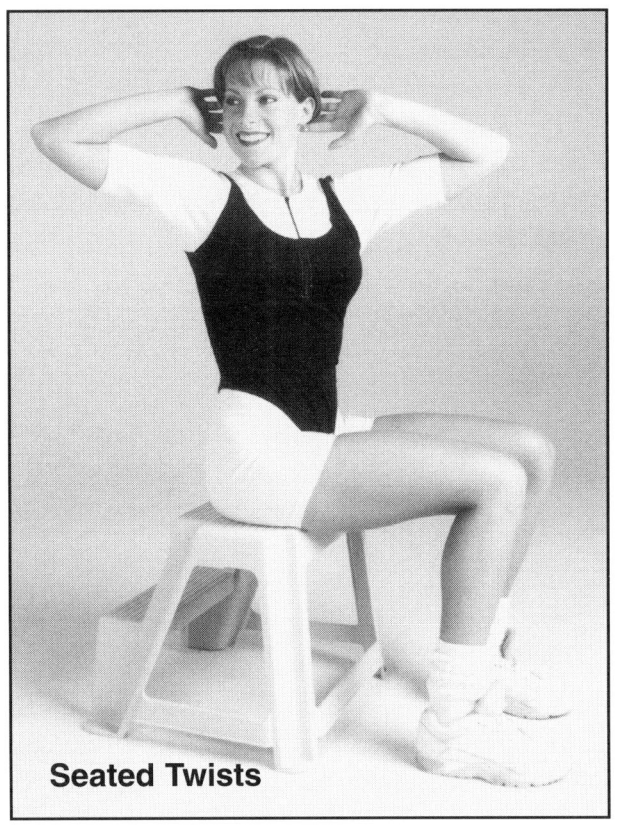

Seated Twists

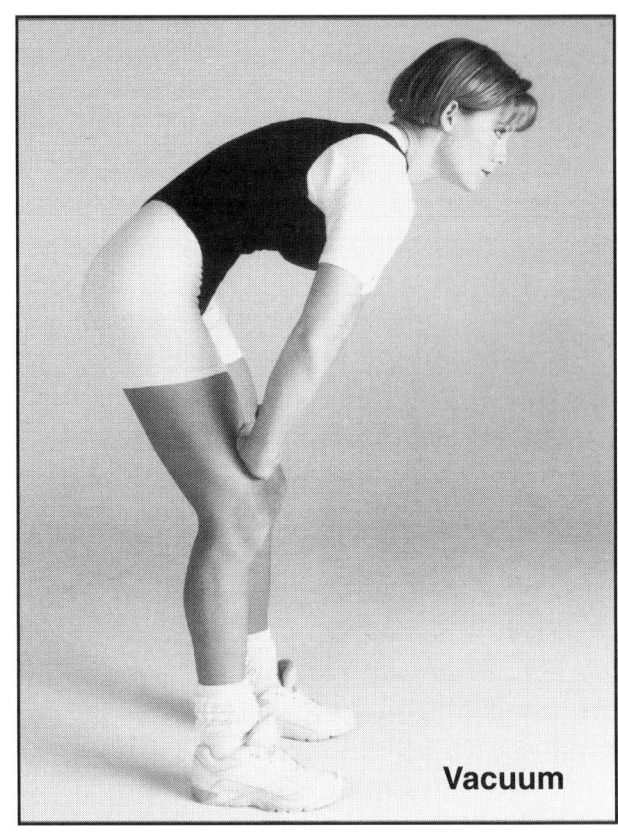

Vacuum

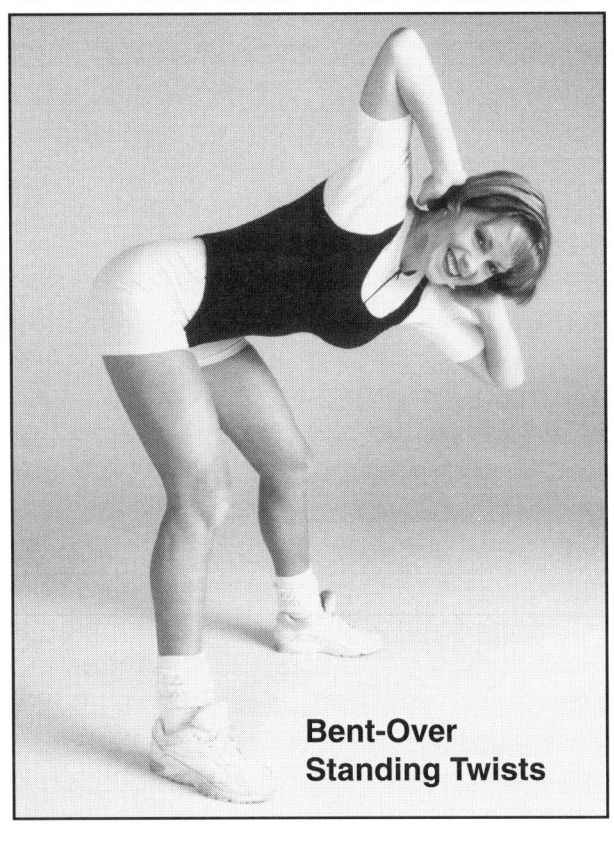

**Bent-Over
Standing Twists**

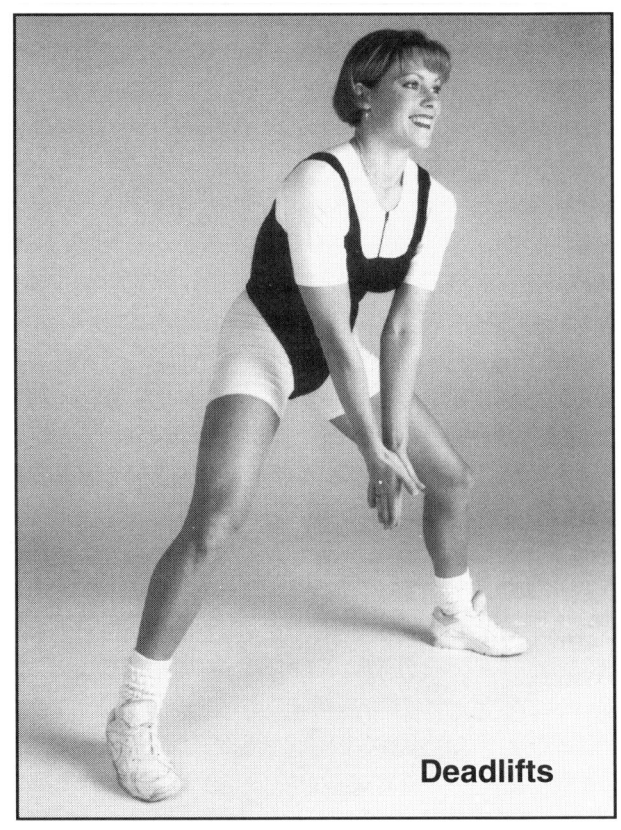

Deadlifts

7. Vacuum

This exercise is best performed early in the day, before putting anything into your stomach. It works your internal abdominal muscles and can help prevent constipation. Standing with knees bent slightly, support your upper body by placing your hands on your thighs. Take a deep breath to fill your lungs with air. Then rapidly blow the air out and hold your breath while attempting to suck your abdomen up into your rib cage. Hold as long as you can, release and breathe in. This movement requires practice at first, but is very effective once mastered.

8. Deadlifts

This exercise is for your glutes, inner thighs, hips and lower back. Stand with your feet wide apart, your toes pointing out, and your hands clasped together in front of your pelvis. Bend your knees as you bend forward from your hips. Make sure you keep your lower back straight. Reach back between your legs and stick out your buttocks. Quickly straighten up, fully extending your hips and knees, and thrust your pelvis forward as you tighten your glutes as hard as you can. Repeat.

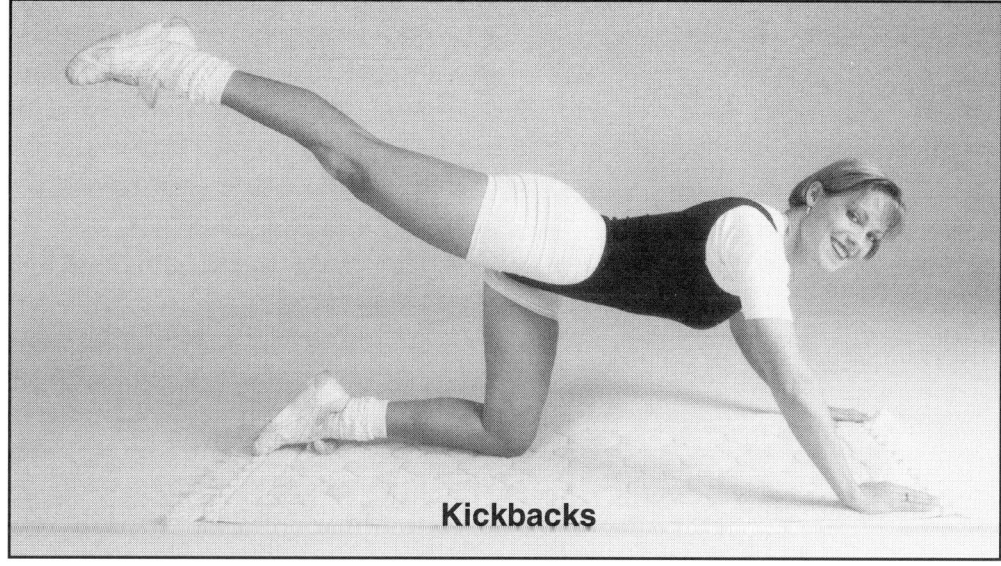

Kickbacks

9. Kneeling Kickbacks

While on your hands and knees, extend one leg straight back and touch your toe to the floor. Raise your leg as high as you can. Lower and repeat. Perform the same movement with your opposite leg.

10. Supine Scissors

For your inner thighs, lie on your back with your feet up in the air. Keep your legs straight as you alternately move your legs apart and close them together.

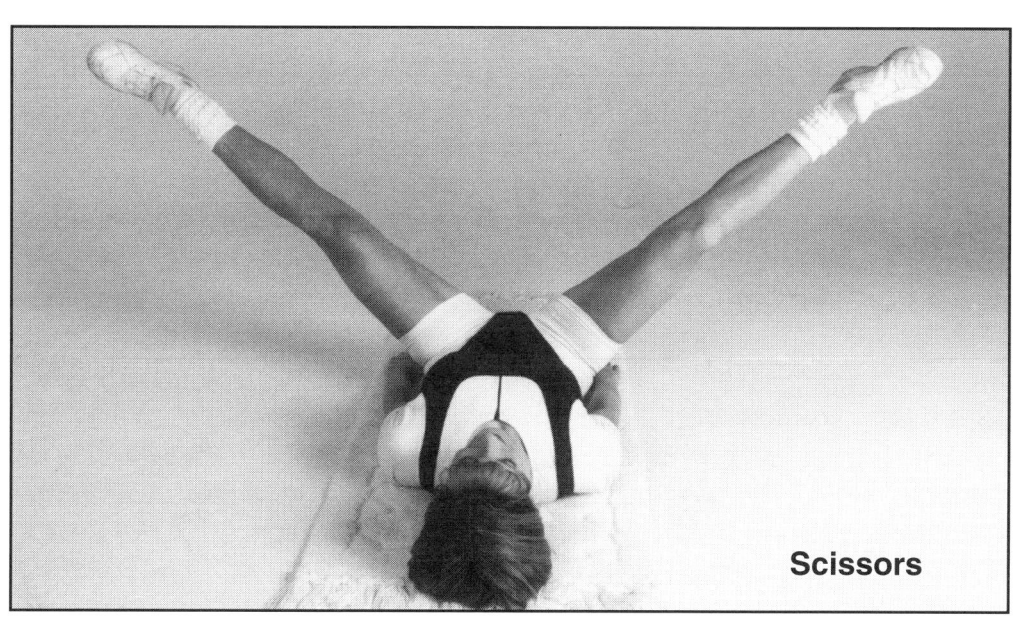

Scissors

Stretching

STRETCHING is great for increasing flexibility and for relieving congestion and tightness of fatigued muscles.

1. Seated One-Leg-Extended Stretch

To stretch your back and thighs, sit on the floor with one leg extended straight out in front of you. Bend your other leg at the knee, bringing the sole of your foot up against the inner thigh of your extended leg, your heel in toward your crotch. Slowly and gently lean forward as you attempt to touch the foot of your extended leg with your hands. Do not strain and do not bounce. Only stretch as far as is comfortable. Hold your position for a short period and release. Stretch again, gradually increasing your stretching distance and holding time. Reverse the position of your legs and repeat.

2. Shoulder Stretch

Place your left arm behind your back and attempt to touch the area between your shoulder blades with the back of your left hand. Raise your right arm and bring your right hand down behind your neck as you stretch to touch   the fingers of both hands together. Only stretch as far as is comfortable, holding your position for a short time and releasing. Reverse the position of your arms and repeat. As your flexibility improves, you will eventually be able to lock the fingers of both hands together.

3. Calf Stretch

Stand with your hands against a wall or chair. Extend one leg back a few inches, touching the floor with your toes. While bending your front knee, lean your body forward at about a 45° angle. Keep your rear leg straight as you gradually stretch your heel towards the floor. Hold, release, reverse positions and repeat with the opposite leg.

Final Word

TO SUM up, make sure you keep body fat gains to a minimum when gaining muscle. Adding body fat while you gain muscle may make you huge, but your appearance and health won't improve if your percentage body fat increases. Also, keep muscle loss to a minimum when losing body fat. Losing as much muscle as body fat may make you smaller, but it won't make you leaner if your percentage body fat doesn't improve. Gaining as much body fat as muscle and losing as much muscle as body fat is a merry-go-round to nowhere!

Remember, always let the actual changes in your body composition be your guide when modifying your energy balance. Also, remember not to go into a panic over small daily fluctuations in your measurements. Pay more attention to changes that last over several days.

The method offered in this book is not difficult, but it requires some effort on your part. Happily, the more effort you put into it, the more you will get out of it. That's all a hard working person like you really wants anyway, isn't it? So don't let this book sit on the shelf unused. Grab a friend, go for a walk, and get down to the business of counting up your calories. You have to eat—you might as well learn how to do it properly. Be patient—you have a lot of meals ahead of you.

You can do it!

R. B.

PART TWO:
BODY COMPOSITION
TABLES

Body Composition   FEMALE   100-131.5 Lb.

Weight: Lb.	Waist: 22 inches Fat: %	Fat: Lb.	LBM: Lb.	RMR: Cal.	22.25 inches Fat: %	Fat: Lb.	LBM: Lb.	RMR: Cal.	22.5 inches Fat: %	Fat: Lb.	LBM: Lb.	RMR: Cal.	22.75 inches Fat: %	Fat: Lb.	LBM: Lb.	RMR: Cal.
100	6.34	6.34	93.66	1295	7.38	7.38	92.62	1281	8.42	8.42	91.59	1267	9.45	9.45	90.55	1252
100.5	6.27	6.30	94.20	1303	7.30	7.34	93.16	1288	8.33	8.37	92.13	1274	9.36	9.41	91.09	1260
101	6.20	6.26	94.74	1310	7.22	7.30	93.70	1296	8.25	8.33	92.67	1282	9.28	9.37	91.63	1267
101.5	6.13	6.22	95.28	1318	7.15	7.25	94.25	1303	8.17	8.29	93.21	1289	9.19	9.33	92.17	1275
102	6.05	6.18	95.82	1325	7.07	7.21	94.79	1311	8.09	8.25	93.75	1297	9.11	9.29	92.71	1282
102.5	5.99	6.14	96.37	1333	7.00	7.17	95.33	1318	8.01	8.21	94.29	1304	9.02	9.25	93.25	1290
103	5.92	6.09	96.91	1340	6.92	7.13	95.87	1326	7.93	8.17	94.83	1312	8.94	9.21	93.79	1297
103.5	5.85	6.05	97.45	1348	6.85	7.09	96.41	1333	7.85	8.13	95.37	1319	8.86	9.17	94.33	1305
104	5.78	6.01	97.99	1355	6.78	7.05	96.95	1341	7.78	8.09	95.91	1326	8.77	9.12	94.88	1312
104.5	5.71	5.97	98.53	1363	6.71	7.01	97.49	1348	7.70	8.05	96.45	1334	8.69	9.08	95.42	1320
105	5.65	5.93	99.07	1370	6.64	6.97	98.03	1356	7.62	8.01	97.00	1341	8.61	9.04	95.96	1327
105.5	5.58	5.89	99.61	1378	6.57	6.93	98.57	1363	7.55	7.96	97.54	1349	8.53	9.00	96.50	1335
106	5.52	5.85	100.15	1385	6.50	6.89	99.11	1371	7.47	7.92	98.08	1356	8.45	8.96	97.04	1342
106.5	5.45	5.81	100.69	1393	6.43	6.84	99.66	1378	7.40	7.88	98.62	1364	8.38	8.92	97.58	1350
107	5.39	5.77	101.23	1400	6.36	6.80	100.20	1386	7.33	7.84	99.16	1371	8.30	8.88	98.12	1357
107.5	5.33	5.72	101.78	1408	6.29	6.76	100.74	1393	7.26	7.80	99.70	1379	8.22	8.84	98.66	1365
108	5.26	5.68	102.32	1415	6.22	6.72	101.28	1401	7.18	7.76	100.24	1386	8.14	8.80	99.20	1372
108.5	5.20	5.64	102.86	1423	6.16	6.68	101.82	1408	7.11	7.72	100.78	1394	8.07	8.76	99.74	1379
109	5.14	5.60	103.40	1430	6.09	6.64	102.36	1416	7.04	7.68	101.32	1401	7.99	8.71	100.29	1387
109.5	5.08	5.56	103.94	1437	6.03	6.60	102.90	1423	6.97	7.64	101.86	1409	7.92	8.67	100.83	1394
110	5.02	5.52	104.48	1445	5.96	6.56	103.44	1431	6.90	7.60	102.41	1416	7.85	8.63	101.37	1402
110.5	4.96	5.48	105.02	1452	5.90	6.52	103.98	1438	6.84	7.55	102.95	1424	7.78	8.59	101.91	1409
111	4.90	5.44	105.56	1460	5.83	6.48	104.52	1446	6.77	7.51	103.49	1431	7.70	8.55	102.45	1417
111.5	4.84	5.40	106.10	1467	5.77	6.43	105.07	1453	6.70	7.47	104.03	1439	7.63	8.51	102.99	1424
112	4.78	5.36	106.64	1475	5.71	6.39	105.61	1461	6.63	7.43	104.57	1446	7.56	8.47	103.53	1432
112.5	4.72	5.32	107.19	1482	5.65	6.35	106.15	1468	6.57	7.39	105.11	1454	7.49	8.43	104.07	1439
113	4.67	5.27	107.73	1490	5.59	6.31	106.69	1476	6.50	7.35	105.65	1461	7.42	8.39	104.61	1447
113.5	4.61	5.23	108.27	1497	5.52	6.27	107.23	1483	6.44	7.31	106.19	1469	7.35	8.35	105.15	1454
114	4.55	5.19	108.81	1505	5.46	6.23	107.77	1490	6.37	7.27	106.73	1476	7.28	8.30	105.70	1462
114.5	4.50	5.15	109.35	1512	5.40	6.19	108.31	1498	6.31	7.23	107.27	1484	7.22	8.26	106.24	1469
115	4.44	5.11	109.89	1520	5.35	6.15	108.85	1505	6.25	7.19	107.82	1491	7.15	8.22	106.78	1477
115.5	4.39	5.07	110.43	1527	5.29	6.11	109.39	1513	6.19	7.14	108.36	1499	7.08	8.18	107.32	1484
116	4.33	5.03	110.97	1535	5.23	6.07	109.93	1520	6.12	7.10	108.90	1506	7.02	8.14	107.86	1492
116.5	4.28	4.99	111.51	1542	5.17	6.02	110.48	1528	6.06	7.06	109.44	1514	6.95	8.10	108.40	1499
117	4.23	4.95	112.05	1550	5.11	5.98	111.02	1535	6.00	7.02	109.98	1521	6.89	8.06	108.94	1507
117.5	4.17	4.91	112.60	1557	5.06	5.94	111.56	1543	5.94	6.98	110.52	1528	6.82	8.02	109.48	1514
118	4.12	4.86	113.14	1565	5.00	5.90	112.10	1550	5.88	6.94	111.06	1536	6.76	7.98	110.02	1522
118.5	4.07	4.82	113.68	1572	4.95	5.86	112.64	1558	5.82	6.90	111.60	1543	6.70	7.94	110.56	1529
119	4.02	4.78	114.22	1580	4.89	5.82	113.18	1565	5.76	6.86	112.14	1551	6.63	7.89	111.11	1537
119.5	3.97	4.74	114.76	1587	4.84	5.78	113.72	1573	5.70	6.82	112.68	1558	6.57	7.85	111.65	1544
120	3.92	4.70	115.30	1595	4.78	5.74	114.26	1580	5.65	6.78	113.23	1566	6.51	7.81	112.19	1552
120.5	3.87	4.66	115.84	1602	4.73	5.70	114.80	1588	5.59	6.73	113.77	1573	6.45	7.77	112.73	1559
121	3.82	4.62	116.38	1610	4.67	5.66	115.34	1595	5.53	6.69	114.31	1581	6.39	7.73	113.27	1567
121.5	3.77	4.58	116.92	1617	4.62	5.61	115.89	1603	5.47	6.65	114.85	1588	6.33	7.69	113.81	1574
122	3.72	4.54	117.46	1625	4.57	5.57	116.43	1610	5.42	6.61	115.39	1596	6.27	7.65	114.35	1581
122.5	3.67	4.49	118.01	1632	4.52	5.53	116.97	1618	5.36	6.57	115.93	1603	6.21	7.61	114.89	1589
123	3.62	4.45	118.55	1639	4.46	5.49	117.51	1625	5.31	6.53	116.47	1611	6.15	7.57	115.43	1596
123.5	3.57	4.41	119.09	1647	4.41	5.45	118.05	1633	5.25	6.49	117.01	1618	6.09	7.53	115.97	1604
124	3.53	4.37	119.63	1654	4.36	5.41	118.59	1640	5.20	6.45	117.55	1626	6.04	7.48	116.52	1611
124.5	3.48	4.33	120.17	1662	4.31	5.37	119.13	1648	5.15	6.41	118.09	1633	5.98	7.44	117.06	1619
125	3.43	4.29	120.71	1669	4.26	5.33	119.67	1655	5.09	6.37	118.64	1641	5.92	7.40	117.60	1626
125.5	3.39	4.25	121.25	1677	4.21	5.29	120.21	1663	5.04	6.32	119.18	1648	5.87	7.36	118.14	1634
126	3.34	4.21	121.79	1684	4.16	5.25	120.75	1670	4.99	6.28	119.72	1656	5.81	7.32	118.68	1641
126.5	3.29	4.17	122.33	1692	4.11	5.20	121.30	1678	4.93	6.24	120.26	1663	5.75	7.28	119.22	1649
127	3.25	4.13	122.87	1699	4.07	5.16	121.84	1685	4.88	6.20	120.80	1671	5.70	7.24	119.76	1656
127.5	3.20	4.08	123.42	1707	4.02	5.12	122.38	1692	4.83	6.16	121.34	1678	5.65	7.20	120.30	1664
128	3.16	4.04	123.96	1714	3.97	5.08	122.92	1700	4.78	6.12	121.88	1686	5.59	7.16	120.84	1671
128.5	3.12	4.00	124.50	1722	3.92	5.04	123.46	1707	4.73	6.08	122.42	1693	5.54	7.12	121.38	1679
129	3.07	3.96	125.04	1729	3.88	5.00	124.00	1715	4.68	6.04	122.96	1701	5.48	7.07	121.93	1686
129.5	3.03	3.92	125.58	1737	3.83	4.96	124.54	1722	4.63	6.00	123.50	1708	5.43	7.03	122.47	1694
130	2.98	3.88	126.12	1744	3.78	4.92	125.08	1730	4.58	5.96	124.05	1716	5.38	6.99	123.01	1701
130.5	2.94	3.84	126.66	1752	3.74	4.88	125.62	1737	4.53	5.91	124.59	1723	5.33	6.95	123.55	1709
131	2.90	3.80	127.20	1759	3.69	4.84	126.16	1745	4.48	5.87	125.13	1731	5.28	6.91	124.09	1716
131.5	2.86	3.76	127.74	1767	3.65	4.79	126.71	1752	4.43	5.83	125.67	1738	5.22	6.87	124.63	1724

Body Composition FEMALE 100-131.5 Lb.

Weight: Lb.	Waist: 23 inches				23.25 inches				23.5 inches				23.75 inches			
	Fat: %	Fat: Lb.	LBM: Lb.	RMR: Cal.	Fat: %	Fat: Lb.	LBM: Lb.	RMR: Cal.	Fat: %	Fat: Lb.	LBM: Lb.	RMR: Cal.	Fat: %	Fat: Lb.	LBM: Lb.	RMR: Cal.
100	10.49	10.49	89.51	1238	11.53	11.53	88.47	1224	12.57	12.57	87.44	1209	13.60	13.60	86.40	1195
100.5	10.40	10.45	90.05	1245	11.43	11.49	89.01	1231	12.46	12.52	87.98	1217	13.49	13.56	86.94	1202
101	10.30	10.41	90.59	1253	11.33	11.45	89.55	1239	12.36	12.48	88.52	1224	13.39	13.52	87.48	1210
101.5	10.21	10.37	91.13	1260	11.24	11.40	90.10	1246	12.26	12.44	89.06	1232	13.28	13.48	88.02	1217
102	10.12	10.33	91.67	1268	11.14	11.36	90.64	1254	12.16	12.40	89.60	1239	13.18	13.44	88.56	1225
102.5	10.03	10.29	92.22	1275	11.05	11.32	91.18	1261	12.06	12.36	90.14	1247	13.07	13.40	89.10	1232
103	9.95	10.24	92.76	1283	10.95	11.28	91.72	1268	11.96	12.32	90.68	1254	12.97	13.36	89.64	1240
103.5	9.86	10.20	93.30	1290	10.86	11.24	92.26	1276	11.86	12.28	91.22	1262	12.87	13.32	90.18	1247
104	9.77	10.16	93.84	1298	10.77	11.20	92.80	1283	11.77	12.24	91.76	1269	12.76	13.27	90.73	1255
104.5	9.69	10.12	94.38	1305	10.68	11.16	93.34	1291	11.67	12.20	92.30	1277	12.66	13.23	91.27	1262
105	9.60	10.08	94.92	1313	10.59	11.12	93.88	1298	11.58	12.16	92.85	1284	12.56	13.19	91.81	1270
105.5	9.52	10.04	95.46	1320	10.50	11.08	94.42	1306	11.48	12.11	93.39	1292	12.47	13.15	92.35	1277
106	9.43	10.00	96.00	1328	10.41	11.04	94.96	1313	11.39	12.07	93.93	1299	12.37	13.11	92.89	1285
106.5	9.35	9.96	96.54	1335	10.32	10.99	95.51	1321	11.30	12.03	94.47	1306	12.27	13.07	93.43	1292
107	9.27	9.92	97.08	1343	10.24	10.95	96.05	1328	11.21	11.99	95.01	1314	12.18	13.03	93.97	1300
107.5	9.19	9.87	97.63	1350	10.15	10.91	96.59	1336	11.12	11.95	95.55	1321	12.08	12.99	94.51	1307
108	9.11	9.83	98.17	1358	10.07	10.87	97.13	1343	11.03	11.91	96.09	1329	11.99	12.95	95.05	1315
108.5	9.03	9.79	98.71	1365	9.98	10.83	97.67	1351	10.94	11.87	96.63	1336	11.89	12.91	95.59	1322
109	8.95	9.75	99.25	1373	9.90	10.79	98.21	1358	10.85	11.83	97.17	1344	11.80	12.86	96.14	1330
109.5	8.87	9.71	99.79	1380	9.82	10.75	98.75	1366	10.76	11.79	97.71	1351	11.71	12.82	96.68	1337
110	8.79	9.67	100.33	1388	9.73	10.71	99.29	1373	10.68	11.75	98.26	1359	11.62	12.78	97.22	1345
110.5	8.71	9.63	100.87	1395	9.65	10.67	99.83	1381	10.59	11.70	98.80	1366	11.53	12.74	97.76	1352
111	8.64	9.59	101.41	1403	9.57	10.63	100.37	1388	10.51	11.66	99.34	1374	11.44	12.70	98.30	1359
111.5	8.56	9.55	101.95	1410	9.49	10.58	100.92	1396	10.42	11.62	99.88	1381	11.35	12.66	98.84	1367
112	8.49	9.51	102.49	1417	9.41	10.54	101.46	1403	10.34	11.58	100.42	1389	11.27	12.62	99.38	1374
112.5	8.41	9.46	103.04	1425	9.34	10.50	102.00	1411	10.26	11.54	100.96	1396	11.18	12.58	99.92	1382
113	8.34	9.42	103.58	1432	9.26	10.46	102.54	1418	10.18	11.50	101.50	1404	11.09	12.54	100.46	1389
113.5	8.27	9.38	104.12	1440	9.18	10.42	103.08	1426	10.10	11.46	102.04	1411	11.01	12.50	101.00	1397
114	8.19	9.34	104.66	1447	9.10	10.38	103.62	1433	10.01	11.42	102.58	1419	10.93	12.45	101.55	1404
114.5	8.12	9.30	105.20	1455	9.03	10.34	104.16	1441	9.94	11.38	103.12	1426	10.84	12.41	102.09	1412
115	8.05	9.26	105.74	1462	8.95	10.30	104.70	1448	9.86	11.34	103.67	1434	10.76	12.37	102.63	1419
115.5	7.98	9.22	106.28	1470	8.88	10.26	105.24	1456	9.78	11.29	104.21	1441	10.68	12.33	103.17	1427
116	7.91	9.18	106.82	1477	8.81	10.22	105.78	1463	9.70	11.25	104.75	1449	10.60	12.29	103.71	1434
116.5	7.84	9.14	107.36	1485	8.73	10.17	106.33	1470	9.62	11.21	105.29	1456	10.51	12.25	104.25	1442
117	7.77	9.10	107.90	1492	8.66	10.13	106.87	1478	9.55	11.17	105.83	1464	10.43	12.21	104.79	1449
117.5	7.71	9.05	108.45	1500	8.59	10.09	107.41	1485	9.47	11.13	106.37	1471	10.36	12.17	105.33	1457
118	7.64	9.01	108.99	1507	8.52	10.05	107.95	1493	9.40	11.09	106.91	1479	10.28	12.13	105.87	1464
118.5	7.57	8.97	109.53	1515	8.45	10.01	108.49	1500	9.32	11.05	107.45	1486	10.20	12.09	106.41	1472
119	7.51	8.93	110.07	1522	8.38	9.97	109.03	1508	9.25	11.01	107.99	1494	10.12	12.04	106.96	1479
119.5	7.44	8.89	110.61	1530	8.31	9.93	109.57	1515	9.18	10.97	108.53	1501	10.04	12.00	107.50	1487
120	7.38	8.85	111.15	1537	8.24	9.89	110.11	1523	9.10	10.93	109.08	1509	9.97	11.96	108.04	1494
120.5	7.31	8.81	111.69	1545	8.17	9.85	110.65	1530	9.03	10.88	109.62	1516	9.89	11.92	108.58	1502
121	7.25	8.77	112.23	1552	8.10	9.81	111.19	1538	8.96	10.84	110.16	1523	9.82	11.88	109.12	1509
121.5	7.18	8.73	112.77	1560	8.04	9.76	111.74	1545	8.89	10.80	110.70	1531	9.74	11.84	109.66	1517
122	7.12	8.69	113.31	1567	7.97	9.72	112.28	1553	8.82	10.76	111.24	1538	9.67	11.80	110.20	1524
122.5	7.06	8.64	113.86	1575	7.90	9.68	112.82	1560	8.75	10.72	111.78	1546	9.60	11.76	110.74	1532
123	7.00	8.60	114.40	1582	7.84	9.64	113.36	1568	8.68	10.68	112.32	1553	9.53	11.72	111.28	1539
123.5	6.93	8.56	114.94	1590	7.77	9.60	113.90	1575	8.61	10.64	112.86	1561	9.45	11.68	111.82	1547
124	6.87	8.52	115.48	1597	7.71	9.56	114.44	1583	8.55	10.60	113.40	1568	9.38	11.63	112.37	1554
124.5	6.81	8.48	116.02	1605	7.65	9.52	114.98	1590	8.48	10.56	113.94	1576	9.31	11.59	112.91	1561
125	6.75	8.44	116.56	1612	7.58	9.48	115.52	1598	8.41	10.52	114.49	1583	9.24	11.55	113.45	1569
125.5	6.69	8.40	117.10	1620	7.52	9.44	116.06	1605	8.35	10.47	115.03	1591	9.17	11.51	113.99	1576
126	6.63	8.36	117.64	1627	7.46	9.40	116.60	1613	8.28	10.43	115.57	1598	9.10	11.47	114.53	1584
126.5	6.57	8.32	118.18	1634	7.39	9.35	117.15	1620	8.22	10.39	116.11	1606	9.04	11.43	115.07	1591
127	6.52	8.28	118.72	1642	7.33	9.31	117.69	1628	8.15	10.35	116.65	1613	8.97	11.39	115.61	1599
127.5	6.46	8.23	119.27	1649	7.27	9.27	118.23	1635	8.09	10.31	117.19	1621	8.90	11.35	116.15	1606
128	6.40	8.19	119.81	1657	7.21	9.23	118.77	1643	8.02	10.27	117.73	1628	8.83	11.31	116.69	1614
128.5	6.34	8.15	120.35	1664	7.15	9.19	119.31	1650	7.96	10.23	118.27	1636	8.77	11.27	117.23	1621
129	6.29	8.11	120.89	1672	7.09	9.15	119.85	1658	7.90	10.19	118.81	1643	8.70	11.22	117.78	1629
129.5	6.23	8.07	121.43	1679	7.03	9.11	120.39	1665	7.83	10.15	119.35	1651	8.64	11.18	118.32	1636
130	6.18	8.03	121.97	1687	6.98	9.07	120.93	1672	7.77	10.11	119.90	1658	8.57	11.14	118.86	1644
130.5	6.12	7.99	122.51	1694	6.92	9.03	121.47	1680	7.71	10.06	120.44	1666	8.51	11.10	119.40	1651
131	6.07	7.95	123.05	1702	6.86	8.99	122.01	1687	7.65	10.02	120.98	1673	8.44	11.06	119.94	1659
131.5	6.01	7.91	123.59	1709	6.80	8.94	122.56	1695	7.59	9.98	121.52	1681	8.38	11.02	120.48	1666

Body Composition FEMALE 100-131.5 Lb.

Weight: Lb.	Waist: 24 inches Fat: %	Fat: Lb.	LBM: Lb.	RMR: Cal.	24.25 inches Fat: %	Fat: Lb.	LBM: Lb.	RMR: Cal.	24.5 inches Fat: %	Fat: Lb.	LBM: Lb.	RMR: Cal.	24.75 inches Fat: %	Fat: Lb.	LBM: Lb.	RMR: Cal.
100	14.64	14.64	85.36	1181	15.68	15.68	84.32	1166	16.72	16.72	83.29	1152	17.75	17.75	82.25	1137
100.5	14.53	14.60	85.90	1188	15.56	15.64	84.86	1174	16.59	16.67	83.83	1159	17.62	17.71	82.79	1145
101	14.41	14.56	86.44	1195	15.44	15.60	85.40	1181	16.47	16.63	84.37	1167	17.50	17.67	83.33	1152
101.5	14.30	14.52	86.98	1203	15.32	15.55	85.95	1189	16.35	16.59	84.91	1174	17.37	17.63	83.87	1160
102	14.19	14.48	87.52	1210	15.21	15.51	86.49	1196	16.23	16.55	85.45	1182	17.24	17.59	84.41	1167
102.5	14.08	14.44	88.07	1218	15.10	15.47	87.03	1204	16.11	16.51	85.99	1189	17.12	17.55	84.95	1175
103	13.97	14.39	88.61	1225	14.98	15.43	87.57	1211	15.99	16.47	86.53	1197	17.00	17.51	85.49	1182
103.5	13.87	14.35	89.15	1233	14.87	15.39	88.11	1219	15.87	16.43	87.07	1204	16.87	17.47	86.03	1190
104	13.76	14.31	89.69	1240	14.76	15.35	88.65	1226	15.76	16.39	87.61	1212	16.75	17.42	86.58	1197
104.5	13.66	14.27	90.23	1248	14.65	15.31	89.19	1234	15.64	16.35	88.15	1219	16.63	17.38	87.12	1205
105	13.55	14.23	90.77	1255	14.54	15.27	89.73	1241	15.53	16.31	88.70	1227	16.52	17.34	87.66	1212
105.5	13.45	14.19	91.31	1263	14.43	15.23	90.27	1248	15.42	16.26	89.24	1234	16.40	17.30	88.20	1220
106	13.35	14.15	91.85	1270	14.33	15.19	90.81	1256	15.30	16.22	89.78	1242	16.28	17.26	88.74	1227
106.5	13.25	14.11	92.39	1278	14.22	15.14	91.36	1263	15.19	16.18	90.32	1249	16.17	17.22	89.28	1235
107	13.15	14.07	92.93	1285	14.12	15.10	91.90	1271	15.09	16.14	90.86	1257	16.05	17.18	89.82	1242
107.5	13.05	14.03	93.48	1293	14.01	15.06	92.44	1278	14.98	16.10	91.40	1264	15.94	17.14	90.36	1250
108	12.95	13.98	94.02	1300	13.91	15.02	92.98	1286	14.87	16.06	91.94	1272	15.83	17.10	90.90	1257
108.5	12.85	13.94	94.56	1308	13.81	14.98	93.52	1293	14.76	16.02	92.48	1279	15.72	17.06	91.44	1265
109	12.75	13.90	95.10	1315	13.71	14.94	94.06	1301	14.66	15.98	93.02	1287	15.61	17.01	91.99	1272
109.5	12.66	13.86	95.64	1323	13.61	14.90	94.60	1308	14.55	15.94	93.56	1294	15.50	16.97	92.53	1280
110	12.56	13.82	96.18	1330	13.51	14.86	95.14	1316	14.45	15.90	94.11	1301	15.39	16.93	93.07	1287
110.5	12.47	13.78	96.72	1338	13.41	14.82	95.68	1323	14.35	15.85	94.65	1309	15.29	16.89	93.61	1295
111	12.38	13.74	97.26	1345	13.31	14.78	96.22	1331	14.25	15.81	95.19	1316	15.18	16.85	94.15	1302
111.5	12.28	13.70	97.80	1353	13.21	14.73	96.77	1338	14.15	15.77	95.73	1324	15.08	16.81	94.69	1310
112	12.19	13.66	98.34	1360	13.12	14.69	97.31	1346	14.05	15.73	96.27	1331	14.97	16.77	95.23	1317
112.5	12.10	13.62	98.89	1368	13.02	14.65	97.85	1353	13.95	15.69	96.81	1339	14.87	16.73	95.77	1325
113	12.01	13.57	99.43	1375	12.93	14.61	98.39	1361	13.85	15.65	97.35	1346	14.77	16.69	96.31	1332
113.5	11.92	13.53	99.97	1383	12.84	14.57	98.93	1368	13.75	15.61	97.89	1354	14.67	16.65	96.85	1339
114	11.84	13.49	100.51	1390	12.75	14.53	99.47	1376	13.66	15.57	98.43	1361	14.57	16.60	97.40	1347
114.5	11.75	13.45	101.05	1398	12.65	14.49	100.01	1383	13.56	15.53	98.97	1369	14.47	16.56	97.94	1354
115	11.66	13.41	101.59	1405	12.56	14.45	100.55	1391	13.47	15.49	99.52	1376	14.37	16.52	98.48	1362
115.5	11.57	13.37	102.13	1412	12.47	14.41	101.09	1398	13.37	15.44	100.06	1384	14.27	16.48	99.02	1369
116	11.49	13.33	102.67	1420	12.38	14.37	101.63	1406	13.28	15.40	100.60	1391	14.17	16.44	99.56	1377
116.5	11.41	13.29	103.21	1427	12.30	14.32	102.18	1413	13.19	15.36	101.14	1399	14.08	16.40	100.10	1384
117	11.32	13.25	103.75	1435	12.21	14.28	102.72	1421	13.09	15.32	101.68	1406	13.98	16.36	100.64	1392
117.5	11.24	13.21	104.30	1442	12.12	14.24	103.26	1428	13.00	15.28	102.22	1414	13.89	16.32	101.18	1399
118	11.16	13.16	104.84	1450	12.04	14.20	103.80	1436	12.91	15.24	102.76	1421	13.79	16.28	101.72	1407
118.5	11.07	13.12	105.38	1457	11.95	14.16	104.34	1443	12.83	15.20	103.30	1429	13.70	16.24	102.26	1414
119	10.99	13.08	105.92	1465	11.87	14.12	104.88	1450	12.74	15.16	103.84	1436	13.61	16.19	102.81	1422
119.5	10.91	13.04	106.46	1472	11.78	14.08	105.42	1458	12.65	15.12	104.38	1444	13.52	16.15	103.35	1429
120	10.83	13.00	107.00	1480	11.70	14.04	105.96	1465	12.56	15.08	104.93	1451	13.43	16.11	103.89	1437
120.5	10.75	12.96	107.54	1487	11.62	14.00	106.50	1473	12.48	15.03	105.47	1459	13.34	16.07	104.43	1444
121	10.68	12.92	108.08	1495	11.53	13.96	107.04	1480	12.39	14.99	106.01	1466	13.25	16.03	104.97	1452
121.5	10.60	12.88	108.62	1502	11.45	13.91	107.59	1488	12.31	14.95	106.55	1474	13.16	15.99	105.51	1459
122	10.52	12.84	109.16	1510	11.37	13.87	108.13	1495	12.22	14.91	107.09	1481	13.07	15.95	106.05	1467
122.5	10.44	12.80	109.71	1517	11.29	13.83	108.67	1503	12.14	14.87	107.63	1489	12.99	15.91	106.59	1474
123	10.37	12.75	110.25	1525	11.21	13.79	109.21	1510	12.06	14.83	108.17	1496	12.90	15.87	107.13	1482
123.5	10.29	12.71	110.79	1532	11.13	13.75	109.75	1518	11.97	14.79	108.71	1503	12.81	15.83	107.67	1489
124	10.22	12.67	111.33	1540	11.06	13.71	110.29	1525	11.89	14.75	109.25	1511	12.73	15.78	108.22	1497
124.5	10.15	12.63	111.87	1547	10.98	13.67	110.83	1533	11.81	14.71	109.79	1518	12.65	15.74	108.76	1504
125	10.07	12.59	112.41	1555	10.90	13.63	111.37	1540	11.73	14.67	110.34	1526	12.56	15.70	109.30	1512
125.5	10.00	12.55	112.95	1562	10.83	13.59	111.91	1548	11.65	14.62	110.88	1533	12.48	15.66	109.84	1519
126	9.93	12.51	113.49	1570	10.75	13.55	112.45	1555	11.57	14.58	111.42	1541	12.40	15.62	110.38	1527
126.5	9.86	12.47	114.03	1577	10.68	13.50	113.00	1563	11.50	14.54	111.96	1548	12.32	15.58	110.92	1534
127	9.78	12.43	114.57	1585	10.60	13.46	113.54	1570	11.42	14.50	112.50	1556	12.24	15.54	111.46	1542
127.5	9.71	12.39	115.12	1592	10.53	13.42	114.08	1578	11.34	14.46	113.04	1563	12.15	15.50	112.00	1549
128	9.64	12.34	115.66	1600	10.45	13.38	114.62	1585	11.26	14.42	113.58	1571	12.08	15.46	112.54	1556
128.5	9.57	12.30	116.20	1607	10.38	13.34	115.16	1593	11.19	14.38	114.12	1578	12.00	15.42	113.08	1564
129	9.51	12.26	116.74	1614	10.31	13.30	115.70	1600	11.11	14.34	114.66	1586	11.92	15.37	113.63	1571
129.5	9.44	12.22	117.28	1622	10.24	13.26	116.24	1608	11.04	14.30	115.20	1593	11.84	15.33	114.17	1579
130	9.37	12.18	117.82	1629	10.17	13.22	116.78	1615	10.97	14.26	115.75	1601	11.76	15.29	114.71	1586
130.5	9.30	12.14	118.36	1637	10.10	13.18	117.32	1623	10.89	14.21	116.29	1608	11.69	15.25	115.25	1594
131	9.24	12.10	118.90	1644	10.03	13.14	117.86	1630	10.82	14.17	116.83	1616	11.61	15.21	115.79	1601
131.5	9.17	12.06	119.44	1652	9.96	13.09	118.41	1638	10.75	14.13	117.37	1623	11.54	15.17	116.33	1609

Body Composition FEMALE 100-131.5 Lb.

Weight: Lb.	Waist: 25 inches				25.25 inches				25.5 inches				25.75 inches			
	Fat: %	Fat: Lb.	LBM: Lb.	RMR: Cal.	Fat: %	Fat: Lb.	LBM: Lb.	RMR: Cal.	Fat: %	Fat: Lb.	LBM: Lb.	RMR: Cal.	Fat: %	Fat: Lb.	LBM: Lb.	RMR: Cal.
100	18.79	18.79	81.21	1123	19.83	19.83	80.17	1109	20.87	20.87	79.14	1094	21.90	21.90	78.10	1080
100.5	18.66	18.75	81.75	1131	19.69	19.79	80.71	1116	20.72	20.82	79.68	1102	21.75	21.86	78.64	1088
101	18.52	18.71	82.29	1138	19.55	19.75	81.25	1124	20.58	20.78	80.22	1109	21.60	21.82	79.18	1095
101.5	18.39	18.67	82.83	1146	19.41	19.70	81.80	1131	20.44	20.74	80.76	1117	21.46	21.78	79.72	1103
102	18.26	18.63	83.37	1153	19.28	19.66	82.34	1139	20.30	20.70	81.30	1124	21.31	21.74	80.26	1110
102.5	18.13	18.59	83.92	1161	19.14	19.62	82.88	1146	20.16	20.66	81.84	1132	21.17	21.70	80.80	1117
103	18.00	18.54	84.46	1168	19.01	19.58	83.42	1154	20.02	20.62	82.38	1139	21.03	21.66	81.34	1125
103.5	17.88	18.50	85.00	1176	18.88	19.54	83.96	1161	19.88	20.58	82.92	1147	20.88	21.62	81.88	1132
104	17.75	18.46	85.54	1183	18.75	19.50	84.50	1169	19.75	20.54	83.46	1154	20.74	21.57	82.43	1140
104.5	17.63	18.42	86.08	1190	18.62	19.46	85.04	1176	19.61	20.50	84.00	1162	20.61	21.53	82.97	1147
105	17.50	18.38	86.62	1198	18.49	19.42	85.58	1184	19.48	20.46	84.55	1169	20.47	21.49	83.51	1155
105.5	17.38	18.34	87.16	1205	18.37	19.38	86.12	1191	19.35	20.41	85.09	1177	20.33	21.45	84.05	1162
106	17.26	18.30	87.70	1213	18.24	19.34	86.66	1199	19.22	20.37	85.63	1184	20.20	21.41	84.59	1170
106.5	17.14	18.26	88.24	1220	18.12	19.29	87.21	1206	19.09	20.33	86.17	1192	20.07	21.37	85.13	1177
107	17.02	18.22	88.78	1228	17.99	19.25	87.75	1214	18.96	20.29	86.71	1199	19.93	21.33	85.67	1185
107.5	16.91	18.18	89.33	1235	17.87	19.21	88.29	1221	18.84	20.25	87.25	1207	19.80	21.29	86.21	1192
108	16.79	18.13	89.87	1243	17.75	19.17	88.83	1228	18.71	20.21	87.79	1214	19.67	21.25	86.75	1200
108.5	16.68	18.09	90.41	1250	17.63	19.13	89.37	1236	18.59	20.17	88.33	1222	19.54	21.21	87.29	1207
109	16.56	18.05	90.95	1258	17.51	19.09	89.91	1243	18.47	20.13	88.87	1229	19.42	21.16	87.84	1215
109.5	16.45	18.01	91.49	1265	17.40	19.05	90.45	1251	18.34	20.09	89.41	1237	19.29	21.12	88.38	1222
110	16.34	17.97	92.03	1273	17.28	19.01	90.99	1258	18.22	20.05	89.96	1244	19.17	21.08	88.92	1230
110.5	16.23	17.93	92.57	1280	17.16	18.97	91.53	1266	18.10	20.00	90.50	1252	19.04	21.04	89.46	1237
111	16.12	17.89	93.11	1288	17.05	18.93	92.07	1273	17.98	19.96	91.04	1259	18.92	21.00	90.00	1245
111.5	16.01	17.85	93.65	1295	16.94	18.88	92.62	1281	17.87	19.92	91.58	1267	18.80	20.96	90.54	1252
112	15.90	17.81	94.19	1303	16.82	18.84	93.16	1288	17.75	19.88	92.12	1274	18.68	20.92	91.08	1260
112.5	15.79	17.77	94.74	1310	16.71	18.80	93.70	1296	17.64	19.84	92.66	1281	18.56	20.88	91.62	1267
113	15.68	17.72	95.28	1318	16.60	18.76	94.24	1303	17.52	19.80	93.20	1289	18.44	20.84	92.16	1275
113.5	15.58	17.68	95.82	1325	16.49	18.72	94.78	1311	17.41	19.76	93.74	1296	18.32	20.80	92.70	1282
114	15.48	17.64	96.36	1333	16.39	18.68	95.32	1318	17.30	19.72	94.28	1304	18.21	20.75	93.25	1290
114.5	15.37	17.60	96.90	1340	16.28	18.64	95.86	1326	17.18	19.68	94.82	1311	18.09	20.71	93.79	1297
115	15.27	17.56	97.44	1348	16.17	18.60	96.40	1333	17.07	19.64	95.37	1319	17.98	20.67	94.33	1305
115.5	15.17	17.52	97.98	1355	16.07	18.56	96.94	1341	16.96	19.59	95.91	1326	17.86	20.63	94.87	1312
116	15.07	17.48	98.52	1363	15.96	18.52	97.48	1348	16.86	19.55	96.45	1334	17.75	20.59	95.41	1320
116.5	14.97	17.44	99.06	1370	15.86	18.47	98.03	1356	16.75	19.51	96.99	1341	17.64	20.55	95.95	1327
117	14.87	17.40	99.60	1378	15.76	18.43	98.57	1363	16.64	19.47	97.53	1349	17.53	20.51	96.49	1334
117.5	14.77	17.36	100.15	1385	15.65	18.39	99.11	1371	16.54	19.43	98.07	1356	17.42	20.47	97.03	1342
118	14.67	17.31	100.69	1392	15.55	18.35	99.65	1378	16.43	19.39	98.61	1364	17.31	20.43	97.57	1349
118.5	14.58	17.27	101.23	1400	15.45	18.31	100.19	1386	16.33	19.35	99.15	1371	17.20	20.39	98.11	1357
119	14.48	17.23	101.77	1407	15.35	18.27	100.73	1393	16.22	19.31	99.69	1379	17.10	20.34	98.66	1364
119.5	14.39	17.19	102.31	1415	15.25	18.23	101.27	1401	16.12	19.27	100.23	1386	16.99	20.30	99.20	1372
120	14.29	17.15	102.85	1422	15.16	18.19	101.81	1408	16.02	19.23	100.78	1394	16.89	20.26	99.74	1379
120.5	14.20	17.11	103.39	1430	15.06	18.15	102.35	1416	15.92	19.18	101.32	1401	16.78	20.22	100.28	1387
121	14.11	17.07	103.93	1437	14.96	18.11	102.89	1423	15.82	19.14	101.86	1409	16.68	20.18	100.82	1394
121.5	14.01	17.03	104.47	1445	14.87	18.06	103.44	1431	15.72	19.10	102.40	1416	16.58	20.14	101.36	1402
122	13.92	16.99	105.01	1452	14.77	18.02	103.98	1438	15.62	19.06	102.94	1424	16.47	20.10	101.90	1409
122.5	13.83	16.95	105.56	1460	14.68	17.98	104.52	1445	15.53	19.02	103.48	1431	16.37	20.06	102.44	1417
123	13.74	16.90	106.10	1467	14.59	17.94	105.06	1453	15.43	18.98	104.02	1439	16.27	20.02	102.98	1424
123.5	13.65	16.86	106.64	1475	14.49	17.90	105.60	1460	15.33	18.94	104.56	1446	16.17	19.98	103.52	1432
124	13.57	16.82	107.18	1482	14.40	17.86	106.14	1468	15.24	18.90	105.10	1454	16.08	19.93	104.07	1439
124.5	13.48	16.78	107.72	1490	14.31	17.82	106.68	1475	15.15	18.86	105.64	1461	15.98	19.89	104.61	1447
125	13.39	16.74	108.26	1497	14.22	17.78	107.22	1483	15.05	18.82	106.19	1469	15.88	19.85	105.15	1454
125.5	13.31	16.70	108.80	1505	14.13	17.74	107.76	1490	14.96	18.77	106.73	1476	15.79	19.81	105.69	1462
126	13.22	16.66	109.34	1512	14.04	17.70	108.30	1498	14.87	18.73	107.27	1484	15.69	19.77	106.23	1469
126.5	13.14	16.62	109.88	1520	13.96	17.65	108.85	1505	14.78	18.69	107.81	1491	15.60	19.73	106.77	1477
127	13.05	16.58	110.42	1527	13.87	17.61	109.39	1513	14.69	18.65	108.35	1498	15.50	19.69	107.31	1484
127.5	12.97	16.54	110.97	1535	13.78	17.57	109.93	1520	14.60	18.61	108.89	1506	15.41	19.65	107.85	1492
128	12.89	16.49	111.51	1542	13.70	17.53	110.47	1528	14.51	18.57	109.43	1513	15.32	19.61	108.39	1499
128.5	12.80	16.45	112.05	1550	13.61	17.49	111.01	1535	14.42	18.53	109.97	1521	15.23	19.57	108.93	1507
129	12.72	16.41	112.59	1557	13.53	17.45	111.55	1543	14.33	18.49	110.51	1528	15.14	19.52	109.48	1514
129.5	12.64	16.37	113.13	1565	13.44	17.41	112.09	1550	14.24	18.45	111.05	1536	15.05	19.48	110.02	1522
130	12.56	16.33	113.67	1572	13.36	17.37	112.63	1558	14.16	18.41	111.60	1543	14.96	19.44	110.56	1529
130.5	12.48	16.29	114.21	1580	13.28	17.33	113.17	1565	14.07	18.36	112.14	1551	14.87	19.40	111.10	1536
131	12.40	16.25	114.75	1587	13.20	17.29	113.71	1573	13.99	18.32	112.68	1558	14.78	19.36	111.64	1544
131.5	12.32	16.21	115.29	1595	13.11	17.24	114.26	1580	13.90	18.28	113.22	1566	14.69	19.32	112.18	1551

Body Composition FEMALE 100-131.5 Lb.

Weight: Lb.	Waist: 26 inches Fat: %	Fat: Lb.	LBM: Lb.	RMR: Cal.	26.25 inches Fat: %	Fat: Lb.	LBM: Lb.	RMR: Cal.	26.5 inches Fat: %	Fat: Lb.	LBM: Lb.	RMR: Cal.	26.75 inches Fat: %	Fat: Lb.	LBM: Lb.	RMR: Cal.
100	22.94	22.94	77.06	1066	23.98	23.98	76.02	1051	25.02	25.02	74.99	1037	26.05	26.05	73.95	1023
100.5	22.79	22.90	77.60	1073	23.82	23.94	76.56	1059	24.85	24.97	75.53	1045	25.88	26.01	74.49	1030
101	22.63	22.86	78.14	1081	23.66	23.90	77.10	1066	24.69	24.93	76.07	1052	25.71	25.97	75.03	1038
101.5	22.48	22.82	78.68	1088	23.50	23.85	77.65	1074	24.52	24.89	76.61	1059	25.55	25.93	75.57	1045
102	22.33	22.78	79.22	1096	23.35	23.81	78.19	1081	24.36	24.85	77.15	1067	25.38	25.89	76.11	1053
102.5	22.18	22.74	79.77	1103	23.19	23.77	78.73	1089	24.20	24.81	77.69	1074	25.22	25.85	76.65	1060
103	22.03	22.69	80.31	1111	23.04	23.73	79.27	1096	24.05	24.77	78.23	1082	25.05	25.81	77.19	1068
103.5	21.89	22.65	80.85	1118	22.89	23.69	79.81	1104	23.89	24.73	78.77	1089	24.89	25.77	77.73	1075
104	21.74	22.61	81.39	1126	22.74	23.65	80.35	1111	23.74	24.69	79.31	1097	24.74	25.72	78.28	1083
104.5	21.60	22.57	81.93	1133	22.59	23.61	80.89	1119	23.58	24.65	79.85	1104	24.58	25.68	78.82	1090
105	21.46	22.53	82.47	1141	22.45	23.57	81.43	1126	23.43	24.61	80.40	1112	24.42	25.64	79.36	1098
105.5	21.32	22.49	83.01	1148	22.30	23.53	81.97	1134	23.28	24.56	80.94	1119	24.27	25.60	79.90	1105
106	21.18	22.45	83.55	1156	22.16	23.49	82.51	1141	23.13	24.52	81.48	1127	24.11	25.56	80.44	1112
106.5	21.04	22.41	84.09	1163	22.01	23.44	83.06	1149	22.99	24.48	82.02	1134	23.96	25.52	80.98	1120
107	20.90	22.37	84.63	1170	21.87	23.40	83.60	1156	22.84	24.44	82.56	1142	23.81	25.48	81.52	1127
107.5	20.77	22.33	85.18	1178	21.73	23.36	84.14	1164	22.70	24.40	83.10	1149	23.66	25.44	82.06	1135
108	20.63	22.28	85.72	1185	21.59	23.32	84.68	1171	22.55	24.36	83.64	1157	23.52	25.40	82.60	1142
108.5	20.50	22.24	86.26	1193	21.46	23.28	85.22	1179	22.41	24.32	84.18	1164	23.37	25.36	83.14	1150
109	20.37	22.20	86.80	1200	21.32	23.24	85.76	1186	22.27	24.28	84.72	1172	23.22	25.31	83.69	1157
109.5	20.24	22.16	87.34	1208	21.19	23.20	86.30	1194	22.13	24.24	85.26	1179	23.08	25.27	84.23	1165
110	20.11	22.12	87.88	1215	21.05	23.16	86.84	1201	22.00	24.20	85.81	1187	22.94	25.23	84.77	1172
110.5	19.98	22.08	88.42	1223	20.92	23.12	87.38	1209	21.86	24.15	86.35	1194	22.80	25.19	85.31	1180
111	19.85	22.04	88.96	1230	20.79	23.08	87.92	1216	21.72	24.11	86.89	1202	22.66	25.15	85.85	1187
111.5	19.73	22.00	89.50	1238	20.66	23.03	88.47	1223	21.59	24.07	87.43	1209	22.52	25.11	86.39	1195
112	19.60	21.96	90.04	1245	20.53	22.99	89.01	1231	21.46	24.03	87.97	1217	22.38	25.07	86.93	1202
112.5	19.48	21.92	90.59	1253	20.40	22.95	89.55	1238	21.32	23.99	88.51	1224	22.25	25.03	87.47	1210
113	19.36	21.87	91.13	1260	20.28	22.91	90.09	1246	21.19	23.95	89.05	1232	22.11	24.99	88.01	1217
113.5	19.24	21.83	91.67	1268	20.15	22.87	90.63	1253	21.06	23.91	89.59	1239	21.98	24.95	88.55	1225
114	19.12	21.79	92.21	1275	20.03	22.83	91.17	1261	20.94	23.87	90.13	1247	21.85	24.90	89.10	1232
114.5	19.00	21.75	92.75	1283	19.90	22.79	91.71	1268	20.81	23.83	90.67	1254	21.71	24.86	89.64	1240
115	18.88	21.71	93.29	1290	19.78	22.75	92.25	1276	20.68	23.79	91.22	1262	21.58	24.82	90.18	1247
115.5	18.76	21.67	93.83	1298	19.66	22.71	92.79	1283	20.56	23.74	91.76	1269	21.46	24.78	90.72	1255
116	18.64	21.63	94.37	1305	19.54	22.67	93.33	1291	20.43	23.70	92.30	1276	21.33	24.74	91.26	1262
116.5	18.53	21.59	94.91	1313	19.42	22.62	93.88	1298	20.31	23.66	92.84	1284	21.20	24.70	91.80	1270
117	18.42	21.55	95.45	1320	19.30	22.58	94.42	1306	20.19	23.62	93.38	1291	21.08	24.66	92.34	1277
117.5	18.30	21.51	96.00	1328	19.19	22.54	94.96	1313	20.07	23.58	93.92	1299	20.95	24.62	92.88	1285
118	18.19	21.46	96.54	1335	19.07	22.50	95.50	1321	19.95	23.54	94.46	1306	20.83	24.58	93.42	1292
118.5	18.08	21.42	97.08	1343	18.95	22.46	96.04	1328	19.83	23.50	95.00	1314	20.71	24.54	93.96	1300
119	17.97	21.38	97.62	1350	18.84	22.42	96.58	1336	19.71	23.46	95.54	1321	20.58	24.49	94.51	1307
119.5	17.86	21.34	98.16	1358	18.73	22.38	97.12	1343	19.59	23.42	96.08	1329	20.46	24.45	95.05	1314
120	17.75	21.30	98.70	1365	18.61	22.34	97.66	1351	19.48	23.38	96.63	1336	20.34	24.41	95.59	1322
120.5	17.64	21.26	99.24	1373	18.50	22.30	98.20	1358	19.36	23.33	97.17	1344	20.23	24.37	96.13	1329
121	17.54	21.22	99.78	1380	18.39	22.26	98.74	1366	19.25	23.29	97.71	1351	20.11	24.33	96.67	1337
121.5	17.43	21.18	100.32	1387	18.28	22.21	99.29	1373	19.14	23.25	98.25	1359	19.99	24.29	97.21	1344
122	17.32	21.14	100.86	1395	18.18	22.17	99.83	1381	19.03	23.21	98.79	1366	19.88	24.25	97.75	1352
122.5	17.22	21.10	101.41	1402	18.07	22.13	100.37	1388	18.91	23.17	99.33	1374	19.76	24.21	98.29	1359
123	17.12	21.05	101.95	1410	17.96	22.09	100.91	1396	18.80	23.13	99.87	1381	19.65	24.17	98.83	1367
123.5	17.01	21.01	102.49	1417	17.85	22.05	101.45	1403	18.69	23.09	100.41	1389	19.53	24.13	99.37	1374
124	16.91	20.97	103.03	1425	17.75	22.01	101.99	1411	18.59	23.05	100.95	1396	19.42	24.08	99.92	1382
124.5	16.81	20.93	103.57	1432	17.65	21.97	102.53	1418	18.48	23.01	101.49	1404	19.31	24.04	100.46	1389
125	16.71	20.89	104.11	1440	17.54	21.93	103.07	1425	18.37	22.97	102.04	1411	19.20	24.00	101.00	1397
125.5	16.61	20.85	104.65	1447	17.44	21.89	103.61	1433	18.27	22.92	102.58	1419	19.09	23.96	101.54	1404
126	16.51	20.81	105.19	1455	17.34	21.85	104.15	1440	18.16	22.88	103.12	1426	18.98	23.92	102.08	1412
126.5	16.42	20.77	105.73	1462	17.24	21.80	104.70	1448	18.06	22.84	103.66	1434	18.88	23.88	102.62	1419
127	16.32	20.73	106.27	1470	17.14	21.76	105.24	1455	17.95	22.80	104.20	1441	18.77	23.84	103.16	1427
127.5	16.22	20.69	106.82	1477	17.04	21.72	105.78	1463	17.85	22.76	104.74	1449	18.66	23.80	103.70	1434
128	16.13	20.64	107.36	1485	16.94	21.68	106.32	1470	17.75	22.72	105.28	1456	18.56	23.76	104.24	1442
128.5	16.03	20.60	107.90	1492	16.84	21.64	106.86	1478	17.65	22.68	105.82	1464	18.46	23.72	104.78	1449
129	15.94	20.56	108.44	1500	16.74	21.60	107.40	1485	17.55	22.64	106.36	1471	18.35	23.67	105.33	1457
129.5	15.85	20.52	108.98	1507	16.65	21.56	107.94	1493	17.45	22.60	106.90	1478	18.25	23.63	105.87	1464
130	15.75	20.48	109.52	1515	16.55	21.52	108.48	1500	17.35	22.56	107.45	1486	18.15	23.59	106.41	1472
130.5	15.66	20.44	110.06	1522	16.46	21.48	109.02	1508	17.25	22.51	107.99	1493	18.05	23.55	106.95	1479
131	15.57	20.40	110.60	1530	16.36	21.44	109.56	1515	17.15	22.47	108.53	1501	17.95	23.51	107.49	1487
131.5	15.48	20.36	111.14	1537	16.27	21.39	110.11	1523	17.06	22.43	109.07	1508	17.85	23.47	108.03	1494

Body Composition FEMALE 100-131.5 Lb.

Weight: Lb.	Waist: 27 inches Fat: %	Fat: Lb.	LBM: Lb.	RMR: Cal.	27.25 inches Fat: %	Fat: Lb.	LBM: Lb.	RMR: Cal.	27.5 inches Fat: %	Fat: Lb.	LBM: Lb.	RMR: Cal.	27.75 inches Fat: %	Fat: Lb.	LBM: Lb.	RMR: Cal.
100	27.09	27.09	72.91	1008	28.13	28.13	71.87	994	29.17	29.17	70.84	980	30.20	30.20	69.80	965
100.5	26.91	27.05	73.45	1016	27.95	28.09	72.41	1001	28.98	29.12	71.38	987	30.01	30.16	70.34	973
101	26.74	27.01	73.99	1023	27.77	28.05	72.95	1009	28.80	29.08	71.92	995	29.82	30.12	70.88	980
101.5	26.57	26.97	74.53	1031	27.59	28.00	73.50	1016	28.61	29.04	72.46	1002	29.63	30.08	71.42	988
102	26.40	26.93	75.07	1038	27.42	27.96	74.04	1024	28.43	29.00	73.00	1010	29.45	30.04	71.96	995
102.5	26.23	26.89	75.62	1046	27.24	27.92	74.58	1031	28.25	28.96	73.54	1017	29.27	30.00	72.50	1003
103	26.06	26.84	76.16	1053	27.07	27.88	75.12	1039	28.08	28.92	74.08	1025	29.08	29.96	73.04	1010
103.5	25.90	26.80	76.70	1061	26.90	27.84	75.66	1046	27.90	28.88	74.62	1032	28.90	29.92	73.58	1018
104	25.73	26.76	77.24	1068	26.73	27.80	76.20	1054	27.73	28.84	75.16	1040	28.73	29.87	74.13	1025
104.5	25.57	26.72	77.78	1076	26.56	27.76	76.74	1061	27.56	28.80	75.70	1047	28.55	29.83	74.67	1033
105	25.41	26.68	78.32	1083	26.40	27.72	77.28	1069	27.39	28.76	76.25	1054	28.37	29.79	75.21	1040
105.5	25.25	26.64	78.86	1091	26.23	27.68	77.82	1076	27.22	28.71	76.79	1062	28.20	29.75	75.75	1048
106	25.09	26.60	79.40	1098	26.07	27.64	78.36	1084	27.05	28.67	77.33	1069	28.03	29.71	76.29	1055
106.5	24.94	26.56	79.94	1106	25.91	27.59	78.91	1091	26.88	28.63	77.87	1077	27.86	29.67	76.83	1063
107	24.78	26.52	80.48	1113	25.75	27.55	79.45	1099	26.72	28.59	78.41	1084	27.69	29.63	77.37	1070
107.5	24.63	26.48	81.03	1121	25.59	27.51	79.99	1106	26.56	28.55	78.95	1092	27.52	29.59	77.91	1078
108	24.48	26.43	81.57	1128	25.44	27.47	80.53	1114	26.40	28.51	79.49	1099	27.36	29.55	78.45	1085
108.5	24.33	26.39	82.11	1136	25.28	27.43	81.07	1121	26.24	28.47	80.03	1107	27.19	29.51	78.99	1092
109	24.18	26.35	82.65	1143	25.13	27.39	81.61	1129	26.08	28.43	80.57	1114	27.03	29.46	79.54	1100
109.5	24.03	26.31	83.19	1151	24.98	27.35	82.15	1136	25.92	28.39	81.11	1122	26.87	29.42	80.08	1107
110	23.88	26.27	83.73	1158	24.83	27.31	82.69	1144	25.77	28.35	81.66	1129	26.71	29.38	80.62	1115
110.5	23.74	26.23	84.27	1165	24.68	27.27	83.23	1151	25.61	28.30	82.20	1137	26.55	29.34	81.16	1122
111	23.59	26.19	84.81	1173	24.53	27.23	83.77	1159	25.46	28.26	82.74	1144	26.40	29.30	81.70	1130
111.5	23.45	26.15	85.35	1180	24.38	27.18	84.32	1166	25.31	28.22	83.28	1152	26.24	29.26	82.24	1137
112	23.31	26.11	85.89	1188	24.24	27.14	84.86	1174	25.16	28.18	83.82	1159	26.09	29.22	82.78	1145
112.5	23.17	26.07	86.44	1195	24.09	27.10	85.40	1181	25.01	28.14	84.36	1167	25.94	29.18	83.32	1152
113	23.03	26.02	86.98	1203	23.95	27.06	85.94	1189	24.87	28.10	84.90	1174	25.78	29.14	83.86	1160
113.5	22.89	25.98	87.52	1210	23.81	27.02	86.48	1196	24.72	28.06	85.44	1182	25.63	29.10	84.40	1167
114	22.76	25.94	88.06	1218	23.67	26.98	87.02	1203	24.58	28.02	85.98	1189	25.49	29.05	84.95	1175
114.5	22.62	25.90	88.60	1225	23.53	26.94	87.56	1211	24.43	27.98	86.52	1197	25.34	29.01	85.49	1182
115	22.49	25.86	89.14	1233	23.39	26.90	88.10	1218	24.29	27.94	87.07	1204	25.19	28.97	86.03	1190
115.5	22.35	25.82	89.68	1240	23.25	26.86	88.64	1226	24.15	27.89	87.61	1212	25.05	28.93	86.57	1197
116	22.22	25.78	90.22	1248	23.12	26.82	89.18	1233	24.01	27.85	88.15	1219	24.91	28.89	87.11	1205
116.5	22.09	25.74	90.76	1255	22.98	26.77	89.73	1241	23.87	27.81	88.69	1227	24.76	28.85	87.65	1212
117	21.96	25.70	91.30	1263	22.85	26.73	90.27	1248	23.74	27.77	89.23	1234	24.62	28.81	88.19	1220
117.5	21.83	25.66	91.85	1270	22.72	26.69	90.81	1256	23.60	27.73	89.77	1242	24.48	28.77	88.73	1227
118	21.71	25.61	92.39	1278	22.59	26.65	91.35	1263	23.47	27.69	90.31	1249	24.34	28.73	89.27	1235
118.5	21.58	25.57	92.93	1285	22.46	26.61	91.89	1271	23.33	27.65	90.85	1256	24.21	28.69	89.81	1242
119	21.46	25.53	93.47	1293	22.33	26.57	92.43	1278	23.20	27.61	91.39	1264	24.07	28.64	90.36	1250
119.5	21.33	25.49	94.01	1300	22.20	26.53	92.97	1286	23.07	27.57	91.93	1271	23.94	28.60	90.90	1257
120	21.21	25.45	94.55	1308	22.07	26.49	93.51	1293	22.94	27.53	92.48	1279	23.80	28.56	91.44	1265
120.5	21.09	25.41	95.09	1315	21.95	26.45	94.05	1301	22.81	27.48	93.02	1286	23.67	28.52	91.98	1272
121	20.97	25.37	95.63	1323	21.82	26.41	94.59	1308	22.68	27.44	93.56	1294	23.54	28.48	92.52	1280
121.5	20.85	25.33	96.17	1330	21.70	26.36	95.14	1316	22.55	27.40	94.10	1301	23.41	28.44	93.06	1287
122	20.73	25.29	96.71	1338	21.58	26.32	95.68	1323	22.43	27.36	94.64	1309	23.28	28.40	93.60	1295
122.5	20.61	25.25	97.26	1345	21.46	26.28	96.22	1331	22.30	27.32	95.18	1316	23.15	28.36	94.14	1302
123	20.49	25.20	97.80	1353	21.33	26.24	96.76	1338	22.18	27.28	95.72	1324	23.02	28.32	94.68	1309
123.5	20.37	25.16	98.34	1360	21.21	26.20	97.30	1346	22.06	27.24	96.26	1331	22.90	28.28	95.22	1317
124	20.26	25.12	98.88	1367	21.10	26.16	97.84	1353	21.93	27.20	96.80	1339	22.77	28.23	95.77	1324
124.5	20.15	25.08	99.42	1375	20.98	26.12	98.38	1361	21.81	27.16	97.34	1346	22.65	28.19	96.31	1332
125	20.03	25.04	99.96	1382	20.86	26.08	98.92	1368	21.69	27.12	97.89	1354	22.52	28.15	96.85	1339
125.5	19.92	25.00	100.50	1390	20.75	26.04	99.46	1376	21.57	27.07	98.43	1361	22.40	28.11	97.39	1347
126	19.81	24.96	101.04	1397	20.63	26.00	100.00	1383	21.45	27.03	98.97	1369	22.28	28.07	97.93	1354
126.5	19.70	24.92	101.58	1405	20.52	25.95	100.55	1391	21.34	26.99	99.51	1376	22.16	28.03	98.47	1362
127	19.59	24.88	102.12	1412	20.40	25.91	101.09	1398	21.22	26.95	100.05	1384	22.04	27.99	99.01	1369
127.5	19.48	24.84	102.67	1420	20.29	25.87	101.63	1406	21.11	26.91	100.59	1391	21.92	27.95	99.55	1377
128	19.37	24.79	103.21	1427	20.18	25.83	102.17	1413	20.99	26.87	101.13	1399	21.80	27.91	100.09	1384
128.5	19.26	24.75	103.75	1435	20.07	25.79	102.71	1420	20.88	26.83	101.67	1406	21.69	27.87	100.63	1392
129	19.16	24.71	104.29	1442	19.96	25.75	103.25	1428	20.77	26.79	102.21	1414	21.57	27.82	101.18	1399
129.5	19.05	24.67	104.83	1450	19.85	25.71	103.79	1435	20.65	26.75	102.75	1421	21.45	27.78	101.72	1407
130	18.95	24.63	105.37	1457	19.74	25.67	104.33	1443	20.54	26.71	103.30	1429	21.34	27.74	102.26	1414
130.5	18.84	24.59	105.91	1465	19.64	25.63	104.87	1450	20.43	26.66	103.84	1436	21.23	27.70	102.80	1422
131	18.74	24.55	106.45	1472	19.53	25.59	105.41	1458	20.32	26.62	104.38	1444	21.11	27.66	103.34	1429
131.5	18.64	24.51	106.99	1480	19.43	25.54	105.96	1465	20.21	26.58	104.92	1451	21.00	27.62	103.88	1437

Body Composition FEMALE 100-131.5 Lb.

Weight: Lb.	Waist: 28 inches Fat: %	Fat: Lb.	LBM: Lb.	RMR: Cal.	28.25 inches Fat: %	Fat: Lb.	LBM: Lb.	RMR: Cal.	28.5 inches Fat: %	Fat: Lb.	LBM: Lb.	RMR: Cal.	28.75 inches Fat: %	Fat: Lb.	LBM: Lb.	RMR: Cal.
100	31.24	31.24	68.76	951	32.28	32.28	67.72	937	33.32	33.32	66.69	922	34.35	34.35	65.65	908
100.5	31.04	31.20	69.30	958	32.08	32.24	68.26	944	33.11	33.27	67.23	930	34.14	34.31	66.19	915
101	30.85	31.16	69.84	966	31.88	32.20	68.80	952	32.90	33.23	67.77	937	33.93	34.27	66.73	923
101.5	30.66	31.12	70.38	973	31.68	32.15	69.35	959	32.70	33.19	68.31	945	33.72	34.23	67.27	930
102	30.47	31.08	70.92	981	31.48	32.11	69.89	967	32.50	33.15	68.85	952	33.52	34.19	67.81	938
102.5	30.28	31.04	71.47	988	31.29	32.07	70.43	974	32.30	33.11	69.39	960	33.31	34.15	68.35	945
103	30.09	30.99	72.01	996	31.10	32.03	70.97	981	32.11	33.07	69.93	967	33.11	34.11	68.89	953
103.5	29.91	30.95	72.55	1003	30.91	31.99	71.51	989	31.91	33.03	70.47	975	32.91	34.07	69.43	960
104	29.72	30.91	73.09	1011	30.72	31.95	72.05	996	31.72	32.99	71.01	982	32.72	34.02	69.98	968
104.5	29.54	30.87	73.63	1018	30.53	31.91	72.59	1004	31.53	32.95	71.55	990	32.52	33.98	70.52	975
105	29.36	30.83	74.17	1026	30.35	31.87	73.13	1011	31.34	32.91	72.10	997	32.33	33.94	71.06	983
105.5	29.18	30.79	74.71	1033	30.17	31.83	73.67	1019	31.15	32.86	72.64	1005	32.13	33.90	71.60	990
106	29.01	30.75	75.25	1041	29.99	31.79	74.21	1026	30.97	32.82	73.18	1012	31.94	33.86	72.14	998
106.5	28.83	30.71	75.79	1048	29.81	31.74	74.76	1034	30.78	32.78	73.72	1020	31.76	33.82	72.68	1005
107	28.66	30.67	76.33	1056	29.63	31.70	75.30	1041	30.60	32.74	74.26	1027	31.57	33.78	73.22	1013
107.5	28.49	30.63	76.88	1063	29.45	31.66	75.84	1049	30.42	32.70	74.80	1034	31.38	33.74	73.76	1020
108	28.32	30.58	77.42	1071	29.28	31.62	76.38	1056	30.24	32.66	75.34	1042	31.20	33.70	74.30	1028
108.5	28.15	30.54	77.96	1078	29.11	31.58	76.92	1064	30.06	32.62	75.88	1049	31.02	33.66	74.84	1035
109	27.98	30.50	78.50	1086	28.94	31.54	77.46	1071	29.89	32.58	76.42	1057	30.84	33.61	75.39	1043
109.5	27.82	30.46	79.04	1093	28.77	31.50	78.00	1079	29.71	32.54	76.96	1064	30.66	33.57	75.93	1050
110	27.65	30.42	79.58	1101	28.60	31.46	78.54	1086	29.54	32.50	77.51	1072	30.48	33.53	76.47	1058
110.5	27.49	30.38	80.12	1108	28.43	31.42	79.08	1094	29.37	32.45	78.05	1079	30.31	33.49	77.01	1065
111	27.33	30.34	80.66	1116	28.27	31.38	79.62	1101	29.20	32.41	78.59	1087	30.14	33.45	77.55	1073
111.5	27.17	30.30	81.20	1123	28.10	31.33	80.17	1109	29.03	32.37	79.13	1094	29.96	33.41	78.09	1080
112	27.01	30.26	81.74	1131	27.94	31.29	80.71	1116	28.87	32.33	79.67	1102	29.79	33.37	78.63	1087
112.5	26.86	30.22	82.29	1138	27.78	31.25	81.25	1124	28.70	32.29	80.21	1109	29.62	33.33	79.17	1095
113	26.70	30.17	82.83	1145	27.62	31.21	81.79	1131	28.54	32.25	80.75	1117	29.46	33.29	79.71	1102
113.5	26.55	30.13	83.37	1153	27.46	31.17	82.33	1139	28.38	32.21	81.29	1124	29.29	33.25	80.25	1110
114	26.40	30.09	83.91	1160	27.31	31.13	82.87	1146	28.22	32.17	81.83	1132	29.13	33.20	80.80	1117
114.5	26.25	30.05	84.45	1168	27.15	31.09	83.41	1154	28.06	32.13	82.37	1139	28.96	33.16	81.34	1125
115	26.10	30.01	84.99	1175	27.00	31.05	83.95	1161	27.90	32.09	82.92	1147	28.80	33.12	81.88	1132
115.5	25.95	29.97	85.53	1183	26.85	31.01	84.49	1169	27.74	32.04	83.46	1154	28.64	33.08	82.42	1140
116	25.80	29.93	86.07	1190	26.69	30.97	85.03	1176	27.59	32.00	84.00	1162	28.48	33.04	82.96	1147
116.5	25.65	29.89	86.61	1198	26.54	30.92	85.58	1184	27.44	31.96	84.54	1169	28.33	33.00	83.50	1155
117	25.51	29.85	87.15	1205	26.40	30.88	86.12	1191	27.28	31.92	85.08	1177	28.17	32.96	84.04	1162
117.5	25.37	29.81	87.70	1213	26.25	30.84	86.66	1198	27.13	31.88	85.62	1184	28.01	32.92	84.58	1170
118	25.22	29.76	88.24	1220	26.10	30.80	87.20	1206	26.98	31.84	86.16	1192	27.86	32.88	85.12	1177
118.5	25.08	29.72	88.78	1228	25.96	30.76	87.74	1213	26.83	31.80	86.70	1199	27.71	32.84	85.66	1185
119	24.94	29.68	89.32	1235	25.81	30.72	88.28	1221	26.69	31.76	87.24	1207	27.56	32.79	86.21	1192
119.5	24.80	29.64	89.86	1243	25.67	30.68	88.82	1228	26.54	31.72	87.78	1214	27.41	32.75	86.75	1200
120	24.67	29.60	90.40	1250	25.53	30.64	89.36	1236	26.40	31.68	88.33	1222	27.26	32.71	87.29	1207
120.5	24.53	29.56	90.94	1258	25.39	30.60	89.90	1243	26.25	31.63	88.87	1229	27.11	32.67	87.83	1215
121	24.40	29.52	91.48	1265	25.25	30.56	90.44	1251	26.11	31.59	89.41	1236	26.97	32.63	88.37	1222
121.5	24.26	29.48	92.02	1273	25.11	30.51	90.99	1258	25.97	31.55	89.95	1244	26.82	32.59	88.91	1230
122	24.13	29.44	92.56	1280	24.98	30.47	91.53	1266	25.83	31.51	90.49	1251	26.68	32.55	89.45	1237
122.5	24.00	29.40	93.11	1288	24.84	30.43	92.07	1273	25.69	31.47	91.03	1259	26.54	32.51	89.99	1245
123	23.87	29.35	93.65	1295	24.71	30.39	92.61	1281	25.55	31.43	91.57	1266	26.40	32.47	90.53	1252
123.5	23.74	29.31	94.19	1303	24.58	30.35	93.15	1288	25.42	31.39	92.11	1274	26.26	32.43	91.07	1260
124	23.61	29.27	94.73	1310	24.44	30.31	93.69	1296	25.28	31.35	92.65	1281	26.12	32.38	91.62	1267
124.5	23.48	29.23	95.27	1318	24.31	30.27	94.23	1303	25.15	31.31	93.19	1289	25.98	32.34	92.16	1275
125	23.35	29.19	95.81	1325	24.18	30.23	94.77	1311	25.01	31.27	93.74	1296	25.84	32.30	92.70	1282
125.5	23.23	29.15	96.35	1333	24.05	30.19	95.31	1318	24.88	31.22	94.28	1304	25.71	32.26	93.24	1289
126	23.10	29.11	96.89	1340	23.93	30.15	95.85	1326	24.75	31.18	94.82	1311	25.57	32.22	93.78	1297
126.5	22.98	29.07	97.43	1347	23.80	30.10	96.40	1333	24.62	31.14	95.36	1319	25.44	32.18	94.32	1304
127	22.86	29.03	97.97	1355	23.67	30.06	96.94	1341	24.49	31.10	95.90	1326	25.31	32.14	94.86	1312
127.5	22.73	28.99	98.52	1362	23.55	30.02	97.48	1348	24.36	31.06	96.44	1334	25.17	32.10	95.40	1319
128	22.61	28.94	99.06	1370	23.42	29.98	98.02	1356	24.23	31.02	96.98	1341	25.04	32.06	95.94	1327
128.5	22.49	28.90	99.60	1377	23.30	29.94	98.56	1363	24.11	30.98	97.52	1349	24.91	32.02	96.48	1334
129	22.37	28.86	100.14	1385	23.18	29.90	99.10	1371	23.98	30.94	98.06	1356	24.79	31.97	97.03	1342
129.5	22.26	28.82	100.68	1392	23.06	29.86	99.64	1378	23.86	30.90	98.60	1364	24.66	31.93	97.57	1349
130	22.14	28.78	101.22	1400	22.94	29.82	100.18	1386	23.73	30.86	99.15	1371	24.53	31.89	98.11	1357
130.5	22.02	28.74	101.76	1407	22.82	29.78	100.72	1393	23.61	30.81	99.69	1379	24.41	31.85	98.65	1364
131	21.91	28.70	102.30	1415	22.70	29.74	101.26	1400	23.49	30.77	100.23	1386	24.28	31.81	99.19	1372
131.5	21.79	28.66	102.84	1422	22.58	29.69	101.81	1408	23.37	30.73	100.77	1394	24.16	31.77	99.73	1379

Body Composition FEMALE 100-131.5 Lb.

Weight: Lb.	Waist: 29 inches				29.25 inches				29.5 inches				29.75 inches			
	Fat: %	Fat: Lb.	LBM: Lb.	RMR: Cal.	Fat: %	Fat: Lb.	LBM: Lb.	RMR: Cal.	Fat: %	Fat: Lb.	LBM: Lb.	RMR: Cal.	Fat: %	Fat: Lb.	LBM: Lb.	RMR: Cal.
100	35.39	35.39	64.61	894	36.43	36.43	63.57	879	37.47	37.47	62.54	865	38.50	38.50	61.50	851
100.5	35.17	35.35	65.15	901	36.21	36.39	64.11	887	37.24	37.42	63.08	872	38.27	38.46	62.04	858
101	34.96	35.31	65.69	909	35.99	36.35	64.65	894	37.01	37.38	63.62	880	38.04	38.42	62.58	865
101.5	34.75	35.27	66.23	916	35.77	36.30	65.20	902	36.79	37.34	64.16	887	37.81	38.38	63.12	873
102	34.54	35.23	66.77	923	35.55	36.26	65.74	909	36.57	37.30	64.70	895	37.59	38.34	63.66	880
102.5	34.33	35.19	67.32	931	35.34	36.22	66.28	917	36.35	37.26	65.24	902	37.36	38.30	64.20	888
103	34.12	35.14	67.86	938	35.13	36.18	66.82	924	36.13	37.22	65.78	910	37.14	38.26	64.74	895
103.5	33.92	35.10	68.40	946	34.92	36.14	67.36	932	35.92	37.18	66.32	917	36.92	38.22	65.28	903
104	33.71	35.06	68.94	953	34.71	36.10	67.90	939	35.71	37.14	66.86	925	36.71	38.17	65.83	910
104.5	33.51	35.02	69.48	961	34.51	36.06	68.44	947	35.50	37.10	67.40	932	36.49	38.13	66.37	918
105	33.31	34.98	70.02	968	34.30	36.02	68.98	954	35.29	37.06	67.95	940	36.28	38.09	66.91	925
105.5	33.12	34.94	70.56	976	34.10	35.98	69.52	962	35.08	37.01	68.49	947	36.07	38.05	67.45	933
106	32.92	34.90	71.10	983	33.90	35.94	70.06	969	34.88	36.97	69.03	955	35.86	38.01	67.99	940
106.5	32.73	34.86	71.64	991	33.70	35.89	70.61	976	34.68	36.93	69.57	962	35.65	37.97	68.53	948
107	32.54	34.82	72.18	998	33.51	35.85	71.15	984	34.48	36.89	70.11	970	35.45	37.93	69.07	955
107.5	32.35	34.78	72.73	1006	33.31	35.81	71.69	991	34.28	36.85	70.65	977	35.24	37.89	69.61	963
108	32.16	34.73	73.27	1013	33.12	35.77	72.23	999	34.08	36.81	71.19	985	35.04	37.85	70.15	970
108.5	31.98	34.69	73.81	1021	32.93	35.73	72.77	1006	33.89	36.77	71.73	992	34.84	37.81	70.69	978
109	31.79	34.65	74.35	1028	32.74	35.69	73.31	1014	33.69	36.73	72.27	1000	34.65	37.76	71.24	985
109.5	31.61	34.61	74.89	1036	32.56	35.65	73.85	1021	33.50	36.69	72.81	1007	34.45	37.72	71.78	993
110	31.43	34.57	75.43	1043	32.37	35.61	74.39	1029	33.31	36.65	73.36	1014	34.26	37.68	72.32	1000
110.5	31.25	34.53	75.97	1051	32.19	35.57	74.93	1036	33.13	36.60	73.90	1022	34.06	37.64	72.86	1008
111	31.07	34.49	76.51	1058	32.00	35.53	75.47	1044	32.94	36.56	74.44	1029	33.87	37.60	73.40	1015
111.5	30.89	34.45	77.05	1066	31.82	35.48	76.02	1051	32.76	36.52	74.98	1037	33.69	37.56	73.94	1023
112	30.72	34.41	77.59	1073	31.65	35.44	76.56	1059	32.57	36.48	75.52	1044	33.50	37.52	74.48	1030
112.5	30.55	34.37	78.14	1081	31.47	35.40	77.10	1066	32.39	36.44	76.06	1052	33.31	37.48	75.02	1038
113	30.38	34.32	78.68	1088	31.29	35.36	77.64	1074	32.21	36.40	76.60	1059	33.13	37.44	75.56	1045
113.5	30.21	34.28	79.22	1096	31.12	35.32	78.18	1081	32.03	36.36	77.14	1067	32.95	37.40	76.10	1053
114	30.04	34.24	79.76	1103	30.95	35.28	78.72	1089	31.86	36.32	77.68	1074	32.77	37.35	76.65	1060
114.5	29.87	34.20	80.30	1111	30.78	35.24	79.26	1096	31.68	36.28	78.22	1082	32.59	37.31	77.19	1067
115	29.70	34.16	80.84	1118	30.61	35.20	79.80	1104	31.51	36.24	78.77	1089	32.41	37.27	77.73	1075
115.5	29.54	34.12	81.38	1125	30.44	35.16	80.34	1111	31.34	36.19	79.31	1097	32.24	37.23	78.27	1082
116	29.38	34.08	81.92	1133	30.27	35.12	80.88	1119	31.17	36.15	79.85	1104	32.06	37.19	78.81	1090
116.5	29.22	34.04	82.46	1140	30.11	35.07	81.43	1126	31.00	36.11	80.39	1112	31.89	37.15	79.35	1097
117	29.06	34.00	83.00	1148	29.94	35.03	81.97	1134	30.83	36.07	80.93	1119	31.72	37.11	79.89	1105
117.5	28.90	33.96	83.55	1155	29.78	34.99	82.51	1141	30.66	36.03	81.47	1127	31.55	37.07	80.43	1112
118	28.74	33.91	84.09	1163	29.62	34.95	83.05	1149	30.50	35.99	82.01	1134	31.38	37.03	80.97	1120
118.5	28.58	33.87	84.63	1170	29.46	34.91	83.59	1156	30.34	35.95	82.55	1142	31.21	36.99	81.51	1127
119	28.43	33.83	85.17	1178	29.30	34.87	84.13	1164	30.17	35.91	83.09	1149	31.05	36.94	82.06	1135
119.5	28.28	33.79	85.71	1185	29.15	34.83	84.67	1171	30.01	35.87	83.63	1157	30.88	36.90	82.60	1142
120	28.13	33.75	86.25	1193	28.99	34.79	85.21	1178	29.85	35.83	84.18	1164	30.72	36.86	83.14	1150
120.5	27.97	33.71	86.79	1200	28.84	34.75	85.75	1186	29.70	35.78	84.72	1172	30.56	36.82	83.68	1157
121	27.82	33.67	87.33	1208	28.68	34.71	86.29	1193	29.54	35.74	85.26	1179	30.40	36.78	84.22	1165
121.5	27.68	33.63	87.87	1215	28.53	34.66	86.84	1201	29.38	35.70	85.80	1187	30.24	36.74	84.76	1172
122	27.53	33.59	88.41	1223	28.38	34.62	87.38	1208	29.23	35.66	86.34	1194	30.08	36.70	85.30	1180
122.5	27.38	33.55	88.96	1230	28.23	34.58	87.92	1216	29.08	35.62	86.88	1202	29.92	36.65	85.84	1187
123	27.24	33.50	89.50	1238	28.08	34.54	88.46	1223	28.93	35.58	87.42	1209	29.77	36.62	86.38	1195
123.5	27.10	33.46	90.04	1245	27.94	34.50	89.00	1231	28.78	35.54	87.96	1217	29.62	36.58	86.92	1202
124	26.95	33.42	90.58	1253	27.79	34.46	89.54	1238	28.63	35.50	88.50	1224	29.46	36.53	87.47	1210
124.5	26.81	33.38	91.12	1260	27.65	34.42	90.08	1246	28.48	35.46	89.04	1231	29.31	36.49	88.01	1217
125	26.67	33.34	91.66	1268	27.50	34.38	90.62	1253	28.33	35.42	89.59	1239	29.16	36.45	88.55	1225
125.5	26.53	33.30	92.20	1275	27.36	34.34	91.16	1261	28.19	35.37	90.13	1246	29.01	36.41	89.09	1232
126	26.40	33.26	92.74	1283	27.22	34.30	91.70	1268	28.04	35.33	90.67	1254	28.87	36.37	89.63	1240
126.5	26.26	33.22	93.28	1290	27.08	34.25	92.25	1276	27.90	35.29	91.21	1261	28.72	36.33	90.17	1247
127	26.12	33.18	93.82	1298	26.94	34.21	92.79	1283	27.76	35.25	91.75	1269	28.57	36.29	90.71	1255
127.5	25.99	33.14	94.37	1305	26.80	34.17	93.33	1291	27.62	35.21	92.29	1276	28.43	36.25	91.25	1262
128	25.85	33.09	94.91	1313	26.67	34.13	93.87	1298	27.48	35.17	92.83	1284	28.29	36.21	91.79	1270
128.5	25.72	33.05	95.45	1320	26.53	34.09	94.41	1306	27.34	35.13	93.37	1291	28.14	36.17	92.33	1277
129	25.59	33.01	95.99	1328	26.39	34.05	94.95	1313	27.20	35.09	93.91	1299	28.00	36.12	92.88	1284
129.5	25.46	32.97	96.53	1335	26.26	34.01	95.49	1321	27.06	35.05	94.45	1306	27.86	36.08	93.42	1292
130	25.33	32.93	97.07	1342	26.13	33.97	96.03	1328	26.93	35.01	95.00	1314	27.73	36.04	93.96	1299
130.5	25.20	32.89	97.61	1350	26.00	33.93	96.57	1336	26.79	34.96	95.54	1321	27.59	36.00	94.50	1307
131	25.07	32.85	98.15	1357	25.87	33.89	97.11	1343	26.66	34.92	96.08	1329	27.45	35.96	95.04	1314
131.5	24.95	32.81	98.69	1365	25.74	33.84	97.66	1351	26.53	34.88	96.62	1336	27.32	35.92	95.58	1322

Body Composition FEMALE 100-131.5 Lb.

Weight: Lb.	Waist: 30 inches				30.25 inches				30.5 inches				30.75 inches			
	Fat: %	Fat: Lb.	LBM: Lb.	RMR: Cal.	Fat: %	Fat: Lb.	LBM: Lb.	RMR: Cal.	Fat: %	Fat: Lb.	LBM: Lb.	RMR: Cal.	Fat: %	Fat: Lb.	LBM: Lb.	RMR: Cal.
100	39.54	39.54	60.46	836	40.58	40.58	59.42	822	41.62	41.62	58.39	807	42.65	42.65	57.35	793
100.5	39.30	39.50	61.00	844	40.33	40.54	59.96	829	41.37	41.57	58.93	815	42.40	42.61	57.89	801
101	39.07	39.46	61.54	851	40.09	40.50	60.50	837	41.12	41.53	59.47	822	42.15	42.57	58.43	808
101.5	38.83	39.42	62.08	859	39.86	40.45	61.05	844	40.88	41.49	60.01	830	41.90	42.53	58.97	816
102	38.60	39.38	62.62	866	39.62	40.41	61.59	852	40.64	41.45	60.55	837	41.66	42.49	59.51	823
102.5	38.38	39.34	63.17	874	39.39	40.37	62.13	859	40.40	41.41	61.09	845	41.41	42.45	60.05	831
103	38.15	39.29	63.71	881	39.16	40.33	62.67	867	40.16	41.37	61.63	852	41.17	42.41	60.59	838
103.5	37.93	39.25	64.25	889	38.93	40.29	63.21	874	39.93	41.33	62.17	860	40.93	42.37	61.13	845
104	37.70	39.21	64.79	896	38.70	40.25	63.75	882	39.70	41.29	62.71	867	40.70	42.32	61.68	853
104.5	37.48	39.17	65.33	904	38.48	40.21	64.29	889	39.47	41.25	63.25	875	40.46	42.28	62.22	860
105	37.27	39.13	65.87	911	38.25	40.17	64.83	897	39.24	41.21	63.80	882	40.23	42.24	62.76	868
105.5	37.05	39.09	66.41	918	38.03	40.13	65.37	904	39.02	41.16	64.34	890	40.00	42.20	63.30	875
106	36.84	39.05	66.95	926	37.82	40.09	65.91	912	38.80	41.12	64.88	897	39.77	42.16	63.84	883
106.5	36.63	39.01	67.49	933	37.60	40.04	66.46	919	38.57	41.08	65.42	905	39.55	42.12	64.38	890
107	36.42	38.97	68.03	941	37.39	40.00	67.00	927	38.36	41.04	65.96	912	39.33	42.08	64.92	898
107.5	36.21	38.93	68.58	948	37.17	39.96	67.54	934	38.14	41.00	66.50	920	39.10	42.04	65.46	905
108	36.00	38.88	69.12	956	36.96	39.92	68.08	942	37.91	40.96	67.04	927	38.89	42.00	66.00	913
108.5	35.80	38.84	69.66	963	36.76	39.88	68.62	949	37.71	40.92	67.58	935	38.67	41.96	66.54	920
109	35.60	38.80	70.20	971	36.55	39.84	69.16	956	37.50	40.88	68.12	942	38.45	41.91	67.09	928
109.5	35.40	38.76	70.74	978	36.35	39.80	69.70	964	37.29	40.84	68.66	950	38.24	41.87	67.63	935
110	35.20	38.72	71.28	986	36.14	39.76	70.24	971	37.09	40.80	69.21	957	38.03	41.83	68.17	943
110.5	35.00	38.68	71.82	993	35.94	39.72	70.78	979	36.88	40.75	69.75	965	37.82	41.79	68.71	950
111	34.81	38.64	72.36	1001	35.74	39.68	71.32	986	36.68	40.71	70.29	972	37.61	41.75	69.25	958
111.5	34.62	38.60	72.90	1008	35.55	39.63	71.87	994	36.48	40.67	70.83	980	37.41	41.71	69.79	965
112	34.43	38.56	73.44	1016	35.35	39.59	72.41	1001	36.28	40.63	71.37	987	37.20	41.67	70.33	973
112.5	34.24	38.52	73.99	1023	35.16	39.55	72.95	1009	36.08	40.59	71.91	995	37.00	41.63	70.87	980
113	34.05	38.47	74.53	1031	34.97	39.51	73.49	1016	35.88	40.55	72.45	1002	36.80	41.59	71.41	988
113.5	33.86	38.43	75.07	1038	34.78	39.47	74.03	1024	35.69	40.51	72.99	1009	36.60	41.55	71.95	995
114	33.68	38.39	75.61	1046	34.59	39.43	74.57	1031	35.50	40.47	73.53	1017	36.41	41.50	72.50	1003
114.5	33.49	38.35	76.15	1053	34.40	39.39	75.11	1039	35.31	40.43	74.07	1024	36.21	41.46	73.04	1010
115	33.31	38.31	76.69	1061	34.22	39.35	75.65	1046	35.12	40.39	74.62	1032	36.02	41.42	73.58	1018
115.5	33.13	38.27	77.23	1068	34.03	39.31	76.19	1054	34.93	40.34	75.16	1039	35.83	41.38	74.12	1025
116	32.96	38.23	77.77	1076	33.85	39.27	76.73	1061	34.74	40.30	75.70	1047	35.64	41.34	74.66	1033
116.5	32.78	38.19	78.31	1083	33.67	39.22	77.28	1069	34.56	40.26	76.24	1054	35.45	41.30	75.20	1040
117	32.60	38.15	78.85	1091	33.49	39.18	77.82	1076	34.38	40.22	76.78	1062	35.26	41.26	75.74	1048
117.5	32.43	38.11	79.40	1098	33.31	39.14	78.36	1084	34.20	40.18	77.32	1069	35.08	41.22	76.28	1055
118	32.26	38.06	79.94	1106	33.14	39.10	78.90	1091	34.02	40.14	77.86	1077	34.90	41.18	76.82	1062
118.5	32.09	38.02	80.48	1113	32.96	39.06	79.44	1099	33.84	40.10	78.40	1084	34.71	41.14	77.36	1070
119	31.92	37.98	81.02	1120	32.79	39.02	79.98	1106	33.66	40.06	78.94	1092	34.53	41.09	77.91	1077
119.5	31.75	37.94	81.56	1128	32.62	38.98	80.52	1114	33.49	40.02	79.48	1099	34.35	41.05	78.45	1085
120	31.58	37.90	82.10	1135	32.45	38.94	81.06	1121	33.31	39.98	80.03	1107	34.18	41.01	78.99	1092
120.5	31.42	37.86	82.64	1143	32.28	38.90	81.60	1129	33.14	39.93	80.57	1114	34.00	40.97	79.53	1100
121	31.25	37.82	83.18	1150	32.11	38.86	82.14	1136	32.97	39.89	81.11	1122	33.83	40.93	80.07	1107
121.5	31.09	37.78	83.72	1158	31.95	38.81	82.69	1144	32.80	39.85	81.65	1129	33.65	40.89	80.61	1115
122	30.93	37.74	84.26	1165	31.78	38.77	83.23	1151	32.63	39.81	82.19	1137	33.48	40.85	81.15	1122
122.5	30.77	37.70	84.81	1173	31.62	38.73	83.77	1159	32.47	39.77	82.73	1144	33.31	40.81	81.69	1130
123	30.61	37.65	85.35	1180	31.46	38.69	84.31	1166	32.30	39.73	83.27	1152	33.14	40.77	82.23	1137
123.5	30.46	37.61	85.89	1188	31.30	38.65	84.85	1173	32.14	39.69	83.81	1159	32.98	40.73	82.77	1145
124	30.30	37.57	86.43	1195	31.14	38.61	85.39	1181	31.97	39.65	84.35	1167	32.81	40.68	83.32	1152
124.5	30.15	37.53	86.97	1203	30.98	38.57	85.93	1188	31.81	39.61	84.89	1174	32.65	40.64	83.86	1160
125	29.99	37.49	87.51	1210	30.82	38.53	86.47	1196	31.65	39.57	85.44	1182	32.48	40.60	84.40	1167
125.5	29.84	37.45	88.05	1218	30.67	38.49	87.01	1203	31.49	39.52	85.98	1189	32.32	40.56	84.94	1175
126	29.69	37.41	88.59	1225	30.51	38.45	87.55	1211	31.34	39.48	86.52	1197	32.16	40.52	85.48	1182
126.5	29.54	37.37	89.13	1233	30.36	38.40	88.10	1218	31.18	39.44	87.06	1204	32.00	40.48	86.02	1190
127	29.39	37.33	89.67	1240	30.21	38.36	88.64	1226	31.02	39.40	87.60	1211	31.84	40.44	86.56	1197
127.5	29.24	37.29	90.22	1248	30.06	38.32	89.18	1233	30.87	39.36	88.14	1219	31.68	40.40	87.10	1205
128	29.10	37.24	90.76	1255	29.91	38.28	89.72	1241	30.72	39.32	88.68	1226	31.53	40.36	87.64	1212
128.5	28.95	37.20	91.30	1263	29.76	38.24	90.26	1248	30.57	39.28	89.22	1234	31.37	40.32	88.18	1220
129	28.81	37.16	91.84	1270	29.61	38.20	90.80	1256	30.42	39.24	89.76	1241	31.22	40.27	88.73	1227
129.5	28.66	37.12	92.38	1278	29.47	38.16	91.34	1263	30.27	39.20	90.30	1249	31.07	40.23	89.27	1235
130	28.52	37.08	92.92	1285	29.32	38.12	91.88	1271	30.12	39.16	90.85	1256	30.92	40.19	89.81	1242
130.5	28.38	37.04	93.46	1293	29.18	38.08	92.42	1278	29.97	39.11	91.39	1264	30.77	40.15	90.35	1250
131	28.24	37.00	94.00	1300	29.03	38.04	92.96	1286	29.83	39.07	91.93	1271	30.62	40.11	90.89	1257
131.5	28.10	36.96	94.54	1308	28.89	37.99	93.51	1293	29.68	39.03	92.47	1279	30.47	40.07	91.43	1264

Body Composition FEMALE 100-131.5 Lb.

Weight: Lb.	Waist: 31 inches Fat: %	Fat: Lb.	LBM: Lb.	RMR: Cal.	31.25 inches Fat: %	Fat: Lb.	LBM: Lb.	RMR: Cal.	31.5 inches Fat: %	Fat: Lb.	LBM: Lb.	RMR: Cal.	31.75 inches Fat: %	Fat: Lb.	LBM: Lb.	RMR: Cal.
100	43.69	43.69	56.31	779	44.73	44.73	55.27	764	45.77	45.77	54.24	750	46.80	46.80	53.20	736
100.5	43.43	43.65	56.85	786	44.46	44.69	55.81	772	45.50	45.72	54.78	758	46.53	46.76	53.74	743
101	43.18	43.61	57.39	794	44.20	44.65	56.35	779	45.23	45.68	55.32	765	46.26	46.72	54.28	751
101.5	42.92	43.57	57.93	801	43.95	44.60	56.90	787	44.97	45.64	55.86	773	45.99	46.68	54.82	758
102	42.67	43.53	58.47	809	43.69	44.56	57.44	794	44.71	45.60	56.40	780	45.72	46.64	55.36	766
102.5	42.42	43.49	59.02	816	43.44	44.52	57.98	802	44.45	45.56	56.94	787	45.46	46.60	55.90	773
103	42.18	43.44	59.56	824	43.19	44.48	58.52	809	44.19	45.52	57.48	795	45.20	46.56	56.44	781
103.5	41.94	43.40	60.10	831	42.94	44.44	59.06	817	43.94	45.48	58.02	802	44.94	46.52	56.98	788
104	41.69	43.36	60.64	839	42.69	44.40	59.60	824	43.69	45.44	58.56	810	44.69	46.47	57.53	796
104.5	41.46	43.32	61.18	846	42.45	44.36	60.14	832	43.44	45.40	59.10	817	44.43	46.43	58.07	803
105	41.22	43.28	61.72	854	42.21	44.32	60.68	839	43.20	45.36	59.65	825	44.18	46.39	58.61	811
105.5	40.98	43.24	62.26	861	41.97	44.28	61.22	847	42.95	45.31	60.19	832	43.94	46.35	59.15	818
106	40.75	43.20	62.80	869	41.73	44.24	61.76	854	42.71	45.27	60.73	840	43.69	46.31	59.69	826
106.5	40.52	43.16	63.34	876	41.50	44.19	62.31	862	42.47	45.23	61.27	847	43.45	46.27	60.23	833
107	40.30	43.12	63.88	884	41.26	44.15	62.85	869	42.23	45.19	61.81	855	43.20	46.23	60.77	840
107.5	40.07	43.08	64.43	891	41.03	44.11	63.39	877	42.00	45.15	62.35	862	42.97	46.19	61.31	848
108	39.85	43.03	64.97	898	40.81	44.07	63.93	884	41.77	45.11	62.89	870	42.73	46.15	61.85	855
108.5	39.62	42.99	65.51	906	40.58	44.03	64.47	892	41.54	45.07	63.43	877	42.49	46.11	62.39	863
109	39.41	42.95	66.05	913	40.36	43.99	65.01	899	41.31	45.03	63.97	885	42.26	46.06	62.94	870
109.5	39.19	42.91	66.59	921	40.14	43.95	65.55	907	41.08	44.99	64.51	892	42.03	46.02	63.48	878
110	38.97	42.87	67.13	928	39.92	43.91	66.09	914	40.86	44.95	65.06	900	41.80	45.98	64.02	885
110.5	38.76	42.83	67.67	936	39.70	43.87	66.63	922	40.64	44.90	65.60	907	41.58	45.94	64.56	893
111	38.55	42.79	68.21	943	39.48	43.83	67.17	929	40.42	44.86	66.14	915	41.35	45.90	65.10	900
111.5	38.34	42.75	68.75	951	39.27	43.78	67.72	937	40.20	44.82	66.68	922	41.13	45.86	65.64	908
112	38.13	42.71	69.29	958	39.06	43.74	68.26	944	39.98	44.78	67.22	930	40.91	45.82	66.18	915
112.5	37.92	42.67	69.84	966	38.85	43.70	68.80	951	39.77	44.74	67.76	937	40.69	45.78	66.72	923
113	37.72	42.62	70.38	973	38.64	43.66	69.34	959	39.56	44.70	68.30	945	40.47	45.74	67.26	930
113.5	37.52	42.58	70.92	981	38.43	43.62	69.88	966	39.35	44.66	68.84	952	40.26	45.70	67.80	938
114	37.32	42.54	71.46	988	38.23	43.58	70.42	974	39.14	44.62	69.38	960	40.05	45.65	68.35	945
114.5	37.12	42.50	72.00	996	38.02	43.54	70.96	981	38.93	44.58	69.92	967	39.84	45.61	68.89	953
115	36.92	42.46	72.54	1003	37.82	43.50	71.50	989	38.73	44.54	70.47	975	39.63	45.57	69.43	960
115.5	36.73	42.42	73.08	1011	37.62	43.46	72.04	996	38.52	44.49	71.01	982	39.42	45.53	69.97	968
116	36.53	42.38	73.62	1018	37.43	43.42	72.58	1004	38.32	44.45	71.55	989	39.22	45.49	70.51	975
116.5	36.34	42.34	74.16	1026	37.23	43.37	73.13	1011	38.12	44.41	72.09	997	39.01	45.45	71.05	983
117	36.15	42.30	74.70	1033	37.04	43.33	73.67	1019	37.92	44.37	72.63	1004	38.81	45.41	71.59	990
117.5	35.96	42.26	75.25	1041	36.84	43.29	74.21	1026	37.73	44.33	73.17	1012	38.61	45.37	72.13	998
118	35.77	42.21	75.79	1048	36.65	43.25	74.75	1034	37.53	44.29	73.71	1019	38.41	45.33	72.67	1005
118.5	35.59	42.17	76.33	1056	36.46	43.21	75.29	1041	37.34	44.25	74.25	1027	38.22	45.29	73.21	1013
119	35.41	42.13	76.87	1063	36.28	43.17	75.83	1049	37.15	44.21	74.79	1034	38.02	45.24	73.76	1020
119.5	35.22	42.09	77.41	1071	36.09	43.13	76.37	1056	36.96	44.17	75.33	1042	37.83	45.20	74.30	1028
120	35.04	42.05	77.95	1078	35.91	43.09	76.91	1064	36.77	44.13	75.88	1049	37.64	45.16	74.84	1035
120.5	34.86	42.01	78.49	1086	35.72	43.05	77.45	1071	36.58	44.08	76.42	1057	37.45	45.12	75.38	1042
121	34.68	41.97	79.03	1093	35.54	43.01	77.99	1079	36.40	44.04	76.96	1064	37.26	45.08	75.92	1050
121.5	34.51	41.93	79.57	1100	35.36	42.96	78.54	1086	36.22	44.00	77.50	1072	37.07	45.04	76.46	1057
122	34.33	41.89	80.11	1108	35.18	42.92	79.08	1094	36.03	43.96	78.04	1079	36.88	45.00	77.00	1065
122.5	34.16	41.85	80.66	1115	35.01	42.88	79.62	1101	35.85	43.92	78.58	1087	36.70	44.96	77.54	1072
123	33.99	41.80	81.20	1123	34.83	42.84	80.16	1109	35.67	43.88	79.12	1094	36.52	44.92	78.08	1080
123.5	33.82	41.76	81.74	1130	34.66	42.80	80.70	1116	35.50	43.84	79.66	1102	36.34	44.88	78.62	1087
124	33.65	41.72	82.28	1138	34.48	42.76	81.24	1124	35.32	43.80	80.20	1109	36.16	44.83	79.17	1095
124.5	33.48	41.68	82.82	1145	34.31	42.72	81.78	1131	35.15	43.76	80.74	1117	35.98	44.79	79.71	1102
125	33.31	41.64	83.36	1153	34.14	42.68	82.32	1139	34.97	43.72	81.29	1124	35.80	44.75	80.25	1110
125.5	33.15	41.60	83.90	1160	33.97	42.64	82.86	1146	34.80	43.67	81.83	1132	35.63	44.71	80.79	1117
126	32.98	41.56	84.44	1168	33.81	42.60	83.40	1153	34.63	43.63	82.37	1139	35.45	44.67	81.33	1125
126.5	32.82	41.52	84.98	1175	33.64	42.55	83.95	1161	34.46	43.59	82.91	1147	35.28	44.63	81.87	1132
127	32.66	41.48	85.52	1183	33.48	42.51	84.49	1168	34.29	43.55	83.45	1154	35.11	44.59	82.41	1140
127.5	32.50	41.44	86.07	1190	33.31	42.47	85.03	1176	34.13	43.51	83.99	1162	34.94	44.55	82.95	1147
128	32.34	41.39	86.61	1198	33.15	42.43	85.57	1183	33.96	43.47	84.53	1169	34.77	44.51	83.49	1155
128.5	32.18	41.35	87.15	1205	32.99	42.39	86.11	1191	33.80	43.43	85.07	1177	34.60	44.47	84.03	1162
129	32.02	41.31	87.69	1213	32.83	42.35	86.65	1198	33.63	43.39	85.61	1184	34.44	44.42	84.58	1170
129.5	31.87	41.27	88.23	1220	32.67	42.31	87.19	1206	33.47	43.35	86.15	1192	34.27	44.38	85.12	1177
130	31.72	41.23	88.77	1228	32.51	42.27	87.73	1213	33.31	43.31	86.70	1199	34.11	44.34	85.66	1185
130.5	31.56	41.19	89.31	1235	32.36	42.23	88.27	1221	33.15	43.26	87.24	1206	33.95	44.30	86.20	1192
131	31.41	41.15	89.85	1243	32.20	42.19	88.81	1228	32.99	43.22	87.78	1214	33.79	44.26	86.74	1200
131.5	31.26	41.11	90.39	1250	32.05	42.14	89.36	1236	32.84	43.18	88.32	1221	33.63	44.22	87.28	1207

Body Composition FEMALE 100-131.5 Lb.

Weight: Lb.	Waist: 32 inches Fat: %	Fat: Lb.	LBM: Lb.	RMR: Cal.	32.25 inches Fat: %	Fat: Lb.	LBM: Lb.	RMR: Cal.	32.5 inches Fat: %	Fat: Lb.	LBM: Lb.	RMR: Cal.	32.75 inches Fat: %	Fat: Lb.	LBM: Lb.	RMR: Cal.
100	47.84	47.84	52.16	721	48.88	48.88	51.12	707	49.92	49.92	50.09	693	50.95	50.95	49.05	678
100.5	47.56	47.80	52.70	729	48.59	48.84	51.66	715	49.63	49.87	50.63	700	50.66	50.91	49.59	686
101	47.29	47.76	53.24	736	48.31	48.80	52.20	722	49.34	49.83	51.17	708	50.37	50.87	50.13	693
101.5	47.01	47.72	53.78	744	48.03	48.75	52.75	729	49.06	49.79	51.71	715	50.08	50.83	50.67	701
102	46.74	47.68	54.32	751	47.76	48.71	53.29	737	48.78	49.75	52.25	723	49.79	50.79	51.21	708
102.5	46.47	47.64	54.87	759	47.49	48.67	53.83	744	48.50	49.71	52.79	730	49.51	50.75	51.75	716
103	46.21	47.59	55.41	766	47.22	48.63	54.37	752	48.22	49.67	53.33	738	49.23	50.71	52.29	723
103.5	45.94	47.55	55.95	774	46.95	48.59	54.91	759	47.95	49.63	53.87	745	48.95	50.67	52.83	731
104	45.68	47.51	56.49	781	46.68	48.55	55.45	767	47.68	49.59	54.41	753	48.68	50.62	53.38	738
104.5	45.43	47.47	57.03	789	46.42	48.51	55.99	774	47.41	49.55	54.95	760	48.41	50.58	53.92	746
105	45.17	47.43	57.57	796	46.16	48.47	56.53	782	47.15	49.51	55.50	767	48.14	50.54	54.46	753
105.5	44.92	47.39	58.11	804	45.90	48.43	57.07	789	46.89	49.46	56.04	775	47.87	50.50	55.00	761
106	44.67	47.35	58.65	811	45.65	48.39	57.61	797	46.63	49.42	56.58	782	47.60	50.46	55.54	768
106.5	44.42	47.31	59.19	819	45.39	48.34	58.16	804	46.37	49.38	57.12	790	47.34	50.42	56.08	776
107	44.17	47.27	59.73	826	45.14	48.30	58.70	812	46.11	49.34	57.66	797	47.08	50.38	56.62	783
107.5	43.93	47.23	60.28	834	44.90	48.26	59.24	819	45.86	49.30	58.20	805	46.83	50.34	57.16	791
108	43.69	47.18	60.82	841	44.65	48.22	59.78	827	45.61	49.26	58.74	812	46.57	50.30	57.70	798
108.5	43.45	47.14	61.36	849	44.41	48.18	60.32	834	45.36	49.22	59.28	820	46.32	50.26	58.24	806
109	43.21	47.10	61.90	856	44.16	48.14	60.86	842	45.12	49.18	59.82	827	46.07	50.21	58.79	813
109.5	42.98	47.06	62.44	864	43.93	48.10	61.40	849	44.87	49.14	60.36	835	45.82	50.17	59.33	820
110	42.75	47.02	62.98	871	43.69	48.06	61.94	857	44.63	49.10	60.91	842	45.58	50.13	59.87	828
110.5	42.51	46.98	63.52	878	43.45	48.02	62.48	864	44.39	49.05	61.45	850	45.33	50.09	60.41	835
111	42.29	46.94	64.06	886	43.22	47.98	63.02	872	44.16	49.01	61.99	857	45.09	50.05	60.95	843
111.5	42.06	46.90	64.60	893	42.99	47.93	63.57	879	43.92	48.97	62.53	865	44.85	50.01	61.49	850
112	41.84	46.86	65.14	901	42.76	47.89	64.11	887	43.69	48.93	63.07	872	44.61	49.97	62.03	858
112.5	41.61	46.82	65.69	908	42.54	47.85	64.65	894	43.46	48.89	63.61	880	44.38	49.93	62.57	865
113	41.39	46.77	66.23	916	42.31	47.81	65.19	902	43.23	48.85	64.15	887	44.15	49.89	63.11	873
113.5	41.17	46.73	66.77	923	42.09	47.77	65.73	909	43.00	48.81	64.69	895	43.92	49.85	63.65	880
114	40.96	46.69	67.31	931	41.87	47.73	66.27	917	42.78	48.77	65.23	902	43.69	49.80	64.20	888
114.5	40.74	46.65	67.85	938	41.65	47.69	66.81	924	42.56	48.73	65.77	910	43.46	49.76	64.74	895
115	40.53	46.61	68.39	946	41.43	47.65	67.35	931	42.33	48.69	66.32	917	43.24	49.72	65.28	903
115.5	40.32	46.57	68.93	953	41.22	47.61	67.89	939	42.12	48.64	66.86	925	43.01	49.68	65.82	910
116	40.11	46.53	69.47	961	41.00	47.57	68.43	946	41.90	48.60	67.40	932	42.79	49.64	66.36	918
116.5	39.90	46.49	70.01	968	40.79	47.52	68.98	954	41.68	48.56	67.94	940	42.57	49.60	66.90	925
117	39.70	46.45	70.55	976	40.58	47.48	69.52	961	41.47	48.52	68.48	947	42.36	49.56	67.44	933
117.5	39.49	46.41	71.10	983	40.38	47.44	70.06	969	41.26	48.48	69.02	955	42.14	49.52	67.98	940
118	39.29	46.36	71.64	991	40.17	47.40	70.60	976	41.05	48.44	69.56	962	41.93	49.48	68.52	948
118.5	39.09	46.32	72.18	998	39.97	47.36	71.14	984	40.84	48.40	70.10	970	41.72	49.44	69.06	955
119	38.89	46.28	72.72	1006	39.76	47.32	71.68	991	40.64	48.36	70.64	977	41.51	49.39	69.61	963
119.5	38.70	46.24	73.26	1013	39.56	47.28	72.22	999	40.43	48.32	71.18	984	41.30	49.35	70.15	970
120	38.50	46.20	73.80	1021	39.36	47.24	72.76	1006	40.23	48.28	71.73	992	41.09	49.31	70.69	978
120.5	38.31	46.16	74.34	1028	39.17	47.20	73.30	1014	40.03	48.23	72.27	999	40.89	49.27	71.23	985
121	38.11	46.12	74.88	1036	38.97	47.16	73.84	1021	39.83	48.19	72.81	1007	40.69	49.23	71.77	993
121.5	37.92	46.08	75.42	1043	38.78	47.11	74.39	1029	39.63	48.15	73.35	1014	40.49	49.19	72.31	1000
122	37.73	46.04	75.96	1051	38.58	47.07	74.93	1036	39.44	48.11	73.89	1022	40.29	49.15	72.85	1008
122.5	37.55	46.00	76.51	1058	38.39	47.03	75.47	1044	39.24	48.07	74.43	1029	40.09	49.11	73.39	1015
123	37.36	45.95	77.05	1066	38.20	46.99	76.01	1051	39.05	48.03	74.97	1037	39.89	49.07	73.93	1023
123.5	37.18	45.91	77.59	1073	38.02	46.95	76.55	1059	38.86	47.99	75.51	1044	39.70	49.03	74.47	1030
124	36.99	45.87	78.13	1081	37.83	46.91	77.09	1066	38.67	47.95	76.05	1052	39.50	48.98	75.02	1037
124.5	36.81	45.83	78.67	1088	37.65	46.87	77.63	1074	38.48	47.91	76.59	1059	39.31	48.94	75.56	1045
125	36.63	45.79	79.21	1095	37.46	46.83	78.17	1081	38.29	47.87	77.14	1067	39.12	48.90	76.10	1052
125.5	36.45	45.75	79.75	1103	37.28	46.79	78.71	1089	38.11	47.82	77.68	1074	38.93	48.86	76.64	1060
126	36.28	45.71	80.29	1110	37.10	46.75	79.25	1096	37.92	47.78	78.22	1082	38.75	48.82	77.18	1067
126.5	36.10	45.67	80.83	1118	36.92	46.70	79.80	1104	37.74	47.74	78.76	1089	38.56	48.78	77.72	1075
127	35.93	45.63	81.37	1125	36.74	46.66	80.34	1111	37.56	47.70	79.30	1097	38.38	48.74	78.26	1082
127.5	35.75	45.59	81.92	1133	36.57	46.62	80.88	1119	37.38	47.66	79.84	1104	38.19	48.70	78.80	1090
128	35.58	45.54	82.46	1140	36.39	46.58	81.42	1126	37.20	47.62	80.38	1112	38.01	48.66	79.34	1097
128.5	35.41	45.50	83.00	1148	36.22	46.54	81.96	1133	37.03	47.58	80.92	1119	37.83	48.62	79.88	1105
129	35.24	45.46	83.54	1155	36.05	46.50	82.50	1141	36.85	47.54	81.46	1127	37.65	48.57	80.43	1112
129.5	35.07	45.42	84.08	1163	35.88	46.46	83.04	1148	36.68	47.50	82.00	1134	37.48	48.53	80.97	1120
130	34.91	45.38	84.62	1170	35.71	46.42	83.58	1156	36.50	47.46	82.55	1142	37.30	48.49	81.51	1127
130.5	34.74	45.34	85.16	1178	35.54	46.38	84.12	1163	36.33	47.41	83.09	1149	37.13	48.45	82.05	1135
131	34.58	45.30	85.70	1185	35.37	46.34	84.66	1171	36.16	47.37	83.63	1157	36.95	48.41	82.59	1142
131.5	34.42	45.26	86.24	1193	35.20	46.29	85.21	1178	35.99	47.33	84.17	1164	36.78	48.37	83.13	1150

Body Composition FEMALE 132-163.5 Lb.

Weight: Lb.	Waist: 25 inches Fat: %	Fat: Lb.	LBM: Lb.	RMR: Cal.	25.25 inches Fat: %	Fat: Lb.	LBM: Lb.	RMR: Cal.	25.5 inches Fat: %	Fat: Lb.	LBM: Lb.	RMR: Cal.	25.75 inches Fat: %	Fat: Lb.	LBM: Lb.	RMR: Cal.
132	12.25	16.17	115.83	1602	13.03	17.20	114.80	1588	13.82	18.24	113.76	1573	14.60	19.28	112.72	1559
132.5	12.17	16.13	116.38	1609	12.95	17.16	115.34	1595	13.74	18.20	114.30	1581	14.52	19.24	113.26	1566
133	12.09	16.08	116.92	1617	12.87	17.12	115.88	1603	13.65	18.16	114.84	1588	14.43	19.20	113.80	1574
133.5	12.02	16.04	117.46	1624	12.79	17.08	116.42	1610	13.57	18.12	115.38	1596	14.35	19.16	114.34	1581
134	11.94	16.00	118.00	1632	12.72	17.04	116.96	1618	13.49	18.08	115.92	1603	14.26	19.11	114.89	1589
134.5	11.87	15.96	118.54	1639	12.64	17.00	117.50	1625	13.41	18.04	116.46	1611	14.18	19.07	115.43	1596
135	11.79	15.92	119.08	1647	12.56	16.96	118.04	1633	13.33	18.00	117.01	1618	14.10	19.03	115.97	1604
135.5	11.72	15.88	119.62	1654	12.48	16.92	118.58	1640	13.25	17.95	117.55	1626	14.02	18.99	116.51	1611
136	11.65	15.84	120.16	1662	12.41	16.88	119.12	1647	13.17	17.91	118.09	1633	13.93	18.95	117.05	1619
136.5	11.57	15.80	120.70	1669	12.33	16.83	119.67	1655	13.09	17.87	118.63	1641	13.85	18.91	117.59	1626
137	11.50	15.76	121.24	1677	12.26	16.79	120.21	1662	13.02	17.83	119.17	1648	13.77	18.87	118.13	1634
137.5	11.43	15.72	121.79	1684	12.18	16.75	120.75	1670	12.94	17.79	119.71	1656	13.69	18.83	118.67	1641
138	11.36	15.67	122.33	1692	12.11	16.71	121.29	1677	12.86	17.75	120.25	1663	13.61	18.79	119.21	1649
138.5	11.29	15.63	122.87	1699	12.04	16.67	121.83	1685	12.79	17.71	120.79	1671	13.53	18.75	119.75	1656
139	11.22	15.59	123.41	1707	11.96	16.63	122.37	1692	12.71	17.67	121.33	1678	13.46	18.70	120.30	1664
139.5	11.15	15.55	123.95	1714	11.89	16.59	122.91	1700	12.64	17.63	121.87	1686	13.38	18.66	120.84	1671
140	11.08	15.51	124.49	1722	11.82	16.55	123.45	1707	12.56	17.59	122.42	1693	13.30	18.62	121.38	1679
140.5	11.01	15.47	125.03	1729	11.75	16.51	123.99	1715	12.49	17.54	122.96	1700	13.23	18.58	121.92	1686
141	10.94	15.43	125.57	1737	11.68	16.47	124.53	1722	12.41	17.50	123.50	1708	13.15	18.54	122.46	1694
141.5	10.87	15.39	126.11	1744	11.61	16.42	125.08	1730	12.34	17.46	124.04	1715	13.07	18.50	123.00	1701
142	10.81	15.35	126.65	1752	11.54	16.38	125.62	1737	12.27	17.42	124.58	1723	13.00	18.46	123.54	1709
142.5	10.74	15.31	127.20	1759	11.47	16.34	126.16	1745	12.20	17.38	125.12	1730	12.92	18.42	124.08	1716
143	10.67	15.26	127.74	1767	11.40	16.30	126.70	1752	12.13	17.34	125.66	1738	12.85	18.38	124.62	1724
143.5	10.61	15.22	128.28	1774	11.33	16.26	127.24	1760	12.05	17.30	126.20	1745	12.78	18.34	125.16	1731
144	10.54	15.18	128.82	1782	11.26	16.22	127.78	1767	11.98	17.26	126.74	1753	12.70	18.29	125.71	1739
144.5	10.48	15.14	129.36	1789	11.20	16.18	128.32	1775	11.91	17.22	127.28	1760	12.63	18.25	126.25	1746
145	10.41	15.10	129.90	1797	11.13	16.14	128.86	1782	11.84	17.18	127.83	1768	12.56	18.21	126.79	1753
145.5	10.35	15.06	130.44	1804	11.06	16.10	129.40	1790	11.78	17.13	128.37	1775	12.49	18.17	127.33	1761
146	10.29	15.02	130.98	1811	11.00	16.06	129.94	1797	11.71	17.09	128.91	1783	12.42	18.13	127.87	1768
146.5	10.22	14.98	131.52	1819	10.93	16.01	130.49	1805	11.64	17.05	129.45	1790	12.35	18.09	128.41	1776
147	10.16	14.94	132.06	1826	10.87	15.97	131.03	1812	11.57	17.01	129.99	1798	12.28	18.05	128.95	1783
147.5	10.10	14.90	132.61	1834	10.80	15.93	131.57	1820	11.51	16.97	130.53	1805	12.21	18.01	129.49	1791
148	10.04	14.85	133.15	1841	10.74	15.89	132.11	1827	11.44	16.93	131.07	1813	12.14	17.97	130.03	1798
148.5	9.98	14.81	133.69	1849	10.67	15.85	132.65	1835	11.37	16.89	131.61	1820	12.07	17.93	130.57	1806
149	9.91	14.77	134.23	1856	10.61	15.81	133.19	1842	11.31	16.85	132.15	1828	12.00	17.88	131.12	1813
149.5	9.85	14.73	134.77	1864	10.55	15.77	133.73	1850	11.24	16.81	132.69	1835	11.94	17.84	131.66	1821
150	9.79	14.69	135.31	1871	10.49	15.73	134.27	1857	11.18	16.77	133.24	1843	11.87	17.80	132.20	1828
150.5	9.73	14.65	135.85	1879	10.42	15.69	134.81	1864	11.11	16.72	133.78	1850	11.80	17.76	132.74	1836
151	9.67	14.61	136.39	1886	10.36	15.65	135.35	1872	11.05	16.68	134.32	1858	11.74	17.72	133.28	1843
151.5	9.62	14.57	136.93	1894	10.30	15.60	135.90	1879	10.98	16.64	134.86	1865	11.67	17.68	133.82	1851
152	9.56	14.53	137.47	1901	10.24	15.56	136.44	1887	10.92	16.60	135.40	1873	11.60	17.64	134.36	1858
152.5	9.50	14.49	138.02	1909	10.18	15.52	136.98	1894	10.86	16.56	135.94	1880	11.54	17.60	134.90	1866
153	9.44	14.44	138.56	1916	10.12	15.48	137.52	1902	10.80	16.52	136.48	1888	11.47	17.56	135.44	1873
153.5	9.38	14.40	139.10	1924	10.06	15.44	138.06	1909	10.73	16.48	137.02	1895	11.41	17.52	135.98	1881
154	9.33	14.36	139.64	1931	10.00	15.40	138.60	1917	10.67	16.44	137.56	1902	11.35	17.47	136.53	1888
154.5	9.27	14.32	140.18	1939	9.94	15.36	139.14	1924	10.61	16.40	138.10	1910	11.28	17.43	137.07	1896
155	9.21	14.28	140.72	1946	9.88	15.32	139.68	1932	10.55	16.36	138.65	1917	11.22	17.39	137.61	1903
155.5	9.16	14.24	141.26	1954	9.82	15.28	140.22	1939	10.49	16.31	139.19	1925	11.16	17.35	138.15	1911
156	9.10	14.20	141.80	1961	9.77	15.24	140.76	1947	10.43	16.27	139.73	1932	11.10	17.31	138.69	1918
156.5	9.05	14.16	142.34	1969	9.71	15.19	141.31	1954	10.37	16.23	140.27	1940	11.03	17.27	139.23	1926
157	8.99	14.12	142.88	1976	9.65	15.15	141.85	1962	10.31	16.19	140.81	1947	10.97	17.23	139.77	1933
157.5	8.94	14.08	143.43	1984	9.60	15.11	142.39	1969	10.25	16.15	141.35	1955	10.91	17.19	140.31	1941
158	8.88	14.03	143.97	1991	9.54	15.07	142.93	1977	10.20	16.11	141.89	1962	10.85	17.15	140.85	1948
158.5	8.83	13.99	144.51	1999	9.48	15.03	143.47	1984	10.14	16.07	142.43	1970	10.79	17.11	141.39	1955
159	8.77	13.95	145.05	2006	9.43	14.99	144.01	1992	10.08	16.03	142.97	1977	10.73	17.06	141.94	1963
159.5	8.72	13.91	145.59	2013	9.37	14.95	144.55	1999	10.02	15.99	143.51	1985	10.67	17.02	142.48	1970
160	8.67	13.87	146.13	2021	9.32	14.91	145.09	2007	9.97	15.95	144.06	1992	10.61	16.98	143.02	1978
160.5	8.62	13.83	146.67	2028	9.26	14.87	145.63	2014	9.91	15.90	144.60	2000	10.56	16.94	143.56	1985
161	8.56	13.79	147.21	2036	9.21	14.83	146.17	2022	9.85	15.86	145.14	2007	10.50	16.90	144.10	1993
161.5	8.51	13.75	147.75	2043	9.15	14.78	146.72	2029	9.80	15.82	145.68	2015	10.44	16.86	144.64	2000
162	8.46	13.71	148.29	2051	9.10	14.74	147.26	2037	9.74	15.78	146.22	2022	10.38	16.82	145.18	2008
162.5	8.41	13.67	148.84	2058	9.05	14.70	147.80	2044	9.69	15.74	146.76	2030	10.32	16.78	145.72	2015
163	8.36	13.62	149.38	2066	8.99	14.66	148.34	2052	9.63	15.70	147.30	2037	10.27	16.74	146.26	2023
163.5	8.31	13.58	149.92	2073	8.94	14.62	148.88	2059	9.58	15.66	147.84	2045	10.21	16.70	146.80	2030

Body Composition   FEMALE   132-163.5 Lb.

Weight: Lb.	Waist: 26 inches Fat:%	Fat:Lb.	LBM:Lb.	RMR:Cal.	26.25 inches Fat:%	Fat:Lb.	LBM:Lb.	RMR:Cal.	26.5 inches Fat:%	Fat:Lb.	LBM:Lb.	RMR:Cal.	26.75 inches Fat:%	Fat:Lb.	LBM:Lb.	RMR:Cal.
132	15.39	20.32	111.68	1545	16.18	21.35	110.65	1530	16.96	22.39	109.61	1516	17.75	23.43	108.57	1502
132.5	15.30	20.28	112.23	1552	16.08	21.31	111.19	1538	16.87	22.35	110.15	1523	17.65	23.39	109.11	1509
133	15.21	20.23	112.77	1560	15.99	21.27	111.73	1545	16.77	22.31	110.69	1531	17.55	23.35	109.65	1517
133.5	15.13	20.19	113.31	1567	15.90	21.23	112.27	1553	16.68	22.27	111.23	1538	17.46	23.31	110.19	1524
134	15.04	20.15	113.85	1575	15.81	21.19	112.81	1560	16.59	22.23	111.77	1546	17.36	23.26	110.74	1531
134.5	14.95	20.11	114.39	1582	15.72	21.15	113.35	1568	16.50	22.19	112.31	1553	17.27	23.22	111.28	1539
135	14.87	20.07	114.93	1589	15.64	21.11	113.89	1575	16.40	22.15	112.86	1561	17.17	23.18	111.82	1546
135.5	14.78	20.03	115.47	1597	15.55	21.07	114.43	1583	16.31	22.10	113.40	1568	17.08	23.14	112.36	1554
136	14.70	19.99	116.01	1604	15.46	21.03	114.97	1590	16.22	22.06	113.94	1576	16.99	23.10	112.90	1561
136.5	14.61	19.95	116.55	1612	15.37	20.98	115.52	1598	16.13	22.02	114.48	1583	16.89	23.06	113.44	1569
137	14.53	19.91	117.09	1619	15.29	20.94	116.06	1605	16.04	21.98	115.02	1591	16.80	23.02	113.98	1576
137.5	14.45	19.87	117.64	1627	15.20	20.90	116.60	1613	15.96	21.94	115.56	1598	16.71	22.98	114.52	1584
138	14.37	19.82	118.18	1634	15.12	20.86	117.14	1620	15.87	21.90	116.10	1606	16.62	22.94	115.06	1591
138.5	14.28	19.78	118.72	1642	15.03	20.82	117.68	1628	15.78	21.86	116.64	1613	16.53	22.90	115.60	1599
139	14.20	19.74	119.26	1649	14.95	20.78	118.22	1635	15.70	21.82	117.18	1621	16.44	22.85	116.15	1606
139.5	14.12	19.70	119.80	1657	14.87	20.74	118.76	1642	15.61	21.78	117.72	1628	16.35	22.81	116.69	1614
140	14.04	19.66	120.34	1664	14.78	20.70	119.30	1650	15.53	21.74	118.27	1636	16.27	22.77	117.23	1621
140.5	13.96	19.62	120.88	1672	14.70	20.66	119.84	1657	15.44	21.69	118.81	1643	16.18	22.73	117.77	1629
141	13.89	19.58	121.42	1679	14.62	20.62	120.38	1665	15.36	21.65	119.35	1651	16.09	22.69	118.31	1636
141.5	13.81	19.54	121.96	1687	14.54	20.57	120.93	1672	15.27	21.61	119.89	1658	16.01	22.65	118.85	1644
142	13.73	19.50	122.50	1694	14.46	20.53	121.47	1680	15.19	21.57	120.43	1666	15.92	22.61	119.39	1651
142.5	13.65	19.46	123.05	1702	14.38	20.49	122.01	1687	15.11	21.53	120.97	1673	15.84	22.57	119.93	1659
143	13.58	19.41	123.59	1709	14.30	20.45	122.55	1695	15.03	21.49	121.51	1680	15.75	22.53	120.47	1666
143.5	13.50	19.37	124.13	1717	14.22	20.41	123.09	1702	14.95	21.45	122.05	1688	15.67	22.49	121.01	1674
144	13.43	19.33	124.67	1724	14.15	20.37	123.63	1710	14.87	21.41	122.59	1695	15.59	22.44	121.56	1681
144.5	13.35	19.29	125.21	1732	14.07	20.33	124.17	1717	14.79	21.37	123.13	1703	15.50	22.40	122.10	1689
145	13.28	19.25	125.75	1739	13.99	20.29	124.71	1725	14.71	21.33	123.68	1710	15.42	22.36	122.64	1696
145.5	13.20	19.21	126.29	1747	13.92	20.25	125.25	1732	14.63	21.28	124.22	1718	15.34	22.32	123.18	1704
146	13.13	19.17	126.83	1754	13.84	20.21	125.79	1740	14.55	21.24	124.76	1725	15.26	22.28	123.72	1711
146.5	13.06	19.13	127.37	1762	13.76	20.16	126.34	1747	14.47	21.20	125.30	1733	15.18	22.24	124.26	1719
147	12.98	19.09	127.91	1769	13.69	20.12	126.88	1755	14.40	21.16	125.84	1740	15.10	22.20	124.80	1726
147.5	12.91	19.05	128.46	1777	13.62	20.08	127.42	1762	14.32	21.12	126.38	1748	15.02	22.16	125.34	1733
148	12.84	19.00	129.00	1784	13.54	20.04	127.96	1770	14.24	21.08	126.92	1755	14.94	22.12	125.88	1741
148.5	12.77	18.96	129.54	1791	13.47	20.00	128.50	1777	14.17	21.04	127.46	1763	14.87	22.08	126.42	1748
149	12.70	18.92	130.08	1799	13.40	19.96	129.04	1785	14.09	21.00	128.00	1770	14.79	22.03	126.97	1756
149.5	12.63	18.88	130.62	1806	13.32	19.92	129.58	1792	14.02	20.96	128.54	1778	14.71	21.99	127.51	1763
150	12.56	18.84	131.16	1814	13.25	19.88	130.12	1800	13.94	20.92	129.09	1785	14.64	21.95	128.05	1771
150.5	12.49	18.80	131.70	1821	13.18	19.84	130.66	1807	13.87	20.87	129.63	1793	14.56	21.91	128.59	1778
151	12.42	18.76	132.24	1829	13.11	19.80	131.20	1815	13.80	20.83	130.17	1800	14.48	21.87	129.13	1786
151.5	12.35	18.72	132.78	1836	13.04	19.75	131.75	1822	13.72	20.79	130.71	1808	14.41	21.83	129.67	1793
152	12.29	18.68	133.32	1844	12.97	19.71	132.29	1830	13.65	20.75	131.25	1815	14.33	21.79	130.21	1801
152.5	12.22	18.64	133.87	1851	12.90	19.67	132.83	1837	13.58	20.71	131.79	1823	14.26	21.75	130.75	1808
153	12.15	18.59	134.41	1859	12.83	19.63	133.37	1844	13.51	20.67	132.33	1830	14.19	21.71	131.29	1816
153.5	12.09	18.55	134.95	1866	12.76	19.59	133.91	1852	13.44	20.63	132.87	1838	14.11	21.67	131.83	1823
154	12.02	18.51	135.49	1874	12.69	19.55	134.45	1859	13.37	20.59	133.41	1845	14.04	21.62	132.38	1831
154.5	11.96	18.47	136.03	1881	12.63	19.51	134.99	1867	13.30	20.55	133.95	1853	13.97	21.58	132.92	1838
155	11.89	18.43	136.57	1889	12.56	19.47	135.53	1874	13.23	20.51	134.50	1860	13.90	21.54	133.46	1846
155.5	11.83	18.39	137.11	1896	12.49	19.43	136.07	1882	13.16	20.46	135.04	1868	13.83	21.50	134.00	1853
156	11.76	18.35	137.65	1904	12.43	19.39	136.61	1889	13.09	20.42	135.58	1875	13.76	21.46	134.54	1861
156.5	11.70	18.31	138.19	1911	12.36	19.34	137.16	1897	13.02	20.38	136.12	1883	13.69	21.42	135.08	1868
157	11.63	18.27	138.73	1919	12.30	19.30	137.70	1904	12.96	20.34	136.66	1890	13.62	21.38	135.62	1876
157.5	11.57	18.23	139.28	1926	12.23	19.26	138.24	1912	12.89	20.30	137.20	1897	13.55	21.34	136.16	1883
158	11.51	18.18	139.82	1934	12.17	19.22	138.78	1919	12.82	20.26	137.74	1905	13.48	21.30	136.70	1891
158.5	11.45	18.14	140.36	1941	12.10	19.18	139.32	1927	12.76	20.22	138.28	1912	13.41	21.26	137.24	1898
159	11.38	18.10	140.90	1949	12.04	19.14	139.86	1934	12.69	20.18	138.82	1920	13.34	21.21	137.79	1906
159.5	11.32	18.06	141.44	1956	11.97	19.10	140.40	1942	12.62	20.14	139.36	1927	13.27	21.17	138.33	1913
160	11.26	18.02	141.98	1964	11.91	19.06	140.94	1949	12.56	20.10	139.91	1935	13.21	21.13	138.87	1921
160.5	11.20	17.98	142.52	1971	11.85	19.02	141.48	1957	12.49	20.05	140.45	1942	13.14	21.09	139.41	1928
161	11.14	17.94	143.06	1979	11.79	18.98	142.02	1964	12.43	20.01	140.99	1950	13.07	21.05	139.95	1936
161.5	11.08	17.90	143.60	1986	11.72	18.93	142.57	1972	12.37	19.97	141.53	1957	13.01	21.01	140.49	1943
162	11.02	17.86	144.14	1994	11.66	18.89	143.11	1979	12.30	19.93	142.07	1965	12.94	20.97	141.03	1950
162.5	10.96	17.82	144.69	2001	11.60	18.85	143.65	1987	12.24	19.89	142.61	1972	12.88	20.93	141.57	1958
163	10.90	17.77	145.23	2008	11.54	18.81	144.19	1994	12.18	19.85	143.15	1980	12.81	20.89	142.11	1965
163.5	10.85	17.73	145.77	2016	11.48	18.77	144.73	2002	12.11	19.81	143.69	1987	12.75	20.85	142.65	1973

Body Composition FEMALE 132-163.5 Lb.

Weight: Lb.	Waist: 27 inches Fat: %	Fat: Lb.	LBM: Lb.	RMR: Cal.	27.25 inches Fat: %	Fat: Lb.	LBM: Lb.	RMR: Cal.	27.5 inches Fat: %	Fat: Lb.	LBM: Lb.	RMR: Cal.	27.75 inches Fat: %	Fat: Lb.	LBM: Lb.	RMR: Cal.
132	18.53	24.47	107.53	1487	19.32	25.50	106.50	1473	20.11	26.54	105.46	1458	20.89	27.58	104.42	1444
132.5	18.43	24.43	108.08	1495	19.22	25.46	107.04	1480	20.00	26.50	106.00	1466	20.78	27.54	104.96	1452
133	18.33	24.38	108.62	1502	19.11	25.42	107.58	1488	19.89	26.46	106.54	1473	20.67	27.50	105.50	1459
133.5	18.23	24.34	109.16	1510	19.01	25.38	108.12	1495	19.79	26.42	107.08	1481	20.57	27.46	106.04	1467
134	18.14	24.30	109.70	1517	18.91	25.34	108.66	1503	19.68	26.38	107.62	1488	20.46	27.41	106.59	1474
134.5	18.04	24.26	110.24	1525	18.81	25.30	109.20	1510	19.58	26.34	108.16	1496	20.35	27.37	107.13	1482
135	17.94	24.22	110.78	1532	18.71	25.26	109.74	1518	19.48	26.30	108.71	1503	20.25	27.33	107.67	1489
135.5	17.84	24.18	111.32	1540	18.61	25.22	110.28	1525	19.38	26.25	109.25	1511	20.14	27.29	108.21	1497
136	17.75	24.14	111.86	1547	18.51	25.18	110.82	1533	19.27	26.21	109.79	1518	20.04	27.25	108.75	1504
136.5	17.65	24.10	112.40	1555	18.41	25.13	111.37	1540	19.17	26.17	110.33	1526	19.93	27.21	109.29	1511
137	17.56	24.06	112.94	1562	18.32	25.09	111.91	1548	19.07	26.13	110.87	1533	19.83	27.17	109.83	1519
137.5	17.47	24.02	113.49	1569	18.22	25.05	112.45	1555	18.97	26.09	111.41	1541	19.73	27.13	110.37	1526
138	17.37	23.97	114.03	1577	18.12	25.01	112.99	1563	18.88	26.05	111.95	1548	19.63	27.09	110.91	1534
138.5	17.28	23.93	114.57	1584	18.03	24.97	113.53	1570	18.78	26.01	112.49	1556	19.53	27.05	111.45	1541
139	17.19	23.89	115.11	1592	17.93	24.93	114.07	1578	18.68	25.97	113.03	1563	19.43	27.00	112.00	1549
139.5	17.10	23.85	115.65	1599	17.84	24.89	114.61	1585	18.58	25.93	113.57	1571	19.33	26.96	112.54	1556
140	17.01	23.81	116.19	1607	17.75	24.85	115.15	1593	18.49	25.89	114.12	1578	19.23	26.92	113.08	1564
140.5	16.92	23.77	116.73	1614	17.66	24.81	115.69	1600	18.39	25.84	114.66	1586	19.13	26.88	113.62	1571
141	16.83	23.73	117.27	1622	17.56	24.77	116.23	1608	18.30	25.80	115.20	1593	19.04	26.84	114.16	1579
141.5	16.74	23.69	117.81	1629	17.47	24.72	116.78	1615	18.21	25.76	115.74	1601	18.94	26.80	114.70	1586
142	16.65	23.65	118.35	1637	17.38	24.68	117.32	1622	18.11	25.72	116.28	1608	18.84	26.76	115.24	1594
142.5	16.56	23.61	118.90	1644	17.29	24.64	117.86	1630	18.02	25.68	116.82	1616	18.75	26.72	115.78	1601
143	16.48	23.56	119.44	1652	17.20	24.60	118.40	1637	17.93	25.64	117.36	1623	18.65	26.68	116.32	1609
143.5	16.39	23.52	119.98	1659	17.12	24.56	118.94	1645	17.84	25.60	117.90	1631	18.56	26.64	116.86	1616
144	16.31	23.48	120.52	1667	17.03	24.52	119.48	1652	17.75	25.56	118.44	1638	18.47	26.59	117.41	1624
144.5	16.22	23.44	121.06	1674	16.94	24.48	120.02	1660	17.66	25.52	118.98	1646	18.38	26.55	117.95	1631
145	16.14	23.40	121.60	1682	16.85	24.44	120.56	1667	17.57	25.48	119.53	1653	18.28	26.51	118.49	1639
145.5	16.05	23.36	122.14	1689	16.77	24.40	121.10	1675	17.48	25.43	120.07	1661	18.19	26.47	119.03	1646
146	15.97	23.32	122.68	1697	16.68	24.36	121.64	1682	17.39	25.39	120.61	1668	18.10	26.43	119.57	1654
146.5	15.89	23.28	123.22	1704	16.60	24.31	122.19	1690	17.31	25.35	121.15	1675	18.01	26.39	120.11	1661
147	15.81	23.24	123.76	1712	16.51	24.27	122.73	1697	17.22	25.31	121.69	1683	17.92	26.35	120.65	1669
147.5	15.73	23.20	124.31	1719	16.43	24.23	123.27	1705	17.13	25.27	122.23	1690	17.84	26.31	121.19	1676
148	15.64	23.15	124.85	1727	16.35	24.19	123.81	1712	17.05	25.23	122.77	1698	17.75	26.27	121.73	1684
148.5	15.56	23.11	125.39	1734	16.26	24.15	124.35	1720	16.96	25.19	123.31	1705	17.66	26.23	122.27	1691
149	15.48	23.07	125.93	1742	16.18	24.11	124.89	1727	16.88	25.15	123.85	1713	17.57	26.18	122.82	1699
149.5	15.41	23.03	126.47	1749	16.10	24.07	125.43	1735	16.79	25.11	124.39	1720	17.49	26.14	123.36	1706
150	15.33	22.99	127.01	1757	16.02	24.03	125.97	1742	16.71	25.07	124.94	1728	17.40	26.10	123.90	1714
150.5	15.25	22.95	127.55	1764	15.94	23.99	126.51	1750	16.63	25.02	125.48	1735	17.32	26.06	124.44	1721
151	15.17	22.91	128.09	1772	15.86	23.95	127.05	1757	16.55	24.98	126.02	1743	17.23	26.02	124.98	1728
151.5	15.09	22.87	128.63	1779	15.78	23.90	127.60	1765	16.46	24.94	126.56	1750	17.15	25.98	125.52	1736
152	15.02	22.83	129.17	1786	15.70	23.86	128.14	1772	16.38	24.90	127.10	1758	17.06	25.94	126.06	1743
152.5	14.94	22.79	129.72	1794	15.62	23.82	128.68	1780	16.30	24.86	127.64	1765	16.98	25.90	126.60	1751
153	14.87	22.74	130.26	1801	15.54	23.78	129.22	1787	16.22	24.82	128.18	1773	16.90	25.86	127.14	1758
153.5	14.79	22.70	130.80	1809	15.47	23.74	129.76	1795	16.14	24.78	128.72	1780	16.82	25.82	127.68	1766
154	14.72	22.66	131.34	1816	15.39	23.70	130.30	1802	16.06	24.74	129.26	1788	16.74	25.77	128.23	1773
154.5	14.64	22.62	131.88	1824	15.31	23.66	130.84	1810	15.98	24.70	129.80	1795	16.66	25.73	128.77	1781
155	14.57	22.58	132.42	1831	15.24	23.62	131.38	1817	15.91	24.66	130.35	1803	16.58	25.69	129.31	1788
155.5	14.49	22.54	132.96	1839	15.16	23.58	131.92	1825	15.83	24.61	130.89	1810	16.50	25.65	129.85	1796
156	14.42	22.50	133.50	1846	15.09	23.54	132.46	1832	15.75	24.57	131.43	1818	16.42	25.61	130.39	1803
156.5	14.35	22.46	134.04	1854	15.01	23.49	133.01	1839	15.68	24.53	131.97	1825	16.34	25.57	130.93	1811
157	14.28	22.42	134.58	1861	14.94	23.45	133.55	1847	15.60	24.49	132.51	1833	16.26	25.53	131.47	1818
157.5	14.21	22.38	135.13	1869	14.87	23.41	134.09	1854	15.52	24.45	133.05	1840	16.18	25.49	132.01	1826
158	14.14	22.33	135.67	1876	14.79	23.37	134.63	1862	15.45	24.41	133.59	1848	16.11	25.45	132.55	1833
158.5	14.06	22.29	136.21	1884	14.72	23.33	135.17	1869	15.37	24.37	134.13	1855	16.03	25.41	133.09	1841
159	13.99	22.25	136.75	1891	14.65	23.29	135.71	1877	15.30	24.33	134.67	1863	15.95	25.36	133.64	1848
159.5	13.93	22.21	137.29	1899	14.58	23.25	136.25	1884	15.23	24.29	135.21	1870	15.88	25.32	134.18	1856
160	13.86	22.17	137.83	1906	14.50	23.21	136.79	1892	15.15	24.25	135.76	1877	15.80	25.28	134.72	1863
160.5	13.79	22.13	138.37	1914	14.43	23.17	137.33	1899	15.08	24.20	136.30	1885	15.73	25.24	135.26	1871
161	13.72	22.09	138.91	1921	14.36	23.13	137.87	1907	15.01	24.16	136.84	1892	15.65	25.20	135.80	1878
161.5	13.65	22.05	139.45	1929	14.29	23.08	138.42	1914	14.94	24.12	137.38	1900	15.58	25.16	136.34	1886
162	13.58	22.01	139.99	1936	14.22	23.04	138.96	1922	14.86	24.08	137.92	1907	15.51	25.12	136.88	1893
162.5	13.52	21.97	140.54	1944	14.16	23.00	139.50	1929	14.79	24.04	138.46	1915	15.43	25.08	137.42	1901
163	13.45	21.92	141.08	1951	14.09	22.96	140.04	1937	14.72	24.00	139.00	1922	15.36	25.04	137.96	1908
163.5	13.38	21.88	141.62	1959	14.02	22.92	140.58	1944	14.65	23.96	139.54	1930	15.29	25.00	138.50	1916

Body Composition FEMALE 132-163.5 Lb.

Weight: Lb.	Waist: 28 inches				28.25 inches				28.5 inches				28.75 inches			
	Fat: %	Fat: Lb.	LBM: Lb.	RMR: Cal.	Fat: %	Fat: Lb.	LBM: Lb.	RMR: Cal.	Fat: %	Fat: Lb.	LBM: Lb.	RMR: Cal.	Fat: %	Fat: Lb.	LBM: Lb.	RMR: Cal.
132	21.68	28.62	103.38	1430	22.46	29.65	102.35	1415	23.25	30.69	101.31	1401	24.04	31.73	100.27	1387
132.5	21.57	28.58	103.93	1437	22.35	29.61	102.89	1423	23.13	30.65	101.85	1409	23.92	31.69	100.81	1394
133	21.45	28.53	104.47	1445	22.23	29.57	103.43	1430	23.01	30.61	102.39	1416	23.79	31.65	101.35	1402
133.5	21.34	28.49	105.01	1452	22.12	29.53	103.97	1438	22.90	30.57	102.93	1424	23.67	31.61	101.89	1409
134	21.23	28.45	105.55	1460	22.01	29.49	104.51	1445	22.78	30.53	103.47	1431	23.56	31.56	102.44	1417
134.5	21.12	28.41	106.09	1467	21.89	29.45	105.05	1453	22.67	30.49	104.01	1439	23.44	31.52	102.98	1424
135	21.01	28.37	106.63	1475	21.78	29.41	105.59	1460	22.55	30.45	104.56	1446	23.32	31.48	103.52	1432
135.5	20.91	28.33	107.17	1482	21.67	29.37	106.13	1468	22.44	30.40	105.10	1453	23.20	31.44	104.06	1439
136	20.80	28.29	107.71	1490	21.56	29.33	106.67	1475	22.33	30.36	105.64	1461	23.09	31.40	104.60	1447
136.5	20.69	28.25	108.25	1497	21.45	29.28	107.22	1483	22.21	30.32	106.18	1468	22.97	31.36	105.14	1454
137	20.59	28.21	108.79	1505	21.35	29.24	107.76	1490	22.10	30.28	106.72	1476	22.86	31.32	105.68	1462
137.5	20.48	28.17	109.34	1512	21.24	29.20	108.30	1498	21.99	30.24	107.26	1483	22.75	31.28	106.22	1469
138	20.38	28.12	109.88	1520	21.13	29.16	108.84	1505	21.88	30.20	107.80	1491	22.64	31.24	106.76	1477
138.5	20.28	28.08	110.42	1527	21.03	29.12	109.38	1513	21.77	30.16	108.34	1498	22.52	31.20	107.30	1484
139	20.17	28.04	110.96	1535	20.92	29.08	109.92	1520	21.67	30.12	108.88	1506	22.41	31.15	107.85	1492
139.5	20.07	28.00	111.50	1542	20.82	29.04	110.46	1528	21.56	30.08	109.42	1513	22.30	31.11	108.39	1499
140	19.97	27.96	112.04	1550	20.71	29.00	111.00	1535	21.45	30.04	109.96	1521	22.19	31.07	108.93	1506
140.5	19.87	27.92	112.58	1557	20.61	28.96	111.54	1543	21.35	29.99	110.51	1528	22.09	31.03	109.47	1514
141	19.77	27.88	113.12	1564	20.51	28.92	112.08	1550	21.24	29.95	111.05	1536	21.98	30.99	110.01	1521
141.5	19.67	27.84	113.66	1572	20.41	28.87	112.63	1558	21.14	29.91	111.59	1543	21.87	30.95	110.55	1529
142	19.57	27.80	114.20	1579	20.31	28.83	113.17	1565	21.04	29.87	112.13	1551	21.77	30.91	111.09	1536
142.5	19.48	27.76	114.75	1587	20.21	28.79	113.71	1573	20.93	29.83	112.67	1558	21.66	30.87	111.63	1544
143	19.38	27.71	115.29	1594	20.11	28.75	114.25	1580	20.83	29.79	113.21	1566	21.56	30.83	112.17	1551
143.5	19.28	27.67	115.83	1602	20.01	28.71	114.79	1588	20.73	29.75	113.75	1573	21.45	30.79	112.71	1559
144	19.19	27.63	116.37	1609	19.91	28.67	115.33	1595	20.63	29.71	114.29	1581	21.35	30.74	113.26	1566
144.5	19.09	27.59	116.91	1617	19.81	28.63	115.87	1603	20.53	29.67	114.83	1588	21.25	30.70	113.80	1574
145	19.00	27.55	117.45	1624	19.72	28.59	116.41	1610	20.43	29.63	115.38	1596	21.15	30.66	114.34	1581
145.5	18.91	27.51	117.99	1632	19.62	28.55	116.95	1617	20.33	29.58	115.92	1603	21.05	30.62	114.88	1589
146	18.81	27.47	118.53	1639	19.52	28.51	117.49	1625	20.23	29.54	116.46	1611	20.95	30.58	115.42	1596
146.5	18.72	27.43	119.07	1647	19.43	28.46	118.04	1632	20.14	29.50	117.00	1618	20.85	30.54	115.96	1604
147	18.63	27.39	119.61	1654	19.34	28.42	118.58	1640	20.04	29.46	117.54	1626	20.75	30.50	116.50	1611
147.5	18.54	27.35	120.16	1662	19.24	28.38	119.12	1647	19.95	29.42	118.08	1633	20.65	30.46	117.04	1619
148	18.45	27.30	120.70	1669	19.15	28.34	119.66	1655	19.85	29.38	118.62	1641	20.55	30.42	117.58	1626
148.5	18.36	27.26	121.24	1677	19.06	28.30	120.20	1662	19.76	29.34	119.16	1648	20.45	30.38	118.12	1634
149	18.27	27.22	121.78	1684	18.97	28.26	120.74	1670	19.66	29.30	119.70	1655	20.36	30.33	118.67	1641
149.5	18.18	27.18	122.32	1692	18.88	28.22	121.28	1677	19.57	29.26	120.24	1663	20.26	30.29	119.21	1649
150	18.09	27.14	122.86	1699	18.79	28.18	121.82	1685	19.48	29.22	120.79	1670	20.17	30.25	119.75	1656
150.5	18.01	27.10	123.40	1707	18.70	28.14	122.36	1692	19.38	29.17	121.33	1678	20.07	30.21	120.29	1664
151	17.92	27.06	123.94	1714	18.61	28.10	122.90	1700	19.29	29.13	121.87	1685	19.98	30.17	120.83	1671
151.5	17.83	27.02	124.48	1722	18.52	28.05	123.45	1707	19.20	29.09	122.41	1693	19.89	30.13	121.37	1679
152	17.75	26.98	125.02	1729	18.43	28.01	123.99	1715	19.11	29.05	122.95	1700	19.80	30.09	121.91	1686
152.5	17.66	26.94	125.57	1737	18.34	27.97	124.53	1722	19.02	29.01	123.49	1708	19.70	30.05	122.45	1694
153	17.58	26.89	126.11	1744	18.26	27.93	125.07	1730	18.93	28.97	124.03	1715	19.61	30.01	122.99	1701
153.5	17.49	26.85	126.65	1752	18.17	27.89	125.61	1737	18.85	28.93	124.57	1723	19.52	29.97	123.53	1708
154	17.41	26.81	127.19	1759	18.08	27.85	126.15	1745	18.76	28.89	125.11	1730	19.43	29.92	124.08	1716
154.5	17.33	26.77	127.73	1766	18.00	27.81	126.69	1752	18.67	28.85	125.65	1738	19.34	29.88	124.62	1723
155	17.25	26.73	128.27	1774	17.91	27.77	127.23	1760	18.58	28.81	126.20	1745	19.25	29.84	125.16	1731
155.5	17.16	26.69	128.81	1781	17.83	27.73	127.77	1767	18.50	28.76	126.74	1753	19.16	29.80	125.70	1738
156	17.08	26.65	129.35	1789	17.75	27.69	128.31	1775	18.41	28.72	127.28	1760	19.08	29.76	126.24	1746
156.5	17.00	26.61	129.89	1796	17.66	27.64	128.86	1782	18.33	28.68	127.82	1768	18.99	29.72	126.78	1753
157	16.92	26.57	130.43	1804	17.58	27.60	129.40	1790	18.24	28.64	128.36	1775	18.90	29.68	127.32	1761
157.5	16.84	26.53	130.98	1811	17.50	27.56	129.94	1797	18.16	28.60	128.90	1783	18.82	29.64	127.86	1768
158	16.76	26.48	131.52	1819	17.42	27.52	130.48	1805	18.08	28.56	129.44	1790	18.73	29.60	128.40	1776
158.5	16.68	26.44	132.06	1826	17.34	27.48	131.02	1812	17.99	28.52	129.98	1798	18.65	29.56	128.94	1783
159	16.61	26.40	132.60	1834	17.26	27.44	131.56	1819	17.91	28.48	130.52	1805	18.56	29.51	129.49	1791
159.5	16.53	26.36	133.14	1841	17.18	27.40	132.10	1827	17.83	28.44	131.06	1813	18.48	29.47	130.03	1798
160	16.45	26.32	133.68	1849	17.10	27.36	132.64	1834	17.75	28.40	131.61	1820	18.40	29.43	130.57	1806
160.5	16.37	26.28	134.22	1856	17.02	27.32	133.18	1842	17.67	28.35	132.15	1828	18.31	29.39	131.11	1813
161	16.30	26.24	134.76	1864	16.94	27.28	133.72	1849	17.59	28.31	132.69	1835	18.23	29.35	131.65	1821
161.5	16.22	26.20	135.30	1871	16.86	27.23	134.27	1857	17.51	28.27	133.23	1843	18.15	29.31	132.19	1828
162	16.15	26.16	135.84	1879	16.79	27.19	134.81	1864	17.43	28.23	133.77	1850	18.07	29.27	132.73	1836
162.5	16.07	26.12	136.39	1886	16.71	27.15	135.35	1872	17.35	28.19	134.31	1858	17.99	29.23	133.27	1843
163	16.00	26.07	136.93	1894	16.63	27.11	135.89	1879	17.27	28.15	134.85	1865	17.91	29.19	133.81	1851
163.5	15.92	26.03	137.47	1901	16.56	27.07	136.43	1887	17.19	28.11	135.39	1872	17.83	29.15	134.35	1858

Body Composition FEMALE 132-163.5 Lb.

Weight: Lb.	Waist: 29 inches				29.25 inches				29.5 inches				29.75 inches			
	Fat: %	Fat: Lb.	LBM: Lb.	RMR: Cal.	Fat: %	Fat: Lb.	LBM: Lb.	RMR: Cal.	Fat: %	Fat: Lb.	LBM: Lb.	RMR: Cal.	Fat: %	Fat: Lb.	LBM: Lb.	RMR: Cal.
132	24.82	32.77	99.23	1372	25.61	33.80	98.20	1358	26.39	34.84	97.16	1344	27.18	35.88	96.12	1329
132.5	24.70	32.73	99.78	1380	25.48	33.76	98.74	1366	26.26	34.80	97.70	1351	27.05	35.84	96.66	1337
133	24.57	32.68	100.32	1387	25.35	33.72	99.28	1373	26.13	34.76	98.24	1359	26.91	35.80	97.20	1344
133.5	24.45	32.64	100.86	1395	25.23	33.68	99.82	1381	26.01	34.72	98.78	1366	26.78	35.76	97.74	1352
134	24.33	32.60	101.40	1402	25.10	33.64	100.36	1388	25.88	34.68	99.32	1374	26.65	35.71	98.29	1359
134.5	24.21	32.56	101.94	1410	24.98	33.60	100.90	1395	25.75	34.64	99.86	1381	26.52	35.67	98.83	1367
135	24.09	32.52	102.48	1417	24.86	33.56	101.44	1403	25.63	34.60	100.41	1389	26.39	35.63	99.37	1374
135.5	23.97	32.48	103.02	1425	24.74	33.52	101.98	1410	25.50	34.55	100.95	1396	26.27	35.59	99.91	1382
136	23.85	32.44	103.56	1432	24.61	33.48	102.52	1418	25.38	34.51	101.49	1404	26.14	35.55	100.45	1389
136.5	23.73	32.40	104.10	1440	24.49	33.43	103.07	1425	25.25	34.47	102.03	1411	26.01	35.51	100.99	1397
137	23.62	32.36	104.64	1447	24.37	33.39	103.61	1433	25.13	34.43	102.57	1419	25.89	35.47	101.53	1404
137.5	23.50	32.32	105.19	1455	24.26	33.35	104.15	1440	25.01	34.39	103.11	1426	25.77	35.43	102.07	1412
138	23.39	32.27	105.73	1462	24.14	33.31	104.69	1448	24.89	34.35	103.65	1433	25.64	35.39	102.61	1419
138.5	23.27	32.23	106.27	1470	24.02	33.27	105.23	1455	24.77	34.31	104.19	1441	25.52	35.35	103.15	1427
139	23.16	32.19	106.81	1477	23.91	33.23	105.77	1463	24.65	34.27	104.73	1448	25.40	35.30	103.70	1434
139.5	23.05	32.15	107.35	1485	23.79	33.19	106.31	1470	24.53	34.23	105.27	1456	25.28	35.26	104.24	1442
140	22.94	32.11	107.89	1492	23.68	33.15	106.85	1478	24.42	34.19	105.82	1463	25.16	35.22	104.78	1449
140.5	22.82	32.07	108.43	1500	23.56	33.11	107.39	1485	24.30	34.14	106.36	1471	25.04	35.18	105.32	1457
141	22.71	32.03	108.97	1507	23.45	33.07	107.93	1493	24.19	34.10	106.90	1478	24.92	35.14	105.86	1464
141.5	22.61	31.99	109.51	1515	23.34	33.02	108.48	1500	24.07	34.06	107.44	1486	24.81	35.10	106.40	1472
142	22.50	31.95	110.05	1522	23.23	32.98	109.02	1508	23.96	34.02	107.98	1493	24.69	35.06	106.94	1479
142.5	22.39	31.91	110.60	1530	23.12	32.94	109.56	1515	23.85	33.98	108.52	1501	24.57	35.02	107.48	1486
143	22.28	31.86	111.14	1537	23.01	32.90	110.10	1523	23.73	33.94	109.06	1508	24.46	34.98	108.02	1494
143.5	22.18	31.82	111.68	1544	22.90	32.86	110.64	1530	23.62	33.90	109.60	1516	24.35	34.94	108.56	1501
144	22.07	31.78	112.22	1552	22.79	32.82	111.18	1538	23.51	33.86	110.14	1523	24.23	34.89	109.11	1509
144.5	21.97	31.74	112.76	1559	22.68	32.78	111.72	1545	23.40	33.82	110.68	1531	24.12	34.85	109.65	1516
145	21.86	31.70	113.30	1567	22.58	32.74	112.26	1553	23.29	33.78	111.23	1538	24.01	34.81	110.19	1524
145.5	21.76	31.66	113.84	1574	22.47	32.70	112.80	1560	23.18	33.73	111.77	1546	23.90	34.77	110.73	1531
146	21.66	31.62	114.38	1582	22.37	32.66	113.34	1568	23.08	33.69	112.31	1553	23.79	34.73	111.27	1539
146.5	21.55	31.58	114.92	1589	22.26	32.61	113.89	1575	22.97	33.65	112.85	1561	23.68	34.69	111.81	1546
147	21.45	31.54	115.46	1597	22.16	32.57	114.43	1583	22.86	33.61	113.39	1568	23.57	34.65	112.35	1554
147.5	21.35	31.50	116.01	1604	22.06	32.53	114.97	1590	22.76	33.57	113.93	1576	23.46	34.61	112.89	1561
148	21.25	31.45	116.55	1612	21.95	32.49	115.51	1597	22.65	33.53	114.47	1583	23.36	34.57	113.43	1569
148.5	21.15	31.41	117.09	1619	21.85	32.45	116.05	1605	22.55	33.49	115.01	1591	23.25	34.53	113.97	1576
149	21.06	31.37	117.63	1627	21.75	32.41	116.59	1612	22.45	33.45	115.55	1598	23.14	34.48	114.52	1584
149.5	20.96	31.33	118.17	1634	21.65	32.37	117.13	1620	22.35	33.41	116.09	1606	23.04	34.44	115.06	1591
150	20.86	31.29	118.71	1642	21.55	32.33	117.67	1627	22.24	33.37	116.64	1613	22.94	34.40	115.60	1599
150.5	20.76	31.25	119.25	1649	21.45	32.29	118.21	1635	22.14	33.32	117.18	1621	22.83	34.36	116.14	1606
151	20.67	31.21	119.79	1657	21.35	32.25	118.75	1642	22.04	33.28	117.72	1628	22.73	34.32	116.68	1614
151.5	20.57	31.17	120.33	1664	21.26	32.20	119.30	1650	21.94	33.24	118.26	1636	22.63	34.28	117.22	1621
152	20.48	31.13	120.87	1672	21.16	32.16	119.84	1657	21.84	33.20	118.80	1643	22.53	34.24	117.76	1629
152.5	20.38	31.09	121.42	1679	21.06	32.12	120.38	1665	21.74	33.16	119.34	1650	22.42	34.20	118.30	1636
153	20.29	31.04	121.96	1687	20.97	32.08	120.92	1672	21.65	33.12	119.88	1658	22.32	34.16	118.84	1644
153.5	20.20	31.00	122.50	1694	20.87	32.04	121.46	1680	21.55	33.08	120.42	1665	22.23	34.12	119.38	1651
154	20.11	30.96	123.04	1702	20.78	32.00	122.00	1687	21.45	33.04	120.96	1673	22.13	34.07	119.93	1659
154.5	20.01	30.92	123.58	1709	20.69	31.96	122.54	1695	21.36	33.00	121.50	1680	22.03	34.03	120.47	1666
155	19.92	30.88	124.12	1717	20.59	31.92	123.08	1702	21.26	32.96	122.05	1688	21.93	33.99	121.01	1674
155.5	19.83	30.84	124.66	1724	20.50	31.88	123.62	1710	21.17	32.91	122.59	1695	21.83	33.95	121.55	1681
156	19.74	30.80	125.20	1732	20.41	31.84	124.16	1717	21.07	32.87	123.13	1703	21.74	33.91	122.09	1688
156.5	19.65	30.76	125.74	1739	20.32	31.79	124.71	1725	20.98	32.83	123.67	1710	21.64	33.87	122.63	1696
157	19.56	30.72	126.28	1747	20.23	31.75	125.25	1732	20.89	32.79	124.21	1718	21.55	33.83	123.17	1703
157.5	19.48	30.68	126.83	1754	20.13	31.71	125.79	1740	20.79	32.75	124.75	1725	21.45	33.79	123.71	1711
158	19.39	30.63	127.37	1761	20.05	31.67	126.33	1747	20.70	32.71	125.29	1733	21.36	33.75	124.25	1718
158.5	19.30	30.59	127.91	1769	19.96	31.63	126.87	1755	20.61	32.67	125.83	1740	21.27	33.71	124.79	1726
159	19.22	30.55	128.45	1776	19.87	31.59	127.41	1762	20.52	32.63	126.37	1748	21.17	33.66	125.34	1733
159.5	19.13	30.51	128.99	1784	19.78	31.55	127.95	1770	20.43	32.59	126.91	1755	21.08	33.62	125.88	1741
160	19.04	30.47	129.53	1791	19.69	31.51	128.49	1777	20.34	32.55	127.46	1763	20.99	33.58	126.42	1748
160.5	18.96	30.43	130.07	1799	19.61	31.47	129.03	1785	20.25	32.50	128.00	1770	20.90	33.54	126.96	1756
161	18.87	30.39	130.61	1806	19.52	31.43	129.57	1792	20.16	32.46	128.54	1778	20.81	33.50	127.50	1763
161.5	18.79	30.35	131.15	1814	19.43	31.38	130.12	1799	20.08	32.42	129.08	1785	20.72	33.46	128.04	1771
162	18.71	30.31	131.69	1821	19.35	31.34	130.66	1807	19.99	32.38	129.62	1793	20.63	33.42	128.58	1778
162.5	18.62	30.27	132.24	1829	19.26	31.30	131.20	1814	19.90	32.34	130.16	1800	20.54	33.38	129.12	1786
163	18.54	30.22	132.78	1836	19.18	31.26	131.74	1822	19.82	32.30	130.70	1808	20.45	33.34	129.66	1793
163.5	18.46	30.18	133.32	1844	19.10	31.22	132.28	1829	19.73	32.26	131.24	1815	20.36	33.30	130.20	1801

Body Composition FEMALE 132-163.5 Lb.

Weight: Lb.	Waist: 30 inches Fat: %	Fat: Lb.	LBM: Lb.	RMR: Cal.	30.25 inches Fat: %	Fat: Lb.	LBM: Lb.	RMR: Cal.	30.5 inches Fat: %	Fat: Lb.	LBM: Lb.	RMR: Cal.	30.75 inches Fat: %	Fat: Lb.	LBM: Lb.	RMR: Cal.
132	27.97	36.92	95.08	1315	28.75	37.95	94.05	1301	29.54	38.99	93.01	1286	30.32	40.03	91.97	1272
132.5	27.83	36.88	95.63	1322	28.61	37.91	94.59	1308	29.40	38.95	93.55	1294	30.18	39.99	92.51	1279
133	27.69	36.83	96.17	1330	28.47	37.87	95.13	1316	29.25	38.91	94.09	1301	30.03	39.95	93.05	1287
133.5	27.56	36.79	96.71	1337	28.34	37.83	95.67	1323	29.11	38.87	94.63	1309	29.89	39.91	93.59	1294
134	27.43	36.75	97.25	1345	28.20	37.79	96.21	1331	28.98	38.83	95.17	1316	29.75	39.86	94.14	1302
134.5	27.29	36.71	97.79	1352	28.07	37.75	96.75	1338	28.84	38.79	95.71	1324	29.61	39.82	94.68	1309
135	27.16	36.67	98.33	1360	27.93	37.71	97.29	1346	28.70	38.75	96.26	1331	29.47	39.78	95.22	1317
135.5	27.03	36.63	98.87	1367	27.80	37.67	97.83	1353	28.56	38.70	96.80	1339	29.33	39.74	95.76	1324
136	26.90	36.59	99.41	1375	27.67	37.63	98.37	1361	28.43	38.66	97.34	1346	29.19	39.70	96.30	1332
136.5	26.77	36.55	99.95	1382	27.53	37.58	98.92	1368	28.29	38.62	97.88	1354	29.05	39.66	96.84	1339
137	26.65	36.51	100.49	1390	27.40	37.54	99.46	1375	28.16	38.58	98.42	1361	28.92	39.62	97.38	1347
137.5	26.52	36.47	101.04	1397	27.27	37.50	100.00	1383	28.03	38.54	98.96	1369	28.78	39.58	97.92	1354
138	26.39	36.42	101.58	1405	27.15	37.46	100.54	1390	27.90	38.50	99.50	1376	28.65	39.54	98.46	1362
138.5	26.27	36.38	102.12	1412	27.02	37.42	101.08	1398	27.77	38.46	100.04	1384	28.52	39.50	99.00	1369
139	26.15	36.34	102.66	1420	26.89	37.38	101.62	1405	27.64	38.42	100.58	1391	28.38	39.45	99.55	1377
139.5	26.02	36.30	103.20	1427	26.77	37.34	102.16	1413	27.51	38.38	101.12	1399	28.25	39.41	100.09	1384
140	25.90	36.26	103.74	1435	26.64	37.30	102.70	1420	27.38	38.34	101.67	1406	28.12	39.37	100.63	1392
140.5	25.78	36.22	104.28	1442	26.52	37.26	103.24	1428	27.26	38.29	102.21	1414	27.99	39.33	101.17	1399
141	25.66	36.18	104.82	1450	26.39	37.22	103.78	1435	27.13	38.25	102.75	1421	27.87	39.29	101.71	1407
141.5	25.54	36.14	105.36	1457	26.27	37.17	104.33	1443	27.00	38.21	103.29	1428	27.74	39.25	102.25	1414
142	25.42	36.10	105.90	1465	26.15	37.13	104.87	1450	26.88	38.17	103.83	1436	27.61	39.21	102.79	1422
142.5	25.30	36.06	106.45	1472	26.03	37.09	105.41	1458	26.76	38.13	104.37	1443	27.49	39.17	103.33	1429
143	25.18	36.01	106.99	1480	25.91	37.05	105.95	1465	26.64	38.09	104.91	1451	27.36	39.13	103.87	1437
143.5	25.07	35.97	107.53	1487	25.79	37.01	106.49	1473	26.51	38.05	105.45	1458	27.24	39.09	104.41	1444
144	24.95	35.93	108.07	1495	25.67	36.97	107.03	1480	26.39	38.01	105.99	1466	27.11	39.04	104.96	1452
144.5	24.84	35.89	108.61	1502	25.56	36.93	107.57	1488	26.27	37.97	106.53	1473	26.99	39.00	105.50	1459
145	24.72	35.85	109.15	1510	25.44	36.89	108.11	1495	26.16	37.93	107.08	1481	26.87	38.96	106.04	1466
145.5	24.61	35.81	109.69	1517	25.32	36.85	108.65	1503	26.04	37.88	107.62	1488	26.75	38.92	106.58	1474
146	24.50	35.77	110.23	1525	25.21	36.81	109.19	1510	25.92	37.84	108.16	1496	26.63	38.88	107.12	1481
146.5	24.39	35.73	110.77	1532	25.10	36.76	109.74	1518	25.80	37.80	108.70	1503	26.51	38.84	107.66	1489
147	24.28	35.69	111.31	1539	24.98	36.72	110.28	1525	25.69	37.76	109.24	1511	26.39	38.80	108.20	1496
147.5	24.17	35.65	111.86	1547	24.87	36.68	110.82	1533	25.57	37.72	109.78	1518	26.28	38.76	108.74	1504
148	24.06	35.60	112.40	1554	24.76	36.64	111.36	1540	25.46	37.68	110.32	1526	26.16	38.72	109.28	1511
148.5	23.95	35.56	112.94	1562	24.65	36.60	111.90	1548	25.35	37.64	110.86	1533	26.04	38.68	109.82	1519
149	23.84	35.52	113.48	1569	24.54	36.56	112.44	1555	25.23	37.60	111.40	1541	25.93	38.63	110.37	1526
149.5	23.73	35.48	114.02	1577	24.43	36.52	112.98	1563	25.12	37.56	111.94	1548	25.82	38.59	110.91	1534
150	23.63	35.44	114.56	1584	24.32	36.48	113.52	1570	25.01	37.52	112.49	1556	25.70	38.55	111.45	1541
150.5	23.52	35.40	115.10	1592	24.21	36.44	114.06	1577	24.90	37.47	113.03	1563	25.59	38.51	111.99	1549
151	23.42	35.36	115.64	1599	24.10	36.40	114.60	1585	24.79	37.43	113.57	1571	25.48	38.47	112.53	1556
151.5	23.31	35.32	116.18	1607	24.00	36.35	115.15	1592	24.68	37.39	114.11	1578	25.37	38.43	113.07	1564
152	23.21	35.28	116.72	1614	23.89	36.31	115.69	1600	24.57	37.35	114.65	1586	25.26	38.39	113.61	1571
152.5	23.10	35.24	117.27	1622	23.79	36.27	116.23	1607	24.47	37.31	115.19	1593	25.15	38.35	114.15	1579
153	23.00	35.19	117.81	1629	23.68	36.23	116.77	1615	24.36	37.27	115.73	1601	25.04	38.31	114.69	1586
153.5	22.90	35.15	118.35	1637	23.58	36.19	117.31	1622	24.25	37.23	116.27	1608	24.93	38.27	115.23	1594
154	22.80	35.11	118.89	1644	23.47	36.15	117.85	1630	24.15	37.19	116.81	1616	24.82	38.22	115.78	1601
154.5	22.70	35.07	119.43	1652	23.37	36.11	118.39	1637	24.04	37.15	117.35	1623	24.71	38.18	116.32	1609
155	22.60	35.03	119.97	1659	23.27	36.07	118.93	1645	23.94	37.11	117.90	1630	24.61	38.14	116.86	1616
155.5	22.50	34.99	120.51	1667	23.17	36.03	119.47	1652	23.84	37.06	118.44	1638	24.50	38.10	117.40	1624
156	22.40	34.95	121.05	1674	23.07	35.99	120.01	1660	23.73	37.02	118.98	1645	24.40	38.06	117.94	1631
156.5	22.30	34.91	121.59	1682	22.97	35.94	120.56	1667	23.63	36.98	119.52	1653	24.29	38.02	118.48	1639
157	22.21	34.87	122.13	1689	22.87	35.90	121.10	1675	23.53	36.94	120.06	1660	24.19	37.98	119.02	1646
157.5	22.11	34.83	122.68	1697	22.77	35.86	121.64	1682	23.43	36.90	120.60	1668	24.09	37.94	119.56	1654
158	22.02	34.78	123.22	1704	22.67	35.82	122.18	1690	23.33	36.86	121.14	1675	23.99	37.90	120.10	1661
158.5	21.92	34.74	123.76	1712	22.57	35.78	122.72	1697	23.23	36.82	121.68	1683	23.88	37.86	120.64	1669
159	21.83	34.70	124.30	1719	22.48	35.74	123.26	1705	23.13	36.78	122.22	1690	23.78	37.81	121.19	1676
159.5	21.73	34.66	124.84	1727	22.38	35.70	123.80	1712	23.03	36.74	122.76	1698	23.68	37.77	121.73	1683
160	21.64	34.62	125.38	1734	22.29	35.66	124.34	1720	22.93	36.70	123.31	1705	23.58	37.73	122.27	1691
160.5	21.54	34.58	125.92	1741	22.19	35.62	124.88	1727	22.84	36.65	123.85	1713	23.48	37.69	122.81	1698
161	21.45	34.54	126.46	1749	22.10	35.58	125.42	1735	22.74	36.61	124.39	1720	23.39	37.65	123.35	1706
161.5	21.36	34.50	127.00	1756	22.00	35.53	125.97	1742	22.65	36.57	124.93	1728	23.29	37.61	123.89	1713
162	21.27	34.46	127.54	1764	21.91	35.49	126.51	1750	22.55	36.53	125.47	1735	23.19	37.57	124.43	1721
162.5	21.18	34.42	128.09	1771	21.82	35.45	127.05	1757	22.46	36.49	126.01	1743	23.09	37.53	124.97	1728
163	21.09	34.37	128.63	1779	21.72	35.41	127.59	1765	22.36	36.45	126.55	1750	23.00	37.49	125.51	1736
163.5	21.00	34.33	129.17	1786	21.63	35.37	128.13	1772	22.27	36.41	127.09	1758	22.90	37.45	126.05	1743

Body Composition FEMALE 132-163.5 Lb.

Weight: Lb.	Waist: 31 inches Fat: %	Fat: Lb.	LBM: Lb.	RMR: Cal.	31.25 inches Fat: %	Fat: Lb.	LBM: Lb.	RMR: Cal.	31.5 inches Fat: %	Fat: Lb.	LBM: Lb.	RMR: Cal.	31.75 inches Fat: %	Fat: Lb.	LBM: Lb.	RMR: Cal.
132	31.11	41.07	90.93	1258	31.90	42.10	89.90	1243	32.68	43.14	88.86	1229	33.47	44.18	87.82	1215
132.5	30.96	41.03	91.48	1265	31.75	42.06	90.44	1251	32.53	43.10	89.40	1236	33.31	44.14	88.36	1222
133	30.82	40.98	92.02	1273	31.60	42.02	90.98	1258	32.38	43.06	89.94	1244	33.16	44.10	88.90	1230
133.5	30.67	40.94	92.56	1280	31.45	41.98	91.52	1266	32.22	43.02	90.48	1251	33.00	44.06	89.44	1237
134	30.52	40.90	93.10	1288	31.30	41.94	92.06	1273	32.07	42.98	91.02	1259	32.85	44.01	89.99	1244
134.5	30.38	40.86	93.64	1295	31.15	41.90	92.60	1281	31.92	42.94	91.56	1266	32.69	43.97	90.53	1252
135	30.24	40.82	94.18	1303	31.01	41.86	93.14	1288	31.77	42.90	92.11	1274	32.54	43.93	91.07	1259
135.5	30.10	40.78	94.72	1310	30.86	41.82	93.68	1296	31.63	42.85	92.65	1281	32.39	43.89	91.61	1267
136	29.95	40.74	95.26	1317	30.72	41.78	94.22	1303	31.48	42.81	93.19	1289	32.24	43.85	92.15	1274
136.5	29.81	40.70	95.80	1325	30.57	41.73	94.77	1311	31.33	42.77	93.73	1296	32.09	43.81	92.69	1282
137	29.68	40.66	96.34	1332	30.43	41.69	95.31	1318	31.19	42.73	94.27	1304	31.95	43.77	93.23	1289
137.5	29.54	40.62	96.89	1340	30.29	41.65	95.85	1326	31.05	42.69	94.81	1311	31.80	43.73	93.77	1297
138	29.40	40.57	97.43	1347	30.15	41.61	96.39	1333	30.91	42.65	95.35	1319	31.66	43.69	94.31	1304
138.5	29.27	40.53	97.97	1355	30.01	41.57	96.93	1341	30.76	42.61	95.89	1326	31.51	43.65	94.85	1312
139	29.13	40.49	98.51	1362	29.88	41.53	97.47	1348	30.62	42.57	96.43	1334	31.37	43.60	95.40	1319
139.5	29.00	40.45	99.05	1370	29.74	41.49	98.01	1355	30.48	42.53	96.97	1341	31.23	43.56	95.94	1327
140	28.86	40.41	99.59	1377	29.61	41.45	98.55	1363	30.35	42.49	97.52	1349	31.09	43.52	96.48	1334
140.5	28.73	40.37	100.13	1385	29.47	41.41	99.09	1370	30.21	42.44	98.06	1356	30.95	43.48	97.02	1342
141	28.60	40.33	100.67	1392	29.34	41.37	99.63	1378	30.07	42.40	98.60	1364	30.81	43.44	97.56	1349
141.5	28.47	40.29	101.21	1400	29.20	41.32	100.18	1385	29.94	42.36	99.14	1371	30.67	43.40	98.10	1357
142	28.34	40.25	101.75	1407	29.07	41.28	100.72	1393	29.80	42.32	99.68	1379	30.53	43.36	98.64	1364
142.5	28.21	40.21	102.30	1415	28.94	41.24	101.26	1400	29.67	42.28	100.22	1386	30.40	43.32	99.18	1372
143	28.09	40.16	102.84	1422	28.81	41.20	101.80	1408	29.54	42.24	100.76	1394	30.26	43.28	99.72	1379
143.5	27.96	40.12	103.38	1430	28.68	41.16	102.34	1415	29.41	42.20	101.30	1401	30.13	43.24	100.26	1387
144	27.83	40.08	103.92	1437	28.56	41.12	102.88	1423	29.28	42.16	101.84	1408	30.00	43.19	100.81	1394
144.5	27.71	40.04	104.46	1445	28.43	41.08	103.42	1430	29.15	42.12	102.38	1416	29.86	43.15	101.35	1402
145	27.59	40.00	105.00	1452	28.30	41.04	103.96	1438	29.02	42.08	102.93	1423	29.73	43.11	101.89	1409
145.5	27.46	39.96	105.54	1460	28.18	41.00	104.50	1445	28.89	42.03	103.47	1431	29.60	43.07	102.43	1417
146	27.34	39.92	106.08	1467	28.05	40.96	105.04	1453	28.76	41.99	104.01	1438	29.47	43.03	102.97	1424
146.5	27.22	39.88	106.62	1475	27.93	40.91	105.59	1460	28.64	41.95	104.55	1446	29.34	42.99	103.51	1432
147	27.10	39.84	107.16	1482	27.81	40.87	106.13	1468	28.51	41.91	105.09	1453	29.22	42.95	104.05	1439
147.5	26.98	39.80	107.71	1490	27.68	40.83	106.67	1475	28.39	41.87	105.63	1461	29.09	42.91	104.59	1447
148	26.86	39.75	108.25	1497	27.56	40.79	107.21	1483	28.26	41.83	106.17	1468	28.96	42.87	105.13	1454
148.5	26.74	39.71	108.79	1505	27.44	40.75	107.75	1490	28.14	41.79	106.71	1476	28.84	42.83	105.67	1461
149	26.63	39.67	109.33	1512	27.32	40.71	108.29	1498	28.02	41.75	107.25	1483	28.71	42.78	106.22	1469
149.5	26.51	39.63	109.87	1519	27.20	40.67	108.83	1505	27.90	41.71	107.79	1491	28.59	42.74	106.76	1476
150	26.39	39.59	110.41	1527	27.09	40.63	109.37	1513	27.78	41.67	108.34	1498	28.47	42.70	107.30	1484
150.5	26.28	39.55	110.95	1534	26.97	40.59	109.91	1520	27.66	41.62	108.88	1506	28.35	42.66	107.84	1491
151	26.16	39.51	111.49	1542	26.85	40.55	110.45	1528	27.54	41.58	109.42	1513	28.23	42.62	108.38	1499
151.5	26.05	39.47	112.03	1549	26.74	40.50	111.00	1535	27.42	41.54	109.96	1521	28.11	42.58	108.92	1506
152	25.94	39.43	112.57	1557	26.62	40.46	111.54	1543	27.30	41.50	110.50	1528	27.99	42.54	109.46	1514
152.5	25.83	39.39	113.12	1564	26.51	40.42	112.08	1550	27.19	41.46	111.04	1536	27.87	42.50	110.00	1521
153	25.72	39.34	113.66	1572	26.39	40.38	112.62	1558	27.07	41.42	111.58	1543	27.75	42.46	110.54	1529
153.5	25.60	39.30	114.20	1579	26.28	40.34	113.16	1565	26.96	41.38	112.12	1551	27.63	42.42	111.08	1536
154	25.49	39.26	114.74	1587	26.17	40.30	113.70	1572	26.84	41.34	112.66	1558	27.52	42.37	111.63	1544
154.5	25.39	39.22	115.28	1594	26.06	40.26	114.24	1580	26.73	41.30	113.20	1566	27.40	42.33	112.17	1551
155	25.28	39.18	115.82	1602	25.95	40.22	114.78	1587	26.62	41.26	113.75	1573	27.29	42.29	112.71	1559
155.5	25.17	39.14	116.36	1609	25.84	40.18	115.32	1595	26.50	41.21	114.29	1581	27.17	42.25	113.25	1566
156	25.06	39.10	116.90	1617	25.73	40.14	115.86	1602	26.39	41.17	114.83	1588	27.06	42.21	113.79	1574
156.5	24.96	39.06	117.44	1624	25.62	40.09	116.41	1610	26.28	41.13	115.37	1596	26.95	42.17	114.33	1581
157	24.85	39.02	117.98	1632	25.51	40.05	116.95	1617	26.17	41.09	115.91	1603	26.83	42.13	114.87	1589
157.5	24.75	38.98	118.53	1639	25.40	40.01	117.49	1625	26.06	41.05	116.45	1611	26.72	42.09	115.41	1596
158	24.64	38.93	119.07	1647	25.30	39.97	118.03	1632	25.96	41.01	116.99	1618	26.61	42.05	115.95	1604
158.5	24.54	38.89	119.61	1654	25.19	39.93	118.57	1640	25.85	40.97	117.53	1625	26.50	42.01	116.49	1611
159	24.44	38.85	120.15	1662	25.09	39.89	119.11	1647	25.74	40.93	118.07	1633	26.39	41.96	117.04	1619
159.5	24.33	38.81	120.69	1669	24.98	39.85	119.65	1655	25.63	40.89	118.61	1640	26.28	41.92	117.58	1626
160	24.23	38.77	121.23	1677	24.88	39.81	120.19	1662	25.53	40.85	119.16	1648	26.18	41.88	118.12	1634
160.5	24.13	38.73	121.77	1684	24.78	39.77	120.73	1670	25.42	40.80	119.70	1655	26.07	41.84	118.66	1641
161	24.03	38.69	122.31	1692	24.67	39.73	121.27	1677	25.32	40.76	120.24	1663	25.96	41.80	119.20	1649
161.5	23.93	38.65	122.85	1699	24.57	39.68	121.82	1685	25.21	40.72	120.78	1670	25.86	41.76	119.74	1656
162	23.83	38.61	123.39	1707	24.47	39.64	122.36	1692	25.11	40.68	121.32	1678	25.75	41.72	120.28	1663
162.5	23.73	38.57	123.94	1714	24.37	39.60	122.90	1700	25.01	40.64	121.86	1685	25.65	41.68	120.82	1671
163	23.63	38.52	124.48	1722	24.27	39.56	123.44	1707	24.91	40.60	122.40	1693	25.54	41.64	121.36	1678
163.5	23.54	38.48	125.02	1729	24.17	39.52	123.98	1715	24.81	40.56	122.94	1700	25.44	41.60	121.90	1686

Body Composition FEMALE 132-163.5 Lb.

Weight: Lb.	Waist: 32 inches				32.25 inches				32.5 inches				32.75 inches			
	Fat: %	Fat: Lb.	LBM: Lb.	RMR: Cal.	Fat: %	Fat: Lb.	LBM: Lb.	RMR: Cal.	Fat: %	Fat: Lb.	LBM: Lb.	RMR: Cal.	Fat: %	Fat: Lb.	LBM: Lb.	RMR: Cal.
132	34.25	45.22	86.78	1200	35.04	46.25	85.75	1186	35.83	47.29	84.71	1172	36.61	48.33	83.67	1157
132.5	34.09	45.18	87.33	1208	34.88	46.21	86.29	1193	35.66	47.25	85.25	1179	36.44	48.29	84.21	1165
133	33.94	45.13	87.87	1215	34.72	46.17	86.83	1201	35.50	47.21	85.79	1186	36.28	48.25	84.75	1172
133.5	33.78	45.09	88.41	1223	34.55	46.13	87.37	1208	35.33	47.17	86.33	1194	36.11	48.21	85.29	1180
134	33.62	45.05	88.95	1230	34.40	46.09	87.91	1216	35.17	47.13	86.87	1201	35.94	48.16	85.84	1187
134.5	33.47	45.01	89.49	1238	34.24	46.05	88.45	1223	35.01	47.09	87.41	1209	35.78	48.12	86.38	1195
135	33.31	44.97	90.03	1245	34.08	46.01	88.99	1231	34.85	47.05	87.96	1216	35.62	48.08	86.92	1202
135.5	33.16	44.93	90.57	1253	33.92	45.97	89.53	1238	34.69	47.00	88.50	1224	35.45	48.04	87.46	1210
136	33.01	44.89	91.11	1260	33.77	45.93	90.07	1246	34.53	46.96	89.04	1231	35.29	48.00	88.00	1217
136.5	32.85	44.85	91.65	1268	33.62	45.88	90.62	1253	34.38	46.92	89.58	1239	35.14	47.96	88.54	1225
137	32.71	44.81	92.19	1275	33.46	45.84	91.16	1261	34.22	46.88	90.12	1246	34.98	47.92	89.08	1232
137.5	32.56	44.77	92.74	1283	33.31	45.80	91.70	1268	34.07	46.84	90.66	1254	34.82	47.88	89.62	1239
138	32.41	44.72	93.28	1290	33.16	45.76	92.24	1276	33.91	46.80	91.20	1261	34.66	47.84	90.16	1247
138.5	32.26	44.68	93.82	1297	33.01	45.72	92.78	1283	33.76	46.76	91.74	1269	34.51	47.80	90.70	1254
139	32.12	44.64	94.36	1305	32.86	45.68	93.32	1291	33.61	46.72	92.28	1276	34.36	47.75	91.25	1262
139.5	31.97	44.60	94.90	1312	32.72	45.64	93.86	1298	33.46	46.68	92.82	1284	34.20	47.71	91.79	1269
140	31.83	44.56	95.44	1320	32.57	45.60	94.40	1306	33.31	46.64	93.37	1291	34.05	47.67	92.33	1277
140.5	31.69	44.52	95.98	1327	32.42	45.56	94.94	1313	33.16	46.59	93.91	1299	33.90	47.63	92.87	1284
141	31.54	44.48	96.52	1335	32.28	45.52	95.48	1321	33.02	46.55	94.45	1306	33.75	47.59	93.41	1292
141.5	31.40	44.44	97.06	1342	32.14	45.47	96.03	1328	32.87	46.51	94.99	1314	33.60	47.55	93.95	1299
142	31.26	44.40	97.60	1350	32.00	45.43	96.57	1336	32.73	46.47	95.53	1321	33.46	47.51	94.49	1307
142.5	31.13	44.36	98.15	1357	31.85	45.39	97.11	1343	32.58	46.43	96.07	1329	33.31	47.47	95.03	1314
143	30.99	44.31	98.69	1365	31.71	45.35	97.65	1350	32.44	46.39	96.61	1336	33.17	47.43	95.57	1322
143.5	30.85	44.27	99.23	1372	31.58	45.31	98.19	1358	32.30	46.35	97.15	1344	33.02	47.39	96.11	1329
144	30.72	44.23	99.77	1380	31.44	45.27	98.73	1365	32.16	46.31	97.69	1351	32.88	47.34	96.66	1337
144.5	30.58	44.19	100.31	1387	31.30	45.23	99.27	1373	32.02	46.27	98.23	1359	32.74	47.30	97.20	1344
145	30.45	44.15	100.85	1395	31.16	45.19	99.81	1380	31.88	46.23	98.78	1366	32.59	47.26	97.74	1352
145.5	30.32	44.11	101.39	1402	31.03	45.15	100.35	1388	31.74	46.18	99.32	1374	32.45	47.22	98.28	1359
146	30.18	44.07	101.93	1410	30.89	45.11	100.89	1395	31.60	46.14	99.86	1381	32.32	47.18	98.82	1367
146.5	30.05	44.03	102.47	1417	30.76	45.06	101.44	1403	31.47	46.10	100.40	1389	32.18	47.14	99.36	1374
147	29.92	43.99	103.01	1425	30.63	45.02	101.98	1410	31.33	46.06	100.94	1396	32.04	47.10	99.90	1382
147.5	29.79	43.95	103.56	1432	30.50	44.98	102.52	1418	31.20	46.02	101.48	1403	31.90	47.06	100.44	1389
148	29.66	43.90	104.10	1440	30.37	44.94	103.06	1425	31.07	45.98	102.02	1411	31.77	47.02	100.98	1397
148.5	29.54	43.86	104.64	1447	30.24	44.90	103.60	1433	30.93	45.94	102.56	1418	31.63	46.98	101.52	1404
149	29.41	43.82	105.18	1455	30.11	44.86	104.14	1440	30.80	45.90	103.10	1426	31.50	46.93	102.07	1412
149.5	29.28	43.78	105.72	1462	29.98	44.82	104.68	1448	30.67	45.86	103.64	1433	31.37	46.89	102.61	1419
150	29.16	43.74	106.26	1470	29.85	44.78	105.22	1455	30.54	45.82	104.19	1441	31.24	46.85	103.15	1427
150.5	29.04	43.70	106.80	1477	29.73	44.74	105.76	1463	30.41	45.77	104.73	1448	31.10	46.81	103.69	1434
151	28.91	43.66	107.34	1485	29.60	44.70	106.30	1470	30.29	45.73	105.27	1456	30.97	46.77	104.23	1441
151.5	28.79	43.62	107.88	1492	29.47	44.65	106.85	1478	30.16	45.69	105.81	1463	30.84	46.73	104.77	1449
152	28.67	43.58	108.42	1500	29.35	44.61	107.39	1485	30.03	45.65	106.35	1471	30.72	46.69	105.31	1456
152.5	28.55	43.54	108.97	1507	29.23	44.57	107.93	1493	29.91	45.61	106.89	1478	30.59	46.65	105.85	1464
153	28.43	43.49	109.51	1514	29.11	44.53	108.47	1500	29.78	45.57	107.43	1486	30.46	46.61	106.39	1471
153.5	28.31	43.45	110.05	1522	28.98	44.49	109.01	1508	29.66	45.53	107.97	1493	30.34	46.57	106.93	1479
154	28.19	43.41	110.59	1529	28.86	44.45	109.55	1515	29.54	45.49	108.51	1501	30.21	46.52	107.48	1486
154.5	28.07	43.37	111.13	1537	28.74	44.41	110.09	1523	29.41	45.45	109.05	1508	30.09	46.48	108.02	1494
155	27.95	43.33	111.67	1544	28.62	44.37	110.63	1530	29.29	45.41	109.60	1516	29.96	46.44	108.56	1501
155.5	27.84	43.29	112.21	1552	28.51	44.33	111.17	1538	29.17	45.36	110.14	1523	29.84	46.40	109.10	1509
156	27.72	43.25	112.75	1559	28.39	44.29	111.71	1545	29.05	45.32	110.68	1531	29.72	46.36	109.64	1516
156.5	27.61	43.21	113.29	1567	28.27	44.24	112.26	1552	28.93	45.28	111.22	1538	29.60	46.32	110.18	1524
157	27.49	43.17	113.83	1574	28.16	44.20	112.80	1560	28.82	45.24	111.76	1546	29.48	46.28	110.72	1531
157.5	27.38	43.13	114.38	1582	28.04	44.16	113.34	1567	28.70	45.20	112.30	1553	29.36	46.24	111.26	1539
158	27.27	43.08	114.92	1589	27.93	44.12	113.88	1575	28.58	45.16	112.84	1561	29.24	46.20	111.80	1546
158.5	27.16	43.04	115.46	1597	27.81	44.08	114.42	1582	28.47	45.12	113.38	1568	29.12	46.16	112.34	1554
159	27.05	43.00	116.00	1604	27.70	44.04	114.96	1590	28.35	45.08	113.92	1576	29.00	46.11	112.89	1561
159.5	26.93	42.96	116.54	1612	27.59	44.00	115.50	1597	28.24	45.04	114.46	1583	28.89	46.07	113.43	1569
160	26.83	42.92	117.08	1619	27.47	43.96	116.04	1605	28.12	45.00	115.01	1591	28.77	46.03	113.97	1576
160.5	26.72	42.88	117.62	1627	27.36	43.92	116.58	1612	28.01	44.95	115.55	1598	28.66	45.99	114.51	1584
161	26.61	42.84	118.16	1634	27.25	43.88	117.12	1620	27.90	44.91	116.09	1605	28.54	45.95	115.05	1591
161.5	26.50	42.80	118.70	1642	27.14	43.83	117.67	1627	27.78	44.87	116.63	1613	28.43	45.91	115.59	1599
162	26.39	42.76	119.24	1649	27.03	43.79	118.21	1635	27.67	44.83	117.17	1620	28.31	45.87	116.13	1606
162.5	26.29	42.72	119.79	1657	26.92	43.75	118.75	1642	27.56	44.79	117.71	1628	28.20	45.83	116.67	1614
163	26.18	42.67	120.33	1664	26.82	43.71	119.29	1650	27.45	44.75	118.25	1635	28.09	45.79	117.21	1621
163.5	26.08	42.63	120.87	1672	26.71	43.67	119.83	1657	27.34	44.71	118.79	1643	27.98	45.75	117.75	1629

Body Composition　FEMALE　132-163.5 Lb.

Weight: Lb.	Waist: 33 inches				33.25 inches				33.5 inches				33.75 inches			
	Fat: %	Fat: Lb.	LBM: Lb.	RMR: Cal.	Fat: %	Fat: Lb.	LBM: Lb.	RMR: Cal.	Fat: %	Fat: Lb.	LBM: Lb.	RMR: Cal.	Fat: %	Fat: Lb.	LBM: Lb.	RMR: Cal.
132	37.40	49.37	82.63	1143	38.18	50.40	81.60	1128	38.97	51.44	80.56	1114	39.76	52.48	79.52	1100
132.5	37.23	49.33	83.18	1150	38.01	50.36	82.14	1136	38.79	51.40	81.10	1122	39.58	52.44	80.06	1107
133	37.06	49.28	83.72	1158	37.84	50.32	82.68	1143	38.62	51.36	81.64	1129	39.40	52.40	80.60	1115
133.5	36.89	49.24	84.26	1165	37.66	50.28	83.22	1151	38.44	51.32	82.18	1137	39.22	52.36	81.14	1122
134	36.72	49.20	84.80	1173	37.49	50.24	83.76	1158	38.27	51.28	82.72	1144	39.04	52.31	81.69	1130
134.5	36.55	49.16	85.34	1180	37.32	50.20	84.30	1166	38.09	51.24	83.26	1152	38.87	52.27	82.23	1137
135	36.39	49.12	85.88	1188	37.15	50.16	84.84	1173	37.92	51.20	83.81	1159	38.69	52.23	82.77	1145
135.5	36.22	49.08	86.42	1195	36.99	50.12	85.38	1181	37.75	51.15	84.35	1167	38.52	52.19	83.31	1152
136	36.06	49.04	86.96	1203	36.82	50.08	85.92	1188	37.58	51.11	84.89	1174	38.35	52.15	83.85	1160
136.5	35.90	49.00	87.50	1210	36.66	50.03	86.47	1196	37.42	51.07	85.43	1181	38.18	52.11	84.39	1167
137	35.73	48.96	88.04	1218	36.49	49.99	87.01	1203	37.25	51.03	85.97	1189	38.01	52.07	84.93	1175
137.5	35.57	48.92	88.59	1225	36.33	49.95	87.55	1211	37.08	50.99	86.51	1196	37.84	52.03	85.47	1182
138	35.42	48.87	89.13	1233	36.17	49.91	88.09	1218	36.92	50.95	87.05	1204	37.67	51.99	86.01	1190
138.5	35.26	48.83	89.67	1240	36.01	49.87	88.63	1226	36.76	50.91	87.59	1211	37.51	51.95	86.55	1197
139	35.10	48.79	90.21	1248	35.85	49.83	89.17	1233	36.59	50.87	88.13	1219	37.34	51.90	87.10	1205
139.5	34.95	48.75	90.75	1255	35.69	49.79	89.71	1241	36.43	50.83	88.67	1226	37.18	51.86	87.64	1212
140	34.79	48.71	91.29	1263	35.53	49.75	90.25	1248	36.28	50.79	89.22	1234	37.02	51.82	88.18	1219
140.5	34.64	48.67	91.83	1270	35.38	49.71	90.79	1256	36.12	50.74	89.76	1241	36.86	51.78	88.72	1227
141	34.49	48.63	92.37	1278	35.22	49.67	91.33	1263	35.96	50.70	90.30	1249	36.70	51.74	89.26	1234
141.5	34.34	48.59	92.91	1285	35.07	49.62	91.88	1271	35.80	50.66	90.84	1256	36.54	51.70	89.80	1242
142	34.19	48.55	93.45	1292	34.92	49.58	92.42	1278	35.65	50.62	91.38	1264	36.38	51.66	90.34	1249
142.5	34.04	48.51	94.00	1300	34.77	49.54	92.96	1286	35.49	50.58	91.92	1271	36.22	51.62	90.88	1257
143	33.89	48.46	94.54	1307	34.62	49.50	93.50	1293	35.34	50.54	92.46	1279	36.07	51.58	91.42	1264
143.5	33.74	48.42	95.08	1315	34.47	49.46	94.04	1301	35.19	50.50	93.00	1286	35.91	51.54	91.96	1272
144	33.60	48.38	95.62	1322	34.32	49.42	94.58	1308	35.04	50.46	93.54	1294	35.76	51.49	92.51	1279
144.5	33.45	48.34	96.16	1330	34.17	49.38	95.12	1316	34.89	50.42	94.08	1301	35.61	51.45	93.05	1287
145	33.31	48.30	96.70	1337	34.03	49.34	95.66	1323	34.74	50.38	94.63	1309	35.46	51.41	93.59	1294
145.5	33.17	48.26	97.24	1345	33.88	49.30	96.20	1330	34.59	50.33	95.17	1316	35.31	51.37	94.13	1302
146	33.03	48.22	97.78	1352	33.74	49.26	96.74	1338	34.45	50.29	95.71	1324	35.16	51.33	94.67	1309
146.5	32.89	48.18	98.32	1360	33.59	49.21	97.29	1345	34.30	50.25	96.25	1331	35.01	51.29	95.21	1317
147	32.75	48.14	98.86	1367	33.45	49.17	97.83	1353	34.16	50.21	96.79	1339	34.86	51.25	95.75	1324
147.5	32.61	48.10	99.41	1375	33.31	49.13	98.37	1360	34.01	50.17	97.33	1346	34.72	51.21	96.29	1332
148	32.47	48.05	99.95	1382	33.17	49.09	98.91	1368	33.87	50.13	97.87	1354	34.57	51.17	96.83	1339
148.5	32.33	48.01	100.49	1390	33.03	49.05	99.45	1375	33.73	50.09	98.41	1361	34.43	51.13	97.37	1347
149	32.20	47.97	101.03	1397	32.89	49.01	99.99	1383	33.59	50.05	98.95	1369	34.28	51.08	97.92	1354
149.5	32.06	47.93	101.57	1405	32.75	48.97	100.53	1390	33.45	50.01	99.49	1376	34.14	51.04	98.46	1362
150	31.93	47.89	102.11	1412	32.62	48.93	101.07	1398	33.31	49.97	100.04	1383	34.00	51.00	99.00	1369
150.5	31.79	47.85	102.65	1420	32.48	48.89	101.61	1405	33.17	49.92	100.58	1391	33.86	50.96	99.54	1377
151	31.66	47.81	103.19	1427	32.35	48.85	102.15	1413	33.04	49.88	101.12	1398	33.72	50.92	100.08	1384
151.5	31.53	47.77	103.73	1435	32.21	48.80	102.70	1420	32.90	49.84	101.66	1406	33.58	50.88	100.62	1392
152	31.40	47.73	104.27	1442	32.08	48.76	103.24	1428	32.76	49.80	102.20	1413	33.45	50.84	101.16	1399
152.5	31.27	47.69	104.82	1450	31.95	48.72	103.78	1435	32.63	49.76	102.74	1421	33.31	50.80	101.70	1407
153	31.14	47.64	105.36	1457	31.82	48.68	104.32	1443	32.50	49.72	103.28	1428	33.17	50.76	102.24	1414
153.5	31.01	47.60	105.90	1465	31.69	48.64	104.86	1450	32.36	49.68	103.82	1436	33.04	50.72	102.78	1422
154	30.88	47.56	106.44	1472	31.56	48.60	105.40	1458	32.23	49.64	104.36	1443	32.91	50.67	103.33	1429
154.5	30.76	47.52	106.98	1480	31.43	48.56	105.94	1465	32.10	49.60	104.90	1451	32.77	50.63	103.87	1436
155	30.63	47.48	107.52	1487	31.30	48.52	106.48	1473	31.97	49.56	105.45	1458	32.64	50.59	104.41	1444
155.5	30.51	47.44	108.06	1494	31.17	48.48	107.02	1480	31.84	49.51	105.99	1466	32.51	50.55	104.95	1451
156	30.38	47.40	108.60	1502	31.05	48.44	107.56	1488	31.71	49.47	106.53	1473	32.38	50.51	105.49	1459
156.5	30.26	47.36	109.14	1509	30.92	48.39	108.11	1495	31.59	49.43	107.07	1481	32.25	50.47	106.03	1466
157	30.14	47.32	109.68	1517	30.80	48.35	108.65	1503	31.46	49.39	107.61	1488	32.12	50.43	106.57	1474
157.5	30.02	47.28	110.23	1524	30.67	48.31	109.19	1510	31.33	49.35	108.15	1496	31.99	50.39	107.11	1481
158	29.89	47.23	110.77	1532	30.55	48.27	109.73	1518	31.21	49.31	108.69	1503	31.86	50.35	107.65	1489
158.5	29.77	47.19	111.31	1539	30.43	48.23	110.27	1525	31.08	49.27	109.23	1511	31.74	50.31	108.19	1496
159	29.66	47.15	111.85	1547	30.31	48.19	110.81	1533	30.96	49.23	109.77	1518	31.61	50.26	108.74	1504
159.5	29.54	47.11	112.39	1554	30.19	48.15	111.35	1540	30.84	49.19	110.31	1526	31.49	50.22	109.28	1511
160	29.42	47.07	112.93	1562	30.07	48.11	111.89	1547	30.72	49.15	110.86	1533	31.36	50.18	109.82	1519
160.5	29.30	47.03	113.47	1569	29.95	48.07	112.43	1555	30.59	49.10	111.40	1541	31.24	50.14	110.36	1526
161	29.19	46.99	114.01	1577	29.83	48.03	112.97	1562	30.47	49.06	111.94	1548	31.12	50.10	110.90	1534
161.5	29.07	46.95	114.55	1584	29.71	47.98	113.52	1570	30.35	49.02	112.48	1556	31.00	50.06	111.44	1541
162	28.95	46.91	115.09	1592	29.59	47.94	114.06	1577	30.24	48.98	113.02	1563	30.88	50.02	111.98	1549
162.5	28.84	46.87	115.64	1599	29.48	47.90	114.60	1585	30.12	48.94	113.56	1571	30.76	49.98	112.52	1556
163	28.73	46.82	116.18	1607	29.36	47.86	115.14	1592	30.00	48.90	114.10	1578	30.64	49.94	113.06	1564
163.5	28.61	46.78	116.72	1614	29.25	47.82	115.68	1600	29.88	48.86	114.64	1585	30.52	49.90	113.60	1571

Body Composition FEMALE 132-163.5 Lb.

Weight: Lb.	Waist: 34 inches Fat: %	Fat: Lb.	LBM: Lb.	RMR: Cal.	34.25 inches Fat: %	Fat: Lb.	LBM: Lb.	RMR: Cal.	34.5 inches Fat: %	Fat: Lb.	LBM: Lb.	RMR: Cal.	34.75 inches Fat: %	Fat: Lb.	LBM: Lb.	RMR: Cal.
132	40.54	53.52	78.48	1085	41.33	54.55	77.45	1071	42.11	55.59	76.41	1057	42.90	56.63	75.37	1042
132.5	40.36	53.48	79.03	1093	41.14	54.51	77.99	1079	41.92	55.55	76.95	1064	42.71	56.59	75.91	1050
133	40.18	53.43	79.57	1100	40.96	54.47	78.53	1086	41.74	55.51	77.49	1072	42.52	56.55	76.45	1057
133.5	39.99	53.39	80.11	1108	40.77	54.43	79.07	1094	41.55	55.47	78.03	1079	42.33	56.51	76.99	1065
134	39.81	53.35	80.65	1115	40.59	54.39	79.61	1101	41.36	55.43	78.57	1087	42.14	56.46	77.54	1072
134.5	39.64	53.31	81.19	1123	40.41	54.35	80.15	1108	41.18	55.39	79.11	1094	41.95	56.42	78.08	1080
135	39.46	53.27	81.73	1130	40.23	54.31	80.69	1116	41.00	55.35	79.66	1102	41.76	56.38	78.62	1087
135.5	39.28	53.23	82.27	1138	40.05	54.27	81.23	1123	40.81	55.30	80.20	1109	41.58	56.34	79.16	1095
136	39.11	53.19	82.81	1145	39.87	54.23	81.77	1131	40.63	55.26	80.74	1117	41.40	56.30	79.70	1102
136.5	38.94	53.15	83.35	1153	39.70	54.18	82.32	1138	40.46	55.22	81.28	1124	41.22	56.26	80.24	1110
137	38.76	53.11	83.89	1160	39.52	54.14	82.86	1146	40.28	55.18	81.82	1132	41.04	56.22	80.78	1117
137.5	38.59	53.07	84.44	1168	39.35	54.10	83.40	1153	40.10	55.14	82.36	1139	40.86	56.18	81.32	1125
138	38.42	53.02	84.98	1175	39.18	54.06	83.94	1161	39.93	55.10	82.90	1147	40.68	56.14	81.86	1132
138.5	38.25	52.98	85.52	1183	39.00	54.02	84.48	1168	39.75	55.06	83.44	1154	40.50	56.10	82.40	1140
139	38.09	52.94	86.06	1190	38.83	53.98	85.02	1176	39.58	55.02	83.98	1161	40.33	56.05	82.95	1147
139.5	37.92	52.90	86.60	1198	38.67	53.94	85.56	1183	39.41	54.98	84.52	1169	40.15	56.01	83.49	1155
140	37.76	52.86	87.14	1205	38.50	53.90	86.10	1191	39.24	54.94	85.07	1176	39.98	55.97	84.03	1162
140.5	37.59	52.82	87.68	1213	38.33	53.86	86.64	1198	39.07	54.89	85.61	1184	39.81	55.93	84.57	1170
141	37.43	52.78	88.22	1220	38.17	53.82	87.18	1206	38.90	54.85	86.15	1191	39.64	55.89	85.11	1177
141.5	37.27	52.74	88.76	1228	38.00	53.77	87.73	1213	38.74	54.81	86.69	1199	39.47	55.85	85.65	1185
142	37.11	52.70	89.30	1235	37.84	53.73	88.27	1221	38.57	54.77	87.23	1206	39.30	55.81	86.19	1192
142.5	36.95	52.66	89.85	1243	37.68	53.69	88.81	1228	38.41	54.73	87.77	1214	39.14	55.77	86.73	1200
143	36.79	52.61	90.39	1250	37.52	53.65	89.35	1236	38.24	54.69	88.31	1221	38.97	55.73	87.27	1207
143.5	36.64	52.57	90.93	1258	37.36	53.61	89.89	1243	38.08	54.65	88.85	1229	38.81	55.69	87.81	1214
144	36.48	52.53	91.47	1265	37.20	53.57	90.43	1251	37.92	54.61	89.39	1236	38.64	55.64	88.36	1222
144.5	36.33	52.49	92.01	1272	37.04	53.53	90.97	1258	37.76	54.57	89.93	1244	38.48	55.60	88.90	1229
145	36.17	52.45	92.55	1280	36.89	53.49	91.51	1266	37.60	54.53	90.48	1251	38.32	55.56	89.44	1237
145.5	36.02	52.41	93.09	1287	36.73	53.45	92.05	1273	37.45	54.48	91.02	1259	38.16	55.52	89.98	1244
146	35.87	52.37	93.63	1295	36.58	53.41	92.59	1281	37.29	54.44	91.56	1266	38.00	55.48	90.52	1252
146.5	35.72	52.33	94.17	1302	36.43	53.36	93.14	1288	37.13	54.40	92.10	1274	37.84	55.44	91.06	1259
147	35.57	52.29	94.71	1310	36.27	53.32	93.68	1296	36.98	54.36	92.64	1281	37.69	55.40	91.60	1267
147.5	35.42	52.25	95.26	1317	36.12	53.28	94.22	1303	36.83	54.32	93.18	1289	37.53	55.36	92.14	1274
148	35.27	52.20	95.80	1325	35.97	53.24	94.76	1311	36.68	54.28	93.72	1296	37.38	55.32	92.68	1282
148.5	35.13	52.16	96.34	1332	35.83	53.20	95.30	1318	36.52	54.24	94.26	1304	37.22	55.28	93.22	1289
149	34.98	52.12	96.88	1340	35.68	53.16	95.84	1325	36.37	54.20	94.80	1311	37.07	55.23	93.77	1297
149.5	34.84	52.08	97.42	1347	35.53	53.12	96.38	1333	36.22	54.16	95.34	1319	36.92	55.19	94.31	1304
150	34.69	52.04	97.96	1355	35.39	53.08	96.92	1340	36.08	54.12	95.89	1326	36.77	55.15	94.85	1312
150.5	34.55	52.00	98.50	1362	35.24	53.04	97.46	1348	35.93	54.07	96.43	1334	36.62	55.11	95.39	1319
151	34.41	51.96	99.04	1370	35.10	53.00	98.00	1355	35.78	54.03	96.97	1341	36.47	55.07	95.93	1327
151.5	34.27	51.92	99.58	1377	34.95	52.95	98.55	1363	35.64	53.99	97.51	1349	36.32	55.03	96.47	1334
152	34.13	51.88	100.12	1385	34.81	52.91	99.09	1370	35.49	53.95	98.05	1356	36.18	54.99	97.01	1342
152.5	33.99	51.84	100.67	1392	34.67	52.87	99.63	1378	35.35	53.91	98.59	1363	36.03	54.95	97.55	1349
153	33.85	51.79	101.21	1400	34.53	52.83	100.17	1385	35.21	53.87	99.13	1371	35.89	54.91	98.09	1357
153.5	33.72	51.75	101.75	1407	34.39	52.79	100.71	1393	35.07	53.83	99.67	1378	35.74	54.87	98.63	1364
154	33.58	51.71	102.29	1415	34.25	52.75	101.25	1400	34.93	53.79	100.21	1386	35.60	54.82	99.18	1372
154.5	33.44	51.67	102.83	1422	34.12	52.71	101.79	1408	34.79	53.75	100.75	1393	35.46	54.78	99.72	1379
155	33.31	51.63	103.37	1430	33.98	52.67	102.33	1415	34.65	53.71	101.30	1401	35.32	54.74	100.26	1387
155.5	33.18	51.59	103.91	1437	33.84	52.63	102.87	1423	34.51	53.66	101.84	1408	35.18	54.70	100.80	1394
156	33.04	51.55	104.45	1445	33.71	52.59	103.41	1430	34.37	53.62	102.38	1416	35.04	54.66	101.34	1402
156.5	32.91	51.51	104.99	1452	33.57	52.54	103.96	1438	34.24	53.58	102.92	1423	34.90	54.62	101.88	1409
157	32.78	51.47	105.53	1460	33.44	52.50	104.50	1445	34.10	53.54	103.46	1431	34.76	54.58	102.42	1416
157.5	32.65	51.43	106.08	1467	33.31	52.46	105.04	1453	33.97	53.50	104.00	1438	34.63	54.54	102.96	1424
158	32.52	51.38	106.62	1474	33.18	52.42	105.58	1460	33.83	53.46	104.54	1446	34.49	54.50	103.50	1431
158.5	32.39	51.34	107.16	1482	33.05	52.38	106.12	1468	33.70	53.42	105.08	1453	34.36	54.46	104.04	1439
159	32.27	51.30	107.70	1489	32.92	52.34	106.66	1475	33.57	53.38	105.62	1461	34.22	54.41	104.59	1446
159.5	32.14	51.26	108.24	1497	32.79	52.30	107.20	1483	33.44	53.34	106.16	1468	34.09	54.37	105.13	1454
160	32.01	51.22	108.78	1504	32.66	52.26	107.74	1490	33.31	53.30	106.71	1476	33.96	54.33	105.67	1461
160.5	31.89	51.18	109.32	1512	32.53	52.22	108.28	1498	33.18	53.25	107.25	1483	33.83	54.29	106.21	1469
161	31.76	51.14	109.86	1519	32.41	52.18	108.82	1505	33.05	53.21	107.79	1491	33.70	54.25	106.75	1476
161.5	31.64	51.10	110.40	1527	32.28	52.13	109.37	1513	32.92	53.17	108.33	1498	33.57	54.21	107.29	1484
162	31.52	51.06	110.94	1534	32.16	52.09	109.91	1520	32.80	53.13	108.87	1506	33.44	54.17	107.83	1491
162.5	31.39	51.02	111.49	1542	32.03	52.05	110.45	1527	32.67	53.09	109.41	1513	33.31	54.13	108.37	1499
163	31.27	50.97	112.03	1549	31.91	52.01	110.99	1535	32.55	53.05	109.95	1521	33.18	54.09	108.91	1506
163.5	31.15	50.93	112.57	1557	31.79	51.97	111.53	1542	32.42	53.01	110.49	1528	33.06	54.05	109.45	1514

THE BODY FAT GUIDE

Body Composition   FEMALE   132-163.5 Lb.

Weight: Lb.	Waist: 35 inches				35.25 inches				35.5 inches				35.75 inches			
	Fat: %	Fat: Lb.	LBM: Lb.	RMR: Cal.	Fat: %	Fat: Lb.	LBM: Lb.	RMR: Cal.	Fat: %	Fat: Lb.	LBM: Lb.	RMR: Cal.	Fat: %	Fat: Lb.	LBM: Lb.	RMR: Cal.
132	43.69	57.67	74.33	1028	44.47	58.70	73.30	1014	45.26	59.74	72.26	999	46.04	60.78	71.22	985
132.5	43.49	57.63	74.88	1036	44.27	58.66	73.84	1021	45.06	59.70	72.80	1007	45.84	60.74	71.76	992
133	43.30	57.58	75.42	1043	44.08	58.62	74.38	1029	44.86	59.66	73.34	1014	45.64	60.70	72.30	1000
133.5	43.10	57.54	75.96	1050	43.88	58.58	74.92	1036	44.66	59.62	73.88	1022	45.43	60.66	72.84	1007
134	42.91	57.50	76.50	1058	43.69	58.54	75.46	1044	44.46	59.58	74.42	1029	45.23	60.61	73.39	1015
134.5	42.72	57.46	77.04	1065	43.49	58.50	76.00	1051	44.26	59.54	74.96	1037	45.04	60.57	73.93	1022
135	42.53	57.42	77.58	1073	43.30	58.46	76.54	1059	44.07	59.50	75.51	1044	44.84	60.53	74.47	1030
135.5	42.35	57.38	78.12	1080	43.11	58.42	77.08	1066	43.88	59.45	76.05	1052	44.64	60.49	75.01	1037
136	42.16	57.34	78.66	1088	42.92	58.38	77.62	1074	43.69	59.41	76.59	1059	44.45	60.45	75.55	1045
136.5	41.98	57.30	79.20	1095	42.74	58.33	78.17	1081	43.50	59.37	77.13	1067	44.26	60.41	76.09	1052
137	41.79	57.26	79.74	1103	42.55	58.29	78.71	1089	43.31	59.33	77.67	1074	44.06	60.37	76.63	1060
137.5	41.61	57.22	80.29	1110	42.37	58.25	79.25	1096	43.12	59.29	78.21	1082	43.87	60.33	77.17	1067
138	41.43	57.17	80.83	1118	42.18	58.21	79.79	1103	42.93	59.25	78.75	1089	43.69	60.29	77.71	1075
138.5	41.25	57.13	81.37	1125	42.00	58.17	80.33	1111	42.75	59.21	79.29	1097	43.50	60.25	78.25	1082
139	41.07	57.09	81.91	1133	41.82	58.13	80.87	1118	42.57	59.17	79.83	1104	43.31	60.20	78.80	1090
139.5	40.90	57.05	82.45	1140	41.64	58.09	81.41	1126	42.38	59.13	80.37	1112	43.13	60.16	79.34	1097
140	40.72	57.01	82.99	1148	41.46	58.05	81.95	1133	42.20	59.09	80.92	1119	42.94	60.12	79.88	1105
140.5	40.55	56.97	83.53	1155	41.29	58.01	82.49	1141	42.02	59.04	81.46	1127	42.76	60.08	80.42	1112
141	40.37	56.93	84.07	1163	41.11	57.97	83.03	1148	41.85	59.00	82.00	1134	42.58	60.04	80.96	1120
141.5	40.20	56.89	84.61	1170	40.94	57.92	83.58	1156	41.67	58.96	82.54	1142	42.40	60.00	81.50	1127
142	40.03	56.85	85.15	1178	40.76	57.88	84.12	1163	41.49	58.92	83.08	1149	42.22	59.96	82.04	1135
142.5	39.86	56.81	85.70	1185	40.59	57.84	84.66	1171	41.32	58.88	83.62	1156	42.05	59.92	82.58	1142
143	39.70	56.76	86.24	1193	40.42	57.80	85.20	1178	41.15	58.84	84.16	1164	41.87	59.88	83.12	1150
143.5	39.53	56.72	86.78	1200	40.25	57.76	85.74	1186	40.97	58.80	84.70	1171	41.70	59.84	83.66	1157
144	39.36	56.68	87.32	1208	40.08	57.72	86.28	1193	40.80	58.76	85.24	1179	41.52	59.79	84.21	1165
144.5	39.20	56.64	87.86	1215	39.92	57.68	86.82	1201	40.63	58.72	85.78	1186	41.35	59.75	84.75	1172
145	39.03	56.60	88.40	1223	39.75	57.64	87.36	1208	40.47	58.68	86.33	1194	41.18	59.71	85.29	1180
145.5	38.87	56.56	88.94	1230	39.59	57.60	87.90	1216	40.30	58.63	86.87	1201	41.01	59.67	85.83	1187
146	38.71	56.52	89.48	1238	39.42	57.56	88.44	1223	40.13	58.59	87.41	1209	40.84	59.63	86.37	1194
146.5	38.55	56.48	90.02	1245	39.26	57.51	88.99	1231	39.97	58.55	87.95	1216	40.68	59.59	86.91	1202
147	38.39	56.44	90.56	1253	39.10	57.47	89.53	1238	39.80	58.51	88.49	1224	40.51	59.55	87.45	1209
147.5	38.23	56.40	91.11	1260	38.94	57.43	90.07	1246	39.64	58.47	89.03	1231	40.34	59.51	87.99	1217
148	38.08	56.35	91.65	1267	38.78	57.39	90.61	1253	39.48	58.43	89.57	1239	40.18	59.47	88.53	1224
148.5	37.92	56.31	92.19	1275	38.62	57.35	91.15	1261	39.32	58.39	90.11	1246	40.02	59.43	89.07	1232
149	37.77	56.27	92.73	1282	38.46	57.31	91.69	1268	39.16	58.35	90.65	1254	39.86	59.38	89.62	1239
149.5	37.61	56.23	93.27	1290	38.31	57.27	92.23	1276	39.00	58.31	91.19	1261	39.69	59.34	90.16	1247
150	37.46	56.19	93.81	1297	38.15	57.23	92.77	1283	38.84	58.27	91.74	1269	39.54	59.30	90.70	1254
150.5	37.31	56.15	94.35	1305	38.00	57.19	93.31	1291	38.69	58.22	92.28	1276	39.38	59.26	91.24	1262
151	37.16	56.11	94.89	1312	37.84	57.15	93.85	1298	38.53	58.18	92.82	1284	39.22	59.22	91.78	1269
151.5	37.01	56.07	95.43	1320	37.69	57.10	94.40	1305	38.38	58.14	93.36	1291	39.06	59.18	92.32	1277
152	36.86	56.03	95.97	1327	37.54	57.06	94.94	1313	38.22	58.10	93.90	1299	38.91	59.14	92.86	1284
152.5	36.71	55.99	96.52	1335	37.39	57.02	95.48	1320	38.07	58.06	94.44	1306	38.75	59.10	93.40	1292
153	36.56	55.94	97.06	1342	37.24	56.98	96.02	1328	37.92	58.02	94.98	1314	38.60	59.06	93.94	1299
153.5	36.42	55.90	97.60	1350	37.09	56.94	96.56	1335	37.77	57.98	95.52	1321	38.45	59.02	94.48	1307
154	36.27	55.86	98.14	1357	36.95	56.90	97.10	1343	37.62	57.94	96.06	1329	38.30	58.97	95.03	1314
154.5	36.13	55.82	98.68	1365	36.80	56.86	97.64	1350	37.47	57.90	96.60	1336	38.14	58.93	95.57	1322
155	35.99	55.78	99.22	1372	36.66	56.82	98.18	1358	37.33	57.86	97.15	1344	38.00	58.89	96.11	1329
155.5	35.85	55.74	99.76	1380	36.51	56.78	98.72	1365	37.18	57.81	97.69	1351	37.85	58.85	96.65	1337
156	35.70	55.70	100.30	1387	36.37	56.74	99.26	1373	37.03	57.77	98.23	1358	37.70	58.81	97.19	1344
156.5	35.56	55.66	100.84	1395	36.23	56.69	99.81	1380	36.89	57.73	98.77	1366	37.55	58.77	97.73	1352
157	35.42	55.62	101.38	1402	36.09	56.65	100.35	1388	36.75	57.69	99.31	1373	37.41	58.73	98.27	1359
157.5	35.29	55.58	101.93	1410	35.94	56.61	100.89	1395	36.60	57.65	99.85	1381	37.26	58.69	98.81	1367
158	35.15	55.53	102.47	1417	35.80	56.57	101.43	1403	36.46	57.61	100.39	1388	37.12	58.65	99.35	1374
158.5	35.01	55.49	103.01	1425	35.67	56.53	101.97	1410	36.32	57.57	100.93	1396	36.98	58.61	99.89	1382
159	34.88	55.45	103.55	1432	35.53	56.49	102.51	1418	36.18	57.53	101.47	1403	36.83	58.56	100.44	1389
159.5	34.74	55.41	104.09	1440	35.39	56.45	103.05	1425	36.04	57.49	102.01	1411	36.69	58.52	100.98	1397
160	34.61	55.37	104.63	1447	35.25	56.41	103.59	1433	35.90	57.45	102.56	1418	36.55	58.48	101.52	1404
160.5	34.47	55.33	105.17	1455	35.12	56.37	104.13	1440	35.77	57.40	103.10	1426	36.41	58.44	102.06	1411
161	34.34	55.29	105.71	1462	34.98	56.33	104.67	1448	35.63	57.36	103.64	1433	36.27	58.40	102.60	1419
161.5	34.21	55.25	106.25	1469	34.85	56.28	105.22	1455	35.49	57.32	104.18	1441	36.14	58.36	103.14	1426
162	34.08	55.21	106.79	1477	34.72	56.24	105.76	1463	35.36	57.28	104.72	1448	36.00	58.32	103.68	1434
162.5	33.95	55.17	107.34	1484	34.59	56.20	106.30	1470	35.22	57.24	105.26	1456	35.86	58.28	104.22	1441
163	33.82	55.12	107.88	1492	34.45	56.16	106.84	1478	35.09	57.20	105.80	1463	35.73	58.24	104.76	1449
163.5	33.69	55.08	108.42	1499	34.32	56.12	107.38	1485	34.96	57.16	106.34	1471	35.59	58.20	105.30	1456

Body Composition FEMALE 132-163.5 Lb.

Weight: Lb.	Waist: 36 inches Fat: %	Fat: Lb.	LBM: Lb.	RMR: Cal.	36.25 inches Fat: %	Fat: Lb.	LBM: Lb.	RMR: Cal.	36.5 inches Fat: %	Fat: Lb.	LBM: Lb.	RMR: Cal.	36.75 inches Fat: %	Fat: Lb.	LBM: Lb.	RMR: Cal.
132	46.83	61.82	70.18	971	47.62	62.85	69.15	956	48.40	63.89	68.11	942	49.19	64.93	67.07	928
132.5	46.62	61.78	70.73	978	47.41	62.81	69.69	964	48.19	63.85	68.65	949	48.97	64.89	67.61	935
133	46.42	61.73	71.27	986	47.20	62.77	70.23	971	47.98	63.81	69.19	957	48.76	64.85	68.15	943
133.5	46.21	61.69	71.81	993	46.99	62.73	70.77	979	47.77	63.77	69.73	964	48.54	64.81	68.69	950
134	46.01	61.65	72.35	1001	46.78	62.69	71.31	986	47.56	63.73	70.27	972	48.33	64.76	69.24	958
134.5	45.81	61.61	72.89	1008	46.58	62.65	71.85	994	47.35	63.69	70.81	979	48.12	64.72	69.78	965
135	45.61	61.57	73.43	1016	46.38	62.61	72.39	1001	47.14	63.65	71.36	987	47.91	64.68	70.32	972
135.5	45.41	61.53	73.97	1023	46.17	62.57	72.93	1009	46.94	63.60	71.90	994	47.71	64.64	70.86	980
136	45.21	61.49	74.51	1031	45.97	62.53	73.47	1016	46.74	63.56	72.44	1002	47.50	64.60	71.40	987
136.5	45.02	61.45	75.05	1038	45.78	62.48	74.02	1024	46.54	63.52	72.98	1009	47.30	64.56	71.94	995
137	44.82	61.41	75.59	1045	45.58	62.44	74.56	1031	46.34	63.48	73.52	1017	47.09	64.52	72.48	1002
137.5	44.63	61.37	76.14	1053	45.38	62.40	75.10	1039	46.14	63.44	74.06	1024	46.89	64.48	73.02	1010
138	44.44	61.32	76.68	1060	45.19	62.36	75.64	1046	45.94	63.40	74.60	1032	46.69	64.44	73.56	1017
138.5	44.25	61.28	77.22	1068	45.00	62.32	76.18	1054	45.75	63.36	75.14	1039	46.49	64.40	74.10	1025
139	44.06	61.24	77.76	1075	44.81	62.28	76.72	1061	45.55	63.32	75.68	1047	46.30	64.35	74.65	1032
139.5	43.87	61.20	78.30	1083	44.62	62.24	77.26	1069	45.36	63.28	76.22	1054	46.10	64.31	75.19	1040
140	43.69	61.16	78.84	1090	44.43	62.20	77.80	1076	45.17	63.24	76.77	1062	45.91	64.27	75.73	1047
140.5	43.50	61.12	79.38	1098	44.24	62.16	78.34	1083	44.98	63.19	77.31	1069	45.72	64.23	76.27	1055
141	43.32	61.08	79.92	1105	44.05	62.12	78.88	1091	44.79	63.15	77.85	1077	45.53	64.19	76.81	1062
141.5	43.14	61.04	80.46	1113	43.87	62.07	79.43	1098	44.60	63.11	78.39	1084	45.34	64.15	77.35	1070
142	42.95	61.00	81.00	1120	43.69	62.03	79.97	1106	44.42	63.07	78.93	1092	45.15	64.11	77.89	1077
142.5	42.78	60.96	81.55	1128	43.50	61.99	80.51	1113	44.23	63.03	79.47	1099	44.96	64.07	78.43	1085
143	42.60	60.91	82.09	1135	43.32	61.95	81.05	1121	44.05	62.99	80.01	1107	44.77	64.03	78.97	1092
143.5	42.42	60.87	82.63	1143	43.14	61.91	81.59	1128	43.87	62.95	80.55	1114	44.59	63.99	79.51	1100
144	42.24	60.83	83.17	1150	42.96	61.87	82.13	1136	43.69	62.91	81.09	1122	44.41	63.94	80.06	1107
144.5	42.07	60.79	83.71	1158	42.79	61.83	82.67	1143	43.51	62.87	81.63	1129	44.22	63.90	80.60	1115
145	41.90	60.75	84.25	1165	42.61	61.79	83.21	1151	43.33	62.83	82.18	1136	44.04	63.86	81.14	1122
145.5	41.72	60.71	84.79	1173	42.44	61.75	83.75	1158	43.15	62.78	82.72	1144	43.86	63.82	81.68	1130
146	41.55	60.67	85.33	1180	42.26	61.71	84.29	1166	42.97	62.74	83.26	1151	43.69	63.78	82.22	1137
146.5	41.38	60.63	85.87	1188	42.09	61.66	84.84	1173	42.80	62.70	83.80	1159	43.51	63.74	82.76	1145
147	41.21	60.59	86.41	1195	41.92	61.62	85.38	1181	42.63	62.66	84.34	1166	43.33	63.70	83.30	1152
147.5	41.05	60.55	86.96	1203	41.75	61.58	85.92	1188	42.45	62.62	84.88	1174	43.16	63.66	83.84	1160
148	40.88	60.50	87.50	1210	41.58	61.54	86.46	1196	42.28	62.58	85.42	1181	42.98	63.62	84.38	1167
148.5	40.72	60.46	88.04	1218	41.41	61.50	87.00	1203	42.11	62.54	85.96	1189	42.81	63.58	84.92	1175
149	40.55	60.42	88.58	1225	41.25	61.46	87.54	1211	41.94	62.50	86.50	1196	42.64	63.53	85.47	1182
149.5	40.39	60.38	89.12	1233	41.08	61.42	88.08	1218	41.78	62.46	87.04	1204	42.47	63.49	86.01	1189
150	40.23	60.34	89.66	1240	40.92	61.38	88.62	1226	41.61	62.42	87.59	1211	42.30	63.45	86.55	1197
150.5	40.07	60.30	90.20	1247	40.76	61.34	89.16	1233	41.44	62.37	88.13	1219	42.13	63.41	87.09	1204
151	39.91	60.26	90.74	1255	40.59	61.30	89.70	1241	41.28	62.33	88.67	1226	41.97	63.37	87.63	1212
151.5	39.75	60.22	91.28	1262	40.43	61.25	90.25	1248	41.12	62.29	89.21	1234	41.80	63.33	88.17	1219
152	39.59	60.18	91.82	1270	40.27	61.21	90.79	1256	40.95	62.25	89.75	1241	41.64	63.29	88.71	1227
152.5	39.43	60.14	92.37	1277	40.11	61.17	91.33	1263	40.79	62.21	90.29	1249	41.47	63.25	89.25	1234
153	39.28	60.09	92.91	1285	39.96	61.13	91.87	1271	40.63	62.17	90.83	1256	41.31	63.21	89.79	1242
153.5	39.12	60.05	93.45	1292	39.80	61.09	92.41	1278	40.47	62.13	91.37	1264	41.15	63.17	90.33	1249
154	38.97	60.01	93.99	1300	39.64	61.05	92.95	1286	40.32	62.09	91.91	1271	40.99	63.12	90.88	1257
154.5	38.82	59.97	94.53	1307	39.49	61.01	93.49	1293	40.16	62.05	92.45	1279	40.83	63.08	91.42	1264
155	38.66	59.93	95.07	1315	39.33	60.97	94.03	1300	40.00	62.01	93.00	1286	40.67	63.04	91.96	1272
155.5	38.51	59.89	95.61	1322	39.18	60.93	94.57	1308	39.85	61.96	93.54	1294	40.52	63.00	92.50	1279
156	38.36	59.85	96.15	1330	39.03	60.89	95.11	1315	39.69	61.92	94.08	1301	40.36	62.96	93.04	1287
156.5	38.22	59.81	96.69	1337	38.88	60.84	95.66	1323	39.54	61.88	94.62	1309	40.20	62.92	93.58	1294
157	38.07	59.77	97.23	1345	38.73	60.80	96.20	1330	39.39	61.84	95.16	1316	40.05	62.88	94.12	1302
157.5	37.92	59.73	97.78	1352	38.58	60.76	96.74	1338	39.24	61.80	95.70	1324	39.90	62.84	94.66	1309
158	37.77	59.68	98.32	1360	38.43	60.72	97.28	1345	39.09	61.76	96.24	1331	39.74	62.80	95.20	1317
158.5	37.63	59.64	98.86	1367	38.28	60.68	97.82	1353	38.94	61.72	96.78	1338	39.59	62.76	95.74	1324
159	37.49	59.60	99.40	1375	38.14	60.64	98.36	1360	38.79	61.68	97.32	1346	39.44	62.71	96.29	1332
159.5	37.34	59.56	99.94	1382	37.99	60.60	98.90	1368	38.64	61.64	97.86	1353	39.29	62.67	96.83	1339
160	37.20	59.52	100.48	1390	37.85	60.56	99.44	1375	38.50	61.60	98.41	1361	39.15	62.63	97.37	1347
160.5	37.06	59.48	101.02	1397	37.70	60.52	99.98	1383	38.35	61.55	98.95	1368	39.00	62.59	97.91	1354
161	36.92	59.44	101.56	1405	37.56	60.48	100.52	1390	38.21	61.51	99.49	1376	38.85	62.55	98.45	1362
161.5	36.78	59.40	102.10	1412	37.42	60.43	101.07	1398	38.06	61.47	100.03	1383	38.71	62.51	98.99	1369
162	36.64	59.36	102.64	1420	37.28	60.39	101.61	1405	37.92	61.43	100.57	1391	38.56	62.47	99.53	1377
162.5	36.50	59.32	103.19	1427	37.14	60.35	102.15	1413	37.78	61.39	101.11	1398	38.42	62.43	100.07	1384
163	36.36	59.27	103.73	1435	37.00	60.31	102.69	1420	37.64	61.35	101.65	1406	38.27	62.39	100.61	1391
163.5	36.23	59.23	104.27	1442	36.86	60.27	103.23	1428	37.50	61.31	102.19	1413	38.13	62.35	101.15	1399

Body Composition FEMALE 164-195.5 Lb.

Weight: Lb.	Waist: 30 inches Fat: %	Fat: Lb.	LBM: Lb.	RMR: Cal.	30.25 inches Fat: %	Fat: Lb.	LBM: Lb.	RMR: Cal.	30.5 inches Fat: %	Fat: Lb.	LBM: Lb.	RMR: Cal.	30.75 inches Fat: %	Fat: Lb.	LBM: Lb.	RMR: Cal.
164	20.91	34.29	129.71	1794	21.54	35.33	128.67	1780	22.18	36.37	127.63	1765	22.81	37.40	126.60	1751
164.5	20.82	34.25	130.25	1801	21.45	35.29	129.21	1787	22.08	36.33	128.17	1773	22.71	37.36	127.14	1758
165	20.73	34.21	130.79	1809	21.36	35.25	129.75	1794	21.99	36.29	128.72	1780	22.62	37.32	127.68	1766
165.5	20.65	34.17	131.33	1816	21.27	35.21	130.29	1802	21.90	36.24	129.26	1788	22.53	37.28	128.22	1773
166	20.56	34.13	131.87	1824	21.18	35.17	130.83	1809	21.81	36.20	129.80	1795	22.43	37.24	128.76	1781
166.5	20.47	34.09	132.41	1831	21.10	35.12	131.38	1817	21.72	36.16	130.34	1803	22.34	37.20	129.30	1788
167	20.39	34.05	132.95	1839	21.01	35.08	131.92	1824	21.63	36.12	130.88	1810	22.25	37.16	129.84	1796
167.5	20.30	34.01	133.50	1846	20.92	35.04	132.46	1832	21.54	36.08	131.42	1818	22.16	37.12	130.38	1803
168	20.22	33.96	134.04	1854	20.83	35.00	133.00	1839	21.45	36.04	131.96	1825	22.07	37.08	130.92	1811
168.5	20.13	33.92	134.58	1861	20.75	34.96	133.54	1847	21.36	36.00	132.50	1833	21.98	37.04	131.46	1818
169	20.05	33.88	135.12	1869	20.66	34.92	134.08	1854	21.28	35.96	133.04	1840	21.89	36.99	132.01	1826
169.5	19.97	33.84	135.66	1876	20.58	34.88	134.62	1862	21.19	35.92	133.58	1847	21.80	36.95	132.55	1833
170	19.88	33.80	136.20	1884	20.49	34.84	135.16	1869	21.10	35.88	134.13	1855	21.71	36.91	133.09	1841
170.5	19.80	33.76	136.74	1891	20.41	34.80	135.70	1877	21.02	35.83	134.67	1862	21.63	36.87	133.63	1848
171	19.72	33.72	137.28	1899	20.32	34.76	136.24	1884	20.93	35.79	135.21	1870	21.54	36.83	134.17	1856
171.5	19.64	33.68	137.82	1906	20.24	34.71	136.79	1892	20.85	35.75	135.75	1877	21.45	36.79	134.71	1863
172	19.56	33.64	138.36	1914	20.16	34.67	137.33	1899	20.76	35.71	136.29	1885	21.37	36.75	135.25	1871
172.5	19.48	33.60	138.91	1921	20.08	34.63	137.87	1907	20.68	35.67	136.83	1892	21.28	36.71	135.79	1878
173	19.40	33.55	139.45	1929	20.00	34.59	138.41	1914	20.59	35.63	137.37	1900	21.19	36.67	136.33	1885
173.5	19.32	33.51	139.99	1936	19.91	34.55	138.95	1922	20.51	35.59	137.91	1907	21.11	36.63	136.87	1893
174	19.24	33.47	140.53	1944	19.83	34.51	139.49	1929	20.43	35.55	138.45	1915	21.03	36.58	137.42	1900
174.5	19.16	33.43	141.07	1951	19.75	34.47	140.03	1937	20.35	35.51	138.99	1922	20.94	36.54	137.96	1908
175	19.08	33.39	141.61	1958	19.67	34.43	140.57	1944	20.27	35.47	139.54	1930	20.86	36.50	138.50	1915
175.5	19.00	33.35	142.15	1966	19.59	34.39	141.11	1952	20.18	35.42	140.08	1937	20.78	36.46	139.04	1923
176	18.93	33.31	142.69	1973	19.51	34.35	141.65	1959	20.10	35.38	140.62	1945	20.69	36.42	139.58	1930
176.5	18.85	33.27	143.23	1981	19.44	34.30	142.20	1967	20.02	35.34	141.16	1952	20.61	36.38	140.12	1938
177	18.77	33.23	143.77	1988	19.36	34.26	142.74	1974	19.94	35.30	141.70	1960	20.53	36.34	140.66	1945
177.5	18.70	33.19	144.32	1996	19.28	34.22	143.28	1982	19.86	35.26	142.24	1967	20.45	36.30	141.20	1953
178	18.62	33.14	144.86	2003	19.20	34.18	143.82	1989	19.79	35.22	142.78	1975	20.37	36.26	141.74	1960
178.5	18.55	33.10	145.40	2011	19.13	34.14	144.36	1996	19.71	35.18	143.32	1982	20.29	36.22	142.28	1968
179	18.47	33.06	145.94	2018	19.05	34.10	144.90	2004	19.63	35.14	143.86	1990	20.21	36.17	142.83	1975
179.5	18.40	33.02	146.48	2026	18.97	34.06	145.44	2011	19.55	35.10	144.40	1997	20.13	36.13	143.37	1983
180	18.32	32.98	147.02	2033	18.90	34.02	145.98	2019	19.48	35.06	144.95	2005	20.05	36.09	143.91	1990
180.5	18.25	32.94	147.56	2041	18.82	33.98	146.52	2026	19.40	35.01	145.49	2012	19.97	36.05	144.45	1998
181	18.18	32.90	148.10	2048	18.75	33.94	147.06	2034	19.32	34.97	146.03	2020	19.90	36.01	144.99	2005
181.5	18.10	32.86	148.64	2056	18.67	33.89	147.61	2041	19.25	34.93	146.57	2027	19.82	35.97	145.53	2013
182	18.03	32.82	149.18	2063	18.60	33.85	148.15	2049	19.17	34.89	147.11	2035	19.74	35.93	146.07	2020
182.5	17.96	32.78	149.73	2071	18.53	33.81	148.69	2056	19.10	34.85	147.65	2042	19.66	35.89	146.61	2028
183	17.89	32.73	150.27	2078	18.45	33.77	149.23	2064	19.02	34.81	148.19	2049	19.59	35.85	147.15	2035
183.5	17.82	32.69	150.81	2086	18.38	33.73	149.77	2071	18.95	34.77	148.73	2057	19.51	35.81	147.69	2043
184	17.75	32.65	151.35	2093	18.31	33.69	150.31	2079	18.87	34.73	149.27	2064	19.44	35.76	148.24	2050
184.5	17.68	32.61	151.89	2101	18.24	33.65	150.85	2086	18.80	34.69	149.81	2072	19.36	35.72	148.78	2058
185	17.61	32.57	152.43	2108	18.17	33.61	151.39	2094	18.73	34.65	150.36	2079	19.29	35.68	149.32	2065
185.5	17.54	32.53	152.97	2116	18.10	33.57	151.93	2101	18.65	34.60	150.90	2087	19.21	35.64	149.86	2073
186	17.47	32.49	153.51	2123	18.02	33.53	152.47	2109	18.58	34.56	151.44	2094	19.14	35.60	150.40	2080
186.5	17.40	32.45	154.05	2131	17.95	33.48	153.02	2116	18.51	34.52	151.98	2102	19.07	35.56	150.94	2088
187	17.33	32.41	154.59	2138	17.88	33.44	153.56	2124	18.44	34.48	152.52	2109	18.99	35.52	151.48	2095
187.5	17.26	32.37	155.14	2146	17.81	33.40	154.10	2131	18.37	34.44	153.06	2117	18.92	35.48	152.02	2102
188	17.19	32.32	155.68	2153	17.75	33.36	154.64	2139	18.30	34.40	153.60	2124	18.85	35.44	152.56	2110
188.5	17.13	32.28	156.22	2160	17.68	33.32	155.18	2146	18.23	34.36	154.14	2132	18.78	35.40	153.10	2117
189	17.06	32.24	156.76	2168	17.61	33.28	155.72	2154	18.16	34.32	154.68	2139	18.71	35.35	153.65	2125
189.5	16.99	32.20	157.30	2175	17.54	33.24	156.26	2161	18.09	34.28	155.22	2147	18.64	35.31	154.19	2132
190	16.93	32.16	157.84	2183	17.47	33.20	156.80	2169	18.02	34.24	155.77	2154	18.56	35.27	154.73	2140
190.5	16.86	32.12	158.38	2190	17.40	33.16	157.34	2176	17.95	34.19	156.31	2162	18.49	35.23	155.27	2147
191	16.79	32.08	158.92	2198	17.34	33.12	157.88	2184	17.88	34.15	156.85	2169	18.42	35.19	155.81	2155
191.5	16.73	32.04	159.46	2205	17.27	33.07	158.43	2191	17.81	34.11	157.39	2177	18.35	35.15	156.35	2162
192	16.66	32.00	160.00	2213	17.20	33.03	158.97	2199	17.75	34.07	157.93	2184	18.29	35.11	156.89	2170
192.5	16.60	31.96	160.55	2220	17.14	32.99	159.51	2206	17.68	34.03	158.47	2192	18.22	35.07	157.43	2177
193	16.54	31.91	161.09	2228	17.07	32.95	160.05	2213	17.61	33.99	159.01	2199	18.15	35.03	157.97	2185
193.5	16.47	31.87	161.63	2235	17.01	32.91	160.59	2221	17.54	33.95	159.55	2207	18.08	34.99	158.51	2192
194	16.41	31.83	162.17	2243	16.94	32.87	161.13	2228	17.48	33.91	160.09	2214	18.01	34.94	159.06	2200
194.5	16.34	31.79	162.71	2250	16.88	32.83	161.67	2236	17.41	33.87	160.63	2222	17.95	34.90	159.60	2207
195	16.28	31.75	163.25	2258	16.81	32.79	162.21	2243	17.35	33.83	161.18	2229	17.88	34.86	160.14	2215
195.5	16.22	31.71	163.79	2265	16.75	32.75	162.75	2251	17.28	33.78	161.72	2237	17.81	34.82	160.68	2222

Body Composition FEMALE 164-195.5 Lb.

Weight: Lb.	Waist: 31 inches Fat: %	Fat: Lb.	LBM: Lb.	RMR: Cal.	31.25 inches Fat: %	Fat: Lb.	LBM: Lb.	RMR: Cal.	31.5 inches Fat: %	Fat: Lb.	LBM: Lb.	RMR: Cal.	31.75 inches Fat: %	Fat: Lb.	LBM: Lb.	RMR: Cal.
164	23.44	38.44	125.56	1736	24.07	39.48	124.52	1722	24.71	40.52	123.48	1708	25.34	41.55	122.45	1693
164.5	23.34	38.40	126.10	1744	23.97	39.44	125.06	1730	24.61	40.48	124.02	1715	25.24	41.51	122.99	1701
165	23.25	38.36	126.64	1751	23.88	39.40	125.60	1737	24.51	40.44	124.57	1723	25.13	41.47	123.53	1708
165.5	23.15	38.32	127.18	1759	23.78	39.36	126.14	1745	24.41	40.39	125.11	1730	25.03	41.43	124.07	1716
166	23.06	38.28	127.72	1766	23.68	39.32	126.68	1752	24.31	40.35	125.65	1738	24.93	41.39	124.61	1723
166.5	22.97	38.24	128.26	1774	23.59	39.27	127.23	1760	24.21	40.31	126.19	1745	24.83	41.35	125.15	1731
167	22.87	38.20	128.80	1781	23.49	39.23	127.77	1767	24.11	40.27	126.73	1753	24.74	41.31	125.69	1738
167.5	22.78	38.16	129.35	1789	23.40	39.19	128.31	1774	24.02	40.23	127.27	1760	24.64	41.27	126.23	1746
168	22.69	38.11	129.89	1796	23.30	39.15	128.85	1782	23.92	40.19	127.81	1768	24.54	41.23	126.77	1753
168.5	22.60	38.07	130.43	1804	23.21	39.11	129.39	1789	23.83	40.15	128.35	1775	24.44	41.19	127.31	1761
169	22.50	38.03	130.97	1811	23.12	39.07	129.93	1797	23.73	40.11	128.89	1783	24.35	41.14	127.86	1768
169.5	22.41	37.99	131.51	1819	23.03	39.03	130.47	1804	23.64	40.07	129.43	1790	24.25	41.10	128.40	1776
170	22.32	37.95	132.05	1826	22.93	38.99	131.01	1812	23.54	40.03	129.98	1798	24.15	41.06	128.94	1783
170.5	22.23	37.91	132.59	1834	22.84	38.95	131.55	1819	23.45	39.98	130.52	1805	24.06	41.02	129.48	1791
171	22.15	37.87	133.13	1841	22.75	38.91	132.09	1827	23.36	39.94	131.06	1813	23.97	40.98	130.02	1798
171.5	22.06	37.83	133.67	1849	22.66	38.86	132.64	1834	23.27	39.90	131.60	1820	23.87	40.94	130.56	1806
172	21.97	37.79	134.21	1856	22.57	38.82	133.18	1842	23.18	39.86	132.14	1827	23.78	40.90	131.10	1813
172.5	21.88	37.75	134.76	1864	22.48	38.78	133.72	1849	23.08	39.82	132.68	1835	23.69	40.86	131.64	1821
173	21.79	37.70	135.30	1871	22.39	38.74	134.26	1857	22.99	39.78	133.22	1842	23.59	40.82	132.18	1828
173.5	21.71	37.66	135.84	1879	22.31	38.70	134.80	1864	22.90	39.74	133.76	1850	23.50	40.78	132.72	1836
174	21.62	37.62	136.38	1886	22.22	38.66	135.34	1872	22.81	39.70	134.30	1857	23.41	40.73	133.27	1843
174.5	21.54	37.58	136.92	1894	22.13	38.62	135.88	1879	22.73	39.66	134.84	1865	23.32	40.69	133.81	1851
175	21.45	37.54	137.46	1901	22.04	38.58	136.42	1887	22.64	39.62	135.39	1872	23.23	40.65	134.35	1858
175.5	21.37	37.50	138.00	1909	21.96	38.54	136.96	1894	22.55	39.57	135.93	1880	23.14	40.61	134.89	1866
176	21.28	37.46	138.54	1916	21.87	38.50	137.50	1902	22.46	39.53	136.47	1887	23.05	40.57	135.43	1873
176.5	21.20	37.42	139.08	1924	21.79	38.45	138.05	1909	22.38	39.49	137.01	1895	22.96	40.53	135.97	1880
177	21.12	37.38	139.62	1931	21.70	38.41	138.59	1917	22.29	39.45	137.55	1902	22.87	40.49	136.51	1888
177.5	21.03	37.34	140.17	1938	21.62	38.37	139.13	1924	22.20	39.41	138.09	1910	22.79	40.45	137.05	1895
178	20.95	37.29	140.71	1946	21.53	38.33	139.67	1932	22.12	39.37	138.63	1917	22.70	40.41	137.59	1903
178.5	20.87	37.25	141.25	1953	21.45	38.29	140.21	1939	22.03	39.33	139.17	1925	22.61	40.37	138.13	1910
179	20.79	37.21	141.79	1961	21.37	38.25	140.75	1947	21.95	39.29	139.71	1932	22.53	40.32	138.68	1918
179.5	20.71	37.17	142.33	1968	21.29	38.21	141.29	1954	21.86	39.25	140.25	1940	22.44	40.28	139.22	1925
180	20.63	37.13	142.87	1976	21.20	38.17	141.83	1962	21.78	39.21	140.80	1947	22.36	40.24	139.76	1933
180.5	20.55	37.09	143.41	1983	21.12	38.13	142.37	1969	21.70	39.16	141.34	1955	22.27	40.20	140.30	1940
181	20.47	37.05	143.95	1991	21.04	38.09	142.91	1977	21.61	39.12	141.88	1962	22.19	40.16	140.84	1948
181.5	20.39	37.01	144.49	1998	20.96	38.04	143.46	1984	21.53	39.08	142.42	1970	22.10	40.12	141.38	1955
182	20.31	36.97	145.03	2006	20.88	38.00	144.00	1991	21.45	39.04	142.96	1977	22.02	40.08	141.92	1963
182.5	20.23	36.93	145.58	2013	20.80	37.96	144.54	1999	21.37	39.00	143.50	1985	21.94	40.04	142.46	1970
183	20.16	36.88	146.12	2021	20.72	37.92	145.08	2006	21.29	38.96	144.04	1992	21.86	40.00	143.00	1978
183.5	20.08	36.84	146.66	2028	20.64	37.88	145.62	2014	21.21	38.92	144.58	2000	21.77	39.96	143.54	1985
184	20.00	36.80	147.20	2036	20.56	37.84	146.16	2021	21.13	38.88	145.12	2007	21.69	39.91	144.09	1993
184.5	19.92	36.76	147.74	2043	20.49	37.80	146.70	2029	21.05	38.84	145.66	2015	21.61	39.87	144.63	2000
185	19.85	36.72	148.28	2051	20.41	37.76	147.24	2036	20.97	38.80	146.21	2022	21.53	39.83	145.17	2008
185.5	19.77	36.68	148.82	2058	20.33	37.72	147.78	2044	20.89	38.75	146.75	2029	21.45	39.79	145.71	2015
186	19.70	36.64	149.36	2066	20.26	37.68	148.32	2051	20.81	38.71	147.29	2037	21.37	39.75	146.25	2023
186.5	19.62	36.60	149.90	2073	20.18	37.63	148.87	2059	20.74	38.67	147.83	2044	21.29	39.71	146.79	2030
187	19.55	36.56	150.44	2081	20.10	37.59	149.41	2066	20.66	38.63	148.37	2052	21.21	39.67	147.33	2038
187.5	19.47	36.52	150.99	2088	20.03	37.55	149.95	2074	20.58	38.59	148.91	2059	21.13	39.63	147.87	2045
188	19.40	36.47	151.53	2096	19.95	37.51	150.49	2081	20.50	38.55	149.45	2067	21.06	39.59	148.41	2053
188.5	19.33	36.43	152.07	2103	19.88	37.47	151.03	2089	20.43	38.51	149.99	2074	20.98	39.55	148.95	2060
189	19.26	36.39	152.61	2111	19.80	37.43	151.57	2096	20.35	38.47	150.53	2082	20.90	39.50	149.50	2068
189.5	19.18	36.35	153.15	2118	19.73	37.39	152.11	2104	20.28	38.43	151.07	2089	20.83	39.46	150.04	2075
190	19.11	36.31	153.69	2126	19.66	37.35	152.65	2111	20.20	38.39	151.62	2097	20.75	39.42	150.58	2082
190.5	19.04	36.27	154.23	2133	19.58	37.31	153.19	2119	20.13	38.34	152.16	2104	20.67	39.38	151.12	2090
191	18.97	36.23	154.77	2140	19.51	37.27	153.73	2126	20.05	38.30	152.70	2112	20.60	39.34	151.66	2097
191.5	18.90	36.19	155.31	2148	19.44	37.22	154.28	2134	19.98	38.26	153.24	2119	20.52	39.30	152.20	2105
192	18.83	36.15	155.85	2155	19.37	37.18	154.82	2141	19.91	38.22	153.78	2127	20.45	39.26	152.74	2112
192.5	18.76	36.11	156.40	2163	19.29	37.14	155.36	2149	19.83	38.18	154.32	2134	20.37	39.22	153.28	2120
193	18.69	36.06	156.94	2170	19.22	37.10	155.90	2156	19.76	38.14	154.86	2142	20.30	39.18	153.82	2127
193.5	18.62	36.02	157.48	2178	19.15	37.06	156.44	2164	19.69	38.10	155.40	2149	20.23	39.14	154.36	2135
194	18.55	35.98	158.02	2185	19.08	37.02	156.98	2171	19.62	38.06	155.94	2157	20.15	39.09	154.91	2142
194.5	18.48	35.94	158.56	2193	19.01	36.98	157.52	2179	19.55	38.02	156.48	2164	20.08	39.05	155.45	2150
195	18.41	35.90	159.10	2200	18.94	36.94	158.06	2186	19.47	37.98	157.03	2172	20.01	39.01	155.99	2157
195.5	18.34	35.86	159.64	2208	18.87	36.90	158.60	2193	19.40	37.93	157.57	2179	19.93	38.97	156.53	2165

Body Composition FEMALE 164-195.5 Lb.

Weight: Lb.	Waist: 32 inches Fat: %	Fat: Lb.	LBM: Lb.	RMR: Cal.	32.25 inches Fat: %	Fat: Lb.	LBM: Lb.	RMR: Cal.	32.5 inches Fat: %	Fat: Lb.	LBM: Lb.	RMR: Cal.	32.75 inches Fat: %	Fat: Lb.	LBM: Lb.	RMR: Cal.
164	25.97	42.59	121.41	1679	26.60	43.63	120.37	1665	27.24	44.67	119.33	1650	27.87	45.70	118.30	1636
164.5	25.87	42.55	121.95	1687	26.50	43.59	120.91	1672	27.13	44.63	119.87	1658	27.76	45.66	118.84	1644
165	25.76	42.51	122.49	1694	26.39	43.55	121.45	1680	27.02	44.59	120.42	1665	27.65	45.62	119.38	1651
165.5	25.66	42.47	123.03	1702	26.29	43.51	121.99	1687	26.91	44.54	120.96	1673	27.54	45.58	119.92	1658
166	25.56	42.43	123.57	1709	26.18	43.47	122.53	1695	26.81	44.50	121.50	1680	27.43	45.54	120.46	1666
166.5	25.46	42.39	124.11	1716	26.08	43.42	123.08	1702	26.70	44.46	122.04	1688	27.33	45.50	121.00	1673
167	25.36	42.35	124.65	1724	25.98	43.38	123.62	1710	26.60	44.42	122.58	1695	27.22	45.46	121.54	1681
167.5	25.26	42.31	125.20	1731	25.88	43.34	124.16	1717	26.50	44.38	123.12	1703	27.11	45.42	122.08	1688
168	25.16	42.26	125.74	1739	25.77	43.30	124.70	1725	26.39	44.34	123.66	1710	27.01	45.38	122.62	1696
168.5	25.06	42.22	126.28	1746	25.67	43.26	125.24	1732	26.29	44.30	124.20	1718	26.91	45.34	123.16	1703
169	24.96	42.18	126.82	1754	25.57	43.22	125.78	1740	26.19	44.26	124.74	1725	26.80	45.29	123.71	1711
169.5	24.86	42.14	127.36	1761	25.47	43.18	126.32	1747	26.09	44.22	125.28	1733	26.70	45.25	124.25	1718
170	24.76	42.10	127.90	1769	25.38	43.14	126.86	1755	25.99	44.18	125.83	1740	26.60	45.21	124.79	1726
170.5	24.67	42.06	128.44	1776	25.28	43.10	127.40	1762	25.89	44.13	126.37	1748	26.49	45.17	125.33	1733
171	24.57	42.02	128.98	1784	25.18	43.06	127.94	1769	25.79	44.09	126.91	1755	26.39	45.13	125.87	1741
171.5	24.48	41.98	129.52	1791	25.08	43.01	128.49	1777	25.69	44.05	127.45	1763	26.29	45.09	126.41	1748
172	24.38	41.94	130.06	1799	24.98	42.97	129.03	1784	25.59	44.01	127.99	1770	26.19	45.05	126.95	1756
172.5	24.29	41.90	130.61	1806	24.89	42.93	129.57	1792	25.49	43.97	128.53	1778	26.09	45.01	127.49	1763
173	24.19	41.85	131.15	1814	24.79	42.89	130.11	1799	25.39	43.93	129.07	1785	25.99	44.97	128.03	1771
173.5	24.10	41.81	131.69	1821	24.70	42.85	130.65	1807	25.30	43.89	129.61	1793	25.89	44.93	128.57	1778
174	24.01	41.77	132.23	1829	24.60	42.81	131.19	1814	25.20	43.85	130.15	1800	25.80	44.88	129.12	1786
174.5	23.91	41.73	132.77	1836	24.51	42.77	131.73	1822	25.10	43.81	130.69	1807	25.70	44.84	129.66	1793
175	23.82	41.69	133.31	1844	24.42	42.73	132.27	1829	25.01	43.77	131.24	1815	25.60	44.80	130.20	1801
175.5	23.73	41.65	133.85	1851	24.32	42.69	132.81	1837	24.91	43.72	131.78	1822	25.51	44.76	130.74	1808
176	23.64	41.61	134.39	1859	24.23	42.65	133.35	1844	24.82	43.68	132.32	1830	25.41	44.72	131.28	1816
176.5	23.55	41.57	134.93	1866	24.14	42.60	133.90	1852	24.73	43.64	132.86	1837	25.31	44.68	131.82	1823
177	23.46	41.53	135.47	1874	24.05	42.56	134.44	1859	24.63	43.60	133.40	1845	25.22	44.64	132.36	1831
177.5	23.37	41.49	136.02	1881	23.96	42.52	134.98	1867	24.54	43.56	133.94	1852	25.13	44.60	132.90	1838
178	23.28	41.44	136.56	1889	23.87	42.48	135.52	1874	24.45	43.52	134.48	1860	25.03	44.56	133.44	1846
178.5	23.19	41.40	137.10	1896	23.78	42.44	136.06	1882	24.36	43.48	135.02	1867	24.94	44.52	133.98	1853
179	23.11	41.36	137.64	1904	23.69	42.40	136.60	1889	24.27	43.44	135.56	1875	24.85	44.47	134.53	1860
179.5	23.02	41.32	138.18	1911	23.60	42.36	137.14	1897	24.18	43.40	136.10	1882	24.75	44.43	135.07	1868
180	22.93	41.28	138.72	1918	23.51	42.32	137.68	1904	24.09	43.36	136.65	1890	24.66	44.39	135.61	1875
180.5	22.85	41.24	139.26	1926	23.42	42.28	138.22	1912	24.00	43.31	137.19	1897	24.57	44.35	136.15	1883
181	22.76	41.20	139.80	1933	23.33	42.24	138.76	1919	23.91	43.27	137.73	1905	24.48	44.31	136.69	1890
181.5	22.68	41.16	140.34	1941	23.25	42.19	139.31	1927	23.82	43.23	138.27	1912	24.39	44.27	137.23	1898
182	22.59	41.12	140.88	1948	23.16	42.15	139.85	1934	23.73	43.19	138.81	1920	24.30	44.23	137.77	1905
182.5	22.51	41.08	141.43	1956	23.08	42.11	140.39	1942	23.64	43.15	139.35	1927	24.21	44.19	138.31	1913
183	22.42	41.03	141.97	1963	22.99	42.07	140.93	1949	23.56	43.11	139.89	1935	24.12	44.15	138.85	1920
183.5	22.34	40.99	142.51	1971	22.90	42.03	141.47	1957	23.47	43.07	140.43	1942	24.04	44.11	139.39	1928
184	22.26	40.95	143.05	1978	22.82	41.99	142.01	1964	23.38	43.03	140.97	1950	23.95	44.06	139.94	1935
184.5	22.17	40.91	143.59	1986	22.74	41.95	142.55	1971	23.30	42.99	141.51	1957	23.86	44.02	140.48	1943
185	22.09	40.87	144.13	1993	22.65	41.91	143.09	1979	23.21	42.95	142.06	1965	23.77	43.98	141.02	1950
185.5	22.01	40.83	144.67	2001	22.57	41.87	143.63	1986	23.13	42.90	142.60	1972	23.69	43.94	141.56	1958
186	21.93	40.79	145.21	2008	22.49	41.83	144.17	1994	23.04	42.86	143.14	1980	23.60	43.90	142.10	1965
186.5	21.85	40.75	145.75	2016	22.40	41.78	144.72	2001	22.96	42.82	143.68	1987	23.52	43.86	142.64	1973
187	21.77	40.71	146.29	2023	22.32	41.74	145.26	2009	22.88	42.78	144.22	1995	23.43	43.82	143.18	1980
187.5	21.69	40.67	146.84	2031	22.24	41.70	145.80	2016	22.79	42.74	144.76	2002	23.35	43.78	143.72	1988
188	21.61	40.62	147.38	2038	22.16	41.66	146.34	2024	22.71	42.70	145.30	2010	23.26	43.74	144.26	1995
188.5	21.53	40.58	147.92	2046	22.08	41.62	146.88	2031	22.63	42.66	145.84	2017	23.18	43.70	144.80	2003
189	21.45	40.54	148.46	2053	22.00	41.58	147.42	2039	22.55	42.62	146.38	2024	23.10	43.65	145.35	2010
189.5	21.37	40.50	149.00	2061	21.92	41.54	147.96	2046	22.47	42.58	146.92	2032	23.02	43.61	145.89	2018
190	21.29	40.46	149.54	2068	21.84	41.50	148.50	2054	22.39	42.54	147.47	2039	22.93	43.57	146.43	2025
190.5	21.22	40.42	150.08	2076	21.76	41.46	149.04	2061	22.31	42.49	148.01	2047	22.85	43.53	146.97	2033
191	21.14	40.38	150.62	2083	21.68	41.42	149.58	2069	22.23	42.45	148.55	2054	22.77	43.49	147.51	2040
191.5	21.06	40.34	151.16	2091	21.61	41.37	150.13	2076	22.15	42.41	149.09	2062	22.69	43.45	148.05	2048
192	20.99	40.30	151.70	2098	21.53	41.33	150.67	2084	22.07	42.37	149.63	2069	22.61	43.41	148.59	2055
192.5	20.91	40.26	152.25	2106	21.45	41.29	151.21	2091	21.99	42.33	150.17	2077	22.53	43.37	149.13	2063
193	20.84	40.21	152.79	2113	21.37	41.25	151.75	2099	21.91	42.29	150.71	2084	22.45	43.33	149.67	2070
193.5	20.76	40.17	153.33	2121	21.30	41.21	152.29	2106	21.83	42.25	151.25	2092	22.37	43.29	150.21	2077
194	20.69	40.13	153.87	2128	21.22	41.17	152.83	2114	21.76	42.21	151.79	2099	22.29	43.24	150.76	2085
194.5	20.61	40.09	154.41	2135	21.15	41.13	153.37	2121	21.68	42.17	152.33	2107	22.21	43.20	151.30	2092
195	20.54	40.05	154.95	2143	21.07	41.09	153.91	2129	21.60	42.13	152.88	2114	22.13	43.16	151.84	2100
195.5	20.46	40.01	155.49	2150	21.00	41.05	154.45	2136	21.53	42.08	153.42	2122	22.06	43.12	152.38	2107

Body Composition   FEMALE   164-195.5 Lb.

Weight: Lb.	Waist: 33 inches Fat: %	Fat: Lb.	LBM: Lb.	RMR: Cal.	33.25 inches Fat: %	Fat: Lb.	LBM: Lb.	RMR: Cal.	33.5 inches Fat: %	Fat: Lb.	LBM: Lb.	RMR: Cal.	33.75 inches Fat: %	Fat: Lb.	LBM: Lb.	RMR: Cal.
164	28.50	46.74	117.26	1622	29.13	47.78	116.22	1607	29.77	48.82	115.18	1593	30.40	49.85	114.15	1579
164.5	28.39	46.70	117.80	1629	29.02	47.74	116.76	1615	29.65	48.78	115.72	1600	30.28	49.81	114.69	1586
165	28.28	46.66	118.34	1637	28.91	47.70	117.30	1622	29.54	48.74	116.27	1608	30.17	49.77	115.23	1594
165.5	28.17	46.62	118.88	1644	28.80	47.66	117.84	1630	29.42	48.69	116.81	1615	30.05	49.73	115.77	1601
166	28.06	46.58	119.42	1652	28.68	47.62	118.38	1637	29.31	48.65	117.35	1623	29.93	49.69	116.31	1609
166.5	27.95	46.54	119.96	1659	28.57	47.57	118.93	1645	29.20	48.61	117.89	1630	29.82	49.65	116.85	1616
167	27.84	46.50	120.50	1667	28.46	47.53	119.47	1652	29.08	48.57	118.43	1638	29.71	49.61	117.39	1624
167.5	27.73	46.46	121.05	1674	28.35	47.49	120.01	1660	28.97	48.53	118.97	1645	29.59	49.57	117.93	1631
168	27.63	46.41	121.59	1682	28.24	47.45	120.55	1667	28.86	48.49	119.51	1653	29.48	49.53	118.47	1638
168.5	27.52	46.37	122.13	1689	28.14	47.41	121.09	1675	28.75	48.45	120.05	1660	29.37	49.49	119.01	1646
169	27.42	46.33	122.67	1696	28.03	47.37	121.63	1682	28.64	48.41	120.59	1668	29.26	49.44	119.56	1653
169.5	27.31	46.29	123.21	1704	27.92	47.33	122.17	1690	28.53	48.37	121.13	1675	29.15	49.40	120.10	1661
170	27.21	46.25	123.75	1711	27.82	47.29	122.71	1697	28.43	48.33	121.68	1683	29.04	49.36	120.64	1668
170.5	27.10	46.21	124.29	1719	27.71	47.25	123.25	1705	28.32	48.28	122.22	1690	28.93	49.32	121.18	1676
171	27.00	46.17	124.83	1726	27.61	47.21	123.79	1712	28.21	48.24	122.76	1698	28.82	49.28	121.72	1683
171.5	26.90	46.13	125.37	1734	27.50	47.16	124.34	1720	28.11	48.20	123.30	1705	28.71	49.24	122.26	1691
172	26.79	46.09	125.91	1741	27.40	47.12	124.88	1727	28.00	48.16	123.84	1713	28.60	49.20	122.80	1698
172.5	26.69	46.05	126.46	1749	27.29	47.08	125.42	1735	27.90	48.12	124.38	1720	28.50	49.16	123.34	1706
173	26.59	46.00	127.00	1756	27.19	47.04	125.96	1742	27.79	48.08	124.92	1728	28.39	49.12	123.88	1713
173.5	26.49	45.96	127.54	1764	27.09	47.00	126.50	1749	27.69	48.04	125.46	1735	28.29	49.08	124.42	1721
174	26.39	45.92	128.08	1771	26.99	46.96	127.04	1757	27.58	48.00	126.00	1743	28.18	49.03	124.97	1728
174.5	26.29	45.88	128.62	1779	26.89	46.92	127.58	1764	27.48	47.96	126.54	1750	28.08	48.99	125.51	1736
175	26.19	45.84	129.16	1786	26.79	46.88	128.12	1772	27.38	47.92	127.09	1758	27.97	48.95	126.05	1743
175.5	26.10	45.80	129.70	1794	26.69	46.84	128.66	1779	27.28	47.87	127.63	1765	27.87	48.91	126.59	1751
176	26.00	45.76	130.24	1801	26.59	46.80	129.20	1787	27.18	47.83	128.17	1773	27.77	48.87	127.13	1758
176.5	25.90	45.72	130.78	1809	26.49	46.75	129.75	1794	27.08	47.79	128.71	1780	27.67	48.83	127.67	1766
177	25.81	45.68	131.32	1816	26.39	46.71	130.29	1802	26.98	47.75	129.25	1788	27.56	48.79	128.21	1773
177.5	25.71	45.64	131.87	1824	26.29	46.67	130.83	1809	26.88	47.71	129.79	1795	27.46	48.75	128.75	1781
178	25.61	45.59	132.41	1831	26.20	46.63	131.37	1817	26.78	47.67	130.33	1802	27.36	48.71	129.29	1788
178.5	25.52	45.55	132.95	1839	26.10	46.59	131.91	1824	26.68	47.63	130.87	1810	27.26	48.67	129.83	1796
179	25.43	45.51	133.49	1846	26.01	46.55	132.45	1832	26.58	47.59	131.41	1817	27.16	48.62	130.38	1803
179.5	25.33	45.47	134.03	1854	25.91	46.51	132.99	1839	26.49	47.55	131.95	1825	27.07	48.58	130.92	1811
180	25.24	45.43	134.57	1861	25.82	46.47	133.53	1847	26.39	47.51	132.50	1832	26.97	48.54	131.46	1818
180.5	25.15	45.39	135.11	1869	25.72	46.43	134.07	1854	26.30	47.46	133.04	1840	26.87	48.50	132.00	1826
181	25.05	45.35	135.65	1876	25.63	46.39	134.61	1862	26.20	47.42	133.58	1847	26.77	48.46	132.54	1833
181.5	24.96	45.31	136.19	1884	25.53	46.34	135.16	1869	26.11	47.38	134.12	1855	26.68	48.42	133.08	1841
182	24.87	45.27	136.73	1891	25.44	46.30	135.70	1877	26.01	47.34	134.66	1862	26.58	48.38	133.62	1848
182.5	24.78	45.23	137.28	1899	25.35	46.26	136.24	1884	25.92	47.30	135.20	1870	26.49	48.34	134.16	1855
183	24.69	45.18	137.82	1906	25.26	46.22	136.78	1892	25.82	47.26	135.74	1877	26.39	48.30	134.70	1863
183.5	24.60	45.14	138.36	1913	25.17	46.18	137.32	1899	25.73	47.22	136.28	1885	26.30	48.26	135.24	1870
184	24.51	45.10	138.90	1921	25.08	46.14	137.86	1907	25.64	47.18	136.82	1892	26.20	48.21	135.79	1878
184.5	24.42	45.06	139.44	1928	24.99	46.10	138.40	1914	25.55	47.14	137.36	1900	26.11	48.17	136.33	1885
185	24.34	45.02	139.98	1936	24.90	46.06	138.94	1922	25.46	47.10	137.91	1907	26.02	48.13	136.87	1893
185.5	24.25	44.98	140.52	1943	24.81	46.02	139.48	1929	25.37	47.05	138.45	1915	25.93	48.09	137.41	1900
186	24.16	44.94	141.06	1951	24.72	45.98	140.02	1937	25.28	47.01	138.99	1922	25.83	48.05	137.95	1908
186.5	24.07	44.90	141.60	1958	24.63	45.93	140.57	1944	25.19	46.97	139.53	1930	25.74	48.01	138.49	1915
187	23.99	44.86	142.14	1966	24.54	45.89	141.11	1952	25.10	46.93	140.07	1937	25.65	47.97	139.03	1923
187.5	23.90	44.82	142.69	1973	24.45	45.85	141.65	1959	25.01	46.89	140.61	1945	25.56	47.93	139.57	1930
188	23.82	44.77	143.23	1981	24.37	45.81	142.19	1966	24.92	46.85	141.15	1952	25.47	47.89	140.11	1938
188.5	23.73	44.73	143.77	1988	24.28	45.77	142.73	1974	24.83	46.81	141.69	1960	25.38	47.85	140.65	1945
189	23.65	44.69	144.31	1996	24.20	45.73	143.27	1981	24.74	46.77	142.23	1967	25.29	47.80	141.20	1953
189.5	23.56	44.65	144.85	2003	24.11	45.69	143.81	1989	24.66	46.73	142.77	1975	25.21	47.76	141.74	1960
190	23.48	44.61	145.39	2011	24.03	45.65	144.35	1996	24.57	46.69	143.32	1982	25.12	47.72	142.28	1968
190.5	23.40	44.57	145.93	2018	23.94	45.61	144.89	2004	24.49	46.64	143.86	1990	25.03	47.68	142.82	1975
191	23.31	44.53	146.47	2026	23.86	45.57	145.43	2011	24.40	46.60	144.40	1997	24.94	47.64	143.36	1983
191.5	23.23	44.49	147.01	2033	23.77	45.52	145.98	2019	24.31	46.56	144.94	2004	24.86	47.60	143.90	1990
192	23.15	44.45	147.55	2041	23.69	45.48	146.52	2026	24.23	46.52	145.48	2012	24.77	47.56	144.44	1998
192.5	23.07	44.41	148.10	2048	23.61	45.44	147.06	2034	24.15	46.48	146.02	2019	24.68	47.52	144.98	2005
193	22.99	44.36	148.64	2056	23.52	45.40	147.60	2041	24.06	46.44	146.56	2027	24.60	47.48	145.52	2013
193.5	22.91	44.32	149.18	2063	23.44	45.36	148.14	2049	23.98	46.40	147.10	2034	24.51	47.44	146.06	2020
194	22.83	44.28	149.72	2071	23.36	45.32	148.68	2056	23.90	46.36	147.64	2042	24.43	47.39	146.61	2028
194.5	22.75	44.24	150.26	2078	23.28	45.28	149.22	2064	23.81	46.32	148.18	2049	24.35	47.35	147.15	2035
195	22.67	44.20	150.80	2086	23.20	45.24	149.76	2071	23.73	46.28	148.73	2057	24.26	47.31	147.69	2043
195.5	22.59	44.16	151.34	2093	23.12	45.20	150.30	2079	23.65	46.23	149.27	2064	24.18	47.27	148.23	2050

Body Composition   FEMALE   164-195.5 Lb.

Weight: Lb.	Waist: 34 inches				34.25 inches				34.5 inches				34.75 inches			
	Fat: %	Fat: Lb.	LBM: Lb.	RMR: Cal.	Fat: %	Fat: Lb.	LBM: Lb.	RMR: Cal.	Fat: %	Fat: Lb.	LBM: Lb.	RMR: Cal.	Fat: %	Fat: Lb.	LBM: Lb.	RMR: Cal.
164	31.03	50.89	113.11	1564	31.66	51.93	112.07	1550	32.30	52.97	111.03	1536	32.93	54.00	110.00	1521
164.5	30.91	50.85	113.65	1572	31.54	51.89	112.61	1557	32.17	52.93	111.57	1543	32.80	53.96	110.54	1529
165	30.79	50.81	114.19	1579	31.42	51.85	113.15	1565	32.05	52.89	112.12	1551	32.68	53.92	111.08	1536
165.5	30.68	50.77	114.73	1587	31.30	51.81	113.69	1572	31.93	52.84	112.66	1558	32.56	53.88	111.62	1544
166	30.56	50.73	115.27	1594	31.18	51.77	114.23	1580	31.81	52.80	113.20	1566	32.43	53.84	112.16	1551
166.5	30.44	50.69	115.81	1602	31.07	51.72	114.78	1587	31.69	52.76	113.74	1573	32.31	53.80	112.70	1559
167	30.33	50.65	116.35	1609	30.95	51.68	115.32	1595	31.57	52.72	114.28	1580	32.19	53.76	113.24	1566
167.5	30.21	50.61	116.90	1617	30.83	51.64	115.86	1602	31.45	52.68	114.82	1588	32.07	53.72	113.78	1574
168	30.10	50.56	117.44	1624	30.72	51.60	116.40	1610	31.33	52.64	115.36	1595	31.95	53.68	114.32	1581
168.5	29.98	50.52	117.98	1632	30.60	51.56	116.94	1617	31.22	52.60	115.90	1603	31.83	53.64	114.86	1589
169	29.87	50.48	118.52	1639	30.48	51.52	117.48	1625	31.10	52.56	116.44	1610	31.71	53.59	115.41	1596
169.5	29.76	50.44	119.06	1647	30.37	51.48	118.02	1632	30.98	52.52	116.98	1618	31.59	53.55	115.95	1604
170	29.65	50.40	119.60	1654	30.26	51.44	118.56	1640	30.87	52.48	117.53	1625	31.48	53.51	116.49	1611
170.5	29.54	50.36	120.14	1662	30.14	51.40	119.10	1647	30.75	52.43	118.07	1633	31.36	53.47	117.03	1619
171	29.43	50.32	120.68	1669	30.03	51.36	119.64	1655	30.64	52.39	118.61	1640	31.25	53.43	117.57	1626
171.5	29.32	50.28	121.22	1677	29.92	51.31	120.19	1662	30.53	52.35	119.15	1648	31.13	53.39	118.11	1633
172	29.21	50.24	121.76	1684	29.81	51.27	120.73	1670	30.41	52.31	119.69	1655	31.02	53.35	118.65	1641
172.5	29.10	50.20	122.31	1691	29.70	51.23	121.27	1677	30.30	52.27	120.23	1663	30.90	53.31	119.19	1648
173	28.99	50.15	122.85	1699	29.59	51.19	121.81	1685	30.19	52.23	120.77	1670	30.79	53.27	119.73	1656
173.5	28.88	50.11	123.39	1706	29.48	51.15	122.35	1692	30.08	52.19	121.31	1678	30.68	53.23	120.27	1663
174	28.78	50.07	123.93	1714	29.37	51.11	122.89	1700	29.97	52.15	121.85	1685	30.57	53.18	120.82	1671
174.5	28.67	50.03	124.47	1721	29.27	51.07	123.43	1707	29.86	52.11	122.39	1693	30.45	53.14	121.36	1678
175	28.57	49.99	125.01	1729	29.16	51.03	123.97	1715	29.75	52.07	122.94	1700	30.34	53.10	121.90	1686
175.5	28.46	49.95	125.55	1736	29.05	50.99	124.51	1722	29.64	52.02	123.48	1708	30.23	53.06	122.44	1693
176	28.36	49.91	126.09	1744	28.95	50.95	125.05	1730	29.54	51.98	124.02	1715	30.13	53.02	122.98	1701
176.5	28.25	49.87	126.63	1751	28.84	50.90	125.60	1737	29.43	51.94	124.56	1723	30.02	52.98	123.52	1708
177	28.15	49.83	127.17	1759	28.74	50.86	126.14	1744	29.32	51.90	125.10	1730	29.91	52.94	124.06	1716
177.5	28.05	49.79	127.72	1766	28.63	50.82	126.68	1752	29.22	51.86	125.64	1738	29.80	52.90	124.60	1723
178	27.95	49.74	128.26	1774	28.53	50.78	127.22	1759	29.11	51.82	126.18	1745	29.69	52.86	125.14	1731
178.5	27.84	49.70	128.80	1781	28.43	50.74	127.76	1767	29.01	51.78	126.72	1753	29.59	52.82	125.68	1738
179	27.74	49.66	129.34	1789	28.32	50.70	128.30	1774	28.90	51.74	127.26	1760	29.48	52.77	126.23	1746
179.5	27.64	49.62	129.88	1796	28.22	50.66	128.84	1782	28.80	51.70	127.80	1768	29.38	52.73	126.77	1753
180	27.54	49.58	130.42	1804	28.12	50.62	129.38	1789	28.70	51.66	128.35	1775	29.27	52.69	127.31	1761
180.5	27.45	49.54	130.96	1811	28.02	50.58	129.92	1797	28.60	51.61	128.89	1782	29.17	52.65	127.85	1768
181	27.35	49.50	131.50	1819	27.92	50.54	130.46	1804	28.49	51.57	129.43	1790	29.07	52.61	128.39	1776
181.5	27.25	49.46	132.04	1826	27.82	50.49	131.01	1812	28.39	51.53	129.97	1797	28.96	52.57	128.93	1783
182	27.15	49.42	132.58	1834	27.72	50.45	131.55	1819	28.29	51.49	130.51	1805	28.86	52.53	129.47	1791
182.5	27.05	49.38	133.13	1841	27.62	50.41	132.09	1827	28.19	51.45	131.05	1812	28.76	52.49	130.01	1798
183	26.96	49.33	133.67	1849	27.53	50.37	132.63	1834	28.09	51.41	131.59	1820	28.66	52.45	130.55	1806
183.5	26.86	49.29	134.21	1856	27.43	50.33	133.17	1842	27.99	51.37	132.13	1827	28.56	52.41	131.09	1813
184	26.77	49.25	134.75	1864	27.33	50.29	133.71	1849	27.90	51.33	132.67	1835	28.46	52.36	131.64	1821
184.5	26.67	49.21	135.29	1871	27.23	50.25	134.25	1857	27.80	51.29	133.21	1842	28.36	52.32	132.18	1828
185	26.58	49.17	135.83	1879	27.14	50.21	134.79	1864	27.70	51.25	133.76	1850	28.26	52.28	132.72	1835
185.5	26.48	49.13	136.37	1886	27.04	50.17	135.33	1872	27.60	51.20	134.30	1857	28.16	52.24	133.26	1843
186	26.39	49.09	136.91	1893	26.95	50.13	135.87	1879	27.51	51.16	134.84	1865	28.06	52.20	133.80	1850
186.5	26.30	49.05	137.45	1901	26.85	50.08	136.42	1887	27.41	51.12	135.38	1872	27.97	52.16	134.34	1858
187	26.21	49.01	137.99	1908	26.76	50.04	136.96	1894	27.32	51.08	135.92	1880	27.87	52.12	134.88	1865
187.5	26.11	48.97	138.54	1916	26.67	50.00	137.50	1902	27.22	51.04	136.46	1887	27.77	52.08	135.42	1873
188	26.02	48.92	139.08	1923	26.58	49.96	138.04	1909	27.13	51.00	137.00	1895	27.68	52.04	135.96	1880
188.5	25.93	48.88	139.62	1931	26.48	49.92	138.58	1917	27.03	50.96	137.54	1902	27.58	52.00	136.50	1888
189	25.84	48.84	140.16	1938	26.39	49.88	139.12	1924	26.94	50.92	138.08	1910	27.49	51.95	137.05	1895
189.5	25.75	48.80	140.70	1946	26.30	49.84	139.66	1932	26.85	50.88	138.62	1917	27.39	51.91	137.59	1903
190	25.66	48.76	141.24	1953	26.21	49.80	140.20	1939	26.76	50.84	139.17	1925	27.30	51.87	138.13	1910
190.5	25.57	48.72	141.78	1961	26.12	49.76	140.74	1946	26.66	50.79	139.71	1932	27.21	51.83	138.67	1918
191	25.49	48.68	142.32	1968	26.03	49.72	141.28	1954	26.57	50.75	140.25	1940	27.12	51.79	139.21	1925
191.5	25.40	48.64	142.86	1976	25.94	49.67	141.83	1961	26.48	50.71	140.79	1947	27.02	51.75	139.75	1933
192	25.31	48.60	143.40	1983	25.85	49.63	142.37	1969	26.39	50.67	141.33	1955	26.93	51.71	140.29	1940
192.5	25.22	48.56	143.95	1991	25.76	49.59	142.91	1976	26.30	50.63	141.87	1962	26.84	51.67	140.83	1948
193	25.14	48.51	144.49	1998	25.67	49.55	143.45	1984	26.21	50.59	142.41	1970	26.75	51.63	141.37	1955
193.5	25.05	48.47	145.03	2006	25.59	49.51	143.99	1991	26.12	50.55	142.95	1977	26.66	51.59	141.91	1963
194	24.96	48.43	145.57	2013	25.50	49.47	144.53	1999	26.03	50.51	143.49	1985	26.57	51.54	142.46	1970
194.5	24.88	48.39	146.11	2021	25.41	49.43	145.07	2006	25.95	50.47	144.03	1992	26.48	51.50	143.00	1978
195	24.79	48.35	146.65	2028	25.33	49.39	145.61	2014	25.86	50.43	144.58	1999	26.39	51.46	143.54	1985
195.5	24.71	48.31	147.19	2036	25.24	49.35	146.15	2021	25.77	50.38	145.12	2007	26.30	51.42	144.08	1993

Body Composition FEMALE 164-195.5 Lb.

Weight: Lb.	Waist: 35 inches				35.25 inches				35.5 inches				35.75 inches			
	Fat: %	Fat: Lb.	LBM: Lb.	RMR: Cal.	Fat: %	Fat: Lb.	LBM: Lb.	RMR: Cal.	Fat: %	Fat: Lb.	LBM: Lb.	RMR: Cal.	Fat: %	Fat: Lb.	LBM: Lb.	RMR: Cal.
164	33.56	55.04	108.96	1507	34.19	56.08	107.92	1493	34.83	57.12	106.88	1478	35.46	58.15	105.85	1464
164.5	33.44	55.00	109.50	1514	34.07	56.04	108.46	1500	34.70	57.08	107.42	1486	35.33	58.11	106.39	1471
165	33.31	54.96	110.04	1522	33.94	56.00	109.00	1508	34.57	57.04	107.97	1493	35.20	58.07	106.93	1479
165.5	33.18	54.92	110.58	1529	33.81	55.96	109.54	1515	34.44	56.99	108.51	1501	35.06	58.03	107.47	1486
166	33.06	54.88	111.12	1537	33.68	55.92	110.08	1522	34.31	56.95	109.05	1508	34.93	57.99	108.01	1494
166.5	32.94	54.84	111.66	1544	33.56	55.87	110.63	1530	34.18	56.91	109.59	1516	34.80	57.95	108.55	1501
167	32.81	54.80	112.20	1552	33.43	55.83	111.17	1537	34.05	56.87	110.13	1523	34.68	57.91	109.09	1509
167.5	32.69	54.76	112.75	1559	33.31	55.79	111.71	1545	33.93	56.83	110.67	1531	34.55	57.87	109.63	1516
168	32.57	54.71	113.29	1567	33.19	55.75	112.25	1552	33.80	56.79	111.21	1538	34.42	57.83	110.17	1524
168.5	32.45	54.67	113.83	1574	33.06	55.71	112.79	1560	33.68	56.75	111.75	1546	34.29	57.79	110.71	1531
169	32.33	54.63	114.37	1582	32.94	55.67	113.33	1567	33.55	56.71	112.29	1553	34.17	57.74	111.26	1539
169.5	32.21	54.59	114.91	1589	32.82	55.63	113.87	1575	33.43	56.67	112.83	1560	34.04	57.70	111.80	1546
170	32.09	54.55	115.45	1597	32.70	55.59	114.41	1582	33.31	56.63	113.38	1568	33.92	57.66	112.34	1554
170.5	31.97	54.51	115.99	1604	32.58	55.55	114.95	1590	33.19	56.58	113.92	1575	33.80	57.62	112.88	1561
171	31.85	54.47	116.53	1612	32.46	55.51	115.49	1597	33.07	56.54	114.46	1583	33.67	57.58	113.42	1569
171.5	31.74	54.43	117.07	1619	32.34	55.46	116.04	1605	32.95	56.50	115.00	1590	33.55	57.54	113.96	1576
172	31.62	54.39	117.61	1627	32.22	55.42	116.58	1612	32.83	56.46	115.54	1598	33.43	57.50	114.50	1584
172.5	31.50	54.35	118.16	1634	32.11	55.38	117.12	1620	32.71	56.42	116.08	1605	33.31	57.46	115.04	1591
173	31.39	54.30	118.70	1642	31.99	55.34	117.66	1627	32.59	56.38	116.62	1613	33.19	57.42	115.58	1599
173.5	31.28	54.26	119.24	1649	31.87	55.30	118.20	1635	32.47	56.34	117.16	1620	33.07	57.38	116.12	1606
174	31.16	54.22	119.78	1657	31.76	55.26	118.74	1642	32.35	56.30	117.70	1628	32.95	57.33	116.67	1613
174.5	31.05	54.18	120.32	1664	31.64	55.22	119.28	1650	32.24	56.26	118.24	1635	32.83	57.29	117.21	1621
175	30.94	54.14	120.86	1671	31.53	55.18	119.82	1657	32.12	56.22	118.79	1643	32.72	57.25	117.75	1628
175.5	30.83	54.10	121.40	1679	31.42	55.14	120.36	1665	32.01	56.17	119.33	1650	32.60	57.21	118.29	1636
176	30.71	54.06	121.94	1686	31.30	55.10	120.90	1672	31.89	56.13	119.87	1658	32.48	57.17	118.83	1643
176.5	30.60	54.02	122.48	1694	31.19	55.05	121.45	1680	31.78	56.09	120.41	1665	32.37	57.13	119.37	1651
177	30.49	53.98	123.02	1701	31.08	55.01	121.99	1687	31.67	56.05	120.95	1673	32.25	57.09	119.91	1658
177.5	30.39	53.94	123.57	1709	30.97	54.97	122.53	1695	31.55	56.01	121.49	1680	32.14	57.05	120.45	1666
178	30.28	53.89	124.11	1716	30.86	54.93	123.07	1702	31.44	55.97	122.03	1688	32.03	57.01	120.99	1673
178.5	30.17	53.85	124.65	1724	30.75	54.89	123.61	1710	31.33	55.93	122.57	1695	31.91	56.97	121.53	1681
179	30.06	53.81	125.19	1731	30.64	54.85	124.15	1717	31.22	55.89	123.11	1703	31.80	56.92	122.08	1688
179.5	29.96	53.77	125.73	1739	30.53	54.81	124.69	1724	31.11	55.85	123.65	1710	31.69	56.88	122.62	1696
180	29.85	53.73	126.27	1746	30.43	54.77	125.23	1732	31.00	55.81	124.20	1718	31.58	56.84	123.16	1703
180.5	29.74	53.69	126.81	1754	30.32	54.73	125.77	1739	30.89	55.76	124.74	1725	31.47	56.80	123.70	1711
181	29.64	53.65	127.35	1761	30.21	54.69	126.31	1747	30.79	55.72	125.28	1733	31.36	56.76	124.24	1718
181.5	29.54	53.61	127.89	1769	30.11	54.64	126.86	1754	30.68	55.68	125.82	1740	31.25	56.72	124.78	1726
182	29.43	53.57	128.43	1776	30.00	54.60	127.40	1762	30.57	55.64	126.36	1748	31.14	56.68	125.32	1733
182.5	29.33	53.53	128.98	1784	29.90	54.56	127.94	1769	30.47	55.60	126.90	1755	31.03	56.64	125.86	1741
183	29.23	53.48	129.52	1791	29.79	54.52	128.48	1777	30.36	55.56	127.44	1763	30.93	56.60	126.40	1748
183.5	29.12	53.44	130.06	1799	29.69	54.48	129.02	1784	30.26	55.52	127.98	1770	30.82	56.56	126.94	1756
184	29.02	53.40	130.60	1806	29.59	54.44	129.56	1792	30.15	55.48	128.52	1777	30.71	56.51	127.49	1763
184.5	28.92	53.36	131.14	1814	29.48	54.40	130.10	1799	30.05	55.44	129.06	1785	30.61	56.47	128.03	1771
185	28.82	53.32	131.68	1821	29.38	54.36	130.64	1807	29.94	55.40	129.61	1792	30.50	56.43	128.57	1778
185.5	28.72	53.28	132.22	1829	29.28	54.32	131.18	1814	29.84	55.35	130.15	1800	30.40	56.39	129.11	1786
186	28.62	53.24	132.76	1836	29.18	54.28	131.72	1822	29.74	55.31	130.69	1807	30.30	56.35	129.65	1793
186.5	28.52	53.20	133.30	1844	29.08	54.23	132.27	1829	29.64	55.27	131.23	1815	30.19	56.31	130.19	1801
187	28.43	53.16	133.84	1851	28.98	54.19	132.81	1837	29.54	55.23	131.77	1822	30.09	56.27	130.73	1808
187.5	28.33	53.12	134.39	1859	28.88	54.15	133.35	1844	29.43	55.19	132.31	1830	29.99	56.23	131.27	1815
188	28.23	53.07	134.93	1866	28.78	54.11	133.89	1852	29.33	55.15	132.85	1837	29.89	56.19	131.81	1823
188.5	28.13	53.03	135.47	1874	28.68	54.07	134.43	1859	29.24	55.11	133.39	1845	29.79	56.15	132.35	1830
189	28.04	52.99	136.01	1881	28.59	54.03	134.97	1867	29.14	55.07	133.93	1852	29.68	56.10	132.90	1838
189.5	27.94	52.95	136.55	1888	28.49	53.99	135.51	1874	29.04	55.03	134.47	1860	29.58	56.06	133.44	1845
190	27.85	52.91	137.09	1896	28.39	53.95	136.05	1882	28.94	54.99	135.02	1867	29.49	56.02	133.98	1853
190.5	27.75	52.87	137.63	1903	28.30	53.91	136.59	1889	28.84	54.94	135.56	1875	29.39	55.98	134.52	1860
191	27.66	52.83	138.17	1911	28.20	53.87	137.13	1897	28.75	54.90	136.10	1882	29.29	55.94	135.06	1868
191.5	27.57	52.79	138.71	1918	28.11	53.82	137.68	1904	28.65	54.86	136.64	1890	29.19	55.90	135.60	1875
192	27.47	52.75	139.25	1926	28.01	53.78	138.22	1912	28.55	54.82	137.18	1897	29.09	55.86	136.14	1883
192.5	27.38	52.71	139.80	1933	27.92	53.74	138.76	1919	28.46	54.78	137.72	1905	29.00	55.82	136.68	1890
193	27.29	52.66	140.34	1941	27.82	53.70	139.30	1926	28.36	54.74	138.26	1912	28.90	55.78	137.22	1898
193.5	27.20	52.62	140.88	1948	27.73	53.66	139.84	1934	28.27	54.70	138.80	1920	28.80	55.74	137.76	1905
194	27.10	52.58	141.42	1956	27.64	53.62	140.38	1941	28.17	54.66	139.34	1927	28.71	55.69	138.31	1913
194.5	27.01	52.54	141.96	1963	27.55	53.58	140.92	1949	28.08	54.62	139.88	1935	28.61	55.65	138.85	1920
195	26.92	52.50	142.50	1971	27.46	53.54	141.46	1956	27.99	54.58	140.43	1942	28.52	55.61	139.39	1928
195.5	26.83	52.46	143.04	1978	27.36	53.50	142.00	1964	27.89	54.53	140.97	1950	28.43	55.57	139.93	1935

Body Composition FEMALE 164-195.5 Lb.

Weight: Lb.	Waist: 36 inches Fat: %	Fat: Lb.	LBM: Lb.	RMR: Cal.	36.25 inches Fat: %	Fat: Lb.	LBM: Lb.	RMR: Cal.	36.5 inches Fat: %	Fat: Lb.	LBM: Lb.	RMR: Cal.	36.75 inches Fat: %	Fat: Lb.	LBM: Lb.	RMR: Cal.
164	36.09	59.19	104.81	1449	36.73	60.23	103.77	1435	37.36	61.27	102.73	1421	37.99	62.30	101.70	1406
164.5	35.96	59.15	105.35	1457	36.59	60.19	104.31	1443	37.22	61.23	103.27	1428	37.85	62.26	102.24	1414
165	35.82	59.11	105.89	1464	36.45	60.15	104.85	1450	37.08	61.19	103.82	1436	37.71	62.22	102.78	1421
165.5	35.69	59.07	106.43	1472	36.32	60.11	105.39	1458	36.95	61.14	104.36	1443	37.57	62.18	103.32	1429
166	35.56	59.03	106.97	1479	36.18	60.07	105.93	1465	36.81	61.10	104.90	1451	37.43	62.14	103.86	1436
166.5	35.43	58.99	107.51	1487	36.05	60.02	106.48	1473	36.67	61.06	105.44	1458	37.30	62.10	104.40	1444
167	35.30	58.95	108.05	1494	35.92	59.98	107.02	1480	36.54	61.02	105.98	1466	37.16	62.06	104.94	1451
167.5	35.17	58.91	108.60	1502	35.79	59.94	107.56	1488	36.41	60.98	106.52	1473	37.03	62.02	105.48	1459
168	35.04	58.86	109.14	1509	35.66	59.90	108.10	1495	36.27	60.94	107.06	1481	36.89	61.98	106.02	1466
168.5	34.91	58.82	109.68	1517	35.53	59.86	108.64	1502	36.14	60.90	107.60	1488	36.76	61.94	106.56	1474
169	34.78	58.78	110.22	1524	35.40	59.82	109.18	1510	36.01	60.86	108.14	1496	36.62	61.89	107.11	1481
169.5	34.66	58.74	110.76	1532	35.27	59.78	109.72	1517	35.88	60.82	108.68	1503	36.49	61.85	107.65	1489
170	34.53	58.70	111.30	1539	35.14	59.74	110.26	1525	35.75	60.78	109.23	1511	36.36	61.81	108.19	1496
170.5	34.40	58.66	111.84	1547	35.01	59.70	110.80	1532	35.62	60.73	109.77	1518	36.23	61.77	108.73	1504
171	34.28	58.62	112.38	1554	34.89	59.66	111.34	1540	35.49	60.69	110.31	1526	36.10	61.73	109.27	1511
171.5	34.16	58.58	112.92	1562	34.76	59.61	111.89	1547	35.37	60.65	110.85	1533	35.97	61.69	109.81	1519
172	34.03	58.54	113.46	1569	34.64	59.57	112.43	1555	35.24	60.61	111.39	1541	35.84	61.65	110.35	1526
172.5	33.91	58.50	114.01	1577	34.51	59.53	112.97	1562	35.11	60.57	111.93	1548	35.71	61.61	110.89	1534
173	33.79	58.45	114.55	1584	34.39	59.49	113.51	1570	34.99	60.53	112.47	1555	35.59	61.57	111.43	1541
173.5	33.67	58.41	115.09	1592	34.27	59.45	114.05	1577	34.86	60.49	113.01	1563	35.46	61.53	111.97	1549
174	33.55	58.37	115.63	1599	34.14	59.41	114.59	1585	34.74	60.45	113.55	1570	35.34	61.48	112.52	1556
174.5	33.43	58.33	116.17	1607	34.02	59.37	115.13	1592	34.62	60.41	114.09	1578	35.21	61.44	113.06	1564
175	33.31	58.29	116.71	1614	33.90	59.33	115.67	1600	34.49	60.37	114.64	1585	35.09	61.40	113.60	1571
175.5	33.19	58.25	117.25	1622	33.78	59.29	116.21	1607	34.37	60.32	115.18	1593	34.96	61.36	114.14	1579
176	33.07	58.21	117.79	1629	33.66	59.25	116.75	1615	34.25	60.28	115.72	1600	34.84	61.32	114.68	1586
176.5	32.96	58.17	118.33	1637	33.54	59.20	117.30	1622	34.13	60.24	116.26	1608	34.72	61.28	115.22	1593
177	32.84	58.13	118.87	1644	33.43	59.16	117.84	1630	34.01	60.20	116.80	1615	34.60	61.24	115.76	1601
177.5	32.72	58.09	119.42	1652	33.31	59.12	118.38	1637	33.89	60.16	117.34	1623	34.48	61.20	116.30	1608
178	32.61	58.04	119.96	1659	33.19	59.08	118.92	1645	33.77	60.12	117.88	1630	34.36	61.16	116.84	1616
178.5	32.49	58.00	120.50	1666	33.08	59.04	119.46	1652	33.66	60.08	118.42	1638	34.24	61.12	117.38	1623
179	32.38	57.96	121.04	1674	32.96	59.00	120.00	1660	33.54	60.04	118.96	1645	34.12	61.07	117.93	1631
179.5	32.27	57.92	121.58	1681	32.85	58.96	120.54	1667	33.42	60.00	119.50	1653	34.00	61.03	118.47	1638
180	32.16	57.88	122.12	1689	32.73	58.92	121.08	1675	33.31	59.96	120.05	1660	33.88	60.99	119.01	1646
180.5	32.04	57.84	122.66	1696	32.62	58.88	121.62	1682	33.19	59.91	120.59	1668	33.77	60.95	119.55	1653
181	31.93	57.80	123.20	1704	32.51	58.84	122.16	1690	33.08	59.87	121.13	1675	33.65	60.91	120.09	1661
181.5	31.82	57.76	123.74	1711	32.39	58.80	122.71	1697	32.97	59.83	121.67	1683	33.54	60.87	120.63	1668
182	31.71	57.72	124.28	1719	32.28	58.75	123.25	1704	32.85	59.79	122.21	1690	33.42	60.83	121.17	1676
182.5	31.60	57.68	124.83	1726	32.17	58.71	123.79	1712	32.74	59.75	122.75	1698	33.31	60.79	121.71	1683
183	31.49	57.63	125.37	1734	32.06	58.67	124.33	1719	32.63	59.71	123.29	1705	33.19	60.75	122.25	1691
183.5	31.39	57.59	125.91	1741	31.95	58.63	124.87	1727	32.52	59.67	123.83	1713	33.08	60.71	122.79	1698
184	31.28	57.55	126.45	1749	31.84	58.59	125.41	1734	32.41	59.63	124.37	1720	32.97	60.66	123.34	1706
184.5	31.17	57.51	126.99	1756	31.73	58.55	125.95	1742	32.30	59.59	124.91	1728	32.86	60.62	123.88	1713
185	31.06	57.47	127.53	1764	31.63	58.51	126.49	1749	32.19	59.55	125.46	1735	32.75	60.58	124.42	1721
185.5	30.96	57.43	128.07	1771	31.52	58.47	127.03	1757	32.08	59.50	126.00	1743	32.64	60.54	124.96	1728
186	30.85	57.39	128.61	1779	31.41	58.43	127.57	1764	31.97	59.46	126.54	1750	32.53	60.50	125.50	1736
186.5	30.75	57.35	129.15	1786	31.31	58.38	128.12	1772	31.86	59.42	127.08	1757	32.42	60.46	126.04	1743
187	30.64	57.31	129.69	1794	31.20	58.34	128.66	1779	31.75	59.38	127.62	1765	32.31	60.42	126.58	1751
187.5	30.54	57.27	130.24	1801	31.09	58.30	129.20	1787	31.65	59.34	128.16	1772	32.20	60.38	127.12	1758
188	30.44	57.22	130.78	1809	30.99	58.26	129.74	1794	31.54	59.30	128.70	1780	32.09	60.34	127.66	1766
188.5	30.34	57.18	131.32	1816	30.89	58.22	130.28	1802	31.44	59.26	129.24	1787	31.99	60.30	128.20	1773
189	30.23	57.14	131.86	1824	30.78	58.18	130.82	1809	31.33	59.22	129.78	1795	31.88	60.25	128.75	1781
189.5	30.13	57.10	132.40	1831	30.68	58.14	131.36	1817	31.23	59.18	130.32	1802	31.77	60.21	129.29	1788
190	30.03	57.06	132.94	1839	30.58	58.10	131.90	1824	31.12	59.14	130.87	1810	31.67	60.17	129.83	1796
190.5	29.93	57.02	133.48	1846	30.48	58.06	132.44	1832	31.02	59.09	131.41	1817	31.57	60.13	130.37	1803
191	29.83	56.98	134.02	1854	30.37	58.02	132.98	1839	30.92	59.05	131.95	1825	31.46	60.09	130.91	1810
191.5	29.73	56.94	134.56	1861	30.27	57.97	133.53	1847	30.82	59.01	132.49	1832	31.36	60.05	131.45	1818
192	29.63	56.90	135.10	1868	30.17	57.93	134.07	1854	30.71	58.97	133.03	1840	31.25	60.01	131.99	1825
192.5	29.54	56.86	135.65	1876	30.07	57.89	134.61	1862	30.61	58.93	133.57	1847	31.15	59.97	132.53	1833
193	29.44	56.81	136.19	1883	29.97	57.85	135.15	1869	30.51	58.89	134.11	1855	31.05	59.93	133.07	1840
193.5	29.34	56.77	136.73	1891	29.88	57.81	135.69	1877	30.41	58.85	134.65	1862	30.95	59.89	133.61	1848
194	29.24	56.73	137.27	1898	29.78	57.77	136.23	1884	30.31	58.81	135.19	1870	30.85	59.84	134.16	1855
194.5	29.15	56.69	137.81	1906	29.68	57.73	136.77	1892	30.21	58.77	135.73	1877	30.75	59.80	134.70	1863
195	29.05	56.65	138.35	1913	29.58	57.69	137.31	1899	30.12	58.73	136.28	1885	30.65	59.76	135.24	1870
195.5	28.96	56.61	138.89	1921	29.49	57.65	137.85	1907	30.02	58.68	136.82	1892	30.55	59.72	135.78	1878

Body Composition FEMALE 164-195.5 Lb.

Weight: Lb.	Waist: 37 inches Fat: %	Fat: Lb.	LBM: Lb.	RMR: Cal.	37.25 inches Fat: %	Fat: Lb.	LBM: Lb.	RMR: Cal.	37.5 inches Fat: %	Fat: Lb.	LBM: Lb.	RMR: Cal.	37.75 inches Fat: %	Fat: Lb.	LBM: Lb.	RMR: Cal.
164	38.62	63.34	100.66	1392	39.26	64.38	99.62	1378	39.89	65.42	98.58	1363	40.52	66.45	97.55	1349
164.5	38.48	63.30	101.20	1400	39.11	64.34	100.16	1385	39.74	65.38	99.12	1371	40.37	66.41	98.09	1357
165	38.34	63.26	101.74	1407	38.97	64.30	100.70	1393	39.60	65.34	99.67	1378	40.23	66.37	98.63	1364
165.5	38.20	63.22	102.28	1415	38.83	64.26	101.24	1400	39.45	65.29	100.21	1386	40.08	66.33	99.17	1372
166	38.06	63.18	102.82	1422	38.68	64.22	101.78	1408	39.31	65.25	100.75	1393	39.93	66.29	99.71	1379
166.5	37.92	63.14	103.36	1430	38.54	64.17	102.33	1415	39.17	65.21	101.29	1401	39.79	66.25	100.25	1386
167	37.78	63.10	103.90	1437	38.40	64.13	102.87	1423	39.02	65.17	101.83	1408	39.65	66.21	100.79	1394
167.5	37.64	63.06	104.45	1444	38.26	64.09	103.41	1430	38.88	65.13	102.37	1416	39.50	66.17	101.33	1401
168	37.51	63.01	104.99	1452	38.13	64.05	103.95	1438	38.74	65.09	102.91	1423	39.36	66.13	101.87	1409
168.5	37.37	62.97	105.53	1459	37.99	64.01	104.49	1445	38.60	65.05	103.45	1431	39.22	66.09	102.41	1416
169	37.24	62.93	106.07	1467	37.85	63.97	105.03	1453	38.47	65.01	103.99	1438	39.08	66.04	102.96	1424
169.5	37.10	62.89	106.61	1474	37.72	63.93	105.57	1460	38.33	64.97	104.53	1446	38.94	66.00	103.50	1431
170	36.97	62.85	107.15	1482	37.58	63.89	106.11	1468	38.19	64.93	105.08	1453	38.80	65.96	104.04	1439
170.5	36.84	62.81	107.69	1489	37.45	63.85	106.65	1475	38.06	64.88	105.62	1461	38.66	65.92	104.58	1446
171	36.71	62.77	108.23	1497	37.31	63.81	107.19	1482	37.92	64.84	106.16	1468	38.53	65.88	105.12	1454
171.5	36.58	62.73	108.77	1504	37.18	63.76	107.74	1490	37.79	64.80	106.70	1476	38.39	65.84	105.66	1461
172	36.45	62.69	109.31	1512	37.05	63.72	108.28	1497	37.65	64.76	107.24	1483	38.25	65.80	106.20	1469
172.5	36.32	62.65	109.86	1519	36.92	63.68	108.82	1505	37.52	64.72	107.78	1491	38.12	65.76	106.74	1476
173	36.19	62.60	110.40	1527	36.79	63.64	109.36	1512	37.39	64.68	108.32	1498	37.99	65.72	107.28	1484
173.5	36.06	62.56	110.94	1534	36.66	63.60	109.90	1520	37.26	64.64	108.86	1506	37.85	65.68	107.82	1491
174	35.93	62.52	111.48	1542	36.53	63.56	110.44	1527	37.12	64.60	109.40	1513	37.72	65.63	108.37	1499
174.5	35.81	62.48	112.02	1549	36.40	63.52	110.98	1535	36.99	64.56	109.94	1521	37.59	65.59	108.91	1506
175	35.68	62.44	112.56	1557	36.27	63.48	111.52	1542	36.87	64.52	110.49	1528	37.46	65.55	109.45	1514
175.5	35.55	62.40	113.10	1564	36.15	63.44	112.06	1550	36.74	64.47	111.03	1535	37.33	65.51	109.99	1521
176	35.43	62.36	113.64	1572	36.02	63.40	112.60	1557	36.61	64.43	111.57	1543	37.20	65.47	110.53	1529
176.5	35.31	62.32	114.18	1579	35.89	63.35	113.15	1565	36.48	64.39	112.11	1550	37.07	65.43	111.07	1536
177	35.18	62.28	114.72	1587	35.77	63.31	113.69	1572	36.36	64.35	112.65	1558	36.94	65.39	111.61	1544
177.5	35.06	62.24	115.27	1594	35.65	63.27	114.23	1580	36.23	64.31	113.19	1565	36.82	65.35	112.15	1551
178	34.94	62.19	115.81	1602	35.52	63.23	114.77	1587	36.11	64.27	113.73	1573	36.69	65.31	112.69	1559
178.5	34.82	62.15	116.35	1609	35.40	63.19	115.31	1595	35.98	64.23	114.27	1580	36.56	65.27	113.23	1566
179	34.70	62.11	116.89	1617	35.28	63.15	115.85	1602	35.86	64.19	114.81	1588	36.44	65.22	113.78	1574
179.5	34.58	62.07	117.43	1624	35.16	63.11	116.39	1610	35.74	64.15	115.35	1595	36.31	65.18	114.32	1581
180	34.46	62.03	117.97	1632	35.04	63.07	116.93	1617	35.61	64.11	115.90	1603	36.19	65.14	114.86	1588
180.5	34.34	61.99	118.51	1639	34.92	63.03	117.47	1625	35.49	64.06	116.44	1610	36.07	65.10	115.40	1596
181	34.23	61.95	119.05	1646	34.80	62.99	118.01	1632	35.37	64.02	116.98	1618	35.95	65.06	115.94	1603
181.5	34.11	61.91	119.59	1654	34.68	62.94	118.56	1640	35.25	63.98	117.52	1625	35.82	65.02	116.48	1611
182	33.99	61.87	120.13	1661	34.56	62.90	119.10	1647	35.13	63.94	118.06	1633	35.70	64.98	117.02	1618
182.5	33.88	61.83	120.68	1669	34.45	62.86	119.64	1655	35.01	63.90	118.60	1640	35.58	64.94	117.56	1626
183	33.76	61.78	121.22	1676	34.33	62.82	120.18	1662	34.90	63.86	119.14	1648	35.46	64.90	118.10	1633
183.5	33.65	61.74	121.76	1684	34.21	62.78	120.72	1670	34.78	63.82	119.68	1655	35.34	64.86	118.64	1641
184	33.53	61.70	122.30	1691	34.10	62.74	121.26	1677	34.66	63.78	120.22	1663	35.23	64.81	119.19	1648
184.5	33.42	61.66	122.84	1699	33.98	62.70	121.80	1685	34.55	63.74	120.76	1670	35.11	64.77	119.73	1656
185	33.31	61.62	123.38	1706	33.87	62.66	122.34	1692	34.43	63.70	121.31	1678	34.99	64.73	120.27	1663
185.5	33.20	61.58	123.92	1714	33.76	62.62	122.88	1699	34.31	63.65	121.85	1685	34.87	64.69	120.81	1671
186	33.08	61.54	124.46	1721	33.64	62.58	123.42	1707	34.20	63.61	122.39	1693	34.76	64.65	121.35	1678
186.5	32.97	61.50	125.00	1729	33.53	62.53	123.97	1714	34.09	63.57	122.93	1700	34.64	64.61	121.89	1686
187	32.86	61.46	125.54	1736	33.42	62.49	124.51	1722	33.97	63.53	123.47	1708	34.53	64.57	122.43	1693
187.5	32.75	61.42	126.09	1744	33.31	62.45	125.05	1729	33.86	63.49	124.01	1715	34.41	64.53	122.97	1701
188	32.65	61.37	126.63	1751	33.20	62.41	125.59	1737	33.75	63.45	124.55	1723	34.30	64.49	123.51	1708
188.5	32.54	61.33	127.17	1759	33.09	62.37	126.13	1744	33.64	63.41	125.09	1730	34.19	64.45	124.05	1716
189	32.43	61.29	127.71	1766	32.98	62.33	126.67	1752	33.53	63.37	125.63	1738	34.08	64.40	124.60	1723
189.5	32.32	61.25	128.25	1774	32.87	62.29	127.21	1759	33.42	63.33	126.17	1745	33.96	64.36	125.14	1731
190	32.22	61.21	128.79	1781	32.76	62.25	127.75	1767	33.31	63.29	126.72	1752	33.85	64.32	125.68	1738
190.5	32.11	61.17	129.33	1789	32.65	62.21	128.29	1774	33.20	63.24	127.26	1760	33.74	64.28	126.22	1746
191	32.00	61.13	129.87	1796	32.55	62.17	128.83	1782	33.09	63.20	127.80	1767	33.63	64.24	126.76	1753
191.5	31.90	61.09	130.41	1804	32.44	62.12	129.38	1789	32.98	63.16	128.34	1775	33.52	64.20	127.30	1761
192	31.79	61.05	130.95	1811	32.34	62.08	129.92	1797	32.88	63.12	128.88	1782	33.42	64.16	127.84	1768
192.5	31.69	61.01	131.50	1819	32.23	62.04	130.46	1804	32.77	63.08	129.42	1790	33.31	64.12	128.38	1776
193	31.59	60.96	132.04	1826	32.13	62.00	131.00	1812	32.66	63.04	129.96	1797	33.20	64.08	128.92	1783
193.5	31.48	60.92	132.58	1834	32.02	61.96	131.54	1819	32.56	63.00	130.50	1805	33.09	64.04	129.46	1790
194	31.38	60.88	133.12	1841	31.92	61.92	132.08	1827	32.45	62.96	131.04	1812	32.99	63.99	130.01	1798
194.5	31.28	60.84	133.66	1849	31.81	61.88	132.62	1834	32.35	62.92	131.58	1820	32.88	63.95	130.55	1805
195	31.18	60.80	134.20	1856	31.71	61.84	133.16	1842	32.24	62.88	132.13	1827	32.78	63.91	131.09	1813
195.5	31.08	60.76	134.74	1863	31.61	61.80	133.70	1849	32.14	62.83	132.67	1835	32.67	63.87	131.63	1820

Body Composition FEMALE 164-195.5 Lb.

Weight: Lb.	Waist: 38 inches Fat: %	Fat: Lb.	LBM: Lb.	RMR: Cal.	38.25 inches Fat: %	Fat: Lb.	LBM: Lb.	RMR: Cal.	38.5 inches Fat: %	Fat: Lb.	LBM: Lb.	RMR: Cal.	38.75 inches Fat: %	Fat: Lb.	LBM: Lb.	RMR: Cal.
164	41.15	67.49	96.51	1335	41.79	68.53	95.47	1320	42.42	69.57	94.43	1306	43.05	70.60	93.40	1292
164.5	41.00	67.45	97.05	1342	41.63	68.49	96.01	1328	42.27	69.53	94.97	1313	42.90	70.56	93.94	1299
165	40.85	67.41	97.59	1350	41.48	68.45	96.55	1335	42.11	69.49	95.52	1321	42.74	70.52	94.48	1307
165.5	40.71	67.37	98.13	1357	41.33	68.41	97.09	1343	41.96	69.44	96.06	1328	42.59	70.48	95.02	1314
166	40.56	67.33	98.67	1365	41.18	68.37	97.63	1350	41.81	69.40	96.60	1336	42.43	70.44	95.56	1322
166.5	40.41	67.29	99.21	1372	41.04	68.32	98.18	1358	41.66	69.36	97.14	1343	42.28	70.40	96.10	1329
167	40.27	67.25	99.75	1380	40.89	68.28	98.72	1365	41.51	69.32	97.68	1351	42.13	70.36	96.64	1337
167.5	40.12	67.21	100.30	1387	40.74	68.24	99.26	1373	41.36	69.28	98.22	1358	41.98	70.32	97.18	1344
168	39.98	67.16	100.84	1395	40.60	68.20	99.80	1380	41.21	69.24	98.76	1366	41.83	70.28	97.72	1352
168.5	39.84	67.12	101.38	1402	40.45	68.16	100.34	1388	41.07	69.20	99.30	1373	41.68	70.24	98.26	1359
169	39.69	67.08	101.92	1410	40.31	68.12	100.88	1395	40.92	69.16	99.84	1381	41.54	70.19	98.81	1366
169.5	39.55	67.04	102.46	1417	40.16	68.08	101.42	1403	40.78	69.12	100.38	1388	41.39	70.15	99.35	1374
170	39.41	67.00	103.00	1424	40.02	68.04	101.96	1410	40.63	69.08	100.93	1396	41.24	70.11	99.89	1381
170.5	39.27	66.96	103.54	1432	39.88	68.00	102.50	1418	40.49	69.03	101.47	1403	41.10	70.07	100.43	1389
171	39.13	66.92	104.08	1439	39.74	67.96	103.04	1425	40.35	68.99	102.01	1411	40.95	70.03	100.97	1396
171.5	39.00	66.88	104.62	1447	39.60	67.91	103.59	1433	40.21	68.95	102.55	1418	40.81	69.99	101.51	1404
172	38.86	66.84	105.16	1454	39.46	67.87	104.13	1440	40.06	68.91	103.09	1426	40.67	69.95	102.05	1411
172.5	38.72	66.80	105.71	1462	39.32	67.83	104.67	1448	39.92	68.87	103.63	1433	40.53	69.91	102.59	1419
173	38.59	66.75	106.25	1469	39.19	67.79	105.21	1455	39.79	68.83	104.17	1441	40.39	69.87	103.13	1426
173.5	38.45	66.71	106.79	1477	39.05	67.75	105.75	1463	39.65	68.79	104.71	1448	40.25	69.83	103.67	1434
174	38.32	66.67	107.33	1484	38.91	67.71	106.29	1470	39.51	68.75	105.25	1456	40.11	69.78	104.22	1441
174.5	38.18	66.63	107.87	1492	38.78	67.67	106.83	1477	39.37	68.71	105.79	1463	39.97	69.74	104.76	1449
175	38.05	66.59	108.41	1499	38.64	67.63	107.37	1485	39.24	68.67	106.34	1471	39.83	69.70	105.30	1456
175.5	37.92	66.55	108.95	1507	38.51	67.59	107.91	1492	39.10	68.62	106.88	1478	39.69	69.66	105.84	1464
176	37.79	66.51	109.49	1514	38.38	67.55	108.45	1500	38.97	68.58	107.42	1486	39.56	69.62	106.38	1471
176.5	37.66	66.47	110.03	1522	38.25	67.50	109.00	1507	38.83	68.54	107.96	1493	39.42	69.58	106.92	1479
177	37.53	66.43	110.57	1529	38.11	67.46	109.54	1515	38.70	68.50	108.50	1501	39.29	69.54	107.46	1486
177.5	37.40	66.39	111.12	1537	37.98	67.42	110.08	1522	38.57	68.46	109.04	1508	39.15	69.50	108.00	1494
178	37.27	66.34	111.66	1544	37.85	67.38	110.62	1530	38.44	68.42	109.58	1516	39.02	69.46	108.54	1501
178.5	37.14	66.30	112.20	1552	37.73	67.34	111.16	1537	38.31	68.38	110.12	1523	38.89	69.42	109.08	1509
179	37.02	66.26	112.74	1559	37.60	67.30	111.70	1545	38.18	68.34	110.66	1530	38.76	69.37	109.63	1516
179.5	36.89	66.22	113.28	1567	37.47	67.26	112.24	1552	38.05	68.30	111.20	1538	38.63	69.33	110.17	1524
180	36.77	66.18	113.82	1574	37.34	67.22	112.78	1560	37.92	68.26	111.75	1545	38.50	69.29	110.71	1531
180.5	36.64	66.14	114.36	1582	37.22	67.18	113.32	1567	37.79	68.21	112.29	1553	38.37	69.25	111.25	1539
181	36.52	66.10	114.90	1589	37.09	67.14	113.86	1575	37.66	68.17	112.83	1560	38.24	69.21	111.79	1546
181.5	36.40	66.06	115.44	1597	36.97	67.09	114.41	1582	37.54	68.13	113.37	1568	38.11	69.17	112.33	1554
182	36.27	66.02	115.98	1604	36.84	67.05	114.95	1590	37.41	68.09	113.91	1575	37.98	69.13	112.87	1561
182.5	36.15	65.98	116.53	1612	36.72	67.01	115.49	1597	37.29	68.05	114.45	1583	37.86	69.09	113.41	1568
183	36.03	65.93	117.07	1619	36.60	66.97	116.03	1605	37.16	68.01	114.99	1590	37.73	69.05	113.95	1576
183.5	35.91	65.89	117.61	1627	36.47	66.93	116.57	1612	37.04	67.97	115.53	1598	37.61	69.01	114.49	1583
184	35.79	65.85	118.15	1634	36.35	66.89	117.11	1620	36.92	67.93	116.07	1605	37.48	68.96	115.04	1591
184.5	35.67	65.81	118.69	1641	36.23	66.85	117.65	1627	36.79	67.89	116.61	1613	37.36	68.92	115.58	1598
185	35.55	65.77	119.23	1649	36.11	66.81	118.19	1635	36.67	67.85	117.16	1620	37.23	68.88	116.12	1606
185.5	35.43	65.73	119.77	1656	35.99	66.77	118.73	1642	36.55	67.80	117.70	1628	37.11	68.84	116.66	1613
186	35.32	65.69	120.31	1664	35.87	66.73	119.27	1650	36.43	67.76	118.24	1635	36.99	68.80	117.20	1621
186.5	35.20	65.65	120.85	1671	35.76	66.68	119.82	1657	36.31	67.72	118.78	1643	36.87	68.76	117.74	1628
187	35.08	65.61	121.39	1679	35.64	66.64	120.36	1665	36.19	67.68	119.32	1650	36.75	68.72	118.28	1636
187.5	34.97	65.57	121.94	1686	35.52	66.60	120.90	1672	36.07	67.64	119.86	1658	36.63	68.68	118.82	1643
188	34.85	65.52	122.48	1694	35.41	66.56	121.44	1679	35.96	67.60	120.40	1665	36.51	68.64	119.36	1651
188.5	34.74	65.48	123.02	1701	35.29	66.52	121.98	1687	35.84	67.56	120.94	1673	36.39	68.60	119.90	1658
189	34.63	65.44	123.56	1709	35.17	66.48	122.52	1694	35.72	67.52	121.48	1680	36.27	68.55	120.45	1666
189.5	34.51	65.40	124.10	1716	35.06	66.44	123.06	1702	35.61	67.48	122.02	1688	36.15	68.51	120.99	1673
190	34.40	65.36	124.64	1724	34.95	66.40	123.60	1709	35.49	67.44	122.57	1695	36.04	68.47	121.53	1681
190.5	34.29	65.32	125.18	1731	34.83	66.36	124.14	1717	35.38	67.39	123.11	1703	35.92	68.43	122.07	1688
191	34.18	65.28	125.72	1739	34.72	66.32	124.68	1724	35.26	67.35	123.65	1710	35.81	68.39	122.61	1696
191.5	34.07	65.24	126.26	1746	34.61	66.27	125.23	1732	35.15	67.31	124.19	1718	35.69	68.35	123.15	1703
192	33.96	65.20	126.80	1754	34.50	66.23	125.77	1739	35.04	67.27	124.73	1725	35.58	68.31	123.69	1711
192.5	33.85	65.16	127.35	1761	34.39	66.19	126.31	1747	34.92	67.23	125.27	1732	35.46	68.27	124.23	1718
193	33.74	65.11	127.89	1769	34.28	66.15	126.85	1754	34.81	67.19	125.81	1740	35.35	68.23	124.77	1726
193.5	33.63	65.07	128.43	1776	34.17	66.11	127.39	1762	34.70	67.15	126.35	1747	35.24	68.19	125.31	1733
194	33.52	65.03	128.97	1784	34.06	66.07	127.93	1769	34.59	67.11	126.89	1755	35.13	68.14	125.86	1741
194.5	33.41	64.99	129.51	1791	33.95	66.03	128.47	1777	34.48	67.07	127.43	1762	35.01	68.10	126.40	1748
195	33.31	64.95	130.05	1799	33.84	65.99	129.01	1784	34.37	67.03	127.98	1770	34.90	68.06	126.94	1756
195.5	33.20	64.91	130.59	1806	33.73	65.95	129.55	1792	34.26	66.98	128.52	1777	34.79	68.02	127.48	1763

Body Composition   FEMALE   164-195.5 Lb.

Weight: Lb.	Waist: 39 inches Fat: %	Fat: Lb.	LBM: Lb.	RMR: Cal.	39.25 inches Fat: %	Fat: Lb.	LBM: Lb.	RMR: Cal.	39.5 inches Fat: %	Fat: Lb.	LBM: Lb.	RMR: Cal.	39.75 inches Fat: %	Fat: Lb.	LBM: Lb.	RMR: Cal.
164	43.68	71.64	92.36	1277	44.32	72.68	91.32	1263	44.95	73.72	90.28	1249	45.58	74.75	89.25	1234
164.5	43.53	71.60	92.90	1285	44.16	72.64	91.86	1270	44.79	73.68	90.82	1256	45.42	74.71	89.79	1242
165	43.37	71.56	93.44	1292	44.00	72.60	92.40	1278	44.63	73.64	91.37	1264	45.26	74.67	90.33	1249
165.5	43.21	71.52	93.98	1300	43.84	72.56	92.94	1285	44.47	73.59	91.91	1271	45.09	74.63	90.87	1257
166	43.06	71.48	94.52	1307	43.68	72.52	93.48	1293	44.31	73.55	92.45	1279	44.93	74.59	91.41	1264
166.5	42.91	71.44	95.06	1315	43.53	72.47	94.03	1300	44.15	73.51	92.99	1286	44.77	74.55	91.95	1272
167	42.75	71.40	95.60	1322	43.37	72.43	94.57	1308	43.99	73.47	93.53	1294	44.62	74.51	92.49	1279
167.5	42.60	71.36	96.15	1330	43.22	72.39	95.11	1315	43.84	73.43	94.07	1301	44.46	74.47	93.03	1287
168	42.45	71.31	96.69	1337	43.07	72.35	95.65	1323	43.68	73.39	94.61	1308	44.30	74.43	93.57	1294
168.5	42.30	71.27	97.23	1345	42.91	72.31	96.19	1330	43.53	73.35	95.15	1316	44.15	74.39	94.11	1302
169	42.15	71.23	97.77	1352	42.76	72.27	96.73	1338	43.38	73.31	95.69	1323	43.99	74.34	94.66	1309
169.5	42.00	71.19	98.31	1360	42.61	72.23	97.27	1345	43.22	73.27	96.23	1331	43.84	74.30	95.20	1317
170	41.85	71.15	98.85	1367	42.46	72.19	97.81	1353	43.07	73.23	96.78	1338	43.68	74.26	95.74	1324
170.5	41.71	71.11	99.39	1375	42.31	72.15	98.35	1360	42.92	73.18	97.32	1346	43.53	74.22	96.28	1332
171	41.56	71.07	99.93	1382	42.17	72.11	98.89	1368	42.77	73.14	97.86	1353	43.38	74.18	96.82	1339
171.5	41.42	71.03	100.47	1390	42.02	72.06	99.44	1375	42.63	73.10	98.40	1361	43.23	74.14	97.36	1346
172	41.27	70.99	101.01	1397	41.87	72.02	99.98	1383	42.48	73.06	98.94	1368	43.08	74.10	97.90	1354
172.5	41.13	70.95	101.56	1405	41.73	71.98	100.52	1390	42.33	73.02	99.48	1376	42.93	74.06	98.44	1361
173	40.98	70.90	102.10	1412	41.58	71.94	101.06	1398	42.18	72.98	100.02	1383	42.78	74.02	98.98	1369
173.5	40.84	70.86	102.64	1419	41.44	71.90	101.60	1405	42.04	72.94	100.56	1391	42.64	73.98	99.52	1376
174	40.70	70.82	103.18	1427	41.30	71.86	102.14	1413	41.89	72.90	101.10	1398	42.49	73.93	100.07	1384
174.5	40.56	70.78	103.72	1434	41.16	71.82	102.68	1420	41.75	72.86	101.64	1406	42.35	73.89	100.61	1391
175	40.42	70.74	104.26	1442	41.02	71.78	103.22	1428	41.61	72.82	102.19	1413	42.20	73.85	101.15	1399
175.5	40.28	70.70	104.80	1449	40.88	71.74	103.76	1435	41.47	72.77	102.73	1421	42.06	73.81	101.69	1406
176	40.15	70.66	105.34	1457	40.74	71.70	104.30	1443	41.33	72.73	103.27	1428	41.92	73.77	102.23	1414
176.5	40.01	70.62	105.88	1464	40.60	71.65	104.85	1450	41.19	72.69	103.81	1436	41.77	73.73	102.77	1421
177	39.87	70.58	106.42	1472	40.46	71.61	105.39	1457	41.05	72.65	104.35	1443	41.63	73.69	103.31	1429
177.5	39.74	70.54	106.97	1479	40.32	71.57	105.93	1465	40.91	72.61	104.89	1451	41.49	73.65	103.85	1436
178	39.60	70.49	107.51	1487	40.19	71.53	106.47	1472	40.77	72.57	105.43	1458	41.35	73.61	104.39	1444
178.5	39.47	70.45	108.05	1494	40.05	71.49	107.01	1480	40.63	72.53	105.97	1466	41.21	73.57	104.93	1451
179	39.34	70.41	108.59	1502	39.92	71.45	107.55	1487	40.50	72.49	106.51	1473	41.08	73.52	105.48	1459
179.5	39.20	70.37	109.13	1509	39.78	71.41	108.09	1495	40.36	72.45	107.05	1481	40.94	73.48	106.02	1466
180	39.07	70.33	109.67	1517	39.65	71.37	108.63	1502	40.23	72.41	107.60	1488	40.80	73.44	106.56	1474
180.5	38.94	70.29	110.21	1524	39.52	71.33	109.17	1510	40.09	72.36	108.14	1496	40.67	73.40	107.10	1481
181	38.81	70.25	110.75	1532	39.38	71.29	109.71	1517	39.96	72.32	108.68	1503	40.53	73.36	107.64	1489
181.5	38.68	70.21	111.29	1539	39.25	71.24	110.26	1525	39.82	72.28	109.22	1510	40.40	73.32	108.18	1496
182	38.55	70.17	111.83	1547	39.12	71.20	110.80	1532	39.69	72.24	109.76	1518	40.26	73.28	108.72	1504
182.5	38.42	70.13	112.38	1554	38.99	71.16	111.34	1540	39.56	72.20	110.30	1525	40.13	73.24	109.26	1511
183	38.30	70.08	112.92	1562	38.86	71.12	111.88	1547	39.43	72.16	110.84	1533	40.00	73.20	109.80	1519
183.5	38.17	70.04	113.46	1569	38.74	71.08	112.42	1555	39.30	72.12	111.38	1540	39.87	73.16	110.34	1526
184	38.04	70.00	114.00	1577	38.61	71.04	112.96	1562	39.17	72.08	111.92	1548	39.74	73.11	110.89	1534
184.5	37.92	69.96	114.54	1584	38.48	71.00	113.50	1570	39.04	72.04	112.46	1555	39.61	73.07	111.43	1541
185	37.79	69.92	115.08	1592	38.36	70.96	114.04	1577	38.92	72.00	113.01	1563	39.48	73.03	111.97	1549
185.5	37.67	69.88	115.62	1599	38.23	70.92	114.58	1585	38.79	71.95	113.55	1570	39.35	72.99	112.51	1556
186	37.55	69.84	116.16	1607	38.11	70.88	115.12	1592	38.66	71.91	114.09	1578	39.22	72.95	113.05	1563
186.5	37.42	69.80	116.70	1614	37.98	70.83	115.67	1600	38.54	71.87	114.63	1585	39.09	72.91	113.59	1571
187	37.30	69.76	117.24	1621	37.86	70.79	116.21	1607	38.41	71.83	115.17	1593	38.97	72.87	114.13	1578
187.5	37.18	69.72	117.79	1629	37.73	70.75	116.75	1615	38.29	71.79	115.71	1600	38.84	72.83	114.67	1586
188	37.06	69.67	118.33	1636	37.61	70.71	117.29	1622	38.16	71.75	116.25	1608	38.72	72.79	115.21	1593
188.5	36.94	69.63	118.87	1644	37.49	70.67	117.83	1630	38.04	71.71	116.79	1615	38.59	72.75	115.75	1601
189	36.82	69.59	119.41	1651	37.37	70.63	118.37	1637	37.92	71.67	117.33	1623	38.47	72.70	116.30	1608
189.5	36.70	69.55	119.95	1659	37.25	70.59	118.91	1645	37.80	71.63	117.87	1630	38.34	72.66	116.84	1616
190	36.58	69.51	120.49	1666	37.13	70.55	119.45	1652	37.68	71.59	118.42	1638	38.22	72.62	117.38	1623
190.5	36.47	69.47	121.03	1674	37.01	70.51	119.99	1660	37.56	71.54	118.96	1645	38.10	72.58	117.92	1631
191	36.35	69.43	121.57	1681	36.89	70.47	120.53	1667	37.44	71.50	119.50	1653	37.98	72.54	118.46	1638
191.5	36.23	69.39	122.11	1689	36.78	70.42	121.08	1674	37.32	71.46	120.04	1660	37.86	72.50	119.00	1646
192	36.12	69.35	122.65	1696	36.66	70.38	121.62	1682	37.20	71.42	120.58	1668	37.74	72.46	119.54	1653
192.5	36.00	69.31	123.20	1704	36.54	70.34	122.16	1689	37.08	71.38	121.12	1675	37.62	72.42	120.08	1661
193	35.89	69.26	123.74	1711	36.43	70.30	122.70	1697	36.96	71.34	121.66	1683	37.50	72.38	120.62	1668
193.5	35.77	69.22	124.28	1719	36.31	70.26	123.24	1704	36.85	71.30	122.20	1690	37.38	72.34	121.16	1676
194	35.66	69.18	124.82	1726	36.20	70.22	123.78	1712	36.73	71.26	122.74	1698	37.27	72.29	121.71	1683
194.5	35.55	69.14	125.36	1734	36.08	70.18	124.32	1719	36.61	71.22	123.28	1705	37.15	72.25	122.25	1691
195	35.44	69.10	125.90	1741	35.97	70.14	124.86	1727	36.50	71.18	123.83	1712	37.03	72.21	122.79	1698
195.5	35.32	69.06	126.44	1749	35.85	70.10	125.40	1734	36.39	71.13	124.37	1720	36.92	72.17	123.33	1706

Body Composition FEMALE 164-195.5 Lb.

Weight: Lb.	Waist: 40 inches Fat: %	Fat: Lb.	LBM: Lb.	RMR: Cal.	40.25 inches Fat: %	Fat: Lb.	LBM: Lb.	RMR: Cal.	40.5 inches Fat: %	Fat: Lb.	LBM: Lb.	RMR: Cal.	40.75 inches Fat: %	Fat: Lb.	LBM: Lb.	RMR: Cal.
164	46.21	75.79	88.21	1220	46.85	76.83	87.17	1206	47.48	77.87	86.13	1191	48.11	78.90	85.10	1177
164.5	46.05	75.75	88.75	1227	46.68	76.79	87.71	1213	47.31	77.83	86.67	1199	47.94	78.86	85.64	1184
165	45.88	75.71	89.29	1235	46.51	76.75	88.25	1221	47.14	77.79	87.22	1206	47.77	78.82	86.18	1192
165.5	45.72	75.67	89.83	1242	46.35	76.71	88.79	1228	46.98	77.74	87.76	1214	47.60	78.78	86.72	1199
166	45.56	75.63	90.37	1250	46.18	76.67	89.33	1235	46.81	77.70	88.30	1221	47.43	78.74	87.26	1207
166.5	45.40	75.59	90.91	1257	46.02	76.62	89.88	1243	46.64	77.66	88.84	1229	47.27	78.70	87.80	1214
167	45.24	75.55	91.45	1265	45.86	76.58	90.42	1250	46.48	77.62	89.38	1236	47.10	78.66	88.34	1222
167.5	45.08	75.51	92.00	1272	45.70	76.54	90.96	1258	46.32	77.58	89.92	1244	46.94	78.62	88.88	1229
168	44.92	75.46	92.54	1280	45.54	76.50	91.50	1265	46.15	77.54	90.46	1251	46.77	78.58	89.42	1237
168.5	44.76	75.42	93.08	1287	45.38	76.46	92.04	1273	45.99	77.50	91.00	1259	46.61	78.54	89.96	1244
169	44.60	75.38	93.62	1295	45.22	76.42	92.58	1280	45.83	77.46	91.54	1266	46.45	78.49	90.51	1252
169.5	44.45	75.34	94.16	1302	45.06	76.38	93.12	1288	45.67	77.42	92.08	1274	46.29	78.45	91.05	1259
170	44.29	75.30	94.70	1310	44.90	76.34	93.66	1295	45.51	77.38	92.63	1281	46.13	78.41	91.59	1267
170.5	44.14	75.26	95.24	1317	44.75	76.30	94.20	1303	45.36	77.33	93.17	1288	45.97	78.37	92.13	1274
171	43.99	75.22	95.78	1325	44.59	76.26	94.74	1310	45.20	77.29	93.71	1296	45.81	78.33	92.67	1282
171.5	43.83	75.18	96.32	1332	44.44	76.21	95.29	1318	45.04	77.25	94.25	1303	45.65	78.29	93.21	1289
172	43.68	75.14	96.86	1340	44.29	76.17	95.83	1325	44.89	77.21	94.79	1311	45.49	78.25	93.75	1297
172.5	43.53	75.10	97.41	1347	44.13	76.13	96.37	1333	44.74	77.17	95.33	1318	45.34	78.21	94.29	1304
173	43.38	75.05	97.95	1355	43.98	76.09	96.91	1340	44.58	77.13	95.87	1326	45.18	78.17	94.83	1312
173.5	43.24	75.01	98.49	1362	43.83	76.05	97.45	1348	44.43	77.09	96.41	1333	45.03	78.13	95.37	1319
174	43.09	74.97	99.03	1370	43.68	76.01	97.99	1355	44.28	77.05	96.95	1341	44.88	78.08	95.92	1327
174.5	42.94	74.93	99.57	1377	43.53	75.97	98.53	1363	44.13	77.01	97.49	1348	44.72	78.04	96.46	1334
175	42.79	74.89	100.11	1385	43.39	75.93	99.07	1370	43.98	76.97	98.04	1356	44.57	78.00	97.00	1341
175.5	42.65	74.85	100.65	1392	43.24	75.89	99.61	1378	43.83	76.92	98.58	1363	44.42	77.96	97.54	1349
176	42.50	74.81	101.19	1399	43.09	75.85	100.15	1385	43.68	76.88	99.12	1371	44.27	77.92	98.08	1356
176.5	42.36	74.77	101.73	1407	42.95	75.80	100.70	1393	43.54	76.84	99.66	1378	44.12	77.88	98.62	1364
177	42.22	74.73	102.27	1414	42.80	75.76	101.24	1400	43.39	76.80	100.20	1386	43.98	77.84	99.16	1371
177.5	42.08	74.69	102.82	1422	42.66	75.72	101.78	1408	43.25	76.76	100.74	1393	43.83	77.80	99.70	1379
178	41.93	74.64	103.36	1429	42.52	75.68	102.32	1415	43.10	76.72	101.28	1401	43.68	77.76	100.24	1386
178.5	41.79	74.60	103.90	1437	42.38	75.64	102.86	1423	42.96	76.68	101.82	1408	43.54	77.72	100.78	1394
179	41.65	74.56	104.44	1444	42.23	75.60	103.40	1430	42.81	76.64	102.36	1416	43.39	77.67	101.33	1401
179.5	41.52	74.52	104.98	1452	42.09	75.56	103.94	1438	42.67	76.60	102.90	1423	43.25	77.63	101.87	1409
180	41.38	74.48	105.52	1459	41.95	75.52	104.48	1445	42.53	76.56	103.45	1431	43.11	77.59	102.41	1416
180.5	41.24	74.44	106.06	1467	41.82	75.48	105.02	1452	42.39	76.51	103.99	1438	42.96	77.55	102.95	1424
181	41.10	74.40	106.60	1474	41.68	75.44	105.56	1460	42.25	76.47	104.53	1446	42.82	77.51	103.49	1431
181.5	40.97	74.36	107.14	1482	41.54	75.39	106.11	1467	42.11	76.43	105.07	1453	42.68	77.47	104.03	1439
182	40.83	74.32	107.68	1489	41.40	75.35	106.65	1475	41.97	76.39	105.61	1461	42.54	77.43	104.57	1446
182.5	40.70	74.28	108.23	1497	41.27	75.31	107.19	1482	41.84	76.35	106.15	1468	42.40	77.39	105.11	1454
183	40.57	74.23	108.77	1504	41.13	75.27	107.73	1490	41.70	76.31	106.69	1476	42.27	77.35	105.65	1461
183.5	40.43	74.19	109.31	1512	41.00	75.23	108.27	1497	41.56	76.27	107.23	1483	42.13	77.31	106.19	1469
184	40.30	74.15	109.85	1519	40.86	75.19	108.81	1505	41.43	76.23	107.77	1491	41.99	77.26	106.74	1476
184.5	40.17	74.11	110.39	1527	40.73	75.15	109.35	1512	41.29	76.19	108.31	1498	41.86	77.22	107.28	1484
185	40.04	74.07	110.93	1534	40.60	75.11	109.89	1520	41.16	76.15	108.86	1505	41.72	77.18	107.82	1491
185.5	39.91	74.03	111.47	1542	40.47	75.07	110.43	1527	41.03	76.10	109.40	1513	41.59	77.14	108.36	1499
186	39.78	73.99	112.01	1549	40.34	75.03	110.97	1535	40.89	76.06	109.94	1520	41.45	77.10	108.90	1506
186.5	39.65	73.95	112.55	1557	40.21	74.98	111.52	1542	40.76	76.02	110.48	1528	41.32	77.06	109.44	1514
187	39.52	73.91	113.09	1564	40.08	74.94	112.06	1550	40.63	75.98	111.02	1535	41.19	77.02	109.98	1521
187.5	39.39	73.87	113.64	1572	39.95	74.90	112.60	1557	40.50	75.94	111.56	1543	41.05	76.98	110.52	1529
188	39.27	73.82	114.18	1579	39.82	74.86	113.14	1565	40.37	75.90	112.10	1550	40.92	76.94	111.06	1536
188.5	39.14	73.78	114.72	1587	39.69	74.82	113.68	1572	40.24	75.86	112.64	1558	40.79	76.90	111.60	1543
189	39.02	73.74	115.26	1594	39.57	74.78	114.22	1580	40.11	75.82	113.18	1565	40.66	76.85	112.15	1551
189.5	38.89	73.70	115.80	1602	39.44	74.74	114.76	1587	39.99	75.78	113.72	1573	40.53	76.81	112.69	1558
190	38.77	73.66	116.34	1609	39.31	74.70	115.30	1595	39.86	75.74	114.27	1580	40.41	76.77	113.23	1566
190.5	38.65	73.62	116.88	1616	39.19	74.66	115.84	1602	39.73	75.69	114.81	1588	40.28	76.73	113.77	1573
191	38.52	73.58	117.42	1624	39.07	74.62	116.38	1610	39.61	75.65	115.35	1595	40.15	76.69	114.31	1581
191.5	38.40	73.54	117.96	1631	38.94	74.57	116.93	1617	39.48	75.61	115.89	1603	40.03	76.65	114.85	1588
192	38.28	73.50	118.50	1639	38.82	74.53	117.47	1625	39.36	75.57	116.43	1610	39.90	76.61	115.39	1596
192.5	38.16	73.46	119.05	1646	38.70	74.49	118.01	1632	39.24	75.53	116.97	1618	39.78	76.57	115.93	1603
193	38.04	73.41	119.59	1654	38.58	74.45	118.55	1640	39.11	75.49	117.51	1625	39.65	76.53	116.47	1611
193.5	37.92	73.37	120.13	1661	38.46	74.41	119.09	1647	38.99	75.45	118.05	1633	39.53	76.49	117.01	1618
194	37.80	73.33	120.67	1669	38.33	74.37	119.63	1654	38.87	75.41	118.59	1640	39.40	76.44	117.56	1626
194.5	37.68	73.29	121.21	1676	38.22	74.33	120.17	1662	38.75	75.37	119.13	1648	39.28	76.40	118.10	1633
195	37.56	73.25	121.75	1684	38.10	74.29	120.71	1669	38.63	75.33	119.68	1655	39.16	76.36	118.64	1641
195.5	37.45	73.21	122.29	1691	37.98	74.25	121.25	1677	38.51	75.28	120.22	1663	39.04	76.32	119.18	1648

Body Composition FEMALE 196-227.5 Lb.

Weight: Lb.	Waist: 35 inches Fat: %	Fat: Lb.	LBM: Lb.	RMR: Cal.	35.25 inches Fat: %	Fat: Lb.	LBM: Lb.	RMR: Cal.	35.5 inches Fat: %	Fat: Lb.	LBM: Lb.	RMR: Cal.	35.75 inches Fat: %	Fat: Lb.	LBM: Lb.	RMR: Cal.
196	26.74	52.42	143.58	1986	27.27	53.46	142.54	1971	27.80	54.49	141.51	1957	28.33	55.53	140.47	1943
196.5	26.65	52.38	144.12	1993	27.18	53.41	143.09	1979	27.71	54.45	142.05	1965	28.24	55.49	141.01	1950
197	26.57	52.34	144.66	2001	27.09	53.37	143.63	1986	27.62	54.41	142.59	1972	28.15	55.45	141.55	1958
197.5	26.48	52.30	145.21	2008	27.00	53.33	144.17	1994	27.53	54.37	143.13	1979	28.05	55.41	142.09	1965
198	26.39	52.25	145.75	2016	26.91	53.29	144.71	2001	27.44	54.33	143.67	1987	27.96	55.37	142.63	1973
198.5	26.30	52.21	146.29	2023	26.83	53.25	145.25	2009	27.35	54.29	144.21	1994	27.87	55.33	143.17	1980
199	26.22	52.17	146.83	2031	26.74	53.21	145.79	2016	27.26	54.25	144.75	2002	27.78	55.28	143.72	1988
199.5	26.13	52.13	147.37	2038	26.65	53.17	146.33	2024	27.17	54.21	145.29	2009	27.69	55.24	144.26	1995
200	26.05	52.09	147.91	2046	26.56	53.13	146.87	2031	27.08	54.17	145.84	2017	27.60	55.20	144.80	2003
200.5	25.96	52.05	148.45	2053	26.48	53.09	147.41	2039	26.99	54.12	146.38	2024	27.51	55.16	145.34	2010
201	25.87	52.01	148.99	2061	26.39	53.05	147.95	2046	26.91	54.08	146.92	2032	27.42	55.12	145.88	2018
201.5	25.79	51.97	149.53	2068	26.30	53.00	148.50	2054	26.82	54.04	147.46	2039	27.33	55.08	146.42	2025
202	25.71	51.93	150.07	2076	26.22	52.96	149.04	2061	26.73	54.00	148.00	2047	27.25	55.04	146.96	2032
202.5	25.62	51.89	150.62	2083	26.13	52.92	149.58	2069	26.65	53.96	148.54	2054	27.16	55.00	147.50	2040
203	25.54	51.84	151.16	2090	26.05	52.88	150.12	2076	26.56	53.92	149.08	2062	27.07	54.96	148.04	2047
203.5	25.46	51.80	151.70	2098	25.97	52.84	150.66	2084	26.48	53.88	149.62	2069	26.99	54.92	148.58	2055
204	25.37	51.76	152.24	2105	25.88	52.80	151.20	2091	26.39	53.84	150.16	2077	26.90	54.87	149.13	2062
204.5	25.29	51.72	152.78	2113	25.80	52.76	151.74	2099	26.31	53.80	150.70	2084	26.81	54.83	149.67	2070
205	25.21	51.68	153.32	2120	25.72	52.72	152.28	2106	26.22	53.76	151.25	2092	26.73	54.79	150.21	2077
205.5	25.13	51.64	153.86	2128	25.63	52.68	152.82	2114	26.14	53.71	151.79	2099	26.64	54.75	150.75	2085
206	25.05	51.60	154.40	2135	25.55	52.64	153.36	2121	26.05	53.67	152.33	2107	26.56	54.71	151.29	2092
206.5	24.97	51.56	154.94	2143	25.47	52.59	153.91	2129	25.97	53.63	152.87	2114	26.47	54.67	151.83	2100
207	24.89	51.52	155.48	2150	25.39	52.55	154.45	2136	25.89	53.59	153.41	2122	26.39	54.63	152.37	2107
207.5	24.81	51.48	156.03	2158	25.31	52.51	154.99	2143	25.81	53.55	153.95	2129	26.31	54.59	152.91	2115
208	24.73	51.43	156.57	2165	25.23	52.47	155.53	2151	25.73	53.51	154.49	2137	26.22	54.55	153.45	2122
208.5	24.65	51.39	157.11	2173	25.15	52.43	156.07	2158	25.64	53.47	155.03	2144	26.14	54.51	153.99	2130
209	24.57	51.35	157.65	2180	25.07	52.39	156.61	2166	25.56	53.43	155.57	2152	26.06	54.46	154.54	2137
209.5	24.49	51.31	158.19	2188	24.99	52.35	157.15	2173	25.48	53.39	156.11	2159	25.98	54.42	155.08	2145
210	24.41	51.27	158.73	2195	24.91	52.31	157.69	2181	25.40	53.35	156.66	2167	25.90	54.38	155.62	2152
210.5	24.34	51.23	159.27	2203	24.83	52.27	158.23	2188	25.32	53.30	157.20	2174	25.82	54.34	156.16	2160
211	24.26	51.19	159.81	2210	24.75	52.23	158.77	2196	25.24	53.26	157.74	2182	25.73	54.30	156.70	2167
211.5	24.18	51.15	160.35	2218	24.67	52.18	159.32	2203	25.16	53.22	158.28	2189	25.65	54.26	157.24	2175
212	24.11	51.11	160.89	2225	24.60	52.14	159.86	2211	25.09	53.18	158.82	2196	25.57	54.22	157.78	2182
212.5	24.03	51.07	161.44	2233	24.52	52.10	160.40	2218	25.01	53.14	159.36	2204	25.50	54.18	158.32	2190
213	23.95	51.02	161.98	2240	24.44	52.06	160.94	2226	24.93	53.10	159.90	2211	25.42	54.14	158.86	2197
213.5	23.88	50.98	162.52	2248	24.37	52.02	161.48	2233	24.85	53.06	160.44	2219	25.34	54.10	159.40	2205
214	23.80	50.94	163.06	2255	24.29	51.98	162.02	2241	24.77	53.02	160.98	2226	25.26	54.05	159.95	2212
214.5	23.73	50.90	163.60	2263	24.21	51.94	162.56	2248	24.70	52.98	161.52	2234	25.18	54.01	160.49	2220
215	23.66	50.86	164.14	2270	24.14	51.90	163.10	2256	24.62	52.94	162.07	2241	25.10	53.97	161.03	2227
215.5	23.58	50.82	164.68	2278	24.06	51.86	163.64	2263	24.54	52.89	162.61	2249	25.03	53.93	161.57	2234
216	23.51	50.78	165.22	2285	23.99	51.82	164.18	2271	24.47	52.85	163.15	2256	24.95	53.89	162.11	2242
216.5	23.44	50.74	165.76	2293	23.91	51.77	164.73	2278	24.39	52.81	163.69	2264	24.87	53.85	162.65	2249
217	23.36	50.70	166.30	2300	23.84	51.73	165.27	2286	24.32	52.77	164.23	2271	24.80	53.81	163.19	2257
217.5	23.29	50.66	166.85	2307	23.77	51.69	165.81	2293	24.24	52.73	164.77	2279	24.72	53.77	163.73	2264
218	23.22	50.61	167.39	2315	23.69	51.65	166.35	2301	24.17	52.69	165.31	2286	24.65	53.73	164.27	2272
218.5	23.15	50.57	167.93	2322	23.62	51.61	166.89	2308	24.10	52.65	165.85	2294	24.57	53.69	164.81	2279
219	23.07	50.53	168.47	2330	23.55	51.57	167.43	2316	24.02	52.61	166.39	2301	24.50	53.64	165.36	2287
219.5	23.00	50.49	169.01	2337	23.48	51.53	167.97	2323	23.95	52.57	166.93	2309	24.42	53.60	165.90	2294
220	22.93	50.45	169.55	2345	23.40	51.49	168.51	2331	23.88	52.53	167.48	2316	24.35	53.56	166.44	2302
220.5	22.86	50.41	170.09	2352	23.33	51.45	169.05	2338	23.80	52.48	168.02	2324	24.27	53.52	166.98	2309
221	22.79	50.37	170.63	2360	23.26	51.41	169.59	2345	23.73	52.44	168.56	2331	24.20	53.48	167.52	2317
221.5	22.72	50.33	171.17	2367	23.19	51.36	170.14	2353	23.66	52.40	169.10	2339	24.13	53.44	168.06	2324
222	22.65	50.29	171.71	2375	23.12	51.32	170.68	2360	23.59	52.36	169.64	2346	24.05	53.40	168.60	2332
222.5	22.58	50.25	172.26	2382	23.05	51.28	171.22	2368	23.51	52.32	170.18	2354	23.98	53.36	169.14	2339
223	22.51	50.20	172.80	2390	22.98	51.24	171.76	2375	23.44	52.28	170.72	2361	23.91	53.32	169.68	2347
223.5	22.44	50.16	173.34	2397	22.91	51.20	172.30	2383	23.37	52.24	171.26	2369	23.84	53.28	170.22	2354
224	22.38	50.12	173.88	2405	22.84	51.16	172.84	2390	23.30	52.20	171.80	2376	23.77	53.23	170.77	2362
224.5	22.31	50.08	174.42	2412	22.77	51.12	173.38	2398	23.23	52.16	172.34	2384	23.69	53.19	171.31	2369
225	22.24	50.04	174.96	2420	22.70	51.08	173.92	2405	23.16	52.12	172.89	2391	23.62	53.15	171.85	2377
225.5	22.17	50.00	175.50	2427	22.63	51.04	174.46	2413	23.09	52.07	173.43	2398	23.55	53.11	172.39	2384
226	22.11	49.96	176.04	2435	22.56	51.00	175.00	2420	23.02	52.03	173.97	2406	23.48	53.07	172.93	2392
226.5	22.04	49.92	176.58	2442	22.50	50.95	175.55	2428	22.95	51.99	174.51	2413	23.41	53.03	173.47	2399
227	21.97	49.88	177.12	2450	22.43	50.91	176.09	2435	22.89	51.95	175.05	2421	23.34	52.99	174.01	2407
227.5	21.91	49.84	177.67	2457	22.36	50.87	176.63	2443	22.82	51.91	175.59	2428	23.27	52.95	174.55	2414

Body Composition   FEMALE   196-227.5 Lb.

Weight: Lb.	Waist: 36 inches				36.25 inches				36.5 inches				36.75 inches			
	Fat: %	Fat: Lb.	LBM: Lb.	RMR: Cal.	Fat: %	Fat: Lb.	LBM: Lb.	RMR: Cal.	Fat: %	Fat: Lb.	LBM: Lb.	RMR: Cal.	Fat: %	Fat: Lb.	LBM: Lb.	RMR: Cal.
196	28.86	56.57	139.43	1928	29.39	57.61	138.39	1914	29.92	58.64	137.36	1900	30.45	59.68	136.32	1885
196.5	28.77	56.53	139.97	1936	29.29	57.56	138.94	1921	29.82	58.60	137.90	1907	30.35	59.64	136.86	1893
197	28.67	56.49	140.51	1943	29.20	57.52	139.48	1929	29.73	58.56	138.44	1915	30.25	59.60	137.40	1900
197.5	28.58	56.45	141.06	1951	29.11	57.48	140.02	1936	29.63	58.52	138.98	1922	30.16	59.56	137.94	1908
198	28.49	56.40	141.60	1958	29.01	57.44	140.56	1944	29.53	58.48	139.52	1930	30.06	59.52	138.48	1915
198.5	28.39	56.36	142.14	1966	28.92	57.40	141.10	1951	29.44	58.44	140.06	1937	29.96	59.48	139.02	1923
199	28.30	56.32	142.68	1973	28.82	57.36	141.64	1959	29.35	58.40	140.60	1945	29.87	59.43	139.57	1930
199.5	28.21	56.28	143.22	1981	28.73	57.32	142.18	1966	29.25	58.36	141.14	1952	29.77	59.39	140.11	1938
200	28.12	56.24	143.76	1988	28.64	57.28	142.72	1974	29.16	58.32	141.69	1960	29.68	59.35	140.65	1945
200.5	28.03	56.20	144.30	1996	28.55	57.24	143.26	1981	29.06	58.27	142.23	1967	29.58	59.31	141.19	1953
201	27.94	56.16	144.84	2003	28.46	57.20	143.80	1989	28.97	58.23	142.77	1974	29.49	59.27	141.73	1960
201.5	27.85	56.12	145.38	2011	28.36	57.15	144.35	1996	28.88	58.19	143.31	1982	29.39	59.23	142.27	1968
202	27.76	56.08	145.92	2018	28.27	57.11	144.89	2004	28.79	58.15	143.85	1989	29.30	59.19	142.81	1975
202.5	27.67	56.04	146.47	2026	28.18	57.07	145.43	2011	28.70	58.11	144.39	1997	29.21	59.15	143.35	1983
203	27.58	55.99	147.01	2033	28.09	57.03	145.97	2019	28.61	58.07	144.93	2004	29.12	59.11	143.89	1990
203.5	27.50	55.95	147.55	2041	28.01	56.99	146.51	2026	28.51	58.03	145.47	2012	29.02	59.07	144.43	1998
204	27.41	55.91	148.09	2048	27.92	56.95	147.05	2034	28.43	57.99	146.01	2019	28.93	59.02	144.98	2005
204.5	27.32	55.87	148.63	2056	27.83	56.91	147.59	2041	28.34	57.95	146.55	2027	28.84	58.98	145.52	2012
205	27.23	55.83	149.17	2063	27.74	56.87	148.13	2049	28.25	57.91	147.10	2034	28.75	58.94	146.06	2020
205.5	27.15	55.79	149.71	2071	27.65	56.83	148.67	2056	28.16	57.86	147.64	2042	28.66	58.90	146.60	2027
206	27.06	55.75	150.25	2078	27.57	56.79	149.21	2064	28.07	57.82	148.18	2049	28.57	58.86	147.14	2035
206.5	26.98	55.71	150.79	2085	27.48	56.74	149.76	2071	27.98	57.78	148.72	2057	28.48	58.82	147.68	2042
207	26.89	55.67	151.33	2093	27.39	56.70	150.30	2079	27.89	57.74	149.26	2064	28.40	58.78	148.22	2050
207.5	26.81	55.63	151.88	2100	27.31	56.66	150.84	2086	27.81	57.70	149.80	2072	28.31	58.74	148.76	2057
208	26.72	55.58	152.42	2108	27.22	56.62	151.38	2094	27.72	57.66	150.34	2079	28.22	58.70	149.30	2065
208.5	26.64	55.54	152.96	2115	27.14	56.58	151.92	2101	27.63	57.62	150.88	2087	28.13	58.66	149.84	2072
209	26.56	55.50	153.50	2123	27.05	56.54	152.46	2109	27.55	57.58	151.42	2094	28.05	58.61	150.39	2080
209.5	26.47	55.46	154.04	2130	26.97	56.50	153.00	2116	27.46	57.54	151.96	2102	27.96	58.57	150.93	2087
210	26.39	55.42	154.58	2138	26.88	56.46	153.54	2123	27.38	57.50	152.51	2109	27.87	58.53	151.47	2095
210.5	26.31	55.38	155.12	2145	26.80	56.42	154.08	2131	27.29	57.45	153.05	2117	27.79	58.49	152.01	2102
211	26.23	55.34	155.66	2153	26.72	56.38	154.62	2138	27.21	57.41	153.59	2124	27.70	58.45	152.55	2110
211.5	26.15	55.30	156.20	2160	26.64	56.33	155.17	2146	27.13	57.37	154.13	2132	27.62	58.41	153.09	2117
212	26.06	55.26	156.74	2168	26.55	56.29	155.71	2153	27.04	57.33	154.67	2139	27.53	58.37	153.63	2125
212.5	25.98	55.22	157.29	2175	26.47	56.25	156.25	2161	26.96	57.29	155.21	2147	27.45	58.33	154.17	2132
213	25.90	55.17	157.83	2183	26.39	56.21	156.79	2168	26.88	57.25	155.75	2154	27.36	58.29	154.71	2140
213.5	25.82	55.13	158.37	2190	26.31	56.17	157.33	2176	26.80	57.21	156.29	2162	27.28	58.25	155.25	2147
214	25.74	55.09	158.91	2198	26.23	56.13	157.87	2183	26.71	57.17	156.83	2169	27.20	58.20	155.80	2155
214.5	25.66	55.05	159.45	2205	26.15	56.09	158.41	2191	26.63	57.13	157.37	2176	27.12	58.16	156.34	2162
215	25.59	55.01	159.99	2213	26.07	56.05	158.95	2198	26.55	57.09	157.92	2184	27.03	58.12	156.88	2170
215.5	25.51	54.97	160.53	2220	25.99	56.01	159.49	2206	26.47	57.04	158.46	2191	26.95	58.08	157.42	2177
216	25.43	54.93	161.07	2228	25.91	55.97	160.03	2213	26.39	57.00	159.00	2199	26.87	58.04	157.96	2185
216.5	25.35	54.89	161.61	2235	25.83	55.92	160.58	2221	26.31	56.96	159.54	2206	26.79	58.00	158.50	2192
217	25.27	54.85	162.15	2243	25.75	55.88	161.12	2228	26.23	56.92	160.08	2214	26.71	57.96	159.04	2200
217.5	25.20	54.81	162.70	2250	25.67	55.84	161.66	2236	26.15	56.88	160.62	2221	26.63	57.92	159.58	2207
218	25.12	54.76	163.24	2258	25.60	55.80	162.20	2243	26.07	56.84	161.16	2229	26.55	57.88	160.12	2215
218.5	25.04	54.72	163.78	2265	25.52	55.76	162.74	2251	25.99	56.80	161.70	2236	26.47	57.84	160.66	2222
219	24.97	54.68	164.32	2273	25.44	55.72	163.28	2258	25.92	56.76	162.24	2244	26.39	57.79	161.21	2229
219.5	24.89	54.64	164.86	2280	25.37	55.68	163.82	2266	25.84	56.72	162.78	2251	26.31	57.75	161.75	2237
220	24.82	54.60	165.40	2287	25.29	55.64	164.36	2273	25.76	56.68	163.33	2259	26.23	57.71	162.29	2244
220.5	24.74	54.56	165.94	2295	25.21	55.60	164.90	2281	25.68	56.63	163.87	2266	26.15	57.67	162.83	2252
221	24.67	54.52	166.48	2302	25.14	55.56	165.44	2288	25.61	56.59	164.41	2274	26.08	57.63	163.37	2259
221.5	24.59	54.48	167.02	2310	25.06	55.51	165.99	2296	25.53	56.55	164.95	2281	26.00	57.59	163.91	2267
222	24.52	54.44	167.56	2317	24.99	55.47	166.53	2303	25.46	56.51	165.49	2289	25.92	57.55	164.45	2274
222.5	24.45	54.40	168.11	2325	24.91	55.43	167.07	2311	25.38	56.47	166.03	2296	25.85	57.51	164.99	2282
223	24.37	54.35	168.65	2332	24.84	55.39	167.61	2318	25.30	56.43	166.57	2304	25.77	57.47	165.53	2289
223.5	24.30	54.31	169.19	2340	24.77	55.35	168.15	2326	25.23	56.39	167.11	2311	25.69	57.43	166.07	2297
224	24.23	54.27	169.73	2347	24.69	55.31	168.69	2333	25.15	56.35	167.65	2319	25.62	57.38	166.62	2304
224.5	24.16	54.23	170.27	2355	24.62	55.27	169.23	2340	25.08	56.31	168.19	2326	25.54	57.34	167.16	2312
225	24.08	54.19	170.81	2362	24.55	55.23	169.77	2348	25.01	56.27	168.74	2334	25.47	57.30	167.70	2319
225.5	24.01	54.15	171.35	2370	24.47	55.19	170.31	2355	24.93	56.22	169.28	2341	25.39	57.26	168.24	2327
226	23.94	54.11	171.89	2377	24.40	55.15	170.85	2363	24.86	56.18	169.82	2349	25.32	57.22	168.78	2334
226.5	23.87	54.07	172.43	2385	24.33	55.10	171.40	2370	24.79	56.14	170.36	2356	25.24	57.18	169.32	2342
227	23.80	54.03	172.97	2392	24.26	55.06	171.94	2378	24.71	56.10	170.90	2364	25.17	57.14	169.86	2349
227.5	23.73	53.99	173.52	2400	24.19	55.02	172.48	2385	24.64	56.06	171.44	2371	25.10	57.10	170.40	2357

Body Composition FEMALE 196-227.5 Lb.

Weight: Lb.	Waist: 37 inches Fat: %	Fat: Lb.	LBM: Lb.	RMR: Cal.	37.25 inches Fat: %	Fat: Lb.	LBM: Lb.	RMR: Cal.	37.5 inches Fat: %	Fat: Lb.	LBM: Lb.	RMR: Cal.	37.75 inches Fat: %	Fat: Lb.	LBM: Lb.	RMR: Cal.
196	30.98	60.72	135.28	1871	31.51	61.76	134.24	1857	32.04	62.79	133.21	1842	32.57	63.83	132.17	1828
196.5	30.88	60.68	135.82	1878	31.41	61.71	134.79	1864	31.93	62.75	133.75	1850	32.46	63.79	132.71	1835
197	30.78	60.64	136.36	1886	31.31	61.67	135.33	1872	31.83	62.71	134.29	1857	32.36	63.75	133.25	1843
197.5	30.68	60.60	136.91	1893	31.21	61.63	135.87	1879	31.73	62.67	134.83	1865	32.26	63.71	133.79	1850
198	30.58	60.55	137.45	1901	31.11	61.59	136.41	1887	31.63	62.63	135.37	1872	32.15	63.67	134.33	1858
198.5	30.49	60.51	137.99	1908	31.01	61.55	136.95	1894	31.53	62.59	135.91	1880	32.05	63.63	134.87	1865
199	30.39	60.47	138.53	1916	30.91	61.51	137.49	1901	31.43	62.55	136.45	1887	31.95	63.58	135.42	1873
199.5	30.29	60.43	139.07	1923	30.81	61.47	138.03	1909	31.33	62.51	136.99	1895	31.85	63.54	135.96	1880
200	30.20	60.39	139.61	1931	30.71	61.43	138.57	1916	31.23	62.47	137.54	1902	31.75	63.50	136.50	1888
200.5	30.10	60.35	140.15	1938	30.62	61.39	139.11	1924	31.13	62.42	138.08	1910	31.65	63.46	137.04	1895
201	30.00	60.31	140.69	1946	30.52	61.35	139.65	1931	31.04	62.38	138.62	1917	31.55	63.42	137.58	1903
201.5	29.91	60.27	141.23	1953	30.42	61.30	140.20	1939	30.94	62.34	139.16	1925	31.45	63.38	138.12	1910
202	29.81	60.23	141.77	1961	30.33	61.26	140.74	1946	30.84	62.30	139.70	1932	31.36	63.34	138.66	1918
202.5	29.72	60.19	142.32	1968	30.23	61.22	141.28	1954	30.75	62.26	140.24	1940	31.26	63.30	139.20	1925
203	29.63	60.14	142.86	1976	30.14	61.18	141.82	1961	30.65	62.22	140.78	1947	31.16	63.26	139.74	1933
203.5	29.53	60.10	143.40	1983	30.04	61.14	142.36	1969	30.55	62.18	141.32	1954	31.06	63.22	140.28	1940
204	29.44	60.06	143.94	1991	29.95	61.10	142.90	1976	30.46	62.14	141.86	1962	30.97	63.17	140.83	1948
204.5	29.35	60.02	144.48	1998	29.86	61.06	143.44	1984	30.36	62.10	142.40	1969	30.87	63.13	141.37	1955
205	29.26	59.98	145.02	2006	29.76	61.02	143.98	1991	30.27	62.06	142.95	1977	30.78	63.09	141.91	1963
205.5	29.17	59.94	145.56	2013	29.67	60.98	144.52	1999	30.18	62.01	143.49	1984	30.68	63.05	142.45	1970
206	29.08	59.90	146.10	2021	29.58	60.94	145.06	2006	30.08	61.97	144.03	1992	30.59	63.01	142.99	1978
206.5	28.99	59.86	146.64	2028	29.49	60.89	145.61	2014	29.99	61.93	144.57	1999	30.49	62.97	143.53	1985
207	28.90	59.82	147.18	2036	29.40	60.85	146.15	2021	29.90	61.89	145.11	2007	30.40	62.93	144.07	1993
207.5	28.81	59.78	147.73	2043	29.31	60.81	146.69	2029	29.81	61.85	145.65	2014	30.31	62.89	144.61	2000
208	28.72	59.73	148.27	2051	29.22	60.77	147.23	2036	29.72	61.81	146.19	2022	30.21	62.85	145.15	2007
208.5	28.63	59.69	148.81	2058	29.13	60.73	147.77	2044	29.62	61.77	146.73	2029	30.12	62.81	145.69	2015
209	28.54	59.65	149.35	2065	29.04	60.69	148.31	2051	29.53	61.73	147.27	2037	30.03	62.76	146.24	2022
209.5	28.45	59.61	149.89	2073	28.95	60.65	148.85	2059	29.44	61.69	147.81	2044	29.94	62.72	146.78	2030
210	28.37	59.57	150.43	2080	28.86	60.61	149.39	2066	29.35	61.65	148.36	2052	29.85	62.68	147.32	2037
210.5	28.28	59.53	150.97	2088	28.77	60.57	149.93	2074	29.27	61.60	148.90	2059	29.76	62.64	147.86	2045
211	28.19	59.49	151.51	2095	28.69	60.53	150.47	2081	29.18	61.56	149.44	2067	29.67	62.60	148.40	2052
211.5	28.11	59.45	152.05	2103	28.60	60.48	151.02	2089	29.09	61.52	149.98	2074	29.58	62.56	148.94	2060
212	28.02	59.41	152.59	2110	28.51	60.44	151.56	2096	29.00	61.48	150.52	2082	29.49	62.52	149.48	2067
212.5	27.94	59.37	153.14	2118	28.42	60.40	152.10	2104	28.91	61.44	151.06	2089	29.40	62.48	150.02	2075
213	27.85	59.32	153.68	2125	28.34	60.36	152.64	2111	28.83	61.40	151.60	2097	29.31	62.44	150.56	2082
213.5	27.77	59.28	154.22	2133	28.25	60.32	153.18	2118	28.74	61.36	152.14	2104	29.23	62.40	151.10	2090
214	27.68	59.24	154.76	2140	28.17	60.28	153.72	2126	28.65	61.32	152.68	2112	29.14	62.35	151.65	2097
214.5	27.60	59.20	155.30	2148	28.08	60.24	154.26	2133	28.57	61.28	153.22	2119	29.05	62.31	152.19	2105
215	27.52	59.16	155.84	2155	28.00	60.20	154.80	2141	28.48	61.24	153.77	2127	28.96	62.27	152.73	2112
215.5	27.43	59.12	156.38	2163	27.91	60.16	155.34	2148	28.40	61.19	154.31	2134	28.88	62.23	153.27	2120
216	27.35	59.08	156.92	2170	27.83	60.12	155.88	2156	28.31	61.15	154.85	2142	28.79	62.19	153.81	2127
216.5	27.27	59.04	157.46	2178	27.75	60.07	156.43	2163	28.23	61.11	155.39	2149	28.71	62.15	154.35	2135
217	27.19	59.00	158.00	2185	27.67	60.03	156.97	2171	28.14	61.07	155.93	2156	28.62	62.11	154.89	2142
217.5	27.11	58.96	158.55	2193	27.58	59.99	157.51	2178	28.06	61.03	156.47	2164	28.54	62.07	155.43	2150
218	27.02	58.91	159.09	2200	27.50	59.95	158.05	2186	27.98	60.99	157.01	2171	28.45	62.03	155.97	2157
218.5	26.94	58.87	159.63	2208	27.42	59.91	158.59	2193	27.89	60.95	157.55	2179	28.37	61.99	156.51	2165
219	26.86	58.83	160.17	2215	27.34	59.87	159.13	2201	27.81	60.91	158.09	2186	28.29	61.94	157.06	2172
219.5	26.78	58.79	160.71	2223	27.26	59.83	159.67	2208	27.73	60.87	158.63	2194	28.20	61.90	157.60	2180
220	26.70	58.75	161.25	2230	27.18	59.79	160.21	2216	27.65	60.83	159.18	2201	28.12	61.86	158.14	2187
220.5	26.63	58.71	161.79	2238	27.10	59.75	160.75	2223	27.57	60.78	159.72	2209	28.04	61.82	158.68	2195
221	26.55	58.67	162.33	2245	27.02	59.71	161.29	2231	27.49	60.74	160.26	2216	27.95	61.78	159.22	2202
221.5	26.47	58.63	162.87	2253	26.94	59.66	161.84	2238	27.40	60.70	160.80	2224	27.87	61.74	159.76	2209
222	26.39	58.59	163.41	2260	26.86	59.62	162.38	2246	27.32	60.66	161.34	2231	27.79	61.70	160.30	2217
222.5	26.31	58.55	163.96	2267	26.78	59.58	162.92	2253	27.24	60.62	161.88	2239	27.71	61.66	160.84	2224
223	26.23	58.50	164.50	2275	26.70	59.54	163.46	2261	27.17	60.58	162.42	2246	27.63	61.62	161.38	2232
223.5	26.16	58.46	165.04	2282	26.62	59.50	164.00	2268	27.09	60.54	162.96	2254	27.55	61.58	161.92	2239
224	26.08	58.42	165.58	2290	26.54	59.46	164.54	2276	27.01	60.50	163.50	2261	27.47	61.53	162.47	2247
224.5	26.00	58.38	166.12	2297	26.47	59.42	165.08	2283	26.93	60.46	164.04	2269	27.39	61.49	163.01	2254
225	25.93	58.34	166.66	2305	26.39	59.38	165.62	2291	26.85	60.42	164.59	2276	27.31	61.45	163.55	2262
225.5	25.85	58.30	167.20	2312	26.31	59.34	166.16	2298	26.77	60.37	165.13	2284	27.23	61.41	164.09	2269
226	25.78	58.26	167.74	2320	26.24	59.30	166.70	2306	26.70	60.33	165.67	2291	27.16	61.37	164.63	2277
226.5	25.70	58.22	168.28	2327	26.16	59.25	167.25	2313	26.62	60.29	166.21	2299	27.08	61.33	165.17	2284
227	25.63	58.18	168.82	2335	26.09	59.21	167.79	2320	26.54	60.25	166.75	2306	27.00	61.29	165.71	2292
227.5	25.55	58.14	169.37	2342	26.01	59.17	168.33	2328	26.47	60.21	167.29	2314	26.92	61.25	166.25	2299

THE BODY FAT GUIDE

Body Composition FEMALE 196-227.5 Lb.

Weight: Lb.	Waist: 38 inches Fat: %	Fat: Lb.	LBM: Lb.	RMR: Cal.	38.25 inches Fat: %	Fat: Lb.	LBM: Lb.	RMR: Cal.	38.5 inches Fat: %	Fat: Lb.	LBM: Lb.	RMR: Cal.	38.75 inches Fat: %	Fat: Lb.	LBM: Lb.	RMR: Cal.
196	33.10	64.87	131.13	1814	33.63	65.91	130.09	1799	34.15	66.94	129.06	1785	34.68	67.98	128.02	1771
196.5	32.99	64.83	131.67	1821	33.52	65.86	130.64	1807	34.05	66.90	129.60	1792	34.57	67.94	128.56	1778
197	32.89	64.79	132.21	1829	33.41	65.82	131.18	1814	33.94	66.86	130.14	1800	34.47	67.90	129.10	1785
197.5	32.78	64.75	132.76	1836	33.31	65.78	131.72	1822	33.83	66.82	130.68	1807	34.36	67.86	129.64	1793
198	32.68	64.70	133.30	1843	33.20	65.74	132.26	1829	33.73	66.78	131.22	1815	34.25	67.82	130.18	1800
198.5	32.58	64.66	133.84	1851	33.10	65.70	132.80	1837	33.62	66.74	131.76	1822	34.14	67.78	130.72	1808
199	32.47	64.62	134.38	1858	32.99	65.66	133.34	1844	33.52	66.70	132.30	1830	34.04	67.73	131.27	1815
199.5	32.37	64.58	134.92	1866	32.89	65.62	133.88	1852	33.41	66.66	132.84	1837	33.93	67.69	131.81	1823
200	32.27	64.54	135.46	1873	32.79	65.58	134.42	1859	33.31	66.62	133.39	1845	33.83	67.65	132.35	1830
200.5	32.17	64.50	136.00	1881	32.69	65.54	134.96	1867	33.20	66.57	133.93	1852	33.72	67.61	132.89	1838
201	32.07	64.46	136.54	1888	32.58	65.50	135.50	1874	33.10	66.53	134.47	1860	33.62	67.57	133.43	1845
201.5	31.97	64.42	137.08	1896	32.48	65.45	136.05	1882	33.00	66.49	135.01	1867	33.51	67.53	133.97	1853
202	31.87	64.38	137.62	1903	32.38	65.41	136.59	1889	32.90	66.45	135.55	1875	33.41	67.49	134.51	1860
202.5	31.77	64.34	138.17	1911	32.28	65.37	137.13	1896	32.80	66.41	136.09	1882	33.31	67.45	135.05	1868
203	31.67	64.29	138.71	1918	32.18	65.33	137.67	1904	32.69	66.37	136.63	1890	33.21	67.41	135.59	1875
203.5	31.57	64.25	139.25	1926	32.08	65.29	138.21	1911	32.59	66.33	137.17	1897	33.10	67.37	136.13	1883
204	31.48	64.21	139.79	1933	31.99	65.25	138.75	1919	32.49	66.29	137.71	1905	33.00	67.32	136.68	1890
204.5	31.38	64.17	140.33	1941	31.89	65.21	139.29	1926	32.39	66.25	138.25	1912	32.90	67.28	137.22	1898
205	31.28	64.13	140.87	1948	31.79	65.17	139.83	1934	32.30	66.21	138.80	1920	32.80	67.24	137.76	1905
205.5	31.19	64.09	141.41	1956	31.69	65.13	140.37	1941	32.20	66.16	139.34	1927	32.70	67.20	138.30	1913
206	31.09	64.05	141.95	1963	31.59	65.09	140.91	1949	32.10	66.12	139.88	1934	32.60	67.16	138.84	1920
206.5	31.00	64.01	142.49	1971	31.50	65.04	141.46	1956	32.00	66.08	140.42	1942	32.50	67.12	139.38	1928
207	30.90	63.97	143.03	1978	31.40	65.00	142.00	1964	31.90	66.04	140.96	1949	32.41	67.08	139.92	1935
207.5	30.81	63.93	143.58	1986	31.31	64.96	142.54	1971	31.81	66.00	141.50	1957	32.31	67.04	140.46	1943
208	30.71	63.88	144.12	1993	31.21	64.92	143.08	1979	31.71	65.96	142.04	1964	32.21	67.00	141.00	1950
208.5	30.62	63.84	144.66	2001	31.12	64.88	143.62	1986	31.62	65.92	142.58	1972	32.11	66.96	141.54	1958
209	30.53	63.80	145.20	2008	31.02	64.84	144.16	1994	31.52	65.88	143.12	1979	32.02	66.91	142.09	1965
209.5	30.43	63.76	145.74	2016	30.93	64.80	144.70	2001	31.43	65.84	143.66	1987	31.92	66.87	142.63	1973
210	30.34	63.72	146.28	2023	30.84	64.76	145.24	2009	31.33	65.80	144.21	1994	31.83	66.83	143.17	1980
210.5	30.25	63.68	146.82	2031	30.74	64.72	145.78	2016	31.24	65.75	144.75	2002	31.73	66.79	143.71	1987
211	30.16	63.64	147.36	2038	30.65	64.68	146.32	2024	31.14	65.71	145.29	2009	31.64	66.75	144.25	1995
211.5	30.07	63.60	147.90	2045	30.56	64.63	146.87	2031	31.05	65.67	145.83	2017	31.54	66.71	144.79	2002
212	29.98	63.56	148.44	2053	30.47	64.59	147.41	2039	30.96	65.63	146.37	2024	31.45	66.67	145.33	2010
212.5	29.89	63.52	148.99	2060	30.38	64.55	147.95	2046	30.87	65.59	146.91	2032	31.35	66.63	145.87	2017
213	29.80	63.47	149.53	2068	30.29	64.51	148.49	2054	30.77	65.55	147.45	2039	31.26	66.59	146.41	2025
213.5	29.71	63.43	150.07	2075	30.20	64.47	149.03	2061	30.68	65.51	147.99	2047	31.17	66.55	146.95	2032
214	29.62	63.39	150.61	2083	30.11	64.43	149.57	2069	30.59	65.47	148.53	2054	31.08	66.50	147.50	2040
214.5	29.53	63.35	151.15	2090	30.02	64.39	150.11	2076	30.50	65.43	149.07	2062	30.99	66.46	148.04	2047
215	29.45	63.31	151.69	2098	29.93	64.35	150.65	2084	30.41	65.39	149.62	2069	30.89	66.42	148.58	2055
215.5	29.36	63.27	152.23	2105	29.84	64.31	151.19	2091	30.32	65.34	150.16	2077	30.80	66.38	149.12	2062
216	29.27	63.23	152.77	2113	29.75	64.27	151.73	2098	30.23	65.30	150.70	2084	30.71	66.34	149.66	2070
216.5	29.19	63.19	153.31	2120	29.66	64.22	152.28	2106	30.14	65.26	151.24	2092	30.62	66.30	150.20	2077
217	29.10	63.15	153.85	2128	29.58	64.18	152.82	2113	30.06	65.22	151.78	2099	30.53	66.26	150.74	2085
217.5	29.01	63.11	154.40	2135	29.49	64.14	153.36	2121	29.97	65.18	152.32	2107	30.44	66.22	151.28	2092
218	28.93	63.06	154.94	2143	29.40	64.10	153.90	2128	29.88	65.14	152.86	2114	30.36	66.18	151.82	2100
218.5	28.84	63.02	155.48	2150	29.32	64.06	154.44	2136	29.79	65.10	153.40	2122	30.27	66.14	152.36	2107
219	28.76	62.98	156.02	2158	29.23	64.02	154.98	2143	29.71	65.06	153.94	2129	30.18	66.09	152.91	2115
219.5	28.67	62.94	156.56	2165	29.15	63.98	155.52	2151	29.62	65.02	154.48	2137	30.09	66.05	153.45	2122
220	28.59	62.90	157.10	2173	29.06	63.94	156.06	2158	29.53	64.98	155.03	2144	30.01	66.01	153.99	2130
220.5	28.51	62.86	157.64	2180	28.98	63.90	156.60	2166	29.45	64.93	155.57	2151	29.92	65.97	154.53	2137
221	28.42	62.82	158.18	2188	28.89	63.86	157.14	2173	29.36	64.89	156.11	2159	29.83	65.93	155.07	2145
221.5	28.34	62.78	158.72	2195	28.81	63.81	157.69	2181	29.28	64.85	156.65	2166	29.75	65.89	155.61	2152
222	28.26	62.74	159.26	2203	28.73	63.77	158.23	2188	29.19	64.81	157.19	2174	29.66	65.85	156.15	2160
222.5	28.18	62.70	159.81	2210	28.64	63.73	158.77	2196	29.11	64.77	157.73	2181	29.58	65.81	156.69	2167
223	28.10	62.65	160.35	2218	28.56	63.69	159.31	2203	29.03	64.73	158.27	2189	29.49	65.77	157.23	2175
223.5	28.01	62.61	160.89	2225	28.48	63.65	159.85	2211	28.94	64.69	158.81	2196	29.41	65.73	157.77	2182
224	27.93	62.57	161.43	2233	28.40	63.61	160.39	2218	28.86	64.65	159.35	2204	29.32	65.68	158.32	2190
224.5	27.85	62.53	161.97	2240	28.32	63.57	160.93	2226	28.78	64.61	159.89	2211	29.24	65.64	158.86	2197
225	27.77	62.49	162.51	2248	28.23	63.53	161.47	2233	28.70	64.57	160.44	2219	29.16	65.60	159.40	2204
225.5	27.69	62.45	163.05	2255	28.15	63.49	162.01	2241	28.61	64.52	160.98	2226	29.07	65.56	159.94	2212
226	27.61	62.41	163.59	2262	28.07	63.45	162.55	2248	28.53	64.48	161.52	2234	28.99	65.52	160.48	2219
226.5	27.54	62.37	164.13	2270	27.99	63.40	163.10	2256	28.45	64.44	162.06	2241	28.91	65.48	161.02	2227
227	27.46	62.33	164.67	2277	27.91	63.36	163.64	2263	28.37	64.40	162.60	2249	28.83	65.44	161.56	2234
227.5	27.38	62.29	165.22	2285	27.83	63.32	164.18	2271	28.29	64.36	163.14	2256	28.75	65.40	162.10	2242

Body Composition FEMALE 196-227.5 Lb.

Weight: Lb.	Waist: 39 inches				39.25 inches				39.5 inches				39.75 inches			
	Fat: %	Fat: Lb.	LBM: Lb.	RMR: Cal.	Fat: %	Fat: Lb.	LBM: Lb.	RMR: Cal.	Fat: %	Fat: Lb.	LBM: Lb.	RMR: Cal.	Fat: %	Fat: Lb.	LBM: Lb.	RMR: Cal.
196	35.21	69.02	126.98	1756	35.74	70.06	125.94	1742	36.27	71.09	124.91	1727	36.80	72.13	123.87	1713
196.5	35.10	68.98	127.52	1764	35.63	70.01	126.49	1749	36.16	71.05	125.45	1735	36.69	72.09	124.41	1721
197	34.99	68.94	128.06	1771	35.52	69.97	127.03	1757	36.05	71.01	125.99	1742	36.57	72.05	124.95	1728
197.5	34.88	68.90	128.61	1779	35.41	69.93	127.57	1764	35.93	70.97	126.53	1750	36.46	72.01	125.49	1736
198	34.77	68.85	129.15	1786	35.30	69.89	128.11	1772	35.82	70.93	127.07	1757	36.35	71.97	126.03	1743
198.5	34.67	68.81	129.69	1794	35.19	69.85	128.65	1779	35.71	70.89	127.61	1765	36.23	71.93	126.57	1751
199	34.56	68.77	130.23	1801	35.08	69.81	129.19	1787	35.60	70.85	128.15	1772	36.12	71.88	127.12	1758
199.5	34.45	68.73	130.77	1809	34.97	69.77	129.73	1794	35.49	70.81	128.69	1780	36.01	71.84	127.66	1765
200	34.35	68.69	131.31	1816	34.86	69.73	130.27	1802	35.38	70.77	129.24	1787	35.90	71.80	128.20	1773
200.5	34.24	68.65	131.85	1823	34.76	69.69	130.81	1809	35.27	70.72	129.78	1795	35.79	71.76	128.74	1780
201	34.13	68.61	132.39	1831	34.65	69.65	131.35	1817	35.17	70.68	130.32	1802	35.68	71.72	129.28	1788
201.5	34.03	68.57	132.93	1838	34.54	69.60	131.90	1824	35.06	70.64	130.86	1810	35.57	71.68	129.82	1795
202	33.92	68.53	133.47	1846	34.44	69.56	132.44	1832	34.95	70.60	131.40	1817	35.46	71.64	130.36	1803
202.5	33.82	68.49	134.02	1853	34.33	69.52	132.98	1839	34.84	70.56	131.94	1825	35.36	71.60	130.90	1810
203	33.72	68.44	134.56	1861	34.23	69.48	133.52	1847	34.74	70.52	132.48	1832	35.25	71.56	131.44	1818
203.5	33.61	68.40	135.10	1868	34.12	69.44	134.06	1854	34.63	70.48	133.02	1840	35.14	71.52	131.98	1825
204	33.51	68.36	135.64	1876	34.02	69.40	134.60	1862	34.53	70.44	133.56	1847	35.04	71.47	132.53	1833
204.5	33.41	68.32	136.18	1883	33.92	69.36	135.14	1869	34.42	70.40	134.10	1855	34.93	71.43	133.07	1840
205	33.31	68.28	136.72	1891	33.81	69.32	135.68	1876	34.32	70.36	134.65	1862	34.83	71.39	133.61	1848
205.5	33.21	68.24	137.26	1898	33.71	69.28	136.22	1884	34.22	70.31	135.19	1870	34.72	71.35	134.15	1855
206	33.11	68.20	137.80	1906	33.61	69.24	136.76	1891	34.11	70.27	135.73	1877	34.62	71.31	134.69	1863
206.5	33.01	68.16	138.34	1913	33.51	69.19	137.31	1899	34.01	70.23	136.27	1885	34.51	71.27	135.23	1870
207	32.91	68.12	138.88	1921	33.41	69.15	137.85	1906	33.91	70.19	136.81	1892	34.41	71.23	135.77	1878
207.5	32.81	68.08	139.43	1928	33.31	69.11	138.39	1914	33.81	70.15	137.35	1900	34.31	71.19	136.31	1885
208	32.71	68.03	139.97	1936	33.21	69.07	138.93	1921	33.71	70.11	137.89	1907	34.21	71.15	136.85	1893
208.5	32.61	67.99	140.51	1943	33.11	69.03	139.47	1929	33.61	70.07	138.43	1915	34.10	71.11	137.39	1900
209	32.51	67.95	141.05	1951	33.01	68.99	140.01	1936	33.51	70.03	138.97	1922	34.00	71.06	137.94	1908
209.5	32.42	67.91	141.59	1958	32.91	68.95	140.55	1944	33.41	69.99	139.51	1929	33.90	71.02	138.48	1915
210	32.32	67.87	142.13	1966	32.81	68.91	141.09	1951	33.31	69.95	140.06	1937	33.80	70.98	139.02	1923
210.5	32.22	67.83	142.67	1973	32.72	68.87	141.63	1959	33.21	69.90	140.60	1944	33.70	70.94	139.56	1930
211	32.13	67.79	143.21	1981	32.62	68.83	142.17	1966	33.11	69.86	141.14	1952	33.60	70.90	140.10	1938
211.5	32.03	67.75	143.75	1988	32.52	68.78	142.72	1974	33.01	69.82	141.68	1959	33.50	70.86	140.64	1945
212	31.94	67.71	144.29	1996	32.43	68.74	143.26	1981	32.92	69.78	142.22	1967	33.40	70.82	141.18	1953
212.5	31.84	67.67	144.84	2003	32.33	68.70	143.80	1989	32.82	69.74	142.76	1974	33.31	70.78	141.72	1960
213	31.75	67.62	145.38	2011	32.24	68.66	144.34	1996	32.72	69.70	143.30	1982	33.21	70.74	142.26	1968
213.5	31.65	67.58	145.92	2018	32.14	68.62	144.88	2004	32.63	69.66	143.84	1989	33.11	70.70	142.80	1975
214	31.56	67.54	146.46	2026	32.05	68.58	145.42	2011	32.53	69.62	144.38	1997	33.02	70.65	143.35	1982
214.5	31.47	67.50	147.00	2033	31.95	68.54	145.96	2019	32.44	69.58	144.92	2004	32.92	70.61	143.89	1990
215	31.38	67.46	147.54	2040	31.86	68.50	146.50	2026	32.34	69.54	145.47	2012	32.82	70.57	144.43	1997
215.5	31.28	67.42	148.08	2048	31.77	68.46	147.04	2034	32.25	69.49	146.01	2019	32.73	70.53	144.97	2005
216	31.19	67.38	148.62	2055	31.67	68.42	147.58	2041	32.15	69.45	146.55	2027	32.63	70.49	145.51	2012
216.5	31.10	67.34	149.16	2063	31.58	68.37	148.13	2049	32.06	69.41	147.09	2034	32.54	70.45	146.05	2020
217	31.01	67.30	149.70	2070	31.49	68.33	148.67	2056	31.97	69.37	147.63	2042	32.45	70.41	146.59	2027
217.5	30.92	67.26	150.25	2078	31.40	68.29	149.21	2064	31.88	69.33	148.17	2049	32.35	70.37	147.13	2035
218	30.83	67.21	150.79	2085	31.31	68.25	149.75	2071	31.78	69.29	148.71	2057	32.26	70.33	147.67	2042
218.5	30.74	67.17	151.33	2093	31.22	68.21	150.29	2079	31.69	69.25	149.25	2064	32.17	70.29	148.21	2050
219	30.65	67.13	151.87	2100	31.13	68.17	150.83	2086	31.60	69.21	149.79	2072	32.08	70.24	148.76	2057
219.5	30.57	67.09	152.41	2108	31.04	68.13	151.37	2093	31.51	69.17	150.33	2079	31.98	70.20	149.30	2065
220	30.48	67.05	152.95	2115	30.95	68.09	151.91	2101	31.42	69.13	150.88	2087	31.89	70.16	149.84	2072
220.5	30.39	67.01	153.49	2123	30.86	68.05	152.45	2108	31.33	69.08	151.42	2094	31.80	70.12	150.38	2080
221	30.30	66.97	154.03	2130	30.77	68.01	152.99	2116	31.24	69.04	151.96	2102	31.71	70.08	150.92	2087
221.5	30.22	66.93	154.57	2138	30.68	67.96	153.54	2123	31.15	69.00	152.50	2109	31.62	70.04	151.46	2095
222	30.13	66.89	155.11	2145	30.60	67.92	154.08	2131	31.06	68.96	153.04	2117	31.53	70.00	152.00	2102
222.5	30.04	66.85	155.66	2153	30.51	67.88	154.62	2138	30.98	68.92	153.58	2124	31.44	69.96	152.54	2110
223	29.96	66.80	156.20	2160	30.42	67.84	155.16	2146	30.89	68.88	154.12	2131	31.35	69.92	153.08	2117
223.5	29.87	66.76	156.74	2168	30.34	67.80	155.70	2153	30.80	68.84	154.66	2139	31.26	69.88	153.62	2125
224	29.79	66.72	157.28	2175	30.25	67.76	156.24	2161	30.71	68.80	155.20	2146	31.18	69.83	154.17	2132
224.5	29.70	66.68	157.82	2183	30.16	67.72	156.78	2168	30.63	68.76	155.74	2154	31.09	69.79	154.71	2140
225	29.62	66.64	158.36	2190	30.08	67.68	157.32	2176	30.54	68.72	156.29	2161	31.00	69.75	155.25	2147
225.5	29.53	66.60	158.90	2198	29.99	67.64	157.86	2183	30.45	68.67	156.83	2169	30.91	69.71	155.79	2155
226	29.45	66.56	159.44	2205	29.91	67.60	158.40	2191	30.37	68.63	157.37	2176	30.83	69.67	156.33	2162
226.5	29.37	66.52	159.98	2213	29.83	67.55	158.95	2198	30.28	68.59	157.91	2184	30.74	69.63	156.87	2170
227	29.28	66.48	160.52	2220	29.74	67.51	159.49	2206	30.20	68.55	158.45	2191	30.66	69.59	157.41	2177
227.5	29.20	66.44	161.07	2228	29.66	67.47	160.03	2213	30.11	68.51	158.99	2199	30.57	69.55	157.95	2184

Body Composition FEMALE 196-227.5 Lb.

Weight: Lb.	Waist: 40 inches				40.25 inches				40.5 inches				40.75 inches			
	Fat: %	Fat: Lb.	LBM: Lb.	RMR: Cal.	Fat: %	Fat: Lb.	LBM: Lb.	RMR: Cal.	Fat: %	Fat: Lb.	LBM: Lb.	RMR: Cal.	Fat: %	Fat: Lb.	LBM: Lb.	RMR: Cal.
196	37.33	73.17	122.83	1699	37.86	74.21	121.79	1684	38.39	75.24	120.76	1670	38.92	76.28	119.72	1656
196.5	37.21	73.13	123.37	1706	37.74	74.16	122.34	1692	38.27	75.20	121.30	1678	38.80	76.24	120.26	1663
197	37.10	73.09	123.91	1714	37.63	74.12	122.88	1699	38.15	75.16	121.84	1685	38.68	76.20	120.80	1671
197.5	36.98	73.05	124.46	1721	37.51	74.08	123.42	1707	38.04	75.12	122.38	1693	38.56	76.16	121.34	1678
198	36.87	73.00	125.00	1729	37.39	74.04	123.96	1714	37.92	75.08	122.92	1700	38.44	76.12	121.88	1686
198.5	36.76	72.96	125.54	1736	37.28	74.00	124.50	1722	37.80	75.04	123.46	1707	38.33	76.08	122.42	1693
199	36.64	72.92	126.08	1744	37.17	73.96	125.04	1729	37.69	75.00	124.00	1715	38.21	76.03	122.97	1701
199.5	36.53	72.88	126.62	1751	37.05	73.92	125.58	1737	37.57	74.96	124.54	1722	38.09	75.99	123.51	1708
200	36.42	72.84	127.16	1759	36.94	73.88	126.12	1744	37.46	74.92	125.09	1730	37.98	75.95	124.05	1716
200.5	36.31	72.80	127.70	1766	36.83	73.84	126.66	1752	37.34	74.87	125.63	1737	37.86	75.91	124.59	1723
201	36.20	72.76	128.24	1774	36.71	73.80	127.20	1759	37.23	74.83	126.17	1745	37.75	75.87	125.13	1731
201.5	36.09	72.72	128.78	1781	36.60	73.75	127.75	1767	37.12	74.79	126.71	1752	37.63	75.83	125.67	1738
202	35.98	72.68	129.32	1789	36.49	73.71	128.29	1774	37.01	74.75	127.25	1760	37.52	75.79	126.21	1746
202.5	35.87	72.64	129.87	1796	36.38	73.67	128.83	1782	36.89	74.71	127.79	1767	37.41	75.75	126.75	1753
203	35.76	72.59	130.41	1804	36.27	73.63	129.37	1789	36.78	74.67	128.33	1775	37.29	75.71	127.29	1760
203.5	35.65	72.55	130.95	1811	36.16	73.59	129.91	1797	36.67	74.63	128.87	1782	37.18	75.67	127.83	1768
204	35.55	72.51	131.49	1818	36.05	73.55	130.45	1804	36.56	74.59	129.41	1790	37.07	75.62	128.38	1775
204.5	35.44	72.47	132.03	1826	35.95	73.51	130.99	1812	36.45	74.55	129.95	1797	36.96	75.58	128.92	1783
205	35.33	72.43	132.57	1833	35.84	73.47	131.53	1819	36.34	74.51	130.50	1805	36.85	75.54	129.46	1790
205.5	35.23	72.39	133.11	1841	35.73	73.43	132.07	1827	36.24	74.46	131.04	1812	36.74	75.50	130.00	1798
206	35.12	72.35	133.65	1848	35.62	73.39	132.61	1834	36.13	74.42	131.58	1820	36.63	75.46	130.54	1805
206.5	35.02	72.31	134.19	1856	35.52	73.34	133.16	1842	36.02	74.38	132.12	1827	36.52	75.42	131.08	1813
207	34.91	72.27	134.73	1863	35.41	73.30	133.70	1849	35.91	74.34	132.66	1835	36.41	75.38	131.62	1820
207.5	34.81	72.23	135.28	1871	35.31	73.26	134.24	1857	35.81	74.30	133.20	1842	36.31	75.34	132.16	1828
208	34.70	72.18	135.82	1878	35.20	73.22	134.78	1864	35.70	74.26	133.74	1850	36.20	75.30	132.70	1835
208.5	34.60	72.14	136.36	1886	35.10	73.18	135.32	1871	35.60	74.22	134.28	1857	36.09	75.26	133.24	1843
209	34.50	72.10	136.90	1893	34.99	73.14	135.86	1879	35.49	74.18	134.82	1865	35.99	75.21	133.79	1850
209.5	34.40	72.06	137.44	1901	34.89	73.10	136.40	1886	35.39	74.14	135.36	1872	35.88	75.17	134.33	1858
210	34.30	72.02	137.98	1908	34.79	73.06	136.94	1894	35.28	74.10	135.91	1880	35.78	75.13	134.87	1865
210.5	34.19	71.98	138.52	1916	34.69	73.02	137.48	1901	35.18	74.05	136.45	1887	35.67	75.09	135.41	1873
211	34.09	71.94	139.06	1923	34.59	72.98	138.02	1909	35.08	74.01	136.99	1895	35.57	75.05	135.95	1880
211.5	33.99	71.90	139.60	1931	34.48	72.93	138.57	1916	34.97	73.97	137.53	1902	35.47	75.01	136.49	1888
212	33.89	71.86	140.14	1938	34.38	72.89	139.11	1924	34.87	73.93	138.07	1909	35.36	74.97	137.03	1895
212.5	33.80	71.82	140.69	1946	34.28	72.85	139.65	1931	34.77	73.89	138.61	1917	35.26	74.93	137.57	1903
213	33.70	71.77	141.23	1953	34.18	72.81	140.19	1939	34.67	73.85	139.15	1924	35.16	74.89	138.11	1910
213.5	33.60	71.73	141.77	1961	34.08	72.77	140.73	1946	34.57	73.81	139.69	1932	35.06	74.85	138.65	1918
214	33.50	71.69	142.31	1968	33.99	72.73	141.27	1954	34.47	73.77	140.23	1939	34.96	74.80	139.20	1925
214.5	33.40	71.65	142.85	1976	33.89	72.69	141.81	1961	34.37	73.73	140.77	1947	34.85	74.76	139.74	1933
215	33.31	71.61	143.39	1983	33.79	72.65	142.35	1969	34.27	73.69	141.32	1954	34.75	74.72	140.28	1940
215.5	33.21	71.57	143.93	1991	33.69	72.61	142.89	1976	34.17	73.64	141.86	1962	34.65	74.68	140.82	1948
216	33.11	71.53	144.47	1998	33.60	72.57	143.43	1984	34.08	73.60	142.40	1969	34.56	74.64	141.36	1955
216.5	33.02	71.49	145.01	2006	33.50	72.52	143.98	1991	33.98	73.56	142.94	1977	34.46	74.60	141.90	1962
217	32.92	71.45	145.55	2013	33.40	72.48	144.52	1999	33.88	73.52	143.48	1984	34.36	74.56	142.44	1970
217.5	32.83	71.41	146.10	2020	33.31	72.44	145.06	2006	33.78	73.48	144.02	1992	34.26	74.52	142.98	1977
218	32.74	71.36	146.64	2028	33.21	72.40	145.60	2014	33.69	73.44	144.56	1999	34.16	74.48	143.52	1985
218.5	32.64	71.32	147.18	2035	33.12	72.36	146.14	2021	33.59	73.40	145.10	2007	34.07	74.44	144.06	1992
219	32.55	71.28	147.72	2043	33.02	72.32	146.68	2029	33.50	73.36	145.64	2014	33.97	74.39	144.61	2000
219.5	32.46	71.24	148.26	2050	32.93	72.28	147.22	2036	33.40	73.32	146.18	2022	33.87	74.35	145.15	2007
220	32.36	71.20	148.80	2058	32.84	72.24	147.76	2044	33.31	73.28	146.73	2029	33.78	74.31	145.69	2015
220.5	32.27	71.16	149.34	2065	32.74	72.20	148.30	2051	33.21	73.23	147.27	2037	33.68	74.27	146.23	2022
221	32.18	71.12	149.88	2073	32.65	72.16	148.84	2059	33.12	73.19	147.81	2044	33.59	74.23	146.77	2030
221.5	32.09	71.08	150.42	2080	32.56	72.11	149.39	2066	33.03	73.15	148.35	2052	33.49	74.19	147.31	2037
222	32.00	71.04	150.96	2088	32.47	72.07	149.93	2073	32.93	73.11	148.89	2059	33.40	74.15	147.85	2045
222.5	31.91	71.00	151.51	2095	32.37	72.03	150.47	2081	32.84	73.07	149.43	2067	33.31	74.11	148.39	2052
223	31.82	70.95	152.05	2103	32.28	71.99	151.01	2088	32.75	73.03	149.97	2074	33.21	74.07	148.93	2060
223.5	31.73	70.91	152.59	2110	32.19	71.95	151.55	2096	32.66	72.99	150.51	2082	33.12	74.03	149.47	2067
224	31.64	70.87	153.13	2118	32.10	71.91	152.09	2103	32.57	72.95	151.05	2089	33.03	73.98	150.02	2075
224.5	31.55	70.83	153.67	2125	32.01	71.87	152.63	2111	32.47	72.91	151.59	2097	32.94	73.94	150.56	2082
225	31.46	70.79	154.21	2133	31.92	71.83	153.17	2118	32.38	72.87	152.14	2104	32.85	73.90	151.10	2090
225.5	31.37	70.75	154.75	2140	31.83	71.79	153.71	2126	32.29	72.82	152.68	2112	32.75	73.86	151.64	2097
226	31.29	70.71	155.29	2148	31.75	71.75	154.25	2133	32.20	72.78	153.22	2119	32.66	73.82	152.18	2105
226.5	31.20	70.67	155.83	2155	31.66	71.70	154.80	2141	32.12	72.74	153.76	2126	32.57	73.78	152.72	2112
227	31.11	70.63	156.37	2163	31.57	71.66	155.34	2148	32.03	72.70	154.30	2134	32.48	73.74	153.26	2120
227.5	31.03	70.59	156.92	2170	31.48	71.62	155.88	2156	31.94	72.66	154.84	2141	32.39	73.70	153.80	2127

Body Composition   FEMALE   196-227.5 Lb.

Weight: Lb.	Waist: 41 inches Fat: %	Fat: Lb.	LBM: Lb.	RMR: Cal.	41.25 inches Fat: %	Fat: Lb.	LBM: Lb.	RMR: Cal.	41.5 inches Fat: %	Fat: Lb.	LBM: Lb.	RMR: Cal.	41.75 inches Fat: %	Fat: Lb.	LBM: Lb.	RMR: Cal.
196	39.45	77.32	118.68	1641	39.98	78.36	117.64	1627	40.51	79.39	116.61	1613	41.04	80.43	115.57	1598
196.5	39.33	77.28	119.22	1649	39.85	78.31	118.19	1635	40.38	79.35	117.15	1620	40.91	80.39	116.11	1606
197	39.21	77.24	119.76	1656	39.73	78.27	118.73	1642	40.26	79.31	117.69	1628	40.79	80.35	116.65	1613
197.5	39.09	77.20	120.31	1664	39.61	78.23	119.27	1649	40.14	79.27	118.23	1635	40.66	80.31	117.19	1621
198	38.97	77.15	120.85	1671	39.49	78.19	119.81	1657	40.01	79.23	118.77	1643	40.54	80.27	117.73	1628
198.5	38.85	77.11	121.39	1679	39.37	78.15	120.35	1664	39.89	79.19	119.31	1650	40.42	80.23	118.27	1636
199	38.73	77.07	121.93	1686	39.25	78.11	120.89	1672	39.77	79.15	119.85	1658	40.29	80.18	118.82	1643
199.5	38.61	77.03	122.47	1694	39.13	78.07	121.43	1679	39.65	79.11	120.39	1665	40.17	80.14	119.36	1651
200	38.50	76.99	123.01	1701	39.01	78.03	121.97	1687	39.53	79.07	120.94	1673	40.05	80.10	119.90	1658
200.5	38.38	76.95	123.55	1709	38.90	77.99	122.51	1694	39.41	79.02	121.48	1680	39.93	80.06	120.44	1666
201	38.26	76.91	124.09	1716	38.78	77.95	123.05	1702	39.30	78.98	122.02	1687	39.81	80.02	120.98	1673
201.5	38.15	76.87	124.63	1724	38.66	77.90	123.60	1709	39.18	78.94	122.56	1695	39.69	79.98	121.52	1681
202	38.03	76.83	125.17	1731	38.55	77.86	124.14	1717	39.06	78.90	123.10	1702	39.57	79.94	122.06	1688
202.5	37.92	76.79	125.72	1739	38.43	77.82	124.68	1724	38.94	78.86	123.64	1710	39.46	79.90	122.60	1696
203	37.80	76.74	126.26	1746	38.32	77.78	125.22	1732	38.83	78.82	124.18	1717	39.34	79.86	123.14	1703
203.5	37.69	76.70	126.80	1754	38.20	77.74	125.76	1739	38.71	78.78	124.72	1725	39.22	79.82	123.68	1711
204	37.58	76.66	127.34	1761	38.09	77.70	126.30	1747	38.60	78.74	125.26	1732	39.11	79.77	124.23	1718
204.5	37.47	76.62	127.88	1769	37.97	77.66	126.84	1754	38.48	78.70	125.80	1740	38.99	79.73	124.77	1726
205	37.36	76.58	128.42	1776	37.86	77.62	127.38	1762	38.37	78.66	126.35	1747	38.87	79.69	125.31	1733
205.5	37.25	76.54	128.96	1784	37.75	77.58	127.92	1769	38.25	78.61	126.89	1755	38.76	79.65	125.85	1740
206	37.13	76.50	129.50	1791	37.64	77.54	128.46	1777	38.14	78.57	127.43	1762	38.65	79.61	126.39	1748
206.5	37.03	76.46	130.04	1798	37.53	77.49	129.01	1784	38.03	78.53	127.97	1770	38.53	79.57	126.93	1755
207	36.92	76.42	130.58	1806	37.42	77.45	129.55	1792	37.92	78.49	128.51	1777	38.42	79.53	127.47	1763
207.5	36.81	76.38	131.13	1813	37.31	77.41	130.09	1799	37.81	78.45	129.05	1785	38.31	79.49	128.01	1770
208	36.70	76.33	131.67	1821	37.20	77.37	130.63	1807	37.70	78.41	129.59	1792	38.20	79.45	128.55	1778
208.5	36.59	76.29	132.21	1828	37.09	77.33	131.17	1814	37.59	78.37	130.13	1800	38.08	79.41	129.09	1785
209	36.48	76.25	132.75	1836	36.98	77.29	131.71	1822	37.48	78.33	130.67	1807	37.97	79.36	129.64	1793
209.5	36.38	76.21	133.29	1843	36.87	77.25	132.25	1829	37.37	78.29	131.21	1815	37.86	79.32	130.18	1800
210	36.27	76.17	133.83	1851	36.77	77.21	132.79	1837	37.26	78.25	131.76	1822	37.75	79.28	130.72	1808
210.5	36.17	76.13	134.37	1858	36.66	77.17	133.33	1844	37.15	78.20	132.30	1830	37.64	79.24	131.26	1815
211	36.06	76.09	134.91	1866	36.55	77.13	133.87	1851	37.04	78.16	132.84	1837	37.54	79.20	131.80	1823
211.5	35.96	76.05	135.45	1873	36.45	77.08	134.42	1859	36.94	78.12	133.38	1845	37.43	79.16	132.34	1830
212	35.85	76.01	135.99	1881	36.34	77.04	134.96	1866	36.83	78.08	133.92	1852	37.32	79.12	132.88	1838
212.5	35.75	75.97	136.54	1888	36.24	77.00	135.50	1874	36.72	78.04	134.46	1860	37.21	79.08	133.42	1845
213	35.65	75.92	137.08	1896	36.13	76.96	136.04	1881	36.62	78.00	135.00	1867	37.11	79.04	133.96	1853
213.5	35.54	75.88	137.62	1903	36.03	76.92	136.58	1889	36.51	77.96	135.54	1875	37.00	79.00	134.50	1860
214	35.44	75.84	138.16	1911	35.93	76.88	137.12	1896	36.41	77.92	136.08	1882	36.89	78.95	135.05	1868
214.5	35.34	75.80	138.70	1918	35.82	76.84	137.66	1904	36.31	77.88	136.62	1890	36.79	78.91	135.59	1875
215	35.24	75.76	139.24	1926	35.72	76.80	138.20	1911	36.20	77.84	137.17	1897	36.68	78.87	136.13	1883
215.5	35.14	75.72	139.78	1933	35.62	76.76	138.74	1919	36.10	77.79	137.71	1904	36.58	78.83	136.67	1890
216	35.04	75.68	140.32	1941	35.52	76.72	139.28	1926	36.00	77.75	138.25	1912	36.48	78.79	137.21	1898
216.5	34.94	75.64	140.86	1948	35.42	76.67	139.83	1934	35.89	77.71	138.79	1919	36.37	78.75	137.75	1905
217	34.84	75.60	141.40	1956	35.31	76.63	140.37	1941	35.79	77.67	139.33	1927	36.27	78.71	138.29	1913
217.5	34.74	75.56	141.95	1963	35.21	76.59	140.91	1949	35.69	77.63	139.87	1934	36.17	78.67	138.83	1920
218	34.64	75.51	142.49	1971	35.12	76.55	141.45	1956	35.59	77.59	140.41	1942	36.07	78.63	139.37	1928
218.5	34.54	75.47	143.03	1978	35.02	76.51	141.99	1964	35.49	77.55	140.95	1949	35.97	78.59	139.91	1935
219	34.44	75.43	143.57	1986	34.92	76.47	142.53	1971	35.39	77.51	141.49	1957	35.87	78.54	140.46	1942
219.5	34.35	75.39	144.11	1993	34.82	76.43	143.07	1979	35.29	77.47	142.03	1964	35.76	78.50	141.00	1950
220	34.25	75.35	144.65	2001	34.72	76.39	143.61	1986	35.19	77.43	142.58	1972	35.66	78.46	141.54	1957
220.5	34.15	75.31	145.19	2008	34.62	76.35	144.15	1994	35.09	77.38	143.12	1979	35.57	78.42	142.08	1965
221	34.06	75.27	145.73	2015	34.53	76.31	144.69	2001	35.00	77.34	143.66	1987	35.47	78.38	142.62	1972
221.5	33.96	75.23	146.27	2023	34.43	76.26	145.24	2009	34.90	77.30	144.20	1994	35.37	78.34	143.16	1980
222	33.87	75.19	146.81	2030	34.33	76.22	145.78	2016	34.80	77.26	144.74	2002	35.27	78.30	143.70	1987
222.5	33.77	75.15	147.36	2038	34.24	76.18	146.32	2024	34.71	77.22	145.28	2009	35.17	78.26	144.24	1995
223	33.68	75.10	147.90	2045	34.14	76.14	146.86	2031	34.61	77.18	145.82	2017	35.07	78.22	144.78	2002
223.5	33.59	75.06	148.44	2053	34.05	76.10	147.40	2039	34.51	77.14	146.36	2024	34.98	78.18	145.32	2010
224	33.49	75.02	148.98	2060	33.96	76.06	147.94	2046	34.42	77.10	146.90	2032	34.88	78.13	145.87	2017
224.5	33.40	74.98	149.52	2068	33.86	76.02	148.48	2053	34.32	77.06	147.44	2039	34.79	78.09	146.41	2025
225	33.31	74.94	150.06	2075	33.77	75.98	149.02	2061	34.23	77.02	147.99	2047	34.69	78.05	146.95	2032
225.5	33.21	74.90	150.60	2083	33.67	75.94	149.56	2068	34.13	76.97	148.53	2054	34.59	78.01	147.49	2040
226	33.12	74.86	151.14	2090	33.58	75.90	150.10	2076	34.04	76.93	149.07	2062	34.50	77.97	148.03	2047
226.5	33.03	74.82	151.68	2098	33.49	75.85	150.65	2083	33.95	76.89	149.61	2069	34.41	77.93	148.57	2055
227	32.94	74.78	152.22	2105	33.40	75.81	151.19	2091	33.86	76.85	150.15	2077	34.31	77.89	149.11	2062
227.5	32.85	74.74	152.77	2113	33.31	75.77	151.73	2098	33.76	76.81	150.69	2084	34.22	77.85	149.65	2070

Body Composition FEMALE 196-227.5 Lb.

Weight: Lb.	Waist: 42 inches Fat: %	Fat: Lb.	LBM: Lb.	RMR: Cal.	42.25 inches Fat: %	Fat: Lb.	LBM: Lb.	RMR: Cal.	42.5 inches Fat: %	Fat: Lb.	LBM: Lb.	RMR: Cal.	42.75 inches Fat: %	Fat: Lb.	LBM: Lb.	RMR: Cal.
196	41.57	81.47	114.53	1584	42.09	82.51	113.49	1570	42.62	83.54	112.46	1555	43.15	84.58	111.42	1541
196.5	41.44	81.43	115.07	1591	41.97	82.46	114.04	1577	42.49	83.50	113.00	1563	43.02	84.54	111.96	1548
197	41.31	81.39	115.61	1599	41.84	82.42	114.58	1585	42.37	83.46	113.54	1570	42.89	84.50	112.50	1556
197.5	41.19	81.35	116.16	1606	41.71	82.38	115.12	1592	42.24	83.42	114.08	1578	42.76	84.46	113.04	1563
198	41.06	81.30	116.70	1614	41.59	82.34	115.66	1600	42.11	83.38	114.62	1585	42.63	84.42	113.58	1571
198.5	40.94	81.26	117.24	1621	41.46	82.30	116.20	1607	41.98	83.34	115.16	1593	42.51	84.38	114.12	1578
199	40.82	81.22	117.78	1629	41.34	82.26	116.74	1615	41.86	83.30	115.70	1600	42.38	84.33	114.67	1586
199.5	40.69	81.18	118.32	1636	41.21	82.22	117.28	1622	41.73	83.26	116.24	1608	42.25	84.29	115.21	1593
200	40.57	81.14	118.86	1644	41.09	82.18	117.82	1629	41.61	83.22	116.79	1615	42.13	84.25	115.75	1601
200.5	40.45	81.10	119.40	1651	40.97	82.14	118.36	1637	41.48	83.17	117.33	1623	42.00	84.21	116.29	1608
201	40.33	81.06	119.94	1659	40.84	82.10	118.90	1644	41.36	83.13	117.87	1630	41.88	84.17	116.83	1616
201.5	40.21	81.02	120.48	1666	40.72	82.05	119.45	1652	41.24	83.09	118.41	1638	41.75	84.13	117.37	1623
202	40.09	80.98	121.02	1674	40.60	82.01	119.99	1659	41.11	83.05	118.95	1645	41.63	84.09	117.91	1631
202.5	39.97	80.94	121.57	1681	40.48	81.97	120.53	1667	40.99	83.01	119.49	1653	41.50	84.05	118.45	1638
203	39.85	80.89	122.11	1689	40.36	81.93	121.07	1674	40.87	82.97	120.03	1660	41.38	84.01	118.99	1646
203.5	39.73	80.85	122.65	1696	40.24	81.89	121.61	1682	40.75	82.93	120.57	1668	41.26	83.97	119.53	1653
204	39.61	80.81	123.19	1704	40.12	81.85	122.15	1689	40.63	82.89	121.11	1675	41.14	83.92	120.08	1661
204.5	39.50	80.77	123.73	1711	40.00	81.81	122.69	1697	40.51	82.85	121.65	1682	41.02	83.88	120.62	1668
205	39.38	80.73	124.27	1719	39.89	81.77	123.23	1704	40.39	82.81	122.20	1690	40.90	83.84	121.16	1676
205.5	39.26	80.69	124.81	1726	39.77	81.73	123.77	1712	40.27	82.76	122.74	1697	40.78	83.80	121.70	1683
206	39.15	80.65	125.35	1734	39.65	81.69	124.31	1719	40.16	82.72	123.28	1705	40.66	83.76	122.24	1691
206.5	39.03	80.61	125.89	1741	39.54	81.64	124.86	1727	40.04	82.68	123.82	1712	40.54	83.72	122.78	1698
207	38.92	80.57	126.43	1749	39.42	81.60	125.40	1734	39.92	82.64	124.36	1720	40.42	83.68	123.32	1706
207.5	38.81	80.53	126.98	1756	39.31	81.56	125.94	1742	39.81	82.60	124.90	1727	40.31	83.64	123.86	1713
208	38.69	80.48	127.52	1764	39.19	81.52	126.48	1749	39.69	82.56	125.44	1735	40.19	83.60	124.40	1721
208.5	38.58	80.44	128.06	1771	39.08	81.48	127.02	1757	39.58	82.52	125.98	1742	40.07	83.56	124.94	1728
209	38.47	80.40	128.60	1779	38.97	81.44	127.56	1764	39.46	82.48	126.52	1750	39.96	83.51	125.49	1735
209.5	38.36	80.36	129.14	1786	38.85	81.40	128.10	1772	39.35	82.44	127.06	1757	39.84	83.47	126.03	1743
210	38.25	80.32	129.68	1793	38.74	81.36	128.64	1779	39.24	82.40	127.61	1765	39.73	83.43	126.57	1750
210.5	38.14	80.28	130.22	1801	38.63	81.32	129.18	1787	39.12	82.35	128.15	1772	39.62	83.39	127.11	1758
211	38.03	80.24	130.76	1808	38.52	81.28	129.72	1794	39.01	82.31	128.69	1780	39.50	83.35	127.65	1765
211.5	37.92	80.20	131.30	1816	38.41	81.23	130.27	1802	38.90	82.27	129.23	1787	39.39	83.31	128.19	1773
212	37.81	80.16	131.84	1823	38.30	81.19	130.81	1809	38.79	82.23	129.77	1795	39.28	83.27	128.73	1780
212.5	37.70	80.12	132.39	1831	38.19	81.15	131.35	1817	38.68	82.19	130.31	1802	39.17	83.23	129.27	1788
213	37.59	80.07	132.93	1838	38.08	81.11	131.89	1824	38.57	82.15	130.85	1810	39.05	83.19	129.81	1795
213.5	37.49	80.03	133.47	1846	37.97	81.07	132.43	1831	38.46	82.11	131.39	1817	38.94	83.15	130.35	1803
214	37.38	79.99	134.01	1853	37.86	81.03	132.97	1839	38.35	82.07	131.93	1825	38.83	83.10	130.90	1810
214.5	37.27	79.95	134.55	1861	37.76	80.99	133.51	1846	38.24	82.03	132.47	1832	38.72	83.06	131.44	1818
215	37.17	79.91	135.09	1868	37.65	80.95	134.05	1854	38.13	81.99	133.02	1840	38.62	83.02	131.98	1825
215.5	37.06	79.87	135.63	1876	37.54	80.91	134.59	1861	38.03	81.94	133.56	1847	38.51	82.98	132.52	1833
216	36.96	79.83	136.17	1883	37.44	80.87	135.13	1869	37.92	81.90	134.10	1855	38.40	82.94	133.06	1840
216.5	36.85	79.79	136.71	1891	37.33	80.82	135.68	1876	37.81	81.86	134.64	1862	38.29	82.90	133.60	1848
217	36.75	79.75	137.25	1898	37.23	80.78	136.22	1884	37.71	81.82	135.18	1870	38.18	82.86	134.14	1855
217.5	36.65	79.71	137.80	1906	37.12	80.74	136.76	1891	37.60	81.78	135.72	1877	38.08	82.82	134.68	1863
218	36.54	79.66	138.34	1913	37.02	80.70	137.30	1899	37.49	81.74	136.26	1884	37.97	82.78	135.22	1870
218.5	36.44	79.62	138.88	1921	36.92	80.66	137.84	1906	37.39	81.70	136.80	1892	37.87	82.74	135.76	1878
219	36.34	79.58	139.42	1928	36.81	80.62	138.38	1914	37.29	81.66	137.34	1899	37.76	82.69	136.31	1885
219.5	36.24	79.54	139.96	1936	36.71	80.58	138.92	1921	37.18	81.62	137.88	1907	37.66	82.65	136.85	1893
220	36.14	79.50	140.50	1943	36.61	80.54	139.46	1929	37.08	81.58	138.43	1914	37.55	82.61	137.39	1900
220.5	36.04	79.46	141.04	1951	36.51	80.50	140.00	1936	36.98	81.53	138.97	1922	37.45	82.57	137.93	1908
221	35.94	79.42	141.58	1958	36.41	80.46	140.54	1944	36.87	81.49	139.51	1929	37.34	82.53	138.47	1915
221.5	35.84	79.38	142.12	1966	36.30	80.41	141.09	1951	36.77	81.45	140.05	1937	37.24	82.49	139.01	1923
222	35.74	79.34	142.66	1973	36.20	80.37	141.63	1959	36.67	81.41	140.59	1944	37.14	82.45	139.55	1930
222.5	35.64	79.30	143.21	1981	36.10	80.33	142.17	1966	36.57	81.37	141.13	1952	37.04	82.41	140.09	1937
223	35.54	79.25	143.75	1988	36.01	80.29	142.71	1974	36.47	81.33	141.67	1959	36.94	82.37	140.63	1945
223.5	35.44	79.21	144.29	1995	35.91	80.25	143.25	1981	36.37	81.29	142.21	1967	36.83	82.33	141.17	1952
224	35.34	79.17	144.83	2003	35.81	80.21	143.79	1989	36.27	81.25	142.75	1974	36.73	82.28	141.72	1960
224.5	35.25	79.13	145.37	2010	35.71	80.17	144.33	1996	36.17	81.21	143.29	1982	36.63	82.24	142.26	1967
225	35.15	79.09	145.91	2018	35.61	80.13	144.87	2004	36.07	81.17	143.84	1989	36.53	82.20	142.80	1975
225.5	35.05	79.05	146.45	2025	35.52	80.09	145.41	2011	35.98	81.12	144.38	1997	36.44	82.16	143.34	1982
226	34.96	79.01	146.99	2033	35.42	80.05	145.95	2019	35.88	81.08	144.92	2004	36.34	82.12	143.88	1990
226.5	34.86	78.97	147.53	2040	35.32	80.00	146.50	2026	35.78	81.04	145.46	2012	36.24	82.08	144.42	1997
227	34.77	78.93	148.07	2048	35.23	79.96	147.04	2034	35.68	81.00	146.00	2019	36.14	82.04	144.96	2005
227.5	34.67	78.89	148.62	2055	35.13	79.92	147.58	2041	35.59	80.96	146.54	2027	36.04	82.00	145.50	2012

Body Composition FEMALE 196-227.5 Lb.

Weight: Lb.	Waist: 43 inches				43.25 inches				43.5 inches				43.75 inches			
	Fat: %	Fat: Lb.	LBM: Lb.	RMR: Cal.	Fat: %	Fat: Lb.	LBM: Lb.	RMR: Cal.	Fat: %	Fat: Lb.	LBM: Lb.	RMR: Cal.	Fat: %	Fat: Lb.	LBM: Lb.	RMR: Cal.
196	43.68	85.62	110.38	1527	44.21	86.66	109.34	1512	44.74	87.69	108.31	1498	45.27	88.73	107.27	1484
196.5	43.55	85.58	110.92	1534	44.08	86.61	109.89	1520	44.61	87.65	108.85	1505	45.13	88.69	107.81	1491
197	43.42	85.54	111.46	1542	43.95	86.57	110.43	1527	44.47	87.61	109.39	1513	45.00	88.65	108.35	1499
197.5	43.29	85.50	112.01	1549	43.81	86.53	110.97	1535	44.34	87.57	109.93	1520	44.86	88.61	108.89	1506
198	43.16	85.45	112.55	1557	43.68	86.49	111.51	1542	44.21	87.53	110.47	1528	44.73	88.57	109.43	1513
198.5	43.03	85.41	113.09	1564	43.55	86.45	112.05	1550	44.07	87.49	111.01	1535	44.60	88.53	109.97	1521
199	42.90	85.37	113.63	1571	43.42	86.41	112.59	1557	43.94	87.45	111.55	1543	44.46	88.48	110.52	1528
199.5	42.77	85.33	114.17	1579	43.29	86.37	113.13	1565	43.81	87.41	112.09	1550	44.33	88.44	111.06	1536
200	42.65	85.29	114.71	1586	43.16	86.33	113.67	1572	43.68	87.37	112.64	1558	44.20	88.40	111.60	1543
200.5	42.52	85.25	115.25	1594	43.04	86.29	114.21	1580	43.55	87.32	113.18	1565	44.07	88.36	112.14	1551
201	42.39	85.21	115.79	1601	42.91	86.25	114.75	1587	43.42	87.28	113.72	1573	43.94	88.32	112.68	1558
201.5	42.27	85.17	116.33	1609	42.78	86.20	115.30	1595	43.30	87.24	114.26	1580	43.81	88.28	113.22	1566
202	42.14	85.13	116.87	1616	42.66	86.16	115.84	1602	43.17	87.20	114.80	1588	43.68	88.24	113.76	1573
202.5	42.02	85.09	117.42	1624	42.53	86.12	116.38	1610	43.04	87.16	115.34	1595	43.55	88.20	114.30	1581
203	41.89	85.04	117.96	1631	42.40	86.08	116.92	1617	42.92	87.12	115.88	1603	43.43	88.16	114.84	1588
203.5	41.77	85.00	118.50	1639	42.28	86.04	117.46	1624	42.79	87.08	116.42	1610	43.30	88.12	115.38	1596
204	41.65	84.96	119.04	1646	42.16	86.00	118.00	1632	42.67	87.04	116.96	1618	43.17	88.07	115.93	1603
204.5	41.53	84.92	119.58	1654	42.03	85.96	118.54	1639	42.54	87.00	117.50	1625	43.05	88.03	116.47	1611
205	41.40	84.88	120.12	1661	41.91	85.92	119.08	1647	42.42	86.96	118.05	1633	42.92	87.99	117.01	1618
205.5	41.28	84.84	120.66	1669	41.79	85.88	119.62	1654	42.29	86.91	118.59	1640	42.80	87.95	117.55	1626
206	41.16	84.80	121.20	1676	41.67	85.84	120.16	1662	42.17	86.87	119.13	1648	42.68	87.91	118.09	1633
206.5	41.04	84.76	121.74	1684	41.55	85.79	120.71	1669	42.05	86.83	119.67	1655	42.55	87.87	118.63	1641
207	40.93	84.72	122.28	1691	41.43	85.75	121.25	1677	41.93	86.79	120.21	1662	42.43	87.83	119.17	1648
207.5	40.81	84.68	122.83	1699	41.31	85.71	121.79	1684	41.81	86.75	120.75	1670	42.31	87.79	119.71	1656
208	40.69	84.63	123.37	1706	41.19	85.67	122.33	1692	41.69	86.71	121.29	1677	42.19	87.75	120.25	1663
208.5	40.57	84.59	123.91	1714	41.07	85.63	122.87	1699	41.57	86.67	121.83	1685	42.06	87.71	120.79	1671
209	40.46	84.55	124.45	1721	40.95	85.59	123.41	1707	41.45	86.63	122.37	1692	41.94	87.66	121.34	1678
209.5	40.34	84.51	124.99	1729	40.83	85.55	123.95	1714	41.33	86.59	122.91	1700	41.83	87.62	121.88	1686
210	40.22	84.47	125.53	1736	40.72	85.51	124.49	1722	41.21	86.55	123.46	1707	41.71	87.58	122.42	1693
210.5	40.11	84.43	126.07	1744	40.60	85.47	125.03	1729	41.09	86.50	124.00	1715	41.59	87.54	122.96	1701
211	39.99	84.39	126.61	1751	40.49	85.43	125.57	1737	40.98	86.46	124.54	1722	41.47	87.50	123.50	1708
211.5	39.88	84.35	127.15	1759	40.37	85.38	126.12	1744	40.86	86.42	125.08	1730	41.35	87.46	124.04	1715
212	39.77	84.31	127.69	1766	40.26	85.34	126.66	1752	40.75	86.38	125.62	1737	41.24	87.42	124.58	1723
212.5	39.65	84.27	128.24	1773	40.14	85.30	127.20	1759	40.63	86.34	126.16	1745	41.12	87.38	125.12	1730
213	39.54	84.22	128.78	1781	40.03	85.26	127.74	1767	40.52	86.30	126.70	1752	41.00	87.34	125.66	1738
213.5	39.43	84.18	129.32	1788	39.92	85.22	128.28	1774	40.40	86.26	127.24	1760	40.89	87.30	126.20	1745
214	39.32	84.14	129.86	1796	39.80	85.18	128.82	1782	40.29	86.22	127.78	1767	40.77	87.25	126.75	1753
214.5	39.21	84.10	130.40	1803	39.69	85.14	129.36	1789	40.18	86.18	128.32	1775	40.66	87.21	127.29	1760
215	39.10	84.06	130.94	1811	39.58	85.10	129.90	1797	40.06	86.14	128.87	1782	40.55	87.17	127.83	1768
215.5	38.99	84.02	131.48	1818	39.47	85.06	130.44	1804	39.95	86.09	129.41	1790	40.43	87.13	128.37	1775
216	38.88	83.98	132.02	1826	39.36	85.02	130.98	1812	39.84	86.05	129.95	1797	40.32	87.09	128.91	1783
216.5	38.77	83.94	132.56	1833	39.25	84.97	131.53	1819	39.73	86.01	130.49	1805	40.21	87.05	129.45	1790
217	38.66	83.90	133.10	1841	39.14	84.93	132.07	1826	39.62	85.97	131.03	1812	40.10	87.01	129.99	1798
217.5	38.55	83.86	133.65	1848	39.03	84.89	132.61	1834	39.51	85.93	131.57	1820	39.99	86.97	130.53	1805
218	38.45	83.81	134.19	1856	38.92	84.85	133.15	1841	39.40	85.89	132.11	1827	39.87	86.93	131.07	1813
218.5	38.34	83.77	134.73	1863	38.81	84.81	133.69	1849	39.29	85.85	132.65	1835	39.76	86.89	131.61	1820
219	38.23	83.73	135.27	1871	38.71	84.77	134.23	1856	39.18	85.81	133.19	1842	39.66	86.84	132.16	1828
219.5	38.13	83.69	135.81	1878	38.60	84.73	134.77	1864	39.07	85.77	133.73	1850	39.55	86.80	132.70	1835
220	38.02	83.65	136.35	1886	38.49	84.69	135.31	1871	38.97	85.73	134.28	1857	39.44	86.76	133.24	1843
220.5	37.92	83.61	136.89	1893	38.39	84.65	135.85	1879	38.86	85.68	134.82	1865	39.33	86.72	133.78	1850
221	37.81	83.57	137.43	1901	38.28	84.61	136.39	1886	38.75	85.64	135.36	1872	39.22	86.68	134.32	1858
221.5	37.71	83.53	137.97	1908	38.18	84.56	136.94	1894	38.65	85.60	135.90	1879	39.11	86.64	134.86	1865
222	37.61	83.49	138.51	1916	38.07	84.52	137.48	1901	38.54	85.56	136.44	1887	39.01	86.60	135.40	1873
222.5	37.50	83.45	139.06	1923	37.97	84.48	138.02	1909	38.44	85.52	136.98	1894	38.90	86.56	135.94	1880
223	37.40	83.40	139.60	1931	37.87	84.44	138.56	1916	38.33	85.48	137.52	1902	38.80	86.52	136.48	1888
223.5	37.30	83.36	140.14	1938	37.76	84.40	139.10	1924	38.23	85.44	138.06	1909	38.69	86.48	137.02	1895
224	37.20	83.32	140.68	1946	37.66	84.36	139.64	1931	38.12	85.40	138.60	1917	38.59	86.43	137.57	1903
224.5	37.10	83.28	141.22	1953	37.56	84.32	140.18	1939	38.02	85.36	139.14	1924	38.48	86.39	138.11	1910
225	37.00	83.24	141.76	1961	37.46	84.28	140.72	1946	37.92	85.32	139.69	1932	38.38	86.35	138.65	1917
225.5	36.90	83.20	142.30	1968	37.36	84.24	141.26	1954	37.82	85.27	140.23	1939	38.28	86.31	139.19	1925
226	36.80	83.16	142.84	1976	37.25	84.20	141.80	1961	37.71	85.23	140.77	1947	38.17	86.27	139.73	1932
226.5	36.70	83.12	143.38	1983	37.15	84.15	142.35	1969	37.61	85.19	141.31	1954	38.07	86.23	140.27	1940
227	36.60	83.08	143.92	1990	37.05	84.11	142.89	1976	37.51	85.15	141.85	1962	37.97	86.19	140.81	1947
227.5	36.50	83.04	144.47	1998	36.95	84.07	143.43	1984	37.41	85.11	142.39	1969	37.87	86.15	141.35	1955

Body Composition FEMALE 196-227.5 Lb.

Weight: Lb.	Waist: 44 inches Fat: %	Fat: Lb.	LBM: Lb.	RMR: Cal.	44.25 inches Fat: %	Fat: Lb.	LBM: Lb.	RMR: Cal.	44.5 inches Fat: %	Fat: Lb.	LBM: Lb.	RMR: Cal.	44.75 inches Fat: %	Fat: Lb.	LBM: Lb.	RMR: Cal.
196	45.80	89.77	106.23	1469	46.33	90.81	105.19	1455	46.86	91.84	104.16	1440	47.39	92.88	103.12	1426
196.5	45.66	89.73	106.77	1477	46.19	90.76	105.74	1462	46.72	91.80	104.70	1448	47.25	92.84	103.66	1434
197	45.53	89.69	107.31	1484	46.05	90.72	106.28	1470	46.58	91.76	105.24	1455	47.11	92.80	104.20	1441
197.5	45.39	89.65	107.86	1492	45.92	90.68	106.82	1477	46.44	91.72	105.78	1463	46.97	92.76	104.74	1449
198	45.25	89.60	108.40	1499	45.78	90.64	107.36	1485	46.30	91.68	106.32	1470	46.83	92.72	105.28	1456
198.5	45.12	89.56	108.94	1507	45.64	90.60	107.90	1492	46.17	91.64	106.86	1478	46.69	92.68	105.82	1464
199	44.99	89.52	109.48	1514	45.51	90.56	108.44	1500	46.03	91.60	107.40	1485	46.55	92.63	106.37	1471
199.5	44.85	89.48	110.02	1522	45.37	90.52	108.98	1507	45.89	91.56	107.94	1493	46.41	92.59	106.91	1479
200	44.72	89.44	110.56	1529	45.24	90.48	109.52	1515	45.76	91.52	108.49	1500	46.28	92.55	107.45	1486
200.5	44.59	89.40	111.10	1537	45.11	90.44	110.06	1522	45.62	91.47	109.03	1508	46.14	92.51	107.99	1493
201	44.46	89.36	111.64	1544	44.97	90.40	110.60	1530	45.49	91.43	109.57	1515	46.01	92.47	108.53	1501
201.5	44.33	89.32	112.18	1551	44.84	90.35	111.15	1537	45.36	91.39	110.11	1523	45.87	92.43	109.07	1508
202	44.20	89.28	112.72	1559	44.71	90.31	111.69	1545	45.22	91.35	110.65	1530	45.74	92.39	109.61	1516
202.5	44.07	89.24	113.27	1566	44.58	90.27	112.23	1552	45.09	91.31	111.19	1538	45.60	92.35	110.15	1523
203	43.94	89.19	113.81	1574	44.45	90.23	112.77	1560	44.96	91.27	111.73	1545	45.47	92.31	110.69	1531
203.5	43.81	89.15	114.35	1581	44.32	90.19	113.31	1567	44.83	91.23	112.27	1553	45.34	92.27	111.23	1538
204	43.68	89.11	114.89	1589	44.19	90.15	113.85	1575	44.70	91.19	112.81	1560	45.21	92.22	111.78	1546
204.5	43.56	89.07	115.43	1596	44.06	90.11	114.39	1582	44.57	91.15	113.35	1568	45.08	92.18	112.32	1553
205	43.43	89.03	115.97	1604	43.94	90.07	114.93	1590	44.44	91.11	113.90	1575	44.95	92.14	112.86	1561
205.5	43.30	88.99	116.51	1611	43.81	90.03	115.47	1597	44.31	91.06	114.44	1583	44.82	92.10	113.40	1568
206	43.18	88.95	117.05	1619	43.68	89.99	116.01	1604	44.19	91.02	114.98	1590	44.69	92.06	113.94	1576
206.5	43.05	88.91	117.59	1626	43.56	89.94	116.56	1612	44.06	90.98	115.52	1598	44.56	92.02	114.48	1583
207	42.93	88.87	118.13	1634	43.43	89.90	117.10	1619	43.93	90.94	116.06	1605	44.43	91.98	115.02	1591
207.5	42.81	88.83	118.68	1641	43.31	89.86	117.64	1627	43.81	90.90	116.60	1613	44.31	91.94	115.56	1598
208	42.68	88.78	119.22	1649	43.18	89.82	118.18	1634	43.68	90.86	117.14	1620	44.18	91.90	116.10	1606
208.5	42.56	88.74	119.76	1656	43.06	89.78	118.72	1642	43.56	90.82	117.68	1628	44.06	91.86	116.64	1613
209	42.44	88.70	120.30	1664	42.94	89.74	119.26	1649	43.43	90.78	118.22	1635	43.93	91.81	117.19	1621
209.5	42.32	88.66	120.84	1671	42.82	89.70	119.80	1657	43.31	90.74	118.76	1643	43.81	91.77	117.73	1628
210	42.20	88.62	121.38	1679	42.69	89.66	120.34	1664	43.19	90.70	119.31	1650	43.68	91.73	118.27	1636
210.5	42.08	88.58	121.92	1686	42.57	89.62	120.88	1672	43.07	90.65	119.85	1657	43.56	91.69	118.81	1643
211	41.96	88.54	122.46	1694	42.45	89.58	121.42	1679	42.94	90.61	120.39	1665	43.44	91.65	119.35	1651
211.5	41.84	88.50	123.00	1701	42.33	89.53	121.97	1687	42.82	90.57	120.93	1672	43.31	91.61	119.89	1658
212	41.72	88.46	123.54	1709	42.21	89.49	122.51	1694	42.70	90.53	121.47	1680	43.19	91.57	120.43	1666
212.5	41.61	88.42	124.09	1716	42.10	89.45	123.05	1702	42.58	90.49	122.01	1687	43.07	91.53	120.97	1673
213	41.49	88.37	124.63	1724	41.98	89.41	123.59	1709	42.46	90.45	122.55	1695	42.95	91.49	121.51	1681
213.5	41.37	88.33	125.17	1731	41.86	89.37	124.13	1717	42.35	90.41	123.09	1702	42.83	91.45	122.05	1688
214	41.26	88.29	125.71	1739	41.74	89.33	124.67	1724	42.23	90.37	123.63	1710	42.71	91.40	122.60	1695
214.5	41.14	88.25	126.25	1746	41.63	89.29	125.21	1732	42.11	90.33	124.17	1717	42.59	91.36	123.14	1703
215	41.03	88.21	126.79	1754	41.51	89.25	125.75	1739	41.99	90.29	124.72	1725	42.48	91.32	123.68	1710
215.5	40.91	88.17	127.33	1761	41.40	89.21	126.29	1747	41.88	90.24	125.26	1732	42.36	91.28	124.22	1718
216	40.80	88.13	127.87	1768	41.28	89.17	126.83	1754	41.76	90.20	125.80	1740	42.24	91.24	124.76	1725
216.5	40.69	88.09	128.41	1776	41.17	89.12	127.38	1762	41.65	90.16	126.34	1747	42.12	91.20	125.30	1733
217	40.57	88.05	128.95	1783	41.05	89.08	127.92	1769	41.53	90.12	126.88	1755	42.01	91.16	125.84	1740
217.5	40.46	88.01	129.50	1791	40.94	89.04	128.46	1777	41.42	90.08	127.42	1762	41.89	91.12	126.38	1748
218	40.35	87.96	130.04	1798	40.83	89.00	129.00	1784	41.30	90.04	127.96	1770	41.78	91.08	126.92	1755
218.5	40.24	87.92	130.58	1806	40.71	88.96	129.54	1792	41.19	90.00	128.50	1777	41.66	91.04	127.46	1763
219	40.13	87.88	131.12	1813	40.60	88.92	130.08	1799	41.08	89.96	129.04	1785	41.55	90.99	128.01	1770
219.5	40.02	87.84	131.66	1821	40.49	88.88	130.62	1806	40.96	89.92	129.58	1792	41.44	90.95	128.55	1778
220	39.91	87.80	132.20	1828	40.38	88.84	131.16	1814	40.85	89.88	130.13	1800	41.32	90.91	129.09	1785
220.5	39.80	87.76	132.74	1836	40.27	88.80	131.70	1821	40.74	89.83	130.67	1807	41.21	90.87	129.63	1793
221	39.69	87.72	133.28	1843	40.16	88.76	132.24	1829	40.63	89.79	131.21	1815	41.10	90.83	130.17	1800
221.5	39.58	87.68	133.82	1851	40.05	88.71	132.79	1836	40.52	89.75	131.75	1822	40.99	90.79	130.71	1808
222	39.48	87.64	134.36	1858	39.94	88.67	133.33	1844	40.41	89.71	132.29	1830	40.88	90.75	131.25	1815
222.5	39.37	87.60	134.91	1866	39.83	88.63	133.87	1851	40.30	89.67	132.83	1837	40.77	90.71	131.79	1823
223	39.26	87.55	135.45	1873	39.73	88.59	134.41	1859	40.19	89.63	133.37	1845	40.66	90.67	132.33	1830
223.5	39.16	87.51	135.99	1881	39.62	88.55	134.95	1866	40.08	89.59	133.91	1852	40.55	90.63	132.87	1838
224	39.05	87.47	136.53	1888	39.51	88.51	135.49	1874	39.98	89.55	134.45	1859	40.44	90.58	133.42	1845
224.5	38.94	87.43	137.07	1896	39.41	88.47	136.03	1881	39.87	89.51	134.99	1867	40.33	90.54	133.96	1853
225	38.84	87.39	137.61	1903	39.30	88.43	136.57	1889	39.76	89.47	135.54	1874	40.22	90.50	134.50	1860
225.5	38.74	87.35	138.15	1911	39.20	88.39	137.11	1896	39.66	89.42	136.08	1882	40.12	90.46	135.04	1868
226	38.63	87.31	138.69	1918	39.09	88.35	137.65	1904	39.55	89.38	136.62	1889	40.01	90.42	135.58	1875
226.5	38.53	87.27	139.23	1926	38.99	88.30	138.20	1911	39.44	89.34	137.16	1897	39.90	90.38	136.12	1883
227	38.43	87.23	139.77	1933	38.88	88.26	138.74	1919	39.34	89.30	137.70	1904	39.80	90.34	136.66	1890
227.5	38.32	87.19	140.32	1941	38.78	88.22	139.28	1926	39.24	89.26	138.24	1912	39.69	90.30	137.20	1898

Body Composition FEMALE 196-227.5 Lb.

Weight: Lb.	Waist: 45 inches Fat: %	Fat: Lb.	LBM: Lb.	RMR: Cal.	45.25 inches Fat: %	Fat: Lb.	LBM: Lb.	RMR: Cal.	45.5 inches Fat: %	Fat: Lb.	LBM: Lb.	RMR: Cal.	45.75 inches Fat: %	Fat: Lb.	LBM: Lb.	RMR: Cal.
196	47.92	93.92	102.08	1412	48.45	94.96	101.04	1397	48.98	95.99	100.01	1383	49.51	97.03	98.97	1369
196.5	47.77	93.88	102.62	1419	48.30	94.91	101.59	1405	48.83	95.95	100.55	1391	49.36	96.99	99.51	1376
197	47.63	93.84	103.16	1427	48.16	94.87	102.13	1412	48.69	95.91	101.09	1398	49.21	96.95	100.05	1384
197.5	47.49	93.80	103.71	1434	48.02	94.83	102.67	1420	48.54	95.87	101.63	1406	49.07	96.91	100.59	1391
198	47.35	93.75	104.25	1442	47.87	94.79	103.21	1427	48.40	95.83	102.17	1413	48.92	96.87	101.13	1399
198.5	47.21	93.71	104.79	1449	47.73	94.75	103.75	1435	48.26	95.79	102.71	1421	48.78	96.83	101.67	1406
199	47.07	93.67	105.33	1457	47.59	94.71	104.29	1442	48.11	95.75	103.25	1428	48.64	96.78	102.22	1414
199.5	46.93	93.63	105.87	1464	47.45	94.67	104.83	1450	47.97	95.71	103.79	1435	48.49	96.74	102.76	1421
200	46.80	93.59	106.41	1472	47.31	94.63	105.37	1457	47.83	95.67	104.34	1443	48.35	96.70	103.30	1429
200.5	46.66	93.55	106.95	1479	47.18	94.59	105.91	1465	47.69	95.62	104.88	1450	48.21	96.66	103.84	1436
201	46.52	93.51	107.49	1487	47.04	94.55	106.45	1472	47.55	95.58	105.42	1458	48.07	96.62	104.38	1444
201.5	46.39	93.47	108.03	1494	46.90	94.50	107.00	1480	47.42	95.54	105.96	1465	47.93	96.58	104.92	1451
202	46.25	93.43	108.57	1502	46.76	94.46	107.54	1487	47.28	95.50	106.50	1473	47.79	96.54	105.46	1459
202.5	46.12	93.39	109.12	1509	46.63	94.42	108.08	1495	47.14	95.46	107.04	1480	47.65	96.50	106.00	1466
203	45.98	93.34	109.66	1517	46.49	94.38	108.62	1502	47.00	95.42	107.58	1488	47.52	96.46	106.54	1473
203.5	45.85	93.30	110.20	1524	46.36	94.34	109.16	1510	46.87	95.38	108.12	1495	47.38	96.42	107.08	1481
204	45.72	93.26	110.74	1532	46.23	94.30	109.70	1517	46.73	95.34	108.66	1503	47.24	96.37	107.63	1488
204.5	45.58	93.22	111.28	1539	46.09	94.26	110.24	1525	46.60	95.30	109.20	1510	47.11	96.33	108.17	1496
205	45.45	93.18	111.82	1546	45.96	94.22	110.78	1532	46.47	95.26	109.75	1518	46.97	96.29	108.71	1503
205.5	45.32	93.14	112.36	1554	45.83	94.18	111.32	1540	46.33	95.21	110.29	1525	46.84	96.25	109.25	1511
206	45.19	93.10	112.90	1561	45.70	94.14	111.86	1547	46.20	95.17	110.83	1533	46.70	96.21	109.79	1518
206.5	45.06	93.06	113.44	1569	45.57	94.09	112.41	1555	46.07	95.13	111.37	1540	46.57	96.17	110.33	1526
207	44.94	93.02	113.98	1576	45.44	94.05	112.95	1562	45.94	95.09	111.91	1548	46.44	96.13	110.87	1533
207.5	44.81	92.98	114.53	1584	45.31	94.01	113.49	1570	45.81	95.05	112.45	1555	46.31	96.09	111.41	1541
208	44.68	92.93	115.07	1591	45.18	93.97	114.03	1577	45.68	95.01	112.99	1563	46.18	96.05	111.95	1548
208.5	44.55	92.89	115.61	1599	45.05	93.93	114.57	1584	45.55	94.97	113.53	1570	46.05	96.01	112.49	1556
209	44.43	92.85	116.15	1606	44.92	93.89	115.11	1592	45.42	94.93	114.07	1578	45.92	95.96	113.04	1563
209.5	44.30	92.81	116.69	1614	44.80	93.85	115.65	1599	45.29	94.89	114.61	1585	45.79	95.92	113.58	1571
210	44.18	92.77	117.23	1621	44.67	93.81	116.19	1607	45.16	94.85	115.16	1593	45.66	95.88	114.12	1578
210.5	44.05	92.73	117.77	1629	44.54	93.77	116.73	1614	45.04	94.80	115.70	1600	45.53	95.84	114.66	1586
211	43.93	92.69	118.31	1636	44.42	93.73	117.27	1622	44.91	94.76	116.24	1608	45.40	95.80	115.20	1593
211.5	43.80	92.65	118.85	1644	44.30	93.68	117.82	1629	44.79	94.72	116.78	1615	45.28	95.76	115.74	1601
212	43.68	92.61	119.39	1651	44.17	93.64	118.36	1637	44.66	94.68	117.32	1623	45.15	95.72	116.28	1608
212.5	43.56	92.57	119.94	1659	44.05	93.60	118.90	1644	44.54	94.64	117.86	1630	45.02	95.68	116.82	1616
213	43.44	92.52	120.48	1666	43.93	93.56	119.44	1652	44.41	94.60	118.40	1637	44.90	95.64	117.36	1623
213.5	43.32	92.48	121.02	1674	43.80	93.52	119.98	1659	44.29	94.56	118.94	1645	44.78	95.60	117.90	1631
214	43.20	92.44	121.56	1681	43.68	93.48	120.52	1667	44.17	94.52	119.48	1652	44.65	95.55	118.45	1638
214.5	43.08	92.40	122.10	1689	43.56	93.44	121.06	1674	44.04	94.48	120.02	1660	44.53	95.51	118.99	1646
215	42.96	92.36	122.64	1696	43.44	93.40	121.60	1682	43.92	94.44	120.57	1667	44.41	95.47	119.53	1653
215.5	42.84	92.32	123.18	1704	43.32	93.36	122.14	1689	43.80	94.39	121.11	1675	44.28	95.43	120.07	1661
216	42.72	92.28	123.72	1711	43.20	93.32	122.68	1697	43.68	94.35	121.65	1682	44.16	95.39	120.61	1668
216.5	42.60	92.24	124.26	1719	43.08	93.27	123.23	1704	43.56	94.31	122.19	1690	44.04	95.35	121.15	1676
217	42.49	92.20	124.80	1726	42.96	93.23	123.77	1712	43.44	94.27	122.73	1697	43.92	95.31	121.69	1683
217.5	42.37	92.16	125.35	1734	42.85	93.19	124.31	1719	43.32	94.23	123.27	1705	43.80	95.27	122.23	1690
218	42.25	92.11	125.89	1741	42.73	93.15	124.85	1727	43.21	94.19	123.81	1712	43.68	95.23	122.77	1698
218.5	42.14	92.07	126.43	1748	42.61	93.11	125.39	1734	43.09	94.15	124.35	1720	43.56	95.19	123.31	1705
219	42.02	92.03	126.97	1756	42.50	93.07	125.93	1742	42.97	94.11	124.89	1727	43.44	95.14	123.86	1713
219.5	41.91	91.99	127.51	1763	42.38	93.03	126.47	1749	42.85	94.07	125.43	1735	43.33	95.10	124.40	1720
220	41.80	91.95	128.05	1771	42.27	92.99	127.01	1757	42.74	94.03	125.98	1742	43.21	95.06	124.94	1728
220.5	41.68	91.91	128.59	1778	42.15	92.95	127.55	1764	42.62	93.98	126.52	1750	43.09	95.02	125.48	1735
221	41.57	91.87	129.13	1786	42.04	92.91	128.09	1772	42.51	93.94	127.06	1757	42.98	94.98	126.02	1743
221.5	41.46	91.83	129.67	1793	41.93	92.86	128.64	1779	42.39	93.90	127.60	1765	42.86	94.94	126.56	1750
222	41.35	91.79	130.21	1801	41.81	92.82	129.18	1787	42.28	93.86	128.14	1772	42.75	94.90	127.10	1758
222.5	41.23	91.75	130.76	1808	41.70	92.78	129.72	1794	42.17	93.82	128.68	1780	42.63	94.86	127.64	1765
223	41.12	91.70	131.30	1816	41.59	92.74	130.26	1801	42.05	93.78	129.22	1787	42.52	94.82	128.18	1773
223.5	41.01	91.66	131.84	1823	41.48	92.70	130.80	1809	41.94	93.74	129.76	1794	42.41	94.78	128.72	1780
224	40.90	91.62	132.38	1831	41.37	92.66	131.34	1816	41.83	93.70	130.30	1802	42.29	94.73	129.27	1788
224.5	40.79	91.58	132.92	1838	41.26	92.62	131.88	1824	41.72	93.66	130.84	1810	42.18	94.69	129.81	1795
225	40.68	91.54	133.46	1846	41.15	92.58	132.42	1831	41.61	93.62	131.39	1817	42.07	94.65	130.35	1803
225.5	40.58	91.50	134.00	1853	41.04	92.54	132.96	1839	41.50	93.57	131.93	1825	41.96	94.61	130.89	1810
226	40.47	91.46	134.54	1861	40.93	92.50	133.50	1846	41.39	93.53	132.47	1832	41.85	94.57	131.43	1818
226.5	40.36	91.42	135.08	1868	40.82	92.45	134.05	1854	41.28	93.49	133.01	1840	41.73	94.53	131.97	1825
227	40.25	91.38	135.62	1876	40.71	92.41	134.59	1861	41.17	93.45	133.55	1847	41.62	94.49	132.51	1833
227.5	40.15	91.34	136.17	1883	40.60	92.37	135.13	1869	41.06	93.41	134.09	1854	41.52	94.45	133.05	1840

Body Composition FEMALE 196-227.5 Lb.

Weight: Lb.	Waist: 46 inches Fat: %	Fat: Lb.	LBM: Lb.	RMR: Cal.	46.25 inches Fat: %	Fat: Lb.	LBM: Lb.	RMR: Cal.	46.5 inches Fat: %	Fat: Lb.	LBM: Lb.	RMR: Cal.	46.75 inches Fat: %	Fat: Lb.	LBM: Lb.	RMR: Cal.
196	50.03	98.07	97.93	1354	50.56	99.11	96.89	1340	51.09	100.14	95.86	1326	51.62	101.18	94.82	1311
196.5	49.89	98.03	98.47	1362	50.41	99.06	97.44	1348	50.94	100.10	96.40	1333	51.47	101.14	95.36	1319
197	49.74	97.99	99.01	1369	50.27	99.02	97.98	1355	50.79	100.06	96.94	1341	51.32	101.10	95.90	1326
197.5	49.59	97.95	99.56	1377	50.12	98.98	98.52	1362	50.64	100.02	97.48	1348	51.17	101.06	96.44	1334
198	49.45	97.90	100.10	1384	49.97	98.94	99.06	1370	50.49	99.98	98.02	1356	51.02	101.02	96.98	1341
198.5	49.30	97.86	100.64	1392	49.82	98.90	99.60	1377	50.35	99.94	98.56	1363	50.87	100.98	97.52	1349
199	49.16	97.82	101.18	1399	49.68	98.86	100.14	1385	50.20	99.90	99.10	1371	50.72	100.93	98.07	1356
199.5	49.01	97.78	101.72	1407	49.53	98.82	100.68	1392	50.05	99.86	99.64	1378	50.57	100.89	98.61	1364
200	48.87	97.74	102.26	1414	49.39	98.78	101.22	1400	49.91	99.82	100.19	1386	50.43	100.85	99.15	1371
200.5	48.73	97.70	102.80	1422	49.25	98.74	101.76	1407	49.76	99.77	100.73	1393	50.28	100.81	99.69	1379
201	48.59	97.66	103.34	1429	49.10	98.70	102.30	1415	49.62	99.73	101.27	1401	50.13	100.77	100.23	1386
201.5	48.45	97.62	103.88	1437	48.96	98.65	102.85	1422	49.47	99.69	101.81	1408	49.99	100.73	100.77	1394
202	48.30	97.58	104.42	1444	48.82	98.61	103.39	1430	49.33	99.65	102.35	1415	49.85	100.69	101.31	1401
202.5	48.17	97.54	104.97	1452	48.68	98.57	103.93	1437	49.19	99.61	102.89	1423	49.70	100.65	101.85	1409
203	48.03	97.49	105.51	1459	48.54	98.53	104.47	1445	49.05	99.57	103.43	1430	49.56	100.61	102.39	1416
203.5	47.89	97.45	106.05	1467	48.40	98.49	105.01	1452	48.91	99.53	103.97	1438	49.42	100.57	102.93	1424
204	47.75	97.41	106.59	1474	48.26	98.45	105.55	1460	48.77	99.49	104.51	1445	49.28	100.52	103.48	1431
204.5	47.61	97.37	107.13	1482	48.12	98.41	106.09	1467	48.63	99.45	105.05	1453	49.14	100.48	104.02	1439
205	47.48	97.33	107.67	1489	47.98	98.37	106.63	1475	48.49	99.41	105.60	1460	49.00	100.44	104.56	1446
205.5	47.34	97.29	108.21	1497	47.85	98.33	107.17	1482	48.35	99.36	106.14	1468	48.86	100.40	105.10	1454
206	47.21	97.25	108.75	1504	47.71	98.29	107.71	1490	48.22	99.32	106.68	1475	48.72	100.36	105.64	1461
206.5	47.07	97.21	109.29	1512	47.58	98.24	108.26	1497	48.08	99.28	107.22	1483	48.58	100.32	106.18	1468
207	46.94	97.17	109.83	1519	47.44	98.20	108.80	1505	47.94	99.24	107.76	1490	48.44	100.28	106.72	1476
207.5	46.81	97.13	110.38	1526	47.31	98.16	109.34	1512	47.81	99.20	108.30	1498	48.31	100.24	107.26	1483
208	46.68	97.08	110.92	1534	47.17	98.12	109.88	1520	47.67	99.16	108.84	1505	48.17	100.20	107.80	1491
208.5	46.54	97.04	111.46	1541	47.04	98.08	110.42	1527	47.54	99.12	109.38	1513	48.04	100.16	108.34	1498
209	46.41	97.00	112.00	1549	46.91	98.04	110.96	1535	47.41	99.08	109.92	1520	47.90	100.11	108.89	1506
209.5	46.28	96.96	112.54	1556	46.78	98.00	111.50	1542	47.27	99.04	110.46	1528	47.77	100.07	109.43	1513
210	46.15	96.92	113.08	1564	46.65	97.96	112.04	1550	47.14	99.00	111.01	1535	47.63	100.03	109.97	1521
210.5	46.02	96.88	113.62	1571	46.52	97.92	112.58	1557	47.01	98.95	111.55	1543	47.50	99.99	110.51	1528
211	45.89	96.84	114.16	1579	46.39	97.88	113.12	1565	46.88	98.91	112.09	1550	47.37	99.95	111.05	1536
211.5	45.77	96.80	114.70	1586	46.26	97.83	113.67	1572	46.75	98.87	112.63	1558	47.24	99.91	111.59	1543
212	45.64	96.76	115.24	1594	46.13	97.79	114.21	1579	46.62	98.83	113.17	1565	47.11	99.87	112.13	1551
212.5	45.51	96.72	115.79	1601	46.00	97.75	114.75	1587	46.49	98.79	113.71	1573	46.98	99.83	112.67	1558
213	45.39	96.67	116.33	1609	45.87	97.71	115.29	1594	46.36	98.75	114.25	1580	46.85	99.79	113.21	1566
213.5	45.26	96.63	116.87	1616	45.75	97.67	115.83	1602	46.23	98.71	114.79	1588	46.72	99.75	113.75	1573
214	45.14	96.59	117.41	1624	45.62	97.63	116.37	1609	46.11	98.67	115.33	1595	46.59	99.70	114.30	1581
214.5	45.01	96.55	117.95	1631	45.50	97.59	116.91	1617	45.98	98.63	115.87	1603	46.46	99.66	114.84	1588
215	44.89	96.51	118.49	1639	45.37	97.55	117.45	1624	45.85	98.59	116.42	1610	46.34	99.62	115.38	1596
215.5	44.77	96.47	119.03	1646	45.25	97.51	117.99	1632	45.73	98.54	116.96	1618	46.21	99.58	115.92	1603
216	44.64	96.43	119.57	1654	45.12	97.47	118.53	1639	45.60	98.50	117.50	1625	46.08	99.54	116.46	1611
216.5	44.52	96.39	120.11	1661	45.00	97.42	119.08	1647	45.48	98.46	118.04	1632	45.96	99.50	117.00	1618
217	44.40	96.35	120.65	1669	44.88	97.38	119.62	1654	45.36	98.42	118.58	1640	45.83	99.46	117.54	1626
217.5	44.28	96.31	121.20	1676	44.76	97.34	120.16	1662	45.23	98.38	119.12	1647	45.71	99.42	118.08	1633
218	44.16	96.26	121.74	1684	44.63	97.30	120.70	1669	45.11	98.34	119.66	1655	45.59	99.38	118.62	1641
218.5	44.04	96.22	122.28	1691	44.51	97.26	121.24	1677	44.99	98.30	120.20	1662	45.46	99.34	119.16	1648
219	43.92	96.18	122.82	1699	44.39	97.22	121.78	1684	44.87	98.26	120.74	1670	45.34	99.29	119.71	1656
219.5	43.80	96.14	123.36	1706	44.27	97.18	122.32	1692	44.75	98.22	121.28	1677	45.22	99.25	120.25	1663
220	43.68	96.10	123.90	1714	44.15	97.14	122.86	1699	44.63	98.18	121.83	1685	45.10	99.21	120.79	1670
220.5	43.56	96.06	124.44	1721	44.03	97.10	123.40	1707	44.51	98.13	122.37	1692	44.98	99.17	121.33	1678
221	43.45	96.02	124.98	1729	43.92	97.06	123.94	1714	44.39	98.09	122.91	1700	44.86	99.13	121.87	1685
221.5	43.33	95.98	125.52	1736	43.80	97.01	124.49	1722	44.27	98.05	123.45	1707	44.74	99.09	122.41	1693
222	43.21	95.94	126.06	1743	43.68	96.97	125.03	1729	44.15	98.01	123.99	1715	44.62	99.05	122.95	1700
222.5	43.10	95.90	126.61	1751	43.57	96.93	125.57	1737	44.03	97.97	124.53	1722	44.50	99.01	123.49	1708
223	42.98	95.85	127.15	1758	43.45	96.89	126.11	1744	43.91	97.93	125.07	1730	44.38	98.97	124.03	1715
223.5	42.87	95.81	127.69	1766	43.33	96.85	126.65	1752	43.80	97.89	125.61	1737	44.26	98.93	124.57	1723
224	42.76	95.77	128.23	1773	43.22	96.81	127.19	1759	43.68	97.85	126.15	1745	44.14	98.88	125.12	1730
224.5	42.64	95.73	128.77	1781	43.10	96.77	127.73	1767	43.57	97.81	126.69	1752	44.03	98.84	125.66	1738
225	42.53	95.69	129.31	1788	42.99	96.73	128.27	1774	43.45	97.77	127.24	1760	43.91	98.80	126.20	1745
225.5	42.42	95.65	129.85	1796	42.88	96.69	128.81	1781	43.34	97.72	127.78	1767	43.80	98.76	126.74	1753
226	42.30	95.61	130.39	1803	42.76	96.65	129.35	1789	43.22	97.68	128.32	1775	43.68	98.72	127.28	1760
226.5	42.19	95.57	130.93	1811	42.65	96.60	129.90	1796	43.11	97.64	128.86	1782	43.57	98.68	127.82	1768
227	42.08	95.53	131.47	1818	42.54	96.56	130.44	1804	43.00	97.60	129.40	1790	43.45	98.64	128.36	1775
227.5	41.97	95.49	132.02	1826	42.43	96.52	130.98	1811	42.88	97.56	129.94	1797	43.34	98.60	128.90	1783

Body Composition FEMALE 196-227.5 Lb.

Weight: Lb.	Waist: 47 inches Fat: %	Fat: Lb.	LBM: Lb.	RMR: Cal.	47.25 inches Fat: %	Fat: Lb.	LBM: Lb.	RMR: Cal.	47.5 inches Fat: %	Fat: Lb.	LBM: Lb.	RMR: Cal.	47.75 inches Fat: %	Fat: Lb.	LBM: Lb.	RMR: Cal.
196	52.15	102.22	93.78	1297	52.68	103.26	92.74	1283	53.21	104.29	91.71	1268	53.74	105.33	90.67	1254
196.5	52.00	102.18	94.32	1304	52.53	103.21	93.29	1290	53.05	104.25	92.25	1276	53.58	105.29	91.21	1261
197	51.85	102.14	94.86	1312	52.37	103.17	93.83	1298	52.90	104.21	92.79	1283	53.43	105.25	91.75	1269
197.5	51.69	102.10	95.41	1319	52.22	103.13	94.37	1305	52.74	104.17	93.33	1291	53.27	105.21	92.29	1276
198	51.54	102.05	95.95	1327	52.07	103.09	94.91	1313	52.59	104.13	93.87	1298	53.11	105.17	92.83	1284
198.5	51.39	102.01	96.49	1334	51.91	103.05	95.45	1320	52.44	104.09	94.41	1306	52.96	105.13	93.37	1291
199	51.24	101.97	97.03	1342	51.76	103.01	95.99	1328	52.28	104.05	94.95	1313	52.81	105.08	93.92	1299
199.5	51.09	101.93	97.57	1349	51.61	102.97	96.53	1335	52.13	104.01	95.49	1321	52.65	105.04	94.46	1306
200	50.95	101.89	98.11	1357	51.46	102.93	97.07	1343	51.98	103.97	96.04	1328	52.50	105.00	95.00	1314
200.5	50.80	101.85	98.65	1364	51.31	102.89	97.61	1350	51.83	103.92	96.58	1336	52.35	104.96	95.54	1321
201	50.65	101.81	99.19	1372	51.17	102.85	98.15	1357	51.68	103.88	97.12	1343	52.20	104.92	96.08	1329
201.5	50.50	101.77	99.73	1379	51.02	102.80	98.70	1365	51.53	103.84	97.66	1351	52.05	104.88	96.62	1336
202	50.36	101.73	100.27	1387	50.87	102.76	99.24	1372	51.39	103.80	98.20	1358	51.90	104.84	97.16	1344
202.5	50.21	101.69	100.82	1394	50.73	102.72	99.78	1380	51.24	103.76	98.74	1366	51.75	104.80	97.70	1351
203	50.07	101.64	101.36	1402	50.58	102.68	100.32	1387	51.09	103.72	99.28	1373	51.60	104.76	98.24	1359
203.5	49.93	101.60	101.90	1409	50.44	102.64	100.86	1395	50.95	103.68	99.82	1381	51.46	104.72	98.78	1366
204	49.79	101.56	102.44	1417	50.29	102.60	101.40	1402	50.80	103.64	100.36	1388	51.31	104.67	99.33	1374
204.5	49.64	101.52	102.98	1424	50.15	102.56	101.94	1410	50.66	103.60	100.90	1396	51.17	104.63	99.87	1381
205	49.50	101.48	103.52	1432	50.01	102.52	102.48	1417	50.51	103.56	101.45	1403	51.02	104.59	100.41	1389
205.5	49.36	101.44	104.06	1439	49.87	102.48	103.02	1425	50.37	103.51	101.99	1410	50.88	104.55	100.95	1396
206	49.22	101.40	104.60	1447	49.73	102.44	103.56	1432	50.23	103.47	102.53	1418	50.73	104.51	101.49	1404
206.5	49.08	101.36	105.14	1454	49.59	102.39	104.11	1440	50.09	103.43	103.07	1425	50.59	104.47	102.03	1411
207	48.94	101.32	105.68	1462	49.45	102.35	104.65	1447	49.95	103.39	103.61	1433	50.45	104.43	102.57	1419
207.5	48.81	101.28	106.23	1469	49.31	102.31	105.19	1455	49.81	103.35	104.15	1440	50.31	104.39	103.11	1426
208	48.67	101.23	106.77	1477	49.17	102.27	105.73	1462	49.67	103.31	104.69	1448	50.17	104.35	103.65	1434
208.5	48.53	101.19	107.31	1484	49.03	102.23	106.27	1470	49.53	103.27	105.23	1455	50.03	104.31	104.19	1441
209	48.40	101.15	107.85	1492	48.89	102.19	106.81	1477	49.39	103.23	105.77	1463	49.89	104.26	104.74	1448
209.5	48.26	101.11	108.39	1499	48.76	102.15	107.35	1485	49.25	103.19	106.31	1470	49.75	104.22	105.28	1456
210	48.13	101.07	108.93	1507	48.62	102.11	107.89	1492	49.12	103.15	106.86	1478	49.61	104.18	105.82	1463
210.5	47.99	101.03	109.47	1514	48.49	102.07	108.43	1500	48.98	103.10	107.40	1485	49.47	104.14	106.36	1471
211	47.86	100.99	110.01	1521	48.35	102.03	108.97	1507	48.85	103.06	107.94	1493	49.34	104.10	106.90	1478
211.5	47.73	100.95	110.55	1529	48.22	101.98	109.52	1515	48.71	103.02	108.48	1500	49.20	104.06	107.44	1486
212	47.60	100.91	111.09	1536	48.09	101.94	110.06	1522	48.58	102.98	109.02	1508	49.07	104.02	107.98	1493
212.5	47.47	100.87	111.64	1544	47.95	101.90	110.60	1530	48.44	102.94	109.56	1515	48.93	103.98	108.52	1501
213	47.34	100.82	112.18	1551	47.82	101.86	111.14	1537	48.31	102.90	110.10	1523	48.80	103.94	109.06	1508
213.5	47.21	100.78	112.72	1559	47.69	101.82	111.68	1545	48.18	102.86	110.64	1530	48.66	103.90	109.60	1516
214	47.08	100.74	113.26	1566	47.56	101.78	112.22	1552	48.05	102.82	111.18	1538	48.53	103.85	110.15	1523
214.5	46.95	100.70	113.80	1574	47.43	101.74	112.76	1559	47.91	102.78	111.72	1545	48.40	103.81	110.69	1531
215	46.82	100.66	114.34	1581	47.30	101.70	113.30	1567	47.78	102.74	112.27	1553	48.27	103.77	111.23	1538
215.5	46.69	100.62	114.88	1589	47.17	101.66	113.84	1574	47.65	102.69	112.81	1560	48.14	103.73	111.77	1546
216	46.56	100.58	115.42	1596	47.04	101.62	114.38	1582	47.52	102.65	113.35	1568	48.00	103.69	112.31	1553
216.5	46.44	100.54	115.96	1604	46.92	101.57	114.93	1589	47.40	102.61	113.89	1575	47.88	103.65	112.85	1561
217	46.31	100.50	116.50	1611	46.79	101.53	115.47	1597	47.27	102.57	114.43	1583	47.75	103.61	113.39	1568
217.5	46.19	100.46	117.05	1619	46.66	101.49	116.01	1604	47.14	102.53	114.97	1590	47.62	103.57	113.93	1576
218	46.06	100.41	117.59	1626	46.54	101.45	116.55	1612	47.01	102.49	115.51	1598	47.49	103.53	114.47	1583
218.5	45.94	100.37	118.13	1634	46.41	101.41	117.09	1619	46.89	102.45	116.05	1605	47.36	103.49	115.01	1591
219	45.81	100.33	118.67	1641	46.29	101.37	117.63	1627	46.76	102.41	116.59	1612	47.23	103.44	115.56	1598
219.5	45.69	100.29	119.21	1649	46.16	101.33	118.17	1634	46.64	102.37	117.13	1620	47.11	103.40	116.10	1606
220	45.57	100.25	119.75	1656	46.04	101.29	118.71	1642	46.51	102.33	117.68	1627	46.98	103.36	116.64	1613
220.5	45.45	100.21	120.29	1664	45.92	101.25	119.25	1649	46.39	102.28	118.22	1635	46.86	103.32	117.18	1621
221	45.32	100.17	120.83	1671	45.79	101.21	119.79	1657	46.26	102.24	118.76	1642	46.73	103.28	117.72	1628
221.5	45.20	100.13	121.37	1679	45.67	101.16	120.34	1664	46.14	102.20	119.30	1650	46.61	103.24	118.26	1636
222	45.08	100.09	121.91	1686	45.55	101.12	120.88	1672	46.02	102.16	119.84	1657	46.49	103.20	118.80	1643
222.5	44.96	100.05	122.46	1694	45.43	101.08	121.42	1679	45.90	102.12	120.38	1665	46.36	103.16	119.34	1651
223	44.84	100.00	123.00	1701	45.31	101.04	121.96	1687	45.78	102.08	120.92	1672	46.24	103.12	119.88	1658
223.5	44.73	99.96	123.54	1709	45.19	101.00	122.50	1694	45.65	102.04	121.46	1680	46.12	103.08	120.42	1665
224	44.61	99.92	124.08	1716	45.07	100.96	123.04	1702	45.53	102.00	122.00	1687	46.00	103.03	120.97	1673
224.5	44.49	99.88	124.62	1723	44.95	100.92	123.58	1709	45.41	101.96	122.54	1695	45.88	102.99	121.51	1680
225	44.37	99.84	125.16	1731	44.83	100.88	124.12	1717	45.30	101.92	123.09	1702	45.76	102.95	122.05	1688
225.5	44.26	99.80	125.70	1738	44.72	100.84	124.66	1724	45.18	101.87	123.63	1710	45.64	102.91	122.59	1695
226	44.14	99.76	126.24	1746	44.60	100.80	125.20	1732	45.06	101.83	124.17	1717	45.52	102.87	123.13	1703
226.5	44.03	99.72	126.78	1753	44.48	100.75	125.75	1739	44.94	101.79	124.71	1725	45.40	102.83	123.67	1710
227	43.91	99.68	127.32	1761	44.37	100.71	126.29	1747	44.82	101.75	125.25	1732	45.28	102.79	124.21	1718
227.5	43.80	99.64	127.87	1768	44.25	100.67	126.83	1754	44.71	101.71	125.79	1740	45.16	102.75	124.75	1725

THE BODY FAT GUIDE

Body Composition   FEMALE   228-259.5 Lb.

Weight: Lb.	Waist: 41 inches Fat: %	Fat: Lb.	LBM: Lb.	RMR: Cal.	41.25 inches Fat: %	Fat: Lb.	LBM: Lb.	RMR: Cal.	41.5 inches Fat: %	Fat: Lb.	LBM: Lb.	RMR: Cal.	41.75 inches Fat: %	Fat: Lb.	LBM: Lb.	RMR: Cal.
228	32.76	74.69	153.31	2120	33.22	75.73	152.27	2106	33.67	76.77	151.23	2092	34.13	77.81	150.19	2077
228.5	32.67	74.65	153.85	2128	33.12	75.69	152.81	2113	33.58	76.73	151.77	2099	34.03	77.77	150.73	2085
229	32.58	74.61	154.39	2135	33.03	75.65	153.35	2121	33.49	76.69	152.31	2106	33.94	77.72	151.28	2092
229.5	32.49	74.57	154.93	2143	32.94	75.61	153.89	2128	33.40	76.65	152.85	2114	33.85	77.68	151.82	2100
230	32.40	74.53	155.47	2150	32.86	75.57	154.43	2136	33.31	76.61	153.40	2121	33.76	77.64	152.36	2107
230.5	32.32	74.49	156.01	2158	32.77	75.53	154.97	2143	33.22	76.56	153.94	2129	33.67	77.60	152.90	2115
231	32.23	74.45	156.55	2165	32.68	75.49	155.51	2151	33.13	76.52	154.48	2136	33.58	77.56	153.44	2122
231.5	32.14	74.41	157.09	2173	32.59	75.44	156.06	2158	33.04	76.48	155.02	2144	33.49	77.52	153.98	2130
232	32.05	74.37	157.63	2180	32.50	75.40	156.60	2166	32.95	76.44	155.56	2151	33.40	77.48	154.52	2137
232.5	31.97	74.33	158.18	2188	32.41	75.36	157.14	2173	32.86	76.40	156.10	2159	33.31	77.44	155.06	2145
233	31.88	74.28	158.72	2195	32.33	75.32	157.68	2181	32.77	76.36	156.64	2166	33.22	77.40	155.60	2152
233.5	31.80	74.24	159.26	2203	32.24	75.28	158.22	2188	32.68	76.32	157.18	2174	33.13	77.36	156.14	2159
234	31.71	74.20	159.80	2210	32.15	75.24	158.76	2196	32.60	76.28	157.72	2181	33.04	77.31	156.69	2167
234.5	31.63	74.16	160.34	2217	32.07	75.20	159.30	2203	32.51	76.24	158.26	2189	32.95	77.27	157.23	2174
235	31.54	74.12	160.88	2225	31.98	75.16	159.84	2211	32.42	76.20	158.81	2196	32.86	77.23	157.77	2182
235.5	31.46	74.08	161.42	2232	31.90	75.12	160.38	2218	32.34	76.15	159.35	2204	32.78	77.19	158.31	2189
236	31.37	74.04	161.96	2240	31.81	75.08	160.92	2226	32.25	76.11	159.89	2211	32.69	77.15	158.85	2197
236.5	31.29	74.00	162.50	2247	31.73	75.03	161.47	2233	32.17	76.07	160.43	2219	32.60	77.11	159.39	2204
237	31.21	73.96	163.04	2255	31.64	74.99	162.01	2241	32.08	76.03	160.97	2226	32.52	77.07	159.93	2212
237.5	31.12	73.92	163.59	2262	31.56	74.95	162.55	2248	32.00	75.99	161.51	2234	32.43	77.03	160.47	2219
238	31.04	73.87	164.13	2270	31.48	74.91	163.09	2256	31.91	75.95	162.05	2241	32.35	76.99	161.01	2227
238.5	30.96	73.83	164.67	2277	31.39	74.87	163.63	2263	31.83	75.91	162.59	2249	32.26	76.95	161.55	2234
239	30.88	73.79	165.21	2285	31.31	74.83	164.17	2270	31.74	75.87	163.13	2256	32.18	76.90	162.10	2242
239.5	30.79	73.75	165.75	2292	31.23	74.79	164.71	2278	31.66	75.83	163.67	2264	32.09	76.86	162.64	2249
240	30.71	73.71	166.29	2300	31.14	74.75	165.25	2285	31.58	75.79	164.22	2271	32.01	76.82	163.18	2257
240.5	30.63	73.67	166.83	2307	31.06	74.71	165.79	2293	31.49	75.74	164.76	2279	31.93	76.78	163.72	2264
241	30.55	73.63	167.37	2315	30.98	74.67	166.33	2300	31.41	75.70	165.30	2286	31.84	76.74	164.26	2272
241.5	30.47	73.59	167.91	2322	30.90	74.62	166.88	2308	31.33	75.66	165.84	2294	31.76	76.70	164.80	2279
242	30.39	73.55	168.45	2330	30.82	74.58	167.42	2315	31.25	75.62	166.38	2301	31.68	76.66	165.34	2287
242.5	30.31	73.51	169.00	2337	30.74	74.54	167.96	2323	31.17	75.58	166.92	2309	31.59	76.62	165.88	2294
243	30.23	73.46	169.54	2345	30.66	74.50	168.50	2330	31.09	75.54	167.46	2316	31.51	76.58	166.42	2302
243.5	30.15	73.42	170.08	2352	30.58	74.46	169.04	2338	31.01	75.50	168.00	2323	31.43	76.54	166.96	2309
244	30.07	73.38	170.62	2360	30.50	74.42	169.58	2345	30.93	75.46	168.54	2331	31.35	76.49	167.51	2317
244.5	30.00	73.34	171.16	2367	30.42	74.38	170.12	2353	30.84	75.42	169.08	2338	31.27	76.45	168.05	2324
245	29.92	73.30	171.70	2375	30.34	74.34	170.66	2360	30.77	75.38	169.63	2346	31.19	76.41	168.59	2332
245.5	29.84	73.26	172.24	2382	30.26	74.30	171.20	2368	30.69	75.33	170.17	2353	31.11	76.37	169.13	2339
246	29.76	73.22	172.78	2390	30.19	74.26	171.74	2375	30.61	75.29	170.71	2361	31.03	76.33	169.67	2347
246.5	29.69	73.18	173.32	2397	30.11	74.21	172.29	2383	30.53	75.25	171.25	2368	30.95	76.29	170.21	2354
247	29.61	73.14	173.86	2405	30.03	74.17	172.83	2390	30.45	75.21	171.79	2376	30.87	76.25	170.75	2361
247.5	29.53	73.10	174.41	2412	29.95	74.13	173.37	2398	30.37	75.17	172.33	2383	30.79	76.21	171.29	2369
248	29.46	73.05	174.95	2420	29.88	74.09	173.91	2405	30.29	75.13	172.87	2391	30.71	76.17	171.83	2376
248.5	29.38	73.01	175.49	2427	29.80	74.05	174.45	2413	30.22	75.09	173.41	2398	30.63	76.13	172.37	2384
249	29.31	72.97	176.03	2434	29.72	74.01	174.99	2420	30.14	75.05	173.95	2406	30.56	76.08	172.92	2391
249.5	29.23	72.93	176.57	2442	29.65	73.97	175.53	2428	30.06	75.01	174.49	2413	30.48	76.04	173.46	2399
250	29.16	72.89	177.11	2449	29.57	73.93	176.07	2435	29.99	74.97	175.04	2421	30.40	76.00	174.00	2406
250.5	29.08	72.85	177.65	2457	29.50	73.89	176.61	2443	29.91	74.92	175.58	2428	30.32	75.96	174.54	2414
251	29.01	72.81	178.19	2464	29.42	73.85	177.15	2450	29.83	74.88	176.12	2436	30.25	75.92	175.08	2421
251.5	28.93	72.77	178.73	2472	29.35	73.80	177.70	2458	29.76	74.84	176.66	2443	30.17	75.88	175.62	2429
252	28.86	72.73	179.27	2479	29.27	73.76	178.24	2465	29.68	74.80	177.20	2451	30.09	75.84	176.16	2436
252.5	28.79	72.68	179.82	2487	29.20	73.72	178.78	2472	29.61	74.76	177.74	2458	30.02	75.80	176.70	2444
253	28.71	72.64	180.36	2494	29.12	73.68	179.32	2480	29.53	74.72	178.28	2466	29.94	75.76	177.24	2451
253.5	28.64	72.60	180.90	2502	29.05	73.64	179.86	2487	29.46	74.68	178.82	2473	29.87	75.72	177.78	2459
254	28.57	72.56	181.44	2509	28.98	73.60	180.40	2495	29.38	74.64	179.36	2481	29.79	75.67	178.33	2466
254.5	28.50	72.52	181.98	2517	28.90	73.56	180.94	2502	29.31	74.60	179.90	2488	29.72	75.63	178.87	2474
255	28.42	72.48	182.52	2524	28.83	73.52	181.48	2510	29.24	74.56	180.45	2496	29.64	75.59	179.41	2481
255.5	28.35	72.44	183.06	2532	28.76	73.48	182.02	2517	29.16	74.51	180.99	2503	29.57	75.55	179.95	2489
256	28.28	72.40	183.60	2539	28.69	73.44	182.56	2525	29.09	74.47	181.53	2511	29.50	75.51	180.49	2496
256.5	28.21	72.36	184.14	2547	28.61	73.39	183.11	2532	29.02	74.43	182.07	2518	29.42	75.47	181.03	2504
257	28.14	72.32	184.68	2554	28.54	73.35	183.65	2540	28.95	74.39	182.61	2525	29.35	75.43	181.57	2511
257.5	28.07	72.28	185.23	2562	28.47	73.31	184.19	2547	28.87	74.35	183.15	2533	29.28	75.39	182.11	2519
258	28.00	72.23	185.77	2569	28.40	73.27	184.73	2555	28.80	74.31	183.69	2540	29.20	75.35	182.65	2526
258.5	27.93	72.19	186.31	2577	28.33	73.23	185.27	2562	28.73	74.27	184.23	2548	29.13	75.31	183.19	2534
259	27.86	72.15	186.85	2584	28.26	73.19	185.81	2570	28.66	74.23	184.77	2555	29.06	75.26	183.74	2541
259.5	27.79	72.11	187.39	2592	28.19	73.15	186.35	2577	28.59	74.19	185.31	2563	28.99	75.22	184.28	2549

Body Composition   FEMALE   228-259.5 Lb.

Weight: Lb.	Waist: 42 inches Fat: %	Fat: Lb.	LBM: Lb.	RMR: Cal.	42.25 inches Fat: %	Fat: Lb.	LBM: Lb.	RMR: Cal.	42.5 inches Fat: %	Fat: Lb.	LBM: Lb.	RMR: Cal.	42.75 inches Fat: %	Fat: Lb.	LBM: Lb.	RMR: Cal.
228	34.58	78.84	149.16	2063	35.04	79.88	148.12	2048	35.49	80.92	147.08	2034	35.95	81.96	146.04	2020
228.5	34.49	78.80	149.70	2070	34.94	79.84	148.66	2056	35.40	80.88	147.62	2042	35.85	81.92	146.58	2027
229	34.39	78.76	150.24	2078	34.85	79.80	149.20	2063	35.30	80.84	148.16	2049	35.75	81.87	147.13	2035
229.5	34.30	78.72	150.78	2085	34.75	79.76	149.74	2071	35.21	80.80	148.70	2057	35.66	81.83	147.67	2042
230	34.21	78.68	151.32	2093	34.66	79.72	150.28	2078	35.11	80.76	149.25	2064	35.56	81.79	148.21	2050
230.5	34.12	78.64	151.86	2100	34.57	79.68	150.82	2086	35.02	80.71	149.79	2072	35.47	81.75	148.75	2057
231	34.03	78.60	152.40	2108	34.47	79.64	151.36	2093	34.92	80.67	150.33	2079	35.37	81.71	149.29	2065
231.5	33.93	78.56	152.94	2115	34.38	79.59	151.91	2101	34.83	80.63	150.87	2087	35.28	81.67	149.83	2072
232	33.84	78.52	153.48	2123	34.29	79.55	152.45	2108	34.74	80.59	151.41	2094	35.18	81.63	150.37	2080
232.5	33.75	78.48	154.03	2130	34.20	79.51	152.99	2116	34.65	80.55	151.95	2101	35.09	81.59	150.91	2087
233	33.66	78.43	154.57	2138	34.11	79.47	153.53	2123	34.55	80.51	152.49	2109	35.00	81.55	151.45	2095
233.5	33.57	78.39	155.11	2145	34.02	79.43	154.07	2131	34.46	80.47	153.03	2116	34.91	81.51	151.99	2102
234	33.48	78.35	155.65	2153	33.93	79.39	154.61	2138	34.37	80.43	153.57	2124	34.81	81.46	152.54	2110
234.5	33.39	78.31	156.19	2160	33.84	79.35	155.15	2146	34.28	80.39	154.11	2131	34.72	81.42	153.08	2117
235	33.31	78.27	156.73	2168	33.75	79.31	155.69	2153	34.19	80.35	154.66	2139	34.63	81.38	153.62	2125
235.5	33.22	78.23	157.27	2175	33.66	79.27	156.23	2161	34.10	80.30	155.20	2146	34.54	81.34	154.16	2132
236	33.13	78.19	157.81	2183	33.57	79.23	156.77	2168	34.01	80.26	155.74	2154	34.45	81.30	154.70	2139
236.5	33.04	78.15	158.35	2190	33.48	79.18	157.32	2176	33.92	80.22	156.28	2161	34.36	81.26	155.24	2147
237	32.96	78.11	158.89	2198	33.39	79.14	157.86	2183	33.83	80.18	156.82	2169	34.27	81.22	155.78	2154
237.5	32.87	78.07	159.44	2205	33.31	79.10	158.40	2191	33.74	80.14	157.36	2176	34.18	81.18	156.32	2162
238	32.78	78.02	159.98	2212	33.22	79.06	158.94	2198	33.66	80.10	157.90	2184	34.09	81.14	156.86	2169
238.5	32.70	77.98	160.52	2220	33.13	79.02	159.48	2206	33.57	80.06	158.44	2191	34.00	81.10	157.40	2177
239	32.61	77.94	161.06	2227	33.05	78.98	160.02	2213	33.48	80.02	158.98	2199	33.91	81.05	157.95	2184
239.5	32.53	77.90	161.60	2235	32.96	78.94	160.56	2221	33.39	79.98	159.52	2206	33.83	81.01	158.49	2192
240	32.44	77.86	162.14	2242	32.87	78.90	161.10	2228	33.31	79.94	160.07	2214	33.74	80.97	159.03	2199
240.5	32.36	77.82	162.68	2250	32.79	78.86	161.64	2236	33.22	79.89	160.61	2221	33.65	80.93	159.57	2207
241	32.27	77.78	163.22	2257	32.70	78.82	162.18	2243	33.13	79.85	161.15	2229	33.56	80.89	160.11	2214
241.5	32.19	77.74	163.76	2265	32.62	78.77	162.73	2250	33.05	79.81	161.69	2236	33.48	80.85	160.65	2222
242	32.11	77.70	164.30	2272	32.53	78.73	163.27	2258	32.96	79.77	162.23	2244	33.39	80.81	161.19	2229
242.5	32.02	77.66	164.85	2280	32.45	78.69	163.81	2265	32.88	79.73	162.77	2251	33.31	80.77	161.73	2237
243	31.94	77.61	165.39	2287	32.37	78.65	164.35	2273	32.79	79.69	163.31	2259	33.22	80.73	162.27	2244
243.5	31.86	77.57	165.93	2295	32.28	78.61	164.89	2280	32.71	79.65	163.85	2266	33.14	80.69	162.81	2252
244	31.78	77.53	166.47	2302	32.20	78.57	165.43	2288	32.63	79.61	164.39	2274	33.05	80.64	163.36	2259
244.5	31.69	77.49	167.01	2310	32.12	78.53	165.97	2295	32.54	79.57	164.93	2281	32.97	80.60	163.90	2267
245	31.61	77.45	167.55	2317	32.04	78.49	166.51	2303	32.46	79.53	165.48	2289	32.88	80.56	164.44	2274
245.5	31.53	77.41	168.09	2325	31.95	78.45	167.05	2310	32.38	79.48	166.02	2296	32.80	80.52	164.98	2282
246	31.45	77.37	168.63	2332	31.87	78.41	167.59	2318	32.29	79.44	166.56	2303	32.72	80.48	165.52	2289
246.5	31.37	77.33	169.17	2340	31.79	78.36	168.14	2325	32.21	79.40	167.10	2311	32.63	80.44	166.06	2297
247	31.29	77.29	169.71	2347	31.71	78.32	168.68	2333	32.13	79.36	167.64	2318	32.55	80.40	166.60	2304
247.5	31.21	77.25	170.26	2355	31.63	78.28	169.22	2340	32.05	79.32	168.18	2326	32.47	80.36	167.14	2312
248	31.13	77.20	170.80	2362	31.55	78.24	169.76	2348	31.97	79.28	168.72	2333	32.39	80.32	167.68	2319
248.5	31.05	77.16	171.34	2370	31.47	78.20	170.30	2355	31.89	79.24	169.26	2341	32.30	80.28	168.22	2327
249	30.97	77.12	171.88	2377	31.39	78.16	170.84	2363	31.81	79.20	169.80	2348	32.22	80.23	168.77	2334
249.5	30.89	77.08	172.42	2385	31.31	78.12	171.38	2370	31.73	79.16	170.34	2356	32.14	80.19	169.31	2342
250	30.82	77.04	172.96	2392	31.23	78.08	171.92	2378	31.65	79.12	170.89	2363	32.06	80.15	169.85	2349
250.5	30.74	77.00	173.50	2400	31.15	78.04	172.46	2385	31.57	79.07	171.43	2371	31.98	80.11	170.39	2356
251	30.66	76.96	174.04	2407	31.07	78.00	173.00	2393	31.49	79.03	171.97	2378	31.90	80.07	170.93	2364
251.5	30.58	76.92	174.58	2414	31.00	77.95	173.55	2400	31.41	78.99	172.51	2386	31.82	80.03	171.47	2371
252	30.51	76.88	175.12	2422	30.92	77.91	174.09	2408	31.33	78.95	173.05	2393	31.74	79.99	172.01	2379
252.5	30.43	76.84	175.67	2429	30.84	77.87	174.63	2415	31.25	78.91	173.59	2401	31.66	79.95	172.55	2386
253	30.35	76.79	176.21	2437	30.76	77.83	175.17	2423	31.17	78.87	174.13	2408	31.58	79.91	173.09	2394
253.5	30.28	76.75	176.75	2444	30.69	77.79	175.71	2430	31.10	78.83	174.67	2416	31.51	79.87	173.63	2401
254	30.20	76.71	177.29	2452	30.61	77.75	176.25	2438	31.02	78.79	175.21	2423	31.43	79.82	174.18	2409
254.5	30.13	76.67	177.83	2459	30.53	77.71	176.79	2445	30.94	78.75	175.75	2431	31.35	79.78	174.72	2416
255	30.05	76.63	178.37	2467	30.46	77.67	177.33	2453	30.86	78.71	176.30	2438	31.27	79.74	175.26	2424
255.5	29.98	76.59	178.91	2474	30.38	77.63	177.87	2460	30.79	78.66	176.84	2446	31.19	79.70	175.80	2431
256	29.90	76.55	179.45	2482	30.31	77.59	178.41	2467	30.71	78.62	177.38	2453	31.12	79.66	176.34	2439
256.5	29.83	76.51	179.99	2489	30.23	77.54	178.96	2475	30.64	78.58	177.92	2461	31.04	79.62	176.88	2446
257	29.75	76.47	180.53	2497	30.16	77.50	179.50	2482	30.56	78.54	178.46	2468	30.96	79.58	177.42	2454
257.5	29.68	76.43	181.08	2504	30.08	77.46	180.04	2490	30.49	78.50	179.00	2476	30.89	79.54	177.96	2461
258	29.61	76.38	181.62	2512	30.01	77.42	180.58	2497	30.41	78.46	179.54	2483	30.81	79.50	178.50	2469
258.5	29.53	76.34	182.16	2519	29.93	77.38	181.12	2505	30.34	78.42	180.08	2491	30.74	79.46	179.04	2476
259	29.46	76.30	182.70	2527	29.86	77.34	181.66	2512	30.26	78.38	180.62	2498	30.66	79.41	179.59	2484
259.5	29.39	76.26	183.24	2534	29.79	77.30	182.20	2520	30.19	78.34	181.16	2505	30.59	79.37	180.13	2491

Body Composition FEMALE 228-259.5 Lb.

Weight: Lb.	Waist: 43 inches Fat: %	Fat: Lb.	LBM: Lb.	RMR: Cal.	43.25 inches Fat: %	Fat: Lb.	LBM: Lb.	RMR: Cal.	43.5 inches Fat: %	Fat: Lb.	LBM: Lb.	RMR: Cal.	43.75 inches Fat: %	Fat: Lb.	LBM: Lb.	RMR: Cal.
228	36.40	82.99	145.01	2005	36.86	84.03	143.97	1991	37.31	85.07	142.93	1977	37.77	86.11	141.89	1962
228.5	36.30	82.95	145.55	2013	36.76	83.99	144.51	1999	37.21	85.03	143.47	1984	37.67	86.07	142.43	1970
229	36.21	82.91	146.09	2020	36.66	83.95	145.05	2006	37.11	84.99	144.01	1992	37.57	86.02	142.98	1977
229.5	36.11	82.87	146.63	2028	36.56	83.91	145.59	2014	37.01	84.95	144.55	1999	37.47	85.98	143.52	1985
230	36.01	82.83	147.17	2035	36.46	83.87	146.13	2021	36.92	84.91	145.10	2007	37.37	85.94	144.06	1992
230.5	35.92	82.79	147.71	2043	36.37	83.83	146.67	2028	36.82	84.86	145.64	2014	37.27	85.90	144.60	2000
231	35.82	82.75	148.25	2050	36.27	83.79	147.21	2036	36.72	84.82	146.18	2022	37.17	85.86	145.14	2007
231.5	35.73	82.71	148.79	2058	36.17	83.74	147.76	2043	36.62	84.78	146.72	2029	37.07	85.82	145.68	2015
232	35.63	82.67	149.33	2065	36.08	83.70	148.30	2051	36.53	84.74	147.26	2037	36.97	85.78	146.22	2022
232.5	35.54	82.63	149.88	2073	35.98	83.66	148.84	2058	36.43	84.70	147.80	2044	36.88	85.74	146.76	2030
233	35.44	82.58	150.42	2080	35.89	83.62	149.38	2066	36.33	84.66	148.34	2052	36.78	85.70	147.30	2037
233.5	35.35	82.54	150.96	2088	35.79	83.58	149.92	2073	36.24	84.62	148.88	2059	36.68	85.66	147.84	2045
234	35.26	82.50	151.50	2095	35.70	83.54	150.46	2081	36.14	84.58	149.42	2067	36.59	85.61	148.39	2052
234.5	35.16	82.46	152.04	2103	35.61	83.50	151.00	2088	36.05	84.54	149.96	2074	36.49	85.57	148.93	2060
235	35.07	82.42	152.58	2110	35.51	83.46	151.54	2096	35.96	84.50	150.51	2081	36.40	85.53	149.47	2067
235.5	34.98	82.38	153.12	2118	35.42	83.42	152.08	2103	35.86	84.45	151.05	2089	36.30	85.49	150.01	2075
236	34.89	82.34	153.66	2125	35.33	83.38	152.62	2111	35.77	84.41	151.59	2096	36.21	85.45	150.55	2082
236.5	34.80	82.30	154.20	2133	35.24	83.33	153.17	2118	35.68	84.37	152.13	2104	36.11	85.41	151.09	2090
237	34.71	82.26	154.74	2140	35.14	83.29	153.71	2126	35.58	84.33	152.67	2111	36.02	85.37	151.63	2097
237.5	34.62	82.22	155.29	2148	35.05	83.25	154.25	2133	35.49	84.29	153.21	2119	35.93	85.33	152.17	2105
238	34.53	82.17	155.83	2155	34.96	83.21	154.79	2141	35.40	84.25	153.75	2126	35.83	85.29	152.71	2112
238.5	34.44	82.13	156.37	2163	34.87	83.17	155.33	2148	35.31	84.21	154.29	2134	35.74	85.25	153.25	2120
239	34.35	82.09	156.91	2170	34.78	83.13	155.87	2156	35.22	84.17	154.83	2141	35.65	85.20	153.80	2127
239.5	34.26	82.05	157.45	2178	34.69	83.09	156.41	2163	35.13	84.13	155.37	2149	35.56	85.16	154.34	2134
240	34.17	82.01	157.99	2185	34.60	83.05	156.95	2171	35.04	84.09	155.92	2156	35.47	85.12	154.88	2142
240.5	34.08	81.97	158.53	2192	34.51	83.01	157.49	2178	34.95	84.04	156.46	2164	35.38	85.08	155.42	2149
241	34.00	81.93	159.07	2200	34.43	82.97	158.03	2186	34.86	84.00	157.00	2171	35.29	85.04	155.96	2157
241.5	33.91	81.89	159.61	2207	34.34	82.92	158.58	2193	34.77	83.96	157.54	2179	35.20	85.00	156.50	2164
242	33.82	81.85	160.15	2215	34.25	82.88	159.12	2201	34.68	83.92	158.08	2186	35.11	84.96	157.04	2172
242.5	33.73	81.81	160.70	2222	34.16	82.84	159.66	2208	34.59	83.88	158.62	2194	35.02	84.92	157.58	2179
243	33.65	81.76	161.24	2230	34.07	82.80	160.20	2216	34.50	83.84	159.16	2201	34.93	84.88	158.12	2187
243.5	33.56	81.72	161.78	2237	33.99	82.76	160.74	2223	34.41	83.80	159.70	2209	34.84	84.84	158.66	2194
244	33.48	81.68	162.32	2245	33.90	82.72	161.28	2231	34.33	83.76	160.24	2216	34.75	84.79	159.21	2202
244.5	33.39	81.64	162.86	2252	33.82	82.68	161.82	2238	34.24	83.72	160.78	2224	34.66	84.75	159.75	2209
245	33.31	81.60	163.40	2260	33.73	82.64	162.36	2245	34.15	83.68	161.33	2231	34.58	84.71	160.29	2217
245.5	33.22	81.56	163.94	2267	33.64	82.60	162.90	2253	34.07	83.63	161.87	2239	34.49	84.67	160.83	2224
246	33.14	81.52	164.48	2275	33.56	82.56	163.44	2260	33.98	83.59	162.41	2246	34.40	84.63	161.37	2232
246.5	33.05	81.48	165.02	2282	33.47	82.51	163.99	2268	33.90	83.55	162.95	2254	34.32	84.59	161.91	2239
247	32.97	81.44	165.56	2290	33.39	82.47	164.53	2275	33.81	83.51	163.49	2261	34.23	84.55	162.45	2247
247.5	32.89	81.40	166.11	2297	33.31	82.43	165.07	2283	33.73	83.47	164.03	2269	34.14	84.51	162.99	2254
248	32.80	81.35	166.65	2305	33.22	82.39	165.61	2290	33.64	83.43	164.57	2276	34.06	84.47	163.53	2262
248.5	32.72	81.31	167.19	2312	33.14	82.35	166.15	2298	33.56	83.39	165.11	2283	33.97	84.43	164.07	2269
249	32.64	81.27	167.73	2320	33.06	82.31	166.69	2305	33.47	83.35	165.65	2291	33.89	84.38	164.62	2277
249.5	32.56	81.23	168.27	2327	32.97	82.27	167.23	2313	33.39	83.31	166.19	2298	33.81	84.34	165.16	2284
250	32.48	81.19	168.81	2335	32.89	82.23	167.77	2320	33.31	83.27	166.74	2306	33.72	84.30	165.70	2292
250.5	32.39	81.15	169.35	2342	32.81	82.19	168.31	2328	33.22	83.22	167.28	2313	33.64	84.26	166.24	2299
251	32.31	81.11	169.89	2350	32.73	82.15	168.85	2335	33.14	83.18	167.82	2321	33.55	84.22	166.78	2307
251.5	32.23	81.07	170.43	2357	32.65	82.10	169.40	2343	33.06	83.14	168.36	2328	33.47	84.18	167.32	2314
252	32.15	81.03	170.97	2365	32.56	82.06	169.94	2350	32.98	83.10	168.90	2336	33.39	84.14	167.86	2322
252.5	32.07	80.99	171.52	2372	32.48	82.02	170.48	2358	32.90	83.06	169.44	2343	33.31	84.10	168.40	2329
253	31.99	80.94	172.06	2380	32.40	81.98	171.02	2365	32.81	83.02	169.98	2351	33.22	84.06	168.94	2336
253.5	31.91	80.90	172.60	2387	32.32	81.94	171.56	2373	32.73	82.98	170.52	2358	33.14	84.02	169.48	2344
254	31.84	80.86	173.14	2394	32.24	81.90	172.10	2380	32.65	82.94	171.06	2366	33.06	83.97	170.03	2351
254.5	31.76	80.82	173.68	2402	32.16	81.86	172.64	2388	32.57	82.90	171.60	2373	32.98	83.93	170.57	2359
255	31.68	80.78	174.22	2409	32.09	81.82	173.18	2395	32.49	82.86	172.15	2381	32.90	83.89	171.11	2366
255.5	31.60	80.74	174.76	2417	32.01	81.78	173.72	2403	32.41	82.81	172.69	2388	32.82	83.85	171.65	2374
256	31.52	80.70	175.30	2424	31.93	81.74	174.26	2410	32.33	82.77	173.23	2396	32.74	83.81	172.19	2381
256.5	31.45	80.66	175.84	2432	31.85	81.69	174.81	2418	32.25	82.73	173.77	2403	32.66	83.77	172.73	2389
257	31.37	80.62	176.38	2439	31.77	81.65	175.35	2425	32.18	82.69	174.31	2411	32.58	83.73	173.27	2396
257.5	31.29	80.58	176.93	2447	31.69	81.61	175.89	2433	32.10	82.65	174.85	2418	32.50	83.69	173.81	2404
258	31.21	80.53	177.47	2454	31.62	81.57	176.43	2440	32.02	82.61	175.39	2426	32.42	83.65	174.35	2411
258.5	31.14	80.49	178.01	2462	31.54	81.53	176.97	2447	31.94	82.57	175.93	2433	32.34	83.61	174.89	2419
259	31.06	80.45	178.55	2469	31.46	81.49	177.51	2455	31.86	82.53	176.47	2441	32.26	83.56	175.44	2426
259.5	30.99	80.41	179.09	2477	31.39	81.45	178.05	2462	31.79	82.49	177.01	2448	32.19	83.52	175.98	2434

Body Composition FEMALE 228-259.5 Lb.

Weight: Lb.	Waist: 44 inches Fat: %	Fat: Lb.	LBM: Lb.	RMR: Cal.	44.25 inches Fat: %	Fat: Lb.	LBM: Lb.	RMR: Cal.	44.5 inches Fat: %	Fat: Lb.	LBM: Lb.	RMR: Cal.	44.75 inches Fat: %	Fat: Lb.	LBM: Lb.	RMR: Cal.
228	38.22	87.14	140.86	1948	38.68	88.18	139.82	1934	39.13	89.22	138.78	1919	39.59	90.26	137.74	1905
228.5	38.12	87.10	141.40	1956	38.57	88.14	140.36	1941	39.03	89.18	139.32	1927	39.48	90.22	138.28	1912
229	38.02	87.06	141.94	1963	38.47	88.10	140.90	1949	38.92	89.14	139.86	1934	39.38	90.17	138.83	1920
229.5	37.92	87.02	142.48	1970	38.37	88.06	141.44	1956	38.82	89.10	140.40	1942	39.27	90.13	139.37	1927
230	37.82	86.98	143.02	1978	38.27	88.02	141.98	1964	38.72	89.06	140.95	1949	39.17	90.09	139.91	1935
230.5	37.72	86.94	143.56	1985	38.17	87.98	142.52	1971	38.62	89.01	141.49	1957	39.07	90.05	140.45	1942
231	37.62	86.90	144.10	1993	38.07	87.94	143.06	1979	38.52	88.97	142.03	1964	38.97	90.01	140.99	1950
231.5	37.52	86.86	144.64	2000	37.97	87.89	143.61	1986	38.42	88.93	142.57	1972	38.86	89.97	141.53	1957
232	37.42	86.82	145.18	2008	37.87	87.85	144.15	1994	38.32	88.89	143.11	1979	38.76	89.93	142.07	1965
232.5	37.32	86.78	145.73	2015	37.77	87.81	144.69	2001	38.22	88.85	143.65	1987	38.66	89.89	142.61	1972
233	37.22	86.73	146.27	2023	37.67	87.77	145.23	2009	38.12	88.81	144.19	1994	38.56	89.85	143.15	1980
233.5	37.13	86.69	146.81	2030	37.57	87.73	145.77	2016	38.02	88.77	144.73	2002	38.46	89.81	143.69	1987
234	37.03	86.65	147.35	2038	37.47	87.69	146.31	2023	37.92	88.73	145.27	2009	38.36	89.76	144.24	1995
234.5	36.93	86.61	147.89	2045	37.38	87.65	146.85	2031	37.82	88.69	145.81	2017	38.26	89.72	144.78	2002
235	36.84	86.57	148.43	2053	37.28	87.61	147.39	2038	37.72	88.65	146.36	2024	38.16	89.68	145.32	2010
235.5	36.74	86.53	148.97	2060	37.18	87.57	147.93	2046	37.62	88.60	146.90	2032	38.06	89.64	145.86	2017
236	36.65	86.49	149.51	2068	37.09	87.53	148.47	2053	37.53	88.56	147.44	2039	37.97	89.60	146.40	2025
236.5	36.55	86.45	150.05	2075	36.99	87.48	149.02	2061	37.43	88.52	147.98	2047	37.87	89.56	146.94	2032
237	36.46	86.41	150.59	2083	36.90	87.44	149.56	2068	37.33	88.48	148.52	2054	37.77	89.52	147.48	2040
237.5	36.36	86.37	151.14	2090	36.80	87.40	150.10	2076	37.24	88.44	149.06	2061	37.67	89.48	148.02	2047
238	36.27	86.32	151.68	2098	36.71	87.36	150.64	2083	37.14	88.40	149.60	2069	37.58	89.44	148.56	2055
238.5	36.18	86.28	152.22	2105	36.61	87.32	151.18	2091	37.05	88.36	150.14	2076	37.48	89.40	149.10	2062
239	36.08	86.24	152.76	2113	36.52	87.28	151.72	2098	36.95	88.32	150.68	2084	37.39	89.35	149.65	2070
239.5	35.99	86.20	153.30	2120	36.43	87.24	152.26	2106	36.86	88.28	151.22	2091	37.29	89.31	150.19	2077
240	35.90	86.16	153.84	2128	36.33	87.20	152.80	2113	36.76	88.24	151.77	2099	37.20	89.27	150.73	2085
240.5	35.81	86.12	154.38	2135	36.24	87.16	153.34	2121	36.67	88.19	152.31	2106	37.10	89.23	151.27	2092
241	35.72	86.08	154.92	2143	36.15	87.12	153.88	2128	36.58	88.15	152.85	2114	37.01	89.19	151.81	2100
241.5	35.63	86.04	155.46	2150	36.06	87.07	154.43	2136	36.49	88.11	153.39	2121	36.91	89.15	152.35	2107
242	35.54	86.00	156.00	2158	35.96	87.03	154.97	2143	36.39	88.07	153.93	2129	36.82	89.11	152.89	2114
242.5	35.45	85.96	156.55	2165	35.87	86.99	155.51	2151	36.30	88.03	154.47	2136	36.73	89.07	153.43	2122
243	35.36	85.91	157.09	2172	35.78	86.95	156.05	2158	36.21	87.99	155.01	2144	36.64	89.03	153.97	2129
243.5	35.27	85.87	157.63	2180	35.69	86.91	156.59	2166	36.12	87.95	155.55	2151	36.54	88.99	154.51	2137
244	35.18	85.83	158.17	2187	35.60	86.87	157.13	2173	36.03	87.91	156.09	2159	36.45	88.94	155.06	2144
244.5	35.09	85.79	158.71	2195	35.51	86.83	157.67	2181	35.94	87.87	156.63	2166	36.36	88.90	155.60	2152
245	35.00	85.75	159.25	2202	35.42	86.79	158.21	2188	35.85	87.83	157.18	2174	36.27	88.86	156.14	2159
245.5	34.91	85.71	159.79	2210	35.33	86.75	158.75	2196	35.76	87.78	157.72	2181	36.18	88.82	156.68	2167
246	34.82	85.67	160.33	2217	35.25	86.71	159.29	2203	35.67	87.74	158.26	2189	36.09	88.78	157.22	2174
246.5	34.74	85.63	160.87	2225	35.16	86.66	159.84	2211	35.58	87.70	158.80	2196	36.00	88.74	157.76	2182
247	34.65	85.59	161.41	2232	35.07	86.62	160.38	2218	35.49	87.66	159.34	2204	35.91	88.70	158.30	2189
247.5	34.56	85.55	161.96	2240	34.98	86.58	160.92	2225	35.40	87.62	159.88	2211	35.82	88.66	158.84	2197
248	34.48	85.50	162.50	2247	34.90	86.54	161.46	2233	35.31	87.58	160.42	2219	35.73	88.62	159.38	2204
248.5	34.39	85.46	163.04	2255	34.81	86.50	162.00	2240	35.23	87.54	160.96	2226	35.64	88.58	159.92	2212
249	34.31	85.42	163.58	2262	34.72	86.46	162.54	2248	35.14	87.50	161.50	2234	35.56	88.53	160.47	2219
249.5	34.22	85.38	164.12	2270	34.64	86.42	163.08	2255	35.05	87.46	162.04	2241	35.47	88.49	161.01	2227
250	34.14	85.34	164.66	2277	34.55	86.38	163.62	2263	34.97	87.42	162.59	2249	35.38	88.45	161.55	2234
250.5	34.05	85.30	165.20	2285	34.47	86.34	164.16	2270	34.88	87.37	163.13	2256	35.29	88.41	162.09	2242
251	33.97	85.26	165.74	2292	34.38	86.30	164.70	2278	34.79	87.33	163.67	2264	35.21	88.37	162.63	2249
251.5	33.88	85.22	166.28	2300	34.30	86.25	165.25	2285	34.71	87.29	164.21	2271	35.12	88.33	163.17	2257
252	33.80	85.18	166.82	2307	34.21	86.21	165.79	2293	34.62	87.25	164.75	2278	35.04	88.29	163.71	2264
252.5	33.72	85.14	167.37	2315	34.13	86.17	166.33	2300	34.54	87.21	165.29	2286	34.95	88.25	164.25	2272
253	33.63	85.09	167.91	2322	34.04	86.13	166.87	2308	34.45	87.17	165.83	2293	34.86	88.21	164.79	2279
253.5	33.55	85.05	168.45	2330	33.96	86.09	167.41	2315	34.37	87.13	166.37	2301	34.78	88.17	165.33	2287
254	33.47	85.01	168.99	2337	33.88	86.05	167.95	2323	34.29	87.09	166.91	2308	34.69	88.12	165.88	2294
254.5	33.39	84.97	169.53	2345	33.80	86.01	168.49	2330	34.20	87.05	167.45	2316	34.61	88.08	166.42	2302
255	33.31	84.93	170.07	2352	33.71	85.97	169.03	2338	34.12	87.01	168.00	2323	34.53	88.04	166.96	2309
255.5	33.22	84.89	170.61	2360	33.63	85.93	169.57	2345	34.04	86.96	168.54	2331	34.44	88.00	167.50	2317
256	33.14	84.85	171.15	2367	33.55	85.89	170.11	2353	33.95	86.92	169.08	2338	34.36	87.96	168.04	2324
256.5	33.06	84.81	171.69	2375	33.47	85.84	170.66	2360	33.87	86.88	169.62	2346	34.28	87.92	168.58	2331
257	32.98	84.77	172.23	2382	33.39	85.80	171.20	2368	33.79	86.84	170.16	2353	34.19	87.88	169.12	2339
257.5	32.90	84.73	172.78	2389	33.31	85.76	171.74	2375	33.71	86.80	170.70	2361	34.11	87.84	169.66	2346
258	32.82	84.68	173.32	2397	33.23	85.72	172.28	2383	33.63	86.76	171.24	2368	34.03	87.80	170.20	2354
258.5	32.74	84.64	173.86	2404	33.15	85.68	172.82	2390	33.55	86.72	171.78	2376	33.95	87.76	170.74	2361
259	32.66	84.60	174.40	2412	33.07	85.64	173.36	2398	33.47	86.68	172.32	2383	33.87	87.71	171.29	2369
259.5	32.59	84.56	174.94	2419	32.99	85.60	173.90	2405	33.39	86.64	172.86	2391	33.79	87.67	171.83	2376

Body Composition   FEMALE   228-259.5 Lb.

Weight: Lb.	Waist: 45 inches				45.25 inches				45.5 inches				45.75 inches			
	Fat: %	Fat: Lb.	LBM: Lb.	RMR: Cal.	Fat: %	Fat: Lb.	LBM: Lb.	RMR: Cal.	Fat: %	Fat: Lb.	LBM: Lb.	RMR: Cal.	Fat: %	Fat: Lb.	LBM: Lb.	RMR: Cal.
228	40.04	91.29	136.71	1891	40.50	92.33	135.67	1876	40.95	93.37	134.63	1862	41.41	94.41	133.59	1848
228.5	39.94	91.25	137.25	1898	40.39	92.29	136.21	1884	40.84	93.33	135.17	1869	41.30	94.37	134.13	1855
229	39.83	91.21	137.79	1906	40.28	92.25	136.75	1891	40.74	93.29	135.71	1877	41.19	94.32	134.68	1863
229.5	39.73	91.17	138.33	1913	40.18	92.21	137.29	1899	40.63	93.25	136.25	1884	41.08	94.28	135.22	1870
230	39.62	91.13	138.87	1921	40.07	92.17	137.83	1906	40.52	93.21	136.80	1892	40.98	94.24	135.76	1878
230.5	39.52	91.09	139.41	1928	39.97	92.13	138.37	1914	40.42	93.16	137.34	1899	40.87	94.20	136.30	1885
231	39.41	91.05	139.95	1936	39.86	92.09	138.91	1921	40.31	93.12	137.88	1907	40.76	94.16	136.84	1892
231.5	39.31	91.01	140.49	1943	39.76	92.04	139.46	1929	40.21	93.08	138.42	1914	40.66	94.12	137.38	1900
232	39.21	90.97	141.03	1951	39.66	92.00	140.00	1936	40.10	93.04	138.96	1922	40.55	94.08	137.92	1907
232.5	39.11	90.93	141.58	1958	39.55	91.96	140.54	1944	40.00	93.00	139.50	1929	40.45	94.04	138.46	1915
233	39.01	90.88	142.12	1965	39.45	91.92	141.08	1951	39.90	92.96	140.04	1937	40.34	94.00	139.00	1922
233.5	38.90	90.84	142.66	1973	39.35	91.88	141.62	1959	39.79	92.92	140.58	1944	40.24	93.96	139.54	1930
234	38.80	90.80	143.20	1980	39.25	91.84	142.16	1966	39.69	92.88	141.12	1952	40.13	93.91	140.09	1937
234.5	38.70	90.76	143.74	1988	39.15	91.80	142.70	1974	39.59	92.84	141.66	1959	40.03	93.87	140.63	1945
235	38.60	90.72	144.28	1995	39.05	91.76	143.24	1981	39.49	92.80	142.21	1967	39.93	93.83	141.17	1952
235.5	38.50	90.68	144.82	2003	38.95	91.72	143.78	1989	39.39	92.75	142.75	1974	39.83	93.79	141.71	1960
236	38.41	90.64	145.36	2010	38.85	91.68	144.32	1996	39.29	92.71	143.29	1982	39.72	93.75	142.25	1967
236.5	38.31	90.60	145.90	2018	38.75	91.63	144.87	2003	39.18	92.67	143.83	1989	39.62	93.71	142.79	1975
237	38.21	90.56	146.44	2025	38.65	91.59	145.41	2011	39.08	92.63	144.37	1997	39.52	93.67	143.33	1982
237.5	38.11	90.52	146.99	2033	38.55	91.55	145.95	2018	38.99	92.59	144.91	2004	39.42	93.63	143.87	1990
238	38.01	90.47	147.53	2040	38.45	91.51	146.49	2026	38.89	92.55	145.45	2012	39.32	93.59	144.41	1997
238.5	37.92	90.43	148.07	2048	38.35	91.47	147.03	2033	38.79	92.51	145.99	2019	39.22	93.55	144.95	2005
239	37.82	90.39	148.61	2055	38.26	91.43	147.57	2041	38.69	92.47	146.53	2027	39.12	93.50	145.50	2012
239.5	37.72	90.35	149.15	2063	38.16	91.39	148.11	2048	38.59	92.43	147.07	2034	39.02	93.46	146.04	2020
240	37.63	90.31	149.69	2070	38.06	91.35	148.65	2056	38.49	92.39	147.62	2042	38.93	93.42	146.58	2027
240.5	37.53	90.27	150.23	2078	37.97	91.31	149.19	2063	38.40	92.34	148.16	2049	38.83	93.38	147.12	2035
241	37.44	90.23	150.77	2085	37.87	91.27	149.73	2071	38.30	92.30	148.70	2056	38.73	93.34	147.66	2042
241.5	37.34	90.19	151.31	2093	37.77	91.22	150.28	2078	38.20	92.26	149.24	2064	38.63	93.30	148.20	2050
242	37.25	90.15	151.85	2100	37.68	91.18	150.82	2086	38.11	92.22	149.78	2071	38.54	93.26	148.74	2057
242.5	37.16	90.11	152.40	2108	37.58	91.14	151.36	2093	38.01	92.18	150.32	2079	38.44	93.22	149.28	2065
243	37.06	90.06	152.94	2115	37.49	91.10	151.90	2101	37.92	92.14	150.86	2086	38.34	93.18	149.82	2072
243.5	36.97	90.02	153.48	2123	37.40	91.06	152.44	2108	37.82	92.10	151.40	2094	38.25	93.14	150.36	2080
244	36.88	89.98	154.02	2130	37.30	91.02	152.98	2116	37.73	92.06	151.94	2101	38.15	93.09	150.91	2087
244.5	36.79	89.94	154.56	2138	37.21	90.98	153.52	2123	37.63	92.02	152.48	2109	38.06	93.05	151.45	2095
245	36.69	89.90	155.10	2145	37.12	90.94	154.06	2131	37.54	91.98	153.03	2116	37.96	93.01	151.99	2102
245.5	36.60	89.86	155.64	2153	37.03	90.90	154.60	2138	37.45	91.93	153.57	2124	37.87	92.97	152.53	2109
246	36.51	89.82	156.18	2160	36.93	90.86	155.14	2146	37.35	91.89	154.11	2131	37.78	92.93	153.07	2117
246.5	36.42	89.78	156.72	2167	36.84	90.81	155.69	2153	37.26	91.85	154.65	2139	37.68	92.89	153.61	2124
247	36.33	89.74	157.26	2175	36.75	90.77	156.23	2161	37.17	91.81	155.19	2146	37.59	92.85	154.15	2132
247.5	36.24	89.70	157.81	2182	36.66	90.73	156.77	2168	37.08	91.77	155.73	2154	37.50	92.81	154.69	2139
248	36.15	89.65	158.35	2190	36.57	90.69	157.31	2176	36.99	91.73	156.27	2161	37.41	92.77	155.23	2147
248.5	36.06	89.61	158.89	2197	36.48	90.65	157.85	2183	36.90	91.69	156.81	2169	37.31	92.73	155.77	2154
249	35.97	89.57	159.43	2205	36.39	90.61	158.39	2191	36.81	91.65	157.35	2176	37.22	92.68	156.32	2162
249.5	35.88	89.53	159.97	2212	36.30	90.57	158.93	2198	36.72	91.61	157.89	2184	37.13	92.64	156.86	2169
250	35.80	89.49	160.51	2220	36.21	90.53	159.47	2206	36.63	91.57	158.44	2191	37.04	92.60	157.40	2177
250.5	35.71	89.45	161.05	2227	36.12	90.49	160.01	2213	36.54	91.52	158.98	2199	36.95	92.56	157.94	2184
251	35.62	89.41	161.59	2235	36.03	90.45	160.55	2220	36.45	91.48	159.52	2206	36.86	92.52	158.48	2192
251.5	35.53	89.37	162.13	2242	35.95	90.40	161.10	2228	36.36	91.44	160.06	2214	36.77	92.48	159.02	2199
252	35.45	89.33	162.67	2250	35.86	90.36	161.64	2235	36.27	91.40	160.60	2221	36.68	92.44	159.56	2207
252.5	35.36	89.29	163.22	2257	35.77	90.32	162.18	2243	36.18	91.36	161.14	2229	36.59	92.40	160.10	2214
253	35.27	89.24	163.76	2265	35.68	90.28	162.72	2250	36.09	91.32	161.68	2236	36.50	92.36	160.64	2222
253.5	35.19	89.20	164.30	2272	35.60	90.24	163.26	2258	36.01	91.28	162.22	2244	36.42	92.32	161.18	2229
254	35.10	89.16	164.84	2280	35.51	90.20	163.80	2265	35.92	91.24	162.76	2251	36.33	92.27	161.73	2237
254.5	35.02	89.12	165.38	2287	35.43	90.16	164.34	2273	35.83	91.20	163.30	2258	36.24	92.23	162.27	2244
255	34.93	89.08	165.92	2295	35.34	90.12	164.88	2280	35.75	91.16	163.85	2266	36.15	92.19	162.81	2252
255.5	34.85	89.04	166.46	2302	35.25	90.08	165.42	2288	35.66	91.11	164.39	2273	36.07	92.15	163.35	2259
256	34.76	89.00	167.00	2310	35.17	90.04	165.96	2295	35.58	91.07	164.93	2281	35.98	92.11	163.89	2267
256.5	34.68	88.96	167.54	2317	35.09	89.99	166.51	2303	35.49	91.03	165.47	2288	35.89	92.07	164.43	2274
257	34.60	88.92	168.08	2325	35.00	89.95	167.05	2310	35.41	90.99	166.01	2296	35.81	92.03	164.97	2282
257.5	34.51	88.88	168.63	2332	34.92	89.91	167.59	2318	35.32	90.95	166.55	2303	35.72	91.99	165.51	2289
258	34.43	88.83	169.17	2340	34.83	89.87	168.13	2325	35.24	90.91	167.09	2311	35.64	91.95	166.05	2297
258.5	34.35	88.79	169.71	2347	34.75	89.83	168.67	2333	35.15	90.87	167.63	2318	35.55	91.91	166.59	2304
259	34.27	88.75	170.25	2355	34.67	89.79	169.21	2340	35.07	90.83	168.17	2326	35.47	91.86	167.14	2311
259.5	34.19	88.71	170.79	2362	34.59	89.75	169.75	2348	34.98	90.79	168.71	2333	35.38	91.82	167.68	2319

Body Composition FEMALE 228-259.5 Lb.

Weight: Lb.	Waist: 46 inches Fat: %	Fat: Lb.	LBM: Lb.	RMR: Cal.	46.25 inches Fat: %	Fat: Lb.	LBM: Lb.	RMR: Cal.	46.5 inches Fat: %	Fat: Lb.	LBM: Lb.	RMR: Cal.	46.75 inches Fat: %	Fat: Lb.	LBM: Lb.	RMR: Cal.
228	41.86	95.44	132.56	1833	42.32	96.48	131.52	1819	42.77	97.52	130.48	1805	43.23	98.56	129.44	1790
228.5	41.75	95.40	133.10	1841	42.21	96.44	132.06	1826	42.66	97.48	131.02	1812	43.11	98.52	129.98	1798
229	41.64	95.36	133.64	1848	42.10	96.40	132.60	1834	42.55	97.44	131.56	1820	43.00	98.47	130.53	1805
229.5	41.53	95.32	134.18	1856	41.99	96.36	133.14	1841	42.44	97.40	132.10	1827	42.89	98.43	131.07	1813
230	41.43	95.28	134.72	1863	41.88	96.32	133.68	1849	42.33	97.36	132.65	1834	42.78	98.39	131.61	1820
230.5	41.32	95.24	135.26	1871	41.77	96.28	134.22	1856	42.22	97.31	133.19	1842	42.67	98.35	132.15	1828
231	41.21	95.20	135.80	1878	41.66	96.24	134.76	1864	42.11	97.27	133.73	1849	42.56	98.31	132.69	1835
231.5	41.10	95.16	136.34	1886	41.55	96.19	135.31	1871	42.00	97.23	134.27	1857	42.45	98.27	133.23	1843
232	41.00	95.12	136.88	1893	41.45	96.15	135.85	1879	41.89	97.19	134.81	1864	42.34	98.23	133.77	1850
232.5	40.89	95.08	137.43	1901	41.34	96.11	136.39	1886	41.78	97.15	135.35	1872	42.23	98.19	134.31	1858
233	40.79	95.03	137.97	1908	41.23	96.07	136.93	1894	41.68	97.11	135.89	1879	42.12	98.15	134.85	1865
233.5	40.68	94.99	138.51	1916	41.13	96.03	137.47	1901	41.57	97.07	136.43	1887	42.02	98.11	135.39	1873
234	40.58	94.95	139.05	1923	41.02	95.99	138.01	1909	41.46	97.03	136.97	1894	41.91	98.06	135.94	1880
234.5	40.47	94.91	139.59	1931	40.92	95.95	138.55	1916	41.36	96.99	137.51	1902	41.80	98.02	136.48	1887
235	40.37	94.87	140.13	1938	40.81	95.91	139.09	1924	41.25	96.95	138.06	1909	41.69	97.98	137.02	1895
235.5	40.27	94.83	140.67	1945	40.71	95.87	139.63	1931	41.15	96.90	138.60	1917	41.59	97.94	137.56	1902
236	40.16	94.79	141.21	1953	40.60	95.83	140.17	1939	41.04	96.86	139.14	1924	41.48	97.90	138.10	1910
236.5	40.06	94.75	141.75	1960	40.50	95.78	140.72	1946	40.94	96.82	139.68	1932	41.38	97.86	138.64	1917
237	39.96	94.71	142.29	1968	40.40	95.74	141.26	1954	40.84	96.78	140.22	1939	41.27	97.82	139.18	1925
237.5	39.86	94.67	142.84	1975	40.30	95.70	141.80	1961	40.73	96.74	140.76	1947	41.17	97.78	139.72	1932
238	39.76	94.62	143.38	1983	40.19	95.66	142.34	1969	40.63	96.70	141.30	1954	41.07	97.74	140.26	1940
238.5	39.66	94.58	143.92	1990	40.09	95.62	142.88	1976	40.53	96.66	141.84	1962	40.96	97.70	140.80	1947
239	39.56	94.54	144.46	1998	39.99	95.58	143.42	1984	40.43	96.62	142.38	1969	40.86	97.65	141.35	1955
239.5	39.46	94.50	145.00	2005	39.89	95.54	143.96	1991	40.32	96.58	142.92	1977	40.76	97.61	141.89	1962
240	39.36	94.46	145.54	2013	39.79	95.50	144.50	1998	40.22	96.54	143.47	1984	40.66	97.57	142.43	1970
240.5	39.26	94.42	146.08	2020	39.69	95.46	145.04	2006	40.12	96.49	144.01	1992	40.55	97.53	142.97	1977
241	39.16	94.38	146.62	2028	39.59	95.42	145.58	2013	40.02	96.45	144.55	1999	40.45	97.49	143.51	1985
241.5	39.06	94.34	147.16	2035	39.49	95.37	146.13	2021	39.92	96.41	145.09	2007	40.35	97.45	144.05	1992
242	38.97	94.30	147.70	2043	39.39	95.33	146.67	2028	39.82	96.37	145.63	2014	40.25	97.41	144.59	2000
242.5	38.87	94.26	148.25	2050	39.30	95.29	147.21	2036	39.72	96.33	146.17	2022	40.15	97.37	145.13	2007
243	38.77	94.21	148.79	2058	39.20	95.25	147.75	2043	39.63	96.29	146.71	2029	40.05	97.33	145.67	2015
243.5	38.67	94.17	149.33	2065	39.10	95.21	148.29	2051	39.53	96.25	147.25	2036	39.95	97.29	146.21	2022
244	38.58	94.13	149.87	2073	39.00	95.17	148.83	2058	39.43	96.21	147.79	2044	39.85	97.24	146.76	2030
244.5	38.48	94.09	150.41	2080	38.91	95.13	149.37	2066	39.33	96.17	148.33	2051	39.76	97.20	147.30	2037
245	38.39	94.05	150.95	2088	38.81	95.09	149.91	2073	39.23	96.13	148.88	2059	39.66	97.16	147.84	2045
245.5	38.29	94.01	151.49	2095	38.72	95.05	150.45	2081	39.14	96.08	149.42	2066	39.56	97.12	148.38	2052
246	38.20	93.97	152.03	2103	38.62	95.01	150.99	2088	39.04	96.04	149.96	2074	39.46	97.08	148.92	2060
246.5	38.10	93.93	152.57	2110	38.53	94.96	151.54	2096	38.95	96.00	150.50	2081	39.37	97.04	149.46	2067
247	38.01	93.89	153.11	2118	38.43	94.92	152.08	2103	38.85	95.96	151.04	2089	39.27	97.00	150.00	2075
247.5	37.92	93.85	153.66	2125	38.34	94.88	152.62	2111	38.76	95.92	151.58	2096	39.17	96.96	150.54	2082
248	37.82	93.80	154.20	2133	38.24	94.84	153.16	2118	38.66	95.88	152.12	2104	39.08	96.92	151.08	2089
248.5	37.73	93.76	154.74	2140	38.15	94.80	153.70	2126	38.57	95.84	152.66	2111	38.98	96.88	151.62	2097
249	37.64	93.72	155.28	2147	38.06	94.76	154.24	2133	38.47	95.80	153.20	2119	38.89	96.83	152.17	2104
249.5	37.55	93.68	155.82	2155	37.96	94.72	154.78	2141	38.38	95.76	153.74	2126	38.79	96.79	152.71	2112
250	37.46	93.64	156.36	2162	37.87	94.68	155.32	2148	38.29	95.72	154.29	2134	38.70	96.75	153.25	2119
250.5	37.36	93.60	156.90	2170	37.78	94.64	155.86	2156	38.19	95.67	154.83	2141	38.61	96.71	153.79	2127
251	37.27	93.56	157.44	2177	37.69	94.60	156.40	2163	38.10	95.63	155.37	2149	38.51	96.67	154.33	2134
251.5	37.18	93.52	157.98	2185	37.60	94.55	156.95	2171	38.01	95.59	155.91	2156	38.42	96.63	154.87	2142
252	37.09	93.48	158.52	2192	37.51	94.51	157.49	2178	37.92	95.55	156.45	2164	38.33	96.59	155.41	2149
252.5	37.00	93.43	159.07	2200	37.41	94.47	158.03	2186	37.83	95.51	156.99	2171	38.24	96.55	155.95	2157
253	36.91	93.39	159.61	2207	37.32	94.43	158.57	2193	37.73	95.47	157.53	2179	38.14	96.51	156.49	2164
253.5	36.83	93.35	160.15	2215	37.23	94.39	159.11	2200	37.64	95.43	158.07	2186	38.05	96.47	157.03	2172
254	36.74	93.31	160.69	2222	37.15	94.35	159.65	2208	37.55	95.39	158.61	2194	37.96	96.42	157.58	2179
254.5	36.65	93.27	161.23	2230	37.06	94.31	160.19	2215	37.46	95.35	159.15	2201	37.87	96.38	158.12	2187
255	36.56	93.23	161.77	2237	36.97	94.27	160.73	2223	37.37	95.31	159.70	2209	37.78	96.34	158.66	2194
255.5	36.47	93.19	162.31	2245	36.88	94.23	161.27	2230	37.29	95.26	160.24	2216	37.69	96.30	159.20	2202
256	36.39	93.15	162.85	2252	36.79	94.19	161.81	2238	37.20	95.22	160.78	2224	37.60	96.26	159.74	2209
256.5	36.30	93.11	163.39	2260	36.70	94.14	162.36	2245	37.11	95.18	161.32	2231	37.51	96.22	160.28	2217
257	36.21	93.07	163.93	2267	36.62	94.10	162.90	2253	37.02	95.14	161.86	2239	37.42	96.18	160.82	2224
257.5	36.13	93.03	164.48	2275	36.53	94.06	163.44	2260	36.93	95.10	162.40	2246	37.33	96.14	161.36	2232
258	36.04	92.98	165.02	2282	36.44	94.02	163.98	2268	36.84	95.06	162.94	2253	37.25	96.10	161.90	2239
258.5	35.95	92.94	165.56	2290	36.36	93.98	164.52	2275	36.76	95.02	163.48	2261	37.16	96.06	162.44	2247
259	35.87	92.90	166.10	2297	36.27	93.94	165.06	2283	36.67	94.98	164.02	2268	37.07	96.01	162.99	2254
259.5	35.78	92.86	166.64	2305	36.18	93.90	165.60	2290	36.58	94.94	164.56	2276	36.98	95.97	163.53	2262

Body Composition   FEMALE   228-259.5 Lb.

Weight: Lb.	Waist: 47 inches Fat: %	Fat: Lb.	LBM: Lb.	RMR: Cal.	47.25 inches Fat: %	Fat: Lb.	LBM: Lb.	RMR: Cal.	47.5 inches Fat: %	Fat: Lb.	LBM: Lb.	RMR: Cal.	47.75 inches Fat: %	Fat: Lb.	LBM: Lb.	RMR: Cal.
228	43.68	99.59	128.41	1776	44.14	100.63	127.37	1762	44.59	101.67	126.33	1747	45.05	102.71	125.29	1733
228.5	43.57	99.55	128.95	1783	44.02	100.59	127.91	1769	44.48	101.63	126.87	1755	44.93	102.67	125.83	1740
229	43.46	99.51	129.49	1791	43.91	100.55	128.45	1776	44.36	101.59	127.41	1762	44.81	102.62	126.38	1748
229.5	43.34	99.47	130.03	1798	43.79	100.51	128.99	1784	44.25	101.55	127.95	1770	44.70	102.58	126.92	1755
230	43.23	99.43	130.57	1806	43.68	100.47	129.53	1791	44.13	101.51	128.50	1777	44.58	102.54	127.46	1763
230.5	43.12	99.39	131.11	1813	43.57	100.43	130.07	1799	44.02	101.46	129.04	1785	44.47	102.50	128.00	1770
231	43.01	99.35	131.65	1821	43.46	100.39	130.61	1806	43.91	101.42	129.58	1792	44.36	102.46	128.54	1778
231.5	42.90	99.31	132.19	1828	43.35	100.34	131.16	1814	43.79	101.38	130.12	1800	44.24	102.42	129.08	1785
232	42.79	99.27	132.73	1836	43.23	100.30	131.70	1821	43.68	101.34	130.66	1807	44.13	102.38	129.62	1793
232.5	42.68	99.23	133.28	1843	43.12	100.26	132.24	1829	43.57	101.30	131.20	1814	44.02	102.34	130.16	1800
233	42.57	99.18	133.82	1851	43.01	100.22	132.78	1836	43.46	101.26	131.74	1822	43.90	102.30	130.70	1808
233.5	42.46	99.14	134.36	1858	42.90	100.18	133.32	1844	43.35	101.22	132.28	1829	43.79	102.26	131.24	1815
234	42.35	99.10	134.90	1866	42.79	100.14	133.86	1851	43.24	101.18	132.82	1837	43.68	102.21	131.79	1823
234.5	42.24	99.06	135.44	1873	42.69	100.10	134.40	1859	43.13	101.14	133.36	1844	43.57	102.17	132.33	1830
235	42.14	99.02	135.98	1881	42.58	100.06	134.94	1866	43.02	101.10	133.91	1852	43.46	102.13	132.87	1838
235.5	42.03	98.98	136.52	1888	42.47	100.02	135.48	1874	42.91	101.05	134.45	1859	43.35	102.09	133.41	1845
236	41.92	98.94	137.06	1896	42.36	99.98	136.02	1881	42.80	101.01	134.99	1867	43.24	102.05	133.95	1853
236.5	41.82	98.90	137.60	1903	42.26	99.93	136.57	1889	42.69	100.97	135.53	1874	43.13	102.01	134.49	1860
237	41.71	98.86	138.14	1911	42.15	99.89	137.11	1896	42.59	100.93	136.07	1882	43.02	101.97	135.03	1867
237.5	41.61	98.82	138.69	1918	42.04	99.85	137.65	1904	42.48	100.89	136.61	1889	42.92	101.93	135.57	1875
238	41.50	98.77	139.23	1925	41.94	99.81	138.19	1911	42.37	100.85	137.15	1897	42.81	101.89	136.11	1882
238.5	41.40	98.73	139.77	1933	41.83	99.77	138.73	1919	42.27	100.81	137.69	1904	42.70	101.85	136.65	1890
239	41.29	98.69	140.31	1940	41.73	99.73	139.27	1926	42.16	100.77	138.23	1912	42.60	101.80	137.20	1897
239.5	41.19	98.65	140.85	1948	41.62	99.69	139.81	1934	42.06	100.73	138.77	1919	42.49	101.76	137.74	1905
240	41.09	98.61	141.39	1955	41.52	99.65	140.35	1941	41.95	100.69	139.32	1927	42.38	101.72	138.28	1912
240.5	40.99	98.57	141.93	1963	41.42	99.61	140.89	1949	41.85	100.64	139.86	1934	42.28	101.68	138.82	1920
241	40.88	98.53	142.47	1970	41.31	99.57	141.43	1956	41.74	100.60	140.40	1942	42.17	101.64	139.36	1927
241.5	40.78	98.49	143.01	1978	41.21	99.52	141.98	1964	41.64	100.56	140.94	1949	42.07	101.60	139.90	1935
242	40.68	98.45	143.55	1985	41.11	99.48	142.52	1971	41.54	100.52	141.48	1957	41.97	101.56	140.44	1942
242.5	40.58	98.41	144.10	1993	41.01	99.44	143.06	1978	41.44	100.48	142.02	1964	41.86	101.52	140.98	1950
243	40.48	98.36	144.64	2000	40.91	99.40	143.60	1986	41.33	100.44	142.56	1972	41.76	101.48	141.52	1957
243.5	40.38	98.32	145.18	2008	40.81	99.36	144.14	1993	41.23	100.40	143.10	1979	41.66	101.44	142.06	1965
244	40.28	98.28	145.72	2015	40.70	99.32	144.68	2001	41.13	100.36	143.64	1987	41.56	101.39	142.61	1972
244.5	40.18	98.24	146.26	2023	40.60	99.28	145.22	2008	41.03	100.32	144.18	1994	41.45	101.35	143.15	1980
245	40.08	98.20	146.80	2030	40.51	99.24	145.76	2016	40.93	100.28	144.73	2002	41.35	101.31	143.69	1987
245.5	39.98	98.16	147.34	2038	40.41	99.20	146.30	2023	40.83	100.23	145.27	2009	41.25	101.27	144.23	1995
246	39.89	98.12	147.88	2045	40.31	99.16	146.84	2031	40.73	100.19	145.81	2017	41.15	101.23	144.77	2002
246.5	39.79	98.08	148.42	2053	40.21	99.11	147.39	2038	40.63	100.15	146.35	2024	41.05	101.19	145.31	2010
247	39.69	98.04	148.96	2060	40.11	99.07	147.93	2046	40.53	100.11	146.89	2031	40.95	101.15	145.85	2017
247.5	39.59	98.00	149.51	2068	40.01	99.03	148.47	2053	40.43	100.07	147.43	2039	40.85	101.11	146.39	2025
248	39.50	97.95	150.05	2075	39.92	98.99	149.01	2061	40.33	100.03	147.97	2046	40.75	101.07	146.93	2032
248.5	39.40	97.91	150.59	2083	39.82	98.95	149.55	2068	40.24	99.99	148.51	2054	40.65	101.03	147.47	2040
249	39.31	97.87	151.13	2090	39.72	98.91	150.09	2076	40.14	99.95	149.05	2061	40.56	100.98	148.02	2047
249.5	39.21	97.83	151.67	2098	39.63	98.87	150.63	2083	40.04	99.91	149.59	2069	40.46	100.94	148.56	2055
250	39.12	97.79	152.21	2105	39.53	98.83	151.17	2091	39.95	99.87	150.14	2076	40.36	100.90	149.10	2062
250.5	39.02	97.75	152.75	2113	39.44	98.79	151.71	2098	39.85	99.82	150.68	2084	40.26	100.86	149.64	2070
251	38.93	97.71	153.29	2120	39.34	98.75	152.25	2106	39.75	99.78	151.22	2091	40.17	100.82	150.18	2077
251.5	38.83	97.67	153.83	2128	39.25	98.70	152.80	2113	39.66	99.74	151.76	2099	40.07	100.78	150.72	2084
252	38.74	97.63	154.37	2135	39.15	98.66	153.34	2121	39.56	99.70	152.30	2106	39.98	100.74	151.26	2092
252.5	38.65	97.59	154.92	2142	39.06	98.62	153.88	2128	39.47	99.66	152.84	2114	39.88	100.70	151.80	2099
253	38.55	97.54	155.46	2150	38.97	98.58	154.42	2136	39.38	99.62	153.38	2121	39.79	100.66	152.34	2107
253.5	38.46	97.50	156.00	2157	38.87	98.54	154.96	2143	39.28	99.58	153.92	2129	39.69	100.62	152.88	2114
254	38.37	97.46	156.54	2165	38.78	98.50	155.50	2151	39.19	99.54	154.46	2136	39.60	100.57	153.43	2122
254.5	38.28	97.42	157.08	2172	38.69	98.46	156.04	2158	39.09	99.50	155.00	2144	39.50	100.53	153.97	2129
255	38.19	97.38	157.62	2180	38.60	98.42	156.58	2166	39.00	99.46	155.55	2151	39.41	100.49	154.51	2137
255.5	38.10	97.34	158.16	2187	38.50	98.38	157.12	2173	38.91	99.41	156.09	2159	39.32	100.45	155.05	2144
256	38.01	97.30	158.70	2195	38.41	98.34	157.66	2181	38.82	99.37	156.63	2166	39.22	100.41	155.59	2152
256.5	37.92	97.26	159.24	2202	38.32	98.29	158.21	2188	38.73	99.33	157.17	2174	39.13	100.37	156.13	2159
257	37.83	97.22	159.78	2210	38.23	98.25	158.75	2195	38.63	99.29	157.71	2181	39.04	100.33	156.67	2167
257.5	37.74	97.18	160.33	2217	38.14	98.21	159.29	2203	38.54	99.25	158.25	2189	38.95	100.29	157.21	2174
258	37.65	97.13	160.87	2225	38.05	98.17	159.83	2210	38.45	99.21	158.79	2196	38.86	100.25	157.75	2182
258.5	37.56	97.09	161.41	2232	37.96	98.13	160.37	2218	38.36	99.17	159.33	2204	38.76	100.21	158.29	2189
259	37.47	97.05	161.95	2240	37.87	98.09	160.91	2225	38.27	99.13	159.87	2211	38.67	100.16	158.84	2197
259.5	37.38	97.01	162.49	2247	37.78	98.05	161.45	2233	38.18	99.09	160.41	2219	38.58	100.12	159.38	2204

Body Composition FEMALE 228-259.5 Lb.

Waist:	48 inches				48.25 inches				48.5 inches				48.75 inches			
Weight: Lb.	Fat: %	Fat: Lb.	LBM: Lb.	RMR: Cal.	Fat: %	Fat: Lb.	LBM: Lb.	RMR: Cal.	Fat: %	Fat: Lb.	LBM: Lb.	RMR: Cal.	Fat: %	Fat: Lb.	LBM: Lb.	RMR: Cal.
228	45.50	103.74	124.26	1718	45.96	104.78	123.22	1704	46.41	105.82	122.18	1690	46.87	106.86	121.14	1675
228.5	45.38	103.70	124.80	1726	45.84	104.74	123.76	1712	46.29	105.78	122.72	1697	46.75	106.82	121.68	1683
229	45.27	103.66	125.34	1733	45.72	104.70	124.30	1719	46.17	105.74	123.26	1705	46.63	106.77	122.23	1690
229.5	45.15	103.62	125.88	1741	45.60	104.66	124.84	1727	46.05	105.70	123.80	1712	46.51	106.73	122.77	1698
230	45.03	103.58	126.42	1748	45.49	104.62	125.38	1734	45.94	105.66	124.35	1720	46.39	106.69	123.31	1705
230.5	44.92	103.54	126.96	1756	45.37	104.58	125.92	1742	45.82	105.61	124.89	1727	46.27	106.65	123.85	1713
231	44.80	103.50	127.50	1763	45.25	104.54	126.46	1749	45.70	105.57	125.43	1735	46.15	106.61	124.39	1720
231.5	44.69	103.46	128.04	1771	45.14	104.49	127.01	1756	45.59	105.53	125.97	1742	46.03	106.57	124.93	1728
232	44.58	103.42	128.58	1778	45.02	104.45	127.55	1764	45.47	105.49	126.51	1750	45.92	106.53	125.47	1735
232.5	44.46	103.38	129.13	1786	44.91	104.41	128.09	1771	45.35	105.45	127.05	1757	45.80	106.49	126.01	1743
233	44.35	103.33	129.67	1793	44.79	104.37	128.63	1779	45.24	105.41	127.59	1765	45.69	106.45	126.55	1750
233.5	44.24	103.29	130.21	1801	44.68	104.33	129.17	1786	45.13	105.37	128.13	1772	45.57	106.41	127.09	1758
234	44.12	103.25	130.75	1808	44.57	104.29	129.71	1794	45.01	105.33	128.67	1780	45.45	106.36	127.64	1765
234.5	44.01	103.21	131.29	1816	44.46	104.25	130.25	1801	44.90	105.29	129.21	1787	45.34	106.32	128.18	1773
235	43.90	103.17	131.83	1823	44.34	104.21	130.79	1809	44.79	105.25	129.76	1795	45.23	106.28	128.72	1780
235.5	43.79	103.13	132.37	1831	44.23	104.17	131.33	1816	44.67	105.20	130.30	1802	45.11	106.24	129.26	1788
236	43.68	103.09	132.91	1838	44.12	104.13	131.87	1824	44.56	105.16	130.84	1809	45.00	106.20	129.80	1795
236.5	43.57	103.05	133.45	1846	44.01	104.08	132.42	1831	44.45	105.12	131.38	1817	44.89	106.16	130.34	1803
237	43.46	103.01	133.99	1853	43.90	104.04	132.96	1839	44.34	105.08	131.92	1824	44.78	106.12	130.88	1810
237.5	43.35	102.97	134.54	1861	43.79	104.00	133.50	1846	44.23	105.04	132.46	1832	44.66	106.08	131.42	1818
238	43.25	102.92	135.08	1868	43.68	103.96	134.04	1854	44.12	105.00	133.00	1839	44.55	106.04	131.96	1825
238.5	43.14	102.88	135.62	1876	43.57	103.92	134.58	1861	44.01	104.96	133.54	1847	44.44	106.00	132.50	1833
239	43.03	102.84	136.16	1883	43.46	103.88	135.12	1869	43.90	104.92	134.08	1854	44.33	105.95	133.05	1840
239.5	42.92	102.80	136.70	1891	43.36	103.84	135.66	1876	43.79	104.88	134.62	1862	44.22	105.91	133.59	1848
240	42.82	102.76	137.24	1898	43.25	103.80	136.20	1884	43.68	104.84	135.17	1869	44.11	105.87	134.13	1855
240.5	42.71	102.72	137.78	1906	43.14	103.76	136.74	1891	43.57	104.79	135.71	1877	44.00	105.83	134.67	1862
241	42.60	102.68	138.32	1913	43.04	103.72	137.28	1899	43.47	104.75	136.25	1884	43.90	105.79	135.21	1870
241.5	42.50	102.64	138.86	1920	42.93	103.67	137.83	1906	43.36	104.71	136.79	1892	43.79	105.75	135.75	1877
242	42.40	102.60	139.40	1928	42.82	103.63	138.37	1914	43.25	104.67	137.33	1899	43.68	105.71	136.29	1885
242.5	42.29	102.56	139.95	1935	42.72	103.59	138.91	1921	43.15	104.63	137.87	1907	43.57	105.67	136.83	1892
243	42.19	102.51	140.49	1943	42.61	103.55	139.45	1929	43.04	104.59	138.41	1914	43.47	105.63	137.37	1900
243.5	42.08	102.47	141.03	1950	42.51	103.51	139.99	1936	42.94	104.55	138.95	1922	43.36	105.59	137.91	1907
244	41.98	102.43	141.57	1958	42.41	103.47	140.53	1944	42.83	104.51	139.49	1929	43.26	105.54	138.46	1915
244.5	41.88	102.39	142.11	1965	42.30	103.43	141.07	1951	42.73	104.47	140.03	1937	43.15	105.50	139.00	1922
245	41.78	102.35	142.65	1973	42.20	103.39	141.61	1959	42.62	104.43	140.58	1944	43.05	105.46	139.54	1930
245.5	41.67	102.31	143.19	1980	42.10	103.35	142.15	1966	42.52	104.38	141.12	1952	42.94	105.42	140.08	1937
246	41.57	102.27	143.73	1988	41.99	103.31	142.69	1973	42.42	104.34	141.66	1959	42.84	105.38	140.62	1945
246.5	41.47	102.23	144.27	1995	41.89	103.26	143.24	1981	42.31	104.30	142.20	1967	42.73	105.34	141.16	1952
247	41.37	102.19	144.81	2003	41.79	103.22	143.78	1988	42.21	104.26	142.74	1974	42.63	105.30	141.70	1960
247.5	41.27	102.15	145.36	2010	41.69	103.18	144.32	1996	42.11	104.22	143.28	1982	42.53	105.26	142.24	1967
248	41.17	102.10	145.90	2018	41.59	103.14	144.86	2003	42.01	104.18	143.82	1989	42.43	105.22	142.78	1975
248.5	41.07	102.06	146.44	2025	41.49	103.10	145.40	2011	41.91	104.14	144.36	1997	42.32	105.18	143.32	1982
249	40.97	102.02	146.98	2033	41.39	103.06	145.94	2018	41.81	104.10	144.90	2004	42.22	105.13	143.87	1990
249.5	40.87	101.98	147.52	2040	41.29	103.02	146.48	2026	41.71	104.06	145.44	2011	42.12	105.09	144.41	1997
250	40.78	101.94	148.06	2048	41.19	102.98	147.02	2033	41.61	104.02	145.99	2019	42.02	105.05	144.95	2005
250.5	40.68	101.90	148.60	2055	41.09	102.94	147.56	2041	41.51	103.97	146.53	2026	41.92	105.01	145.49	2012
251	40.58	101.86	149.14	2063	40.99	102.90	148.10	2048	41.41	103.93	147.07	2034	41.82	104.97	146.03	2020
251.5	40.48	101.82	149.68	2070	40.90	102.85	148.65	2056	41.31	103.89	147.61	2041	41.72	104.93	146.57	2027
252	40.39	101.78	150.22	2078	40.80	102.81	149.19	2063	41.21	103.85	148.15	2049	41.62	104.89	147.11	2035
252.5	40.29	101.74	150.77	2085	40.70	102.77	149.73	2071	41.11	103.81	148.69	2056	41.52	104.85	147.65	2042
253	40.20	101.69	151.31	2093	40.61	102.73	150.27	2078	41.02	103.77	149.23	2064	41.43	104.81	148.19	2050
253.5	40.10	101.65	151.85	2100	40.51	102.69	150.81	2086	40.92	103.73	149.77	2071	41.33	104.77	148.73	2057
254	40.00	101.61	152.39	2108	40.41	102.65	151.35	2093	40.82	103.69	150.31	2079	41.23	104.72	149.28	2064
254.5	39.91	101.57	152.93	2115	40.32	102.61	151.89	2101	40.73	103.65	150.85	2086	41.13	104.68	149.82	2072
255	39.82	101.53	153.47	2122	40.22	102.57	152.43	2108	40.63	103.61	151.40	2094	41.04	104.64	150.36	2079
255.5	39.72	101.49	154.01	2130	40.13	102.53	152.97	2116	40.53	103.56	151.94	2101	40.94	104.60	150.90	2087
256	39.63	101.45	154.55	2137	40.03	102.49	153.51	2123	40.44	103.52	152.48	2109	40.84	104.56	151.44	2094
256.5	39.53	101.41	155.09	2145	39.94	102.44	154.06	2131	40.34	103.48	153.02	2116	40.75	104.52	151.98	2102
257	39.44	101.37	155.63	2152	39.85	102.40	154.60	2138	40.25	103.44	153.56	2124	40.65	104.48	152.52	2109
257.5	39.35	101.33	156.18	2160	39.75	102.36	155.14	2146	40.16	103.40	154.10	2131	40.56	104.44	153.06	2117
258	39.26	101.28	156.72	2167	39.66	102.32	155.68	2153	40.06	103.36	154.64	2139	40.46	104.40	153.60	2124
258.5	39.17	101.24	157.26	2175	39.57	102.28	156.22	2161	39.97	103.32	155.18	2146	40.37	104.36	154.14	2132
259	39.07	101.20	157.80	2182	39.47	102.24	156.76	2168	39.88	103.28	155.72	2154	40.28	104.31	154.69	2139
259.5	38.98	101.16	158.34	2190	39.38	102.20	157.30	2175	39.78	103.24	156.26	2161	40.18	104.27	155.23	2147

Body Composition FEMALE 228-259.5 Lb.

Waist:	49 inches				49.25 inches				49.5 inches				49.75 inches			
Weight: Lb.	Fat: %	Fat: Lb.	LBM: Lb.	RMR: Cal.	Fat: %	Fat: Lb.	LBM: Lb.	RMR: Cal.	Fat: %	Fat: Lb.	LBM: Lb.	RMR: Cal.	Fat: %	Fat: Lb.	LBM: Lb.	RMR: Cal.
228	47.32	107.89	120.11	1661	47.78	108.93	119.07	1647	48.23	109.97	118.03	1632	48.69	111.01	116.99	1618
228.5	47.20	107.85	120.65	1669	47.65	108.89	119.61	1654	48.11	109.93	118.57	1640	48.56	110.97	117.53	1626
229	47.08	107.81	121.19	1676	47.53	108.85	120.15	1662	47.99	109.89	119.11	1647	48.44	110.92	118.08	1633
229.5	46.96	107.77	121.73	1684	47.41	108.81	120.69	1669	47.86	109.85	119.65	1655	48.32	110.88	118.62	1640
230	46.84	107.73	122.27	1691	47.29	108.77	121.23	1677	47.74	109.81	120.20	1662	48.19	110.84	119.16	1648
230.5	46.72	107.69	122.81	1698	47.17	108.73	121.77	1684	47.62	109.76	120.74	1670	48.07	110.80	119.70	1655
231	46.60	107.65	123.35	1706	47.05	108.69	122.31	1692	47.50	109.72	121.28	1677	47.95	110.76	120.24	1663
231.5	46.48	107.61	123.89	1713	46.93	108.64	122.86	1699	47.38	109.68	121.82	1685	47.83	110.72	120.78	1670
232	46.36	107.57	124.43	1721	46.81	108.60	123.40	1707	47.26	109.64	122.36	1692	47.71	110.68	121.32	1678
232.5	46.25	107.53	124.98	1728	46.69	108.56	123.94	1714	47.14	109.60	122.90	1700	47.59	110.64	121.86	1685
233	46.13	107.48	125.52	1736	46.58	108.52	124.48	1722	47.02	109.56	123.44	1707	47.47	110.60	122.40	1693
233.5	46.01	107.44	126.06	1743	46.46	108.48	125.02	1729	46.90	109.52	123.98	1715	47.35	110.56	122.94	1700
234	45.90	107.40	126.60	1751	46.34	108.44	125.56	1737	46.79	109.48	124.52	1722	47.23	110.51	123.49	1708
234.5	45.78	107.36	127.14	1758	46.23	108.40	126.10	1744	46.67	109.44	125.06	1730	47.11	110.47	124.03	1715
235	45.67	107.32	127.68	1766	46.11	108.36	126.64	1751	46.55	109.40	125.61	1737	46.99	110.43	124.57	1723
235.5	45.55	107.28	128.22	1773	45.99	108.32	127.18	1759	46.43	109.35	126.15	1745	46.88	110.39	125.11	1730
236	45.44	107.24	128.76	1781	45.88	108.28	127.72	1766	46.32	109.31	126.69	1752	46.76	110.35	125.65	1738
236.5	45.33	107.20	129.30	1788	45.77	108.23	128.27	1774	46.20	109.27	127.23	1760	46.64	110.31	126.19	1745
237	45.21	107.16	129.84	1796	45.65	108.19	128.81	1781	46.09	109.23	127.77	1767	46.53	110.27	126.73	1753
237.5	45.10	107.12	130.39	1803	45.54	108.15	129.35	1789	45.97	109.19	128.31	1775	46.41	110.23	127.27	1760
238	44.99	107.07	130.93	1811	45.43	108.11	129.89	1796	45.86	109.15	128.85	1782	46.30	110.19	127.81	1768
238.5	44.88	107.03	131.47	1818	45.31	108.07	130.43	1804	45.75	109.11	129.39	1789	46.18	110.15	128.35	1775
239	44.77	106.99	132.01	1826	45.20	108.03	130.97	1811	45.63	109.07	129.93	1797	46.07	110.10	128.90	1783
239.5	44.66	106.95	132.55	1833	45.09	107.99	131.51	1819	45.52	109.03	130.47	1804	45.96	110.06	129.44	1790
240	44.55	106.91	133.09	1841	44.98	107.95	132.05	1826	45.41	108.99	131.02	1812	45.84	110.02	129.98	1798
240.5	44.44	106.87	133.63	1848	44.87	107.91	132.59	1834	45.30	108.94	131.56	1819	45.73	109.98	130.52	1805
241	44.33	106.83	134.17	1856	44.76	107.87	133.13	1841	45.19	108.90	132.10	1827	45.62	109.94	131.06	1813
241.5	44.22	106.79	134.71	1863	44.65	107.82	133.68	1849	45.08	108.86	132.64	1834	45.51	109.90	131.60	1820
242	44.11	106.75	135.25	1871	44.54	107.78	134.22	1856	44.97	108.82	133.18	1842	45.40	109.86	132.14	1828
242.5	44.00	106.71	135.80	1878	44.43	107.74	134.76	1864	44.86	108.78	133.72	1849	45.29	109.82	132.68	1835
243	43.89	106.66	136.34	1886	44.32	107.70	135.30	1871	44.75	108.74	134.26	1857	45.18	109.78	133.22	1842
243.5	43.79	106.62	136.88	1893	44.21	107.66	135.84	1879	44.64	108.70	134.80	1864	45.07	109.74	133.76	1850
244	43.68	106.58	137.42	1900	44.11	107.62	136.38	1886	44.53	108.66	135.34	1872	44.96	109.69	134.31	1857
244.5	43.58	106.54	137.96	1908	44.00	107.58	136.92	1894	44.42	108.62	135.88	1879	44.85	109.65	134.85	1865
245	43.47	106.50	138.50	1915	43.89	107.54	137.46	1901	44.32	108.58	136.43	1887	44.74	109.61	135.39	1872
245.5	43.36	106.46	139.04	1923	43.79	107.50	138.00	1909	44.21	108.53	136.97	1894	44.63	109.57	135.93	1880
246	43.26	106.42	139.58	1930	43.68	107.46	138.54	1916	44.10	108.49	137.51	1902	44.52	109.53	136.47	1887
246.5	43.15	106.38	140.12	1938	43.58	107.41	139.09	1924	44.00	108.45	138.05	1909	44.42	109.49	137.01	1895
247	43.05	106.34	140.66	1945	43.47	107.37	139.63	1931	43.89	108.41	138.59	1917	44.31	109.45	137.55	1902
247.5	42.95	106.30	141.21	1953	43.37	107.33	140.17	1939	43.79	108.37	139.13	1924	44.21	109.41	138.09	1910
248	42.84	106.25	141.75	1960	43.26	107.29	140.71	1946	43.68	108.33	139.67	1932	44.10	109.37	138.63	1917
248.5	42.74	106.21	142.29	1968	43.16	107.25	141.25	1953	43.58	108.29	140.21	1939	43.99	109.33	139.17	1925
249	42.64	106.17	142.83	1975	43.06	107.21	141.79	1961	43.47	108.25	140.75	1947	43.89	109.28	139.72	1932
249.5	42.54	106.13	143.37	1983	42.95	107.17	142.33	1968	43.37	108.21	141.29	1954	43.78	109.24	140.26	1940
250	42.44	106.09	143.91	1990	42.85	107.13	142.87	1976	43.27	108.17	141.84	1962	43.68	109.20	140.80	1947
250.5	42.33	106.05	144.45	1998	42.75	107.09	143.41	1983	43.16	108.12	142.38	1969	43.58	109.16	141.34	1955
251	42.23	106.01	144.99	2005	42.65	107.05	143.95	1991	43.06	108.08	142.92	1977	43.47	109.12	141.88	1962
251.5	42.13	105.97	145.53	2013	42.55	107.00	144.50	1998	42.96	108.04	143.46	1984	43.37	109.08	142.42	1970
252	42.03	105.93	146.07	2020	42.45	106.96	145.04	2006	42.86	108.00	144.00	1992	43.27	109.04	142.96	1977
252.5	41.93	105.89	146.62	2028	42.35	106.92	145.58	2013	42.76	107.96	144.54	1999	43.17	109.00	143.50	1985
253	41.84	105.84	147.16	2035	42.25	106.88	146.12	2021	42.66	107.92	145.08	2006	43.07	108.96	144.04	1992
253.5	41.74	105.80	147.70	2043	42.15	106.84	146.66	2028	42.56	107.88	145.62	2014	42.96	108.92	144.58	2000
254	41.64	105.76	148.24	2050	42.05	106.80	147.20	2036	42.46	107.84	146.16	2021	42.86	108.87	145.13	2007
254.5	41.54	105.72	148.78	2058	41.95	106.76	147.74	2043	42.36	107.80	146.70	2029	42.76	108.83	145.67	2015
255	41.44	105.68	149.32	2065	41.85	106.72	148.28	2051	42.26	107.76	147.25	2036	42.66	108.79	146.21	2022
255.5	41.35	105.64	149.86	2073	41.75	106.68	148.82	2058	42.16	107.71	147.79	2044	42.56	108.75	146.75	2030
256	41.25	105.60	150.40	2080	41.65	106.64	149.36	2066	42.06	107.67	148.33	2051	42.47	108.71	147.29	2037
256.5	41.15	105.56	150.94	2088	41.56	106.59	149.91	2073	41.96	107.63	148.87	2059	42.37	108.67	147.83	2044
257	41.06	105.52	151.48	2095	41.46	106.55	150.45	2081	41.86	107.59	149.41	2066	42.27	108.63	148.37	2052
257.5	40.96	105.48	152.03	2103	41.36	106.51	150.99	2088	41.77	107.55	149.95	2074	42.17	108.59	148.91	2059
258	40.87	105.43	152.57	2110	41.27	106.47	151.53	2096	41.67	107.51	150.49	2081	42.07	108.55	149.45	2067
258.5	40.77	105.39	153.11	2117	41.17	106.43	152.07	2103	41.57	107.47	151.03	2089	41.98	108.51	149.99	2074
259	40.68	105.35	153.65	2125	41.08	106.39	152.61	2111	41.48	107.43	151.57	2096	41.88	108.46	150.54	2082
259.5	40.58	105.31	154.19	2132	40.98	106.35	153.15	2118	41.38	107.39	152.11	2104	41.78	108.42	151.08	2089

Body Composition FEMALE 228-259.5 Lb.

Weight: Lb.	Waist: 50 inches Fat: %	Fat: Lb.	LBM: Lb.	RMR: Cal.	50.25 inches Fat: %	Fat: Lb.	LBM: Lb.	RMR: Cal.	50.5 inches Fat: %	Fat: Lb.	LBM: Lb.	RMR: Cal.	50.75 inches Fat: %	Fat: Lb.	LBM: Lb.	RMR: Cal.
228	49.14	112.04	115.96	1604	49.60	113.08	114.92	1589	50.05	114.12	113.88	1575	50.51	115.16	112.84	1561
228.5	49.02	112.00	116.50	1611	49.47	113.04	115.46	1597	49.92	114.08	114.42	1582	50.38	115.12	113.38	1568
229	48.89	111.96	117.04	1619	49.34	113.00	116.00	1604	49.80	114.04	114.96	1590	50.25	115.07	113.93	1576
229.5	48.77	111.92	117.58	1626	49.22	112.96	116.54	1612	49.67	114.00	115.50	1597	50.12	115.03	114.47	1583
230	48.64	111.88	118.12	1634	49.09	112.92	117.08	1619	49.55	113.96	116.05	1605	50.00	114.99	115.01	1591
230.5	48.52	111.84	118.66	1641	48.97	112.88	117.62	1627	49.42	113.91	116.59	1612	49.87	114.95	115.55	1598
231	48.40	111.80	119.20	1649	48.85	112.84	118.16	1634	49.30	113.87	117.13	1620	49.74	114.91	116.09	1606
231.5	48.28	111.76	119.74	1656	48.72	112.79	118.71	1642	49.17	113.83	117.67	1627	49.62	114.87	116.63	1613
232	48.15	111.72	120.28	1664	48.60	112.75	119.25	1649	49.05	113.79	118.21	1635	49.50	114.83	117.17	1620
232.5	48.03	111.68	120.83	1671	48.48	112.71	119.79	1657	48.92	113.75	118.75	1642	49.37	114.79	117.71	1628
233	47.91	111.63	121.37	1678	48.36	112.67	120.33	1664	48.80	113.71	119.29	1650	49.25	114.75	118.25	1635
233.5	47.79	111.59	121.91	1686	48.24	112.63	120.87	1672	48.68	113.67	119.83	1657	49.12	114.71	118.79	1643
234	47.67	111.55	122.45	1693	48.12	112.59	121.41	1679	48.56	113.63	120.37	1665	49.00	114.66	119.34	1650
234.5	47.55	111.51	122.99	1701	48.00	112.55	121.95	1687	48.44	113.59	120.91	1672	48.88	114.62	119.88	1658
235	47.43	111.47	123.53	1708	47.88	112.51	122.49	1694	48.32	113.55	121.46	1680	48.76	114.58	120.42	1665
235.5	47.32	111.43	124.07	1716	47.76	112.47	123.03	1702	48.20	113.50	122.00	1687	48.64	114.54	120.96	1673
236	47.20	111.39	124.61	1723	47.64	112.43	123.57	1709	48.08	113.46	122.54	1695	48.52	114.50	121.50	1680
236.5	47.08	111.35	125.15	1731	47.52	112.38	124.12	1717	47.96	113.42	123.08	1702	48.40	114.46	122.04	1688
237	46.96	111.31	125.69	1738	47.40	112.34	124.66	1724	47.84	113.38	123.62	1710	48.28	114.42	122.58	1695
237.5	46.85	111.27	126.24	1746	47.29	112.30	125.20	1731	47.72	113.34	124.16	1717	48.16	114.38	123.12	1703
238	46.73	111.22	126.78	1753	47.17	112.26	125.74	1739	47.60	113.30	124.70	1725	48.04	114.34	123.66	1710
238.5	46.62	111.18	127.32	1761	47.05	112.22	126.28	1746	47.49	113.26	125.24	1732	47.92	114.30	124.20	1718
239	46.50	111.14	127.86	1768	46.94	112.18	126.82	1754	47.37	113.22	125.78	1740	47.81	114.25	124.75	1725
239.5	46.39	111.10	128.40	1776	46.82	112.14	127.36	1761	47.26	113.18	126.32	1747	47.69	114.21	125.29	1733
240	46.28	111.06	128.94	1783	46.71	112.10	127.90	1769	47.14	113.14	126.87	1755	47.57	114.17	125.83	1740
240.5	46.16	111.02	129.48	1791	46.59	112.06	128.44	1776	47.02	113.09	127.41	1762	47.46	114.13	126.37	1748
241	46.05	110.98	130.02	1798	46.48	112.02	128.98	1784	46.91	113.05	127.95	1770	47.34	114.09	126.91	1755
241.5	45.94	110.94	130.56	1806	46.37	111.97	129.53	1791	46.80	113.01	128.49	1777	47.23	114.05	127.45	1763
242	45.82	110.90	131.10	1813	46.25	111.93	130.07	1799	46.68	112.97	129.03	1784	47.11	114.01	127.99	1770
242.5	45.71	110.86	131.65	1821	46.14	111.89	130.61	1806	46.57	112.93	129.57	1792	47.00	113.97	128.53	1778
243	45.60	110.81	132.19	1828	46.03	111.85	131.15	1814	46.46	112.89	130.11	1799	46.88	113.93	129.07	1785
243.5	45.49	110.77	132.73	1836	45.92	111.81	131.69	1821	46.34	112.85	130.65	1807	46.77	113.89	129.61	1793
244	45.38	110.73	133.27	1843	45.81	111.77	132.23	1829	46.23	112.81	131.19	1814	46.66	113.84	130.16	1800
244.5	45.27	110.69	133.81	1851	45.70	111.73	132.77	1836	46.12	112.77	131.73	1822	46.55	113.80	130.70	1808
245	45.16	110.65	134.35	1858	45.59	111.69	133.31	1844	46.01	112.73	132.28	1829	46.43	113.76	131.24	1815
245.5	45.05	110.61	134.89	1866	45.48	111.65	133.85	1851	45.90	112.68	132.82	1837	46.32	113.72	131.78	1822
246	44.95	110.57	135.43	1873	45.37	111.61	134.39	1859	45.79	112.64	133.36	1844	46.21	113.68	132.32	1830
246.5	44.84	110.53	135.97	1881	45.26	111.56	134.94	1866	45.68	112.60	133.90	1852	46.10	113.64	132.86	1837
247	44.73	110.49	136.51	1888	45.15	111.52	135.48	1874	45.57	112.56	134.44	1859	45.99	113.60	133.40	1845
247.5	44.62	110.45	137.06	1895	45.04	111.48	136.02	1881	45.46	112.52	134.98	1867	45.88	113.56	133.94	1852
248	44.52	110.40	137.60	1903	44.94	111.44	136.56	1889	45.35	112.48	135.52	1874	45.77	113.52	134.48	1860
248.5	44.41	110.36	138.14	1910	44.83	111.40	137.10	1896	45.25	112.44	136.06	1882	45.66	113.48	135.02	1867
249	44.31	110.32	138.68	1918	44.72	111.36	137.64	1904	45.14	112.40	136.60	1889	45.56	113.43	135.57	1875
249.5	44.20	110.28	139.22	1925	44.62	111.32	138.18	1911	45.03	112.36	137.14	1897	45.45	113.39	136.11	1882
250	44.10	110.24	139.76	1933	44.51	111.28	138.72	1919	44.93	112.32	137.69	1904	45.34	113.35	136.65	1890
250.5	43.99	110.20	140.30	1940	44.41	111.24	139.26	1926	44.82	112.27	138.23	1912	45.23	113.31	137.19	1897
251	43.89	110.16	140.84	1948	44.30	111.20	139.80	1933	44.71	112.23	138.77	1919	45.13	113.27	137.73	1905
251.5	43.78	110.12	141.38	1955	44.20	111.15	140.35	1941	44.61	112.19	139.31	1927	45.02	113.23	138.27	1912
252	43.68	110.08	141.92	1963	44.09	111.11	140.89	1948	44.50	112.15	139.85	1934	44.92	113.19	138.81	1920
252.5	43.58	110.04	142.47	1970	43.99	111.07	141.43	1956	44.40	112.11	140.39	1942	44.81	113.15	139.35	1927
253	43.48	109.99	143.01	1978	43.89	111.03	141.97	1963	44.30	112.07	140.93	1949	44.71	113.11	139.89	1935
253.5	43.37	109.95	143.55	1985	43.78	110.99	142.51	1971	44.19	112.03	141.47	1957	44.60	113.07	140.43	1942
254	43.27	109.91	144.09	1993	43.68	110.95	143.05	1978	44.09	111.99	142.01	1964	44.50	113.02	140.98	1950
254.5	43.17	109.87	144.63	2000	43.58	110.91	143.59	1986	43.99	111.95	142.55	1972	44.39	112.98	141.52	1957
255	43.07	109.83	145.17	2008	43.48	110.87	144.13	1993	43.88	111.91	143.10	1979	44.29	112.94	142.06	1965
255.5	42.97	109.79	145.71	2015	43.38	110.83	144.67	2001	43.78	111.86	143.64	1986	44.19	112.90	142.60	1972
256	42.87	109.75	146.25	2023	43.28	110.79	145.21	2008	43.68	111.82	144.18	1994	44.09	112.86	143.14	1980
256.5	42.77	109.71	146.79	2030	43.18	110.74	145.76	2016	43.58	111.78	144.72	2001	43.98	112.82	143.68	1987
257	42.67	109.67	147.33	2038	43.08	110.70	146.30	2023	43.48	111.74	145.26	2009	43.88	112.78	144.22	1995
257.5	42.57	109.63	147.88	2045	42.98	110.66	146.84	2031	43.38	111.70	145.80	2016	43.78	112.74	144.76	2002
258	42.47	109.58	148.42	2053	42.88	110.62	147.38	2038	43.28	111.66	146.34	2024	43.68	112.70	145.30	2010
258.5	42.38	109.54	148.96	2060	42.78	110.58	147.92	2046	43.18	111.62	146.88	2031	43.58	112.66	145.84	2017
259	42.28	109.50	149.50	2068	42.68	110.54	148.46	2053	43.08	111.58	147.42	2039	43.48	112.61	146.39	2025
259.5	42.18	109.46	150.04	2075	42.58	110.50	149.00	2061	42.98	111.54	147.96	2046	43.38	112.57	146.93	2032

Body Composition FEMALE 228-259.5 Lb.

Weight: Lb.	Waist: 51 inches				51.25 inches				51.5 inches				51.75 inches			
	Fat: %	Fat: Lb.	LBM: Lb.	RMR: Cal.	Fat: %	Fat: Lb.	LBM: Lb.	RMR: Cal.	Fat: %	Fat: Lb.	LBM: Lb.	RMR: Cal.	Fat: %	Fat: Lb.	LBM: Lb.	RMR: Cal.
228	50.96	116.19	111.81	1546	51.42	117.23	110.77	1532	51.87	118.27	109.73	1518	52.33	119.31	108.69	1503
228.5	50.83	116.15	112.35	1554	51.29	117.19	111.31	1539	51.74	118.23	110.27	1525	52.19	119.27	109.23	1511
229	50.70	116.11	112.89	1561	51.16	117.15	111.85	1547	51.61	118.19	110.81	1533	52.06	119.22	109.78	1518
229.5	50.58	116.07	113.43	1569	51.03	117.11	112.39	1554	51.48	118.15	111.35	1540	51.93	119.18	110.32	1526
230	50.45	116.03	113.97	1576	50.90	117.07	112.93	1562	51.35	118.11	111.90	1548	51.80	119.14	110.86	1533
230.5	50.32	115.99	114.51	1584	50.77	117.03	113.47	1569	51.22	118.06	112.44	1555	51.67	119.10	111.40	1541
231	50.19	115.95	115.05	1591	50.64	116.99	114.01	1577	51.09	118.02	112.98	1562	51.54	119.06	111.94	1548
231.5	50.07	115.91	115.59	1599	50.52	116.94	114.56	1584	50.96	117.98	113.52	1570	51.41	119.02	112.48	1556
232	49.94	115.87	116.13	1606	50.39	116.90	115.10	1592	50.84	117.94	114.06	1577	51.28	118.98	113.02	1563
232.5	49.82	115.83	116.68	1614	50.26	116.86	115.64	1599	50.71	117.90	114.60	1585	51.16	118.94	113.56	1571
233	49.69	115.78	117.22	1621	50.14	116.82	116.18	1607	50.58	117.86	115.14	1592	51.03	118.90	114.10	1578
233.5	49.57	115.74	117.76	1629	50.01	116.78	116.72	1614	50.46	117.82	115.68	1600	50.90	118.86	114.64	1586
234	49.45	115.70	118.30	1636	49.89	116.74	117.26	1622	50.33	117.78	116.22	1607	50.78	118.81	115.19	1593
234.5	49.32	115.66	118.84	1644	49.76	116.70	117.80	1629	50.21	117.74	116.76	1615	50.65	118.77	115.73	1600
235	49.20	115.62	119.38	1651	49.64	116.66	118.34	1637	50.08	117.70	117.31	1622	50.52	118.73	116.27	1608
235.5	49.08	115.58	119.92	1659	49.52	116.62	118.88	1644	49.96	117.65	117.85	1630	50.40	118.69	116.81	1615
236	48.96	115.54	120.46	1666	49.40	116.58	119.42	1652	49.84	117.61	118.39	1637	50.28	118.65	117.35	1623
236.5	48.84	115.50	121.00	1673	49.27	116.53	119.97	1659	49.71	117.57	118.93	1645	50.15	118.61	117.89	1630
237	48.72	115.46	121.54	1681	49.15	116.49	120.51	1667	49.59	117.53	119.47	1652	50.03	118.57	118.43	1638
237.5	48.60	115.42	122.09	1688	49.03	116.45	121.05	1674	49.47	117.49	120.01	1660	49.91	118.53	118.97	1645
238	48.48	115.37	122.63	1696	48.91	116.41	121.59	1682	49.35	117.45	120.55	1667	49.78	118.49	119.51	1653
238.5	48.36	115.33	123.17	1703	48.79	116.37	122.13	1689	49.23	117.41	121.09	1675	49.66	118.45	120.05	1660
239	48.24	115.29	123.71	1711	48.67	116.33	122.67	1697	49.11	117.37	121.63	1682	49.54	118.40	120.60	1668
239.5	48.12	115.25	124.25	1718	48.55	116.29	123.21	1704	48.99	117.33	122.17	1690	49.42	118.36	121.14	1675
240	48.00	115.21	124.79	1726	48.44	116.25	123.75	1711	48.87	117.29	122.72	1697	49.30	118.32	121.68	1683
240.5	47.89	115.17	125.33	1733	48.32	116.21	124.29	1719	48.75	117.24	123.26	1705	49.18	118.28	122.22	1690
241	47.77	115.13	125.87	1741	48.20	116.17	124.83	1726	48.63	117.20	123.80	1712	49.06	118.24	122.76	1698
241.5	47.66	115.09	126.41	1748	48.08	116.12	125.38	1734	48.51	117.16	124.34	1720	48.94	118.20	123.30	1705
242	47.54	115.05	126.95	1756	47.97	116.08	125.92	1741	48.40	117.12	124.88	1727	48.83	118.16	123.84	1713
242.5	47.42	115.01	127.50	1763	47.85	116.04	126.46	1749	48.28	117.08	125.42	1735	48.71	118.12	124.38	1720
243	47.31	114.96	128.04	1771	47.74	116.00	127.00	1756	48.16	117.04	125.96	1742	48.59	118.08	124.92	1728
243.5	47.20	114.92	128.58	1778	47.62	115.96	127.54	1764	48.05	117.00	126.50	1750	48.47	118.04	125.46	1735
244	47.08	114.88	129.12	1786	47.51	115.92	128.08	1771	47.93	116.96	127.04	1757	48.36	117.99	126.01	1743
244.5	46.97	114.84	129.66	1793	47.39	115.88	128.62	1779	47.82	116.92	127.58	1764	48.24	117.95	126.55	1750
245	46.86	114.80	130.20	1801	47.28	115.84	129.16	1786	47.70	116.88	128.13	1772	48.13	117.91	127.09	1758
245.5	46.75	114.76	130.74	1808	47.17	115.80	129.70	1794	47.59	116.83	128.67	1779	48.01	117.87	127.63	1765
246	46.63	114.72	131.28	1816	47.06	115.76	130.24	1801	47.48	116.79	129.21	1787	47.90	117.83	128.17	1773
246.5	46.52	114.68	131.82	1823	46.94	115.71	130.79	1809	47.36	116.75	129.75	1794	47.78	117.79	128.71	1780
247	46.41	114.64	132.36	1831	46.83	115.67	131.33	1816	47.25	116.71	130.29	1802	47.67	117.75	129.25	1788
247.5	46.30	114.60	132.91	1838	46.72	115.63	131.87	1824	47.14	116.67	130.83	1809	47.56	117.71	129.79	1795
248	46.19	114.55	133.45	1846	46.61	115.59	132.41	1831	47.03	116.63	131.37	1817	47.45	117.67	130.33	1803
248.5	46.08	114.51	133.99	1853	46.50	115.55	132.95	1839	46.92	116.59	131.91	1824	47.33	117.63	130.87	1810
249	45.97	114.47	134.53	1861	46.39	115.51	133.49	1846	46.81	116.55	132.45	1832	47.22	117.58	131.42	1817
249.5	45.86	114.43	135.07	1868	46.28	115.47	134.03	1854	46.70	116.51	132.99	1839	47.11	117.54	131.96	1825
250	45.76	114.39	135.61	1875	46.17	115.43	134.57	1861	46.59	116.47	133.54	1847	47.00	117.50	132.50	1832
250.5	45.65	114.35	136.15	1883	46.06	115.39	135.11	1869	46.48	116.42	134.08	1854	46.89	117.46	133.04	1840
251	45.54	114.31	136.69	1890	45.95	115.35	135.65	1876	46.37	116.38	134.62	1862	46.78	117.42	133.58	1847
251.5	45.43	114.27	137.23	1898	45.85	115.30	136.20	1884	46.26	116.34	135.16	1869	46.67	117.38	134.12	1855
252	45.33	114.23	137.77	1905	45.74	115.26	136.74	1891	46.15	116.30	135.70	1877	46.56	117.34	134.66	1862
252.5	45.22	114.19	138.32	1913	45.63	115.22	137.28	1899	46.04	116.26	136.24	1884	46.45	117.30	135.20	1870
253	45.12	114.14	138.86	1920	45.53	115.18	137.82	1906	45.94	116.22	136.78	1892	46.35	117.26	135.74	1877
253.5	45.01	114.10	139.40	1928	45.42	115.14	138.36	1914	45.83	116.18	137.32	1899	46.24	117.22	136.28	1885
254	44.91	114.06	139.94	1935	45.31	115.10	138.90	1921	45.72	116.14	137.86	1907	46.13	117.17	136.83	1892
254.5	44.80	114.02	140.48	1943	45.21	115.06	139.44	1928	45.62	116.10	138.40	1914	46.02	117.13	137.37	1900
255	44.70	113.98	141.02	1950	45.10	115.02	139.98	1936	45.51	116.06	138.95	1922	45.92	117.09	137.91	1907
255.5	44.59	113.94	141.56	1958	45.00	114.98	140.52	1943	45.41	116.01	139.49	1929	45.81	117.05	138.45	1915
256	44.49	113.90	142.10	1965	44.90	114.94	141.06	1951	45.30	115.97	140.03	1937	45.71	117.01	138.99	1922
256.5	44.39	113.86	142.64	1973	44.79	114.89	141.61	1958	45.20	115.93	140.57	1944	45.60	116.97	139.53	1930
257	44.29	113.82	143.18	1980	44.69	114.85	142.15	1966	45.09	115.89	141.11	1952	45.50	116.93	140.07	1937
257.5	44.18	113.78	143.73	1988	44.59	114.81	142.69	1973	44.99	115.85	141.65	1959	45.39	116.89	140.61	1945
258	44.08	113.73	144.27	1995	44.49	114.77	143.23	1981	44.89	115.81	142.19	1967	45.29	116.85	141.15	1952
258.5	43.98	113.69	144.81	2003	44.38	114.73	143.77	1988	44.78	115.77	142.73	1974	45.19	116.81	141.69	1960
259	43.88	113.65	145.35	2010	44.28	114.69	144.31	1996	44.68	115.73	143.27	1981	45.08	116.76	142.24	1967
259.5	43.78	113.61	145.89	2018	44.18	114.65	144.85	2003	44.58	115.69	143.81	1989	44.98	116.72	142.78	1975

Body Composition FEMALE 228-259.5 Lb.

Weight: Lb.	Waist: 52 inches				52.25 inches				52.5 inches				52.75 inches			
	Fat: %	Fat: Lb.	LBM: Lb.	RMR: Cal.	Fat: %	Fat: Lb.	LBM: Lb.	RMR: Cal.	Fat: %	Fat: Lb.	LBM: Lb.	RMR: Cal.	Fat: %	Fat: Lb.	LBM: Lb.	RMR: Cal.
228	52.78	120.34	107.66	1489	53.24	121.38	106.62	1475	53.69	122.42	105.58	1460	54.15	123.46	104.54	1446
228.5	52.65	120.30	108.20	1496	53.10	121.34	107.16	1482	53.56	122.38	106.12	1468	54.01	123.42	105.08	1453
229	52.52	120.26	108.74	1504	52.97	121.30	107.70	1489	53.42	122.34	106.66	1475	53.88	123.37	105.63	1461
229.5	52.38	120.22	109.28	1511	52.84	121.26	108.24	1497	53.29	122.30	107.20	1483	53.74	123.33	106.17	1468
230	52.25	120.18	109.82	1519	52.70	121.22	108.78	1504	53.15	122.26	107.75	1490	53.61	123.29	106.71	1476
230.5	52.12	120.14	110.36	1526	52.57	121.18	109.32	1512	53.02	122.21	108.29	1498	53.47	123.25	107.25	1483
231	51.99	120.10	110.90	1534	52.44	121.14	109.86	1519	52.89	122.17	108.83	1505	53.34	123.21	107.79	1491
231.5	51.86	120.06	111.44	1541	52.31	121.09	110.41	1527	52.76	122.13	109.37	1513	53.20	123.17	108.33	1498
232	51.73	120.02	111.98	1549	52.18	121.05	110.95	1534	52.63	122.09	109.91	1520	53.07	123.13	108.87	1506
232.5	51.60	119.98	112.53	1556	52.05	121.01	111.49	1542	52.49	122.05	110.45	1528	52.94	123.09	109.41	1513
233	51.47	119.93	113.07	1564	51.92	120.97	112.03	1549	52.36	122.01	110.99	1535	52.81	123.05	109.95	1521
233.5	51.35	119.89	113.61	1571	51.79	120.93	112.57	1557	52.23	121.97	111.53	1542	52.68	123.01	110.49	1528
234	51.22	119.85	114.15	1579	51.66	120.89	113.11	1564	52.11	121.93	112.07	1550	52.55	122.96	111.04	1536
234.5	51.09	119.81	114.69	1586	51.53	120.85	113.65	1572	51.98	121.89	112.61	1557	52.42	122.92	111.58	1543
235	50.97	119.77	115.23	1594	51.41	120.81	114.19	1579	51.85	121.85	113.16	1565	52.29	122.88	112.12	1551
235.5	50.84	119.73	115.77	1601	51.28	120.77	114.73	1587	51.72	121.80	113.70	1572	52.16	122.84	112.66	1558
236	50.72	119.69	116.31	1609	51.15	120.73	115.27	1594	51.59	121.76	114.24	1580	52.03	122.80	113.20	1566
236.5	50.59	119.65	116.85	1616	51.03	120.68	115.82	1602	51.47	121.72	114.78	1587	51.91	122.76	113.74	1573
237	50.47	119.61	117.39	1624	50.90	120.64	116.36	1609	51.34	121.68	115.32	1595	51.78	122.72	114.28	1581
237.5	50.34	119.57	117.94	1631	50.78	120.60	116.90	1617	51.22	121.64	115.86	1602	51.65	122.68	114.82	1588
238	50.22	119.52	118.48	1639	50.66	120.56	117.44	1624	51.09	121.60	116.40	1610	51.53	122.64	115.36	1595
238.5	50.10	119.48	119.02	1646	50.53	120.52	117.98	1632	50.97	121.56	116.94	1617	51.40	122.60	115.90	1603
239	49.98	119.44	119.56	1653	50.41	120.48	118.52	1639	50.84	121.52	117.48	1625	51.28	122.55	116.45	1610
239.5	49.85	119.40	120.10	1661	50.29	120.44	119.06	1647	50.72	121.48	118.02	1632	51.15	122.51	116.99	1618
240	49.73	119.36	120.64	1668	50.17	120.40	119.60	1654	50.60	121.44	118.57	1640	51.03	122.47	117.53	1625
240.5	49.61	119.32	121.18	1676	50.04	120.36	120.14	1662	50.48	121.39	119.11	1647	50.91	122.43	118.07	1633
241	49.49	119.28	121.72	1683	49.92	120.32	120.68	1669	50.35	121.35	119.65	1655	50.78	122.39	118.61	1640
241.5	49.37	119.24	122.26	1691	49.80	120.27	121.23	1677	50.23	121.31	120.19	1662	50.66	122.35	119.15	1648
242	49.25	119.20	122.80	1698	49.68	120.23	121.77	1684	50.11	121.27	120.73	1670	50.54	122.31	119.69	1655
242.5	49.14	119.16	123.35	1706	49.56	120.19	122.31	1692	49.99	121.23	121.27	1677	50.42	122.27	120.23	1663
243	49.02	119.11	123.89	1713	49.45	120.15	122.85	1699	49.87	121.19	121.81	1685	50.30	122.23	120.77	1670
243.5	48.90	119.07	124.43	1721	49.33	120.11	123.39	1706	49.75	121.15	122.35	1692	50.18	122.19	121.31	1678
244	48.78	119.03	124.97	1728	49.21	120.07	123.93	1714	49.63	121.11	122.89	1700	50.06	122.14	121.86	1685
244.5	48.67	118.99	125.51	1736	49.09	120.03	124.47	1721	49.52	121.07	123.43	1707	49.94	122.10	122.40	1693
245	48.55	118.95	126.05	1743	48.97	119.99	125.01	1729	49.40	121.03	123.98	1715	49.82	122.06	122.94	1700
245.5	48.44	118.91	126.59	1751	48.86	119.95	125.55	1736	49.28	120.98	124.52	1722	49.70	122.02	123.48	1708
246	48.32	118.87	127.13	1758	48.74	119.91	126.09	1744	49.16	120.94	125.06	1730	49.59	121.98	124.02	1715
246.5	48.21	118.83	127.67	1766	48.63	119.86	126.64	1751	49.05	120.90	125.60	1737	49.47	121.94	124.56	1723
247	48.09	118.79	128.21	1773	48.51	119.82	127.18	1759	48.93	120.86	126.14	1745	49.35	121.90	125.10	1730
247.5	47.98	118.75	128.76	1781	48.40	119.78	127.72	1766	48.82	120.82	126.68	1752	49.24	121.86	125.64	1738
248	47.86	118.70	129.30	1788	48.28	119.74	128.26	1774	48.70	120.78	127.22	1759	49.12	121.82	126.18	1745
248.5	47.75	118.66	129.84	1796	48.17	119.70	128.80	1781	48.59	120.74	127.76	1767	49.00	121.78	126.72	1753
249	47.64	118.62	130.38	1803	48.06	119.66	129.34	1789	48.47	120.70	128.30	1774	48.89	121.73	127.27	1760
249.5	47.53	118.58	130.92	1811	47.94	119.62	129.88	1796	48.36	120.66	128.84	1782	48.77	121.69	127.81	1768
250	47.42	118.54	131.46	1818	47.83	119.58	130.42	1804	48.25	120.62	129.39	1789	48.66	121.65	128.35	1775
250.5	47.30	118.50	132.00	1826	47.72	119.54	130.96	1811	48.13	120.57	129.93	1797	48.55	121.61	128.89	1783
251	47.19	118.46	132.54	1833	47.61	119.50	131.50	1819	48.02	120.53	130.47	1804	48.43	121.57	129.43	1790
251.5	47.08	118.42	133.08	1841	47.50	119.45	132.05	1826	47.91	120.49	131.01	1812	48.32	121.53	129.97	1797
252	46.97	118.38	133.62	1848	47.39	119.41	132.59	1834	47.80	120.45	131.55	1819	48.21	121.49	130.51	1805
252.5	46.87	118.34	134.17	1856	47.28	119.37	133.13	1841	47.69	120.41	132.09	1827	48.10	121.45	131.05	1812
253	46.76	118.29	134.71	1863	47.17	119.33	133.67	1849	47.58	120.37	132.63	1834	47.99	121.41	131.59	1820
253.5	46.65	118.25	135.25	1870	47.06	119.29	134.21	1856	47.47	120.33	133.17	1842	47.88	121.37	132.13	1827
254	46.54	118.21	135.79	1878	46.95	119.25	134.75	1864	47.36	120.29	133.71	1849	47.77	121.32	132.68	1835
254.5	46.43	118.17	136.33	1885	46.84	119.21	135.29	1871	47.25	120.25	134.25	1857	47.66	121.28	133.22	1842
255	46.33	118.13	136.87	1893	46.73	119.17	135.83	1879	47.14	120.21	134.80	1864	47.55	121.24	133.76	1850
255.5	46.22	118.09	137.41	1900	46.62	119.13	136.37	1886	47.03	120.16	135.34	1872	47.44	121.20	134.30	1857
256	46.11	118.05	137.95	1908	46.52	119.09	136.91	1894	46.92	120.12	135.88	1879	47.33	121.16	134.84	1865
256.5	46.01	118.01	138.49	1915	46.41	119.04	137.46	1901	46.82	120.08	136.42	1887	47.22	121.12	135.38	1872
257	45.90	117.97	139.03	1923	46.30	119.00	138.00	1908	46.71	120.04	136.96	1894	47.11	121.08	135.92	1880
257.5	45.80	117.93	139.58	1930	46.20	118.96	138.54	1916	46.60	120.00	137.50	1902	47.00	121.04	136.46	1887
258	45.69	117.88	140.12	1938	46.09	118.92	139.08	1923	46.50	119.96	138.04	1909	46.90	121.00	137.00	1895
258.5	45.59	117.84	140.66	1945	45.99	118.88	139.62	1931	46.39	119.92	138.58	1917	46.79	120.96	137.54	1902
259	45.48	117.80	141.20	1953	45.88	118.84	140.16	1938	46.28	119.88	139.12	1924	46.69	120.91	138.09	1910
259.5	45.38	117.76	141.74	1960	45.78	118.80	140.70	1946	46.18	119.84	139.66	1932	46.58	120.87	138.63	1917

Body Composition FEMALE 228-259.5 Lb.

Weight: Lb.	Waist: 53 inches				53.25 inches				53.5 inches				53.75 inches			
	Fat: %	Fat: Lb.	LBM: Lb.	RMR: Cal.	Fat: %	Fat: Lb.	LBM: Lb.	RMR: Cal.	Fat: %	Fat: Lb.	LBM: Lb.	RMR: Cal.	Fat: %	Fat: Lb.	LBM: Lb.	RMR: Cal.
228	54.60	124.49	103.51	1431	55.06	125.53	102.47	1417	55.51	126.57	101.43	1403	55.97	127.61	100.39	1388
228.5	54.47	124.45	104.05	1439	54.92	125.49	103.01	1425	55.37	126.53	101.97	1410	55.83	127.57	100.93	1396
229	54.33	124.41	104.59	1446	54.78	125.45	103.55	1432	55.23	126.49	102.51	1418	55.69	127.52	101.48	1403
229.5	54.19	124.37	105.13	1454	54.64	125.41	104.09	1440	55.10	126.45	103.05	1425	55.55	127.48	102.02	1411
230	54.06	124.33	105.67	1461	54.51	125.37	104.63	1447	54.96	126.41	103.60	1433	55.41	127.44	102.56	1418
230.5	53.92	124.29	106.21	1469	54.37	125.33	105.17	1455	54.82	126.36	104.14	1440	55.27	127.40	103.10	1426
231	53.79	124.25	106.75	1476	54.24	125.29	105.71	1462	54.69	126.32	104.68	1448	55.13	127.36	103.64	1433
231.5	53.65	124.21	107.29	1484	54.10	125.24	106.26	1470	54.55	126.28	105.22	1455	55.00	127.32	104.18	1441
232	53.52	124.17	107.83	1491	53.97	125.20	106.80	1477	54.41	126.24	105.76	1463	54.86	127.28	104.72	1448
232.5	53.39	124.13	108.38	1499	53.83	125.16	107.34	1484	54.28	126.20	106.30	1470	54.73	127.24	105.26	1456
233	53.25	124.08	108.92	1506	53.70	125.12	107.88	1492	54.15	126.16	106.84	1478	54.59	127.20	105.80	1463
233.5	53.12	124.04	109.46	1514	53.57	125.08	108.42	1499	54.01	126.12	107.38	1485	54.46	127.16	106.34	1471
234	52.99	124.00	110.00	1521	53.44	125.04	108.96	1507	53.88	126.08	107.92	1493	54.32	127.11	106.89	1478
234.5	52.86	123.96	110.54	1529	53.30	125.00	109.50	1514	53.75	126.04	108.46	1500	54.19	127.07	107.43	1486
235	52.73	123.92	111.08	1536	53.17	124.96	110.04	1522	53.61	126.00	109.01	1508	54.06	127.03	107.97	1493
235.5	52.60	123.88	111.62	1544	53.04	124.92	110.58	1529	53.48	125.95	109.55	1515	53.92	126.99	108.51	1501
236	52.47	123.84	112.16	1551	52.91	124.88	111.12	1537	53.35	125.91	110.09	1523	53.79	126.95	109.05	1508
236.5	52.35	123.80	112.70	1559	52.78	124.83	111.67	1544	53.22	125.87	110.63	1530	53.66	126.91	109.59	1516
237	52.22	123.76	113.24	1566	52.66	124.79	112.21	1552	53.09	125.83	111.17	1537	53.53	126.87	110.13	1523
237.5	52.09	123.72	113.79	1574	52.53	124.75	112.75	1559	52.96	125.79	111.71	1545	53.40	126.83	110.67	1531
238	51.96	123.67	114.33	1581	52.40	124.71	113.29	1567	52.84	125.75	112.25	1552	53.27	126.79	111.21	1538
238.5	51.84	123.63	114.87	1589	52.27	124.67	113.83	1574	52.71	125.71	112.79	1560	53.14	126.75	111.75	1546
239	51.71	123.59	115.41	1596	52.15	124.63	114.37	1582	52.58	125.67	113.33	1567	53.01	126.70	112.30	1553
239.5	51.59	123.55	115.95	1604	52.02	124.59	114.91	1589	52.45	125.63	113.87	1575	52.89	126.66	112.84	1561
240	51.46	123.51	116.49	1611	51.89	124.55	115.45	1597	52.33	125.59	114.42	1582	52.76	126.62	113.38	1568
240.5	51.34	123.47	117.03	1619	51.77	124.51	115.99	1604	52.20	125.54	114.96	1590	52.63	126.58	113.92	1575
241	51.21	123.43	117.57	1626	51.65	124.47	116.53	1612	52.08	125.50	115.50	1597	52.51	126.54	114.46	1583
241.5	51.09	123.39	118.11	1634	51.52	124.42	117.08	1619	51.95	125.46	116.04	1605	52.38	126.50	115.00	1590
242	50.97	123.35	118.65	1641	51.40	124.38	117.62	1627	51.83	125.42	116.58	1612	52.26	126.46	115.54	1598
242.5	50.85	123.31	119.20	1648	51.28	124.34	118.16	1634	51.70	125.38	117.12	1620	52.13	126.42	116.08	1605
243	50.73	123.26	119.74	1656	51.15	124.30	118.70	1642	51.58	125.34	117.66	1627	52.01	126.38	116.62	1613
243.5	50.60	123.22	120.28	1663	51.03	124.26	119.24	1649	51.46	125.30	118.20	1635	51.88	126.34	117.16	1620
244	50.48	123.18	120.82	1671	50.91	124.22	119.78	1657	51.33	125.26	118.74	1642	51.76	126.29	117.71	1628
244.5	50.36	123.14	121.36	1678	50.79	124.18	120.32	1664	51.21	125.22	119.28	1650	51.64	126.25	118.25	1635
245	50.24	123.10	121.90	1686	50.67	124.14	120.86	1672	51.09	125.18	119.83	1657	51.52	126.21	118.79	1643
245.5	50.13	123.06	122.44	1693	50.55	124.10	121.40	1679	50.97	125.13	120.37	1665	51.39	126.17	119.33	1650
246	50.01	123.02	122.98	1701	50.43	124.06	121.94	1686	50.85	125.09	120.91	1672	51.27	126.13	119.87	1658
246.5	49.89	122.98	123.52	1708	50.31	124.01	122.49	1694	50.73	125.05	121.45	1680	51.15	126.09	120.41	1665
247	49.77	122.94	124.06	1716	50.19	123.97	123.03	1701	50.61	125.01	121.99	1687	51.03	126.05	120.95	1673
247.5	49.65	122.90	124.61	1723	50.07	123.93	123.57	1709	50.49	124.97	122.53	1695	50.91	126.01	121.49	1680
248	49.54	122.85	125.15	1731	49.96	123.89	124.11	1716	50.37	124.93	123.07	1702	50.79	125.97	122.03	1688
248.5	49.42	122.81	125.69	1738	49.84	123.85	124.65	1724	50.26	124.89	123.61	1710	50.67	125.93	122.57	1695
249	49.31	122.77	126.23	1746	49.72	123.81	125.19	1731	50.14	124.85	124.15	1717	50.56	125.88	123.12	1703
249.5	49.19	122.73	126.77	1753	49.61	123.77	125.73	1739	50.02	124.81	124.69	1725	50.44	125.84	123.66	1710
250	49.08	122.69	127.31	1761	49.49	123.73	126.27	1746	49.91	124.77	125.24	1732	50.32	125.80	124.20	1718
250.5	48.96	122.65	127.85	1768	49.38	123.69	126.81	1754	49.79	124.72	125.78	1739	50.20	125.76	124.74	1725
251	48.85	122.61	128.39	1776	49.26	123.65	127.35	1761	49.67	124.68	126.32	1747	50.09	125.72	125.28	1733
251.5	48.73	122.57	128.93	1783	49.15	123.60	127.90	1769	49.56	124.64	126.86	1754	49.97	125.68	125.82	1740
252	48.62	122.53	129.47	1791	49.03	123.56	128.44	1776	49.44	124.60	127.40	1762	49.86	125.64	126.36	1748
252.5	48.51	122.49	130.02	1798	48.92	123.52	128.98	1784	49.33	124.56	127.94	1769	49.74	125.60	126.90	1755
253	48.40	122.44	130.56	1806	48.81	123.48	129.52	1791	49.22	124.52	128.48	1777	49.63	125.56	127.44	1763
253.5	48.29	122.40	131.10	1813	48.69	123.44	130.06	1799	49.10	124.48	129.02	1784	49.51	125.52	127.98	1770
254	48.17	122.36	131.64	1821	48.58	123.40	130.60	1806	48.99	124.44	129.56	1792	49.40	125.47	128.53	1778
254.5	48.06	122.32	132.18	1828	48.47	123.36	131.14	1814	48.88	124.40	130.10	1799	49.29	125.43	129.07	1785
255	47.95	122.28	132.72	1836	48.36	123.32	131.68	1821	48.77	124.36	130.65	1807	49.17	125.39	129.61	1792
255.5	47.84	122.24	133.26	1843	48.25	123.28	132.22	1829	48.66	124.31	131.19	1814	49.06	125.35	130.15	1800
256	47.73	122.20	133.80	1850	48.14	123.24	132.76	1836	48.54	124.27	131.73	1822	48.95	125.31	130.69	1807
256.5	47.62	122.16	134.34	1858	48.03	123.19	133.31	1844	48.43	124.23	132.27	1829	48.84	125.27	131.23	1815
257	47.52	122.12	134.88	1865	47.92	123.15	133.85	1851	48.32	124.19	132.81	1837	48.73	125.23	131.77	1822
257.5	47.41	122.08	135.43	1873	47.81	123.11	134.39	1859	48.21	124.15	133.35	1844	48.62	125.19	132.31	1830
258	47.30	122.03	135.97	1880	47.70	123.07	134.93	1866	48.10	124.11	133.89	1852	48.51	125.15	132.85	1837
258.5	47.19	121.99	136.51	1888	47.59	123.03	135.47	1874	48.00	124.07	134.43	1859	48.40	125.11	133.39	1845
259	47.09	121.95	137.05	1895	47.49	122.99	136.01	1881	47.89	124.03	134.97	1867	48.29	125.06	133.94	1852
259.5	46.98	121.91	137.59	1903	47.38	122.95	136.55	1889	47.78	123.99	135.51	1874	48.18	125.02	134.48	1860

Body Composition FEMALE 228-259.5 Lb.

Weight: Lb.	Waist: 54 inches Fat: %	Fat: Lb.	LBM: Lb.	RMR: Cal.	54.25 inches Fat: %	Fat: Lb.	LBM: Lb.	RMR: Cal.	54.5 inches Fat: %	Fat: Lb.	LBM: Lb.	RMR: Cal.	54.75 inches Fat: %	Fat: Lb.	LBM: Lb.	RMR: Cal.
228	56.42	128.64	99.36	1374	56.88	129.68	98.32	1360	57.33	130.72	97.28	1345	57.79	131.76	96.24	1331
228.5	56.28	128.60	99.90	1382	56.74	129.64	98.86	1367	57.19	130.68	97.82	1353	57.64	131.72	96.78	1339
229	56.14	128.56	100.44	1389	56.59	129.60	99.40	1375	57.05	130.64	98.36	1360	57.50	131.67	97.33	1346
229.5	56.00	128.52	100.98	1397	56.45	129.56	99.94	1382	56.90	130.60	98.90	1368	57.36	131.63	97.87	1353
230	55.86	128.48	101.52	1404	56.31	129.52	100.48	1390	56.76	130.56	99.45	1375	57.21	131.59	98.41	1361
230.5	55.72	128.44	102.06	1412	56.17	129.48	101.02	1397	56.62	130.51	99.99	1383	57.07	131.55	98.95	1368
231	55.58	128.40	102.60	1419	56.03	129.44	101.56	1405	56.48	130.47	100.53	1390	56.93	131.51	99.49	1376
231.5	55.45	128.36	103.14	1426	55.89	129.39	102.11	1412	56.34	130.43	101.07	1398	56.79	131.47	100.03	1383
232	55.31	128.32	103.68	1434	55.76	129.35	102.65	1420	56.20	130.39	101.61	1405	56.65	131.43	100.57	1391
232.5	55.17	128.28	104.23	1441	55.62	129.31	103.19	1427	56.06	130.35	102.15	1413	56.51	131.39	101.11	1398
233	55.04	128.23	104.77	1449	55.48	129.27	103.73	1435	55.93	130.31	102.69	1420	56.37	131.35	101.65	1406
233.5	54.90	128.19	105.31	1456	55.34	129.23	104.27	1442	55.79	130.27	103.23	1428	56.23	131.31	102.19	1413
234	54.77	128.15	105.85	1464	55.21	129.19	104.81	1450	55.65	130.23	103.77	1435	56.10	131.26	102.74	1421
234.5	54.63	128.11	106.39	1471	55.07	129.15	105.35	1457	55.52	130.19	104.31	1443	55.96	131.22	103.28	1428
235	54.50	128.07	106.93	1479	54.94	129.11	105.89	1464	55.38	130.15	104.86	1450	55.82	131.18	103.82	1436
235.5	54.36	128.03	107.47	1486	54.81	129.07	106.43	1472	55.25	130.10	105.40	1458	55.69	131.14	104.36	1443
236	54.23	127.99	108.01	1494	54.67	129.03	106.97	1479	55.11	130.06	105.94	1465	55.55	131.10	104.90	1451
236.5	54.10	127.95	108.55	1501	54.54	128.98	107.52	1487	54.98	130.02	106.48	1473	55.42	131.06	105.44	1458
237	53.97	127.91	109.09	1509	54.41	128.94	108.06	1494	54.84	129.98	107.02	1480	55.28	131.02	105.98	1466
237.5	53.84	127.87	109.64	1516	54.27	128.90	108.60	1502	54.71	129.94	107.56	1488	55.15	130.98	106.52	1473
238	53.71	127.82	110.18	1524	54.14	128.86	109.14	1509	54.58	129.90	108.10	1495	55.02	130.94	107.06	1481
238.5	53.58	127.78	110.72	1531	54.01	128.82	109.68	1517	54.45	129.86	108.64	1503	54.88	130.90	107.60	1488
239	53.45	127.74	111.26	1539	53.88	128.78	110.22	1524	54.32	129.82	109.18	1510	54.75	130.85	108.15	1496
239.5	53.32	127.70	111.80	1546	53.75	128.74	110.76	1532	54.19	129.78	109.72	1517	54.62	130.81	108.69	1503
240	53.19	127.66	112.34	1554	53.62	128.70	111.30	1539	54.06	129.74	110.27	1525	54.49	130.77	109.23	1511
240.5	53.06	127.62	112.88	1561	53.50	128.66	111.84	1547	53.93	129.69	110.81	1532	54.36	130.73	109.77	1518
241	52.94	127.58	113.42	1569	53.37	128.62	112.38	1554	53.80	129.65	111.35	1540	54.23	130.69	110.31	1526
241.5	52.81	127.54	113.96	1576	53.24	128.57	112.93	1562	53.67	129.61	111.89	1547	54.10	130.65	110.85	1533
242	52.68	127.50	114.50	1584	53.11	128.53	113.47	1569	53.54	129.57	112.43	1555	53.97	130.61	111.39	1541
242.5	52.56	127.46	115.05	1591	52.99	128.49	114.01	1577	53.41	129.53	112.97	1562	53.84	130.57	111.93	1548
243	52.43	127.41	115.59	1599	52.86	128.45	114.55	1584	53.29	129.49	113.51	1570	53.71	130.53	112.47	1556
243.5	52.31	127.37	116.13	1606	52.74	128.41	115.09	1592	53.16	129.45	114.05	1577	53.59	130.49	113.01	1563
244	52.19	127.33	116.67	1614	52.61	128.37	115.63	1599	53.04	129.41	114.59	1585	53.46	130.44	113.56	1570
244.5	52.06	127.29	117.21	1621	52.49	128.33	116.17	1607	52.91	129.37	115.13	1592	53.33	130.40	114.10	1578
245	51.94	127.25	117.75	1628	52.36	128.29	116.71	1614	52.79	129.33	115.68	1600	53.21	130.36	114.64	1585
245.5	51.82	127.21	118.29	1636	52.24	128.25	117.25	1622	52.66	129.28	116.22	1607	53.08	130.32	115.18	1593
246	51.69	127.17	118.83	1643	52.12	128.21	117.79	1629	52.54	129.24	116.76	1615	52.96	130.28	115.72	1600
246.5	51.57	127.13	119.37	1651	51.99	128.16	118.34	1637	52.41	129.20	117.30	1622	52.84	130.24	116.26	1608
247	51.45	127.09	119.91	1658	51.87	128.12	118.88	1644	52.29	129.16	117.84	1630	52.71	130.20	116.80	1615
247.5	51.33	127.05	120.46	1666	51.75	128.08	119.42	1652	52.17	129.12	118.38	1637	52.59	130.16	117.34	1623
248	51.21	127.00	121.00	1673	51.63	128.04	119.96	1659	52.05	129.08	118.92	1645	52.47	130.12	117.88	1630
248.5	51.09	126.96	121.54	1681	51.51	128.00	120.50	1667	51.93	129.04	119.46	1652	52.34	130.08	118.42	1638
249	50.97	126.92	122.08	1688	51.39	127.96	121.04	1674	51.81	129.00	120.00	1660	52.22	130.03	118.97	1645
249.5	50.85	126.88	122.62	1696	51.27	127.92	121.58	1681	51.69	128.96	120.54	1667	52.10	129.99	119.51	1653
250	50.74	126.84	123.16	1703	51.15	127.88	122.12	1689	51.57	128.92	121.09	1675	51.98	129.95	120.05	1660
250.5	50.62	126.80	123.70	1711	51.03	127.84	122.66	1696	51.45	128.87	121.63	1682	51.86	129.91	120.59	1668
251	50.50	126.76	124.24	1718	50.91	127.80	123.20	1704	51.33	128.83	122.17	1690	51.74	129.87	121.13	1675
251.5	50.38	126.72	124.78	1726	50.80	127.75	123.75	1711	51.21	128.79	122.71	1697	51.62	129.83	121.67	1683
252	50.27	126.68	125.32	1733	50.68	127.71	124.29	1719	51.09	128.75	123.25	1705	51.50	129.79	122.21	1690
252.5	50.15	126.64	125.87	1741	50.56	127.67	124.83	1726	50.97	128.71	123.79	1712	51.39	129.75	122.75	1698
253	50.04	126.59	126.41	1748	50.45	127.63	125.37	1734	50.86	128.67	124.33	1719	51.27	129.71	123.29	1705
253.5	49.92	126.55	126.95	1756	50.33	127.59	125.91	1741	50.74	128.63	124.87	1727	51.15	129.67	123.83	1713
254	49.81	126.51	127.49	1763	50.22	127.55	126.45	1749	50.62	128.59	125.41	1734	51.03	129.62	124.38	1720
254.5	49.69	126.47	128.03	1771	50.10	127.51	126.99	1756	50.51	128.55	125.95	1742	50.92	129.58	124.92	1728
255	49.58	126.43	128.57	1778	49.99	127.47	127.53	1764	50.39	128.51	126.50	1749	50.80	129.54	125.46	1735
255.5	49.47	126.39	129.11	1786	49.87	127.43	128.07	1771	50.28	128.46	127.04	1757	50.69	129.50	126.00	1743
256	49.35	126.35	129.65	1793	49.76	127.39	128.61	1779	50.17	128.42	127.58	1764	50.57	129.46	126.54	1750
256.5	49.24	126.31	130.19	1801	49.65	127.34	129.16	1786	50.05	128.38	128.12	1772	50.46	129.42	127.08	1758
257	49.13	126.27	130.73	1808	49.53	127.30	129.70	1794	49.94	128.34	128.66	1779	50.34	129.38	127.62	1765
257.5	49.02	126.23	131.28	1816	49.42	127.26	130.24	1801	49.83	128.30	129.20	1787	50.23	129.34	128.16	1772
258	48.91	126.18	131.82	1823	49.31	127.22	130.78	1809	49.71	128.26	129.74	1794	50.11	129.30	128.70	1780
258.5	48.80	126.14	132.36	1830	49.20	127.18	131.32	1816	49.60	128.22	130.28	1802	50.00	129.26	129.24	1787
259	48.69	126.10	132.90	1838	49.09	127.14	131.86	1824	49.49	128.18	130.82	1809	49.89	129.21	129.79	1795
259.5	48.58	126.06	133.44	1845	48.98	127.10	132.40	1831	49.38	128.14	131.36	1817	49.78	129.17	130.33	1802

Body Composition FEMALE 228-259.5 Lb.

Weight: Lb.	Waist: 55 inches Fat: %	Fat: Lb.	LBM: Lb.	RMR: Cal.	55.25 inches Fat: %	Fat: Lb.	LBM: Lb.	RMR: Cal.	55.5 inches Fat: %	Fat: Lb.	LBM: Lb.	RMR: Cal.	55.75 inches Fat: %	Fat: Lb.	LBM: Lb.	RMR: Cal.
228	58.24	132.79	95.21	1317	58.70	133.83	94.17	1302	59.15	134.87	93.13	1288	59.61	135.91	92.09	1274
228.5	58.10	132.75	95.75	1324	58.55	133.79	94.71	1310	59.01	134.83	93.67	1295	59.46	135.87	92.63	1281
229	57.95	132.71	96.29	1332	58.41	133.75	95.25	1317	58.86	134.79	94.21	1303	59.31	135.82	93.18	1289
229.5	57.81	132.67	96.83	1339	58.26	133.71	95.79	1325	58.71	134.75	94.75	1310	59.16	135.78	93.72	1296
230	57.67	132.63	97.37	1347	58.12	133.67	96.33	1332	58.57	134.71	95.30	1318	59.02	135.74	94.26	1304
230.5	57.52	132.59	97.91	1354	57.97	133.63	96.87	1340	58.42	134.66	95.84	1325	58.87	135.70	94.80	1311
231	57.38	132.55	98.45	1362	57.83	133.59	97.41	1347	58.28	134.62	96.38	1333	58.73	135.66	95.34	1319
231.5	57.24	132.51	98.99	1369	57.69	133.54	97.96	1355	58.13	134.58	96.92	1340	58.58	135.62	95.88	1326
232	57.10	132.47	99.53	1377	57.54	133.50	98.50	1362	57.99	134.54	97.46	1348	58.44	135.58	96.42	1334
232.5	56.96	132.43	100.08	1384	57.40	133.46	99.04	1370	57.85	134.50	98.00	1355	58.30	135.54	96.96	1341
233	56.82	132.38	100.62	1392	57.26	133.42	99.58	1377	57.71	134.46	98.54	1363	58.15	135.50	97.50	1348
233.5	56.68	132.34	101.16	1399	57.12	133.38	100.12	1385	57.57	134.42	99.08	1370	58.01	135.46	98.04	1356
234	56.54	132.30	101.70	1406	56.98	133.34	100.66	1392	57.43	134.38	99.62	1378	57.87	135.41	98.59	1363
234.5	56.40	132.26	102.24	1414	56.84	133.30	101.20	1400	57.29	134.34	100.16	1385	57.73	135.37	99.13	1371
235	56.26	132.22	102.78	1421	56.71	133.26	101.74	1407	57.15	134.30	100.71	1393	57.59	135.33	99.67	1378
235.5	56.13	132.18	103.32	1429	56.57	133.22	102.28	1415	57.01	134.25	101.25	1400	57.45	135.29	100.21	1386
236	55.99	132.14	103.86	1436	56.43	133.18	102.82	1422	56.87	134.21	101.79	1408	57.31	135.25	100.75	1393
236.5	55.85	132.10	104.40	1444	56.29	133.13	103.37	1430	56.73	134.17	102.33	1415	57.17	135.21	101.29	1401
237	55.72	132.06	104.94	1451	56.16	133.09	103.91	1437	56.60	134.13	102.87	1423	57.03	135.17	101.83	1408
237.5	55.59	132.02	105.49	1459	56.02	133.05	104.45	1445	56.46	134.09	103.41	1430	56.90	135.13	102.37	1416
238	55.45	131.97	106.03	1466	55.89	133.01	104.99	1452	56.32	134.05	103.95	1438	56.76	135.09	102.91	1423
238.5	55.32	131.93	106.57	1474	55.75	132.97	105.53	1459	56.19	134.01	104.49	1445	56.62	135.05	103.45	1431
239	55.18	131.89	107.11	1481	55.62	132.93	106.07	1467	56.05	133.97	105.03	1453	56.49	135.00	104.00	1438
239.5	55.05	131.85	107.65	1489	55.49	132.89	106.61	1474	55.92	133.93	105.57	1460	56.35	134.96	104.54	1446
240	54.92	131.81	108.19	1496	55.35	132.85	107.15	1482	55.79	133.89	106.12	1468	56.22	134.92	105.08	1453
240.5	54.79	131.77	108.73	1504	55.22	132.81	107.69	1489	55.65	133.84	106.66	1475	56.08	134.88	105.62	1461
241	54.66	131.73	109.27	1511	55.09	132.77	108.23	1497	55.52	133.80	107.20	1483	55.95	134.84	106.16	1468
241.5	54.53	131.69	109.81	1519	54.96	132.72	108.78	1504	55.39	133.76	107.74	1490	55.82	134.80	106.70	1476
242	54.40	131.65	110.35	1526	54.83	132.68	109.32	1512	55.26	133.72	108.28	1497	55.69	134.76	107.24	1483
242.5	54.27	131.61	110.90	1534	54.70	132.64	109.86	1519	55.13	133.68	108.82	1505	55.55	134.72	107.78	1491
243	54.14	131.56	111.44	1541	54.57	132.60	110.40	1527	55.00	133.64	109.36	1512	55.42	134.68	108.32	1498
243.5	54.01	131.52	111.98	1549	54.44	132.56	110.94	1534	54.87	133.60	109.90	1520	55.29	134.64	108.86	1506
244	53.89	131.48	112.52	1556	54.31	132.52	111.48	1542	54.74	133.56	110.44	1527	55.16	134.59	109.41	1513
244.5	53.76	131.44	113.06	1564	54.18	132.48	112.02	1549	54.61	133.52	110.98	1535	55.03	134.55	109.95	1521
245	53.63	131.40	113.60	1571	54.06	132.44	112.56	1557	54.48	133.48	111.53	1542	54.90	134.51	110.49	1528
245.5	53.51	131.36	114.14	1579	53.93	132.40	113.10	1564	54.35	133.43	112.07	1550	54.77	134.47	111.03	1536
246	53.38	131.32	114.68	1586	53.80	132.36	113.64	1572	54.22	133.39	112.61	1557	54.65	134.43	111.57	1543
246.5	53.26	131.28	115.22	1594	53.68	132.31	114.19	1579	54.10	133.35	113.15	1565	54.52	134.39	112.11	1550
247	53.13	131.24	115.76	1601	53.55	132.27	114.73	1587	53.97	133.31	113.69	1572	54.39	134.35	112.65	1558
247.5	53.01	131.20	116.31	1608	53.43	132.23	115.27	1594	53.85	133.27	114.23	1580	54.27	134.31	113.19	1565
248	52.88	131.15	116.85	1616	53.30	132.19	115.81	1602	53.72	133.23	114.77	1587	54.14	134.27	113.73	1573
248.5	52.76	131.11	117.39	1623	53.18	132.15	116.35	1609	53.60	133.19	115.31	1595	54.01	134.23	114.27	1580
249	52.64	131.07	117.93	1631	53.06	132.11	116.89	1617	53.47	133.15	115.85	1602	53.89	134.18	114.82	1588
249.5	52.52	131.03	118.47	1638	52.93	132.07	117.43	1624	53.35	133.11	116.39	1610	53.76	134.14	115.36	1595
250	52.40	130.99	119.01	1646	52.81	132.03	117.97	1632	53.23	133.07	116.94	1617	53.64	134.10	115.90	1603
250.5	52.28	130.95	119.55	1653	52.69	131.99	118.51	1639	53.10	133.02	117.48	1625	53.52	134.06	116.44	1610
251	52.15	130.91	120.09	1661	52.57	131.95	119.05	1647	52.98	132.98	118.02	1632	53.39	134.02	116.98	1618
251.5	52.03	130.87	120.63	1668	52.45	131.90	119.60	1654	52.86	132.94	118.56	1640	53.27	133.98	117.52	1625
252	51.92	130.83	121.17	1676	52.33	131.86	120.14	1661	52.74	132.90	119.10	1647	53.15	133.94	118.06	1633
252.5	51.80	130.79	121.72	1683	52.21	131.82	120.68	1669	52.62	132.86	119.64	1655	53.03	133.90	118.60	1640
253	51.68	130.74	122.26	1691	52.09	131.78	121.22	1676	52.50	132.82	120.18	1662	52.91	133.86	119.14	1648
253.5	51.56	130.70	122.80	1698	51.97	131.74	121.76	1684	52.38	132.78	120.72	1670	52.79	133.82	119.68	1655
254	51.44	130.66	123.34	1706	51.85	131.70	122.30	1691	52.26	132.74	121.26	1677	52.67	133.77	120.23	1663
254.5	51.32	130.62	123.88	1713	51.73	131.66	122.84	1699	52.14	132.70	121.80	1685	52.55	133.73	120.77	1670
255	51.21	130.58	124.42	1721	51.61	131.62	123.38	1706	52.02	132.66	122.35	1692	52.43	133.69	121.31	1678
255.5	51.09	130.54	124.96	1728	51.50	131.58	123.92	1714	51.90	132.61	122.89	1700	52.31	133.65	121.85	1685
256	50.98	130.50	125.50	1736	51.38	131.54	124.46	1721	51.79	132.57	123.43	1707	52.19	133.61	122.39	1693
256.5	50.86	130.46	126.04	1743	51.26	131.49	125.01	1729	51.67	132.53	123.97	1714	52.07	133.57	122.93	1700
257	50.75	130.42	126.58	1751	51.15	131.45	125.55	1736	51.55	132.49	124.51	1722	51.96	133.53	123.47	1708
257.5	50.63	130.38	127.13	1758	51.03	131.41	126.09	1744	51.44	132.45	125.05	1729	51.84	133.49	124.01	1715
258	50.52	130.33	127.67	1766	50.92	131.37	126.63	1751	51.32	132.41	125.59	1737	51.72	133.45	124.55	1723
258.5	50.40	130.29	128.21	1773	50.80	131.33	127.17	1759	51.21	132.37	126.13	1744	51.61	133.41	125.09	1730
259	50.29	130.25	128.75	1781	50.69	131.29	127.71	1766	51.09	132.33	126.67	1752	51.49	133.36	125.64	1738
259.5	50.18	130.21	129.29	1788	50.58	131.25	128.25	1774	50.98	132.29	127.21	1759	51.38	133.32	126.18	1745

Body Composition FEMALE 260-291.5 Lb.

Weight: Lb.	Waist: 47 inches Fat: %	Fat: Lb.	LBM: Lb.	RMR: Cal.	47.25 inches Fat: %	Fat: Lb.	LBM: Lb.	RMR: Cal.	47.5 inches Fat: %	Fat: Lb.	LBM: Lb.	RMR: Cal.	47.75 inches Fat: %	Fat: Lb.	LBM: Lb.	RMR: Cal.
260	37.30	96.97	163.03	2255	37.70	98.01	161.99	2240	38.09	99.05	160.96	2226	38.49	100.08	159.92	2212
260.5	37.21	96.93	163.57	2262	37.61	97.97	162.53	2248	38.01	99.00	161.50	2233	38.40	100.04	160.46	2219
261	37.12	96.89	164.11	2270	37.52	97.93	163.07	2255	37.92	98.96	162.04	2241	38.31	100.00	161.00	2227
261.5	37.04	96.85	164.65	2277	37.43	97.88	163.62	2263	37.83	98.92	162.58	2248	38.23	99.96	161.54	2234
262	36.95	96.81	165.19	2285	37.34	97.84	164.16	2270	37.74	98.88	163.12	2256	38.14	99.92	162.08	2242
262.5	36.86	96.77	165.74	2292	37.26	97.80	164.70	2278	37.65	98.84	163.66	2263	38.05	99.88	162.62	2249
263	36.78	96.72	166.28	2300	37.17	97.76	165.24	2285	37.57	98.80	164.20	2271	37.96	99.84	163.16	2257
263.5	36.69	96.68	166.82	2307	37.09	97.72	165.78	2293	37.48	98.76	164.74	2278	37.87	99.80	163.70	2264
264	36.61	96.64	167.36	2315	37.00	97.68	166.32	2300	37.39	98.72	165.28	2286	37.79	99.75	164.25	2272
264.5	36.52	96.60	167.90	2322	36.91	97.64	166.86	2308	37.31	98.68	165.82	2293	37.70	99.71	164.79	2279
265	36.44	96.56	168.44	2330	36.83	97.60	167.40	2315	37.22	98.64	166.37	2301	37.61	99.67	165.33	2286
265.5	36.35	96.52	168.98	2337	36.74	97.56	167.94	2323	37.14	98.59	166.91	2308	37.53	99.63	165.87	2294
266	36.27	96.48	169.52	2344	36.66	97.52	168.48	2330	37.05	98.55	167.45	2316	37.44	99.59	166.41	2301
266.5	36.19	96.44	170.06	2352	36.58	97.47	169.03	2338	36.97	98.51	167.99	2323	37.35	99.55	166.95	2309
267	36.10	96.40	170.60	2359	36.49	97.43	169.57	2345	36.88	98.47	168.53	2331	37.27	99.51	167.49	2316
267.5	36.02	96.36	171.15	2367	36.41	97.39	170.11	2353	36.80	98.43	169.07	2338	37.18	99.47	168.03	2324
268	35.94	96.31	171.69	2374	36.33	97.35	170.65	2360	36.71	98.39	169.61	2346	37.10	99.43	168.57	2331
268.5	35.86	96.27	172.23	2382	36.24	97.31	171.19	2368	36.63	98.35	170.15	2353	37.02	99.39	169.11	2339
269	35.77	96.23	172.77	2389	36.16	97.27	171.73	2375	36.55	98.31	170.69	2361	36.93	99.34	169.66	2346
269.5	35.69	96.19	173.31	2397	36.08	97.23	172.27	2383	36.46	98.27	171.23	2368	36.85	99.30	170.20	2354
270	35.61	96.15	173.85	2404	36.00	97.19	172.81	2390	36.38	98.23	171.78	2376	36.76	99.26	170.74	2361
270.5	35.53	96.11	174.39	2412	35.91	97.15	173.35	2397	36.30	98.18	172.32	2383	36.68	99.22	171.28	2369
271	35.45	96.07	174.93	2419	35.83	97.11	173.89	2405	36.22	98.14	172.86	2391	36.60	99.18	171.82	2376
271.5	35.37	96.03	175.47	2427	35.75	97.06	174.44	2412	36.13	98.10	173.40	2398	36.52	99.14	172.36	2384
272	35.29	95.99	176.01	2434	35.67	97.02	174.98	2420	36.05	98.06	173.94	2406	36.43	99.10	172.90	2391
272.5	35.21	95.95	176.56	2442	35.59	96.98	175.52	2427	35.97	98.02	174.48	2413	36.35	99.06	173.44	2399
273	35.13	95.90	177.10	2449	35.51	96.94	176.06	2435	35.89	97.98	175.02	2421	36.27	99.02	173.98	2406
273.5	35.05	95.86	177.64	2457	35.43	96.90	176.60	2442	35.81	97.94	175.56	2428	36.19	98.98	174.52	2414
274	34.97	95.82	178.18	2464	35.35	96.86	177.14	2450	35.73	97.90	176.10	2436	36.11	98.93	175.07	2421
274.5	34.89	95.78	178.72	2472	35.27	96.82	177.68	2457	35.65	97.86	176.64	2443	36.03	98.89	175.61	2429
275	34.81	95.74	179.26	2479	35.19	96.78	178.22	2465	35.57	97.82	177.19	2450	35.95	98.85	176.15	2436
275.5	34.74	95.70	179.80	2487	35.11	96.74	178.76	2472	35.49	97.77	177.73	2458	35.87	98.81	176.69	2444
276	34.66	95.66	180.34	2494	35.03	96.70	179.30	2480	35.41	97.73	178.27	2465	35.79	98.77	177.23	2451
276.5	34.58	95.62	180.88	2502	34.96	96.65	179.85	2487	35.33	97.69	178.81	2473	35.71	98.73	177.77	2459
277	34.50	95.58	181.42	2509	34.88	96.61	180.39	2495	35.25	97.65	179.35	2480	35.63	98.69	178.31	2466
277.5	34.43	95.54	181.97	2517	34.80	96.57	180.93	2502	35.17	97.61	179.89	2488	35.55	98.65	178.85	2474
278	34.35	95.49	182.51	2524	34.72	96.53	181.47	2510	35.10	97.57	180.43	2495	35.47	98.61	179.39	2481
278.5	34.27	95.45	183.05	2532	34.65	96.49	182.01	2517	35.02	97.53	180.97	2503	35.39	98.57	179.93	2488
279	34.20	95.41	183.59	2539	34.57	96.45	182.55	2525	34.94	97.49	181.51	2510	35.31	98.52	180.48	2496
279.5	34.12	95.37	184.13	2547	34.49	96.41	183.09	2532	34.86	97.45	182.05	2518	35.24	98.48	181.02	2503
280	34.05	95.33	184.67	2554	34.42	96.37	183.63	2540	34.79	97.41	182.60	2525	35.16	98.44	181.56	2511
280.5	33.97	95.29	185.21	2561	34.34	96.33	184.17	2547	34.71	97.36	183.14	2533	35.08	98.40	182.10	2518
281	33.90	95.25	185.75	2569	34.27	96.29	184.71	2555	34.63	97.32	183.68	2540	35.00	98.36	182.64	2526
281.5	33.82	95.21	186.29	2576	34.19	96.24	185.26	2562	34.56	97.28	184.22	2548	34.93	98.32	183.18	2533
282	33.75	95.17	186.83	2584	34.11	96.20	185.80	2570	34.48	97.24	184.76	2555	34.85	98.28	183.72	2541
282.5	33.67	95.13	187.38	2591	34.04	96.16	186.34	2577	34.41	97.20	185.30	2563	34.77	98.24	184.26	2548
283	33.60	95.08	187.92	2599	33.97	96.12	186.88	2585	34.33	97.16	185.84	2570	34.70	98.20	184.80	2556
283.5	33.52	95.04	188.46	2606	33.89	96.08	187.42	2592	34.26	97.12	186.38	2578	34.62	98.16	185.34	2563
284	33.45	95.00	189.00	2614	33.82	96.04	187.96	2599	34.18	97.08	186.92	2585	34.55	98.11	185.89	2571
284.5	33.38	94.96	189.54	2621	33.74	96.00	188.50	2607	34.11	97.04	187.46	2593	34.47	98.07	186.43	2578
285	33.31	94.92	190.08	2629	33.67	95.96	189.04	2614	34.03	97.00	188.01	2600	34.40	98.03	186.97	2586
285.5	33.23	94.88	190.62	2636	33.60	95.92	189.58	2622	33.96	96.95	188.55	2608	34.32	97.99	187.51	2593
286	33.16	94.84	191.16	2644	33.52	95.88	190.12	2629	33.89	96.91	189.09	2615	34.25	97.95	188.05	2601
286.5	33.09	94.80	191.70	2651	33.45	95.83	190.67	2637	33.81	96.87	189.63	2623	34.17	97.91	188.59	2608
287	33.02	94.76	192.24	2659	33.38	95.79	191.21	2644	33.74	96.83	190.17	2630	34.10	97.87	189.13	2616
287.5	32.94	94.72	192.79	2666	33.31	95.75	191.75	2652	33.67	96.79	190.71	2638	34.03	97.83	189.67	2623
288	32.87	94.67	193.33	2674	33.23	95.71	192.29	2659	33.59	96.75	191.25	2645	33.95	97.79	190.21	2631
288.5	32.80	94.63	193.87	2681	33.16	95.67	192.83	2667	33.52	96.71	191.79	2652	33.88	97.75	190.75	2638
289	32.73	94.59	194.41	2689	33.09	95.63	193.37	2674	33.45	96.67	192.33	2660	33.81	97.70	191.30	2646
289.5	32.66	94.55	194.95	2696	33.02	95.59	193.91	2682	33.38	96.63	192.87	2667	33.74	97.66	191.84	2653
290	32.59	94.51	195.49	2704	32.95	95.55	194.45	2689	33.31	96.59	193.42	2675	33.66	97.62	192.38	2661
290.5	32.52	94.47	196.03	2711	32.88	95.51	194.99	2697	33.23	96.54	193.96	2682	33.59	97.58	192.92	2668
291	32.45	94.43	196.57	2719	32.81	95.47	195.53	2704	33.16	96.50	194.50	2690	33.52	97.54	193.46	2676
291.5	32.38	94.39	197.11	2726	32.74	95.42	196.08	2712	33.09	96.46	195.04	2697	33.45	97.50	194.00	2683

Body Composition FEMALE 260-291.5 Lb.

Weight: Lb.	Waist: 48 inches				48.25 inches				48.5 inches				48.75 inches			
	Fat: %	Fat: Lb.	LBM: Lb.	RMR: Cal.	Fat: %	Fat: Lb.	LBM: Lb.	RMR: Cal.	Fat: %	Fat: Lb.	LBM: Lb.	RMR: Cal.	Fat: %	Fat: Lb.	LBM: Lb.	RMR: Cal.
260	38.89	101.12	158.88	2197	39.29	102.16	157.84	2183	39.69	103.20	156.81	2169	40.09	104.23	155.77	2154
260.5	38.80	101.08	159.42	2205	39.20	102.12	158.38	2190	39.60	103.15	157.35	2176	40.00	104.19	156.31	2162
261	38.71	101.04	159.96	2212	39.11	102.08	158.92	2198	39.51	103.11	157.89	2184	39.90	104.15	156.85	2169
261.5	38.62	101.00	160.50	2220	39.02	102.03	159.47	2205	39.42	103.07	158.43	2191	39.81	104.11	157.39	2177
262	38.53	100.96	161.04	2227	38.93	101.99	160.01	2213	39.32	103.03	158.97	2199	39.72	104.07	157.93	2184
262.5	38.44	100.92	161.59	2235	38.84	101.95	160.55	2220	39.23	102.99	159.51	2206	39.63	104.03	158.47	2192
263	38.36	100.87	162.13	2242	38.75	101.91	161.09	2228	39.14	102.95	160.05	2214	39.54	103.99	159.01	2199
263.5	38.27	100.83	162.67	2250	38.66	101.87	161.63	2235	39.05	102.91	160.59	2221	39.45	103.95	159.55	2207
264	38.18	100.79	163.21	2257	38.57	101.83	162.17	2243	38.96	102.87	161.13	2228	39.36	103.90	160.10	2214
264.5	38.09	100.75	163.75	2265	38.48	101.79	162.71	2250	38.88	102.83	161.67	2236	39.27	103.86	160.64	2222
265	38.00	100.71	164.29	2272	38.40	101.75	163.25	2258	38.79	102.79	162.22	2243	39.18	103.82	161.18	2229
265.5	37.92	100.67	164.83	2280	38.31	101.71	163.79	2265	38.70	102.74	162.76	2251	39.09	103.78	161.72	2237
266	37.83	100.63	165.37	2287	38.22	101.67	164.33	2273	38.61	102.70	163.30	2258	39.00	103.74	162.26	2244
266.5	37.74	100.59	165.91	2295	38.13	101.62	164.88	2280	38.52	102.66	163.84	2266	38.91	103.70	162.80	2252
267	37.66	100.55	166.45	2302	38.05	101.58	165.42	2288	38.43	102.62	164.38	2273	38.82	103.66	163.34	2259
267.5	37.57	100.51	167.00	2310	37.96	101.54	165.96	2295	38.35	102.58	164.92	2281	38.74	103.62	163.88	2266
268	37.49	100.46	167.54	2317	37.87	101.50	166.50	2303	38.26	102.54	165.46	2288	38.65	103.58	164.42	2274
268.5	37.40	100.42	168.08	2325	37.79	101.46	167.04	2310	38.17	102.50	166.00	2296	38.56	103.54	164.96	2281
269	37.32	100.38	168.62	2332	37.70	101.42	167.58	2318	38.09	102.46	166.54	2303	38.47	103.49	165.51	2289
269.5	37.23	100.34	169.16	2339	37.62	101.38	168.12	2325	38.00	102.42	167.08	2311	38.39	103.45	166.05	2296
270	37.15	100.30	169.70	2347	37.53	101.34	168.66	2333	37.92	102.38	167.63	2318	38.30	103.41	166.59	2304
270.5	37.06	100.26	170.24	2354	37.45	101.30	169.20	2340	37.83	102.33	168.17	2326	38.21	103.37	167.13	2311
271	36.98	100.22	170.78	2362	37.36	101.26	169.74	2348	37.75	102.29	168.71	2333	38.13	103.33	167.67	2319
271.5	36.90	100.18	171.32	2369	37.28	101.21	170.29	2355	37.66	102.25	169.25	2341	38.04	103.29	168.21	2326
272	36.81	100.14	171.86	2377	37.20	101.17	170.83	2363	37.58	102.21	169.79	2348	37.96	103.25	168.75	2334
272.5	36.73	100.10	172.41	2384	37.11	101.13	171.37	2370	37.49	102.17	170.33	2356	37.87	103.21	169.29	2341
273	36.65	100.05	172.95	2392	37.03	101.09	171.91	2377	37.41	102.13	170.87	2363	37.79	103.17	169.83	2349
273.5	36.57	100.01	173.49	2399	36.95	101.05	172.45	2385	37.33	102.09	171.41	2371	37.71	103.13	170.37	2356
274	36.49	99.97	174.03	2407	36.86	101.01	172.99	2392	37.24	102.05	171.95	2378	37.62	103.08	170.92	2364
274.5	36.40	99.93	174.57	2414	36.78	100.97	173.53	2400	37.16	102.01	172.49	2386	37.54	103.04	171.46	2371
275	36.32	99.89	175.11	2422	36.70	100.93	174.07	2407	37.08	101.97	173.04	2393	37.46	103.00	172.00	2379
275.5	36.24	99.85	175.65	2429	36.62	100.89	174.61	2415	37.00	101.92	173.58	2401	37.37	102.96	172.54	2386
276	36.16	99.81	176.19	2437	36.54	100.85	175.15	2422	36.91	101.88	174.12	2408	37.29	102.92	173.08	2394
276.5	36.08	99.77	176.73	2444	36.46	100.80	175.70	2430	36.83	101.84	174.66	2416	37.21	102.88	173.62	2401
277	36.00	99.73	177.27	2452	36.38	100.76	176.24	2437	36.75	101.80	175.20	2423	37.13	102.84	174.16	2409
277.5	35.92	99.69	177.82	2459	36.30	100.72	176.78	2445	36.67	101.76	175.74	2430	37.04	102.80	174.70	2416
278	35.84	99.64	178.36	2467	36.22	100.68	177.32	2452	36.59	101.72	176.28	2438	36.96	102.76	175.24	2424
278.5	35.76	99.60	178.90	2474	36.14	100.64	177.86	2460	36.51	101.68	176.82	2445	36.88	102.72	175.78	2431
279	35.69	99.56	179.44	2482	36.06	100.60	178.40	2467	36.43	101.64	177.36	2453	36.80	102.67	176.33	2439
279.5	35.61	99.52	179.98	2489	35.98	100.56	178.94	2475	36.35	101.60	177.90	2460	36.72	102.63	176.87	2446
280	35.53	99.48	180.52	2497	35.90	100.52	179.48	2482	36.27	101.56	178.45	2468	36.64	102.59	177.41	2454
280.5	35.45	99.44	181.06	2504	35.82	100.48	180.02	2490	36.19	101.51	178.99	2475	36.56	102.55	177.95	2461
281	35.37	99.40	181.60	2512	35.74	100.44	180.56	2497	36.11	101.47	179.53	2483	36.48	102.51	178.49	2469
281.5	35.30	99.36	182.14	2519	35.66	100.39	181.11	2505	36.03	101.43	180.07	2490	36.40	102.47	179.03	2476
282	35.22	99.32	182.68	2527	35.59	100.35	181.65	2512	35.95	101.39	180.61	2498	36.32	102.43	179.57	2483
282.5	35.14	99.28	183.23	2534	35.51	100.31	182.19	2520	35.88	101.35	181.15	2505	36.24	102.39	180.11	2491
283	35.07	99.23	183.77	2541	35.43	100.27	182.73	2527	35.80	101.31	181.69	2513	36.16	102.35	180.65	2498
283.5	34.99	99.19	184.31	2549	35.35	100.23	183.27	2535	35.72	101.27	182.23	2520	36.09	102.31	181.19	2506
284	34.91	99.15	184.85	2556	35.28	100.19	183.81	2542	35.64	101.23	182.77	2528	36.01	102.26	181.74	2513
284.5	34.84	99.11	185.39	2564	35.20	100.15	184.35	2550	35.57	101.19	183.31	2535	35.93	102.22	182.28	2521
285	34.76	99.07	185.93	2571	35.13	100.11	184.89	2557	35.49	101.15	183.86	2543	35.85	102.18	182.82	2528
285.5	34.69	99.03	186.47	2579	35.05	100.07	185.43	2565	35.41	101.10	184.40	2550	35.78	102.14	183.36	2536
286	34.61	98.99	187.01	2586	34.97	100.03	185.97	2572	35.34	101.06	184.94	2558	35.70	102.10	183.90	2543
286.5	34.54	98.95	187.55	2594	34.90	99.98	186.52	2580	35.26	101.02	185.48	2565	35.62	102.06	184.44	2551
287	34.46	98.91	188.09	2601	34.82	99.94	187.06	2587	35.19	100.98	186.02	2573	35.55	102.02	184.98	2558
287.5	34.39	98.87	188.64	2609	34.75	99.90	187.60	2594	35.11	100.94	186.56	2580	35.47	101.98	185.52	2566
288	34.31	98.82	189.18	2616	34.67	99.86	188.14	2602	35.03	100.90	187.10	2588	35.39	101.94	186.06	2573
288.5	34.24	98.78	189.72	2624	34.60	99.82	188.68	2609	34.96	100.86	187.64	2595	35.32	101.90	186.60	2581
289	34.17	98.74	190.26	2631	34.53	99.78	189.22	2617	34.88	100.82	188.18	2603	35.24	101.85	187.15	2588
289.5	34.09	98.70	190.80	2639	34.45	99.74	189.76	2624	34.81	100.78	188.72	2610	35.17	101.81	187.69	2596
290	34.02	98.66	191.34	2646	34.38	99.70	190.30	2632	34.74	100.74	189.27	2618	35.09	101.77	188.23	2603
290.5	33.95	98.62	191.88	2654	34.31	99.66	190.84	2639	34.66	100.69	189.81	2625	35.02	101.73	188.77	2611
291	33.88	98.58	192.42	2661	34.23	99.62	191.38	2647	34.59	100.65	190.35	2632	34.95	101.69	189.31	2618
291.5	33.80	98.54	192.96	2669	34.16	99.57	191.93	2654	34.52	100.61	190.89	2640	34.87	101.65	189.85	2626

Body Composition FEMALE 260-291.5 Lb.

Weight: Lb.	Waist: 49 inches Fat: %	Fat: Lb.	LBM: Lb.	RMR: Cal.	49.25 inches Fat: %	Fat: Lb.	LBM: Lb.	RMR: Cal.	49.5 inches Fat: %	Fat: Lb.	LBM: Lb.	RMR: Cal.	49.75 inches Fat: %	Fat: Lb.	LBM: Lb.	RMR: Cal.
260	40.49	105.27	154.73	2140	40.89	106.31	153.69	2126	41.29	107.35	152.66	2111	41.69	108.38	151.62	2097
260.5	40.40	105.23	155.27	2147	40.79	106.27	154.23	2133	41.19	107.30	153.20	2119	41.59	108.34	152.16	2104
261	40.30	105.19	155.81	2155	40.70	106.23	154.77	2141	41.10	107.26	153.74	2126	41.49	108.30	152.70	2112
261.5	40.21	105.15	156.35	2162	40.61	106.18	155.32	2148	41.00	107.22	154.28	2134	41.40	108.26	153.24	2119
262	40.12	105.11	156.89	2170	40.51	106.14	155.86	2155	40.91	107.18	154.82	2141	41.30	108.22	153.78	2127
262.5	40.02	105.07	157.44	2177	40.42	106.10	156.40	2163	40.82	107.14	155.36	2149	41.21	108.18	154.32	2134
263	39.93	105.02	157.98	2185	40.33	106.06	156.94	2170	40.72	107.10	155.90	2156	41.12	108.14	154.86	2142
263.5	39.84	104.98	158.52	2192	40.24	106.02	157.48	2178	40.63	107.06	156.44	2164	41.02	108.10	155.40	2149
264	39.75	104.94	159.06	2200	40.14	105.98	158.02	2185	40.54	107.02	156.98	2171	40.93	108.05	155.95	2157
264.5	39.66	104.90	159.60	2207	40.05	105.94	158.56	2193	40.44	106.98	157.52	2179	40.84	108.01	156.49	2164
265	39.57	104.86	160.14	2215	39.96	105.90	159.10	2200	40.35	106.94	158.07	2186	40.74	107.97	157.03	2172
265.5	39.48	104.82	160.68	2222	39.87	105.86	159.64	2208	40.26	106.89	158.61	2194	40.65	107.93	157.57	2179
266	39.39	104.78	161.22	2230	39.78	105.82	160.18	2215	40.17	106.85	159.15	2201	40.56	107.89	158.11	2187
266.5	39.30	104.74	161.76	2237	39.69	105.77	160.73	2223	40.08	106.81	159.69	2208	40.47	107.85	158.65	2194
267	39.21	104.70	162.30	2245	39.60	105.73	161.27	2230	39.99	106.77	160.23	2216	40.38	107.81	159.19	2202
267.5	39.12	104.66	162.85	2252	39.51	105.69	161.81	2238	39.90	106.73	160.77	2223	40.29	107.77	159.73	2209
268	39.04	104.61	163.39	2260	39.42	105.65	162.35	2245	39.81	106.69	161.31	2231	40.20	107.73	160.27	2217
268.5	38.95	104.57	163.93	2267	39.33	105.61	162.89	2253	39.72	106.65	161.85	2238	40.11	107.69	160.81	2224
269	38.86	104.53	164.47	2275	39.25	105.57	163.43	2260	39.63	106.61	162.39	2246	40.02	107.64	161.36	2232
269.5	38.77	104.49	165.01	2282	39.16	105.53	163.97	2268	39.54	106.57	162.93	2253	39.93	107.60	161.90	2239
270	38.69	104.45	165.55	2290	39.07	105.49	164.51	2275	39.45	106.53	163.48	2261	39.84	107.56	162.44	2247
270.5	38.60	104.41	166.09	2297	38.98	105.45	165.05	2283	39.37	106.48	164.02	2268	39.75	107.52	162.98	2254
271	38.51	104.37	166.63	2305	38.90	105.41	165.59	2290	39.28	106.44	164.56	2276	39.66	107.48	163.52	2261
271.5	38.43	104.33	167.17	2312	38.81	105.36	166.14	2298	39.19	106.40	165.10	2283	39.57	107.44	164.06	2269
272	38.34	104.29	167.71	2319	38.72	105.32	166.68	2305	39.10	106.36	165.64	2291	39.48	107.40	164.60	2276
272.5	38.26	104.25	168.26	2327	38.64	105.28	167.22	2313	39.02	106.32	166.18	2298	39.40	107.36	165.14	2284
273	38.17	104.20	168.80	2334	38.55	105.24	167.76	2320	38.93	106.28	166.72	2306	39.31	107.32	165.68	2291
273.5	38.09	104.16	169.34	2342	38.46	105.20	168.30	2328	38.84	106.24	167.26	2313	39.22	107.28	166.22	2299
274	38.00	104.12	169.88	2349	38.38	105.16	168.84	2335	38.76	106.20	167.80	2321	39.14	107.23	166.77	2306
274.5	37.92	104.08	170.42	2357	38.29	105.12	169.38	2343	38.67	106.16	168.34	2328	39.05	107.19	167.31	2314
275	37.83	104.04	170.96	2364	38.21	105.08	169.92	2350	38.59	106.12	168.89	2336	38.96	107.15	167.85	2321
275.5	37.75	104.00	171.50	2372	38.13	105.04	170.46	2358	38.50	106.07	169.43	2343	38.88	107.11	168.39	2329
276	37.67	103.96	172.04	2379	38.04	105.00	171.00	2365	38.42	106.03	169.97	2351	38.79	107.07	168.93	2336
276.5	37.58	103.92	172.58	2387	37.96	104.95	171.55	2372	38.33	105.99	170.51	2358	38.71	107.03	169.47	2344
277	37.50	103.88	173.12	2394	37.87	104.91	172.09	2380	38.25	105.95	171.05	2366	38.62	106.99	170.01	2351
277.5	37.42	103.84	173.67	2402	37.79	104.87	172.63	2387	38.17	105.91	171.59	2373	38.54	106.95	170.55	2359
278	37.34	103.79	174.21	2409	37.71	104.83	173.17	2395	38.08	105.87	172.13	2381	38.46	106.91	171.09	2366
278.5	37.25	103.75	174.75	2417	37.63	104.79	173.71	2402	38.00	105.83	172.67	2388	38.37	106.87	171.63	2374
279	37.17	103.71	175.29	2424	37.54	104.75	174.25	2410	37.92	105.79	173.21	2396	38.29	106.82	172.18	2381
279.5	37.09	103.67	175.83	2432	37.46	104.71	174.79	2417	37.83	105.75	173.75	2403	38.21	106.78	172.72	2389
280	37.01	103.63	176.37	2439	37.38	104.67	175.33	2425	37.75	105.71	174.30	2410	38.12	106.74	173.26	2396
280.5	36.93	103.59	176.91	2447	37.30	104.63	175.87	2432	37.67	105.66	174.84	2418	38.04	106.70	173.80	2404
281	36.85	103.55	177.45	2454	37.22	104.59	176.41	2440	37.59	105.62	175.38	2425	37.96	106.66	174.34	2411
281.5	36.77	103.51	177.99	2462	37.14	104.54	176.96	2447	37.51	105.58	175.92	2433	37.88	106.62	174.88	2419
282	36.69	103.47	178.53	2469	37.06	104.50	177.50	2455	37.43	105.54	176.46	2440	37.79	106.58	175.42	2426
282.5	36.61	103.43	179.08	2477	36.98	104.46	178.04	2462	37.35	105.50	177.00	2448	37.71	106.54	175.96	2434
283	36.53	103.38	179.62	2484	36.90	104.42	178.58	2470	37.26	105.46	177.54	2455	37.63	106.50	176.50	2441
283.5	36.45	103.34	180.16	2492	36.82	104.38	179.12	2477	37.18	105.42	178.08	2463	37.55	106.46	177.04	2449
284	36.37	103.30	180.70	2499	36.74	104.34	179.66	2485	37.10	105.38	178.62	2470	37.47	106.41	177.59	2456
284.5	36.30	103.26	181.24	2507	36.66	104.30	180.20	2492	37.02	105.34	179.16	2478	37.39	106.37	178.13	2463
285	36.22	103.22	181.78	2514	36.58	104.26	180.74	2500	36.95	105.30	179.71	2485	37.31	106.33	178.67	2471
285.5	36.14	103.18	182.32	2521	36.50	104.22	181.28	2507	36.87	105.25	180.25	2493	37.23	106.29	179.21	2478
286	36.06	103.14	182.86	2529	36.43	104.18	181.82	2515	36.79	105.21	180.79	2500	37.15	106.25	179.75	2486
286.5	35.98	103.10	183.40	2536	36.35	104.13	182.37	2522	36.71	105.17	181.33	2508	37.07	106.21	180.29	2493
287	35.91	103.06	183.94	2544	36.27	104.09	182.91	2530	36.63	105.13	181.87	2515	36.99	106.17	180.83	2501
287.5	35.83	103.02	184.49	2551	36.19	104.05	183.45	2537	36.55	105.09	182.41	2523	36.91	106.13	181.37	2508
288	35.75	102.97	185.03	2559	36.12	104.01	183.99	2545	36.48	105.05	182.95	2530	36.84	106.09	181.91	2516
288.5	35.68	102.93	185.57	2566	36.04	103.97	184.53	2552	36.40	105.01	183.49	2538	36.76	106.05	182.45	2523
289	35.60	102.89	186.11	2574	35.96	103.93	185.07	2560	36.32	104.97	184.03	2545	36.68	106.00	183.00	2531
289.5	35.53	102.85	186.65	2581	35.89	103.89	185.61	2567	36.24	104.93	184.57	2553	36.60	105.96	183.54	2538
290	35.45	102.81	187.19	2589	35.81	103.85	186.15	2574	36.17	104.89	185.12	2560	36.53	105.92	184.08	2546
290.5	35.38	102.77	187.73	2596	35.73	103.81	186.69	2582	36.09	104.84	185.66	2568	36.45	105.88	184.62	2553
291	35.30	102.73	188.27	2604	35.66	103.77	187.23	2589	36.01	104.80	186.20	2575	36.37	105.84	185.16	2561
291.5	35.23	102.69	188.81	2611	35.58	103.72	187.78	2597	35.94	104.76	186.74	2583	36.29	105.80	185.70	2568

Body Composition   FEMALE   260-291.5 Lb.

Weight: Lb.	Waist: 50 inches Fat: %	Fat: Lb.	LBM: Lb.	RMR: Cal.	50.25 inches Fat: %	Fat: Lb.	LBM: Lb.	RMR: Cal.	50.5 inches Fat: %	Fat: Lb.	LBM: Lb.	RMR: Cal.	50.75 inches Fat: %	Fat: Lb.	LBM: Lb.	RMR: Cal.
260	42.08	109.42	150.58	2083	42.48	110.46	149.54	2068	42.88	111.50	148.51	2054	43.28	112.53	147.47	2039
260.5	41.99	109.38	151.12	2090	42.39	110.42	150.08	2076	42.78	111.45	149.05	2061	43.18	112.49	148.01	2047
261	41.89	109.34	151.66	2097	42.29	110.38	150.62	2083	42.69	111.41	149.59	2069	43.08	112.45	148.55	2054
261.5	41.80	109.30	152.20	2105	42.19	110.33	151.17	2091	42.59	111.37	150.13	2076	42.99	112.41	149.09	2062
262	41.70	109.26	152.74	2112	42.10	110.29	151.71	2098	42.49	111.33	150.67	2084	42.89	112.37	149.63	2069
262.5	41.61	109.22	153.29	2120	42.00	110.25	152.25	2106	42.40	111.29	151.21	2091	42.79	112.33	150.17	2077
263	41.51	109.17	153.83	2127	41.91	110.21	152.79	2113	42.30	111.25	151.75	2099	42.69	112.29	150.71	2084
263.5	41.42	109.13	154.37	2135	41.81	110.17	153.33	2121	42.20	111.21	152.29	2106	42.60	112.25	151.25	2092
264	41.32	109.09	154.91	2142	41.72	110.13	153.87	2128	42.11	111.17	152.83	2114	42.50	112.20	151.80	2099
264.5	41.23	109.05	155.45	2150	41.62	110.09	154.41	2136	42.01	111.13	153.37	2121	42.41	112.16	152.34	2107
265	41.14	109.01	155.99	2157	41.53	110.05	154.95	2143	41.92	111.09	153.92	2129	42.31	112.12	152.88	2114
265.5	41.04	108.97	156.53	2165	41.43	110.01	155.49	2150	41.82	111.04	154.46	2136	42.22	112.08	153.42	2122
266	40.95	108.93	157.07	2172	41.34	109.97	156.03	2158	41.73	111.00	155.00	2144	42.12	112.04	153.96	2129
266.5	40.86	108.89	157.61	2180	41.25	109.92	156.58	2165	41.64	110.96	155.54	2151	42.03	112.00	154.50	2137
267	40.77	108.85	158.15	2187	41.15	109.88	157.12	2173	41.54	110.92	156.08	2159	41.93	111.96	155.04	2144
267.5	40.67	108.81	158.70	2195	41.06	109.84	157.66	2180	41.45	110.88	156.62	2166	41.84	111.92	155.58	2152
268	40.58	108.76	159.24	2202	40.97	109.80	158.20	2188	41.36	110.84	157.16	2174	41.74	111.88	156.12	2159
268.5	40.49	108.72	159.78	2210	40.88	109.76	158.74	2195	41.27	110.80	157.70	2181	41.65	111.84	156.66	2167
269	40.40	108.68	160.32	2217	40.79	109.72	159.28	2203	41.17	110.76	158.24	2189	41.56	111.79	157.21	2174
269.5	40.31	108.64	160.86	2225	40.70	109.68	159.82	2210	41.08	110.72	158.78	2196	41.47	111.75	157.75	2182
270	40.22	108.60	161.40	2232	40.61	109.64	160.36	2218	40.99	110.68	159.33	2203	41.38	111.71	158.29	2189
270.5	40.13	108.56	161.94	2240	40.52	109.60	160.90	2225	40.90	110.63	159.87	2211	41.28	111.67	158.83	2197
271	40.04	108.52	162.48	2247	40.43	109.56	161.44	2233	40.81	110.59	160.41	2218	41.19	111.63	159.37	2204
271.5	39.95	108.48	163.02	2255	40.34	109.51	161.99	2240	40.72	110.55	160.95	2226	41.10	111.59	159.91	2212
272	39.87	108.44	163.56	2262	40.25	109.47	162.53	2248	40.63	110.51	161.49	2233	41.01	111.55	160.45	2219
272.5	39.78	108.40	164.11	2270	40.16	109.43	163.07	2255	40.54	110.47	162.03	2241	40.92	111.51	160.99	2227
273	39.69	108.35	164.65	2277	40.07	109.39	163.61	2263	40.45	110.43	162.57	2248	40.83	111.47	161.53	2234
273.5	39.60	108.31	165.19	2285	39.98	109.35	164.15	2270	40.36	110.39	163.11	2256	40.74	111.43	162.07	2241
274	39.52	108.27	165.73	2292	39.89	109.31	164.69	2278	40.27	110.35	163.65	2263	40.65	111.38	162.62	2249
274.5	39.43	108.23	166.27	2300	39.81	109.27	165.23	2285	40.18	110.31	164.19	2271	40.56	111.34	163.16	2256
275	39.34	108.19	166.81	2307	39.72	109.23	165.77	2293	40.10	110.27	164.74	2278	40.47	111.30	163.70	2264
275.5	39.26	108.15	167.35	2314	39.63	109.19	166.31	2300	40.01	110.22	165.28	2286	40.39	111.26	164.24	2271
276	39.17	108.11	167.89	2322	39.55	109.15	166.85	2308	39.92	110.18	165.82	2293	40.30	111.22	164.78	2279
276.5	39.08	108.07	168.43	2329	39.46	109.10	167.40	2315	39.83	110.14	166.36	2301	40.21	111.18	165.32	2286
277	39.00	108.03	168.97	2337	39.37	109.06	167.94	2323	39.75	110.10	166.90	2308	40.12	111.14	165.86	2294
277.5	38.91	107.99	169.52	2344	39.29	109.02	168.48	2330	39.66	110.06	167.44	2316	40.04	111.10	166.40	2301
278	38.83	107.94	170.06	2352	39.20	108.98	169.02	2338	39.58	110.02	167.98	2323	39.95	111.06	166.94	2309
278.5	38.74	107.90	170.60	2359	39.12	108.94	169.56	2345	39.49	109.98	168.52	2331	39.86	111.02	167.48	2316
279	38.66	107.86	171.14	2367	39.03	108.90	170.10	2352	39.40	109.94	169.06	2338	39.78	110.97	168.03	2324
279.5	38.58	107.82	171.68	2374	38.95	108.86	170.64	2360	39.32	109.90	169.60	2346	39.69	110.93	168.57	2331
280	38.49	107.78	172.22	2382	38.86	108.82	171.18	2367	39.23	109.86	170.15	2353	39.60	110.89	169.11	2339
280.5	38.41	107.74	172.76	2389	38.78	108.78	171.72	2375	39.15	109.81	170.69	2361	39.52	110.85	169.65	2346
281	38.33	107.70	173.30	2397	38.70	108.74	172.26	2382	39.07	109.77	171.23	2368	39.43	110.81	170.19	2354
281.5	38.24	107.66	173.84	2404	38.61	108.69	172.81	2390	38.98	109.73	171.77	2376	39.35	110.77	170.73	2361
282	38.16	107.62	174.38	2412	38.53	108.65	173.35	2397	38.90	109.69	172.31	2383	39.27	110.73	171.27	2369
282.5	38.08	107.58	174.93	2419	38.45	108.61	173.89	2405	38.81	109.65	172.85	2391	39.18	110.69	171.81	2376
283	38.00	107.53	175.47	2427	38.36	108.57	174.43	2412	38.73	109.61	173.39	2398	39.10	110.65	172.35	2384
283.5	37.92	107.49	176.01	2434	38.28	108.53	174.97	2420	38.65	109.57	173.93	2405	39.01	110.61	172.89	2391
284	37.84	107.45	176.55	2442	38.20	108.49	175.51	2427	38.57	109.53	174.47	2413	38.93	110.56	173.44	2399
284.5	37.75	107.41	177.09	2449	38.12	108.45	176.05	2435	38.48	109.49	175.01	2420	38.85	110.52	173.98	2406
285	37.67	107.37	177.63	2457	38.04	108.41	176.59	2442	38.40	109.45	175.56	2428	38.77	110.48	174.52	2414
285.5	37.59	107.33	178.17	2464	37.96	108.37	177.13	2450	38.32	109.40	176.10	2435	38.68	110.44	175.06	2421
286	37.51	107.29	178.71	2472	37.88	108.33	177.67	2457	38.24	109.36	176.64	2443	38.60	110.40	175.60	2429
286.5	37.43	107.25	179.25	2479	37.80	108.28	178.22	2465	38.16	109.32	177.18	2450	38.52	110.36	176.14	2436
287	37.35	107.21	179.79	2487	37.72	108.24	178.76	2472	38.08	109.28	177.72	2458	38.44	110.32	176.68	2444
287.5	37.27	107.17	180.34	2494	37.64	108.20	179.30	2480	38.00	109.24	178.26	2465	38.36	110.28	177.22	2451
288	37.20	107.12	180.88	2502	37.56	108.16	179.84	2487	37.92	109.20	178.80	2473	38.28	110.24	177.76	2458
288.5	37.12	107.08	181.42	2509	37.48	108.12	180.38	2495	37.84	109.16	179.34	2480	38.20	110.20	178.30	2466
289	37.04	107.04	181.96	2516	37.40	108.08	180.92	2502	37.76	109.12	179.88	2488	38.12	110.15	178.85	2473
289.5	36.96	107.00	182.50	2524	37.32	108.04	181.46	2510	37.68	109.08	180.42	2495	38.04	110.11	179.39	2481
290	36.88	106.96	183.04	2531	37.24	108.00	182.00	2517	37.60	109.04	180.97	2503	37.96	110.07	179.93	2488
290.5	36.81	106.92	183.58	2539	37.16	107.96	182.54	2525	37.52	108.99	181.51	2510	37.88	110.03	180.47	2496
291	36.73	106.88	184.12	2546	37.08	107.92	183.08	2532	37.44	108.95	182.05	2518	37.80	109.99	181.01	2503
291.5	36.65	106.84	184.66	2554	37.01	107.87	183.63	2540	37.36	108.91	182.59	2525	37.72	109.95	181.55	2511

Body Composition   FEMALE   260-291.5 Lb.

Weight: Lb.	Waist: 51 inches Fat: %	Fat: Lb.	LBM: Lb.	RMR: Cal.	51.25 inches Fat: %	Fat: Lb.	LBM: Lb.	RMR: Cal.	51.5 inches Fat: %	Fat: Lb.	LBM: Lb.	RMR: Cal.	51.75 inches Fat: %	Fat: Lb.	LBM: Lb.	RMR: Cal.
260	43.68	113.57	146.43	2025	44.08	114.61	145.39	2011	44.48	115.65	144.36	1996	44.88	116.68	143.32	1982
260.5	43.58	113.53	146.97	2033	43.98	114.57	145.93	2018	44.38	115.60	144.90	2004	44.78	116.64	143.86	1990
261	43.48	113.49	147.51	2040	43.88	114.53	146.47	2026	44.28	115.56	145.44	2011	44.67	116.60	144.40	1997
261.5	43.38	113.45	148.05	2048	43.78	114.48	147.02	2033	44.18	115.52	145.98	2019	44.57	116.56	144.94	2005
262	43.28	113.41	148.59	2055	43.68	114.44	147.56	2041	44.08	115.48	146.52	2026	44.47	116.52	145.48	2012
262.5	43.19	113.37	149.14	2063	43.58	114.40	148.10	2048	43.98	115.44	147.06	2034	44.37	116.48	146.02	2019
263	43.09	113.32	149.68	2070	43.48	114.36	148.64	2056	43.88	115.40	147.60	2041	44.27	116.44	146.56	2027
263.5	42.99	113.28	150.22	2078	43.39	114.32	149.18	2063	43.78	115.36	148.14	2049	44.17	116.40	147.10	2034
264	42.89	113.24	150.76	2085	43.29	114.28	149.72	2071	43.68	115.32	148.68	2056	44.07	116.35	147.65	2042
264.5	42.80	113.20	151.30	2092	43.19	114.24	150.26	2078	43.58	115.28	149.22	2064	43.97	116.31	148.19	2049
265	42.70	113.16	151.84	2100	43.09	114.20	150.80	2086	43.48	115.24	149.77	2071	43.88	116.27	148.73	2057
265.5	42.61	113.12	152.38	2107	43.00	114.16	151.34	2093	43.39	115.19	150.31	2079	43.78	116.23	149.27	2064
266	42.51	113.08	152.92	2115	42.90	114.12	151.88	2101	43.29	115.15	150.85	2086	43.68	116.19	149.81	2072
266.5	42.42	113.04	153.46	2122	42.80	114.07	152.43	2108	43.19	115.11	151.39	2094	43.58	116.15	150.35	2079
267	42.32	113.00	154.00	2130	42.71	114.03	152.97	2116	43.10	115.07	151.93	2101	43.49	116.11	150.89	2087
267.5	42.23	112.96	154.55	2137	42.61	113.99	153.51	2123	43.00	115.03	152.47	2109	43.39	116.07	151.43	2094
268	42.13	112.91	155.09	2145	42.52	113.95	154.05	2130	42.91	114.99	153.01	2116	43.29	116.03	151.97	2102
268.5	42.04	112.87	155.63	2152	42.42	113.91	154.59	2138	42.81	114.95	153.55	2124	43.20	115.99	152.51	2109
269	41.94	112.83	156.17	2160	42.33	113.87	155.13	2145	42.72	114.91	154.09	2131	43.10	115.94	153.06	2117
269.5	41.85	112.79	156.71	2167	42.24	113.83	155.67	2153	42.62	114.87	154.63	2139	43.01	115.90	153.60	2124
270	41.76	112.75	157.25	2175	42.14	113.79	156.21	2160	42.53	114.83	155.18	2146	42.91	115.86	154.14	2132
270.5	41.67	112.71	157.79	2182	42.05	113.75	156.75	2168	42.43	114.78	155.72	2154	42.82	115.82	154.68	2139
271	41.57	112.67	158.33	2190	41.96	113.71	157.29	2175	42.34	114.74	156.26	2161	42.72	115.78	155.22	2147
271.5	41.48	112.63	158.87	2197	41.87	113.66	157.84	2183	42.25	114.70	156.80	2169	42.63	115.74	155.76	2154
272	41.39	112.59	159.41	2205	41.77	113.62	158.38	2190	42.15	114.66	157.34	2176	42.54	115.70	156.30	2162
272.5	41.30	112.55	159.96	2212	41.68	113.58	158.92	2198	42.06	114.62	157.88	2183	42.44	115.66	156.84	2169
273	41.21	112.50	160.50	2220	41.59	113.54	159.46	2205	41.97	114.58	158.42	2191	42.35	115.62	157.38	2177
273.5	41.12	112.46	161.04	2227	41.50	113.50	160.00	2213	41.88	114.54	158.96	2198	42.26	115.58	157.92	2184
274	41.03	112.42	161.58	2235	41.41	113.46	160.54	2220	41.79	114.50	159.50	2206	42.17	115.53	158.47	2192
274.5	40.94	112.38	162.12	2242	41.32	113.42	161.08	2228	41.70	114.46	160.04	2213	42.07	115.49	159.01	2199
275	40.85	112.34	162.66	2250	41.23	113.38	161.62	2235	41.61	114.42	160.59	2221	41.98	115.45	159.55	2207
275.5	40.76	112.30	163.20	2257	41.14	113.34	162.16	2243	41.52	114.37	161.13	2228	41.89	115.41	160.09	2214
276	40.67	112.26	163.74	2265	41.05	113.30	162.70	2250	41.43	114.33	161.67	2236	41.80	115.37	160.63	2222
276.5	40.58	112.22	164.28	2272	40.96	113.25	163.25	2258	41.34	114.29	162.21	2243	41.71	115.33	161.17	2229
277	40.50	112.18	164.82	2280	40.87	113.21	163.79	2265	41.25	114.25	162.75	2251	41.62	115.29	161.71	2236
277.5	40.41	112.14	165.37	2287	40.78	113.17	164.33	2273	41.16	114.21	163.29	2258	41.53	115.25	162.25	2244
278	40.32	112.09	165.91	2294	40.69	113.13	164.87	2280	41.07	114.17	163.83	2266	41.44	115.21	162.79	2251
278.5	40.23	112.05	166.45	2302	40.61	113.09	165.41	2288	40.98	114.13	164.37	2273	41.35	115.17	163.33	2259
279	40.15	112.01	166.99	2309	40.52	113.05	165.95	2295	40.89	114.09	164.91	2281	41.26	115.12	163.88	2266
279.5	40.06	111.97	167.53	2317	40.43	113.01	166.49	2303	40.80	114.05	165.45	2288	41.17	115.08	164.42	2274
280	39.98	111.93	168.07	2324	40.35	112.97	167.03	2310	40.72	114.01	166.00	2296	41.09	115.04	164.96	2281
280.5	39.89	111.89	168.61	2332	40.26	112.93	167.57	2318	40.63	113.96	166.54	2303	41.00	115.00	165.50	2289
281	39.80	111.85	169.15	2339	40.17	112.89	168.11	2325	40.54	113.92	167.08	2311	40.91	114.96	166.04	2296
281.5	39.72	111.81	169.69	2347	40.09	112.84	168.66	2333	40.46	113.88	167.62	2318	40.82	114.92	166.58	2304
282	39.63	111.77	170.23	2354	40.00	112.80	169.20	2340	40.37	113.84	168.16	2326	40.74	114.88	167.12	2311
282.5	39.55	111.73	170.78	2362	39.92	112.76	169.74	2347	40.28	113.80	168.70	2333	40.65	114.84	167.66	2319
283	39.46	111.68	171.32	2369	39.83	112.72	170.28	2355	40.20	113.76	169.24	2341	40.56	114.80	168.20	2326
283.5	39.38	111.64	171.86	2377	39.75	112.68	170.82	2362	40.11	113.72	169.78	2348	40.48	114.76	168.74	2334
284	39.30	111.60	172.40	2384	39.66	112.64	171.36	2370	40.03	113.68	170.32	2356	40.39	114.71	169.29	2341
284.5	39.21	111.56	172.94	2392	39.58	112.60	171.90	2377	39.94	113.64	170.86	2363	40.31	114.67	169.83	2349
285	39.13	111.52	173.48	2399	39.49	112.56	172.44	2385	39.86	113.60	171.41	2371	40.22	114.63	170.37	2356
285.5	39.05	111.48	174.02	2407	39.41	112.52	172.98	2392	39.77	113.55	171.95	2378	40.14	114.59	170.91	2364
286	38.96	111.44	174.56	2414	39.33	112.48	173.52	2400	39.69	113.51	172.49	2385	40.05	114.55	171.45	2371
286.5	38.88	111.40	175.10	2422	39.24	112.43	174.07	2407	39.61	113.47	173.03	2393	39.97	114.51	171.99	2379
287	38.80	111.36	175.64	2429	39.16	112.39	174.61	2415	39.52	113.43	173.57	2400	39.88	114.47	172.53	2386
287.5	38.72	111.32	176.19	2437	39.08	112.35	175.15	2422	39.44	113.39	174.11	2408	39.80	114.43	173.07	2394
288	38.64	111.27	176.73	2444	39.00	112.31	175.69	2430	39.36	113.35	174.65	2415	39.72	114.39	173.61	2401
288.5	38.56	111.23	177.27	2452	38.92	112.27	176.23	2437	39.27	113.31	175.19	2423	39.63	114.35	174.15	2409
289	38.47	111.19	177.81	2459	38.83	112.23	176.77	2445	39.19	113.27	175.73	2430	39.55	114.30	174.70	2416
289.5	38.39	111.15	178.35	2467	38.75	112.19	177.31	2452	39.11	113.23	176.27	2438	39.47	114.26	175.24	2424
290	38.31	111.11	178.89	2474	38.67	112.15	177.85	2460	39.03	113.19	176.82	2445	39.39	114.22	175.78	2431
290.5	38.23	111.07	179.43	2482	38.59	112.11	178.39	2467	38.95	113.14	177.36	2453	39.31	114.18	176.32	2438
291	38.15	111.03	179.97	2489	38.51	112.07	178.93	2475	38.87	113.10	177.90	2460	39.22	114.14	176.86	2446
291.5	38.07	110.99	180.51	2496	38.43	112.02	179.48	2482	38.79	113.06	178.44	2468	39.14	114.10	177.40	2453

Body Composition   FEMALE   260-291.5 Lb.

Weight: Lb.	Waist: 52 inches				52.25 inches				52.5 inches				52.75 inches			
	Fat: %	Fat: Lb.	LBM: Lb.	RMR: Cal.	Fat: %	Fat: Lb.	LBM: Lb.	RMR: Cal.	Fat: %	Fat: Lb.	LBM: Lb.	RMR: Cal.	Fat: %	Fat: Lb.	LBM: Lb.	RMR: Cal.
260	45.28	117.72	142.28	1968	45.68	118.76	141.24	1953	46.08	119.80	140.21	1939	46.47	120.83	139.17	1925
260.5	45.17	117.68	142.82	1975	45.57	118.72	141.78	1961	45.97	119.75	140.75	1947	46.37	120.79	139.71	1932
261	45.07	117.64	143.36	1983	45.47	118.68	142.32	1968	45.87	119.71	141.29	1954	46.26	120.75	140.25	1940
261.5	44.97	117.60	143.90	1990	45.37	118.63	142.87	1976	45.76	119.67	141.83	1961	46.16	120.71	140.79	1947
262	44.87	117.56	144.44	1998	45.26	118.59	143.41	1983	45.66	119.63	142.37	1969	46.06	120.67	141.33	1955
262.5	44.77	117.52	144.99	2005	45.16	118.55	143.95	1991	45.56	119.59	142.91	1976	45.95	120.63	141.87	1962
263	44.67	117.47	145.53	2013	45.06	118.51	144.49	1998	45.46	119.55	143.45	1984	45.85	120.59	142.41	1970
263.5	44.57	117.43	146.07	2020	44.96	118.47	145.03	2006	45.35	119.51	143.99	1991	45.75	120.55	142.95	1977
264	44.47	117.39	146.61	2028	44.86	118.43	145.57	2013	45.25	119.47	144.53	1999	45.65	120.50	143.50	1985
264.5	44.37	117.35	147.15	2035	44.76	118.39	146.11	2021	45.15	119.43	145.07	2006	45.54	120.46	144.04	1992
265	44.27	117.31	147.69	2043	44.66	118.35	146.65	2028	45.05	119.39	145.62	2014	45.44	120.42	144.58	2000
265.5	44.17	117.27	148.23	2050	44.56	118.31	147.19	2036	44.95	119.34	146.16	2021	45.34	120.38	145.12	2007
266	44.07	117.23	148.77	2058	44.46	118.27	147.73	2043	44.85	119.30	146.70	2029	45.24	120.34	145.66	2014
266.5	43.97	117.19	149.31	2065	44.36	118.22	148.28	2051	44.75	119.26	147.24	2036	45.14	120.30	146.20	2022
267	43.87	117.15	149.85	2072	44.26	118.18	148.82	2058	44.65	119.22	147.78	2044	45.04	120.26	146.74	2029
267.5	43.78	117.11	150.40	2080	44.17	118.14	149.36	2066	44.55	119.18	148.32	2051	44.94	120.22	147.28	2037
268	43.68	117.06	150.94	2087	44.07	118.10	149.90	2073	44.45	119.14	148.86	2059	44.84	120.18	147.82	2044
268.5	43.58	117.02	151.48	2095	43.97	118.06	150.44	2081	44.36	119.10	149.40	2066	44.74	120.14	148.36	2052
269	43.49	116.98	152.02	2102	43.87	118.02	150.98	2088	44.26	119.06	149.94	2074	44.64	120.09	148.91	2059
269.5	43.39	116.94	152.56	2110	43.78	117.98	151.52	2096	44.16	119.02	150.48	2081	44.55	120.05	149.45	2067
270	43.30	116.90	153.10	2117	43.68	117.94	152.06	2103	44.06	118.98	151.03	2089	44.45	120.01	149.99	2074
270.5	43.20	116.86	153.64	2125	43.58	117.90	152.60	2111	43.97	118.93	151.57	2096	44.35	119.97	150.53	2082
271	43.11	116.82	154.18	2132	43.49	117.86	153.14	2118	43.87	118.89	152.11	2104	44.25	119.93	151.07	2089
271.5	43.01	116.78	154.72	2140	43.39	117.81	153.69	2125	43.78	118.85	152.65	2111	44.16	119.89	151.61	2097
272	42.92	116.74	155.26	2147	43.30	117.77	154.23	2133	43.68	118.81	153.19	2119	44.06	119.85	152.15	2104
272.5	42.82	116.70	155.81	2155	43.20	117.73	154.77	2140	43.59	118.77	153.73	2126	43.97	119.81	152.69	2112
273	42.73	116.65	156.35	2162	43.11	117.69	155.31	2148	43.49	118.73	154.27	2134	43.87	119.77	153.23	2119
273.5	42.64	116.61	156.89	2170	43.02	117.65	155.85	2155	43.40	118.69	154.81	2141	43.78	119.73	153.77	2127
274	42.54	116.57	157.43	2177	42.92	117.61	156.39	2163	43.30	118.65	155.35	2149	43.68	119.68	154.32	2134
274.5	42.45	116.53	157.97	2185	42.83	117.57	156.93	2170	43.21	118.61	155.89	2156	43.59	119.64	154.86	2142
275	42.36	116.49	158.51	2192	42.74	117.53	157.47	2178	43.11	118.57	156.44	2163	43.49	119.60	155.40	2149
275.5	42.27	116.45	159.05	2200	42.64	117.49	158.01	2185	43.02	118.52	156.98	2171	43.40	119.56	155.94	2157
276	42.18	116.41	159.59	2207	42.55	117.45	158.55	2193	42.93	118.48	157.52	2178	43.30	119.52	156.48	2164
276.5	42.09	116.37	160.13	2215	42.46	117.40	159.10	2200	42.84	118.44	158.06	2186	43.21	119.48	157.02	2172
277	41.99	116.33	160.67	2222	42.37	117.36	159.64	2208	42.74	118.40	158.60	2193	43.12	119.44	157.56	2179
277.5	41.90	116.29	161.22	2230	42.28	117.32	160.18	2215	42.65	118.36	159.14	2201	43.03	119.40	158.10	2187
278	41.81	116.24	161.76	2237	42.19	117.28	160.72	2223	42.56	118.32	159.68	2208	42.93	119.36	158.64	2194
278.5	41.72	116.20	162.30	2245	42.10	117.24	161.26	2230	42.47	118.28	160.22	2216	42.84	119.32	159.18	2202
279	41.64	116.16	162.84	2252	42.01	117.20	161.80	2238	42.38	118.24	160.76	2223	42.75	119.27	159.73	2209
279.5	41.55	116.12	163.38	2260	41.92	117.16	162.34	2245	42.29	118.20	161.30	2231	42.66	119.23	160.27	2216
280	41.46	116.08	163.92	2267	41.83	117.12	162.88	2253	42.20	118.16	161.85	2238	42.57	119.19	160.81	2224
280.5	41.37	116.04	164.46	2274	41.74	117.08	163.42	2260	42.11	118.11	162.39	2246	42.48	119.15	161.35	2231
281	41.28	116.00	165.00	2282	41.65	117.04	163.96	2268	42.02	118.07	162.93	2253	42.39	119.11	161.89	2239
281.5	41.19	115.96	165.54	2289	41.56	116.99	164.51	2275	41.93	118.03	163.47	2261	42.30	119.07	162.43	2246
282	41.10	115.92	166.08	2297	41.47	116.95	165.05	2283	41.84	117.99	164.01	2268	42.21	119.03	162.97	2254
282.5	41.02	115.88	166.63	2304	41.38	116.91	165.59	2290	41.75	117.95	164.55	2276	42.12	118.99	163.51	2261
283	40.93	115.83	167.17	2312	41.30	116.87	166.13	2298	41.66	117.91	165.09	2283	42.03	118.95	164.05	2269
283.5	40.84	115.79	167.71	2319	41.21	116.83	166.67	2305	41.58	117.87	165.63	2291	41.94	118.91	164.59	2276
284	40.76	115.75	168.25	2327	41.12	116.79	167.21	2313	41.49	117.83	166.17	2298	41.85	118.86	165.14	2284
284.5	40.67	115.71	168.79	2334	41.04	116.75	167.75	2320	41.40	117.79	166.71	2306	41.77	118.82	165.68	2291
285	40.59	115.67	169.33	2342	40.95	116.71	168.29	2327	41.31	117.75	167.26	2313	41.68	118.78	166.22	2299
285.5	40.50	115.63	169.87	2349	40.86	116.67	168.83	2335	41.23	117.70	167.80	2321	41.59	118.74	166.76	2306
286	40.42	115.59	170.41	2357	40.78	116.63	169.37	2342	41.14	117.66	168.34	2328	41.50	118.70	167.30	2314
286.5	40.33	115.55	170.95	2364	40.69	116.58	169.92	2350	41.05	117.62	168.88	2336	41.42	118.66	167.84	2321
287	40.25	115.51	171.49	2372	40.61	116.54	170.46	2357	40.97	117.58	169.42	2343	41.33	118.62	168.38	2329
287.5	40.16	115.47	172.04	2379	40.52	116.50	171.00	2365	40.88	117.54	169.96	2351	41.24	118.58	168.92	2336
288	40.08	115.42	172.58	2387	40.44	116.46	171.54	2372	40.80	117.50	170.50	2358	41.16	118.54	169.46	2344
288.5	39.99	115.38	173.12	2394	40.35	116.42	172.08	2380	40.71	117.46	171.04	2366	41.07	118.50	170.00	2351
289	39.91	115.34	173.66	2402	40.27	116.38	172.62	2387	40.63	117.42	171.58	2373	40.99	118.45	170.55	2359
289.5	39.83	115.30	174.20	2409	40.19	116.34	173.16	2395	40.54	117.38	172.12	2380	40.90	118.41	171.09	2366
290	39.74	115.26	174.74	2417	40.10	116.30	173.70	2402	40.46	117.34	172.67	2388	40.82	118.37	171.63	2374
290.5	39.66	115.22	175.28	2424	40.02	116.26	174.24	2410	40.38	117.29	173.21	2395	40.73	118.33	172.17	2381
291	39.58	115.18	175.82	2432	39.94	116.22	174.78	2417	40.29	117.25	173.75	2403	40.65	118.29	172.71	2389
291.5	39.50	115.14	176.36	2439	39.85	116.17	175.33	2425	40.21	117.21	174.29	2410	40.57	118.25	173.25	2396

Body Composition   FEMALE   260-291.5 Lb.

Weight: Lb.	Waist: 53 inches				53.25 inches				53.5 inches				53.75 inches			
	Fat: %	Fat: Lb.	LBM: Lb.	RMR: Cal.	Fat: %	Fat: Lb.	LBM: Lb.	RMR: Cal.	Fat: %	Fat: Lb.	LBM: Lb.	RMR: Cal.	Fat: %	Fat: Lb.	LBM: Lb.	RMR: Cal.
260	46.87	121.87	138.13	1910	47.27	122.91	137.09	1896	47.67	123.95	136.06	1882	48.07	124.98	135.02	1867
260.5	46.77	121.83	138.67	1918	47.17	122.87	137.63	1903	47.56	123.90	136.60	1889	47.96	124.94	135.56	1875
261	46.66	121.79	139.21	1925	47.06	122.83	138.17	1911	47.46	123.86	137.14	1897	47.85	124.90	136.10	1882
261.5	46.56	121.75	139.75	1933	46.95	122.78	138.72	1918	47.35	123.82	137.68	1904	47.75	124.86	136.64	1890
262	46.45	121.71	140.29	1940	46.85	122.74	139.26	1926	47.24	123.78	138.22	1912	47.64	124.82	137.18	1897
262.5	46.35	121.67	140.84	1948	46.74	122.70	139.80	1933	47.14	123.74	138.76	1919	47.53	124.78	137.72	1905
263	46.24	121.62	141.38	1955	46.64	122.66	140.34	1941	47.03	123.70	139.30	1927	47.43	124.74	138.26	1912
263.5	46.14	121.58	141.92	1963	46.54	122.62	140.88	1948	46.93	123.66	139.84	1934	47.32	124.70	138.80	1920
264	46.04	121.54	142.46	1970	46.43	122.58	141.42	1956	46.82	123.62	140.38	1941	47.22	124.65	139.35	1927
264.5	45.94	121.50	143.00	1978	46.33	122.54	141.96	1963	46.72	123.58	140.92	1949	47.11	124.61	139.89	1935
265	45.83	121.46	143.54	1985	46.23	122.50	142.50	1971	46.62	123.54	141.47	1956	47.01	124.57	140.43	1942
265.5	45.73	121.42	144.08	1993	46.12	122.46	143.04	1978	46.51	123.49	142.01	1964	46.90	124.53	140.97	1950
266	45.63	121.38	144.62	2000	46.02	122.42	143.58	1986	46.41	123.45	142.55	1971	46.80	124.49	141.51	1957
266.5	45.53	121.34	145.16	2008	45.92	122.37	144.13	1993	46.31	123.41	143.09	1979	46.70	124.45	142.05	1965
267	45.43	121.30	145.70	2015	45.82	122.33	144.67	2001	46.21	123.37	143.63	1986	46.59	124.41	142.59	1972
267.5	45.33	121.26	146.25	2023	45.72	122.29	145.21	2008	46.10	123.33	144.17	1994	46.49	124.37	143.13	1980
268	45.23	121.21	146.79	2030	45.62	122.25	145.75	2016	46.00	123.29	144.71	2001	46.39	124.33	143.67	1987
268.5	45.13	121.17	147.33	2038	45.52	122.21	146.29	2023	45.90	123.25	145.25	2009	46.29	124.29	144.21	1994
269	45.03	121.13	147.87	2045	45.42	122.17	146.83	2031	45.80	123.21	145.79	2016	46.19	124.24	144.76	2002
269.5	44.93	121.09	148.41	2052	45.32	122.13	147.37	2038	45.70	123.17	146.33	2024	46.09	124.20	145.30	2009
270	44.83	121.05	148.95	2060	45.22	122.09	147.91	2046	45.60	123.13	146.88	2031	45.99	124.16	145.84	2017
270.5	44.74	121.01	149.49	2067	45.12	122.05	148.45	2053	45.50	123.08	147.42	2039	45.89	124.12	146.38	2024
271	44.64	120.97	150.03	2075	45.02	122.01	148.99	2061	45.40	123.04	147.96	2046	45.79	124.08	146.92	2032
271.5	44.54	120.93	150.57	2082	44.92	121.96	149.54	2068	45.30	123.00	148.50	2054	45.69	124.04	147.46	2039
272	44.44	120.89	151.11	2090	44.82	121.92	150.08	2076	45.21	122.96	149.04	2061	45.59	124.00	148.00	2047
272.5	44.35	120.85	151.66	2097	44.73	121.88	150.62	2083	45.11	122.92	149.58	2069	45.49	123.96	148.54	2054
273	44.25	120.80	152.20	2105	44.63	121.84	151.16	2091	45.01	122.88	150.12	2076	45.39	123.92	149.08	2062
273.5	44.15	120.76	152.74	2112	44.53	121.80	151.70	2098	44.91	122.84	150.66	2084	45.29	123.88	149.62	2069
274	44.06	120.72	153.28	2120	44.44	121.76	152.24	2105	44.82	122.80	151.20	2091	45.20	123.83	150.17	2077
274.5	43.96	120.68	153.82	2127	44.34	121.72	152.78	2113	44.72	122.76	151.74	2099	45.10	123.79	150.71	2084
275	43.87	120.64	154.36	2135	44.25	121.68	153.32	2120	44.62	122.72	152.29	2106	45.00	123.75	151.25	2092
275.5	43.77	120.60	154.90	2142	44.15	121.64	153.86	2128	44.53	122.67	152.83	2114	44.90	123.71	151.79	2099
276	43.68	120.56	155.44	2150	44.06	121.60	154.40	2135	44.43	122.63	153.37	2121	44.81	123.67	152.33	2107
276.5	43.59	120.52	155.98	2157	43.96	121.55	154.95	2143	44.34	122.59	153.91	2129	44.71	123.63	152.87	2114
277	43.49	120.48	156.52	2165	43.87	121.51	155.49	2150	44.24	122.55	154.45	2136	44.62	123.59	153.41	2122
277.5	43.40	120.44	157.07	2172	43.77	121.47	156.03	2158	44.15	122.51	154.99	2144	44.52	123.55	153.95	2129
278	43.31	120.39	157.61	2180	43.68	121.43	156.57	2165	44.05	122.47	155.53	2151	44.43	123.51	154.49	2137
278.5	43.21	120.35	158.15	2187	43.59	121.39	157.11	2173	43.96	122.43	156.07	2158	44.33	123.47	155.03	2144
279	43.12	120.31	158.69	2195	43.49	121.35	157.65	2180	43.87	122.39	156.61	2166	44.24	123.42	155.58	2152
279.5	43.03	120.27	159.23	2202	43.40	121.31	158.19	2188	43.77	122.35	157.15	2173	44.14	123.38	156.12	2159
280	42.94	120.23	159.77	2210	43.31	121.27	158.73	2195	43.68	122.31	157.70	2181	44.05	123.34	156.66	2167
280.5	42.85	120.19	160.31	2217	43.22	121.23	159.27	2203	43.59	122.26	158.24	2188	43.96	123.30	157.20	2174
281	42.76	120.15	160.85	2225	43.13	121.19	159.81	2210	43.50	122.22	158.78	2196	43.86	123.26	157.74	2182
281.5	42.67	120.11	161.39	2232	43.04	121.14	160.36	2218	43.40	122.18	159.32	2203	43.77	123.22	158.28	2189
282	42.58	120.07	161.93	2240	42.94	121.10	160.90	2225	43.31	122.14	159.86	2211	43.68	123.18	158.82	2197
282.5	42.49	120.03	162.48	2247	42.85	121.06	161.44	2233	43.22	122.10	160.40	2218	43.59	123.14	159.36	2204
283	42.40	119.98	163.02	2255	42.76	121.02	161.98	2240	43.13	122.06	160.94	2226	43.50	123.10	159.90	2211
283.5	42.31	119.94	163.56	2262	42.67	120.98	162.52	2248	43.04	122.02	161.48	2233	43.41	123.06	160.44	2219
284	42.22	119.90	164.10	2269	42.58	120.94	163.06	2255	42.95	121.98	162.02	2241	43.31	123.01	160.99	2226
284.5	42.13	119.86	164.64	2277	42.50	120.90	163.60	2263	42.86	121.94	162.56	2248	43.22	122.97	161.53	2234
285	42.04	119.82	165.18	2284	42.41	120.86	164.14	2270	42.77	121.90	163.11	2256	43.13	122.93	162.07	2241
285.5	41.95	119.78	165.72	2292	42.32	120.82	164.68	2278	42.68	121.85	163.65	2263	43.04	122.89	162.61	2249
286	41.87	119.74	166.26	2299	42.23	120.78	165.22	2285	42.59	121.81	164.19	2271	42.95	122.85	163.15	2256
286.5	41.78	119.70	166.80	2307	42.14	120.73	165.77	2293	42.50	121.77	164.73	2278	42.87	122.81	163.69	2264
287	41.69	119.66	167.34	2314	42.05	120.69	166.31	2300	42.41	121.73	165.27	2286	42.78	122.77	164.23	2271
287.5	41.61	119.62	167.89	2322	41.97	120.65	166.85	2308	42.33	121.69	165.81	2293	42.69	122.73	164.77	2279
288	41.52	119.57	168.43	2329	41.88	120.61	167.39	2315	42.24	121.65	166.35	2301	42.60	122.69	165.31	2286
288.5	41.43	119.53	168.97	2337	41.79	120.57	167.93	2322	42.15	121.61	166.89	2308	42.51	122.65	165.85	2294
289	41.35	119.49	169.51	2344	41.71	120.53	168.47	2330	42.06	121.57	167.43	2316	42.42	122.60	166.40	2301
289.5	41.26	119.45	170.05	2352	41.62	120.49	169.01	2337	41.98	121.53	167.97	2323	42.34	122.56	166.94	2309
290	41.18	119.41	170.59	2359	41.53	120.45	169.55	2345	41.89	121.49	168.52	2331	42.25	122.52	167.48	2316
290.5	41.09	119.37	171.13	2367	41.45	120.41	170.09	2352	41.81	121.44	169.06	2338	42.16	122.48	168.02	2324
291	41.01	119.33	171.67	2374	41.36	120.37	170.63	2360	41.72	121.40	169.60	2346	42.08	122.44	168.56	2331
291.5	40.92	119.29	172.21	2382	41.28	120.32	171.18	2367	41.63	121.36	170.14	2353	41.99	122.40	169.10	2339

Body Composition FEMALE 260-291.5 Lb.

Weight: Lb.	Waist: 54 inches Fat: %	Fat: Lb.	LBM: Lb.	RMR: Cal.	54.25 inches Fat: %	Fat: Lb.	LBM: Lb.	RMR: Cal.	54.5 inches Fat: %	Fat: Lb.	LBM: Lb.	RMR: Cal.	54.75 inches Fat: %	Fat: Lb.	LBM: Lb.	RMR: Cal.
260	48.47	126.02	133.98	1853	48.87	127.06	132.94	1839	49.27	128.10	131.91	1824	49.67	129.13	130.87	1810
260.5	48.36	125.98	134.52	1860	48.76	127.02	133.48	1846	49.16	128.05	132.45	1832	49.56	129.09	131.41	1817
261	48.25	125.94	135.06	1868	48.65	126.98	134.02	1854	49.05	128.01	132.99	1839	49.44	129.05	131.95	1825
261.5	48.14	125.90	135.60	1875	48.54	126.93	134.57	1861	48.94	127.97	133.53	1847	49.33	129.01	132.49	1832
262	48.04	125.86	136.14	1883	48.43	126.89	135.11	1869	48.83	127.93	134.07	1854	49.22	128.97	133.03	1840
262.5	47.93	125.82	136.69	1890	48.32	126.85	135.65	1876	48.72	127.89	134.61	1862	49.12	128.93	133.57	1847
263	47.82	125.77	137.23	1898	48.22	126.81	136.19	1883	48.61	127.85	135.15	1869	49.01	128.89	134.11	1855
263.5	47.72	125.73	137.77	1905	48.11	126.77	136.73	1891	48.50	127.81	135.69	1877	48.90	128.85	134.65	1862
264	47.61	125.69	138.31	1913	48.00	126.73	137.27	1898	48.40	127.77	136.23	1884	48.79	128.80	135.20	1870
264.5	47.51	125.65	138.85	1920	47.90	126.69	137.81	1906	48.29	127.73	136.77	1892	48.68	128.76	135.74	1877
265	47.40	125.61	139.39	1928	47.79	126.65	138.35	1913	48.18	127.69	137.32	1899	48.57	128.72	136.28	1885
265.5	47.30	125.57	139.93	1935	47.69	126.61	138.89	1921	48.08	127.64	137.86	1907	48.47	128.68	136.82	1892
266	47.19	125.53	140.47	1943	47.58	126.57	139.43	1928	47.97	127.60	138.40	1914	48.36	128.64	137.36	1900
266.5	47.09	125.49	141.01	1950	47.48	126.52	139.98	1936	47.87	127.56	138.94	1922	48.25	128.60	137.90	1907
267	46.98	125.45	141.55	1958	47.37	126.48	140.52	1943	47.76	127.52	139.48	1929	48.15	128.56	138.44	1915
267.5	46.88	125.41	142.10	1965	47.27	126.44	141.06	1951	47.66	127.48	140.02	1936	48.04	128.52	138.98	1922
268	46.78	125.36	142.64	1973	47.16	126.40	141.60	1958	47.55	127.44	140.56	1944	47.94	128.48	139.52	1930
268.5	46.68	125.32	143.18	1980	47.06	126.36	142.14	1966	47.45	127.40	141.10	1951	47.83	128.44	140.06	1937
269	46.57	125.28	143.72	1988	46.96	126.32	142.68	1973	47.34	127.36	141.64	1959	47.73	128.39	140.61	1945
269.5	46.47	125.24	144.26	1995	46.86	126.28	143.22	1981·	47.24	127.32	142.18	1966	47.63	128.35	141.15	1952
270	46.37	125.20	144.80	2003	46.75	126.24	143.76	1988	47.14	127.28	142.73	1974	47.52	128.31	141.69	1960
270.5	46.27	125.16	145.34	2010	46.65	126.20	144.30	1996	47.04	127.23	143.27	1981	47.42	128.27	142.23	1967
271	46.17	125.12	145.88	2018	46.55	126.16	144.84	2003	46.93	127.19	143.81	1989	47.32	128.23	142.77	1975
271.5	46.07	125.08	146.42	2025	46.45	126.11	145.39	2011	46.83	127.15	144.35	1996	47.22	128.19	143.31	1982
272	45.97	125.04	146.96	2033	46.35	126.07	145.93	2018	46.73	127.11	144.89	2004	47.11	128.15	143.85	1989
272.5	45.87	125.00	147.51	2040	46.25	126.03	146.47	2026	46.63	127.07	145.43	2011	47.01	128.11	144.39	1997
273	45.77	124.95	148.05	2047	46.15	125.99	147.01	2033	46.53	127.03	145.97	2019	46.91	128.07	144.93	2004
273.5	45.67	124.91	148.59	2055	46.05	125.95	147.55	2041	46.43	126.99	146.51	2026	46.81	128.03	145.47	2012
274	45.57	124.87	149.13	2062	45.95	125.91	148.09	2048	46.33	126.95	147.05	2034	46.71	127.98	146.02	2019
274.5	45.48	124.83	149.67	2070	45.85	125.87	148.63	2056	46.23	126.91	147.59	2041	46.61	127.94	146.56	2027
275	45.38	124.79	150.21	2077	45.76	125.83	149.17	2063	46.13	126.87	148.14	2049	46.51	127.90	147.10	2034
275.5	45.28	124.75	150.75	2085	45.66	125.79	149.71	2071	46.03	126.82	148.68	2056	46.41	127.86	147.64	2042
276	45.18	124.71	151.29	2092	45.56	125.75	150.25	2078	45.94	126.78	149.22	2064	46.31	127.82	148.18	2049
276.5	45.09	124.67	151.83	2100	45.46	125.70	150.80	2086	45.84	126.74	149.76	2071	46.21	127.78	148.72	2057
277	44.99	124.63	152.37	2107	45.37	125.66	151.34	2093	45.74	126.70	150.30	2079	46.11	127.74	149.26	2064
277.5	44.90	124.59	152.92	2115	45.27	125.62	151.88	2100	45.64	126.66	150.84	2086	46.02	127.70	149.80	2072
278	44.80	124.54	153.46	2122	45.17	125.58	152.42	2108	45.55	126.62	151.38	2094	45.92	127.66	150.34	2079
278.5	44.70	124.50	154.00	2130	45.08	125.54	152.96	2115	45.45	126.58	151.92	2101	45.82	127.62	150.88	2087
279	44.61	124.46	154.54	2137	44.98	125.50	153.50	2123	45.35	126.54	152.46	2109	45.73	127.57	151.43	2094
279.5	44.52	124.42	155.08	2145	44.89	125.46	154.04	2130	45.26	126.50	153.00	2116	45.63	127.53	151.97	2102
280	44.42	124.38	155.62	2152	44.79	125.42	154.58	2138	45.16	126.46	153.55	2124	45.53	127.49	152.51	2109
280.5	44.33	124.34	156.16	2160	44.70	125.38	155.12	2145	45.07	126.41	154.09	2131	45.44	127.45	153.05	2117
281	44.23	124.30	156.70	2167	44.60	125.34	155.66	2153	44.97	126.37	154.63	2138	45.34	127.41	153.59	2124
281.5	44.14	124.26	157.24	2175	44.51	125.29	156.21	2160	44.88	126.33	155.17	2146	45.25	127.37	154.13	2132
282	44.05	124.22	157.78	2182	44.42	125.25	156.75	2168	44.78	126.29	155.71	2153	45.15	127.33	154.67	2139
282.5	43.96	124.18	158.33	2190	44.32	125.21	157.29	2175	44.69	126.25	156.25	2161	45.06	127.29	155.21	2147
283	43.86	124.13	158.87	2197	44.23	125.17	157.83	2183	44.60	126.21	156.79	2168	44.96	127.25	155.75	2154
283.5	43.77	124.09	159.41	2205	44.14	125.13	158.37	2190	44.50	126.17	157.33	2176	44.87	127.21	156.29	2162
284	43.68	124.05	159.95	2212	44.05	125.09	158.91	2198	44.41	126.13	157.87	2183	44.78	127.16	156.84	2169
284.5	43.59	124.01	160.49	2220	43.95	125.05	159.45	2205	44.32	126.09	158.41	2191	44.68	127.12	157.38	2177
285	43.50	123.97	161.03	2227	43.86	125.01	159.99	2213	44.23	126.05	158.96	2198	44.59	127.08	157.92	2184
285.5	43.41	123.93	161.57	2235	43.77	124.97	160.53	2220	44.13	126.00	159.50	2206	44.50	127.04	158.46	2191
286	43.32	123.89	162.11	2242	43.68	124.93	161.07	2228	44.04	125.96	160.04	2213	44.41	127.00	159.00	2199
286.5	43.23	123.85	162.65	2249	43.59	124.88	161.62	2235	43.95	125.92	160.58	2221	44.31	126.96	159.54	2206
287	43.14	123.81	163.19	2257	43.50	124.84	162.16	2243	43.86	125.88	161.12	2228	44.22	126.92	160.08	2214
287.5	43.05	123.77	163.74	2264	43.41	124.80	162.70	2250	43.77	125.84	161.66	2236	44.13	126.88	160.62	2221
288	42.96	123.72	164.28	2272	43.32	124.76	163.24	2258	43.68	125.80	162.20	2243	44.04	126.84	161.16	2229
288.5	42.87	123.68	164.82	2279	43.23	124.72	163.78	2265	43.59	125.76	162.74	2251	43.95	126.80	161.70	2236
289	42.78	123.64	165.36	2287	43.14	124.68	164.32	2273	43.50	125.72	163.28	2258	43.86	126.75	162.25	2244
289.5	42.69	123.60	165.90	2294	43.05	124.64	164.86	2280	43.41	125.68	163.82	2266	43.77	126.71	162.79	2251
290	42.61	123.56	166.44	2302	42.96	124.60	165.40	2288	43.32	125.64	164.37	2273	43.68	126.67	163.33	2259
290.5	42.52	123.52	166.98	2309	42.88	124.56	165.94	2295	43.23	125.59	164.91	2281	43.59	126.63	163.87	2266
291	42.43	123.48	167.52	2317	42.79	124.52	166.48	2302	43.15	125.55	165.45	2288	43.50	126.59	164.41	2274
291.5	42.35	123.44	168.06	2324	42.70	124.47	167.03	2310	43.06	125.51	165.99	2296	43.41	126.55	164.95	2281

Body Composition FEMALE 260-291.5 Lb.

Weight: Lb.	Waist: 55 inches Fat: %	Fat: Lb.	LBM: Lb.	RMR: Cal.	55.25 inches Fat: %	Fat: Lb.	LBM: Lb.	RMR: Cal.	55.5 inches Fat: %	Fat: Lb.	LBM: Lb.	RMR: Cal.	55.75 inches Fat: %	Fat: Lb.	LBM: Lb.	RMR: Cal.
260	50.07	130.17	129.83	1796	50.46	131.21	128.79	1781	50.86	132.25	127.76	1767	51.26	133.28	126.72	1753
260.5	49.95	130.13	130.37	1803	50.35	131.17	129.33	1789	50.75	132.20	128.30	1774	51.15	133.24	127.26	1760
261	49.84	130.09	130.91	1811	50.24	131.13	129.87	1796	50.64	132.16	128.84	1782	51.03	133.20	127.80	1767
261.5	49.73	130.05	131.45	1818	50.13	131.08	130.42	1804	50.52	132.12	129.38	1789	50.92	133.16	128.34	1775
262	49.62	130.01	131.99	1825	50.02	131.04	130.96	1811	50.41	132.08	129.92	1797	50.81	133.12	128.88	1782
262.5	49.51	129.97	132.54	1833	49.91	131.00	131.50	1819	50.30	132.04	130.46	1804	50.70	133.08	129.42	1790
263	49.40	129.92	133.08	1840	49.80	130.96	132.04	1826	50.19	132.00	131.00	1812	50.58	133.04	129.96	1797
263.5	49.29	129.88	133.62	1848	49.69	130.92	132.58	1834	50.08	131.96	131.54	1819	50.47	133.00	130.50	1805
264	49.18	129.84	134.16	1855	49.58	130.88	133.12	1841	49.97	131.92	132.08	1827	50.36	132.95	131.05	1812
264.5	49.07	129.80	134.70	1863	49.47	130.84	133.66	1849	49.86	131.88	132.62	1834	50.25	132.91	131.59	1820
265	48.97	129.76	135.24	1870	49.36	130.80	134.20	1856	49.75	131.84	133.17	1842	50.14	132.87	132.13	1827
265.5	48.86	129.72	135.78	1878	49.25	130.76	134.74	1864	49.64	131.79	133.71	1849	50.03	132.83	132.67	1835
266	48.75	129.68	136.32	1885	49.14	130.72	135.28	1871	49.53	131.75	134.25	1857	49.92	132.79	133.21	1842
266.5	48.64	129.64	136.86	1893	49.03	130.67	135.83	1878	49.42	131.71	134.79	1864	49.81	132.75	133.75	1850
267	48.54	129.60	137.40	1900	48.93	130.63	136.37	1886	49.31	131.67	135.33	1872	49.70	132.71	134.29	1857
267.5	48.43	129.56	137.95	1908	48.82	130.59	136.91	1893	49.21	131.63	135.87	1879	49.60	132.67	134.83	1865
268	48.33	129.51	138.49	1915	48.71	130.55	137.45	1901	49.10	131.59	136.41	1887	49.49	132.63	135.37	1872
268.5	48.22	129.47	139.03	1923	48.61	130.51	137.99	1908	48.99	131.55	136.95	1894	49.38	132.59	135.91	1880
269	48.12	129.43	139.57	1930	48.50	130.47	138.53	1916	48.89	131.51	137.49	1902	49.27	132.54	136.46	1887
269.5	48.01	129.39	140.11	1938	48.40	130.43	139.07	1923	48.78	131.47	138.03	1909	49.17	132.50	137.00	1895
270	47.91	129.35	140.65	1945	48.29	130.39	139.61	1931	48.68	131.43	138.58	1916	49.06	132.46	137.54	1902
270.5	47.80	129.31	141.19	1953	48.19	130.35	140.15	1938	48.57	131.38	139.12	1924	48.95	132.42	138.08	1910
271	47.70	129.27	141.73	1960	48.08	130.31	140.69	1946	48.47	131.34	139.66	1931	48.85	132.38	138.62	1917
271.5	47.60	129.23	142.27	1968	47.98	130.26	141.24	1953	48.36	131.30	140.20	1939	48.74	132.34	139.16	1925
272	47.49	129.19	142.81	1975	47.88	130.22	141.78	1961	48.26	131.26	140.74	1946	48.64	132.30	139.70	1932
272.5	47.39	129.15	143.36	1983	47.77	130.18	142.32	1968	48.15	131.22	141.28	1954	48.53	132.26	140.24	1940
273	47.29	129.10	143.90	1990	47.67	130.14	142.86	1976	48.05	131.18	141.82	1961	48.43	132.22	140.78	1947
273.5	47.19	129.06	144.44	1998	47.57	130.10	143.40	1983	47.95	131.14	142.36	1969	48.33	132.18	141.32	1955
274	47.09	129.02	144.98	2005	47.47	130.06	143.94	1991	47.85	131.10	142.90	1976	48.22	132.13	141.87	1962
274.5	46.99	128.98	145.52	2013	47.37	130.02	144.48	1998	47.74	131.06	143.44	1984	48.12	132.09	142.41	1969
275	46.89	128.94	146.06	2020	47.26	129.98	145.02	2006	47.64	131.02	143.99	1991	48.02	132.05	142.95	1977
275.5	46.79	128.90	146.60	2027	47.16	129.94	145.56	2013	47.54	130.97	144.53	1999	47.92	132.01	143.49	1984
276	46.69	128.86	147.14	2035	47.06	129.90	146.10	2021	47.44	130.93	145.07	2006	47.82	131.97	144.03	1992
276.5	46.59	128.82	147.68	2042	46.96	129.85	146.65	2028	47.34	130.89	145.61	2014	47.71	131.93	144.57	1999
277	46.49	128.78	148.22	2050	46.86	129.81	147.19	2036	47.24	130.85	146.15	2021	47.61	131.89	145.11	2007
277.5	46.39	128.74	148.77	2057	46.76	129.77	147.73	2043	47.14	130.81	146.69	2029	47.51	131.85	145.65	2014
278	46.29	128.69	149.31	2065	46.67	129.73	148.27	2051	47.04	130.77	147.23	2036	47.41	131.81	146.19	2022
278.5	46.19	128.65	149.85	2072	46.57	129.69	148.81	2058	46.94	130.73	147.77	2044	47.31	131.77	146.73	2029
279	46.10	128.61	150.39	2080	46.47	129.65	149.35	2066	46.84	130.69	148.31	2051	47.21	131.72	147.28	2037
279.5	46.00	128.57	150.93	2087	46.37	129.61	149.89	2073	46.74	130.65	148.85	2059	47.11	131.68	147.82	2044
280	45.90	128.53	151.47	2095	46.27	129.57	150.43	2080	46.64	130.61	149.40	2066	47.02	131.64	148.36	2052
280.5	45.81	128.49	152.01	2102	46.18	129.53	150.97	2088	46.55	130.56	149.94	2074	46.92	131.60	148.90	2059
281	45.71	128.45	152.55	2110	46.08	129.49	151.51	2095	46.45	130.52	150.48	2081	46.82	131.56	149.44	2067
281.5	45.62	128.41	153.09	2117	45.98	129.44	152.06	2103	46.35	130.48	151.02	2089	46.72	131.52	149.98	2074
282	45.52	128.37	153.63	2125	45.89	129.40	152.60	2110	46.26	130.44	151.56	2096	46.62	131.48	150.52	2082
282.5	45.42	128.33	154.18	2132	45.79	129.36	153.14	2118	46.16	130.40	152.10	2104	46.53	131.44	151.06	2089
283	45.33	128.28	154.72	2140	45.70	129.32	153.68	2125	46.06	130.36	152.64	2111	46.43	131.40	151.60	2097
283.5	45.24	128.24	155.26	2147	45.60	129.28	154.22	2133	45.97	130.32	153.18	2119	46.33	131.36	152.14	2104
284	45.14	128.20	155.80	2155	45.51	129.24	154.76	2140	45.87	130.28	153.72	2126	46.24	131.31	152.69	2112
284.5	45.05	128.16	156.34	2162	45.41	129.20	155.30	2148	45.78	130.24	154.26	2133	46.14	131.27	153.23	2119
285	44.95	128.12	156.88	2170	45.32	129.16	155.84	2155	45.68	130.20	154.81	2141	46.05	131.23	153.77	2127
285.5	44.86	128.08	157.42	2177	45.22	129.12	156.38	2163	45.59	130.15	155.35	2148	45.95	131.19	154.31	2134
286	44.77	128.04	157.96	2185	45.13	129.08	156.92	2170	45.49	130.11	155.89	2156	45.86	131.15	154.85	2142
286.5	44.68	128.00	158.50	2192	45.04	129.03	157.47	2178	45.40	130.07	156.43	2163	45.76	131.11	155.39	2149
287	44.58	127.96	159.04	2200	44.95	128.99	158.01	2185	45.31	130.03	156.97	2171	45.67	131.07	155.93	2157
287.5	44.49	127.92	159.59	2207	44.85	128.95	158.55	2193	45.21	129.99	157.51	2178	45.57	131.03	156.47	2164
288	44.40	127.87	160.13	2215	44.76	128.91	159.09	2200	45.12	129.95	158.05	2186	45.48	130.99	157.01	2171
288.5	44.31	127.83	160.67	2222	44.67	128.87	159.63	2208	45.03	129.91	158.59	2193	45.39	130.95	157.55	2179
289	44.22	127.79	161.21	2230	44.58	128.83	160.17	2215	44.94	129.87	159.13	2201	45.30	130.90	158.10	2186
289.5	44.13	127.75	161.75	2237	44.49	128.79	160.71	2223	44.84	129.83	159.67	2208	45.20	130.86	158.64	2194
290	44.04	127.71	162.29	2244	44.40	128.75	161.25	2230	44.75	129.79	160.22	2216	45.11	130.82	159.18	2201
290.5	43.95	127.67	162.83	2252	44.31	128.71	161.79	2238	44.66	129.74	160.76	2223	45.02	130.78	159.72	2209
291	43.86	127.63	163.37	2259	44.21	128.67	162.33	2245	44.57	129.70	161.30	2231	44.93	130.74	160.26	2216
291.5	43.77	127.59	163.91	2267	44.13	128.62	162.88	2253	44.48	129.66	161.84	2238	44.84	130.70	160.80	2224

Body Composition FEMALE 260-291.5 Lb.

Weight: Lb.	Waist: 56 inches				56.25 inches				56.5 inches				56.75 inches			
	Fat: %	Fat: Lb.	LBM: Lb.	RMR: Cal.	Fat: %	Fat: Lb.	LBM: Lb.	RMR: Cal.	Fat: %	Fat: Lb.	LBM: Lb.	RMR: Cal.	Fat: %	Fat: Lb.	LBM: Lb.	RMR: Cal.
260	51.66	134.32	125.68	1738	52.06	135.36	124.64	1724	52.46	136.40	123.61	1709	52.86	137.43	122.57	1695
260.5	51.55	134.28	126.22	1746	51.94	135.32	125.18	1731	52.34	136.35	124.15	1717	52.74	137.39	123.11	1703
261	51.43	134.24	126.76	1753	51.83	135.28	125.72	1739	52.23	136.31	124.69	1724	52.62	137.35	123.65	1710
261.5	51.32	134.20	127.30	1761	51.71	135.23	126.27	1746	52.11	136.27	125.23	1732	52.51	137.31	124.19	1718
262	51.20	134.16	127.84	1768	51.60	135.19	126.81	1754	52.00	136.23	125.77	1739	52.39	137.27	124.73	1725
262.5	51.09	134.12	128.39	1776	51.49	135.15	127.35	1761	51.88	136.19	126.31	1747	52.28	137.23	125.27	1733
263	50.98	134.07	128.93	1783	51.37	135.11	127.89	1769	51.77	136.15	126.85	1754	52.16	137.19	125.81	1740
263.5	50.87	134.03	129.47	1791	51.26	135.07	128.43	1776	51.65	136.11	127.39	1762	52.05	137.15	126.35	1747
264	50.75	133.99	130.01	1798	51.15	135.03	128.97	1784	51.54	136.07	127.93	1769	51.93	137.10	126.90	1755
264.5	50.64	133.95	130.55	1805	51.04	134.99	129.51	1791	51.43	136.03	128.47	1777	51.82	137.06	127.44	1762
265	50.53	133.91	131.09	1813	50.92	134.95	130.05	1799	51.32	135.99	129.02	1784	51.71	137.02	127.98	1770
265.5	50.42	133.87	131.63	1820	50.81	134.91	130.59	1806	51.20	135.94	129.56	1792	51.59	136.98	128.52	1777
266	50.31	133.83	132.17	1828	50.70	134.87	131.13	1814	51.09	135.90	130.10	1799	51.48	136.94	129.06	1785
266.5	50.20	133.79	132.71	1835	50.59	134.82	131.68	1821	50.98	135.86	130.64	1807	51.37	136.90	129.60	1792
267	50.09	133.75	133.25	1843	50.48	134.78	132.22	1829	50.87	135.82	131.18	1814	51.26	136.86	130.14	1800
267.5	49.98	133.71	133.80	1850	50.37	134.74	132.76	1836	50.76	135.78	131.72	1822	51.15	136.82	130.68	1807
268	49.87	133.66	134.34	1858	50.26	134.70	133.30	1844	50.65	135.74	132.26	1829	51.04	136.78	131.22	1815
268.5	49.77	133.62	134.88	1865	50.15	134.66	133.84	1851	50.54	135.70	132.80	1837	50.93	136.74	131.76	1822
269	49.66	133.58	135.42	1873	50.04	134.62	134.38	1858	50.43	135.66	133.34	1844	50.82	136.69	132.31	1830
269.5	49.55	133.54	135.96	1880	49.94	134.58	134.92	1866	50.32	135.62	133.88	1852	50.71	136.65	132.85	1837
270	49.44	133.50	136.50	1888	49.83	134.54	135.46	1873	50.21	135.58	134.43	1859	50.60	136.61	133.39	1845
270.5	49.34	133.46	137.04	1895	49.72	134.50	136.00	1881	50.10	135.53	134.97	1867	50.49	136.57	133.93	1852
271	49.23	133.42	137.58	1903	49.61	134.46	136.54	1888	50.00	135.49	135.51	1874	50.38	136.53	134.47	1860
271.5	49.13	133.38	138.12	1910	49.51	134.41	137.09	1896	49.89	135.45	136.05	1882	50.27	136.49	135.01	1867
272	49.02	133.34	138.66	1918	49.40	134.37	137.63	1903	49.78	135.41	136.59	1889	50.16	136.45	135.55	1875
272.5	48.92	133.30	139.21	1925	49.30	134.33	138.17	1911	49.68	135.37	137.13	1897	50.06	136.41	136.09	1882
273	48.81	133.25	139.75	1933	49.19	134.29	138.71	1918	49.57	135.33	137.67	1904	49.95	136.37	136.63	1890
273.5	48.71	133.21	140.29	1940	49.09	134.25	139.25	1926	49.47	135.29	138.21	1911	49.84	136.33	137.17	1897
274	48.60	133.17	140.83	1948	48.98	134.21	139.79	1933	49.36	135.25	138.75	1919	49.74	136.28	137.72	1905
274.5	48.50	133.13	141.37	1955	48.88	134.17	140.33	1941	49.26	135.21	139.29	1926	49.63	136.24	138.26	1912
275	48.40	133.09	141.91	1963	48.77	134.13	140.87	1948	49.15	135.17	139.84	1934	49.53	136.20	138.80	1920
275.5	48.29	133.05	142.45	1970	48.67	134.09	141.41	1956	49.05	135.12	140.38	1941	49.42	136.16	139.34	1927
276	48.19	133.01	142.99	1978	48.57	134.05	141.95	1963	48.94	135.08	140.92	1949	49.32	136.12	139.88	1935
276.5	48.09	132.97	143.53	1985	48.46	134.00	142.50	1971	48.84	135.04	141.46	1956	49.22	136.08	140.42	1942
277	47.99	132.93	144.07	1993	48.36	133.96	143.04	1978	48.74	135.00	142.00	1964	49.11	136.04	140.96	1949
277.5	47.89	132.89	144.62	2000	48.26	133.92	143.58	1986	48.63	134.96	142.54	1971	49.01	136.00	141.50	1957
278	47.79	132.84	145.16	2008	48.16	133.88	144.12	1993	48.53	134.92	143.08	1979	48.91	135.96	142.04	1964
278.5	47.69	132.80	145.70	2015	48.06	133.84	144.66	2001	48.43	134.88	143.62	1986	48.80	135.92	142.58	1972
279	47.58	132.76	146.24	2022	47.96	133.80	145.20	2008	48.33	134.84	144.16	1994	48.70	135.87	143.13	1979
279.5	47.49	132.72	146.78	2030	47.86	133.76	145.74	2016	48.23	134.80	144.70	2001	48.60	135.83	143.67	1987
280	47.39	132.68	147.32	2037	47.76	133.72	146.28	2023	48.13	134.76	145.25	2009	48.50	135.79	144.21	1994
280.5	47.29	132.64	147.86	2045	47.66	133.68	146.82	2031	48.03	134.71	145.79	2016	48.40	135.75	144.75	2002
281	47.19	132.60	148.40	2052	47.56	133.64	147.36	2038	47.93	134.67	146.33	2024	48.30	135.71	145.29	2009
281.5	47.09	132.56	148.94	2060	47.46	133.59	147.91	2046	47.83	134.63	146.87	2031	48.20	135.67	145.83	2017
282	46.99	132.52	149.48	2067	47.36	133.55	148.45	2053	47.73	134.59	147.41	2039	48.10	135.63	146.37	2024
282.5	46.89	132.48	150.03	2075	47.26	133.51	148.99	2060	47.63	134.55	147.95	2046	48.00	135.59	146.91	2032
283	46.80	132.43	150.57	2082	47.16	133.47	149.53	2068	47.53	134.51	148.49	2054	47.90	135.55	147.45	2039
283.5	46.70	132.39	151.11	2090	47.07	133.43	150.07	2075	47.43	134.47	149.03	2061	47.80	135.51	147.99	2047
284	46.60	132.35	151.65	2097	46.97	133.39	150.61	2083	47.33	134.43	149.57	2069	47.70	135.46	148.54	2054
284.5	46.51	132.31	152.19	2105	46.87	133.35	151.15	2090	47.24	134.39	150.11	2076	47.60	135.42	149.08	2062
285	46.41	132.27	152.73	2112	46.77	133.31	151.69	2098	47.14	134.35	150.66	2084	47.50	135.38	149.62	2069
285.5	46.31	132.23	153.27	2120	46.68	133.27	152.23	2105	47.04	134.30	151.20	2091	47.41	135.34	150.16	2077
286	46.22	132.19	153.81	2127	46.58	133.23	152.77	2113	46.95	134.26	151.74	2099	47.31	135.30	150.70	2084
286.5	46.12	132.15	154.35	2135	46.49	133.18	153.32	2120	46.85	134.22	152.28	2106	47.21	135.26	151.24	2092
287	46.03	132.11	154.89	2142	46.39	133.14	153.86	2128	46.75	134.18	152.82	2113	47.11	135.22	151.78	2099
287.5	45.94	132.07	155.44	2150	46.30	133.10	154.40	2135	46.66	134.14	153.36	2121	47.02	135.18	152.32	2107
288	45.84	132.02	155.98	2157	46.20	133.06	154.94	2143	46.56	134.10	153.90	2128	46.92	135.14	152.86	2114
288.5	45.75	131.98	156.52	2165	46.11	133.02	155.48	2150	46.47	134.06	154.44	2136	46.83	135.10	153.40	2122
289	45.65	131.94	157.06	2172	46.01	132.98	156.02	2158	46.37	134.02	154.98	2143	46.73	135.05	153.95	2129
289.5	45.56	131.90	157.60	2180	45.92	132.94	156.56	2165	46.28	133.98	155.52	2151	46.64	135.01	154.49	2137
290	45.47	131.86	158.14	2187	45.83	132.90	157.10	2173	46.18	133.94	156.07	2158	46.54	134.97	155.03	2144
290.5	45.38	131.82	158.68	2195	45.73	132.86	157.64	2180	46.09	133.89	156.61	2166	46.45	134.93	155.57	2152
291	45.28	131.78	159.22	2202	45.64	132.82	158.18	2188	46.00	133.85	157.15	2173	46.35	134.89	156.11	2159
291.5	45.19	131.74	159.76	2210	45.55	132.77	158.73	2195	45.90	133.81	157.69	2181	46.26	134.85	156.65	2166

Body Composition FEMALE 260-291.5 Lb.

Weight: Lb.	Waist: 57 inches Fat: %	Fat: Lb.	LBM: Lb.	RMR: Cal.	57.25 inches Fat: %	Fat: Lb.	LBM: Lb.	RMR: Cal.	57.5 inches Fat: %	Fat: Lb.	LBM: Lb.	RMR: Cal.	57.75 inches Fat: %	Fat: Lb.	LBM: Lb.	RMR: Cal.
260	53.26	138.47	121.53	1681	53.66	139.51	120.49	1666	54.06	140.55	119.46	1652	54.45	141.58	118.42	1638
260.5	53.14	138.43	122.07	1688	53.54	139.47	121.03	1674	53.94	140.50	120.00	1660	54.33	141.54	118.96	1645
261	53.02	138.39	122.61	1696	53.42	139.43	121.57	1681	53.82	140.46	120.54	1667	54.21	141.50	119.50	1653
261.5	52.91	138.35	123.15	1703	53.30	139.38	122.12	1689	53.70	140.42	121.08	1675	54.10	141.46	120.04	1660
262	52.79	138.31	123.69	1711	53.18	139.34	122.66	1696	53.58	140.38	121.62	1682	53.98	141.42	120.58	1668
262.5	52.67	138.27	124.24	1718	53.07	139.30	123.20	1704	53.46	140.34	122.16	1689	53.86	141.38	121.12	1675
263	52.56	138.22	124.78	1726	52.95	139.26	123.74	1711	53.35	140.30	122.70	1697	53.74	141.34	121.66	1683
263.5	52.44	138.18	125.32	1733	52.84	139.22	124.28	1719	53.23	140.26	123.24	1704	53.62	141.30	122.20	1690
264	52.33	138.14	125.86	1741	52.72	139.18	124.82	1726	53.11	140.22	123.78	1712	53.51	141.25	122.75	1698
264.5	52.21	138.10	126.40	1748	52.60	139.14	125.36	1734	53.00	140.18	124.32	1719	53.39	141.21	123.29	1705
265	52.10	138.06	126.94	1756	52.49	139.10	125.90	1741	52.88	140.14	124.87	1727	53.27	141.17	123.83	1713
265.5	51.98	138.02	127.48	1763	52.38	139.06	126.44	1749	52.77	140.09	125.41	1734	53.16	141.13	124.37	1720
266	51.87	137.98	128.02	1771	52.26	139.02	126.98	1756	52.65	140.05	125.95	1742	53.04	141.09	124.91	1727
266.5	51.76	137.94	128.56	1778	52.15	138.97	127.53	1764	52.54	140.01	126.49	1749	52.93	141.05	125.45	1735
267	51.65	137.90	129.10	1786	52.04	138.93	128.07	1771	52.42	139.97	127.03	1757	52.81	141.01	125.99	1742
267.5	51.53	137.86	129.65	1793	51.92	138.89	128.61	1779	52.31	139.93	127.57	1764	52.70	140.97	126.53	1750
268	51.42	137.81	130.19	1800	51.81	138.85	129.15	1786	52.20	139.89	128.11	1772	52.58	140.93	127.07	1757
268.5	51.31	137.77	130.73	1808	51.70	138.81	129.69	1794	52.08	139.85	128.65	1779	52.47	140.89	127.61	1765
269	51.20	137.73	131.27	1815	51.59	138.77	130.23	1801	51.97	139.81	129.19	1787	52.36	140.84	128.16	1772
269.5	51.09	137.69	131.81	1823	51.48	138.73	130.77	1809	51.86	139.77	129.73	1794	52.25	140.80	128.70	1780
270	50.98	137.65	132.35	1830	51.37	138.69	131.31	1816	51.75	139.73	130.28	1802	52.13	140.76	129.24	1787
270.5	50.87	137.61	132.89	1838	51.26	138.65	131.85	1824	51.64	139.68	130.82	1809	52.02	140.72	129.78	1795
271	50.76	137.57	133.43	1845	51.15	138.61	132.39	1831	51.53	139.64	131.36	1817	51.91	140.68	130.32	1802
271.5	50.65	137.53	133.97	1853	51.04	138.56	132.94	1838	51.42	139.60	131.90	1824	51.80	140.64	130.86	1810
272	50.55	137.49	134.51	1860	50.93	138.52	133.48	1846	51.31	139.56	132.44	1832	51.69	140.60	131.40	1817
272.5	50.44	137.45	135.06	1868	50.82	138.48	134.02	1853	51.20	139.52	132.98	1839	51.58	140.56	131.94	1825
273	50.33	137.40	135.60	1875	50.71	138.44	134.56	1861	51.09	139.48	133.52	1847	51.47	140.52	132.48	1832
273.5	50.22	137.36	136.14	1883	50.60	138.40	135.10	1868	50.98	139.44	134.06	1854	51.36	140.48	133.02	1840
274	50.12	137.32	136.68	1890	50.50	138.36	135.64	1876	50.87	139.40	134.60	1862	51.25	140.43	133.57	1847
274.5	50.01	137.28	137.22	1898	50.39	138.32	136.18	1883	50.77	139.36	135.14	1869	51.15	140.39	134.11	1855
275	49.91	137.24	137.76	1905	50.28	138.28	136.72	1891	50.66	139.32	135.69	1877	51.04	140.35	134.65	1862
275.5	49.80	137.20	138.30	1913	50.18	138.24	137.26	1898	50.55	139.27	136.23	1884	50.93	140.31	135.19	1870
276	49.69	137.16	138.84	1920	50.07	138.20	137.80	1906	50.45	139.23	136.77	1891	50.82	140.27	135.73	1877
276.5	49.59	137.12	139.38	1928	49.97	138.15	138.35	1913	50.34	139.19	137.31	1899	50.72	140.23	136.27	1885
277	49.49	137.08	139.92	1935	49.86	138.11	138.89	1921	50.24	139.15	137.85	1906	50.61	140.19	136.81	1892
277.5	49.38	137.04	140.47	1943	49.76	138.07	139.43	1928	50.13	139.11	138.39	1914	50.50	140.15	137.35	1900
278	49.28	136.99	141.01	1950	49.65	138.03	139.97	1936	50.02	139.07	138.93	1921	50.40	140.11	137.89	1907
278.5	49.18	136.95	141.55	1958	49.55	137.99	140.51	1943	49.92	139.03	139.47	1929	50.29	140.07	138.43	1915
279	49.07	136.91	142.09	1965	49.44	137.95	141.05	1951	49.82	138.99	140.01	1936	50.19	140.02	138.98	1922
279.5	48.97	136.87	142.63	1973	49.34	137.91	141.59	1958	49.71	138.95	140.55	1944	50.08	139.98	139.52	1930
280	48.87	136.83	143.17	1980	49.24	137.87	142.13	1966	49.61	138.91	141.10	1951	49.98	139.94	140.06	1937
280.5	48.77	136.79	143.71	1988	49.14	137.83	142.67	1973	49.51	138.86	141.64	1959	49.88	139.90	140.60	1944
281	48.66	136.75	144.25	1995	49.03	137.79	143.21	1981	49.40	138.82	142.18	1966	49.77	139.86	141.14	1952
281.5	48.56	136.71	144.79	2002	48.93	137.74	143.76	1988	49.30	138.78	142.72	1974	49.67	139.82	141.68	1959
282	48.46	136.67	145.33	2010	48.83	137.70	144.30	1996	49.20	138.74	143.26	1981	49.57	139.78	142.22	1967
282.5	48.36	136.63	145.88	2017	48.73	137.66	144.84	2003	49.10	138.70	143.80	1989	49.46	139.74	142.76	1974
283	48.26	136.58	146.42	2025	48.63	137.62	145.38	2011	49.00	138.66	144.34	1996	49.36	139.70	143.30	1982
283.5	48.16	136.54	146.96	2032	48.53	137.58	145.92	2018	48.90	138.62	144.88	2004	49.26	139.66	143.84	1989
284	48.06	136.50	147.50	2040	48.43	137.54	146.46	2026	48.79	138.58	145.42	2011	49.16	139.61	144.39	1997
284.5	47.97	136.46	148.04	2047	48.33	137.50	147.00	2033	48.69	138.54	145.96	2019	49.06	139.57	144.93	2004
285	47.87	136.42	148.58	2055	48.23	137.46	147.54	2041	48.59	138.50	146.51	2026	48.96	139.53	145.47	2012
285.5	47.77	136.38	149.12	2062	48.13	137.42	148.08	2048	48.50	138.45	147.05	2034	48.86	139.49	146.01	2019
286	47.67	136.34	149.66	2070	48.03	137.38	148.62	2055	48.40	138.41	147.59	2041	48.76	139.45	146.55	2027
286.5	47.57	136.30	150.20	2077	47.94	137.33	149.17	2063	48.30	138.37	148.13	2049	48.66	139.41	147.09	2034
287	47.48	136.26	150.74	2085	47.84	137.29	149.71	2070	48.20	138.33	148.67	2056	48.56	139.37	147.63	2042
287.5	47.38	136.22	151.29	2092	47.74	137.25	150.25	2078	48.10	138.29	149.21	2064	48.46	139.33	148.17	2049
288	47.28	136.17	151.83	2100	47.64	137.21	150.79	2085	48.00	138.25	149.75	2071	48.36	139.29	148.71	2057
288.5	47.19	136.13	152.37	2107	47.55	137.17	151.33	2093	47.91	138.21	150.29	2079	48.27	139.25	149.25	2064
289	47.09	136.09	152.91	2115	47.45	137.13	151.87	2100	47.81	138.17	150.83	2086	48.17	139.20	149.80	2072
289.5	47.00	136.05	153.45	2122	47.35	137.09	152.41	2108	47.71	138.13	151.37	2094	48.07	139.16	150.34	2079
290	46.90	136.01	153.99	2130	47.26	137.05	152.95	2115	47.62	138.09	151.92	2101	47.97	139.12	150.88	2087
290.5	46.81	135.97	154.53	2137	47.16	137.01	153.49	2123	47.52	138.04	152.46	2108	47.88	139.08	151.42	2094
291	46.71	135.93	155.07	2145	47.07	136.97	154.03	2130	47.42	138.00	153.00	2116	47.78	139.04	151.96	2102
291.5	46.62	135.89	155.61	2152	46.97	136.92	154.58	2138	47.33	137.96	153.54	2123	47.68	139.00	152.50	2109

Body Composition FEMALE 260-291.5 Lb.

Weight: Lb.	Waist: 58 inches Fat: %	Fat: Lb.	LBM: Lb.	RMR: Cal.	58.25 inches Fat: %	Fat: Lb.	LBM: Lb.	RMR: Cal.	58.5 inches Fat: %	Fat: Lb.	LBM: Lb.	RMR: Cal.	58.75 inches Fat: %	Fat: Lb.	LBM: Lb.	RMR: Cal.
260	54.85	142.62	117.38	1623	55.25	143.66	116.34	1609	55.65	144.70	115.31	1595	56.05	145.73	114.27	1580
260.5	54.73	142.58	117.92	1631	55.13	143.62	116.88	1616	55.53	144.65	115.85	1602	55.93	145.69	114.81	1588
261	54.61	142.54	118.46	1638	55.01	143.58	117.42	1624	55.41	144.61	116.39	1610	55.80	145.65	115.35	1595
261.5	54.49	142.50	119.00	1646	54.89	143.53	117.97	1631	55.29	144.57	116.93	1617	55.68	145.61	115.89	1603
262	54.37	142.46	119.54	1653	54.77	143.49	118.51	1639	55.16	144.53	117.47	1625	55.56	145.57	116.43	1610
262.5	54.25	142.42	120.09	1661	54.65	143.45	119.05	1646	55.04	144.49	118.01	1632	55.44	145.53	116.97	1618
263	54.13	142.37	120.63	1668	54.53	143.41	119.59	1654	54.92	144.45	118.55	1640	55.32	145.49	117.51	1625
263.5	54.02	142.33	121.17	1676	54.41	143.37	120.13	1661	54.80	144.41	119.09	1647	55.20	145.45	118.05	1633
264	53.90	142.29	121.71	1683	54.29	143.33	120.67	1669	54.68	144.37	119.63	1655	55.08	145.40	118.60	1640
264.5	53.78	142.25	122.25	1691	54.17	143.29	121.21	1676	54.57	144.33	120.17	1662	54.96	145.36	119.14	1648
265	53.66	142.21	122.79	1698	54.06	143.25	121.75	1684	54.45	144.29	120.72	1669	54.84	145.32	119.68	1655
265.5	53.55	142.17	123.33	1706	53.94	143.21	122.29	1691	54.33	144.24	121.26	1677	54.72	145.28	120.22	1663
266	53.43	142.13	123.87	1713	53.82	143.17	122.83	1699	54.21	144.20	121.80	1684	54.60	145.24	120.76	1670
266.5	53.32	142.09	124.41	1721	53.71	143.12	123.38	1706	54.09	144.16	122.34	1692	54.48	145.20	121.30	1678
267	53.20	142.05	124.95	1728	53.59	143.08	123.92	1714	53.98	144.12	122.88	1699	54.37	145.16	121.84	1685
267.5	53.09	142.01	125.50	1736	53.47	143.04	124.46	1721	53.86	144.08	123.42	1707	54.25	145.12	122.38	1693
268	52.97	141.96	126.04	1743	53.36	143.00	125.00	1729	53.75	144.04	123.96	1714	54.13	145.08	122.92	1700
268.5	52.86	141.92	126.58	1751	53.24	142.96	125.54	1736	53.63	144.00	124.50	1722	54.02	145.04	123.46	1708
269	52.74	141.88	127.12	1758	53.13	142.92	126.08	1744	53.52	143.96	125.04	1729	53.90	144.99	124.01	1715
269.5	52.63	141.84	127.66	1766	53.02	142.88	126.62	1751	53.40	143.92	125.58	1737	53.79	144.95	124.55	1722
270	52.52	141.80	128.20	1773	52.90	142.84	127.16	1759	53.29	143.88	126.13	1744	53.67	144.91	125.09	1730
270.5	52.41	141.76	128.74	1780	52.79	142.80	127.70	1766	53.17	143.83	126.67	1752	53.56	144.87	125.63	1737
271	52.29	141.72	129.28	1788	52.68	142.76	128.24	1774	53.06	143.79	127.21	1759	53.44	144.83	126.17	1745
271.5	52.18	141.68	129.82	1795	52.57	142.71	128.79	1781	52.95	143.75	127.75	1767	53.33	144.79	126.71	1752
272	52.07	141.64	130.36	1803	52.45	142.67	129.33	1789	52.83	143.71	128.29	1774	53.22	144.75	127.25	1760
272.5	51.96	141.60	130.91	1810	52.34	142.63	129.87	1796	52.72	143.67	128.83	1782	53.10	144.71	127.79	1767
273	51.85	141.55	131.45	1818	52.23	142.59	130.41	1804	52.61	143.63	129.37	1789	52.99	144.67	128.33	1775
273.5	51.74	141.51	131.99	1825	52.12	142.55	130.95	1811	52.50	143.59	129.91	1797	52.88	144.63	128.87	1782
274	51.63	141.47	132.53	1833	52.01	142.51	131.49	1819	52.39	143.55	130.45	1804	52.77	144.58	129.42	1790
274.5	51.52	141.43	133.07	1840	51.90	142.47	132.03	1826	52.28	143.51	130.99	1812	52.66	144.54	129.96	1797
275	51.41	141.39	133.61	1848	51.79	142.43	132.57	1833	52.17	143.47	131.54	1819	52.55	144.50	130.50	1805
275.5	51.31	141.35	134.15	1855	51.68	142.39	133.11	1841	52.06	143.42	132.08	1827	52.44	144.46	131.04	1812
276	51.20	141.31	134.69	1863	51.57	142.35	133.65	1848	51.95	143.38	132.62	1834	52.33	144.42	131.58	1820
276.5	51.09	141.27	135.23	1870	51.47	142.30	134.20	1856	51.84	143.34	133.16	1842	52.22	144.38	132.12	1827
277	50.98	141.23	135.77	1878	51.36	142.26	134.74	1863	51.73	143.30	133.70	1849	52.11	144.34	132.66	1835
277.5	50.88	141.19	136.32	1885	51.25	142.22	135.28	1871	51.63	143.26	134.24	1857	52.00	144.30	133.20	1842
278	50.77	141.14	136.86	1893	51.14	142.18	135.82	1878	51.52	143.22	134.78	1864	51.89	144.26	133.74	1850
278.5	50.67	141.10	137.40	1900	51.04	142.14	136.36	1886	51.41	143.18	135.32	1872	51.78	144.22	134.28	1857
279	50.56	141.06	137.94	1908	50.93	142.10	136.90	1893	51.30	143.14	135.86	1879	51.68	144.17	134.83	1865
279.5	50.45	141.02	138.48	1915	50.83	142.06	137.44	1901	51.20	143.10	136.40	1886	51.57	144.13	135.37	1872
280	50.35	140.98	139.02	1923	50.72	142.02	137.98	1908	51.09	143.06	136.95	1894	51.46	144.09	135.91	1880
280.5	50.25	140.94	139.56	1930	50.62	141.98	138.52	1916	50.99	143.01	137.49	1901	51.36	144.05	136.45	1887
281	50.14	140.90	140.10	1938	50.51	141.94	139.06	1923	50.88	142.97	138.03	1909	51.25	144.01	136.99	1895
281.5	50.04	140.86	140.64	1945	50.41	141.89	139.61	1931	50.78	142.93	138.57	1916	51.14	143.97	137.53	1902
282	49.93	140.82	141.18	1953	50.30	141.85	140.15	1938	50.67	142.89	139.11	1924	51.04	143.93	138.07	1910
282.5	49.83	140.78	141.73	1960	50.20	141.81	140.69	1946	50.57	142.85	139.65	1931	50.93	143.89	138.61	1917
283	49.73	140.73	142.27	1968	50.10	141.77	141.23	1953	50.46	142.81	140.19	1939	50.83	143.85	139.15	1924
283.5	49.63	140.69	142.81	1975	49.99	141.73	141.77	1961	50.36	142.77	140.73	1946	50.73	143.81	139.69	1932
284	49.53	140.65	143.35	1983	49.89	141.69	142.31	1968	50.26	142.73	141.27	1954	50.62	143.76	140.24	1939
284.5	49.42	140.61	143.89	1990	49.79	141.65	142.85	1976	50.15	142.69	141.81	1961	50.52	143.72	140.78	1947
285	49.32	140.57	144.43	1997	49.69	141.61	143.39	1983	50.05	142.65	142.36	1969	50.41	143.68	141.32	1954
285.5	49.22	140.53	144.97	2005	49.59	141.57	143.93	1991	49.95	142.60	142.90	1976	50.31	143.64	141.86	1962
286	49.12	140.49	145.51	2012	49.48	141.53	144.47	1998	49.85	142.56	143.44	1984	50.21	143.60	142.40	1969
286.5	49.02	140.45	146.05	2020	49.38	141.48	145.02	2006	49.75	142.52	143.98	1991	50.11	143.56	142.94	1977
287	48.92	140.41	146.59	2027	49.28	141.44	145.56	2013	49.64	142.48	144.52	1999	50.01	143.52	143.48	1984
287.5	48.82	140.37	147.14	2035	49.18	141.40	146.10	2021	49.54	142.44	145.06	2006	49.91	143.48	144.02	1992
288	48.72	140.32	147.68	2042	49.08	141.36	146.64	2028	49.44	142.40	145.60	2014	49.80	143.44	144.56	1999
288.5	48.62	140.28	148.22	2050	48.98	141.32	147.18	2035	49.34	142.36	146.14	2021	49.70	143.40	145.10	2007
289	48.53	140.24	148.76	2057	48.89	141.28	147.72	2043	49.24	142.32	146.68	2029	49.60	143.35	145.65	2014
289.5	48.43	140.20	149.30	2065	48.79	141.24	148.26	2050	49.15	142.28	147.22	2036	49.50	143.31	146.19	2022
290	48.33	140.16	149.84	2072	48.69	141.20	148.80	2058	49.05	142.24	147.77	2044	49.40	143.27	146.73	2029
290.5	48.23	140.12	150.38	2080	48.59	141.16	149.34	2065	48.95	142.19	148.31	2051	49.31	143.23	147.27	2037
291	48.14	140.08	150.92	2087	48.49	141.12	149.88	2073	48.85	142.15	148.85	2059	49.21	143.19	147.81	2044
291.5	48.04	140.04	151.46	2095	48.40	141.07	150.43	2080	48.75	142.11	149.39	2066	49.11	143.15	148.35	2052

Body Composition FEMALE 260-291.5 Lb.

Weight: Lb.	Waist: 59 inches Fat: %	Fat: Lb.	LBM: Lb.	RMR: Cal.	59.25 inches Fat: %	Fat: Lb.	LBM: Lb.	RMR: Cal.	59.5 inches Fat: %	Fat: Lb.	LBM: Lb.	RMR: Cal.	59.75 inches Fat: %	Fat: Lb.	LBM: Lb.	RMR: Cal.
260	56.45	146.77	113.23	1566	56.85	147.81	112.19	1552	57.25	148.85	111.16	1537	57.65	149.88	110.12	1523
260.5	56.33	146.73	113.77	1573	56.72	147.77	112.73	1559	57.12	148.80	111.70	1545	57.52	149.84	110.66	1530
261	56.20	146.69	114.31	1581	56.60	147.73	113.27	1567	57.00	148.76	112.24	1552	57.39	149.80	111.20	1538
261.5	56.08	146.65	114.85	1588	56.48	147.68	113.82	1574	56.87	148.72	112.78	1560	57.27	149.76	111.74	1545
262	55.96	146.61	115.39	1596	56.35	147.64	114.36	1582	56.75	148.68	113.32	1567	57.14	149.72	112.28	1553
262.5	55.83	146.57	115.94	1603	56.23	147.60	114.90	1589	56.62	148.64	113.86	1575	57.02	149.68	112.82	1560
263	55.71	146.52	116.48	1611	56.11	147.56	115.44	1597	56.50	148.60	114.40	1582	56.90	149.64	113.36	1568
263.5	55.59	146.48	117.02	1618	55.99	147.52	115.98	1604	56.38	148.56	114.94	1590	56.77	149.60	113.90	1575
264	55.47	146.44	117.56	1626	55.86	147.48	116.52	1611	56.26	148.52	115.48	1597	56.65	149.55	114.45	1583
264.5	55.35	146.40	118.10	1633	55.74	147.44	117.06	1619	56.13	148.48	116.02	1605	56.53	149.51	114.99	1590
265	55.23	146.36	118.64	1641	55.62	147.40	117.60	1626	56.01	148.44	116.57	1612	56.40	149.47	115.53	1598
265.5	55.11	146.32	119.18	1648	55.50	147.36	118.14	1634	55.89	148.39	117.11	1620	56.28	149.43	116.07	1605
266	54.99	146.28	119.72	1656	55.38	147.32	118.68	1641	55.77	148.35	117.65	1627	56.16	149.39	116.61	1613
266.5	54.87	146.24	120.26	1663	55.26	147.27	119.23	1649	55.65	148.31	118.19	1635	56.04	149.35	117.15	1620
267	54.76	146.20	120.80	1671	55.14	147.23	119.77	1656	55.53	148.27	118.73	1642	55.92	149.31	117.69	1628
267.5	54.64	146.16	121.35	1678	55.03	147.19	120.31	1664	55.41	148.23	119.27	1650	55.80	149.27	118.23	1635
268	54.52	146.11	121.89	1686	54.91	147.15	120.85	1671	55.29	148.19	119.81	1657	55.68	149.23	118.77	1643
268.5	54.40	146.07	122.43	1693	54.79	147.11	121.39	1679	55.18	148.15	120.35	1664	55.56	149.19	119.31	1650
269	54.29	146.03	122.97	1701	54.67	147.07	121.93	1686	55.06	148.11	120.89	1672	55.44	149.14	119.86	1658
269.5	54.17	145.99	123.51	1708	54.56	147.03	122.47	1694	54.94	148.07	121.43	1679	55.33	149.10	120.40	1665
270	54.06	145.95	124.05	1716	54.44	146.99	123.01	1701	54.82	148.03	121.98	1687	55.21	149.06	120.94	1673
270.5	53.94	145.91	124.59	1723	54.32	146.95	123.55	1709	54.71	147.98	122.52	1694	55.09	149.02	121.48	1680
271	53.83	145.87	125.13	1731	54.21	146.91	124.09	1716	54.59	147.94	123.06	1702	54.97	148.98	122.02	1688
271.5	53.71	145.83	125.67	1738	54.09	146.86	124.64	1724	54.48	147.90	123.60	1709	54.86	148.94	122.56	1695
272	53.60	145.79	126.21	1746	53.98	146.82	125.18	1731	54.36	147.86	124.14	1717	54.74	148.90	123.10	1702
272.5	53.48	145.75	126.76	1753	53.87	146.78	125.72	1739	54.25	147.82	124.68	1724	54.63	148.86	123.64	1710
273	53.37	145.70	127.30	1761	53.75	146.74	126.26	1746	54.13	147.78	125.22	1732	54.51	148.82	124.18	1717
273.5	53.26	145.66	127.84	1768	53.64	146.70	126.80	1754	54.02	147.74	125.76	1739	54.40	148.78	124.72	1725
274	53.15	145.62	128.38	1775	53.53	146.66	127.34	1761	53.90	147.70	126.30	1747	54.28	148.73	125.27	1732
274.5	53.03	145.58	128.92	1783	53.41	146.62	127.88	1769	53.79	147.66	126.84	1754	54.17	148.69	125.81	1740
275	52.92	145.54	129.46	1790	53.30	146.58	128.42	1776	53.68	147.62	127.39	1762	54.06	148.65	126.35	1747
275.5	52.81	145.50	130.00	1798	53.19	146.54	128.96	1784	53.57	147.57	127.93	1769	53.94	148.61	126.89	1755
276	52.70	145.46	130.54	1805	53.08	146.50	129.50	1791	53.45	147.53	128.47	1777	53.83	148.57	127.43	1762
276.5	52.59	145.42	131.08	1813	52.97	146.45	130.05	1799	53.34	147.49	129.01	1784	53.72	148.53	127.97	1770
277	52.48	145.38	131.62	1820	52.86	146.41	130.59	1806	53.23	147.45	129.55	1792	53.61	148.49	128.51	1777
277.5	52.37	145.34	132.17	1828	52.75	146.37	131.13	1813	53.12	147.41	130.09	1799	53.49	148.45	129.05	1785
278	52.26	145.29	132.71	1835	52.64	146.33	131.67	1821	53.01	147.37	130.63	1807	53.38	148.41	129.59	1792
278.5	52.16	145.25	133.25	1843	52.53	146.29	132.21	1828	52.90	147.33	131.17	1814	53.27	148.37	130.13	1800
279	52.05	145.21	133.79	1850	52.42	146.25	132.75	1836	52.79	147.29	131.71	1822	53.16	148.32	130.68	1807
279.5	51.94	145.17	134.33	1858	52.31	146.21	133.29	1843	52.68	147.25	132.25	1829	53.05	148.28	131.22	1815
280	51.83	145.13	134.87	1865	52.20	146.17	133.83	1851	52.57	147.21	132.80	1837	52.94	148.24	131.76	1822
280.5	51.73	145.09	135.41	1873	52.10	146.13	134.37	1858	52.46	147.16	133.34	1844	52.83	148.20	132.30	1830
281	51.62	145.05	135.95	1880	51.99	146.09	134.91	1866	52.36	147.12	133.88	1852	52.73	148.16	132.84	1837
281.5	51.51	145.01	136.49	1888	51.88	146.04	135.46	1873	52.25	147.08	134.42	1859	52.62	148.12	133.38	1845
282	51.41	144.97	137.03	1895	51.77	146.00	136.00	1881	52.14	147.04	134.96	1866	52.51	148.08	133.92	1852
282.5	51.30	144.93	137.58	1903	51.67	145.96	136.54	1888	52.04	147.00	135.50	1874	52.40	148.04	134.46	1860
283	51.20	144.88	138.12	1910	51.56	145.92	137.08	1896	51.93	146.96	136.04	1881	52.30	148.00	135.00	1867
283.5	51.09	144.84	138.66	1918	51.46	145.88	137.62	1903	51.82	146.92	136.58	1889	52.19	147.96	135.54	1875
284	50.99	144.80	139.20	1925	51.35	145.84	138.16	1911	51.72	146.88	137.12	1896	52.08	147.91	136.09	1882
284.5	50.88	144.76	139.74	1933	51.25	145.80	138.70	1918	51.61	146.84	137.66	1904	51.98	147.87	136.63	1890
285	50.78	144.72	140.28	1940	51.14	145.76	139.24	1926	51.51	146.80	138.21	1911	51.87	147.83	137.17	1897
285.5	50.68	144.68	140.82	1948	51.04	145.72	139.78	1933	51.40	146.75	138.75	1919	51.77	147.79	137.71	1905
286	50.57	144.64	141.36	1955	50.94	145.68	140.32	1941	51.30	146.71	139.29	1926	51.66	147.75	138.25	1912
286.5	50.47	144.60	141.90	1963	50.83	145.63	140.87	1948	51.19	146.67	139.83	1934	51.56	147.71	138.79	1919
287	50.37	144.56	142.44	1970	50.73	145.59	141.41	1956	51.09	146.63	140.37	1941	51.45	147.67	139.33	1927
287.5	50.27	144.52	142.99	1977	50.63	145.55	141.95	1963	50.99	146.59	140.91	1949	51.35	147.63	139.87	1934
288	50.16	144.47	143.53	1985	50.52	145.51	142.49	1971	50.89	146.55	141.45	1956	51.25	147.59	140.41	1942
288.5	50.06	144.43	144.07	1992	50.42	145.47	143.03	1978	50.78	146.51	141.99	1964	51.14	147.55	140.95	1949
289	49.96	144.39	144.61	2000	50.32	145.43	143.57	1986	50.68	146.47	142.53	1971	51.04	147.50	141.50	1957
289.5	49.86	144.35	145.15	2007	50.22	145.39	144.11	1993	50.58	146.43	143.07	1979	50.94	147.46	142.04	1964
290	49.76	144.31	145.69	2015	50.12	145.35	144.65	2001	50.48	146.39	143.62	1986	50.84	147.42	142.58	1972
290.5	49.66	144.27	146.23	2022	50.02	145.31	145.19	2008	50.38	146.34	144.16	1994	50.73	147.38	143.12	1979
291	49.56	144.23	146.77	2030	49.92	145.27	145.73	2016	50.28	146.30	144.70	2001	50.63	147.34	143.66	1987
291.5	49.46	144.19	147.31	2037	49.82	145.22	146.28	2023	50.18	146.26	145.24	2009	50.53	147.30	144.20	1994

Body Composition FEMALE 260-291.5 Lb.

Weight: Lb.	Waist: 60 inches				60.25 inches				60.5 inches				60.75 inches			
	Fat: %	Fat: Lb.	LBM: Lb.	RMR: Cal.	Fat: %	Fat: Lb.	LBM: Lb.	RMR: Cal.	Fat: %	Fat: Lb.	LBM: Lb.	RMR: Cal.	Fat: %	Fat: Lb.	LBM: Lb.	RMR: Cal.
260	58.05	150.92	109.08	1509	58.45	151.96	108.04	1494	58.84	153.00	107.01	1480	59.24	154.03	105.97	1466
260.5	57.92	150.88	109.62	1516	58.32	151.92	108.58	1502	58.72	152.95	107.55	1487	59.11	153.99	106.51	1473
261	57.79	150.84	110.16	1524	58.19	151.88	109.12	1509	58.59	152.91	108.09	1495	58.98	153.95	107.05	1480
261.5	57.67	150.80	110.70	1531	58.06	151.83	109.67	1517	58.46	152.87	108.63	1502	58.86	153.91	107.59	1488
262	57.54	150.76	111.24	1539	57.94	151.79	110.21	1524	58.33	152.83	109.17	1510	58.73	153.87	108.13	1495
262.5	57.42	150.72	111.79	1546	57.81	151.75	110.75	1532	58.21	152.79	109.71	1517	58.60	153.83	108.67	1503
263	57.29	150.67	112.33	1553	57.68	151.71	111.29	1539	58.08	152.75	110.25	1525	58.47	153.79	109.21	1510
263.5	57.17	150.63	112.87	1561	57.56	151.67	111.83	1547	57.95	152.71	110.79	1532	58.35	153.75	109.75	1518
264	57.04	150.59	113.41	1568	57.44	151.63	112.37	1554	57.83	152.67	111.33	1540	58.22	153.70	110.30	1525
264.5	56.92	150.55	113.95	1576	57.31	151.59	112.91	1562	57.70	152.63	111.87	1547	58.10	153.66	110.84	1533
265	56.80	150.51	114.49	1583	57.19	151.55	113.45	1569	57.58	152.59	112.42	1555	57.97	153.62	111.38	1540
265.5	56.67	150.47	115.03	1591	57.06	151.51	113.99	1577	57.46	152.54	112.96	1562	57.85	153.58	111.92	1548
266	56.55	150.43	115.57	1598	56.94	151.47	114.53	1584	57.33	152.50	113.50	1570	57.72	153.54	112.46	1555
266.5	56.43	150.39	116.11	1606	56.82	151.42	115.08	1591	57.21	152.46	114.04	1577	57.60	153.50	113.00	1563
267	56.31	150.35	116.65	1613	56.70	151.38	115.62	1599	57.09	152.42	114.58	1585	57.48	153.46	113.54	1570
267.5	56.19	150.31	117.20	1621	56.58	151.34	116.16	1606	56.96	152.38	115.12	1592	57.35	153.42	114.08	1578
268	56.07	150.26	117.74	1628	56.46	151.30	116.70	1614	56.84	152.34	115.66	1600	57.23	153.38	114.62	1585
268.5	55.95	150.22	118.28	1636	56.34	151.26	117.24	1621	56.72	152.30	116.20	1607	57.11	153.34	115.16	1593
269	55.83	150.18	118.82	1643	56.22	151.22	117.78	1629	56.60	152.26	116.74	1615	56.99	153.29	115.71	1600
269.5	55.71	150.14	119.36	1651	56.10	151.18	118.32	1636	56.48	152.22	117.28	1622	56.87	153.25	116.25	1608
270	55.59	150.10	119.90	1658	55.98	151.14	118.86	1644	56.36	152.18	117.83	1630	56.75	153.21	116.79	1615
270.5	55.47	150.06	120.44	1666	55.86	151.10	119.40	1651	56.24	152.13	118.37	1637	56.63	153.17	117.33	1623
271	55.36	150.02	120.98	1673	55.74	151.06	119.94	1659	56.12	152.09	118.91	1644	56.51	153.13	117.87	1630
271.5	55.24	149.98	121.52	1681	55.62	151.01	120.49	1666	56.00	152.05	119.45	1652	56.39	153.09	118.41	1638
272	55.12	149.94	122.06	1688	55.50	150.97	121.03	1674	55.89	152.01	119.99	1659	56.27	153.05	118.95	1645
272.5	55.01	149.90	122.61	1696	55.39	150.93	121.57	1681	55.77	151.97	120.53	1667	56.15	153.01	119.49	1653
273	54.89	149.85	123.15	1703	55.27	150.89	122.11	1689	55.65	151.93	121.07	1674	56.03	152.97	120.03	1660
273.5	54.78	149.81	123.69	1711	55.16	150.85	122.65	1696	55.53	151.89	121.61	1682	55.91	152.93	120.57	1668
274	54.66	149.77	124.23	1718	55.04	150.81	123.19	1704	55.42	151.85	122.15	1689	55.80	152.88	121.12	1675
274.5	54.55	149.73	124.77	1726	54.92	150.77	123.73	1711	55.30	151.81	122.69	1697	55.68	152.84	121.66	1683
275	54.43	149.69	125.31	1733	54.81	150.73	124.27	1719	55.19	151.77	123.24	1704	55.56	152.80	122.20	1690
275.5	54.32	149.65	125.85	1741	54.70	150.69	124.81	1726	55.07	151.72	123.78	1712	55.45	152.76	122.74	1697
276	54.21	149.61	126.39	1748	54.58	150.65	125.35	1734	54.96	151.68	124.32	1719	55.33	152.72	123.28	1705
276.5	54.09	149.57	126.93	1755	54.47	150.60	125.90	1741	54.84	151.64	124.86	1727	55.22	152.68	123.82	1712
277	53.98	149.53	127.47	1763	54.36	150.56	126.44	1749	54.73	151.60	125.40	1734	55.10	152.64	124.36	1720
277.5	53.87	149.49	128.02	1770	54.24	150.52	126.98	1756	54.62	151.56	125.94	1742	54.99	152.60	124.90	1727
278	53.76	149.44	128.56	1778	54.13	150.48	127.52	1764	54.50	151.52	126.48	1749	54.88	152.56	125.44	1735
278.5	53.65	149.40	129.10	1785	54.02	150.44	128.06	1771	54.39	151.48	127.02	1757	54.76	152.52	125.98	1742
279	53.53	149.36	129.64	1793	53.91	150.40	128.60	1779	54.28	151.44	127.56	1764	54.65	152.47	126.53	1750
279.5	53.42	149.32	130.18	1800	53.80	150.36	129.14	1786	54.17	151.40	128.10	1772	54.54	152.43	127.07	1757
280	53.31	149.28	130.72	1808	53.68	150.32	129.68	1794	54.06	151.36	128.65	1779	54.43	152.39	127.61	1765
280.5	53.20	149.24	131.26	1815	53.57	150.28	130.22	1801	53.94	151.31	129.19	1787	54.31	152.35	128.15	1772
281	53.10	149.20	131.80	1823	53.46	150.24	130.76	1808	53.83	151.27	129.73	1794	54.20	152.31	128.69	1780
281.5	52.99	149.16	132.34	1830	53.36	150.19	131.31	1816	53.72	151.23	130.27	1802	54.09	152.27	129.23	1787
282	52.88	149.12	132.88	1838	53.25	150.15	131.85	1823	53.61	151.19	130.81	1809	53.98	152.23	129.77	1795
282.5	52.77	149.08	133.43	1845	53.14	150.11	132.39	1831	53.50	151.15	131.35	1817	53.87	152.19	130.31	1802
283	52.66	149.03	133.97	1853	53.03	150.07	132.93	1838	53.40	151.11	131.89	1824	53.76	152.15	130.85	1810
283.5	52.55	148.99	134.51	1860	52.92	150.03	133.47	1846	53.29	151.07	132.43	1832	53.65	152.11	131.39	1817
284	52.45	148.95	135.05	1868	52.81	149.99	134.01	1853	53.18	151.03	132.97	1839	53.54	152.06	131.94	1825
284.5	52.34	148.91	135.59	1875	52.71	149.95	134.55	1861	53.07	150.99	133.51	1846	53.44	152.02	132.48	1832
285	52.24	148.87	136.13	1883	52.60	149.91	135.09	1868	52.96	150.95	134.06	1854	53.33	151.98	133.02	1840
285.5	52.13	148.83	136.67	1890	52.49	149.87	135.63	1876	52.86	150.90	134.60	1861	53.22	151.94	133.56	1847
286	52.02	148.79	137.21	1898	52.39	149.83	136.17	1883	52.75	150.86	135.14	1869	53.11	151.90	134.10	1855
286.5	51.92	148.75	137.75	1905	52.28	149.78	136.72	1891	52.64	150.82	135.68	1876	53.01	151.86	134.64	1862
287	51.81	148.71	138.29	1913	52.18	149.74	137.26	1898	52.54	150.78	136.22	1884	52.90	151.82	135.18	1870
287.5	51.71	148.67	138.84	1920	52.07	149.70	137.80	1906	52.43	150.74	136.76	1891	52.79	151.78	135.72	1877
288	51.61	148.62	139.38	1928	51.97	149.66	138.34	1913	52.33	150.70	137.30	1899	52.69	151.74	136.26	1885
288.5	51.50	148.58	139.92	1935	51.86	149.62	138.88	1921	52.22	150.66	137.84	1906	52.58	151.70	136.80	1892
289	51.40	148.54	140.46	1943	51.76	149.58	139.42	1928	52.12	150.62	138.38	1914	52.48	151.65	137.35	1899
289.5	51.30	148.50	141.00	1950	51.65	149.54	139.96	1936	52.01	150.58	138.92	1921	52.37	151.61	137.89	1907
290	51.19	148.46	141.54	1957	51.55	149.50	140.50	1943	51.91	150.54	139.47	1929	52.27	151.57	138.43	1914
290.5	51.09	148.42	142.08	1965	51.45	149.46	141.04	1951	51.81	150.49	140.01	1936	52.16	151.53	138.97	1922
291	50.99	148.38	142.62	1972	51.35	149.42	141.58	1958	51.70	150.45	140.55	1944	52.06	151.49	139.51	1929
291.5	50.89	148.34	143.16	1980	51.24	149.37	142.13	1966	51.60	150.41	141.09	1951	51.96	151.45	140.05	1937

Body Composition FEMALE 260-291.5 Lb.

Weight: Lb.	Waist: 61 inches Fat: %	Fat: Lb.	LBM: Lb.	RMR: Cal.	61.25 inches Fat: %	Fat: Lb.	LBM: Lb.	RMR: Cal.	61.5 inches Fat: %	Fat: Lb.	LBM: Lb.	RMR: Cal.	61.75 inches Fat: %	Fat: Lb.	LBM: Lb.	RMR: Cal.
260	59.64	155.07	104.93	1451	60.04	156.11	103.89	1437	60.44	157.15	102.86	1422	60.84	158.18	101.82	1408
260.5	59.51	155.03	105.47	1459	59.91	156.07	104.43	1444	60.31	157.10	103.40	1430	60.71	158.14	102.36	1416
261	59.38	154.99	106.01	1466	59.78	156.03	104.97	1452	60.18	157.06	103.94	1437	60.57	158.10	102.90	1423
261.5	59.25	154.95	106.55	1474	59.65	155.98	105.52	1459	60.05	157.02	104.48	1445	60.44	158.06	103.44	1431
262	59.12	154.91	107.09	1481	59.52	155.94	106.06	1467	59.92	156.98	105.02	1452	60.31	158.02	103.98	1438
262.5	59.00	154.87	107.64	1489	59.39	155.90	106.60	1474	59.79	156.94	105.56	1460	60.18	157.98	104.52	1446
263	58.87	154.82	108.18	1496	59.26	155.86	107.14	1482	59.66	156.90	106.10	1467	60.05	157.94	105.06	1453
263.5	58.74	154.78	108.72	1504	59.13	155.82	107.68	1489	59.53	156.86	106.64	1475	59.92	157.90	105.60	1461
264	58.61	154.74	109.26	1511	59.01	155.78	108.22	1497	59.40	156.82	107.18	1482	59.79	157.85	106.15	1468
264.5	58.49	154.70	109.80	1519	58.88	155.74	108.76	1504	59.27	156.78	107.72	1490	59.66	157.81	106.69	1475
265	58.36	154.66	110.34	1526	58.75	155.70	109.30	1512	59.15	156.74	108.27	1497	59.54	157.77	107.23	1483
265.5	58.24	154.62	110.88	1533	58.63	155.66	109.84	1519	59.02	156.69	108.81	1505	59.41	157.73	107.77	1490
266	58.11	154.58	111.42	1541	58.50	155.62	110.38	1527	58.89	156.65	109.35	1512	59.28	157.69	108.31	1498
266.5	57.99	154.54	111.96	1548	58.38	155.57	110.93	1534	58.77	156.61	109.89	1520	59.16	157.65	108.85	1505
267	57.86	154.50	112.50	1556	58.25	155.53	111.47	1542	58.64	156.57	110.43	1527	59.03	157.61	109.39	1513
267.5	57.74	154.46	113.05	1563	58.13	155.49	112.01	1549	58.52	156.53	110.97	1535	58.90	157.57	109.93	1520
268	57.62	154.41	113.59	1571	58.00	155.45	112.55	1557	58.39	156.49	111.51	1542	58.78	157.53	110.47	1528
268.5	57.49	154.37	114.13	1578	57.88	155.41	113.09	1564	58.27	156.45	112.05	1550	58.65	157.49	111.01	1535
269	57.37	154.33	114.67	1586	57.76	155.37	113.63	1572	58.14	156.41	112.59	1557	58.53	157.44	111.56	1543
269.5	57.25	154.29	115.21	1593	57.64	155.33	114.17	1579	58.02	156.37	113.13	1565	58.41	157.40	112.10	1550
270	57.13	154.25	115.75	1601	57.51	155.29	114.71	1586	57.90	156.33	113.68	1572	58.28	157.36	112.64	1558
270.5	57.01	154.21	116.29	1608	57.39	155.25	115.25	1594	57.78	156.28	114.22	1580	58.16	157.32	113.18	1565
271	56.89	154.17	116.83	1616	57.27	155.21	115.79	1601	57.65	156.24	114.76	1587	58.04	157.28	113.72	1573
271.5	56.77	154.13	117.37	1623	57.15	155.16	116.34	1609	57.53	156.20	115.30	1595	57.92	157.24	114.26	1580
272	56.65	154.09	117.91	1631	57.03	155.12	116.88	1616	57.41	156.16	115.84	1602	57.79	157.20	114.80	1588
272.5	56.53	154.05	118.46	1638	56.91	155.08	117.42	1624	57.29	156.12	116.38	1610	57.67	157.16	115.34	1595
273	56.41	154.00	119.00	1646	56.79	155.04	117.96	1631	57.17	156.08	116.92	1617	57.55	157.12	115.88	1603
273.5	56.29	153.96	119.54	1653	56.67	155.00	118.50	1639	57.05	156.04	117.46	1624	57.43	157.08	116.42	1610
274	56.18	153.92	120.08	1661	56.55	154.96	119.04	1646	56.93	156.00	118.00	1632	57.31	157.03	116.97	1618
274.5	56.06	153.88	120.62	1668	56.44	154.92	119.58	1654	56.81	155.96	118.54	1639	57.19	156.99	117.51	1625
275	55.94	153.84	121.16	1676	56.32	154.88	120.12	1661	56.70	155.92	119.09	1647	57.07	156.95	118.05	1633
275.5	55.83	153.80	121.70	1683	56.20	154.84	120.66	1669	56.58	155.87	119.63	1654	56.96	156.91	118.59	1640
276	55.71	153.76	122.24	1691	56.09	154.80	121.20	1676	56.46	155.83	120.17	1662	56.84	156.87	119.13	1648
276.5	55.59	153.72	122.78	1698	55.97	154.75	121.75	1684	56.34	155.79	120.71	1669	56.72	156.83	119.67	1655
277	55.48	153.68	123.32	1706	55.85	154.71	122.29	1691	56.23	155.75	121.25	1677	56.60	156.79	120.21	1663
277.5	55.36	153.64	123.87	1713	55.74	154.67	122.83	1699	56.11	155.71	121.79	1684	56.49	156.75	120.75	1670
278	55.25	153.59	124.41	1721	55.62	154.63	123.37	1706	56.00	155.67	122.33	1692	56.37	156.71	121.29	1677
278.5	55.14	153.55	124.95	1728	55.51	154.59	123.91	1714	55.88	155.63	122.87	1699	56.25	156.67	121.83	1685
279	55.02	153.51	125.49	1735	55.39	154.55	124.45	1721	55.77	155.59	123.41	1707	56.14	156.62	122.38	1692
279.5	54.91	153.47	126.03	1743	55.28	154.51	124.99	1729	55.65	155.55	123.95	1714	56.02	156.58	122.92	1700
280	54.80	153.43	126.57	1750	55.17	154.47	125.53	1736	55.54	155.51	124.50	1722	55.91	156.54	123.46	1707
280.5	54.68	153.39	127.11	1758	55.05	154.43	126.07	1744	55.42	155.46	125.04	1729	55.79	156.50	124.00	1715
281	54.57	153.35	127.65	1765	54.94	154.39	126.61	1751	55.31	155.42	125.58	1737	55.68	156.46	124.54	1722
281.5	54.46	153.31	128.19	1773	54.83	154.34	127.16	1759	55.20	155.38	126.12	1744	55.57	156.42	125.08	1730
282	54.35	153.27	128.73	1780	54.72	154.30	127.70	1766	55.09	155.34	126.66	1752	55.45	156.38	125.62	1737
282.5	54.24	153.23	129.28	1788	54.61	154.26	128.24	1774	54.97	155.30	127.20	1759	55.34	156.34	126.16	1745
283	54.13	153.18	129.82	1795	54.50	154.22	128.78	1781	54.86	155.26	127.74	1767	55.23	156.30	126.70	1752
283.5	54.02	153.14	130.36	1803	54.38	154.18	129.32	1788	54.75	155.22	128.28	1774	55.12	156.26	127.24	1760
284	53.91	153.10	130.90	1810	54.27	154.14	129.86	1796	54.64	155.18	128.82	1782	55.01	156.21	127.79	1767
284.5	53.80	153.06	131.44	1818	54.16	154.10	130.40	1803	54.53	155.14	129.36	1789	54.89	156.17	128.33	1775
285	53.69	153.02	131.98	1825	54.06	154.06	130.94	1811	54.42	155.10	129.91	1797	54.78	156.13	128.87	1782
285.5	53.58	152.98	132.52	1833	53.95	154.02	131.48	1818	54.31	155.05	130.45	1804	54.67	156.09	129.41	1790
286	53.47	152.94	133.06	1840	53.84	153.98	132.02	1826	54.20	155.01	130.99	1812	54.56	156.05	129.95	1797
286.5	53.37	152.90	133.60	1848	53.73	153.93	132.57	1833	54.09	154.97	131.53	1819	54.45	156.01	130.49	1805
287	53.26	152.86	134.14	1855	53.62	153.89	133.11	1841	53.98	154.93	132.07	1827	54.34	155.97	131.03	1812
287.5	53.15	152.82	134.69	1863	53.51	153.85	133.65	1848	53.87	154.89	132.61	1834	54.24	155.93	131.57	1820
288	53.05	152.77	135.23	1870	53.41	153.81	134.19	1856	53.77	154.85	133.15	1841	54.13	155.89	132.11	1827
288.5	52.94	152.73	135.77	1878	53.30	153.77	134.73	1863	53.66	154.81	133.69	1849	54.02	155.85	132.65	1835
289	52.83	152.69	136.31	1885	53.19	153.73	135.27	1871	53.55	154.77	134.23	1856	53.91	155.80	133.20	1842
289.5	52.73	152.65	136.85	1893	53.09	153.69	135.81	1878	53.45	154.73	134.77	1864	53.80	155.76	133.74	1850
290	52.62	152.61	137.39	1900	52.98	153.65	136.35	1886	53.34	154.69	135.32	1871	53.70	155.72	134.28	1857
290.5	52.52	152.57	137.93	1908	52.88	153.61	136.89	1893	53.23	154.64	135.86	1879	53.59	155.68	134.82	1865
291	52.42	152.53	138.47	1915	52.77	153.57	137.43	1901	53.13	154.60	136.40	1886	53.48	155.64	135.36	1872
291.5	52.31	152.49	139.01	1923	52.67	153.52	137.98	1908	53.02	154.56	136.94	1894	53.38	155.60	135.90	1880

Body Composition   FEMALE   260-291.5 Lb.

Weight: Lb.	Waist: 62 inches				62.25 inches				62.5 inches				62.75 inches			
	Fat: %	Fat: Lb.	LBM: Lb.	RMR: Cal.	Fat: %	Fat: Lb.	LBM: Lb.	RMR: Cal.	Fat: %	Fat: Lb.	LBM: Lb.	RMR: Cal.	Fat: %	Fat: Lb.	LBM: Lb.	RMR: Cal.
260	61.24	159.22	100.78	1394	61.64	160.26	99.74	1379	62.04	161.30	98.71	1365	62.44	162.33	97.67	1351
260.5	61.11	159.18	101.32	1401	61.50	160.22	100.28	1387	61.90	161.25	99.25	1373	62.30	162.29	98.21	1358
261	60.97	159.14	101.86	1409	61.37	160.18	100.82	1394	61.77	161.21	99.79	1380	62.16	162.25	98.75	1366
261.5	60.84	159.10	102.40	1416	61.24	160.13	101.37	1402	61.63	161.17	100.33	1388	62.03	162.21	99.29	1373
262	60.71	159.06	102.94	1424	61.10	160.09	101.91	1409	61.50	161.13	100.87	1395	61.90	162.17	99.83	1381
262.5	60.58	159.02	103.49	1431	60.97	160.05	102.45	1417	61.37	161.09	101.41	1403	61.76	162.13	100.37	1388
263	60.45	158.97	104.03	1439	60.84	160.01	102.99	1424	61.24	161.05	101.95	1410	61.63	162.09	100.91	1396
263.5	60.32	158.93	104.57	1446	60.71	159.97	103.53	1432	61.10	161.01	102.49	1417	61.50	162.05	101.45	1403
264	60.19	158.89	105.11	1454	60.58	159.93	104.07	1439	60.97	160.97	103.03	1425	61.37	162.00	102.00	1411
264.5	60.06	158.85	105.65	1461	60.45	159.89	104.61	1447	60.84	160.93	103.57	1432	61.23	161.96	102.54	1418
265	59.93	158.81	106.19	1469	60.32	159.85	105.15	1454	60.71	160.89	104.12	1440	61.10	161.92	103.08	1426
265.5	59.80	158.77	106.73	1476	60.19	159.81	105.69	1462	60.58	160.84	104.66	1447	60.97	161.88	103.62	1433
266	59.67	158.73	107.27	1484	60.06	159.77	106.23	1469	60.45	160.80	105.20	1455	60.84	161.84	104.16	1441
266.5	59.54	158.69	107.81	1491	59.93	159.72	106.78	1477	60.32	160.76	105.74	1462	60.71	161.80	104.70	1448
267	59.42	158.65	108.35	1499	59.81	159.68	107.32	1484	60.20	160.72	106.28	1470	60.58	161.76	105.24	1455
267.5	59.29	158.61	108.90	1506	59.68	159.64	107.86	1492	60.07	160.68	106.82	1477	60.46	161.72	105.78	1463
268	59.17	158.56	109.44	1513	59.55	159.60	108.40	1499	59.94	160.64	107.36	1485	60.33	161.68	106.32	1470
268.5	59.04	158.52	109.98	1521	59.43	159.56	108.94	1507	59.81	160.60	107.90	1492	60.20	161.64	106.86	1478
269	58.92	158.48	110.52	1528	59.30	159.52	109.48	1514	59.69	160.56	108.44	1500	60.07	161.59	107.41	1485
269.5	58.79	158.44	111.06	1536	59.18	159.48	110.02	1522	59.56	160.52	108.98	1507	59.95	161.55	107.95	1493
270	58.67	158.40	111.60	1543	59.05	159.44	110.56	1529	59.44	160.48	109.53	1515	59.82	161.51	108.49	1500
270.5	58.54	158.36	112.14	1551	58.93	159.40	111.10	1537	59.31	160.43	110.07	1522	59.69	161.47	109.03	1508
271	58.42	158.32	112.68	1558	58.80	159.36	111.64	1544	59.19	160.39	110.61	1530	59.57	161.43	109.57	1515
271.5	58.30	158.28	113.22	1566	58.68	159.31	112.19	1552	59.06	160.35	111.15	1537	59.44	161.39	110.11	1523
272	58.18	158.24	113.76	1573	58.56	159.27	112.73	1559	58.94	160.31	111.69	1545	59.32	161.35	110.65	1530
272.5	58.05	158.20	114.31	1581	58.43	159.23	113.27	1566	58.81	160.27	112.23	1552	59.20	161.31	111.19	1538
273	57.93	158.15	114.85	1588	58.31	159.19	113.81	1574	58.69	160.23	112.77	1560	59.07	161.27	111.73	1545
273.5	57.81	158.11	115.39	1596	58.19	159.15	114.35	1581	58.57	160.19	113.31	1567	58.95	161.23	112.27	1553
274	57.69	158.07	115.93	1603	58.07	159.11	114.89	1589	58.45	160.15	113.85	1575	58.83	161.18	112.82	1560
274.5	57.57	158.03	116.47	1611	57.95	159.07	115.43	1596	58.33	160.11	114.39	1582	58.70	161.14	113.36	1568
275	57.45	157.99	117.01	1618	57.83	159.03	115.97	1604	58.21	160.07	114.94	1590	58.58	161.10	113.90	1575
275.5	57.33	157.95	117.55	1626	57.71	158.99	116.51	1611	58.08	160.02	115.48	1597	58.46	161.06	114.44	1583
276	57.21	157.91	118.09	1633	57.59	158.95	117.05	1619	57.96	159.98	116.02	1605	58.34	161.02	114.98	1590
276.5	57.09	157.87	118.63	1641	57.47	158.91	117.60	1626	57.85	159.94	116.56	1612	58.22	160.98	115.52	1598
277	56.98	157.83	119.17	1648	57.35	158.86	118.14	1634	57.73	159.90	117.10	1619	58.10	160.94	116.06	1605
277.5	56.86	157.79	119.72	1656	57.23	158.82	118.68	1641	57.61	159.86	117.64	1627	57.98	160.90	116.60	1613
278	56.74	157.74	120.26	1663	57.12	158.78	119.22	1649	57.49	159.82	118.18	1634	57.86	160.86	117.14	1620
278.5	56.63	157.70	120.80	1671	57.00	158.74	119.76	1656	57.37	159.78	118.72	1642	57.74	160.82	117.68	1628
279	56.51	157.66	121.34	1678	56.88	158.70	120.30	1664	57.25	159.74	119.26	1649	57.63	160.77	118.23	1635
279.5	56.39	157.62	121.88	1686	56.77	158.66	120.84	1671	57.14	159.70	119.80	1657	57.51	160.73	118.77	1643
280	56.28	157.58	122.42	1693	56.65	158.62	121.38	1679	57.02	159.66	120.35	1664	57.39	160.69	119.31	1650
280.5	56.16	157.54	122.96	1701	56.53	158.58	121.92	1686	56.90	159.61	120.89	1672	57.27	160.65	119.85	1658
281	56.05	157.50	123.50	1708	56.42	158.54	122.46	1694	56.79	159.57	121.43	1679	57.16	160.61	120.39	1665
281.5	55.93	157.46	124.04	1716	56.30	158.49	123.01	1701	56.67	159.53	121.97	1687	57.04	160.57	120.93	1672
282	55.82	157.42	124.58	1723	56.19	158.45	123.55	1709	56.56	159.49	122.51	1694	56.93	160.53	121.47	1680
282.5	55.71	157.38	125.13	1730	56.08	158.41	124.09	1716	56.44	159.45	123.05	1702	56.81	160.49	122.01	1687
283	55.60	157.33	125.67	1738	55.96	158.37	124.63	1724	56.33	159.41	123.59	1709	56.69	160.45	122.55	1695
283.5	55.48	157.29	126.21	1745	55.85	158.33	125.17	1731	56.21	159.37	124.13	1717	56.58	160.41	123.09	1702
284	55.37	157.25	126.75	1753	55.74	158.29	125.71	1739	56.10	159.33	124.67	1724	56.47	160.36	123.64	1710
284.5	55.26	157.21	127.29	1760	55.62	158.25	126.25	1746	55.99	159.29	125.21	1732	56.35	160.32	124.18	1717
285	55.15	157.17	127.83	1768	55.51	158.21	126.79	1754	55.88	159.25	125.76	1739	56.24	160.28	124.72	1725
285.5	55.04	157.13	128.37	1775	55.40	158.17	127.33	1761	55.76	159.20	126.30	1747	56.13	160.24	125.26	1732
286	54.93	157.09	128.91	1783	55.29	158.13	127.87	1769	55.65	159.16	126.84	1754	56.01	160.20	125.80	1740
286.5	54.82	157.05	129.45	1790	55.18	158.08	128.42	1776	55.54	159.12	127.38	1762	55.90	160.16	126.34	1747
287	54.71	157.01	129.99	1798	55.07	158.04	128.96	1783	55.43	159.08	127.92	1769	55.79	160.12	126.88	1755
287.5	54.60	156.97	130.54	1805	54.96	158.00	129.50	1791	55.32	159.04	128.46	1777	55.68	160.08	127.42	1762
288	54.49	156.92	131.08	1813	54.85	157.96	130.04	1798	55.21	159.00	129.00	1784	55.57	160.04	127.96	1770
288.5	54.38	156.88	131.62	1820	54.74	157.92	130.58	1806	55.10	158.96	129.54	1792	55.46	160.00	128.50	1777
289	54.27	156.84	132.16	1828	54.63	157.88	131.12	1813	54.99	158.92	130.08	1799	55.35	159.95	129.05	1785
289.5	54.16	156.80	132.70	1835	54.52	157.84	131.66	1821	54.88	158.88	130.62	1807	55.24	159.91	129.59	1792
290	54.06	156.76	133.24	1843	54.41	157.80	132.20	1828	54.77	158.84	131.17	1814	55.13	159.87	130.13	1800
290.5	53.95	156.72	133.78	1850	54.31	157.76	132.74	1836	54.66	158.79	131.71	1821	55.02	159.83	130.67	1807
291	53.84	156.68	134.32	1858	54.20	157.72	133.28	1843	54.55	158.75	132.25	1829	54.91	159.79	131.21	1815
291.5	53.73	156.64	134.86	1865	54.09	157.67	133.83	1851	54.45	158.71	132.79	1836	54.80	159.75	131.75	1822

Body Composition FEMALE 260-291.5 Lb.

Weight: Lb.	Waist: 63 inches				63.25 inches				63.5 inches				63.75 inches			
	Fat: %	Fat: Lb.	LBM: Lb.	RMR: Cal.	Fat: %	Fat: Lb.	LBM: Lb.	RMR: Cal.	Fat: %	Fat: Lb.	LBM: Lb.	RMR: Cal.	Fat: %	Fat: Lb.	LBM: Lb.	RMR: Cal.
260	62.83	163.37	96.63	1336	63.23	164.41	95.59	1322	63.63	165.45	94.56	1308	64.03	166.48	93.52	1293
260.5	62.70	163.33	97.17	1344	63.10	164.37	96.13	1330	63.49	165.40	95.10	1315	63.89	166.44	94.06	1301
261	62.56	163.29	97.71	1351	62.96	164.33	96.67	1337	63.36	165.36	95.64	1323	63.75	166.40	94.60	1308
261.5	62.43	163.25	98.25	1359	62.82	164.28	97.22	1344	63.22	165.32	96.18	1330	63.62	166.36	95.14	1316
262	62.29	163.21	98.79	1366	62.69	164.24	97.76	1352	63.08	165.28	96.72	1338	63.48	166.32	95.68	1323
262.5	62.16	163.17	99.34	1374	62.55	164.20	98.30	1359	62.95	165.24	97.26	1345	63.34	166.28	96.22	1331
263	62.02	163.12	99.88	1381	62.42	164.16	98.84	1367	62.81	165.20	97.80	1353	63.21	166.24	96.76	1338
263.5	61.89	163.08	100.42	1389	62.28	164.12	99.38	1374	62.68	165.16	98.34	1360	63.07	166.20	97.30	1346
264	61.76	163.04	100.96	1396	62.15	164.08	99.92	1382	62.54	165.12	98.88	1368	62.94	166.15	97.85	1353
264.5	61.63	163.00	101.50	1404	62.02	164.04	100.46	1389	62.41	165.08	99.42	1375	62.80	166.11	98.39	1361
265	61.49	162.96	102.04	1411	61.89	164.00	101.00	1397	62.28	165.04	99.97	1383	62.67	166.07	98.93	1368
265.5	61.36	162.92	102.58	1419	61.75	163.96	101.54	1404	62.14	164.99	100.51	1390	62.54	166.03	99.47	1376
266	61.23	162.88	103.12	1426	61.62	163.92	102.08	1412	62.01	164.95	101.05	1397	62.40	165.99	100.01	1383
266.5	61.10	162.84	103.66	1434	61.49	163.87	102.63	1419	61.88	164.91	101.59	1405	62.27	165.95	100.55	1391
267	60.97	162.80	104.20	1441	61.36	163.83	103.17	1427	61.75	164.87	102.13	1412	62.14	165.91	101.09	1398
267.5	60.84	162.76	104.75	1449	61.23	163.79	103.71	1434	61.62	164.83	102.67	1420	62.01	165.87	101.63	1406
268	60.71	162.71	105.29	1456	61.10	163.75	104.25	1442	61.49	164.79	103.21	1427	61.88	165.83	102.17	1413
268.5	60.59	162.67	105.83	1464	60.97	163.71	104.79	1449	61.36	164.75	103.75	1435	61.75	165.79	102.71	1421
269	60.46	162.63	106.37	1471	60.84	163.67	105.33	1457	61.23	164.71	104.29	1442	61.62	165.74	103.26	1428
269.5	60.33	162.59	106.91	1479	60.72	163.63	105.87	1464	61.10	164.67	104.83	1450	61.49	165.70	103.80	1436
270	60.20	162.55	107.45	1486	60.59	163.59	106.41	1472	60.97	164.63	105.38	1457	61.36	165.66	104.34	1443
270.5	60.08	162.51	107.99	1494	60.46	163.55	106.95	1479	60.84	164.58	105.92	1465	61.23	165.62	104.88	1450
271	59.95	162.47	108.53	1501	60.33	163.51	107.49	1487	60.72	164.54	106.46	1472	61.10	165.58	105.42	1458
271.5	59.83	162.43	109.07	1508	60.21	163.46	108.04	1494	60.59	164.50	107.00	1480	60.97	165.54	105.96	1465
272	59.70	162.39	109.61	1516	60.08	163.42	108.58	1502	60.46	164.46	107.54	1487	60.85	165.50	106.50	1473
272.5	59.58	162.35	110.16	1523	59.96	163.38	109.12	1509	60.34	164.42	108.08	1495	60.72	165.46	107.04	1480
273	59.45	162.30	110.70	1531	59.83	163.34	109.66	1517	60.21	164.38	108.62	1502	60.59	165.42	107.58	1488
273.5	59.33	162.26	111.24	1538	59.71	163.30	110.20	1524	60.09	164.34	109.16	1510	60.47	165.38	108.12	1495
274	59.21	162.22	111.78	1546	59.58	163.26	110.74	1532	59.96	164.30	109.70	1517	60.34	165.33	108.67	1503
274.5	59.08	162.18	112.32	1553	59.46	163.22	111.28	1539	59.84	164.26	110.24	1525	60.22	165.29	109.21	1510
275	58.96	162.14	112.86	1561	59.34	163.18	111.82	1547	59.71	164.22	110.79	1532	60.09	165.25	109.75	1518
275.5	58.84	162.10	113.40	1568	59.21	163.14	112.36	1554	59.59	164.17	111.33	1540	59.97	165.21	110.29	1525
276	58.72	162.06	113.94	1576	59.09	163.10	112.90	1561	59.47	164.13	111.87	1547	59.84	165.17	110.83	1533
276.5	58.60	162.02	114.48	1583	58.97	163.05	113.45	1569	59.35	164.09	112.41	1555	59.72	165.13	111.37	1540
277	58.48	161.98	115.02	1591	58.85	163.01	113.99	1576	59.22	164.05	112.95	1562	59.60	165.09	111.91	1548
277.5	58.35	161.94	115.57	1598	58.73	162.97	114.53	1584	59.10	164.01	113.49	1570	59.48	165.05	112.45	1555
278	58.24	161.89	116.11	1606	58.61	162.93	115.07	1591	58.98	163.97	114.03	1577	59.35	165.01	112.99	1563
278.5	58.12	161.85	116.65	1613	58.49	162.89	115.61	1599	58.86	163.93	114.57	1585	59.23	164.97	113.53	1570
279	58.00	161.81	117.19	1621	58.37	162.85	116.15	1606	58.74	163.89	115.11	1592	59.11	164.92	114.08	1578
279.5	57.88	161.77	117.73	1628	58.25	162.81	116.69	1614	58.62	163.85	115.65	1599	58.99	164.88	114.62	1585
280	57.76	161.73	118.27	1636	58.13	162.77	117.23	1621	58.50	163.81	116.20	1607	58.87	164.84	115.16	1593
280.5	57.64	161.69	118.81	1643	58.01	162.73	117.77	1629	58.38	163.76	116.74	1614	58.75	164.80	115.70	1600
281	57.53	161.65	119.35	1651	57.90	162.69	118.31	1636	58.26	163.72	117.28	1622	58.63	164.76	116.24	1608
281.5	57.41	161.61	119.89	1658	57.78	162.64	118.86	1644	58.15	163.68	117.82	1629	58.51	164.72	116.78	1615
282	57.29	161.57	120.43	1666	57.66	162.60	119.40	1651	58.03	163.64	118.36	1637	58.40	164.68	117.32	1623
282.5	57.18	161.53	120.98	1673	57.54	162.56	119.94	1659	57.91	163.60	118.90	1644	58.28	164.64	117.86	1630
283	57.06	161.48	121.52	1681	57.43	162.52	120.48	1666	57.79	163.56	119.44	1652	58.16	164.60	118.40	1638
283.5	56.95	161.44	122.06	1688	57.31	162.48	121.02	1674	57.68	163.52	119.98	1659	58.04	164.56	118.94	1645
284	56.83	161.40	122.60	1696	57.20	162.44	121.56	1681	57.56	163.48	120.52	1667	57.93	164.51	119.49	1652
284.5	56.72	161.36	123.14	1703	57.08	162.40	122.10	1689	57.45	163.44	121.06	1674	57.81	164.47	120.03	1660
285	56.60	161.32	123.68	1710	56.97	162.36	122.64	1696	57.33	163.40	121.61	1682	57.70	164.43	120.57	1667
285.5	56.49	161.28	124.22	1718	56.85	162.32	123.18	1704	57.22	163.35	122.15	1689	57.58	164.39	121.11	1675
286	56.38	161.24	124.76	1725	56.74	162.28	123.72	1711	57.10	163.31	122.69	1697	57.47	164.35	121.65	1682
286.5	56.26	161.20	125.30	1733	56.63	162.23	124.27	1719	56.99	163.27	123.23	1704	57.35	164.31	122.19	1690
287	56.15	161.16	125.84	1740	56.51	162.19	124.81	1726	56.87	163.23	123.77	1712	57.24	164.27	122.73	1697
287.5	56.04	161.12	126.39	1748	56.40	162.15	125.35	1734	56.76	163.19	124.31	1719	57.12	164.23	123.27	1705
288	55.93	161.07	126.93	1755	56.29	162.11	125.89	1741	56.65	163.15	124.85	1727	57.01	164.19	123.81	1712
288.5	55.82	161.03	127.47	1763	56.18	162.07	126.43	1749	56.54	163.11	125.39	1734	56.90	164.15	124.35	1720
289	55.71	160.99	128.01	1770	56.07	162.03	126.97	1756	56.42	163.07	125.93	1742	56.78	164.10	124.90	1727
289.5	55.60	160.95	128.55	1778	55.95	161.99	127.51	1763	56.31	163.03	126.47	1749	56.67	164.06	125.44	1735
290	55.49	160.91	129.09	1785	55.84	161.95	128.05	1771	56.20	162.99	127.02	1757	56.56	164.02	125.98	1742
290.5	55.38	160.87	129.63	1793	55.73	161.91	128.59	1778	56.09	162.94	127.56	1764	56.45	163.98	126.52	1750
291	55.27	160.83	130.17	1800	55.62	161.87	129.13	1786	55.98	162.90	128.10	1772	56.34	163.94	127.06	1757
291.5	55.16	160.79	130.71	1808	55.51	161.82	129.68	1793	55.87	162.86	128.64	1779	56.23	163.90	127.60	1765

Body Composition　FEMALE　260-291.5 Lb.

Weight: Lb.	Waist: 64 inches Fat: %	Fat: Lb.	LBM: Lb.	RMR: Cal.	64.25 inches Fat: %	Fat: Lb.	LBM: Lb.	RMR: Cal.	64.5 inches Fat: %	Fat: Lb.	LBM: Lb.	RMR: Cal.	64.75 inches Fat: %	Fat: Lb.	LBM: Lb.	RMR: Cal.
260	64.43	167.52	92.48	1279	64.83	168.56	91.44	1265	65.23	169.60	90.41	1250	65.63	170.63	89.37	1236
260.5	64.29	167.48	93.02	1286	64.69	168.52	91.98	1272	65.09	169.55	90.95	1258	65.49	170.59	89.91	1243
261	64.15	167.44	93.56	1294	64.55	168.48	92.52	1280	64.95	169.51	91.49	1265	65.35	170.55	90.45	1251
261.5	64.01	167.40	94.10	1301	64.41	168.43	93.07	1287	64.81	169.47	92.03	1273	65.20	170.51	90.99	1258
262	63.88	167.36	94.64	1309	64.27	168.39	93.61	1295	64.67	169.43	92.57	1280	65.06	170.47	91.53	1266
262.5	63.74	167.32	95.19	1316	64.13	168.35	94.15	1302	64.53	169.39	93.11	1288	64.92	170.43	92.07	1273
263	63.60	167.27	95.73	1324	64.00	168.31	94.69	1310	64.39	169.35	93.65	1295	64.79	170.39	92.61	1281
263.5	63.47	167.23	96.27	1331	63.86	168.27	95.23	1317	64.25	169.31	94.19	1303	64.65	170.35	93.15	1288
264	63.33	167.19	96.81	1339	63.72	168.23	95.77	1325	64.12	169.27	94.73	1310	64.51	170.30	93.70	1296
264.5	63.20	167.15	97.35	1346	63.59	168.19	96.31	1332	63.98	169.23	95.27	1318	64.37	170.26	94.24	1303
265	63.06	167.11	97.89	1354	63.45	168.15	96.85	1339	63.84	169.19	95.82	1325	64.23	170.22	94.78	1311
265.5	62.93	167.07	98.43	1361	63.32	168.11	97.39	1347	63.71	169.14	96.36	1333	64.10	170.18	95.32	1318
266	62.79	167.03	98.97	1369	63.18	168.07	97.93	1354	63.57	169.10	96.90	1340	63.96	170.14	95.86	1326
266.5	62.66	166.99	99.51	1376	63.05	168.02	98.48	1362	63.44	169.06	97.44	1348	63.83	170.10	96.40	1333
267	62.53	166.95	100.05	1384	62.92	167.98	99.02	1369	63.30	169.02	97.98	1355	63.69	170.06	96.94	1341
267.5	62.39	166.91	100.60	1391	62.78	167.94	99.56	1377	63.17	168.98	98.52	1363	63.56	170.02	97.48	1348
268	62.26	166.86	101.14	1399	62.65	167.90	100.10	1384	63.04	168.94	99.06	1370	63.42	169.98	98.02	1356
268.5	62.13	166.82	101.68	1406	62.52	167.86	100.64	1392	62.90	168.90	99.60	1377	63.29	169.94	98.56	1363
269	62.00	166.78	102.22	1414	62.39	167.82	101.18	1399	62.77	168.86	100.14	1385	63.16	169.89	99.11	1371
269.5	61.87	166.74	102.76	1421	62.26	167.78	101.72	1407	62.64	168.82	100.68	1392	63.03	169.85	99.65	1378
270	61.74	166.70	103.30	1429	62.13	167.74	102.26	1414	62.51	168.78	101.23	1400	62.89	169.81	100.19	1386
270.5	61.61	166.66	103.84	1436	62.00	167.70	102.80	1422	62.38	168.73	101.77	1407	62.76	169.77	100.73	1393
271	61.48	166.62	104.38	1444	61.87	167.66	103.34	1429	62.25	168.69	102.31	1415	62.63	169.73	101.27	1401
271.5	61.35	166.58	104.92	1451	61.74	167.61	103.89	1437	62.12	168.65	102.85	1422	62.50	169.69	101.81	1408
272	61.23	166.54	105.46	1459	61.61	167.57	104.43	1444	61.99	168.61	103.39	1430	62.37	169.65	102.35	1416
272.5	61.10	166.50	106.01	1466	61.48	167.53	104.97	1452	61.86	168.57	103.93	1437	62.24	169.61	102.89	1423
273	60.97	166.45	106.55	1474	61.35	167.49	105.51	1459	61.73	168.53	104.47	1445	62.11	169.57	103.43	1430
273.5	60.85	166.41	107.09	1481	61.23	167.45	106.05	1467	61.60	168.49	105.01	1452	61.98	169.53	103.97	1438
274	60.72	166.37	107.63	1488	61.10	167.41	106.59	1474	61.48	168.45	105.55	1460	61.86	169.48	104.52	1445
274.5	60.59	166.33	108.17	1496	60.97	167.37	107.13	1482	61.35	168.41	106.09	1467	61.73	169.44	105.06	1453
275	60.47	166.29	108.71	1503	60.85	167.33	107.67	1489	61.22	168.37	106.64	1475	61.60	169.40	105.60	1460
275.5	60.34	166.25	109.25	1511	60.72	167.29	108.21	1497	61.10	168.32	107.18	1482	61.47	169.36	106.14	1468
276	60.22	166.21	109.79	1518	60.60	167.25	108.75	1504	60.97	168.28	107.72	1490	61.35	169.32	106.68	1475
276.5	60.10	166.17	110.33	1526	60.47	167.20	109.30	1512	60.85	168.24	108.26	1497	61.22	169.28	107.22	1483
277	59.97	166.13	110.87	1533	60.35	167.16	109.84	1519	60.72	168.20	108.80	1505	61.10	169.24	107.76	1490
277.5	59.85	166.09	111.42	1541	60.22	167.12	110.38	1527	60.60	168.16	109.34	1512	60.97	169.20	108.30	1498
278	59.73	166.04	111.96	1548	60.10	167.08	110.92	1534	60.47	168.12	109.88	1520	60.85	169.16	108.84	1505
278.5	59.61	166.00	112.50	1556	59.98	167.04	111.46	1541	60.35	168.08	110.42	1527	60.72	169.12	109.38	1513
279	59.48	165.96	113.04	1563	59.86	167.00	112.00	1549	60.23	168.04	110.96	1535	60.60	169.07	109.93	1520
279.5	59.36	165.92	113.58	1571	59.73	166.96	112.54	1556	60.11	168.00	111.50	1542	60.48	169.03	110.47	1528
280	59.24	165.88	114.12	1578	59.61	166.92	113.08	1564	59.98	167.96	112.05	1550	60.35	168.99	111.01	1535
280.5	59.12	165.84	114.66	1586	59.49	166.88	113.62	1571	59.86	167.91	112.59	1557	60.23	168.95	111.55	1543
281	59.00	165.80	115.20	1593	59.37	166.84	114.16	1579	59.74	167.87	113.13	1565	60.11	168.91	112.09	1550
281.5	58.88	165.76	115.74	1601	59.25	166.79	114.71	1586	59.62	167.83	113.67	1572	59.99	168.87	112.63	1558
282	58.76	165.72	116.28	1608	59.13	166.75	115.25	1594	59.50	167.79	114.21	1580	59.87	168.83	113.17	1565
282.5	58.65	165.68	116.83	1616	59.01	166.71	115.79	1601	59.38	167.75	114.75	1587	59.75	168.79	113.71	1573
283	58.53	165.63	117.37	1623	58.89	166.67	116.33	1609	59.26	167.71	115.29	1594	59.63	168.75	114.25	1580
283.5	58.41	165.59	117.91	1631	58.78	166.63	116.87	1616	59.14	167.67	115.83	1602	59.51	168.71	114.79	1588
284	58.29	165.55	118.45	1638	58.66	166.59	117.41	1624	59.02	167.63	116.37	1609	59.39	168.66	115.34	1595
284.5	58.18	165.51	118.99	1646	58.54	166.55	117.95	1631	58.91	167.59	116.91	1617	59.27	168.62	115.88	1603
285	58.06	165.47	119.53	1653	58.42	166.51	118.49	1639	58.79	167.55	117.46	1624	59.15	168.58	116.42	1610
285.5	57.94	165.43	120.07	1661	58.31	166.47	119.03	1646	58.67	167.50	118.00	1632	59.03	168.54	116.96	1618
286	57.83	165.39	120.61	1668	58.19	166.43	119.57	1654	58.55	167.46	118.54	1639	58.92	168.50	117.50	1625
286.5	57.71	165.35	121.15	1676	58.07	166.38	120.12	1661	58.44	167.42	119.08	1647	58.80	168.46	118.04	1633
287	57.60	165.31	121.69	1683	57.96	166.34	120.66	1669	58.32	167.38	119.62	1654	58.68	168.42	118.58	1640
287.5	57.48	165.27	122.24	1691	57.84	166.30	121.20	1676	58.21	167.34	120.16	1662	58.57	168.38	119.12	1647
288	57.37	165.22	122.78	1698	57.73	166.26	121.74	1684	58.09	167.30	120.70	1669	58.45	168.34	119.66	1655
288.5	57.26	165.18	123.32	1705	57.62	166.22	122.28	1691	57.98	167.26	121.24	1677	58.33	168.30	120.20	1662
289	57.14	165.14	123.86	1713	57.50	166.18	122.82	1699	57.86	167.22	121.78	1684	58.22	168.25	120.75	1670
289.5	57.03	165.10	124.40	1720	57.39	166.14	123.36	1706	57.75	167.18	122.32	1692	58.10	168.21	121.29	1677
290	56.92	165.06	124.94	1728	57.28	166.10	123.90	1714	57.63	167.14	122.87	1699	57.99	168.17	121.83	1685
290.5	56.81	165.02	125.48	1735	57.16	166.06	124.44	1721	57.52	167.09	123.41	1707	57.88	168.13	122.37	1692
291	56.69	164.98	126.02	1743	57.05	166.02	124.98	1729	57.41	167.05	123.95	1714	57.76	168.09	122.91	1700
291.5	56.58	164.94	126.56	1750	56.94	165.97	125.53	1736	57.29	167.01	124.49	1722	57.65	168.05	123.45	1707

Body Composition FEMALE 260-291.5 Lb.

Weight: Lb.	Waist: 65 inches				65.25 inches				65.5 inches				65.75 inches			
	Fat: %	Fat: Lb.	LBM: Lb.	RMR: Cal.	Fat: %	Fat: Lb.	LBM: Lb.	RMR: Cal.	Fat: %	Fat: Lb.	LBM: Lb.	RMR: Cal.	Fat: %	Fat: Lb.	LBM: Lb.	RMR: Cal.
260	66.03	171.67	88.33	1222	66.43	172.71	87.29	1207	66.83	173.75	86.26	1193	67.22	174.78	85.22	1179
260.5	65.88	171.63	88.87	1229	66.28	172.67	87.83	1215	66.68	173.70	86.80	1200	67.08	174.74	85.76	1186
261	65.74	171.59	89.41	1237	66.14	172.63	88.37	1222	66.54	173.66	87.34	1208	66.94	174.70	86.30	1194
261.5	65.60	171.55	89.95	1244	66.00	172.58	88.92	1230	66.39	173.62	87.88	1215	66.79	174.66	86.84	1201
262	65.46	171.51	90.49	1252	65.86	172.54	89.46	1237	66.25	173.58	88.42	1223	66.65	174.62	87.38	1208
262.5	65.32	171.47	91.04	1259	65.72	172.50	90.00	1245	66.11	173.54	88.96	1230	66.51	174.58	87.92	1216
263	65.18	171.42	91.58	1266	65.57	172.46	90.54	1252	65.97	173.50	89.50	1238	66.36	174.54	88.46	1223
263.5	65.04	171.38	92.12	1274	65.43	172.42	91.08	1260	65.83	173.46	90.04	1245	66.22	174.50	89.00	1231
264	64.90	171.34	92.66	1281	65.30	172.38	91.62	1267	65.69	173.42	90.58	1253	66.08	174.45	89.55	1238
264.5	64.76	171.30	93.20	1289	65.16	172.34	92.16	1275	65.55	173.38	91.12	1260	65.94	174.41	90.09	1246
265	64.63	171.26	93.74	1296	65.02	172.30	92.70	1282	65.41	173.34	91.67	1268	65.80	174.37	90.63	1253
265.5	64.49	171.22	94.28	1304	64.88	172.26	93.24	1290	65.27	173.29	92.21	1275	65.66	174.33	91.17	1261
266	64.35	171.18	94.82	1311	64.74	172.22	93.78	1297	65.13	173.25	92.75	1283	65.52	174.29	91.71	1268
266.5	64.22	171.14	95.36	1319	64.61	172.17	94.33	1305	65.00	173.21	93.29	1290	65.38	174.25	92.25	1276
267	64.08	171.10	95.90	1326	64.47	172.13	94.87	1312	64.86	173.17	93.83	1298	65.25	174.21	92.79	1283
267.5	63.95	171.06	96.45	1334	64.33	172.09	95.41	1319	64.72	173.13	94.37	1305	65.11	174.17	93.33	1291
268	63.81	171.01	96.99	1341	64.20	172.05	95.95	1327	64.59	173.09	94.91	1313	64.97	174.13	93.87	1298
268.5	63.68	170.97	97.53	1349	64.06	172.01	96.49	1334	64.45	173.05	95.45	1320	64.84	174.09	94.41	1306
269	63.54	170.93	98.07	1356	63.93	171.97	97.03	1342	64.31	173.01	95.99	1328	64.70	174.04	94.96	1313
269.5	63.41	170.89	98.61	1364	63.80	171.93	97.57	1349	64.18	172.97	96.53	1335	64.57	174.00	95.50	1321
270	63.28	170.85	99.15	1371	63.66	171.89	98.11	1357	64.05	172.93	97.08	1343	64.43	173.96	96.04	1328
270.5	63.15	170.81	99.69	1379	63.53	171.85	98.65	1364	63.91	172.88	97.62	1350	64.30	173.92	96.58	1336
271	63.01	170.77	100.23	1386	63.40	171.81	99.19	1372	63.78	172.84	98.16	1358	64.16	173.88	97.12	1343
271.5	62.88	170.73	100.77	1394	63.27	171.76	99.74	1379	63.65	172.80	98.70	1365	64.03	173.84	97.66	1351
272	62.75	170.69	101.31	1401	63.13	171.72	100.28	1387	63.52	172.76	99.24	1372	63.90	173.80	98.20	1358
272.5	62.62	170.65	101.86	1409	63.00	171.68	100.82	1394	63.38	172.72	99.78	1380	63.76	173.76	98.74	1366
273	62.49	170.60	102.40	1416	62.87	171.64	101.36	1402	63.25	172.68	100.32	1387	63.63	173.72	99.28	1373
273.5	62.36	170.56	102.94	1424	62.74	171.60	101.90	1409	63.12	172.64	100.86	1395	63.50	173.68	99.82	1381
274	62.23	170.52	103.48	1431	62.61	171.56	102.44	1417	62.99	172.60	101.40	1402	63.37	173.63	100.37	1388
274.5	62.11	170.48	104.02	1439	62.48	171.52	102.98	1424	62.86	172.56	101.94	1410	63.24	173.59	100.91	1396
275	61.98	170.44	104.56	1446	62.36	171.48	103.52	1432	62.73	172.52	102.49	1417	63.11	173.55	101.45	1403
275.5	61.85	170.40	105.10	1454	62.23	171.44	104.06	1439	62.60	172.47	103.03	1425	62.98	173.51	101.99	1411
276	61.72	170.36	105.64	1461	62.10	171.40	104.60	1447	62.48	172.43	103.57	1432	62.85	173.47	102.53	1418
276.5	61.60	170.32	106.18	1469	61.97	171.35	105.15	1454	62.35	172.39	104.11	1440	62.72	173.43	103.07	1425
277	61.47	170.28	106.72	1476	61.85	171.31	105.69	1462	62.22	172.35	104.65	1447	62.60	173.39	103.61	1433
277.5	61.35	170.24	107.27	1483	61.72	171.27	106.23	1469	62.09	172.31	105.19	1455	62.47	173.35	104.15	1440
278	61.22	170.19	107.81	1491	61.59	171.23	106.77	1477	61.97	172.27	105.73	1462	62.34	173.31	104.69	1448
278.5	61.10	170.15	108.35	1498	61.47	171.19	107.31	1484	61.84	172.23	106.27	1470	62.21	173.27	105.23	1455
279	60.97	170.11	108.89	1506	61.34	171.15	107.85	1492	61.72	172.19	106.81	1477	62.09	173.22	105.78	1463
279.5	60.85	170.07	109.43	1513	61.22	171.11	108.39	1499	61.59	172.15	107.35	1485	61.96	173.18	106.32	1470
280	60.73	170.03	109.97	1521	61.10	171.07	108.93	1507	61.47	172.11	107.90	1492	61.84	173.14	106.86	1478
280.5	60.60	169.99	110.51	1528	60.97	171.03	109.47	1514	61.34	172.06	108.44	1500	61.71	173.10	107.40	1485
281	60.48	169.95	111.05	1536	60.85	170.99	110.01	1522	61.22	172.02	108.98	1507	61.59	173.06	107.94	1493
281.5	60.36	169.91	111.59	1543	60.73	170.94	110.56	1529	61.09	171.98	109.52	1515	61.46	173.02	108.48	1500
282	60.24	169.87	112.13	1551	60.60	170.90	111.10	1536	60.97	171.94	110.06	1522	61.34	172.98	109.02	1508
282.5	60.12	169.83	112.68	1558	60.48	170.86	111.64	1544	60.85	171.90	110.60	1530	61.22	172.94	109.56	1515
283	59.99	169.78	113.22	1566	60.36	170.82	112.18	1551	60.73	171.86	111.14	1537	61.09	172.90	110.10	1523
283.5	59.87	169.74	113.76	1573	60.24	170.78	112.72	1559	60.61	171.82	111.68	1545	60.97	172.86	110.64	1530
284	59.75	169.70	114.30	1581	60.12	170.74	113.26	1566	60.48	171.78	112.22	1552	60.85	172.81	111.19	1538
284.5	59.63	169.66	114.84	1588	60.00	170.70	113.80	1574	60.36	171.74	112.76	1560	60.73	172.77	111.73	1545
285	59.52	169.62	115.38	1596	59.88	170.66	114.34	1581	60.24	171.70	113.31	1567	60.61	172.73	112.27	1553
285.5	59.40	169.58	115.92	1603	59.76	170.62	114.88	1589	60.12	171.65	113.85	1574	60.49	172.69	112.81	1560
286	59.28	169.54	116.46	1611	59.64	170.58	115.42	1596	60.00	171.61	114.39	1582	60.37	172.65	113.35	1568
286.5	59.16	169.50	117.00	1618	59.52	170.53	115.97	1604	59.89	171.57	114.93	1589	60.25	172.61	113.89	1575
287	59.04	169.46	117.54	1626	59.41	170.49	116.51	1611	59.77	171.53	115.47	1597	60.13	172.57	114.43	1583
287.5	58.93	169.42	118.09	1633	59.29	170.45	117.05	1619	59.65	171.49	116.01	1604	60.01	172.53	114.97	1590
288	58.81	169.37	118.63	1641	59.17	170.41	117.59	1626	59.53	171.45	116.55	1612	59.89	172.49	115.51	1598
288.5	58.69	169.33	119.17	1648	59.05	170.37	118.13	1634	59.41	171.41	117.09	1619	59.77	172.45	116.05	1605
289	58.58	169.29	119.71	1656	58.94	170.33	118.67	1641	59.30	171.37	117.63	1627	59.66	172.40	116.60	1613
289.5	58.46	169.25	120.25	1663	58.82	170.29	119.21	1649	59.18	171.33	118.17	1634	59.54	172.36	117.14	1620
290	58.35	169.21	120.79	1671	58.71	170.25	119.75	1656	59.06	171.29	118.72	1642	59.42	172.32	117.68	1627
290.5	58.23	169.17	121.33	1678	58.59	170.21	120.29	1664	58.95	171.24	119.26	1649	59.31	172.28	118.22	1635
291	58.12	169.13	121.87	1685	58.48	170.17	120.83	1671	58.83	171.20	119.80	1657	59.19	172.24	118.76	1642
291.5	58.01	169.09	122.41	1693	58.36	170.12	121.38	1679	58.72	171.16	120.34	1664	59.07	172.20	119.30	1650

Body Composition FEMALE 260-291.5 Lb.

Weight: Lb.	Waist: 66 inches Fat: %	Fat: Lb.	LBM: Lb.	RMR: Cal.	66.25 inches Fat: %	Fat: Lb.	LBM: Lb.	RMR: Cal.	66.5 inches Fat: %	Fat: Lb.	LBM: Lb.	RMR: Cal.	66.75 inches Fat: %	Fat: Lb.	LBM: Lb.	RMR: Cal.
260	67.62	175.82	84.18	1164	68.02	176.86	83.14	1150	68.42	177.90	82.11	1136	68.82	178.93	81.07	1121
260.5	67.48	175.78	84.72	1172	67.88	176.82	83.68	1157	68.27	177.85	82.65	1143	68.67	178.89	81.61	1129
261	67.33	175.74	85.26	1179	67.73	176.78	84.22	1165	68.13	177.81	83.19	1150	68.53	178.85	82.15	1136
261.5	67.19	175.70	85.80	1187	67.58	176.73	84.77	1172	67.98	177.77	83.73	1158	68.38	178.81	82.69	1144
262	67.04	175.66	86.34	1194	67.44	176.69	85.31	1180	67.84	177.73	84.27	1165	68.23	178.77	83.23	1151
262.5	66.90	175.62	86.89	1202	67.30	176.65	85.85	1187	67.69	177.69	84.81	1173	68.09	178.73	83.77	1159
263	66.76	175.57	87.43	1209	67.15	176.61	86.39	1195	67.55	177.65	85.35	1180	67.94	178.69	84.31	1166
263.5	66.62	175.53	87.97	1217	67.01	176.57	86.93	1202	67.40	177.61	85.89	1188	67.80	178.65	84.85	1174
264	66.47	175.49	88.51	1224	66.87	176.53	87.47	1210	67.26	177.57	86.43	1195	67.65	178.60	85.40	1181
264.5	66.33	175.45	89.05	1232	66.73	176.49	88.01	1217	67.12	177.53	86.97	1203	67.51	178.56	85.94	1189
265	66.19	175.41	89.59	1239	66.58	176.45	88.55	1225	66.98	177.49	87.52	1210	67.37	178.52	86.48	1196
265.5	66.05	175.37	90.13	1247	66.44	176.41	89.09	1232	66.83	177.44	88.06	1218	67.22	178.48	87.02	1203
266	65.91	175.33	90.67	1254	66.30	176.37	89.63	1240	66.69	177.40	88.60	1225	67.08	178.44	87.56	1211
266.5	65.77	175.29	91.21	1261	66.16	176.32	90.18	1247	66.55	177.36	89.14	1233	66.94	178.40	88.10	1218
267	65.64	175.25	91.75	1269	66.02	176.28	90.72	1255	66.41	177.32	89.68	1240	66.80	178.36	88.64	1226
267.5	65.50	175.21	92.30	1276	65.89	176.24	91.26	1262	66.27	177.28	90.22	1248	66.66	178.32	89.18	1233
268	65.36	175.16	92.84	1284	65.75	176.20	91.80	1270	66.13	177.24	90.76	1255	66.52	178.28	89.72	1241
268.5	65.22	175.12	93.38	1291	65.61	176.16	92.34	1277	66.00	177.20	91.30	1263	66.38	178.24	90.26	1248
269	65.09	175.08	93.92	1299	65.47	176.12	92.88	1285	65.86	177.16	91.84	1270	66.24	178.19	90.81	1256
269.5	64.95	175.04	94.46	1306	65.34	176.08	93.42	1292	65.72	177.12	92.38	1278	66.11	178.15	91.35	1263
270	64.81	175.00	95.00	1314	65.20	176.04	93.96	1300	65.58	177.08	92.93	1285	65.97	178.11	91.89	1271
270.5	64.68	174.96	95.54	1321	65.06	176.00	94.50	1307	65.45	177.03	93.47	1293	65.83	178.07	92.43	1278
271	64.55	174.92	96.08	1329	64.93	175.96	95.04	1314	65.31	176.99	94.01	1300	65.69	178.03	92.97	1286
271.5	64.41	174.88	96.62	1336	64.79	175.91	95.59	1322	65.18	176.95	94.55	1308	65.56	177.99	93.51	1293
272	64.28	174.84	97.16	1344	64.66	175.87	96.13	1329	65.04	176.91	95.09	1315	65.42	177.95	94.05	1301
272.5	64.14	174.80	97.71	1351	64.53	175.83	96.67	1337	64.91	176.87	95.63	1323	65.29	177.91	94.59	1308
273	64.01	174.75	98.25	1359	64.39	175.79	97.21	1344	64.77	176.83	96.17	1330	65.15	177.87	95.13	1316
273.5	63.88	174.71	98.79	1366	64.26	175.75	97.75	1352	64.64	176.79	96.71	1338	65.02	177.83	95.67	1323
274	63.75	174.67	99.33	1374	64.13	175.71	98.29	1359	64.51	176.75	97.25	1345	64.88	177.78	96.22	1331
274.5	63.62	174.63	99.87	1381	64.00	175.67	98.83	1367	64.37	176.71	97.79	1352	64.75	177.74	96.76	1338
275	63.49	174.59	100.41	1389	63.86	175.63	99.37	1374	64.24	176.67	98.34	1360	64.62	177.70	97.30	1346
275.5	63.36	174.55	100.95	1396	63.73	175.59	99.91	1382	64.11	176.62	98.88	1367	64.49	177.66	97.84	1353
276	63.23	174.51	101.49	1404	63.60	175.55	100.45	1389	63.98	176.58	99.42	1375	64.36	177.62	98.38	1361
276.5	63.10	174.47	102.03	1411	63.47	175.50	101.00	1397	63.85	176.54	99.96	1382	64.22	177.58	98.92	1368
277	62.97	174.43	102.57	1419	63.34	175.46	101.54	1404	63.72	176.50	100.50	1390	64.09	177.54	99.46	1376
277.5	62.84	174.39	103.12	1426	63.22	175.42	102.08	1412	63.59	176.46	101.04	1397	63.96	177.50	100.00	1383
278	62.71	174.34	103.66	1434	63.09	175.38	102.62	1419	63.46	176.42	101.58	1405	63.83	177.46	100.54	1391
278.5	62.59	174.30	104.20	1441	62.96	175.34	103.16	1427	63.33	176.38	102.12	1412	63.70	177.42	101.08	1398
279	62.46	174.26	104.74	1449	62.83	175.30	103.70	1434	63.20	176.34	102.66	1420	63.58	177.37	101.63	1405
279.5	62.33	174.22	105.28	1456	62.70	175.26	104.24	1442	63.08	176.30	103.20	1427	63.45	177.33	102.17	1413
280	62.21	174.18	105.82	1463	62.58	175.22	104.78	1449	62.95	176.26	103.75	1435	63.32	177.29	102.71	1420
280.5	62.08	174.14	106.36	1471	62.45	175.18	105.32	1457	62.82	176.21	104.29	1442	63.19	177.25	103.25	1428
281	61.96	174.10	106.90	1478	62.33	175.14	105.86	1464	62.70	176.17	104.83	1450	63.06	177.21	103.79	1435
281.5	61.83	174.06	107.44	1486	62.20	175.09	106.41	1472	62.57	176.13	105.37	1457	62.94	177.17	104.33	1443
282	61.71	174.02	107.98	1493	62.08	175.05	106.95	1479	62.44	176.09	105.91	1465	62.81	177.13	104.87	1450
282.5	61.58	173.98	108.53	1501	61.95	175.01	107.49	1487	62.32	176.05	106.45	1472	62.69	177.09	105.41	1458
283	61.46	173.93	109.07	1508	61.83	174.97	108.03	1494	62.19	176.01	106.99	1480	62.56	177.05	105.95	1465
283.5	61.34	173.89	109.61	1516	61.70	174.93	108.57	1502	62.07	175.97	107.53	1487	62.44	177.01	106.49	1473
284	61.22	173.85	110.15	1523	61.58	174.89	109.11	1509	61.95	175.93	108.07	1495	62.31	176.96	107.04	1480
284.5	61.09	173.81	110.69	1531	61.46	174.85	109.65	1516	61.82	175.89	108.61	1502	62.19	176.92	107.58	1488
285	60.97	173.77	111.23	1538	61.34	174.81	110.19	1524	61.70	175.85	109.16	1510	62.06	176.88	108.12	1495
285.5	60.85	173.73	111.77	1546	61.21	174.77	110.73	1531	61.58	175.80	109.70	1517	61.94	176.84	108.66	1503
286	60.73	173.69	112.31	1553	61.09	174.73	111.27	1539	61.46	175.76	110.24	1525	61.82	176.80	109.20	1510
286.5	60.61	173.65	112.85	1561	60.97	174.68	111.82	1546	61.33	175.72	110.78	1532	61.70	176.76	109.74	1518
287	60.49	173.61	113.39	1568	60.85	174.64	112.36	1554	61.21	175.68	111.32	1540	61.57	176.72	110.28	1525
287.5	60.37	173.57	113.94	1576	60.73	174.60	112.90	1561	61.09	175.64	111.86	1547	61.45	176.68	110.82	1533
288	60.25	173.52	114.48	1583	60.61	174.56	113.44	1569	60.97	175.60	112.40	1555	61.33	176.64	111.36	1540
288.5	60.13	173.48	115.02	1591	60.49	174.52	113.98	1576	60.85	175.56	112.94	1562	61.21	176.60	111.90	1548
289	60.01	173.44	115.56	1598	60.37	174.48	114.52	1584	60.73	175.52	113.48	1569	61.09	176.55	112.45	1555
289.5	59.90	173.40	116.10	1606	60.26	174.44	115.06	1591	60.61	175.48	114.02	1577	60.97	176.51	112.99	1563
290	59.78	173.36	116.64	1613	60.14	174.40	115.60	1599	60.49	175.44	114.57	1584	60.85	176.47	113.53	1570
290.5	59.66	173.32	117.18	1621	60.02	174.36	116.14	1606	60.38	175.39	115.11	1592	60.73	176.43	114.07	1578
291	59.55	173.28	117.72	1628	59.90	174.32	116.68	1614	60.26	175.35	115.65	1599	60.62	176.39	114.61	1585
291.5	59.43	173.24	118.26	1636	59.79	174.27	117.23	1621	60.14	175.31	116.19	1607	60.50	176.35	115.15	1593

Body Composition MALE 120-151.5 Lb.

Weight: Lb.	Waist: 27 inches Fat: %	Fat: Lb.	LBM: Lb.	RMR: Cal.	27.25 inches Fat: %	Fat: Lb.	LBM: Lb.	RMR: Cal.	27.5 inches Fat: %	Fat: Lb.	LBM: Lb.	RMR: Cal.	27.75 inches Fat: %	Fat: Lb.	LBM: Lb.	RMR: Cal.
120	3.16	3.79	116.21	1607	4.02	4.83	115.17	1593	4.89	5.87	114.14	1578	5.75	6.90	113.10	1564
120.5	3.11	3.75	116.75	1615	3.97	4.79	115.71	1600	4.83	5.82	114.68	1586	5.69	6.86	113.64	1572
121	3.06	3.71	117.29	1622	3.92	4.75	116.25	1608	4.78	5.78	115.22	1593	5.64	6.82	114.18	1579
121.5	3.02	3.67	117.83	1630	3.87	4.70	116.80	1615	4.73	5.74	115.76	1601	5.58	6.78	114.72	1587
122	2.97	3.63	118.37	1637	3.82	4.66	117.34	1623	4.67	5.70	116.30	1608	5.52	6.74	115.26	1594
122.5	2.93	3.58	118.92	1645	3.77	4.62	117.88	1630	4.62	5.66	116.84	1616	5.47	6.70	115.80	1602
123	2.88	3.54	119.46	1652	3.72	4.58	118.42	1638	4.57	5.62	117.38	1623	5.41	6.66	116.34	1609
123.5	2.84	3.50	120.00	1660	3.68	4.54	118.96	1645	4.52	5.58	117.92	1631	5.36	6.62	116.88	1617
124	2.79	3.46	120.54	1667	3.63	4.50	119.50	1653	4.47	5.54	118.46	1638	5.30	6.57	117.43	1624
124.5	2.75	3.42	121.08	1675	3.58	4.46	120.04	1660	4.41	5.50	119.00	1646	5.25	6.53	117.97	1631
125	2.70	3.38	121.62	1682	3.53	4.42	120.58	1668	4.36	5.46	119.55	1653	5.19	6.49	118.51	1639
125.5	2.66	3.34	122.16	1689	3.49	4.38	121.12	1675	4.31	5.41	120.09	1661	5.14	6.45	119.05	1646
126	2.62	3.30	122.70	1697	3.44	4.34	121.66	1683	4.26	5.37	120.63	1668	5.09	6.41	119.59	1654
126.5	2.57	3.26	123.24	1704	3.39	4.29	122.21	1690	4.22	5.33	121.17	1676	5.04	6.37	120.13	1661
127	2.53	3.22	123.78	1712	3.35	4.25	122.75	1698	4.17	5.29	121.71	1683	4.98	6.33	120.67	1669
127.5	2.49	3.18	124.33	1719	3.30	4.21	123.29	1705	4.12	5.25	122.25	1691	4.93	6.29	121.21	1676
128	2.45	3.13	124.87	1727	3.26	4.17	123.83	1713	4.07	5.21	122.79	1698	4.88	6.25	121.75	1684
128.5	2.41	3.09	125.41	1734	3.21	4.13	124.37	1720	4.02	5.17	123.33	1706	4.83	6.21	122.29	1691
129	2.37	3.05	125.95	1742	3.17	4.09	124.91	1728	3.97	5.13	123.87	1713	4.78	6.16	122.84	1699
129.5	2.33	3.01	126.49	1749	3.13	4.05	125.45	1735	3.93	5.09	124.41	1721	4.73	6.12	123.38	1706
130	2.28	2.97	127.03	1757	3.08	4.01	125.99	1742	3.88	5.05	124.96	1728	4.68	6.08	123.92	1714
130.5	2.24	2.93	127.57	1764	3.04	3.97	126.53	1750	3.83	5.00	125.50	1736	4.63	6.04	124.46	1721
131	2.20	2.89	128.11	1772	3.00	3.93	127.07	1757	3.79	4.96	126.04	1743	4.58	6.00	125.00	1729
131.5	2.17	2.85	128.65	1779	2.95	3.88	127.62	1765	3.74	4.92	126.58	1751	4.53	5.96	125.54	1736
132	2.13	2.81	129.19	1787	2.91	3.84	128.16	1772	3.70	4.88	127.12	1758	4.48	5.92	126.08	1744
132.5	2.09	2.76	129.74	1794	2.87	3.80	128.70	1780	3.65	4.84	127.66	1766	4.44	5.88	126.62	1751
133	2.05	2.72	130.28	1802	2.83	3.76	129.24	1787	3.61	4.80	128.20	1773	4.39	5.84	127.16	1759
133.5	2.01	2.68	130.82	1809	2.79	3.72	129.78	1795	3.56	4.76	128.74	1781	4.34	5.80	127.70	1766
134	1.97	2.64	131.36	1817	2.75	3.68	130.32	1802	3.52	4.72	129.28	1788	4.29	5.75	128.25	1774
134.5	1.93	2.60	131.90	1824	2.71	3.64	130.86	1810	3.48	4.68	129.82	1795	4.25	5.71	128.79	1781
135	1.90	2.56	132.44	1832	2.66	3.60	131.40	1817	3.43	4.63	130.37	1803	4.20	5.67	129.33	1789
135.5	1.86	2.52	132.98	1839	2.62	3.56	131.94	1825	3.39	4.59	130.91	1810	4.16	5.63	129.87	1796
136	1.82	2.48	133.52	1847	2.58	3.52	132.48	1832	3.35	4.55	131.45	1818	4.11	5.59	130.41	1804
136.5	1.79	2.44	134.06	1854	2.55	3.47	133.03	1840	3.31	4.51	131.99	1825	4.07	5.55	130.95	1811
137	1.75	2.40	134.60	1862	2.51	3.43	133.57	1847	3.26	4.47	132.53	1833	4.02	5.51	131.49	1819
137.5	1.71	2.36	135.15	1869	2.47	3.39	134.11	1855	3.22	4.43	133.07	1840	3.98	5.47	132.03	1826
138	1.68	2.31	135.69	1877	2.43	3.35	134.65	1862	3.18	4.39	133.61	1848	3.93	5.43	132.57	1833
138.5	1.64	2.27	136.23	1884	2.39	3.31	135.19	1870	3.14	4.35	134.15	1855	3.89	5.39	133.11	1841
139	1.61	2.23	136.77	1892	2.35	3.27	135.73	1877	3.10	4.31	134.69	1863	3.84	5.34	133.66	1848
139.5	1.57	2.19	137.31	1899	2.31	3.23	136.27	1885	3.06	4.27	135.23	1870	3.80	5.30	134.20	1856
140	1.54	2.15	137.85	1906	2.28	3.19	136.81	1892	3.02	4.22	135.78	1878	3.76	5.26	134.74	1863
140.5	1.50	2.11	138.39	1914	2.24	3.15	137.35	1900	2.98	4.18	136.32	1885	3.72	5.22	135.28	1871
141	1.47	2.07	138.93	1921	2.20	3.11	137.89	1907	2.94	4.14	136.86	1893	3.67	5.18	135.82	1878
141.5	1.43	2.03	139.47	1929	2.17	3.06	138.44	1915	2.90	4.10	137.40	1900	3.63	5.14	136.36	1886
142	1.40	1.99	140.01	1936	2.13	3.02	138.98	1922	2.86	4.06	137.94	1908	3.59	5.10	136.90	1893
142.5	1.36	1.94	140.56	1944	2.09	2.98	139.52	1930	2.82	4.02	138.48	1915	3.55	5.06	137.44	1901
143	1.33	1.90	141.10	1951	2.06	2.94	140.06	1937	2.78	3.98	139.02	1923	3.51	5.02	137.98	1908
143.5	1.30	1.86	141.64	1959	2.02	2.90	140.60	1944	2.74	3.94	139.56	1930	3.47	4.98	138.52	1916
144	1.27	1.82	142.18	1966	1.99	2.86	141.14	1952	2.71	3.90	140.10	1938	3.43	4.93	139.07	1923
144.5	1.23	1.78	142.72	1974	1.95	2.82	141.68	1959	2.67	3.86	140.64	1945	3.39	4.89	139.61	1931
145	1.20	1.74	143.26	1981	1.92	2.78	142.22	1967	2.63	3.82	141.19	1953	3.35	4.85	140.15	1938
145.5	1.17	1.70	143.80	1989	1.88	2.74	142.76	1974	2.59	3.77	141.73	1960	3.31	4.81	140.69	1946
146	1.14	1.66	144.34	1996	1.85	2.70	143.30	1982	2.56	3.73	142.27	1968	3.27	4.77	141.23	1953
146.5	1.10	1.62	144.88	2004	1.81	2.65	143.85	1989	2.52	3.69	142.81	1975	3.23	4.73	141.77	1961
147	1.07	1.58	145.42	2011	1.78	2.61	144.39	1997	2.48	3.65	143.35	1983	3.19	4.69	142.31	1968
147.5	1.04	1.54	145.97	2019	1.74	2.57	144.93	2004	2.45	3.61	143.89	1990	3.15	4.65	142.85	1976
148	1.01	1.49	146.51	2026	1.71	2.53	145.47	2012	2.41	3.57	144.43	1997	3.11	4.61	143.39	1983
148.5	0.98	1.45	147.05	2034	1.68	2.49	146.01	2019	2.38	3.53	144.97	2005	3.07	4.57	143.93	1991
149	0.95	1.41	147.59	2041	1.64	2.45	146.55	2027	2.34	3.49	145.51	2012	3.04	4.52	144.48	1998
149.5	0.92	1.37	148.13	2049	1.61	2.41	147.09	2034	2.31	3.45	146.05	2020	3.00	4.48	145.02	2006
150	0.89	1.33	148.67	2056	1.58	2.37	147.63	2042	2.27	3.41	146.60	2027	2.96	4.44	145.56	2013
150.5	0.86	1.29	149.21	2064	1.55	2.33	148.17	2049	2.24	3.36	147.14	2035	2.92	4.40	146.10	2021
151	0.83	1.25	149.75	2071	1.51	2.29	148.71	2057	2.20	3.32	147.68	2042	2.89	4.36	146.64	2028
151.5	0.80	1.21	150.29	2079	1.48	2.24	149.26	2064	2.17	3.28	148.22	2050	2.85	4.32	147.18	2036

THE BODY FAT GUIDE

Body Composition   MALE   120-151.5 Lb.

Weight: Lb.	Waist: 28 inches Fat: %	Fat: Lb.	LBM: Lb.	RMR: Cal.	28.25 inches Fat: %	Fat: Lb.	LBM: Lb.	RMR: Cal.	28.5 inches Fat: %	Fat: Lb.	LBM: Lb.	RMR: Cal.	28.75 inches Fat: %	Fat: Lb.	LBM: Lb.	RMR: Cal.
120	6.62	7.94	112.06	1550	7.48	8.98	111.02	1535	8.35	10.02	109.99	1521	9.21	11.05	108.95	1507
120.5	6.56	7.90	112.60	1557	7.42	8.94	111.56	1543	8.28	9.97	110.53	1529	9.14	11.01	109.49	1514
121	6.49	7.86	113.14	1565	7.35	8.90	112.10	1550	8.21	9.93	111.07	1536	9.07	10.97	110.03	1522
121.5	6.43	7.82	113.68	1572	7.29	8.85	112.65	1558	8.14	9.89	111.61	1544	9.00	10.93	110.57	1529
122	6.37	7.78	114.22	1580	7.22	8.81	113.19	1565	8.07	9.85	112.15	1551	8.92	10.89	111.11	1537
122.5	6.31	7.74	114.77	1587	7.16	8.77	113.73	1573	8.01	9.81	112.69	1559	8.86	10.85	111.65	1544
123	6.26	7.69	115.31	1595	7.10	8.73	114.27	1580	7.94	9.77	113.23	1566	8.79	10.81	112.19	1552
123.5	6.20	7.65	115.85	1602	7.04	8.69	114.81	1588	7.88	9.73	113.77	1573	8.72	10.77	112.73	1559
124	6.14	7.61	116.39	1610	6.98	8.65	115.35	1595	7.81	9.69	114.31	1581	8.65	10.72	113.28	1567
124.5	6.08	7.57	116.93	1617	6.91	8.61	115.89	1603	7.75	9.65	114.85	1588	8.58	10.68	113.82	1574
125	6.02	7.53	117.47	1625	6.85	8.57	116.43	1610	7.68	9.61	115.40	1596	8.51	10.64	114.36	1582
125.5	5.97	7.49	118.01	1632	6.79	8.53	116.97	1618	7.62	9.56	115.94	1603	8.45	10.60	114.90	1589
126	5.91	7.45	118.55	1640	6.73	8.49	117.51	1625	7.56	9.52	116.48	1611	8.38	10.56	115.44	1597
126.5	5.86	7.41	119.09	1647	6.68	8.44	118.06	1633	7.50	9.48	117.02	1618	8.32	10.52	115.98	1604
127	5.80	7.37	119.63	1655	6.62	8.40	118.60	1640	7.43	9.44	117.56	1626	8.25	10.48	116.52	1611
127.5	5.75	7.33	120.18	1662	6.56	8.36	119.14	1648	7.37	9.40	118.10	1633	8.19	10.44	117.06	1619
128	5.69	7.28	120.72	1670	6.50	8.32	119.68	1655	7.31	9.36	118.64	1641	8.12	10.40	117.60	1626
128.5	5.64	7.24	121.26	1677	6.44	8.28	120.22	1663	7.25	9.32	119.18	1648	8.06	10.36	118.14	1634
129	5.58	7.20	121.80	1684	6.39	8.24	120.76	1670	7.19	9.28	119.72	1656	8.00	10.31	118.69	1641
129.5	5.53	7.16	122.34	1692	6.33	8.20	121.30	1678	7.13	9.24	120.26	1663	7.93	10.27	119.23	1649
130	5.48	7.12	122.88	1699	6.28	8.16	121.84	1685	7.07	9.20	120.81	1671	7.87	10.23	119.77	1656
130.5	5.42	7.08	123.42	1707	6.22	8.12	122.38	1693	7.01	9.15	121.35	1678	7.81	10.19	120.31	1664
131	5.37	7.04	123.96	1714	6.16	8.08	122.92	1700	6.96	9.11	121.89	1686	7.75	10.15	120.85	1671
131.5	5.32	7.00	124.50	1722	6.11	8.03	123.47	1708	6.90	9.07	122.43	1693	7.69	10.11	121.39	1679
132	5.27	6.96	125.04	1729	6.06	7.99	124.01	1715	6.84	9.03	122.97	1701	7.63	10.07	121.93	1686
132.5	5.22	6.92	125.59	1737	6.00	7.95	124.55	1722	6.78	8.99	123.51	1708	7.57	10.03	122.47	1694
133	5.17	6.87	126.13	1744	5.95	7.91	125.09	1730	6.73	8.95	124.05	1716	7.51	9.99	123.01	1701
133.5	5.12	6.83	126.67	1752	5.90	7.87	125.63	1737	6.67	8.91	124.59	1723	7.45	9.95	123.55	1709
134	5.07	6.79	127.21	1759	5.84	7.83	126.17	1745	6.62	8.87	125.13	1731	7.39	9.90	124.10	1716
134.5	5.02	6.75	127.75	1767	5.79	7.79	126.71	1752	6.56	8.83	125.67	1738	7.33	9.86	124.64	1724
135	4.97	6.71	128.29	1774	5.74	7.75	127.25	1760	6.51	8.78	126.22	1746	7.28	9.82	125.18	1731
135.5	4.92	6.67	128.83	1782	5.69	7.71	127.79	1767	6.45	8.74	126.76	1753	7.22	9.78	125.72	1739
136	4.87	6.63	129.37	1789	5.64	7.67	128.33	1775	6.40	8.70	127.30	1761	7.16	9.74	126.26	1746
136.5	4.83	6.59	129.91	1797	5.59	7.62	128.88	1782	6.35	8.66	127.84	1768	7.11	9.70	126.80	1754
137	4.78	6.55	130.45	1804	5.54	7.58	129.42	1790	6.29	8.62	128.38	1775	7.05	9.66	127.34	1761
137.5	4.73	6.51	131.00	1812	5.49	7.54	129.96	1797	6.24	8.58	128.92	1783	6.99	9.62	127.88	1769
138	4.68	6.46	131.54	1819	5.44	7.50	130.50	1805	6.19	8.54	129.46	1790	6.94	9.58	128.42	1776
138.5	4.64	6.42	132.08	1827	5.39	7.46	131.04	1812	6.14	8.50	130.00	1798	6.88	9.54	128.96	1784
139	4.59	6.38	132.62	1834	5.34	7.42	131.58	1820	6.08	8.46	130.54	1805	6.83	9.49	129.51	1791
139.5	4.55	6.34	133.16	1842	5.29	7.38	132.12	1827	6.03	8.42	131.08	1813	6.78	9.45	130.05	1799
140	4.50	6.30	133.70	1849	5.24	7.34	132.66	1835	5.98	8.38	131.63	1820	6.72	9.41	130.59	1806
140.5	4.45	6.26	134.24	1857	5.19	7.30	133.20	1842	5.93	8.33	132.17	1828	6.67	9.37	131.13	1814
141	4.41	6.22	134.78	1864	5.15	7.26	133.74	1850	5.88	8.29	132.71	1835	6.62	9.33	131.67	1821
141.5	4.37	6.18	135.32	1872	5.10	7.21	134.29	1857	5.83	8.25	133.25	1843	6.57	9.29	132.21	1828
142	4.32	6.14	135.86	1879	5.05	7.17	134.83	1865	5.78	8.21	133.79	1850	6.51	9.25	132.75	1836
142.5	4.28	6.10	136.41	1886	5.01	7.13	135.37	1872	5.73	8.17	134.33	1858	6.46	9.21	133.29	1843
143	4.23	6.05	136.95	1894	4.96	7.09	135.91	1880	5.68	8.13	134.87	1865	6.41	9.17	133.83	1851
143.5	4.19	6.01	137.49	1901	4.91	7.05	136.45	1887	5.64	8.09	135.41	1873	6.36	9.13	134.37	1858
144	4.15	5.97	138.03	1909	4.87	7.01	136.99	1895	5.59	8.05	135.95	1880	6.31	9.08	134.92	1866
144.5	4.10	5.93	138.57	1916	4.82	6.97	137.53	1902	5.54	8.01	136.49	1888	6.26	9.04	135.46	1873
145	4.06	5.89	139.11	1924	4.78	6.93	138.07	1910	5.49	7.96	137.04	1895	6.21	9.00	136.00	1881
145.5	4.02	5.85	139.65	1931	4.73	6.89	138.61	1917	5.45	7.92	137.58	1903	6.16	8.96	136.54	1888
146	3.98	5.81	140.19	1939	4.69	6.85	139.15	1925	5.40	7.88	138.12	1910	6.11	8.92	137.08	1896
146.5	3.94	5.77	140.73	1946	4.64	6.80	139.70	1932	5.35	7.84	138.66	1918	6.06	8.88	137.62	1903
147	3.90	5.73	141.27	1954	4.60	6.76	140.24	1939	5.31	7.80	139.20	1925	6.01	8.84	138.16	1911
147.5	3.85	5.69	141.82	1961	4.56	6.72	140.78	1947	5.26	7.76	139.74	1933	5.96	8.80	138.70	1918
148	3.81	5.64	142.36	1969	4.51	6.68	141.32	1954	5.22	7.72	140.28	1940	5.92	8.76	139.24	1926
148.5	3.77	5.60	142.90	1976	4.47	6.64	141.86	1962	5.17	7.68	140.82	1948	5.87	8.72	139.78	1933
149	3.73	5.56	143.44	1984	4.43	6.60	142.40	1969	5.13	7.64	141.36	1955	5.82	8.67	140.33	1941
149.5	3.69	5.52	143.98	1991	4.39	6.56	142.94	1977	5.08	7.60	141.90	1963	5.77	8.63	140.87	1948
150	3.65	5.48	144.52	1999	4.34	6.52	143.48	1984	5.04	7.56	142.45	1970	5.73	8.59	141.41	1956
150.5	3.61	5.44	145.06	2006	4.30	6.48	144.02	1992	4.99	7.51	142.99	1977	5.68	8.55	141.95	1963
151	3.57	5.40	145.60	2014	4.26	6.44	144.56	1999	4.95	7.47	143.53	1985	5.64	8.51	142.49	1971
151.5	3.54	5.36	146.14	2021	4.22	6.39	145.11	2007	4.91	7.43	144.07	1992	5.59	8.47	143.03	1978

Body Composition MALE 120-151.5 Lb.

Weight: Lb.	Waist: 29 in Fat: %	Fat: Lb.	LBM: Lb.	RMR: Cal.	29.25 in Fat: %	Fat: Lb.	LBM: Lb.	RMR: Cal.	29.5 in Fat: %	Fat: Lb.	LBM: Lb.	RMR: Cal.	29.75 in Fat: %	Fat: Lb.	LBM: Lb.	RMR: Cal.
120	10.08	12.09	107.91	1492	10.94	13.13	106.87	1478	11.80	14.17	105.84	1464	12.67	15.20	104.80	1449
120.5	10.00	12.05	108.45	1500	10.86	13.09	107.41	1486	11.72	14.12	106.38	1471	12.58	15.16	105.34	1457
121	9.92	12.01	108.99	1507	10.78	13.05	107.95	1493	11.64	14.08	106.92	1479	12.50	15.12	105.88	1464
121.5	9.85	11.97	109.53	1515	10.70	13.00	108.50	1500	11.56	14.04	107.46	1486	12.41	15.08	106.42	1472
122	9.78	11.93	110.07	1522	10.63	12.96	109.04	1508	11.48	14.00	108.00	1494	12.33	15.04	106.96	1479
122.5	9.70	11.89	110.62	1530	10.55	12.92	109.58	1515	11.40	13.96	108.54	1501	12.24	15.00	107.50	1487
123	9.63	11.84	111.16	1537	10.47	12.88	110.12	1523	11.32	13.92	109.08	1509	12.16	14.96	108.04	1494
123.5	9.56	11.80	111.70	1545	10.40	12.84	110.66	1530	11.24	13.88	109.62	1516	12.08	14.92	108.58	1502
124	9.49	11.76	112.24	1552	10.32	12.80	111.20	1538	11.16	13.84	110.16	1524	12.00	14.87	109.13	1509
124.5	9.41	11.72	112.78	1560	10.25	12.76	111.74	1545	11.08	13.80	110.70	1531	11.91	14.83	109.67	1517
125	9.34	11.68	113.32	1567	10.17	12.72	112.28	1553	11.00	13.76	111.25	1539	11.83	14.79	110.21	1524
125.5	9.27	11.64	113.86	1575	10.10	12.68	112.82	1560	10.93	13.71	111.79	1546	11.75	14.75	110.75	1532
126	9.20	11.60	114.40	1582	10.03	12.64	113.36	1568	10.85	13.67	112.33	1553	11.68	14.71	111.29	1539
126.5	9.14	11.56	114.94	1590	9.96	12.59	113.91	1575	10.78	13.63	112.87	1561	11.60	14.67	111.83	1547
127	9.07	11.52	115.48	1597	9.88	12.55	114.45	1583	10.70	13.59	113.41	1568	11.52	14.63	112.37	1554
127.5	9.00	11.48	116.03	1605	9.81	12.51	114.99	1590	10.63	13.55	113.95	1576	11.44	14.59	112.91	1562
128	8.93	11.43	116.57	1612	9.74	12.47	115.53	1598	10.55	13.51	114.49	1583	11.36	14.55	113.45	1569
128.5	8.87	11.39	117.11	1620	9.67	12.43	116.07	1605	10.48	13.47	115.03	1591	11.29	14.51	113.99	1577
129	8.80	11.35	117.65	1627	9.60	12.39	116.61	1613	10.41	13.43	115.57	1598	11.21	14.46	114.54	1584
129.5	8.73	11.31	118.19	1635	9.54	12.35	117.15	1620	10.34	13.39	116.11	1606	11.14	14.42	115.08	1592
130	8.67	11.27	118.73	1642	9.47	12.31	117.69	1628	10.27	13.35	116.66	1613	11.06	14.38	115.62	1599
130.5	8.60	11.23	119.27	1650	9.40	12.27	118.23	1635	10.19	13.30	117.20	1621	10.99	14.34	116.16	1606
131	8.54	11.19	119.81	1657	9.33	12.23	118.77	1643	10.12	13.26	117.74	1628	10.92	14.30	116.70	1614
131.5	8.48	11.15	120.35	1664	9.27	12.18	119.32	1650	10.05	13.22	118.28	1636	10.84	14.26	117.24	1621
132	8.41	11.11	120.89	1672	9.20	12.14	119.86	1658	9.99	13.18	118.82	1643	10.77	14.22	117.78	1629
132.5	8.35	11.07	121.44	1679	9.13	12.10	120.40	1665	9.92	13.14	119.36	1651	10.70	14.18	118.32	1636
133	8.29	11.02	121.98	1687	9.07	12.06	120.94	1673	9.85	13.10	119.90	1658	10.63	14.14	118.86	1644
133.5	8.23	10.98	122.52	1694	9.00	12.02	121.48	1680	9.78	13.06	120.44	1666	10.56	14.10	119.40	1651
134	8.17	10.94	123.06	1702	8.94	11.98	122.02	1688	9.71	13.02	120.98	1673	10.49	14.05	119.95	1659
134.5	8.10	10.90	123.60	1709	8.88	11.94	122.56	1695	9.65	12.98	121.52	1681	10.42	14.01	120.49	1666
135	8.04	10.86	124.14	1717	8.81	11.90	123.10	1703	9.58	12.94	122.07	1688	10.35	13.97	121.03	1674
135.5	7.98	10.82	124.68	1724	8.75	11.86	123.64	1710	9.52	12.89	122.61	1696	10.28	13.93	121.57	1681
136	7.92	10.78	125.22	1732	8.69	11.82	124.18	1717	9.45	12.85	123.15	1703	10.21	13.89	122.11	1689
136.5	7.87	10.74	125.76	1739	8.63	11.77	124.73	1725	9.39	12.81	123.69	1711	10.15	13.85	122.65	1696
137	7.81	10.70	126.30	1747	8.56	11.73	125.27	1732	9.32	12.77	124.23	1718	10.08	13.81	123.19	1704
137.5	7.75	10.66	126.85	1754	8.50	11.69	125.81	1740	9.26	12.73	124.77	1726	10.01	13.77	123.73	1711
138	7.69	10.61	127.39	1762	8.44	11.65	126.35	1747	9.19	12.69	125.31	1733	9.95	13.73	124.27	1719
138.5	7.63	10.57	127.93	1769	8.38	11.61	126.89	1755	9.13	12.65	125.85	1741	9.88	13.69	124.81	1726
139	7.58	10.53	128.47	1777	8.32	11.57	127.43	1762	9.07	12.61	126.39	1748	9.82	13.64	125.36	1734
139.5	7.52	10.49	129.01	1784	8.26	11.53	127.97	1770	9.01	12.57	126.93	1755	9.75	13.60	125.90	1741
140	7.46	10.45	129.55	1792	8.21	11.49	128.51	1777	8.95	12.53	127.48	1763	9.69	13.56	126.44	1749
140.5	7.41	10.41	130.09	1799	8.15	11.45	129.05	1785	8.89	12.48	128.02	1770	9.62	13.52	126.98	1756
141	7.35	10.37	130.63	1807	8.09	11.41	129.59	1792	8.82	12.44	128.56	1778	9.56	13.48	127.52	1764
141.5	7.30	10.33	131.17	1814	8.03	11.36	130.14	1800	8.76	12.40	129.10	1785	9.50	13.44	128.06	1771
142	7.24	10.29	131.71	1822	7.97	11.32	130.68	1807	8.70	12.36	129.64	1793	9.44	13.40	128.60	1779
142.5	7.19	10.25	132.26	1829	7.92	11.28	131.22	1815	8.65	12.32	130.18	1800	9.37	13.36	129.14	1786
143	7.14	10.20	132.80	1837	7.86	11.24	131.76	1822	8.59	12.28	130.72	1808	9.31	13.32	129.68	1794
143.5	7.08	10.16	133.34	1844	7.81	11.20	132.30	1830	8.53	12.24	131.26	1815	9.25	13.28	130.22	1801
144	7.03	10.12	133.88	1852	7.75	11.16	132.84	1837	8.47	12.20	131.80	1823	9.19	13.23	130.77	1808
144.5	6.98	10.08	134.42	1859	7.69	11.12	133.38	1845	8.41	12.16	132.34	1830	9.13	13.19	131.31	1816
145	6.92	10.04	134.96	1866	7.64	11.08	133.92	1852	8.36	12.12	132.89	1838	9.07	13.15	131.85	1823
145.5	6.87	10.00	135.50	1874	7.59	11.04	134.46	1860	8.30	12.07	133.43	1845	9.01	13.11	132.39	1831
146	6.82	9.96	136.04	1881	7.53	11.00	135.00	1867	8.24	12.03	133.97	1853	8.95	13.07	132.93	1838
146.5	6.77	9.92	136.58	1889	7.48	10.95	135.55	1875	8.19	11.99	134.51	1860	8.89	13.03	133.47	1846
147	6.72	9.88	137.12	1896	7.42	10.91	136.09	1882	8.13	11.95	135.05	1868	8.84	12.99	134.01	1853
147.5	6.67	9.84	137.67	1904	7.37	10.87	136.63	1890	8.07	11.91	135.59	1875	8.78	12.95	134.55	1861
148	6.62	9.79	138.21	1911	7.32	10.83	137.17	1897	8.02	11.87	136.13	1883	8.72	12.91	135.09	1868
148.5	6.57	9.75	138.75	1919	7.27	10.79	137.71	1905	7.96	11.83	136.67	1890	8.66	12.87	135.63	1876
149	6.52	9.71	139.29	1926	7.21	10.75	138.25	1912	7.91	11.79	137.21	1898	8.61	12.82	136.18	1883
149.5	6.47	9.67	139.83	1934	7.16	10.71	138.79	1919	7.86	11.75	137.75	1905	8.55	12.78	136.72	1891
150	6.42	9.63	140.37	1941	7.11	10.67	139.33	1927	7.80	11.71	138.30	1913	8.50	12.74	137.26	1898
150.5	6.37	9.59	140.91	1949	7.06	10.63	139.87	1934	7.75	11.66	138.84	1920	8.44	12.70	137.80	1906
151	6.32	9.55	141.45	1956	7.01	10.59	140.41	1942	7.70	11.62	139.38	1928	8.38	12.66	138.34	1913
151.5	6.28	9.51	141.99	1964	6.96	10.54	140.96	1949	7.64	11.58	139.92	1935	8.33	12.62	138.88	1921

Body Composition MALE 120-151.5 Lb.

Weight: Lb.	Waist: 30 inches Fat: %	Fat: Lb.	LBM: Lb.	RMR: Cal.	30.25 inches Fat: %	Fat: Lb.	LBM: Lb.	RMR: Cal.	30.5 inches Fat: %	Fat: Lb.	LBM: Lb.	RMR: Cal.	30.75 inches Fat: %	Fat: Lb.	LBM: Lb.	RMR: Cal.
120	13.53	16.24	103.76	1435	14.40	17.28	102.72	1421	15.26	18.32	101.69	1406	16.13	19.35	100.65	1392
120.5	13.44	16.20	104.30	1442	14.30	17.24	103.26	1428	15.17	18.27	102.23	1414	16.03	19.31	101.19	1399
121	13.35	16.16	104.84	1450	14.21	17.20	103.80	1436	15.07	18.23	102.77	1421	15.93	19.27	101.73	1407
121.5	13.27	16.12	105.38	1457	14.12	17.15	104.35	1443	14.97	18.19	103.31	1429	15.83	19.23	102.27	1414
122	13.18	16.08	105.92	1465	14.03	17.11	104.89	1451	14.88	18.15	103.85	1436	15.73	19.19	102.81	1422
122.5	13.09	16.04	106.47	1472	13.94	17.07	105.43	1458	14.78	18.11	104.39	1444	15.63	19.15	103.35	1429
123	13.00	15.99	107.01	1480	13.85	17.03	105.97	1466	14.69	18.07	104.93	1451	15.53	19.11	103.89	1437
123.5	12.92	15.95	107.55	1487	13.76	16.99	106.51	1473	14.60	18.03	105.47	1459	15.44	19.07	104.43	1444
124	12.83	15.91	108.09	1495	13.67	16.95	107.05	1481	14.51	17.99	106.01	1466	15.34	19.02	104.98	1452
124.5	12.75	15.87	108.63	1502	13.58	16.91	107.59	1488	14.41	17.95	106.55	1474	15.25	18.98	105.52	1459
125	12.66	15.83	109.17	1510	13.49	16.87	108.13	1495	14.32	17.91	107.10	1481	15.15	18.94	106.06	1467
125.5	12.58	15.79	109.71	1517	13.41	16.83	108.67	1503	14.23	17.86	107.64	1489	15.06	18.90	106.60	1474
126	12.50	15.75	110.25	1525	13.32	16.79	109.21	1510	14.15	17.82	108.18	1496	14.97	18.86	107.14	1482
126.5	12.42	15.71	110.79	1532	13.24	16.74	109.76	1518	14.06	17.78	108.72	1504	14.88	18.82	107.68	1489
127	12.34	15.67	111.33	1540	13.15	16.70	110.30	1525	13.97	17.74	109.26	1511	14.79	18.78	108.22	1497
127.5	12.25	15.63	111.88	1547	13.07	16.66	110.84	1533	13.88	17.70	109.80	1519	14.70	18.74	108.76	1504
128	12.18	15.58	112.42	1555	12.99	16.62	111.38	1540	13.80	17.66	110.34	1526	14.61	18.70	109.30	1512
128.5	12.10	15.54	112.96	1562	12.90	16.58	111.92	1548	13.71	17.62	110.88	1533	14.52	18.66	109.84	1519
129	12.02	15.50	113.50	1570	12.82	16.54	112.46	1555	13.63	17.58	111.42	1541	14.43	18.61	110.39	1527
129.5	11.94	15.46	114.04	1577	12.74	16.50	113.00	1563	13.54	17.54	111.96	1548	14.34	18.57	110.93	1534
130	11.86	15.42	114.58	1585	12.66	16.46	113.54	1570	13.46	17.50	112.51	1556	14.26	18.53	111.47	1542
130.5	11.78	15.38	115.12	1592	12.58	16.42	114.08	1578	13.37	17.45	113.05	1563	14.17	18.49	112.01	1549
131	11.71	15.34	115.66	1600	12.50	16.38	114.62	1585	13.29	17.41	113.59	1571	14.08	18.45	112.55	1557
131.5	11.63	15.30	116.20	1607	12.42	16.33	115.17	1593	13.21	17.37	114.13	1578	14.00	18.41	113.09	1564
132	11.56	15.26	116.74	1615	12.34	16.29	115.71	1600	13.13	17.33	114.67	1586	13.92	18.37	113.63	1572
132.5	11.48	15.22	117.29	1622	12.27	16.25	116.25	1608	13.05	17.29	115.21	1593	13.83	18.33	114.17	1579
133	11.41	15.17	117.83	1630	12.19	16.21	116.79	1615	12.97	17.25	115.75	1601	13.75	18.29	114.71	1586
133.5	11.34	15.13	118.37	1637	12.11	16.17	117.33	1623	12.89	17.21	116.29	1608	13.67	18.25	115.25	1594
134	11.26	15.09	118.91	1644	12.04	16.13	117.87	1630	12.81	17.17	116.83	1616	13.59	18.20	115.80	1601
134.5	11.19	15.05	119.45	1652	11.96	16.09	118.41	1638	12.73	17.13	117.37	1623	13.50	18.16	116.34	1609
135	11.12	15.01	119.99	1659	11.89	16.05	118.95	1645	12.66	17.09	117.92	1631	13.42	18.12	116.88	1616
135.5	11.05	14.97	120.53	1667	11.81	16.01	119.49	1653	12.58	17.04	118.46	1638	13.34	18.08	117.42	1624
136	10.98	14.93	121.07	1674	11.74	15.97	120.03	1660	12.50	17.00	119.00	1646	13.27	18.04	117.96	1631
136.5	10.91	14.89	121.61	1682	11.67	15.92	120.58	1668	12.43	16.96	119.54	1653	13.19	18.00	118.50	1639
137	10.84	14.85	122.15	1689	11.59	15.88	121.12	1675	12.35	16.92	120.08	1661	13.11	17.96	119.04	1646
137.5	10.77	14.81	122.70	1697	11.52	15.84	121.66	1683	12.28	16.88	120.62	1668	13.03	17.92	119.58	1654
138	10.70	14.76	123.24	1704	11.45	15.80	122.20	1690	12.20	16.84	121.16	1676	12.95	17.88	120.12	1661
138.5	10.63	14.72	123.78	1712	11.38	15.76	122.74	1697	12.13	16.80	121.70	1683	12.88	17.84	120.66	1669
139	10.56	14.68	124.32	1719	11.31	15.72	123.28	1705	12.06	16.76	122.24	1691	12.80	17.79	121.21	1676
139.5	10.50	14.64	124.86	1727	11.24	15.68	123.82	1712	11.98	16.72	122.78	1698	12.73	17.75	121.75	1684
140	10.43	14.60	125.40	1734	11.17	15.64	124.36	1720	11.91	16.68	123.33	1706	12.65	17.71	122.29	1691
140.5	10.36	14.56	125.94	1742	11.10	15.60	124.90	1727	11.84	16.63	123.87	1713	12.58	17.67	122.83	1699
141	10.30	14.52	126.48	1749	11.03	15.56	125.44	1735	11.77	16.59	124.41	1721	12.50	17.63	123.37	1706
141.5	10.23	14.48	127.02	1757	10.96	15.51	125.99	1742	11.70	16.55	124.95	1728	12.43	17.59	123.91	1714
142	10.17	14.44	127.56	1764	10.90	15.47	126.53	1750	11.63	16.51	125.49	1736	12.36	17.55	124.45	1721
142.5	10.10	14.40	128.11	1772	10.83	15.43	127.07	1757	11.56	16.47	126.03	1743	12.29	17.51	124.99	1729
143	10.04	14.35	128.65	1779	10.76	15.39	127.61	1765	11.49	16.43	126.57	1750	12.21	17.47	125.53	1736
143.5	9.97	14.31	129.19	1787	10.70	15.35	128.15	1772	11.42	16.39	127.11	1758	12.14	17.43	126.07	1744
144	9.91	14.27	129.73	1794	10.63	15.31	128.69	1780	11.35	16.35	127.65	1765	12.07	17.38	126.62	1751
144.5	9.85	14.23	130.27	1802	10.57	15.27	129.23	1787	11.28	16.31	128.19	1773	12.00	17.34	127.16	1759
145	9.79	14.19	130.81	1809	10.50	15.23	129.77	1795	11.22	16.27	128.74	1780	11.93	17.30	127.70	1766
145.5	9.72	14.15	131.35	1817	10.44	15.19	130.31	1802	11.15	16.22	129.28	1788	11.86	17.26	128.24	1774
146	9.66	14.11	131.89	1824	10.37	15.15	130.85	1810	11.08	16.18	129.82	1795	11.79	17.22	128.78	1781
146.5	9.60	14.07	132.43	1832	10.31	15.10	131.40	1817	11.02	16.14	130.36	1803	11.73	17.18	129.32	1789
147	9.54	14.03	132.97	1839	10.25	15.06	131.94	1825	10.95	16.10	130.90	1810	11.66	17.14	129.86	1796
147.5	9.48	13.99	133.52	1847	10.18	15.02	132.48	1832	10.89	16.06	131.44	1818	11.59	17.10	130.40	1803
148	9.42	13.94	134.06	1854	10.12	14.98	133.02	1840	10.82	16.02	131.98	1825	11.52	17.06	130.94	1811
148.5	9.36	13.90	134.60	1861	10.06	14.94	133.56	1847	10.76	15.98	132.52	1833	11.46	17.02	131.48	1818
149	9.30	13.86	135.14	1869	10.00	14.90	134.10	1855	10.70	15.94	133.06	1840	11.39	16.97	132.03	1826
149.5	9.24	13.82	135.68	1876	9.94	14.86	134.64	1862	10.63	15.90	133.60	1848	11.33	16.93	132.57	1833
150	9.19	13.78	136.22	1884	9.88	14.82	135.18	1870	10.57	15.86	134.15	1855	11.26	16.89	133.11	1841
150.5	9.13	13.74	136.76	1891	9.82	14.78	135.72	1877	10.51	15.81	134.69	1863	11.20	16.85	133.65	1848
151	9.07	13.70	137.30	1899	9.76	14.74	136.26	1885	10.45	15.77	135.23	1870	11.13	16.81	134.19	1856
151.5	9.01	13.66	137.84	1906	9.70	14.69	136.81	1892	10.38	15.73	135.77	1878	11.07	16.77	134.73	1863

Body Composition MALE 120-151.5 Lb.

Weight: Lb.	Waist: 31 inches				31.25 inches				31.5 inches				31.75 inches			
	Fat: %	Fat: Lb.	LBM: Lb.	RMR: Cal.	Fat: %	Fat: Lb.	LBM: Lb.	RMR: Cal.	Fat: %	Fat: Lb.	LBM: Lb.	RMR: Cal.	Fat: %	Fat: Lb.	LBM: Lb.	RMR: Cal.
120	16.99	20.39	99.61	1378	17.86	21.43	98.57	1363	18.72	22.47	97.54	1349	19.59	23.50	96.50	1335
120.5	16.89	20.35	100.15	1385	17.75	21.39	99.11	1371	18.61	22.42	98.08	1356	19.47	23.46	97.04	1342
121	16.78	20.31	100.69	1393	17.64	21.35	99.65	1378	18.50	22.38	98.62	1364	19.36	23.42	97.58	1350
121.5	16.68	20.27	101.23	1400	17.53	21.30	100.20	1386	18.39	22.34	99.16	1371	19.24	23.38	98.12	1357
122	16.58	20.23	101.77	1408	17.43	21.26	100.74	1393	18.28	22.30	99.70	1379	19.13	23.34	98.66	1364
122.5	16.48	20.19	102.32	1415	17.32	21.22	101.28	1401	18.17	22.26	100.24	1386	19.02	23.30	99.20	1372
123	16.38	20.14	102.86	1422	17.22	21.18	101.82	1408	18.06	22.22	100.78	1394	18.91	23.26	99.74	1379
123.5	16.28	20.10	103.40	1430	17.12	21.14	102.36	1416	17.96	22.18	101.32	1401	18.80	23.22	100.28	1387
124	16.18	20.06	103.94	1437	17.02	21.10	102.90	1423	17.85	22.14	101.86	1409	18.69	23.17	100.83	1394
124.5	16.08	20.02	104.48	1445	16.91	21.06	103.44	1431	17.75	22.10	102.40	1416	18.58	23.13	101.37	1402
125	15.98	19.98	105.02	1452	16.81	21.02	103.98	1438	17.64	22.06	102.95	1424	18.47	23.09	101.91	1409
125.5	15.89	19.94	105.56	1460	16.71	20.98	104.52	1446	17.54	22.01	103.49	1431	18.37	23.05	102.45	1417
126	15.79	19.90	106.10	1467	16.62	20.94	105.06	1453	17.44	21.97	104.03	1439	18.26	23.01	102.99	1424
126.5	15.70	19.86	106.64	1475	16.52	20.89	105.61	1461	17.34	21.93	104.57	1446	18.16	22.97	103.53	1432
127	15.60	19.82	107.18	1482	16.42	20.85	106.15	1468	17.24	21.89	105.11	1454	18.05	22.93	104.07	1439
127.5	15.51	19.78	107.73	1490	16.32	20.81	106.69	1475	17.14	21.85	105.65	1461	17.95	22.89	104.61	1447
128	15.42	19.73	108.27	1497	16.23	20.77	107.23	1483	17.04	21.81	106.19	1469	17.85	22.85	105.15	1454
128.5	15.33	19.69	108.81	1505	16.13	20.73	107.77	1490	16.94	21.77	106.73	1476	17.75	22.81	105.69	1462
129	15.23	19.65	109.35	1512	16.04	20.69	108.31	1498	16.84	21.73	107.27	1484	17.65	22.76	106.24	1469
129.5	15.14	19.61	109.89	1520	15.94	20.65	108.85	1505	16.75	21.69	107.81	1491	17.55	22.72	106.78	1477
130	15.05	19.57	110.43	1527	15.85	20.61	109.39	1513	16.65	21.65	108.36	1499	17.45	22.68	107.32	1484
130.5	14.96	19.53	110.97	1535	15.76	20.57	109.93	1520	16.55	21.60	108.90	1506	17.35	22.64	107.86	1492
131	14.88	19.49	111.51	1542	15.67	20.53	110.47	1528	16.46	21.56	109.44	1514	17.25	22.60	108.40	1499
131.5	14.79	19.45	112.05	1550	15.58	20.48	111.02	1535	16.37	21.52	109.98	1521	17.16	22.56	108.94	1507
132	14.70	19.41	112.59	1557	15.49	20.44	111.56	1543	16.27	21.48	110.52	1528	17.06	22.52	109.48	1514
132.5	14.62	19.37	113.14	1565	15.40	20.40	112.10	1550	16.18	21.44	111.06	1536	16.96	22.48	110.02	1522
133	14.53	19.32	113.68	1572	15.31	20.36	112.64	1558	16.09	21.40	111.60	1543	16.87	22.44	110.56	1529
133.5	14.44	19.28	114.22	1580	15.22	20.32	113.18	1565	16.00	21.36	112.14	1551	16.78	22.40	111.10	1537
134	14.36	19.24	114.76	1587	15.13	20.28	113.72	1573	15.91	21.32	112.68	1558	16.68	22.35	111.65	1544
134.5	14.28	19.20	115.30	1595	15.05	20.24	114.26	1580	15.82	21.28	113.22	1566	16.59	22.31	112.19	1552
135	14.19	19.16	115.84	1602	14.96	20.20	114.80	1588	15.73	21.24	113.77	1573	16.50	22.27	112.73	1559
135.5	14.11	19.12	116.38	1610	14.88	20.16	115.34	1595	15.64	21.19	114.31	1581	16.41	22.23	113.27	1567
136	14.03	19.08	116.92	1617	14.79	20.12	115.88	1603	15.55	21.15	114.85	1588	16.32	22.19	113.81	1574
136.5	13.95	19.04	117.46	1625	14.71	20.07	116.43	1610	15.47	21.11	115.39	1596	16.23	22.15	114.35	1581
137	13.87	19.00	118.00	1632	14.62	20.03	116.97	1618	15.38	21.07	115.93	1603	16.14	22.11	114.89	1589
137.5	13.79	18.96	118.55	1639	14.54	19.99	117.51	1625	15.29	21.03	116.47	1611	16.05	22.07	115.43	1596
138	13.71	18.91	119.09	1647	14.46	19.95	118.05	1633	15.21	20.99	117.01	1618	15.96	22.03	115.97	1604
138.5	13.63	18.87	119.63	1654	14.38	19.91	118.59	1640	15.12	20.95	117.55	1626	15.87	21.99	116.51	1611
139	13.55	18.83	120.17	1662	14.29	19.87	119.13	1648	15.04	20.91	118.09	1633	15.79	21.94	117.06	1619
139.5	13.47	18.79	120.71	1669	14.21	19.83	119.67	1655	14.96	20.87	118.63	1641	15.70	21.90	117.60	1626
140	13.39	18.75	121.25	1677	14.13	19.79	120.21	1663	14.88	20.83	119.18	1648	15.62	21.86	118.14	1634
140.5	13.32	18.71	121.79	1684	14.05	19.75	120.75	1670	14.79	20.78	119.72	1656	15.53	21.82	118.68	1641
141	13.24	18.67	122.33	1692	13.98	19.71	121.29	1678	14.71	20.74	120.26	1663	15.45	21.78	119.22	1649
141.5	13.16	18.63	122.87	1699	13.90	19.66	121.84	1685	14.63	20.70	120.80	1671	15.36	21.74	119.76	1656
142	13.09	18.59	123.41	1707	13.82	19.62	122.38	1692	14.55	20.66	121.34	1678	15.28	21.70	120.30	1664
142.5	13.01	18.55	123.96	1714	13.74	19.58	122.92	1700	14.47	20.62	121.88	1686	15.20	21.66	120.84	1671
143	12.94	18.50	124.50	1722	13.67	19.54	123.46	1707	14.39	20.58	122.42	1693	15.12	21.62	121.38	1679
143.5	12.87	18.46	125.04	1729	13.59	19.50	124.00	1715	14.31	20.54	122.96	1701	15.04	21.58	121.92	1686
144	12.79	18.42	125.58	1737	13.51	19.46	124.54	1722	14.23	20.50	123.50	1708	14.95	21.53	122.47	1694
144.5	12.72	18.38	126.12	1744	13.44	19.42	125.08	1730	14.16	20.46	124.04	1716	14.87	21.49	123.01	1701
145	12.65	18.34	126.66	1752	13.36	19.38	125.62	1737	14.08	20.42	124.59	1723	14.79	21.45	123.55	1709
145.5	12.58	18.30	127.20	1759	13.29	19.34	126.16	1745	14.00	20.37	125.13	1730	14.72	21.41	124.09	1716
146	12.51	18.26	127.74	1767	13.22	19.30	126.70	1752	13.93	20.33	125.67	1738	14.64	21.37	124.63	1724
146.5	12.43	18.22	128.28	1774	13.14	19.25	127.25	1760	13.85	20.29	126.21	1745	14.56	21.33	125.17	1731
147	12.36	18.18	128.82	1782	13.07	19.21	127.79	1767	13.78	20.25	126.75	1753	14.48	21.29	125.71	1739
147.5	12.29	18.14	129.37	1789	13.00	19.17	128.33	1775	13.70	20.21	127.29	1760	14.41	21.25	126.25	1746
148	12.23	18.09	129.91	1797	12.93	19.13	128.87	1782	13.63	20.17	127.83	1768	14.33	21.21	126.79	1754
148.5	12.16	18.05	130.45	1804	12.86	19.09	129.41	1790	13.55	20.13	128.37	1775	14.25	21.17	127.33	1761
149	12.09	18.01	130.99	1812	12.78	19.05	129.95	1797	13.48	20.09	128.91	1783	14.18	21.12	127.88	1769
149.5	12.02	17.97	131.53	1819	12.71	19.01	130.49	1805	13.41	20.05	129.45	1790	14.10	21.08	128.42	1776
150	11.95	17.93	132.07	1827	12.65	18.97	131.03	1812	13.34	20.01	130.00	1798	14.03	21.04	128.96	1783
150.5	11.89	17.89	132.61	1834	12.58	18.93	131.57	1820	13.27	19.96	130.54	1805	13.95	21.00	129.50	1791
151	11.82	17.85	133.15	1841	12.51	18.89	132.11	1827	13.19	19.92	131.08	1813	13.88	20.96	130.04	1798
151.5	11.75	17.81	133.69	1849	12.44	18.84	132.66	1835	13.12	19.88	131.62	1820	13.81	20.92	130.58	1806

Body Composition   MALE   120-151.5 Lb.

Weight: Lb.	Waist: 32 inches				32.25 inches				32.5 inches				32.75 inches			
	Fat: %	Fat: Lb.	LBM: Lb.	RMR: Cal.	Fat: %	Fat: Lb.	LBM: Lb.	RMR: Cal.	Fat: %	Fat: Lb.	LBM: Lb.	RMR: Cal.	Fat: %	Fat: Lb.	LBM: Lb.	RMR: Cal.
120	20.45	24.54	95.46	1320	21.31	25.58	94.42	1306	22.18	26.62	93.39	1292	23.04	27.65	92.35	1277
120.5	20.33	24.50	96.00	1328	21.19	25.54	94.96	1313	22.05	26.57	93.93	1299	22.91	27.61	92.89	1285
121	20.21	24.46	96.54	1335	21.07	25.50	95.50	1321	21.93	26.53	94.47	1306	22.79	27.57	93.43	1292
121.5	20.10	24.42	97.08	1343	20.95	25.45	96.05	1328	21.80	26.49	95.01	1314	22.66	27.53	93.97	1300
122	19.98	24.38	97.62	1350	20.83	25.41	96.59	1336	21.68	26.45	95.55	1321	22.53	27.49	94.51	1307
122.5	19.87	24.34	98.17	1358	20.71	25.37	97.13	1343	21.56	26.41	96.09	1329	22.41	27.45	95.05	1315
123	19.75	24.29	98.71	1365	20.59	25.33	97.67	1351	21.44	26.37	96.63	1336	22.28	27.41	95.59	1322
123.5	19.64	24.25	99.25	1373	20.48	25.29	98.21	1358	21.32	26.33	97.17	1344	22.16	27.37	96.13	1330
124	19.53	24.21	99.79	1380	20.36	25.25	98.75	1366	21.20	26.29	97.71	1351	22.04	27.32	96.68	1337
124.5	19.41	24.17	100.33	1388	20.25	25.21	99.29	1373	21.08	26.25	98.25	1359	21.91	27.28	97.22	1345
125	19.30	24.13	100.87	1395	20.13	25.17	99.83	1381	20.96	26.21	98.80	1366	21.79	27.24	97.76	1352
125.5	19.19	24.09	101.41	1403	20.02	25.13	100.37	1388	20.85	26.16	99.34	1374	21.67	27.20	98.30	1359
126	19.09	24.05	101.95	1410	19.91	25.09	100.91	1396	20.73	26.12	99.88	1381	21.56	27.16	98.84	1367
126.5	18.98	24.01	102.49	1417	19.80	25.04	101.46	1403	20.62	26.08	100.42	1389	21.44	27.12	99.38	1374
127	18.87	23.97	103.03	1425	19.69	25.00	102.00	1411	20.50	26.04	100.96	1396	21.32	27.08	99.92	1382
127.5	18.76	23.93	103.58	1432	19.58	24.96	102.54	1418	20.39	26.00	101.50	1404	21.21	27.04	100.46	1389
128	18.66	23.88	104.12	1440	19.47	24.92	103.08	1426	20.28	25.96	102.04	1411	21.09	27.00	101.00	1397
128.5	18.55	23.84	104.66	1447	19.36	24.88	103.62	1433	20.17	25.92	102.58	1419	20.98	26.96	101.54	1404
129	18.45	23.80	105.20	1455	19.26	24.84	104.16	1441	20.06	25.88	103.12	1426	20.86	26.91	102.09	1412
129.5	18.35	23.76	105.74	1462	19.15	24.80	104.70	1448	19.95	25.84	103.66	1434	20.75	26.87	102.63	1419
130	18.25	23.72	106.28	1470	19.04	24.76	105.24	1456	19.84	25.80	104.21	1441	20.64	26.83	103.17	1427
130.5	18.14	23.68	106.82	1477	18.94	24.72	105.78	1463	19.73	25.75	104.75	1449	20.53	26.79	103.71	1434
131	18.04	23.64	107.36	1485	18.84	24.68	106.32	1470	19.63	25.71	105.29	1456	20.42	26.75	104.25	1442
131.5	17.94	23.60	107.90	1492	18.73	24.63	106.87	1478	19.52	25.67	105.83	1464	20.31	26.71	104.79	1449
132	17.85	23.56	108.44	1500	18.63	24.59	107.41	1485	19.42	25.63	106.37	1471	20.20	26.67	105.33	1457
132.5	17.75	23.52	108.99	1507	18.53	24.55	107.95	1493	19.31	25.59	106.91	1479	20.10	26.63	105.87	1464
133	17.65	23.47	109.53	1515	18.43	24.51	108.49	1500	19.21	25.55	107.45	1486	19.99	26.59	106.41	1472
133.5	17.55	23.43	110.07	1522	18.33	24.47	109.03	1508	19.11	25.51	107.99	1494	19.88	26.55	106.95	1479
134	17.46	23.39	110.61	1530	18.23	24.43	109.57	1515	19.01	25.47	108.53	1501	19.78	26.50	107.50	1487
134.5	17.36	23.35	111.15	1537	18.13	24.39	110.11	1523	18.90	25.43	109.07	1508	19.68	26.46	108.04	1494
135	17.27	23.31	111.69	1545	18.04	24.35	110.65	1530	18.80	25.39	109.62	1516	19.57	26.42	108.58	1502
135.5	17.17	23.27	112.23	1552	17.94	24.31	111.19	1538	18.70	25.34	110.16	1523	19.47	26.38	109.12	1509
136	17.08	23.23	112.77	1560	17.84	24.27	111.73	1545	18.61	25.30	110.70	1531	19.37	26.34	109.66	1517
136.5	16.99	23.19	113.31	1567	17.75	24.22	112.28	1553	18.51	25.26	111.24	1538	19.27	26.30	110.20	1524
137	16.89	23.15	113.85	1575	17.65	24.18	112.82	1560	18.41	25.22	111.78	1546	19.17	26.26	110.74	1532
137.5	16.80	23.11	114.40	1582	17.56	24.14	113.36	1568	18.31	25.18	112.32	1553	19.07	26.22	111.28	1539
138	16.71	23.06	114.94	1590	17.46	24.10	113.90	1575	18.22	25.14	112.86	1561	18.97	26.18	111.82	1547
138.5	16.62	23.02	115.48	1597	17.37	24.06	114.44	1583	18.12	25.10	113.40	1568	18.87	26.14	112.36	1554
139	16.53	22.98	116.02	1605	17.28	24.02	114.98	1590	18.03	25.06	113.94	1576	18.77	26.09	112.91	1561
139.5	16.45	22.94	116.56	1612	17.19	23.98	115.52	1598	17.93	25.02	114.48	1583	18.68	26.05	113.45	1569
140	16.36	22.90	117.10	1619	17.10	23.94	116.06	1605	17.84	24.98	115.03	1591	18.58	26.01	113.99	1576
140.5	16.27	22.86	117.64	1627	17.01	23.90	116.60	1613	17.75	24.93	115.57	1598	18.49	25.97	114.53	1584
141	16.18	22.82	118.18	1634	16.92	23.86	117.14	1620	17.65	24.89	116.11	1606	18.39	25.93	115.07	1591
141.5	16.10	22.78	118.72	1642	16.83	23.81	117.69	1628	17.56	24.85	116.65	1613	18.30	25.89	115.61	1599
142	16.01	22.74	119.26	1649	16.74	23.77	118.23	1635	17.47	24.81	117.19	1621	18.20	25.85	116.15	1606
142.5	15.93	22.70	119.81	1657	16.65	23.73	118.77	1643	17.38	24.77	117.73	1628	18.11	25.81	116.69	1614
143	15.84	22.65	120.35	1664	16.57	23.69	119.31	1650	17.29	24.73	118.27	1636	18.02	25.77	117.23	1621
143.5	15.76	22.61	120.89	1672	16.48	23.65	119.85	1658	17.20	24.69	118.81	1643	17.93	25.73	117.77	1629
144	15.68	22.57	121.43	1679	16.40	23.61	120.39	1665	17.12	24.65	119.35	1651	17.84	25.68	118.32	1636
144.5	15.59	22.53	121.97	1687	16.31	23.57	120.93	1672	17.03	24.61	119.89	1658	17.75	25.64	118.86	1644
145	15.51	22.49	122.51	1694	16.23	23.53	121.47	1680	16.94	24.57	120.44	1666	17.66	25.60	119.40	1651
145.5	15.43	22.45	123.05	1702	16.14	23.49	122.01	1687	16.85	24.52	120.98	1673	17.57	25.56	119.94	1659
146	15.35	22.41	123.59	1709	16.06	23.45	122.55	1695	16.77	24.48	121.52	1681	17.48	25.52	120.48	1666
146.5	15.27	22.37	124.13	1717	15.98	23.40	123.10	1702	16.68	24.44	122.06	1688	17.39	25.48	121.02	1674
147	15.19	22.33	124.67	1724	15.89	23.36	123.64	1710	16.60	24.40	122.60	1696	17.31	25.44	121.56	1681
147.5	15.11	22.29	125.22	1732	15.81	23.32	124.18	1717	16.52	24.36	123.14	1703	17.22	25.40	122.10	1689
148	15.03	22.24	125.76	1739	15.73	23.28	124.72	1725	16.43	24.32	123.68	1711	17.13	25.36	122.64	1696
148.5	14.95	22.20	126.30	1747	15.65	23.24	125.26	1732	16.35	24.28	124.22	1718	17.05	25.32	123.18	1704
149	14.87	22.16	126.84	1754	15.57	23.20	125.80	1740	16.27	24.24	124.76	1725	16.96	25.27	123.73	1711
149.5	14.80	22.12	127.38	1762	15.49	23.16	126.34	1747	16.18	24.20	125.30	1733	16.88	25.23	124.27	1719
150	14.72	22.08	127.92	1769	15.41	23.12	126.88	1755	16.10	24.16	125.85	1740	16.80	25.19	124.81	1726
150.5	14.64	22.04	128.46	1777	15.33	23.08	127.42	1762	16.02	24.11	126.39	1748	16.71	25.15	125.35	1734
151	14.57	22.00	129.00	1784	15.26	23.04	127.96	1770	15.94	24.07	126.93	1755	16.63	25.11	125.89	1741
151.5	14.49	21.96	129.54	1792	15.18	22.99	128.51	1777	15.86	24.03	127.47	1763	16.55	25.07	126.43	1749

Body Composition   MALE   120-151.5 Lb.

Weight: Lb.	Waist: 33 inches				33.25 inches				33.5 inches				33.75 inches			
	Fat: %	Fat: Lb.	LBM: Lb.	RMR: Cal.	Fat: %	Fat: Lb.	LBM: Lb.	RMR: Cal.	Fat: %	Fat: Lb.	LBM: Lb.	RMR: Cal.	Fat: %	Fat: Lb.	LBM: Lb.	RMR: Cal.
120	23.91	28.69	91.31	1263	24.77	29.73	90.27	1248	25.64	30.77	89.24	1234	26.50	31.80	88.20	1220
120.5	23.78	28.65	91.85	1270	24.64	29.69	90.81	1256	25.50	30.72	89.78	1242	26.36	31.76	88.74	1227
121	23.64	28.61	92.39	1278	24.50	29.65	91.35	1263	25.36	30.68	90.32	1249	26.22	31.72	89.28	1235
121.5	23.51	28.57	92.93	1285	24.37	29.60	91.90	1271	25.22	30.64	90.86	1257	26.07	31.68	89.82	1242
122	23.38	28.53	93.47	1293	24.23	29.56	92.44	1278	25.08	30.60	91.40	1264	25.93	31.64	90.36	1250
122.5	23.25	28.49	94.02	1300	24.10	29.52	92.98	1286	24.95	30.56	91.94	1272	25.79	31.60	90.90	1257
123	23.13	28.44	94.56	1308	23.97	29.48	93.52	1293	24.81	30.52	92.48	1279	25.66	31.56	91.44	1265
123.5	23.00	28.40	95.10	1315	23.84	29.44	94.06	1301	24.68	30.48	93.02	1286	25.52	31.52	91.98	1272
124	22.87	28.36	95.64	1323	23.71	29.40	94.60	1308	24.55	30.44	93.56	1294	25.38	31.47	92.53	1280
124.5	22.75	28.32	96.18	1330	23.58	29.36	95.14	1316	24.41	30.40	94.10	1301	25.25	31.43	93.07	1287
125	22.62	28.28	96.72	1338	23.45	29.32	95.68	1323	24.28	30.36	94.65	1309	25.11	31.39	93.61	1295
125.5	22.50	28.24	97.26	1345	23.33	29.28	96.22	1331	24.15	30.31	95.19	1316	24.98	31.35	94.15	1302
126	22.38	28.20	97.80	1353	23.20	29.24	96.76	1338	24.03	30.27	95.73	1324	24.85	31.31	94.69	1310
126.5	22.26	28.16	98.34	1360	23.08	29.19	97.31	1346	23.90	30.23	96.27	1331	24.72	31.27	95.23	1317
127	22.14	28.12	98.88	1368	22.96	29.15	97.85	1353	23.77	30.19	96.81	1339	24.59	31.23	95.77	1325
127.5	22.02	28.08	99.43	1375	22.83	29.11	98.39	1361	23.65	30.15	97.35	1346	24.46	31.19	96.31	1332
128	21.90	28.03	99.97	1383	22.71	29.07	98.93	1368	23.52	30.11	97.89	1354	24.33	31.15	96.85	1339
128.5	21.78	27.99	100.51	1390	22.59	29.03	99.47	1376	23.40	30.07	98.43	1361	24.21	31.11	97.39	1347
129	21.67	27.95	101.05	1397	22.47	28.99	100.01	1383	23.28	30.03	98.97	1369	24.08	31.06	97.94	1354
129.5	21.55	27.91	101.59	1405	22.35	28.95	100.55	1391	23.16	29.99	99.51	1376	23.96	31.02	98.48	1362
130	21.44	27.87	102.13	1412	22.24	28.91	101.09	1398	23.03	29.95	100.06	1384	23.83	30.98	99.02	1369
130.5	21.32	27.83	102.67	1420	22.12	28.87	101.63	1406	22.91	29.90	100.60	1391	23.71	30.94	99.56	1377
131	21.21	27.79	103.21	1427	22.00	28.83	102.17	1413	22.80	29.86	101.14	1399	23.59	30.90	100.10	1384
131.5	21.10	27.75	103.75	1435	21.89	28.78	102.72	1421	22.68	29.82	101.68	1406	23.47	30.86	100.64	1392
132	20.99	27.71	104.29	1442	21.78	28.74	103.26	1428	22.56	29.78	102.22	1414	23.35	30.82	101.18	1399
132.5	20.88	27.67	104.84	1450	21.66	28.70	103.80	1436	22.45	29.74	102.76	1421	23.23	30.78	101.72	1407
133	20.77	27.62	105.38	1457	21.55	28.66	104.34	1443	22.33	29.70	103.30	1429	23.11	30.74	102.26	1414
133.5	20.66	27.58	105.92	1465	21.44	28.62	104.88	1450	22.22	29.66	103.84	1436	22.99	30.70	102.80	1422
134	20.55	27.54	106.46	1472	21.33	28.58	105.42	1458	22.10	29.62	104.38	1444	22.88	30.65	103.35	1429
134.5	20.45	27.50	107.00	1480	21.22	28.54	105.96	1465	21.99	29.58	104.92	1451	22.76	30.61	103.89	1437
135	20.34	27.46	107.54	1487	21.11	28.50	106.50	1473	21.88	29.54	105.47	1459	22.65	30.57	104.43	1444
135.5	20.24	27.42	108.08	1495	21.00	28.46	107.04	1480	21.77	29.49	106.01	1466	22.53	30.53	104.97	1452
136	20.13	27.38	108.62	1502	20.89	28.42	107.58	1488	21.66	29.45	106.55	1474	22.42	30.49	105.51	1459
136.5	20.03	27.34	109.16	1510	20.79	28.37	108.13	1495	21.55	29.41	107.09	1481	22.31	30.45	106.05	1467
137	19.92	27.30	109.70	1517	20.68	28.33	108.67	1503	21.44	29.37	107.63	1489	22.20	30.41	106.59	1474
137.5	19.82	27.26	110.25	1525	20.58	28.29	109.21	1510	21.33	29.33	108.17	1496	22.09	30.37	107.13	1482
138	19.72	27.21	110.79	1532	20.47	28.25	109.75	1518	21.22	29.29	108.71	1503	21.98	30.33	107.67	1489
138.5	19.62	27.17	111.33	1540	20.37	28.21	110.29	1525	21.12	29.25	109.25	1511	21.87	30.29	108.21	1497
139	19.52	27.13	111.87	1547	20.27	28.17	110.83	1533	21.01	29.21	109.79	1518	21.76	30.24	108.76	1504
139.5	19.42	27.09	112.41	1555	20.16	28.13	111.37	1540	20.91	29.17	110.33	1526	21.65	30.20	109.30	1512
140	19.32	27.05	112.95	1562	20.06	28.09	111.91	1548	20.80	29.13	110.88	1533	21.54	30.16	109.84	1519
140.5	19.22	27.01	113.49	1570	19.96	28.05	112.45	1555	20.70	29.08	111.42	1541	21.44	30.12	110.38	1527
141	19.13	26.97	114.03	1577	19.86	28.01	112.99	1563	20.60	29.04	111.96	1548	21.33	30.08	110.92	1534
141.5	19.03	26.93	114.57	1585	19.76	27.96	113.54	1570	20.50	29.00	112.50	1556	21.23	30.04	111.46	1541
142	18.93	26.89	115.11	1592	19.66	27.92	114.08	1578	20.40	28.96	113.04	1563	21.13	30.00	112.00	1549
142.5	18.84	26.85	115.66	1600	19.57	27.88	114.62	1585	20.29	28.92	113.58	1571	21.02	29.96	112.54	1556
143	18.74	26.80	116.20	1607	19.47	27.84	115.16	1593	20.20	28.88	114.12	1578	20.92	29.92	113.08	1564
143.5	18.65	26.76	116.74	1614	19.37	27.80	115.70	1600	20.10	28.84	114.66	1586	20.82	29.88	113.62	1571
144	18.56	26.72	117.28	1622	19.28	27.76	116.24	1608	20.00	28.80	115.20	1593	20.72	29.83	114.17	1579
144.5	18.46	26.68	117.82	1629	19.18	27.72	116.78	1615	19.90	28.76	115.74	1601	20.62	29.79	114.71	1586
145	18.37	26.64	118.36	1637	19.09	27.68	117.32	1623	19.80	28.72	116.29	1608	20.52	29.75	115.25	1594
145.5	18.28	26.60	118.90	1644	18.99	27.64	117.86	1630	19.71	28.67	116.83	1616	20.42	29.71	115.79	1601
146	18.19	26.56	119.44	1652	18.90	27.60	118.40	1638	19.61	28.63	117.37	1623	20.32	29.67	116.33	1609
146.5	18.10	26.52	119.98	1659	18.81	27.55	118.95	1645	19.52	28.59	117.91	1631	20.22	29.63	116.87	1616
147	18.01	26.48	120.52	1667	18.72	27.51	119.49	1652	19.42	28.55	118.45	1638	20.13	29.59	117.41	1624
147.5	17.92	26.44	121.07	1674	18.63	27.47	120.03	1660	19.33	28.51	118.99	1646	20.03	29.55	117.95	1631
148	17.83	26.39	121.61	1682	18.53	27.43	120.57	1667	19.24	28.47	119.53	1653	19.94	29.51	118.49	1639
148.5	17.75	26.35	122.15	1689	18.44	27.39	121.11	1675	19.14	28.43	120.07	1661	19.84	29.47	119.03	1646
149	17.66	26.31	122.69	1697	18.36	27.35	121.65	1682	19.05	28.39	120.61	1668	19.75	29.42	119.58	1654
149.5	17.57	26.27	123.23	1704	18.27	27.31	122.19	1690	18.96	28.35	121.15	1676	19.65	29.38	120.12	1661
150	17.49	26.23	123.77	1712	18.18	27.27	122.73	1697	18.87	28.31	121.70	1683	19.56	29.34	120.66	1669
150.5	17.40	26.19	124.31	1719	18.09	27.23	123.27	1705	18.78	28.26	122.24	1691	19.47	29.30	121.20	1676
151	17.32	26.15	124.85	1727	18.00	27.19	123.81	1712	18.69	28.22	122.78	1698	19.38	29.26	121.74	1684
151.5	17.23	26.11	125.39	1734	17.92	27.14	124.36	1720	18.60	28.18	123.32	1705	19.29	29.22	122.28	1691

Body Composition MALE 120-151.5 Lb.

Weight: Lb.	Waist: 34 inches				34.25 inches				34.5 inches				34.75 inches			
	Fat: %	Fat: Lb.	LBM: Lb.	RMR: Cal.	Fat: %	Fat: Lb.	LBM: Lb.	RMR: Cal.	Fat: %	Fat: Lb.	LBM: Lb.	RMR: Cal.	Fat: %	Fat: Lb.	LBM: Lb.	RMR: Cal.
120	27.37	32.84	87.16	1205	28.23	33.88	86.12	1191	29.10	34.92	85.09	1177	29.96	35.95	84.05	1162
120.5	27.22	32.80	87.70	1213	28.08	33.84	86.66	1199	28.94	34.87	85.63	1184	29.80	35.91	84.59	1170
121	27.07	32.76	88.24	1220	27.93	33.80	87.20	1206	28.79	34.83	86.17	1192	29.65	35.87	85.13	1177
121.5	26.93	32.72	88.78	1228	27.78	33.75	87.75	1214	28.64	34.79	86.71	1199	29.49	35.83	85.67	1185
122	26.78	32.68	89.32	1235	27.63	33.71	88.29	1221	28.48	34.75	87.25	1207	29.33	35.79	86.21	1192
122.5	26.64	32.64	89.87	1243	27.49	33.67	88.83	1228	28.33	34.71	87.79	1214	29.18	35.75	86.75	1200
123	26.50	32.59	90.41	1250	27.34	33.63	89.37	1236	28.19	34.67	88.33	1222	29.03	35.71	87.29	1207
123.5	26.36	32.55	90.95	1258	27.20	33.59	89.91	1243	28.04	34.63	88.87	1229	28.88	35.67	87.83	1215
124	26.22	32.51	91.49	1265	27.06	33.55	90.45	1251	27.89	34.59	89.41	1237	28.73	35.62	88.38	1222
124.5	26.08	32.47	92.03	1273	26.91	33.51	90.99	1258	27.75	34.55	89.95	1244	28.58	35.58	88.92	1230
125	25.94	32.43	92.57	1280	26.77	33.47	91.53	1266	27.60	34.51	90.50	1252	28.43	35.54	89.46	1237
125.5	25.81	32.39	93.11	1288	26.63	33.43	92.07	1273	27.46	34.46	91.04	1259	28.29	35.50	90.00	1245
126	25.67	32.35	93.65	1295	26.50	33.39	92.61	1281	27.32	34.42	91.58	1267	28.14	35.46	90.54	1252
126.5	25.54	32.31	94.19	1303	26.36	33.34	93.16	1288	27.18	34.38	92.12	1274	28.00	35.42	91.08	1260
127	25.41	32.27	94.73	1310	26.22	33.30	93.70	1296	27.04	34.34	92.66	1281	27.86	35.38	91.62	1267
127.5	25.27	32.23	95.28	1318	26.09	33.26	94.24	1303	26.90	34.30	93.20	1289	27.72	35.34	92.16	1275
128	25.14	32.18	95.82	1325	25.95	33.22	94.78	1311	26.76	34.26	93.74	1296	27.58	35.30	92.70	1282
128.5	25.01	32.14	96.36	1333	25.82	33.18	95.32	1318	26.63	34.22	94.28	1304	27.44	35.26	93.24	1290
129	24.89	32.10	96.90	1340	25.69	33.14	95.86	1326	26.49	34.18	94.82	1311	27.30	35.21	93.79	1297
129.5	24.76	32.06	97.44	1348	25.56	33.10	96.40	1333	26.36	34.14	95.36	1319	27.16	35.17	94.33	1305
130	24.63	32.02	97.98	1355	25.43	33.06	96.94	1341	26.23	34.10	95.91	1326	27.03	35.13	94.87	1312
130.5	24.50	31.98	98.52	1363	25.30	33.02	97.48	1348	26.10	34.05	96.45	1334	26.89	35.09	95.41	1319
131	24.38	31.94	99.06	1370	25.17	32.98	98.02	1356	25.96	34.01	96.99	1341	26.76	35.05	95.95	1327
131.5	24.26	31.90	99.60	1378	25.05	32.93	98.57	1363	25.83	33.97	97.53	1349	26.62	35.01	96.49	1334
132	24.13	31.86	100.14	1385	24.92	32.89	99.11	1371	25.71	33.93	98.07	1356	26.49	34.97	97.03	1342
132.5	24.01	31.82	100.69	1392	24.79	32.85	99.65	1378	25.58	33.89	98.61	1364	26.36	34.93	97.57	1349
133	23.89	31.77	101.23	1400	24.67	32.81	100.19	1386	25.45	33.85	99.15	1371	26.23	34.89	98.11	1357
133.5	23.77	31.73	101.77	1407	24.55	32.77	100.73	1393	25.32	33.81	99.69	1379	26.10	34.85	98.65	1364
134	23.65	31.69	102.31	1415	24.43	32.73	101.27	1401	25.20	33.77	100.23	1386	25.97	34.80	99.20	1372
134.5	23.53	31.65	102.85	1422	24.30	32.69	101.81	1408	25.08	33.73	100.77	1394	25.85	34.76	99.74	1379
135	23.41	31.61	103.39	1430	24.18	32.65	102.35	1416	24.95	33.69	101.32	1401	25.72	34.72	100.28	1387
135.5	23.30	31.57	103.93	1437	24.06	32.61	102.89	1423	24.83	33.64	101.86	1409	25.60	34.68	100.82	1394
136	23.18	31.53	104.47	1445	23.95	32.57	103.43	1430	24.71	33.60	102.40	1416	25.47	34.64	101.36	1402
136.5	23.07	31.49	105.01	1452	23.83	32.52	103.98	1438	24.59	33.56	102.94	1424	25.35	34.60	101.90	1409
137	22.95	31.45	105.55	1460	23.71	32.48	104.52	1445	24.47	33.52	103.48	1431	25.23	34.56	102.44	1417
137.5	22.84	31.41	106.10	1467	23.59	32.44	105.06	1453	24.35	33.48	104.02	1439	25.10	34.52	102.98	1424
138	22.73	31.36	106.64	1475	23.48	32.40	105.60	1460	24.23	33.44	104.56	1446	24.98	34.48	103.52	1432
138.5	22.62	31.32	107.18	1482	23.36	32.36	106.14	1468	24.11	33.40	105.10	1454	24.86	34.44	104.06	1439
139	22.51	31.28	107.72	1490	23.25	32.32	106.68	1475	24.00	33.36	105.64	1461	24.74	34.39	104.61	1447
139.5	22.39	31.24	108.26	1497	23.14	32.28	107.22	1483	23.88	33.32	106.18	1469	24.63	34.35	105.15	1454
140	22.29	31.20	108.80	1505	23.03	32.24	107.76	1490	23.77	33.28	106.73	1476	24.51	34.31	105.69	1462
140.5	22.18	31.16	109.34	1512	22.92	32.20	108.30	1498	23.65	33.23	107.27	1483	24.39	34.27	106.23	1469
141	22.07	31.12	109.88	1520	22.81	32.16	108.84	1505	23.54	33.19	107.81	1491	24.28	34.23	106.77	1477
141.5	21.96	31.08	110.42	1527	22.70	32.11	109.39	1513	23.43	33.15	108.35	1498	24.16	34.19	107.31	1484
142	21.86	31.04	110.96	1535	22.59	32.07	109.93	1520	23.32	33.11	108.89	1506	24.05	34.15	107.85	1492
142.5	21.75	31.00	111.51	1542	22.48	32.03	110.47	1528	23.21	33.07	109.43	1513	23.94	34.11	108.39	1499
143	21.65	30.95	112.05	1550	22.37	31.99	111.01	1535	23.10	33.03	109.97	1521	23.82	34.07	108.93	1507
143.5	21.54	30.91	112.59	1557	22.27	31.95	111.55	1543	22.99	32.99	110.51	1528	23.71	34.03	109.47	1514
144	21.44	30.87	113.13	1565	22.16	31.91	112.09	1550	22.88	32.95	111.05	1536	23.60	33.98	110.02	1522
144.5	21.34	30.83	113.67	1572	22.05	31.87	112.63	1558	22.77	32.91	111.59	1543	23.49	33.94	110.56	1529
145	21.23	30.79	114.21	1580	21.95	31.83	113.17	1565	22.67	32.87	112.14	1551	23.38	33.90	111.10	1536
145.5	21.13	30.75	114.75	1587	21.85	31.79	113.71	1573	22.56	32.82	112.68	1558	23.27	33.86	111.64	1544
146	21.03	30.71	115.29	1594	21.74	31.75	114.25	1580	22.45	32.78	113.22	1566	23.16	33.82	112.18	1551
146.5	20.93	30.67	115.83	1602	21.64	31.70	114.80	1588	22.35	32.74	113.76	1573	23.06	33.78	112.72	1559
147	20.83	30.63	116.37	1609	21.54	31.66	115.34	1595	22.25	32.70	114.30	1581	22.95	33.74	113.26	1566
147.5	20.74	30.59	116.92	1617	21.44	31.62	115.88	1603	22.14	32.66	114.84	1588	22.85	33.70	113.80	1574
148	20.64	30.54	117.46	1624	21.34	31.58	116.42	1610	22.04	32.62	115.38	1596	22.74	33.66	114.34	1581
148.5	20.54	30.50	118.00	1632	21.24	31.54	116.96	1618	21.94	32.58	115.92	1603	22.64	33.62	114.88	1589
149	20.44	30.46	118.54	1639	21.14	31.50	117.50	1625	21.84	32.54	116.46	1611	22.53	33.57	115.43	1596
149.5	20.35	30.42	119.08	1647	21.04	31.46	118.04	1633	21.74	32.50	117.00	1618	22.43	33.53	115.97	1604
150	20.25	30.38	119.62	1654	20.95	31.42	118.58	1640	21.64	32.46	117.55	1626	22.33	33.49	116.51	1611
150.5	20.16	30.34	120.16	1662	20.85	31.38	119.12	1647	21.54	32.41	118.09	1633	22.23	33.45	117.05	1619
151	20.06	30.30	120.70	1669	20.75	31.34	119.66	1655	21.44	32.37	118.63	1641	22.13	33.41	117.59	1626
151.5	19.97	30.26	121.24	1677	20.66	31.29	120.21	1662	21.34	32.33	119.17	1648	22.03	33.37	118.13	1634

Body Composition MALE 120-151.5 Lb.

Weight: Lb.	Waist: 35 inches Fat: %	Fat: Lb.	LBM: Lb.	RMR: Cal.	35.25 inches Fat: %	Fat: Lb.	LBM: Lb.	RMR: Cal.	35.5 inches Fat: %	Fat: Lb.	LBM: Lb.	RMR: Cal.	35.75 inches Fat: %	Fat: Lb.	LBM: Lb.	RMR: Cal.
120	30.83	36.99	83.01	1148	31.69	38.03	81.97	1134	32.55	39.07	80.94	1119	33.42	40.10	79.90	1105
120.5	30.66	36.95	83.55	1156	31.52	37.99	82.51	1141	32.39	39.02	81.48	1127	33.25	40.06	80.44	1112
121	30.50	36.91	84.09	1163	31.36	37.95	83.05	1149	32.22	38.98	82.02	1134	33.07	40.02	80.98	1120
121.5	30.34	36.87	84.63	1170	31.20	37.90	83.60	1156	32.05	38.94	82.56	1142	32.90	39.98	81.52	1127
122	30.19	36.83	85.17	1178	31.04	37.86	84.14	1164	31.89	38.90	83.10	1149	32.74	39.94	82.06	1135
122.5	30.03	36.79	85.72	1185	30.88	37.82	84.68	1171	31.72	38.86	83.64	1157	32.57	39.90	82.60	1142
123	29.87	36.74	86.26	1193	30.72	37.78	85.22	1179	31.56	38.82	84.18	1164	32.40	39.86	83.14	1150
123.5	29.72	36.70	86.80	1200	30.56	37.74	85.76	1186	31.40	38.78	84.72	1172	32.24	39.82	83.68	1157
124	29.57	36.66	87.34	1208	30.40	37.70	86.30	1194	31.24	38.74	85.26	1179	32.08	39.77	84.23	1165
124.5	29.41	36.62	87.88	1215	30.25	37.66	86.84	1201	31.08	38.70	85.80	1187	31.91	39.73	84.77	1172
125	29.26	36.58	88.42	1223	30.09	37.62	87.38	1208	30.92	38.66	86.35	1194	31.75	39.69	85.31	1180
125.5	29.11	36.54	88.96	1230	29.94	37.58	87.92	1216	30.77	38.61	86.89	1202	31.59	39.65	85.85	1187
126	28.97	36.50	89.50	1238	29.79	37.54	88.46	1223	30.61	38.57	87.43	1209	31.44	39.61	86.39	1195
126.5	28.82	36.46	90.04	1245	29.64	37.49	89.01	1231	30.46	38.53	87.97	1217	31.28	39.57	86.93	1202
127	28.67	36.42	90.58	1253	29.49	37.45	89.55	1238	30.31	38.49	88.51	1224	31.12	39.53	87.47	1210
127.5	28.53	36.38	91.13	1260	29.34	37.41	90.09	1246	30.16	38.45	89.05	1232	30.97	39.49	88.01	1217
128	28.39	36.33	91.67	1268	29.20	37.37	90.63	1253	30.01	38.41	89.59	1239	30.82	39.45	88.55	1225
128.5	28.24	36.29	92.21	1275	29.05	37.33	91.17	1261	29.86	38.37	90.13	1247	30.67	39.41	89.09	1232
129	28.10	36.25	92.75	1283	28.91	37.29	91.71	1268	29.71	38.33	90.67	1254	30.52	39.36	89.64	1240
129.5	27.96	36.21	93.29	1290	28.76	37.25	92.25	1276	29.56	38.29	91.21	1261	30.37	39.32	90.18	1247
130	27.82	36.17	93.83	1298	28.62	37.21	92.79	1283	29.42	38.25	91.76	1269	30.22	39.28	90.72	1255
130.5	27.69	36.13	94.37	1305	28.48	37.17	93.33	1291	29.28	38.20	92.30	1276	30.07	39.24	91.26	1262
131	27.55	36.09	94.91	1313	28.34	37.13	93.87	1298	29.13	38.16	92.84	1284	29.92	39.20	91.80	1270
131.5	27.41	36.05	95.45	1320	28.20	37.08	94.42	1306	28.99	38.12	93.38	1291	29.78	39.16	92.34	1277
132	27.28	36.01	95.99	1328	28.06	37.04	94.96	1313	28.85	38.08	93.92	1299	29.64	39.12	92.88	1285
132.5	27.14	35.97	96.54	1335	27.93	37.00	95.50	1321	28.71	38.04	94.46	1306	29.49	39.08	93.42	1292
133	27.01	35.92	97.08	1343	27.79	36.96	96.04	1328	28.57	38.00	95.00	1314	29.35	39.04	93.96	1300
133.5	26.88	35.88	97.62	1350	27.66	36.92	96.58	1336	28.43	37.96	95.54	1321	29.21	39.00	94.50	1307
134	26.75	35.84	98.16	1358	27.52	36.88	97.12	1343	28.30	37.92	96.08	1329	29.07	38.95	95.05	1314
134.5	26.62	35.80	98.70	1365	27.39	36.84	97.66	1351	28.16	37.88	96.62	1336	28.93	38.91	95.59	1322
135	26.49	35.76	99.24	1372	27.26	36.80	98.20	1358	28.03	37.84	97.17	1344	28.79	38.87	96.13	1329
135.5	26.36	35.72	99.78	1380	27.13	36.76	98.74	1366	27.89	37.79	97.71	1351	28.66	38.83	96.67	1337
136	26.23	35.68	100.32	1387	27.00	36.72	99.28	1373	27.76	37.75	98.25	1359	28.52	38.79	97.21	1344
136.5	26.11	35.64	100.86	1395	26.87	36.67	99.83	1381	27.63	37.71	98.79	1366	28.39	38.75	97.75	1352
137	25.98	35.60	101.40	1402	26.74	36.63	100.37	1388	27.50	37.67	99.33	1374	28.25	38.71	98.29	1359
137.5	25.86	35.56	101.95	1410	26.61	36.59	100.91	1396	27.37	37.63	99.87	1381	28.12	38.67	98.83	1367
138	25.73	35.51	102.49	1417	26.49	36.55	101.45	1403	27.24	37.59	100.41	1389	27.99	38.63	99.37	1374
138.5	25.61	35.47	103.03	1425	26.36	36.51	101.99	1411	27.11	37.55	100.95	1396	27.86	38.59	99.91	1382
139	25.49	35.43	103.57	1432	26.24	36.47	102.53	1418	26.98	37.51	101.49	1404	27.73	38.54	100.46	1389
139.5	25.37	35.39	104.11	1440	26.11	36.43	103.07	1425	26.86	37.47	102.03	1411	27.60	38.50	101.00	1397
140	25.25	35.35	104.65	1447	25.99	36.39	103.61	1433	26.73	37.43	102.58	1419	27.47	38.46	101.54	1404
140.5	25.13	35.31	105.19	1455	25.87	36.35	104.15	1440	26.61	37.38	103.12	1426	27.35	38.42	102.08	1412
141	25.01	35.27	105.73	1462	25.75	36.31	104.69	1448	26.48	37.34	103.66	1434	27.22	38.38	102.62	1419
141.5	24.90	35.23	106.27	1470	25.63	36.26	105.24	1455	26.36	37.30	104.20	1441	27.10	38.34	103.16	1427
142	24.78	35.19	106.81	1477	25.51	36.22	105.78	1463	26.24	37.26	104.74	1449	26.97	38.30	103.70	1434
142.5	24.66	35.15	107.36	1485	25.39	36.18	106.32	1470	26.12	37.22	105.28	1456	26.85	38.26	104.24	1442
143	24.55	35.10	107.90	1492	25.27	36.14	106.86	1478	26.00	37.18	105.82	1464	26.72	38.22	104.78	1449
143.5	24.43	35.06	108.44	1500	25.16	36.10	107.40	1485	25.88	37.14	106.36	1471	26.60	38.18	105.32	1457
144	24.32	35.02	108.98	1507	25.04	36.06	107.94	1493	25.76	37.10	106.90	1478	26.48	38.13	105.87	1464
144.5	24.21	34.98	109.52	1515	24.93	36.02	108.48	1500	25.64	37.06	107.44	1486	26.36	38.09	106.41	1472
145	24.10	34.94	110.06	1522	24.81	35.98	109.02	1508	25.53	37.02	107.99	1493	26.24	38.05	106.95	1479
145.5	23.99	34.90	110.60	1530	24.70	35.94	109.56	1515	25.41	36.97	108.53	1501	26.12	38.01	107.49	1487
146	23.88	34.86	111.14	1537	24.59	35.90	110.10	1523	25.30	36.93	109.07	1508	26.01	37.97	108.03	1494
146.5	23.77	34.82	111.68	1545	24.47	35.85	110.65	1530	25.18	36.89	109.61	1516	25.89	37.93	108.57	1502
147	23.66	34.78	112.22	1552	24.36	35.81	111.19	1538	25.07	36.85	110.15	1523	25.77	37.89	109.11	1509
147.5	23.55	34.74	112.77	1560	24.25	35.77	111.73	1545	24.96	36.81	110.69	1531	25.66	37.85	109.65	1516
148	23.44	34.69	113.31	1567	24.14	35.73	112.27	1553	24.84	36.77	111.23	1538	25.54	37.81	110.19	1524
148.5	23.34	34.65	113.85	1575	24.03	35.69	112.81	1560	24.73	36.73	111.77	1546	25.43	37.77	110.73	1531
149	23.23	34.61	114.39	1582	23.93	35.65	113.35	1568	24.62	36.69	112.31	1553	25.32	37.72	111.28	1539
149.5	23.12	34.57	114.93	1589	23.82	35.61	113.89	1575	24.51	36.65	112.85	1561	25.21	37.68	111.82	1546
150	23.02	34.53	115.47	1597	23.71	35.57	114.43	1583	24.40	36.61	113.40	1568	25.10	37.64	112.36	1554
150.5	22.92	34.49	116.01	1604	23.61	35.53	114.97	1590	24.30	36.56	113.94	1576	24.98	37.60	112.90	1561
151	22.81	34.45	116.55	1612	23.50	35.49	115.51	1598	24.19	36.52	114.48	1583	24.87	37.56	113.44	1569
151.5	22.71	34.41	117.09	1619	23.40	35.44	116.06	1605	24.08	36.48	115.02	1591	24.77	37.52	113.98	1576

Body Composition MALE 120-151.5 Lb.

Weight: Lb.	Waist: 36 inches				36.25 inches				36.5 inches				36.75 inches			
	Fat: %	Fat: Lb.	LBM: Lb.	RMR: Cal.	Fat: %	Fat: Lb.	LBM: Lb.	RMR: Cal.	Fat: %	Fat: Lb.	LBM: Lb.	RMR: Cal.	Fat: %	Fat: Lb.	LBM: Lb.	RMR: Cal.
120	34.28	41.14	78.86	1091	35.15	42.18	77.82	1076	36.01	43.22	76.79	1062	36.88	44.25	75.75	1048
120.5	34.11	41.10	79.40	1098	34.97	42.14	78.36	1084	35.83	43.17	77.33	1069	36.69	44.21	76.29	1055
121	33.93	41.06	79.94	1106	34.79	42.10	78.90	1091	35.65	43.13	77.87	1077	36.50	44.17	76.83	1063
121.5	33.76	41.02	80.48	1113	34.61	42.05	79.45	1099	35.47	43.09	78.41	1084	36.32	44.13	77.37	1070
122	33.59	40.98	81.02	1121	34.44	42.01	79.99	1106	35.29	43.05	78.95	1092	36.14	44.09	77.91	1078
122.5	33.42	40.94	81.57	1128	34.26	41.97	80.53	1114	35.11	43.01	79.49	1099	35.96	44.05	78.45	1085
123	33.25	40.89	82.11	1136	34.09	41.93	81.07	1121	34.93	42.97	80.03	1107	35.78	44.01	78.99	1092
123.5	33.08	40.85	82.65	1143	33.92	41.89	81.61	1129	34.76	42.93	80.57	1114	35.60	43.97	79.53	1100
124	32.91	40.81	83.19	1150	33.75	41.85	82.15	1136	34.59	42.89	81.11	1122	35.42	43.92	80.08	1107
124.5	32.75	40.77	83.73	1158	33.58	41.81	82.69	1144	34.41	42.85	81.65	1129	35.25	43.88	80.62	1115
125	32.58	40.73	84.27	1165	33.41	41.77	83.23	1151	34.24	42.81	82.20	1137	35.07	43.84	81.16	1122
125.5	32.42	40.69	84.81	1173	33.25	41.73	83.77	1159	34.07	42.76	82.74	1144	34.90	43.80	81.70	1130
126	32.26	40.65	85.35	1180	33.08	41.69	84.31	1166	33.91	42.72	83.28	1152	34.73	43.76	82.24	1137
126.5	32.10	40.61	85.89	1188	32.92	41.64	84.86	1174	33.74	42.68	83.82	1159	34.56	43.72	82.78	1145
127	31.94	40.57	86.43	1195	32.76	41.60	85.40	1181	33.58	42.64	84.36	1167	34.39	43.68	83.32	1152
127.5	31.78	40.53	86.98	1203	32.60	41.56	85.94	1189	33.41	42.60	84.90	1174	34.23	43.64	83.86	1160
128	31.63	40.48	87.52	1210	32.44	41.52	86.48	1196	33.25	42.56	85.44	1182	34.06	43.60	84.40	1167
128.5	31.47	40.44	88.06	1218	32.28	41.48	87.02	1203	33.09	42.52	85.98	1189	33.90	43.56	84.94	1175
129	31.32	40.40	88.60	1225	32.12	41.44	87.56	1211	32.93	42.48	86.52	1197	33.73	43.51	85.49	1182
129.5	31.17	40.36	89.14	1233	31.97	41.40	88.10	1218	32.77	42.44	87.06	1204	33.57	43.47	86.03	1190
130	31.02	40.32	89.68	1240	31.81	41.36	88.64	1226	32.61	42.40	87.61	1212	33.41	43.43	86.57	1197
130.5	30.87	40.28	90.22	1248	31.66	41.32	89.18	1233	32.46	42.35	88.15	1219	33.25	43.39	87.11	1205
131	30.72	40.24	90.76	1255	31.51	41.28	89.72	1241	32.30	42.31	88.69	1227	33.09	43.35	87.65	1212
131.5	30.57	40.20	91.30	1263	31.36	41.23	90.27	1248	32.15	42.27	89.23	1234	32.93	43.31	88.19	1220
132	30.42	40.16	91.84	1270	31.21	41.19	90.81	1256	31.99	42.23	89.77	1242	32.78	43.27	88.73	1227
132.5	30.28	40.12	92.39	1278	31.06	41.15	91.35	1263	31.84	42.19	90.31	1249	32.62	43.23	89.27	1235
133	30.13	40.07	92.93	1285	30.91	41.11	91.89	1271	31.69	42.15	90.85	1256	32.47	43.19	89.81	1242
133.5	29.99	40.03	93.47	1293	30.76	41.07	92.43	1278	31.54	42.11	91.39	1264	32.32	43.15	90.35	1250
134	29.84	39.99	94.01	1300	30.62	41.03	92.97	1286	31.39	42.07	91.93	1271	32.17	43.10	90.90	1257
134.5	29.70	39.95	94.55	1308	30.47	40.99	93.51	1293	31.25	42.03	92.47	1279	32.02	43.06	91.44	1265
135	29.56	39.91	95.09	1315	30.33	40.95	94.05	1301	31.10	41.99	93.02	1286	31.87	43.02	91.98	1272
135.5	29.42	39.87	95.63	1323	30.19	40.91	94.59	1308	30.95	41.94	93.56	1294	31.72	42.98	92.52	1280
136	29.29	39.83	96.17	1330	30.05	40.87	95.13	1316	30.81	41.90	94.10	1301	31.57	42.94	93.06	1287
136.5	29.15	39.79	96.71	1338	29.91	40.82	95.68	1323	30.67	41.86	94.64	1309	31.43	42.90	93.60	1294
137	29.01	39.75	97.25	1345	29.77	40.78	96.22	1331	30.53	41.82	95.18	1316	31.28	42.86	94.14	1302
137.5	28.88	39.71	97.80	1353	29.63	40.74	96.76	1338	30.39	41.78	95.72	1324	31.14	42.82	94.68	1309
138	28.74	39.66	98.34	1360	29.49	40.70	97.30	1346	30.25	41.74	96.26	1331	31.00	42.78	95.22	1317
138.5	28.61	39.62	98.88	1367	29.36	40.66	97.84	1353	30.11	41.70	96.80	1339	30.86	42.74	95.76	1324
139	28.48	39.58	99.42	1375	29.22	40.62	98.38	1361	29.97	41.66	97.34	1346	30.72	42.69	96.31	1332
139.5	28.34	39.54	99.96	1382	29.09	40.58	98.92	1368	29.83	41.62	97.88	1354	30.58	42.65	96.85	1339
140	28.21	39.50	100.50	1390	28.96	40.54	99.46	1376	29.70	41.58	98.43	1361	30.44	42.61	97.39	1347
140.5	28.08	39.46	101.04	1397	28.82	40.50	100.00	1383	29.56	41.53	98.97	1369	30.30	42.57	97.93	1354
141	27.96	39.42	101.58	1405	28.69	40.46	100.54	1391	29.43	41.49	99.51	1376	30.16	42.53	98.47	1362
141.5	27.83	39.38	102.12	1412	28.56	40.41	101.09	1398	29.29	41.45	100.05	1384	30.03	42.49	99.01	1369
142	27.70	39.34	102.66	1420	28.43	40.37	101.63	1405	29.16	41.41	100.59	1391	29.89	42.45	99.55	1377
142.5	27.58	39.30	103.21	1427	28.30	40.33	102.17	1413	29.03	41.37	101.13	1399	29.76	42.41	100.09	1384
143	27.45	39.25	103.75	1435	28.18	40.29	102.71	1420	28.90	41.33	101.67	1406	29.63	42.37	100.63	1392
143.5	27.33	39.21	104.29	1442	28.05	40.25	103.25	1428	28.77	41.29	102.21	1414	29.50	42.33	101.17	1399
144	27.20	39.17	104.83	1450	27.92	40.21	103.79	1435	28.64	41.25	102.75	1421	29.36	42.28	101.72	1407
144.5	27.08	39.13	105.37	1457	27.80	40.17	104.33	1443	28.52	41.21	103.29	1429	29.23	42.24	102.26	1414
145	26.96	39.09	105.91	1465	27.67	40.13	104.87	1450	28.39	41.17	103.84	1436	29.11	42.20	102.80	1422
145.5	26.84	39.05	106.45	1472	27.55	40.09	105.41	1458	28.26	41.12	104.38	1444	28.98	42.16	103.34	1429
146	26.72	39.01	106.99	1480	27.43	40.05	105.95	1465	28.14	41.08	104.92	1451	28.85	42.12	103.88	1437
146.5	26.60	38.97	107.53	1487	27.31	40.00	106.50	1473	28.02	41.04	105.46	1458	28.72	42.08	104.42	1444
147	26.48	38.93	108.07	1495	27.19	39.96	107.04	1480	27.89	41.00	106.00	1466	28.60	42.04	104.96	1452
147.5	26.36	38.89	108.62	1502	27.07	39.92	107.58	1488	27.77	40.96	106.54	1473	28.47	42.00	105.50	1459
148	26.25	38.84	109.16	1510	26.95	39.88	108.12	1495	27.65	40.92	107.08	1481	28.35	41.96	106.04	1467
148.5	26.13	38.80	109.70	1517	26.83	39.84	108.66	1503	27.53	40.88	107.62	1488	28.23	41.92	106.58	1474
149	26.01	38.76	110.24	1525	26.71	39.80	109.20	1510	27.41	40.84	108.16	1496	28.10	41.87	107.13	1482
149.5	25.90	38.72	110.78	1532	26.59	39.76	109.74	1518	27.29	40.80	108.70	1503	27.98	41.83	107.67	1489
150	25.79	38.68	111.32	1540	26.48	39.72	110.28	1525	27.17	40.76	109.25	1511	27.86	41.79	108.21	1497
150.5	25.67	38.64	111.86	1547	26.36	39.68	110.82	1533	27.05	40.71	109.79	1518	27.74	41.75	108.75	1504
151	25.56	38.60	112.40	1555	26.25	39.64	111.36	1540	26.94	40.67	110.33	1526	27.62	41.71	109.29	1511
151.5	25.45	38.56	112.94	1562	26.13	39.59	111.91	1548	26.82	40.63	110.87	1533	27.50	41.67	109.83	1519

Body Composition MALE 120-151.5 Lb.

Weight: Lb.	Waist: 37 inches Fat: %	Fat: Lb.	LBM: Lb.	RMR: Cal.	37.25 inches Fat: %	Fat: Lb.	LBM: Lb.	RMR: Cal.	37.5 inches Fat: %	Fat: Lb.	LBM: Lb.	RMR: Cal.	37.75 inches Fat: %	Fat: Lb.	LBM: Lb.	RMR: Cal.
120	37.74	45.29	74.71	1033	38.61	46.33	73.67	1019	39.47	47.37	72.64	1005	40.34	48.40	71.60	990
120.5	37.55	45.25	75.25	1041	38.41	46.29	74.21	1026	39.27	47.32	73.18	1012	40.13	48.36	72.14	998
121	37.36	45.21	75.79	1048	38.22	46.25	74.75	1034	39.08	47.28	73.72	1020	39.93	48.32	72.68	1005
121.5	37.17	45.17	76.33	1056	38.03	46.20	75.30	1041	38.88	47.24	74.26	1027	39.74	48.28	73.22	1013
122	36.99	45.13	76.87	1063	37.84	46.16	75.84	1049	38.69	47.20	74.80	1034	39.54	48.24	73.76	1020
122.5	36.80	45.09	77.42	1071	37.65	46.12	76.38	1056	38.50	47.16	75.34	1042	39.34	48.20	74.30	1028
123	36.62	45.04	77.96	1078	37.46	46.08	76.92	1064	38.31	47.12	75.88	1049	39.15	48.16	74.84	1035
123.5	36.44	45.00	78.50	1086	37.28	46.04	77.46	1071	38.12	47.08	76.42	1057	38.96	48.12	75.38	1043
124	36.26	44.96	79.04	1093	37.10	46.00	78.00	1079	37.93	47.04	76.96	1064	38.77	48.07	75.93	1050
124.5	36.08	44.92	79.58	1101	36.91	45.96	78.54	1086	37.75	47.00	77.50	1072	38.58	48.03	76.47	1058
125	35.90	44.88	80.12	1108	36.73	45.92	79.08	1094	37.56	46.96	78.05	1079	38.39	47.99	77.01	1065
125.5	35.73	44.84	80.66	1116	36.55	45.88	79.62	1101	37.38	46.91	78.59	1087	38.21	47.95	77.55	1072
126	35.55	44.80	81.20	1123	36.38	45.84	80.16	1109	37.20	46.87	79.13	1094	38.02	47.91	78.09	1080
126.5	35.38	44.76	81.74	1131	36.20	45.79	80.71	1116	37.02	46.83	79.67	1102	37.84	47.87	78.63	1087
127	35.21	44.72	82.28	1138	36.03	45.75	81.25	1124	36.84	46.79	80.21	1109	37.66	47.83	79.17	1095
127.5	35.04	44.68	82.83	1145	35.85	45.71	81.79	1131	36.67	46.75	80.75	1117	37.48	47.79	79.71	1102
128	34.87	44.63	83.37	1153	35.68	45.67	82.33	1139	36.49	46.71	81.29	1124	37.30	47.75	80.25	1110
128.5	34.70	44.59	83.91	1160	35.51	45.63	82.87	1146	36.32	46.67	81.83	1132	37.12	47.71	80.79	1117
129	34.54	44.55	84.45	1168	35.34	45.59	83.41	1154	36.14	46.63	82.37	1139	36.95	47.66	81.34	1125
129.5	34.37	44.51	84.99	1175	35.17	45.55	83.95	1161	35.97	46.59	82.91	1147	36.77	47.62	81.88	1132
130	34.21	44.47	85.53	1183	35.01	45.51	84.49	1169	35.80	46.55	83.46	1154	36.60	47.58	82.42	1140
130.5	34.05	44.43	86.07	1190	34.84	45.47	85.03	1176	35.64	46.50	84.00	1162	36.43	47.54	82.96	1147
131	33.88	44.39	86.61	1198	34.68	45.43	85.57	1183	35.47	46.46	84.54	1169	36.26	47.50	83.50	1155
131.5	33.72	44.35	87.15	1205	34.51	45.38	86.12	1191	35.30	46.42	85.08	1177	36.09	47.46	84.04	1162
132	33.57	44.31	87.69	1213	34.35	45.34	86.66	1198	35.14	46.38	85.62	1184	35.92	47.42	84.58	1170
132.5	33.41	44.27	88.24	1220	34.19	45.30	87.20	1206	34.97	46.34	86.16	1192	35.76	47.38	85.12	1177
133	33.25	44.22	88.78	1228	34.03	45.26	87.74	1213	34.81	46.30	86.70	1199	35.59	47.34	85.66	1185
133.5	33.10	44.18	89.32	1235	33.87	45.22	88.28	1221	34.65	46.26	87.24	1207	35.43	47.30	86.20	1192
134	32.94	44.14	89.86	1243	33.72	45.18	88.82	1228	34.49	46.22	87.78	1214	35.26	47.25	86.75	1200
134.5	32.79	44.10	90.40	1250	33.56	45.14	89.36	1236	34.33	46.18	88.32	1222	35.10	47.21	87.29	1207
135	32.64	44.06	90.94	1258	33.41	45.10	89.90	1243	34.17	46.14	88.87	1229	34.94	47.17	87.83	1215
135.5	32.49	44.02	91.48	1265	33.25	45.06	90.44	1251	34.02	46.09	89.41	1236	34.78	47.13	88.37	1222
136	32.34	43.98	92.02	1273	33.10	45.02	90.98	1258	33.86	46.05	89.95	1244	34.63	47.09	88.91	1230
136.5	32.19	43.94	92.56	1280	32.95	44.97	91.53	1266	33.71	46.01	90.49	1251	34.47	47.05	89.45	1237
137	32.04	43.90	93.10	1288	32.80	44.93	92.07	1273	33.56	45.97	91.03	1259	34.31	47.01	89.99	1245
137.5	31.89	43.86	93.65	1295	32.65	44.89	92.61	1281	33.40	45.93	91.57	1266	34.16	46.97	90.53	1252
138	31.75	43.81	94.19	1303	32.50	44.85	93.15	1288	33.25	45.89	92.11	1274	34.00	46.93	91.07	1260
138.5	31.61	43.77	94.73	1310	32.35	44.81	93.69	1296	33.10	45.85	92.65	1281	33.85	46.89	91.61	1267
139	31.46	43.73	95.27	1318	32.21	44.77	94.23	1303	32.95	45.81	93.19	1289	33.70	46.84	92.16	1275
139.5	31.32	43.69	95.81	1325	32.06	44.73	94.77	1311	32.81	45.77	93.73	1296	33.55	46.80	92.70	1282
140	31.18	43.65	96.35	1333	31.92	44.69	95.31	1318	32.66	45.73	94.28	1304	33.40	46.76	93.24	1289
140.5	31.04	43.61	96.89	1340	31.78	44.65	95.85	1326	32.52	45.68	94.82	1311	33.25	46.72	93.78	1297
141	30.90	43.57	97.43	1347	31.64	44.61	96.39	1333	32.37	45.64	95.36	1319	33.11	46.68	94.32	1304
141.5	30.76	43.53	97.97	1355	31.49	44.56	96.94	1341	32.23	45.60	95.90	1326	32.96	46.64	94.86	1312
142	30.62	43.49	98.51	1362	31.35	44.52	97.48	1348	32.09	45.56	96.44	1334	32.82	46.60	95.40	1319
142.5	30.49	43.45	99.06	1370	31.22	44.48	98.02	1356	31.94	45.52	96.98	1341	32.67	46.56	95.94	1327
143	30.35	43.40	99.60	1377	31.08	44.44	98.56	1363	31.80	45.48	97.52	1349	32.53	46.52	96.48	1334
143.5	30.22	43.36	100.14	1385	30.94	44.40	99.10	1371	31.66	45.44	98.06	1356	32.39	46.48	97.02	1342
144	30.08	43.32	100.68	1392	30.81	44.36	99.64	1378	31.53	45.40	98.60	1364	32.25	46.43	97.57	1349
144.5	29.95	43.28	101.22	1400	30.67	44.32	100.18	1386	31.39	45.36	99.14	1371	32.11	46.39	98.11	1357
145	29.82	43.24	101.76	1407	30.54	44.28	100.72	1393	31.25	45.32	99.69	1379	31.97	46.35	98.65	1364
145.5	29.69	43.20	102.30	1415	30.40	44.24	101.26	1400	31.12	45.27	100.23	1386	31.83	46.31	99.19	1372
146	29.56	43.16	102.84	1422	30.27	44.20	101.80	1408	30.98	45.23	100.77	1394	31.69	46.27	99.73	1379
146.5	29.43	43.12	103.38	1430	30.14	44.15	102.35	1415	30.85	45.19	101.31	1401	31.56	46.23	100.27	1387
147	29.30	43.08	103.92	1437	30.01	44.11	102.89	1423	30.71	45.15	101.85	1409	31.42	46.19	100.81	1394
147.5	29.18	43.04	104.47	1445	29.88	44.07	103.43	1430	30.58	45.11	102.39	1416	31.29	46.15	101.35	1402
148	29.05	42.99	105.01	1452	29.75	44.03	103.97	1438	30.45	45.07	102.93	1424	31.15	46.11	101.89	1409
148.5	28.92	42.95	105.55	1460	29.62	43.99	104.51	1445	30.32	45.03	103.47	1431	31.02	46.07	102.43	1417
149	28.80	42.91	106.09	1467	29.50	43.95	105.05	1453	30.19	44.99	104.01	1438	30.89	46.02	102.98	1424
149.5	28.68	42.87	106.63	1475	29.37	43.91	105.59	1460	30.06	44.95	104.55	1446	30.76	45.98	103.52	1432
150	28.55	42.83	107.17	1482	29.25	43.87	106.13	1468	29.94	44.91	105.10	1453	30.63	45.94	104.06	1439
150.5	28.43	42.79	107.71	1490	29.12	43.83	106.67	1475	29.81	44.86	105.64	1461	30.50	45.90	104.60	1447
151	28.31	42.75	108.25	1497	29.00	43.79	107.21	1483	29.68	44.82	106.18	1468	30.37	45.86	105.14	1454
151.5	28.19	42.71	108.79	1505	28.87	43.74	107.76	1490	29.56	44.78	106.72	1476	30.24	45.82	105.68	1462

Body Composition   MALE   120-151.5 Lb.

Weight: Lb.	Waist: 38 inches Fat: %	Fat: Lb.	LBM: Lb.	RMR: Cal.	38.25 inches Fat: %	Fat: Lb.	LBM: Lb.	RMR: Cal.	38.5 inches Fat: %	Fat: Lb.	LBM: Lb.	RMR: Cal.	38.75 inches Fat: %	Fat: Lb.	LBM: Lb.	RMR: Cal.
120	41.20	49.44	70.56	976	42.06	50.48	69.52	961	42.93	51.52	68.49	947	43.79	52.55	67.45	933
120.5	41.00	49.40	71.10	983	41.86	50.44	70.06	969	42.72	51.47	69.03	955	43.58	52.51	67.99	940
121	40.79	49.36	71.64	991	41.65	50.40	70.60	976	42.51	51.43	69.57	962	43.36	52.47	68.53	948
121.5	40.59	49.32	72.18	998	41.44	50.35	71.15	984	42.30	51.39	70.11	970	43.15	52.43	69.07	955
122	40.39	49.28	72.72	1006	41.24	50.31	71.69	991	42.09	51.35	70.65	977	42.94	52.39	69.61	963
122.5	40.19	49.24	73.27	1013	41.04	50.27	72.23	999	41.89	51.31	71.19	985	42.73	52.35	70.15	970
123	40.00	49.19	73.81	1021	40.84	50.23	72.77	1006	41.68	51.27	71.73	992	42.53	52.31	70.69	978
123.5	39.80	49.15	74.35	1028	40.64	50.19	73.31	1014	41.48	51.23	72.27	1000	42.32	52.27	71.23	985
124	39.61	49.11	74.89	1036	40.44	50.15	73.85	1021	41.28	51.19	72.81	1007	42.12	52.22	71.78	993
124.5	39.41	49.07	75.43	1043	40.25	50.11	74.39	1029	41.08	51.15	73.35	1014	41.91	52.18	72.32	1000
125	39.22	49.03	75.97	1051	40.05	50.07	74.93	1036	40.88	51.11	73.90	1022	41.71	52.14	72.86	1008
125.5	39.04	48.99	76.51	1058	39.86	50.03	75.47	1044	40.69	51.06	74.44	1029	41.52	52.10	73.40	1015
126	38.85	48.95	77.05	1066	39.67	49.99	76.01	1051	40.49	51.02	74.98	1037	41.32	52.06	73.94	1023
126.5	38.66	48.91	77.59	1073	39.48	49.94	76.56	1059	40.30	50.98	75.52	1044	41.12	52.02	74.48	1030
127	38.48	48.87	78.13	1081	39.29	49.90	77.10	1066	40.11	50.94	76.06	1052	40.93	51.98	75.02	1038
127.5	38.29	48.83	78.68	1088	39.11	49.86	77.64	1074	39.92	50.90	76.60	1059	40.74	51.94	75.56	1045
128	38.11	48.78	79.22	1096	38.92	49.82	78.18	1081	39.73	50.86	77.14	1067	40.54	51.90	76.10	1053
128.5	37.93	48.74	79.76	1103	38.74	49.78	78.72	1089	39.55	50.82	77.68	1074	40.35	51.86	76.64	1060
129	37.75	48.70	80.30	1111	38.56	49.74	79.26	1096	39.36	50.78	78.22	1082	40.17	51.81	77.19	1067
129.5	37.58	48.66	80.84	1118	38.38	49.70	79.80	1104	39.18	50.74	78.76	1089	39.98	51.77	77.73	1075
130	37.40	48.62	81.38	1125	38.20	49.66	80.34	1111	39.00	50.70	79.31	1097	39.79	51.73	78.27	1082
130.5	37.23	48.58	81.92	1133	38.02	49.62	80.88	1119	38.82	50.65	79.85	1104	39.61	51.69	78.81	1090
131	37.05	48.54	82.46	1140	37.84	49.58	81.42	1126	38.64	50.61	80.39	1112	39.43	51.65	79.35	1097
131.5	36.88	48.50	83.00	1148	37.67	49.53	81.97	1134	38.46	50.57	80.93	1119	39.25	51.61	79.89	1105
132	36.71	48.46	83.54	1155	37.50	49.49	82.51	1141	38.28	50.53	81.47	1127	39.07	51.57	80.43	1112
132.5	36.54	48.42	84.09	1163	37.32	49.45	83.05	1149	38.11	50.49	82.01	1134	38.89	51.53	80.97	1120
133	36.37	48.37	84.63	1170	37.15	49.41	83.59	1156	37.93	50.45	82.55	1142	38.71	51.49	81.51	1127
133.5	36.20	48.33	85.17	1178	36.98	49.37	84.13	1164	37.76	50.41	83.09	1149	38.54	51.45	82.05	1135
134	36.04	48.29	85.71	1185	36.81	49.33	84.67	1171	37.59	50.37	83.63	1157	38.36	51.40	82.60	1142
134.5	35.87	48.25	86.25	1193	36.65	49.29	85.21	1178	37.42	50.33	84.17	1164	38.19	51.36	83.14	1150
135	35.71	48.21	86.79	1200	36.48	49.25	85.75	1186	37.25	50.29	84.72	1172	38.02	51.32	83.68	1157
135.5	35.55	48.17	87.33	1208	36.31	49.21	86.29	1193	37.08	50.24	85.26	1179	37.85	51.28	84.22	1165
136	35.39	48.13	87.87	1215	36.15	49.17	86.83	1201	36.91	50.20	85.80	1187	37.68	51.24	84.76	1172
136.5	35.23	48.09	88.41	1223	35.99	49.12	87.38	1208	36.75	50.16	86.34	1194	37.51	51.20	85.30	1180
137	35.07	48.05	88.95	1230	35.83	49.08	87.92	1216	36.58	50.12	86.88	1202	37.34	51.16	85.84	1187
137.5	34.91	48.01	89.50	1238	35.67	49.04	88.46	1223	36.42	50.08	87.42	1209	37.18	51.12	86.38	1195
138	34.76	47.96	90.04	1245	35.51	49.00	89.00	1231	36.26	50.04	87.96	1217	37.01	51.08	86.92	1202
138.5	34.60	47.92	90.58	1253	35.35	48.96	89.54	1238	36.10	50.00	88.50	1224	36.85	51.04	87.46	1210
139	34.45	47.88	91.12	1260	35.19	48.92	90.08	1246	35.94	49.96	89.04	1231	36.69	50.99	88.01	1217
139.5	34.29	47.84	91.66	1268	35.04	48.88	90.62	1253	35.78	49.92	89.58	1239	36.53	50.95	88.55	1225
140	34.14	47.80	92.20	1275	34.88	48.84	91.16	1261	35.63	49.88	90.13	1246	36.37	50.91	89.09	1232
140.5	33.99	47.76	92.74	1283	34.73	48.80	91.70	1268	35.47	49.83	90.67	1254	36.21	50.87	89.63	1240
141	33.84	47.72	93.28	1290	34.58	48.76	92.24	1276	35.31	49.79	91.21	1261	36.05	50.83	90.17	1247
141.5	33.69	47.68	93.82	1298	34.43	48.71	92.79	1283	35.16	49.75	91.75	1269	35.89	50.79	90.71	1255
142	33.55	47.64	94.36	1305	34.28	48.67	93.33	1291	35.01	49.71	92.29	1276	35.74	50.75	91.25	1262
142.5	33.40	47.60	94.91	1313	34.13	48.63	93.87	1298	34.86	49.67	92.83	1284	35.58	50.71	91.79	1269
143	33.25	47.55	95.45	1320	33.98	48.59	94.41	1306	34.71	49.63	93.37	1291	35.43	50.67	92.33	1277
143.5	33.11	47.51	95.99	1328	33.83	48.55	94.95	1313	34.56	49.59	93.91	1299	35.28	50.63	92.87	1284
144	32.97	47.47	96.53	1335	33.69	48.51	95.49	1321	34.41	49.55	94.45	1306	35.13	50.58	93.42	1292
144.5	32.82	47.43	97.07	1342	33.54	48.47	96.03	1328	34.26	49.51	94.99	1314	34.98	50.54	93.96	1299
145	32.68	47.39	97.61	1350	33.40	48.43	96.57	1336	34.11	49.47	95.54	1321	34.83	50.50	94.50	1307
145.5	32.54	47.35	98.15	1357	33.26	48.39	97.11	1343	33.97	49.42	96.08	1329	34.68	50.46	95.04	1314
146	32.40	47.31	98.69	1365	33.11	48.35	97.65	1351	33.82	49.38	96.62	1336	34.53	50.42	95.58	1322
146.5	32.26	47.27	99.23	1372	32.97	48.30	98.20	1358	33.68	49.34	97.16	1344	34.39	50.38	96.12	1329
147	32.13	47.23	99.77	1380	32.83	48.26	98.74	1366	33.54	49.30	97.70	1351	34.24	50.34	96.66	1337
147.5	31.99	47.19	100.32	1387	32.69	48.22	99.28	1373	33.40	49.26	98.24	1359	34.10	50.30	97.20	1344
148	31.85	47.14	100.86	1395	32.56	48.18	99.82	1380	33.26	49.22	98.78	1366	33.96	50.26	97.74	1352
148.5	31.72	47.10	101.40	1402	32.42	48.14	100.36	1388	33.12	49.18	99.32	1374	33.82	50.22	98.28	1359
149	31.59	47.06	101.94	1410	32.28	48.10	100.90	1395	32.98	49.14	99.86	1381	33.67	50.17	98.83	1367
149.5	31.45	47.02	102.48	1417	32.15	48.06	101.44	1403	32.84	49.10	100.40	1389	33.53	50.13	99.37	1374
150	31.32	46.98	103.02	1425	32.01	48.02	101.98	1410	32.70	49.06	100.95	1396	33.40	50.09	99.91	1382
150.5	31.19	46.94	103.56	1432	31.88	47.98	102.52	1418	32.57	49.01	101.49	1404	33.26	50.05	100.45	1389
151	31.06	46.90	104.10	1440	31.75	47.94	103.06	1425	32.43	48.97	102.03	1411	33.12	50.01	100.99	1397
151.5	30.93	46.86	104.64	1447	31.61	47.89	103.61	1433	32.30	48.93	102.57	1419	32.98	49.97	101.53	1404

Body Composition MALE 152-183.5 Lb.

Weight: Lb.	Waist: 28 inches Fat: %	Fat: Lb.	LBM: Lb.	RMR: Cal.	28.25 inches Fat: %	Fat: Lb.	LBM: Lb.	RMR: Cal.	28.5 inches Fat: %	Fat: Lb.	LBM: Lb.	RMR: Cal.	28.75 inches Fat: %	Fat: Lb.	LBM: Lb.	RMR: Cal.
152	3.50	5.32	146.68	2029	4.18	6.35	145.65	2014	4.86	7.39	144.61	2000	5.55	8.43	143.57	1986
152.5	3.46	5.27	147.23	2036	4.14	6.31	146.19	2022	4.82	7.35	145.15	2007	5.50	8.39	144.11	1993
153	3.42	5.23	147.77	2044	4.10	6.27	146.73	2029	4.78	7.31	145.69	2015	5.46	8.35	144.65	2001
153.5	3.38	5.19	148.31	2051	4.06	6.23	147.27	2037	4.73	7.27	146.23	2022	5.41	8.31	145.19	2008
154	3.35	5.15	148.85	2059	4.02	6.19	147.81	2044	4.69	7.23	146.77	2030	5.37	8.26	145.74	2016
154.5	3.31	5.11	149.39	2066	3.98	6.15	148.35	2052	4.65	7.19	147.31	2037	5.32	8.22	146.28	2023
155	3.27	5.07	149.93	2074	3.94	6.11	148.89	2059	4.61	7.14	147.86	2045	5.28	8.18	146.82	2030
155.5	3.23	5.03	150.47	2081	3.90	6.07	149.43	2067	4.57	7.10	148.40	2052	5.24	8.14	147.36	2038
156	3.20	4.99	151.01	2088	3.86	6.03	149.97	2074	4.53	7.06	148.94	2060	5.19	8.10	147.90	2045
156.5	3.16	4.95	151.55	2096	3.82	5.98	150.52	2082	4.49	7.02	149.48	2067	5.15	8.06	148.44	2053
157	3.12	4.91	152.09	2103	3.79	5.94	151.06	2089	4.45	6.98	150.02	2075	5.11	8.02	148.98	2060
157.5	3.09	4.87	152.64	2111	3.75	5.90	151.60	2097	4.41	6.94	150.56	2082	5.07	7.98	149.52	2068
158	3.05	4.82	153.18	2118	3.71	5.86	152.14	2104	4.37	6.90	151.10	2090	5.02	7.94	150.06	2075
158.5	3.02	4.78	153.72	2126	3.67	5.82	152.68	2112	4.33	6.86	151.64	2097	4.98	7.90	150.60	2083
159	2.98	4.74	154.26	2133	3.63	5.78	153.22	2119	4.29	6.82	152.18	2105	4.94	7.85	151.15	2090
159.5	2.95	4.70	154.80	2141	3.60	5.74	153.76	2127	4.25	6.78	152.72	2112	4.90	7.81	151.69	2098
160	2.91	4.66	155.34	2148	3.56	5.70	154.30	2134	4.21	6.74	153.27	2120	4.86	7.77	152.23	2105
160.5	2.88	4.62	155.88	2156	3.52	5.66	154.84	2141	4.17	6.69	153.81	2127	4.82	7.73	152.77	2113
161	2.84	4.58	156.42	2163	3.49	5.62	155.38	2149	4.13	6.65	154.35	2135	4.78	7.69	153.31	2120
161.5	2.81	4.54	156.96	2171	3.45	5.57	155.93	2156	4.09	6.61	154.89	2142	4.74	7.65	153.85	2128
162	2.78	4.50	157.50	2178	3.42	5.53	156.47	2164	4.06	6.57	155.43	2150	4.70	7.61	154.39	2135
162.5	2.74	4.45	158.05	2186	3.38	5.49	157.01	2171	4.02	6.53	155.97	2157	4.66	7.57	154.93	2143
163	2.71	4.41	158.59	2193	3.34	5.45	157.55	2179	3.98	6.49	156.51	2165	4.62	7.53	155.47	2150
163.5	2.67	4.37	159.13	2201	3.31	5.41	158.09	2186	3.94	6.45	157.05	2172	4.58	7.49	156.01	2158
164	2.64	4.33	159.67	2208	3.27	5.37	158.63	2194	3.91	6.41	157.59	2180	4.54	7.44	156.56	2165
164.5	2.61	4.29	160.21	2216	3.24	5.33	159.17	2201	3.87	6.37	158.13	2187	4.50	7.40	157.10	2173
165	2.58	4.25	160.75	2223	3.20	5.29	159.71	2209	3.83	6.32	158.68	2194	4.46	7.36	157.64	2180
165.5	2.54	4.21	161.29	2231	3.17	5.25	160.25	2216	3.80	6.28	159.22	2202	4.42	7.32	158.18	2188
166	2.51	4.17	161.83	2238	3.14	5.21	160.79	2224	3.76	6.24	159.76	2209	4.39	7.28	158.72	2195
166.5	2.48	4.13	162.37	2246	3.10	5.16	161.34	2231	3.72	6.20	160.30	2217	4.35	7.24	159.26	2203
167	2.45	4.09	162.91	2253	3.07	5.12	161.88	2239	3.69	6.16	160.84	2224	4.31	7.20	159.80	2210
167.5	2.41	4.05	163.46	2261	3.03	5.08	162.42	2246	3.65	6.12	161.38	2232	4.27	7.16	160.34	2218
168	2.38	4.00	164.00	2268	3.00	5.04	162.96	2254	3.62	6.08	161.92	2239	4.24	7.12	160.88	2225
168.5	2.35	3.96	164.54	2276	2.97	5.00	163.50	2261	3.58	6.04	162.46	2247	4.20	7.08	161.42	2233
169	2.32	3.92	165.08	2283	2.93	4.96	164.04	2269	3.55	6.00	163.00	2254	4.16	7.03	161.97	2240
169.5	2.29	3.88	165.62	2291	2.90	4.92	164.58	2276	3.51	5.96	163.54	2262	4.13	6.99	162.51	2247
170	2.26	3.84	166.16	2298	2.87	4.88	165.12	2284	3.48	5.91	164.09	2269	4.09	6.95	163.05	2255
170.5	2.23	3.80	166.70	2305	2.84	4.84	165.66	2291	3.45	5.87	164.63	2277	4.05	6.91	163.59	2262
171	2.20	3.76	167.24	2313	2.80	4.80	166.20	2299	3.41	5.83	165.17	2284	4.02	6.87	164.13	2270
171.5	2.17	3.72	167.78	2320	2.77	4.75	166.75	2306	3.38	5.79	165.71	2292	3.98	6.83	164.67	2277
172	2.14	3.68	168.32	2328	2.74	4.71	167.29	2314	3.34	5.75	166.25	2299	3.95	6.79	165.21	2285
172.5	2.11	3.63	168.87	2335	2.71	4.67	167.83	2321	3.31	5.71	166.79	2307	3.91	6.75	165.75	2292
173	2.08	3.59	169.41	2343	2.68	4.63	168.37	2329	3.28	5.67	167.33	2314	3.88	6.71	166.29	2300
173.5	2.05	3.55	169.95	2350	2.65	4.59	168.91	2336	3.24	5.63	167.87	2322	3.84	6.67	166.83	2307
174	2.02	3.51	170.49	2358	2.61	4.55	169.45	2344	3.21	5.59	168.41	2329	3.81	6.62	167.38	2315
174.5	1.99	3.47	171.03	2365	2.58	4.51	169.99	2351	3.18	5.55	168.95	2337	3.77	6.58	167.92	2322
175	1.96	3.43	171.57	2373	2.55	4.47	170.53	2358	3.15	5.51	169.50	2344	3.74	6.54	168.46	2330
175.5	1.93	3.39	172.11	2380	2.52	4.43	171.07	2366	3.11	5.46	170.04	2352	3.70	6.50	169.00	2337
176	1.90	3.35	172.65	2388	2.49	4.39	171.61	2373	3.08	5.42	170.58	2359	3.67	6.46	169.54	2345
176.5	1.87	3.31	173.19	2395	2.46	4.34	172.16	2381	3.05	5.38	171.12	2367	3.64	6.42	170.08	2352
177	1.85	3.27	173.73	2403	2.43	4.30	172.70	2388	3.02	5.34	171.66	2374	3.60	6.38	170.62	2360
177.5	1.82	3.23	174.28	2410	2.40	4.26	173.24	2396	2.99	5.30	172.20	2382	3.57	6.34	171.16	2367
178	1.79	3.18	174.82	2418	2.37	4.22	173.78	2403	2.95	5.26	172.74	2389	3.54	6.30	171.70	2375
178.5	1.76	3.14	175.36	2425	2.34	4.18	174.32	2411	2.92	5.22	173.28	2396	3.50	6.26	172.24	2382
179	1.73	3.10	175.90	2433	2.31	4.14	174.86	2418	2.89	5.18	173.82	2404	3.47	6.21	172.79	2390
179.5	1.71	3.06	176.44	2440	2.28	4.10	175.40	2426	2.86	5.14	174.36	2411	3.44	6.17	173.33	2397
180	1.68	3.02	176.98	2448	2.25	4.06	175.94	2433	2.83	5.09	174.91	2419	3.41	6.13	173.87	2405
180.5	1.65	2.98	177.52	2455	2.23	4.02	176.48	2441	2.80	5.05	175.45	2426	3.37	6.09	174.41	2412
181	1.62	2.94	178.06	2463	2.20	3.98	177.02	2448	2.77	5.01	175.99	2434	3.34	6.05	174.95	2420
181.5	1.60	2.90	178.60	2470	2.17	3.93	177.57	2456	2.74	4.97	176.53	2441	3.31	6.01	175.49	2427
182	1.57	2.86	179.14	2478	2.14	3.89	178.11	2463	2.71	4.93	177.07	2449	3.28	5.97	176.03	2435
182.5	1.54	2.82	179.69	2485	2.11	3.85	178.65	2471	2.68	4.89	177.61	2456	3.25	5.93	176.57	2442
183	1.52	2.77	180.23	2493	2.08	3.81	179.19	2478	2.65	4.85	178.15	2464	3.22	5.89	177.11	2449
183.5	1.49	2.73	180.77	2500	2.05	3.77	179.73	2486	2.62	4.81	178.69	2471	3.19	5.85	177.65	2457

Body Composition   MALE   152-183.5 Lb.

Weight: Lb.	Waist: 29 inches				29.25 inches				29.5 inches				29.75 inches			
	Fat: %	Fat: Lb.	LBM: Lb.	RMR: Cal.	Fat: %	Fat: Lb.	LBM: Lb.	RMR: Cal.	Fat: %	Fat: Lb.	LBM: Lb.	RMR: Cal.	Fat: %	Fat: Lb.	LBM: Lb.	RMR: Cal.
152	6.23	9.47	142.53	1971	6.91	10.50	141.50	1957	7.59	11.54	140.46	1943	8.28	12.58	139.42	1928
152.5	6.18	9.42	143.08	1979	6.86	10.46	142.04	1964	7.54	11.50	141.00	1950	8.22	12.54	139.96	1936
153	6.13	9.38	143.62	1986	6.81	10.42	142.58	1972	7.49	11.46	141.54	1958	8.17	12.50	140.50	1943
153.5	6.09	9.34	144.16	1994	6.76	10.38	143.12	1979	7.44	11.42	142.08	1965	8.11	12.46	141.04	1951
154	6.04	9.30	144.70	2001	6.71	10.34	143.66	1987	7.39	11.38	142.62	1972	8.06	12.41	141.59	1958
154.5	5.99	9.26	145.24	2009	6.67	10.30	144.20	1994	7.34	11.34	143.16	1980	8.01	12.37	142.13	1966
155	5.95	9.22	145.78	2016	6.62	10.26	144.74	2002	7.29	11.30	143.71	1987	7.96	12.33	142.67	1973
155.5	5.90	9.18	146.32	2024	6.57	10.22	145.28	2009	7.24	11.25	144.25	1995	7.90	12.29	143.21	1981
156	5.86	9.14	146.86	2031	6.52	10.18	145.82	2017	7.19	11.21	144.79	2002	7.85	12.25	143.75	1988
156.5	5.81	9.10	147.40	2039	6.48	10.13	146.37	2024	7.14	11.17	145.33	2010	7.80	12.21	144.29	1996
157	5.77	9.06	147.94	2046	6.43	10.09	146.91	2032	7.09	11.13	145.87	2017	7.75	12.17	144.83	2003
157.5	5.72	9.01	148.49	2054	6.38	10.05	147.45	2039	7.04	11.09	146.41	2025	7.70	12.13	145.37	2011
158	5.68	8.97	149.03	2061	6.34	10.01	147.99	2047	6.99	11.05	146.95	2032	7.65	12.09	145.91	2018
158.5	5.64	8.93	149.57	2069	6.29	9.97	148.53	2054	6.95	11.01	147.49	2040	7.60	12.05	146.45	2025
159	5.59	8.89	150.11	2076	6.24	9.93	149.07	2062	6.90	10.97	148.03	2047	7.55	12.00	147.00	2033
159.5	5.55	8.85	150.65	2083	6.20	9.89	149.61	2069	6.85	10.93	148.57	2055	7.50	11.96	147.54	2040
160	5.51	8.81	151.19	2091	6.15	9.85	150.15	2077	6.80	10.89	149.12	2062	7.45	11.92	148.08	2048
160.5	5.46	8.77	151.73	2098	6.11	9.81	150.69	2084	6.76	10.84	149.66	2070	7.40	11.88	148.62	2055
161	5.42	8.73	152.27	2106	6.07	9.77	151.23	2092	6.71	10.80	150.20	2077	7.35	11.84	149.16	2063
161.5	5.38	8.69	152.81	2113	6.02	9.72	151.78	2099	6.66	10.76	150.74	2085	7.31	11.80	149.70	2070
162	5.34	8.65	153.35	2121	5.98	9.68	152.32	2107	6.62	10.72	151.28	2092	7.26	11.76	150.24	2078
162.5	5.30	8.60	153.90	2128	5.93	9.64	152.86	2114	6.57	10.68	151.82	2100	7.21	11.72	150.78	2085
163	5.25	8.56	154.44	2136	5.89	9.60	153.40	2122	6.53	10.64	152.36	2107	7.16	11.68	151.32	2093
163.5	5.21	8.52	154.98	2143	5.85	9.56	153.94	2129	6.48	10.60	152.90	2115	7.12	11.64	151.86	2100
164	5.17	8.48	155.52	2151	5.80	9.52	154.48	2136	6.44	10.56	153.44	2122	7.07	11.59	152.41	2108
164.5	5.13	8.44	156.06	2158	5.76	9.48	155.02	2144	6.39	10.52	153.98	2130	7.02	11.55	152.95	2115
165	5.09	8.40	156.60	2166	5.72	9.44	155.56	2151	6.35	10.48	154.53	2137	6.98	11.51	153.49	2123
165.5	5.05	8.36	157.14	2173	5.68	9.40	156.10	2159	6.30	10.43	155.07	2145	6.93	11.47	154.03	2130
166	5.01	8.32	157.68	2181	5.64	9.36	156.64	2166	6.26	10.39	155.61	2152	6.89	11.43	154.57	2138
166.5	4.97	8.28	158.22	2188	5.59	9.31	157.19	2174	6.22	10.35	156.15	2160	6.84	11.39	155.11	2145
167	4.93	8.24	158.76	2196	5.55	9.27	157.73	2181	6.17	10.31	156.69	2167	6.80	11.35	155.65	2153
167.5	4.89	8.19	159.31	2203	5.51	9.23	158.27	2189	6.13	10.27	157.23	2174	6.75	11.31	156.19	2160
168	4.85	8.15	159.85	2211	5.47	9.19	158.81	2196	6.09	10.23	157.77	2182	6.71	11.27	156.73	2168
168.5	4.81	8.11	160.39	2218	5.43	9.15	159.35	2204	6.05	10.19	158.31	2189	6.66	11.23	157.27	2175
169	4.78	8.07	160.93	2226	5.39	9.11	159.89	2211	6.00	10.15	158.85	2197	6.62	11.18	157.82	2183
169.5	4.74	8.03	161.47	2233	5.35	9.07	160.43	2219	5.96	10.11	159.39	2204	6.57	11.14	158.36	2190
170	4.70	7.99	162.01	2241	5.31	9.03	160.97	2226	5.92	10.07	159.94	2212	6.53	11.10	158.90	2198
170.5	4.66	7.95	162.55	2248	5.27	8.99	161.51	2234	5.88	10.02	160.48	2219	6.49	11.06	159.44	2205
171	4.62	7.91	163.09	2256	5.23	8.95	162.05	2241	5.84	9.98	161.02	2227	6.44	11.02	159.98	2213
171.5	4.59	7.87	163.63	2263	5.19	8.90	162.60	2249	5.80	9.94	161.56	2234	6.40	10.98	160.52	2220
172	4.55	7.83	164.17	2271	5.15	8.86	163.14	2256	5.76	9.90	162.10	2242	6.36	10.94	161.06	2227
172.5	4.51	7.79	164.72	2278	5.11	8.82	163.68	2264	5.72	9.86	162.64	2249	6.32	10.90	161.60	2235
173	4.48	7.74	165.26	2285	5.08	8.78	164.22	2271	5.68	9.82	163.18	2257	6.28	10.86	162.14	2242
173.5	4.44	7.70	165.80	2293	5.04	8.74	164.76	2279	5.64	9.78	163.72	2264	6.23	10.82	162.68	2250
174	4.40	7.66	166.34	2300	5.00	8.70	165.30	2286	5.60	9.74	164.26	2272	6.19	10.77	163.23	2257
174.5	4.37	7.62	166.88	2308	4.96	8.66	165.84	2294	5.56	9.70	164.80	2279	6.15	10.73	163.77	2265
175	4.33	7.58	167.42	2315	4.92	8.62	166.38	2301	5.52	9.65	165.35	2287	6.11	10.69	164.31	2272
175.5	4.30	7.54	167.96	2323	4.89	8.58	166.92	2309	5.48	9.61	165.89	2294	6.07	10.65	164.85	2280
176	4.26	7.50	168.50	2330	4.85	8.54	167.46	2316	5.44	9.57	166.43	2302	6.03	10.61	165.39	2287
176.5	4.22	7.46	169.04	2338	4.81	8.49	168.01	2324	5.40	9.53	166.97	2309	5.99	10.57	165.93	2295
177	4.19	7.42	169.58	2345	4.78	8.45	168.55	2331	5.36	9.49	167.51	2317	5.95	10.53	166.47	2302
177.5	4.15	7.38	170.13	2353	4.74	8.41	169.09	2338	5.32	9.45	168.05	2324	5.91	10.49	167.01	2310
178	4.12	7.33	170.67	2360	4.70	8.37	169.63	2346	5.29	9.41	168.59	2332	5.87	10.45	167.55	2317
178.5	4.09	7.29	171.21	2368	4.67	8.33	170.17	2353	5.25	9.37	169.13	2339	5.83	10.41	168.09	2325
179	4.05	7.25	171.75	2375	4.63	8.29	170.71	2361	5.21	9.33	169.67	2347	5.79	10.36	168.64	2332
179.5	4.02	7.21	172.29	2383	4.60	8.25	171.25	2368	5.17	9.29	170.21	2354	5.75	10.32	169.18	2340
180	3.98	7.17	172.83	2390	4.56	8.21	171.79	2376	5.14	9.25	170.76	2362	5.71	10.28	169.72	2347
180.5	3.95	7.13	173.37	2398	4.52	8.17	172.33	2383	5.10	9.20	171.30	2369	5.67	10.24	170.26	2355
181	3.92	7.09	173.91	2405	4.49	8.13	172.87	2391	5.06	9.16	171.84	2377	5.64	10.20	170.80	2362
181.5	3.88	7.05	174.45	2413	4.45	8.08	173.42	2398	5.03	9.12	172.38	2384	5.60	10.16	171.34	2370
182	3.85	7.01	174.99	2420	4.42	8.04	173.96	2406	4.99	9.08	172.92	2391	5.56	10.12	171.88	2377
182.5	3.82	6.97	175.54	2428	4.38	8.00	174.50	2413	4.95	9.04	173.46	2399	5.52	10.08	172.42	2385
183	3.78	6.92	176.08	2435	4.35	7.96	175.04	2421	4.92	9.00	174.00	2406	5.48	10.04	172.96	2392
183.5	3.75	6.88	176.62	2443	4.32	7.92	175.58	2428	4.88	8.96	174.54	2414	5.45	10.00	173.50	2400

Body Composition MALE 152-183.5 Lb.

Weight: Lb.	Waist: 30 inches				30.25 inches				30.5 inches				30.75 inches			
	Fat: %	Fat: Lb.	LBM: Lb.	RMR: Cal.	Fat: %	Fat: Lb.	LBM: Lb.	RMR: Cal.	Fat: %	Fat: Lb.	LBM: Lb.	RMR: Cal.	Fat: %	Fat: Lb.	LBM: Lb.	RMR: Cal.
152	8.96	13.62	138.38	1914	9.64	14.65	137.35	1900	10.32	15.69	136.31	1885	11.01	16.73	135.27	1871
152.5	8.90	13.58	138.93	1921	9.58	14.61	137.89	1907	10.26	15.65	136.85	1893	10.94	16.69	135.81	1878
153	8.85	13.53	139.47	1929	9.52	14.57	138.43	1914	10.20	15.61	137.39	1900	10.88	16.65	136.35	1886
153.5	8.79	13.49	140.01	1936	9.47	14.53	138.97	1922	10.14	15.57	137.93	1908	10.82	16.61	136.89	1893
154	8.74	13.45	140.55	1944	9.41	14.49	139.51	1929	10.08	15.53	138.47	1915	10.76	16.56	137.44	1901
154.5	8.68	13.41	141.09	1951	9.35	14.45	140.05	1937	10.02	15.49	139.01	1923	10.69	16.52	137.98	1908
155	8.63	13.37	141.63	1959	9.30	14.41	140.59	1944	9.96	15.45	139.56	1930	10.63	16.48	138.52	1916
155.5	8.57	13.33	142.17	1966	9.24	14.37	141.13	1952	9.91	15.40	140.10	1938	10.57	16.44	139.06	1923
156	8.52	13.29	142.71	1974	9.18	14.33	141.67	1959	9.85	15.36	140.64	1945	10.51	16.40	139.60	1931
156.5	8.46	13.25	143.25	1981	9.13	14.28	142.22	1967	9.79	15.32	141.18	1952	10.45	16.36	140.14	1938
157	8.41	13.21	143.79	1989	9.07	14.24	142.76	1974	9.73	15.28	141.72	1960	10.39	16.32	140.68	1946
157.5	8.36	13.17	144.34	1996	9.02	14.20	143.30	1982	9.68	15.24	142.26	1967	10.33	16.28	141.22	1953
158	8.31	13.12	144.88	2004	8.96	14.16	143.84	1989	9.62	15.20	142.80	1975	10.28	16.24	141.76	1961
158.5	8.25	13.08	145.42	2011	8.91	14.12	144.38	1997	9.56	15.16	143.34	1982	10.22	16.20	142.30	1968
159	8.20	13.04	145.96	2019	8.86	14.08	144.92	2004	9.51	15.12	143.88	1990	10.16	16.15	142.85	1976
159.5	8.15	13.00	146.50	2026	8.80	14.04	145.46	2012	9.45	15.08	144.42	1997	10.10	16.11	143.39	1983
160	8.10	12.96	147.04	2034	8.75	14.00	146.00	2019	9.40	15.04	144.97	2005	10.05	16.07	143.93	1991
160.5	8.05	12.92	147.58	2041	8.70	13.96	146.54	2027	9.34	14.99	145.51	2012	9.99	16.03	144.47	1998
161	8.00	12.88	148.12	2049	8.64	13.92	147.08	2034	9.29	14.95	146.05	2020	9.93	15.99	145.01	2005
161.5	7.95	12.84	148.66	2056	8.59	13.87	147.63	2042	9.23	14.91	146.59	2027	9.88	15.95	145.55	2013
162	7.90	12.80	149.20	2063	8.54	13.83	148.17	2049	9.18	14.87	147.13	2035	9.82	15.91	146.09	2020
162.5	7.85	12.76	149.75	2071	8.49	13.79	148.71	2057	9.13	14.83	147.67	2042	9.76	15.87	146.63	2028
163	7.80	12.71	150.29	2078	8.44	13.75	149.25	2064	9.07	14.79	148.21	2050	9.71	15.83	147.17	2035
163.5	7.75	12.67	150.83	2086	8.39	13.71	149.79	2072	9.02	14.75	148.75	2057	9.65	15.79	147.71	2043
164	7.70	12.63	151.37	2093	8.34	13.67	150.33	2079	8.97	14.71	149.29	2065	9.60	15.74	148.26	2050
164.5	7.65	12.59	151.91	2101	8.28	13.63	150.87	2087	8.92	14.67	149.83	2072	9.55	15.70	148.80	2058
165	7.61	12.55	152.45	2108	8.23	13.59	151.41	2094	8.86	14.63	150.38	2080	9.49	15.66	149.34	2065
165.5	7.56	12.51	152.99	2116	8.19	13.55	151.95	2102	8.81	14.58	150.92	2087	9.44	15.62	149.88	2073
166	7.51	12.47	153.53	2123	8.14	13.51	152.49	2109	8.76	14.54	151.46	2095	9.39	15.58	150.42	2080
166.5	7.46	12.43	154.07	2131	8.09	13.46	153.04	2116	8.71	14.50	152.00	2102	9.33	15.54	150.96	2088
167	7.42	12.39	154.61	2138	8.04	13.42	153.58	2124	8.66	14.46	152.54	2110	9.28	15.50	151.50	2095
167.5	7.37	12.35	155.16	2146	7.99	13.38	154.12	2131	8.61	14.42	153.08	2117	9.23	15.46	152.04	2103
168	7.32	12.30	155.70	2153	7.94	13.34	154.66	2139	8.56	14.38	153.62	2125	9.18	15.42	152.58	2110
168.5	7.28	12.26	156.24	2161	7.89	13.30	155.20	2146	8.51	14.34	154.16	2132	9.12	15.38	153.12	2118
169	7.23	12.22	156.78	2168	7.85	13.26	155.74	2154	8.46	14.30	154.70	2140	9.07	15.33	153.67	2125
169.5	7.19	12.18	157.32	2176	7.80	13.22	156.28	2161	8.41	14.26	155.24	2147	9.02	15.29	154.21	2133
170	7.14	12.14	157.86	2183	7.75	13.18	156.82	2169	8.36	14.22	155.79	2155	8.97	15.25	154.75	2140
170.5	7.10	12.10	158.40	2191	7.70	13.14	157.36	2176	8.31	14.17	156.33	2162	8.92	15.21	155.29	2148
171	7.05	12.06	158.94	2198	7.66	13.10	157.90	2184	8.26	14.13	156.87	2169	8.87	15.17	155.83	2155
171.5	7.01	12.02	159.48	2206	7.61	13.05	158.45	2191	8.22	14.09	157.41	2177	8.82	15.13	156.37	2163
172	6.96	11.98	160.02	2213	7.57	13.01	158.99	2199	8.17	14.05	157.95	2184	8.77	15.09	156.91	2170
172.5	6.92	11.94	160.57	2221	7.52	12.97	159.53	2206	8.12	14.01	158.49	2192	8.72	15.05	157.45	2178
173	6.88	11.89	161.11	2228	7.47	12.93	160.07	2214	8.07	13.97	159.03	2199	8.67	15.01	157.99	2185
173.5	6.83	11.85	161.65	2236	7.43	12.89	160.61	2221	8.03	13.93	159.57	2207	8.63	14.97	158.53	2193
174	6.79	11.81	162.19	2243	7.38	12.85	161.15	2229	7.98	13.89	160.11	2214	8.58	14.92	159.08	2200
174.5	6.75	11.77	162.73	2251	7.34	12.81	161.69	2236	7.93	13.85	160.65	2222	8.53	14.88	159.62	2207
175	6.70	11.73	163.27	2258	7.30	12.77	162.23	2244	7.89	13.81	161.20	2229	8.48	14.84	160.16	2215
175.5	6.66	11.69	163.81	2266	7.25	12.73	162.77	2251	7.84	13.76	161.74	2237	8.43	14.80	160.70	2222
176	6.62	11.65	164.35	2273	7.21	12.69	163.31	2259	7.80	13.72	162.28	2244	8.39	14.76	161.24	2230
176.5	6.58	11.61	164.89	2280	7.16	12.64	163.86	2266	7.75	13.68	162.82	2252	8.34	14.72	161.78	2237
177	6.53	11.57	165.43	2288	7.12	12.60	164.40	2274	7.71	13.64	163.36	2259	8.29	14.68	162.32	2245
177.5	6.49	11.53	165.98	2295	7.08	12.56	164.94	2281	7.66	13.60	163.90	2267	8.25	14.64	162.86	2252
178	6.45	11.48	166.52	2303	7.03	12.52	165.48	2289	7.62	13.56	164.44	2274	8.20	14.60	163.40	2260
178.5	6.41	11.44	167.06	2310	6.99	12.48	166.02	2296	7.57	13.52	164.98	2282	8.15	14.56	163.94	2267
179	6.37	11.40	167.60	2318	6.95	12.44	166.56	2304	7.53	13.48	165.52	2289	8.11	14.51	164.49	2275
179.5	6.33	11.36	168.14	2325	6.91	12.40	167.10	2311	7.49	13.44	166.06	2297	8.06	14.47	165.03	2282
180	6.29	11.32	168.68	2333	6.87	12.36	167.64	2318	7.44	13.40	166.61	2304	8.02	14.43	165.57	2290
180.5	6.25	11.28	169.22	2340	6.82	12.32	168.18	2326	7.40	13.35	167.15	2312	7.97	14.39	166.11	2297
181	6.21	11.24	169.76	2348	6.78	12.28	168.72	2333	7.36	13.31	167.69	2319	7.93	14.35	166.65	2305
181.5	6.17	11.20	170.30	2355	6.74	12.23	169.27	2341	7.31	13.27	168.23	2327	7.88	14.31	167.19	2312
182	6.13	11.16	170.84	2363	6.70	12.19	169.81	2348	7.27	13.23	168.77	2334	7.84	14.27	167.73	2320
182.5	6.09	11.12	171.39	2370	6.66	12.15	170.35	2356	7.23	13.19	169.31	2342	7.80	14.23	168.27	2327
183	6.05	11.07	171.93	2378	6.62	12.11	170.89	2363	7.19	13.15	169.85	2349	7.75	14.19	168.81	2335
183.5	6.01	11.03	172.47	2385	6.58	12.07	171.43	2371	7.14	13.11	170.39	2357	7.71	14.15	169.35	2342

Body Composition MALE 152-183.5 Lb.

Weight: Lb.	Waist: 31 inches Fat: %	Fat: Lb.	LBM: Lb.	RMR: Cal.	31.25 inches Fat: %	Fat: Lb.	LBM: Lb.	RMR: Cal.	31.5 inches Fat: %	Fat: Lb.	LBM: Lb.	RMR: Cal.	31.75 inches Fat: %	Fat: Lb.	LBM: Lb.	RMR: Cal.
152	11.69	17.77	134.23	1856	12.37	18.80	133.20	1842	13.05	19.84	132.16	1828	13.74	20.88	131.12	1813
152.5	11.62	17.73	134.78	1864	12.30	18.76	133.74	1850	12.98	19.80	132.70	1835	13.66	20.84	131.66	1821
153	11.56	17.68	135.32	1871	12.24	18.72	134.28	1857	12.91	19.76	133.24	1843	13.59	20.80	132.20	1828
153.5	11.49	17.64	135.86	1879	12.17	18.68	134.82	1865	12.85	19.72	133.78	1850	13.52	20.76	132.74	1836
154	11.43	17.60	136.40	1886	12.10	18.64	135.36	1872	12.78	19.68	134.32	1858	13.45	20.71	133.29	1843
154.5	11.37	17.56	136.94	1894	12.04	18.60	135.90	1880	12.71	19.64	134.86	1865	13.38	20.67	133.83	1851
155	11.30	17.52	137.48	1901	11.97	18.56	136.44	1887	12.64	19.60	135.41	1873	13.31	20.63	134.37	1858
155.5	11.24	17.48	138.02	1909	11.91	18.52	136.98	1894	12.57	19.55	135.95	1880	13.24	20.59	134.91	1866
156	11.18	17.44	138.56	1916	11.84	18.48	137.52	1902	12.51	19.51	136.49	1888	13.17	20.55	135.45	1873
156.5	11.12	17.40	139.10	1924	11.78	18.43	138.07	1909	12.44	19.47	137.03	1895	13.11	20.51	135.99	1881
157	11.05	17.36	139.64	1931	11.72	18.39	138.61	1917	12.38	19.43	137.57	1903	13.04	20.47	136.53	1888
157.5	10.99	17.32	140.19	1939	11.65	18.35	139.15	1924	12.31	19.39	138.11	1910	12.97	20.43	137.07	1896
158	10.93	17.27	140.73	1946	11.59	18.31	139.69	1932	12.25	19.35	138.65	1918	12.90	20.39	137.61	1903
158.5	10.87	17.23	141.27	1954	11.53	18.27	140.23	1939	12.18	19.31	139.19	1925	12.84	20.35	138.15	1911
159	10.81	17.19	141.81	1961	11.47	18.23	140.77	1947	12.12	19.27	139.73	1933	12.77	20.30	138.70	1918
159.5	10.75	17.15	142.35	1969	11.40	18.19	141.31	1954	12.05	19.23	140.27	1940	12.70	20.26	139.24	1926
160	10.69	17.11	142.89	1976	11.34	18.15	141.85	1962	11.99	19.19	140.82	1947	12.64	20.22	139.78	1933
160.5	10.63	17.07	143.43	1984	11.28	18.11	142.39	1969	11.93	19.14	141.36	1955	12.57	20.18	140.32	1941
161	10.58	17.03	143.97	1991	11.22	18.07	142.93	1977	11.87	19.10	141.90	1962	12.51	20.14	140.86	1948
161.5	10.52	16.99	144.51	1999	11.16	18.02	143.48	1984	11.80	19.06	142.44	1970	12.45	20.10	141.40	1956
162	10.46	16.95	145.05	2006	11.10	17.98	144.02	1992	11.74	19.02	142.98	1977	12.38	20.06	141.94	1963
162.5	10.40	16.91	145.60	2014	11.04	17.94	144.56	1999	11.68	18.98	143.52	1985	12.32	20.02	142.48	1971
163	10.35	16.86	146.14	2021	10.98	17.90	145.10	2007	11.62	18.94	144.06	1992	12.26	19.98	143.02	1978
163.5	10.29	16.82	146.68	2029	10.92	17.86	145.64	2014	11.56	18.90	144.60	2000	12.19	19.94	143.56	1985
164	10.23	16.78	147.22	2036	10.87	17.82	146.18	2022	11.50	18.86	145.14	2007	12.13	19.90	144.11	1993
164.5	10.18	16.74	147.76	2044	10.81	17.78	146.72	2029	11.44	18.82	145.68	2015	12.07	19.85	144.65	2000
165	10.12	16.70	148.30	2051	10.75	17.74	147.26	2037	11.38	18.78	146.23	2022	12.01	19.81	145.19	2008
165.5	10.07	16.66	148.84	2058	10.69	17.70	147.80	2044	11.32	18.73	146.77	2030	11.95	19.77	145.73	2015
166	10.01	16.62	149.38	2066	10.64	17.66	148.34	2052	11.26	18.69	147.31	2037	11.89	19.73	146.27	2023
166.5	9.96	16.58	149.92	2073	10.58	17.61	148.89	2059	11.20	18.65	147.85	2045	11.83	19.69	146.81	2030
167	9.90	16.54	150.46	2081	10.52	17.57	149.43	2067	11.14	18.61	148.39	2052	11.77	19.65	147.35	2038
167.5	9.85	16.50	151.01	2088	10.47	17.53	149.97	2074	11.09	18.57	148.93	2060	11.71	19.61	147.89	2045
168	9.79	16.45	151.55	2096	10.41	17.49	150.51	2082	11.03	18.53	149.47	2067	11.65	19.57	148.43	2053
168.5	9.74	16.41	152.09	2103	10.36	17.45	151.05	2089	10.97	18.49	150.01	2075	11.59	19.53	148.97	2060
169	9.69	16.37	152.63	2111	10.30	17.41	151.59	2096	10.92	18.45	150.55	2082	11.53	19.48	149.52	2068
169.5	9.63	16.33	153.17	2118	10.25	17.37	152.13	2104	10.86	18.41	151.09	2090	11.47	19.44	150.06	2075
170	9.58	16.29	153.71	2126	10.19	17.33	152.67	2111	10.80	18.37	151.64	2097	11.41	19.40	150.60	2083
170.5	9.53	16.25	154.25	2133	10.14	17.29	153.21	2119	10.75	18.32	152.18	2105	11.36	19.36	151.14	2090
171	9.48	16.21	154.79	2141	10.09	17.25	153.75	2126	10.69	18.28	152.72	2112	11.30	19.32	151.68	2098
171.5	9.43	16.17	155.33	2148	10.03	17.20	154.30	2134	10.64	18.24	153.26	2120	11.24	19.28	152.22	2105
172	9.38	16.13	155.87	2156	9.98	17.16	154.84	2141	10.58	18.20	153.80	2127	11.19	19.24	152.76	2113
172.5	9.32	16.09	156.42	2163	9.93	17.12	155.38	2149	10.53	18.16	154.34	2135	11.13	19.20	153.30	2120
173	9.27	16.04	156.96	2171	9.87	17.08	155.92	2156	10.47	18.12	154.88	2142	11.07	19.16	153.84	2128
173.5	9.22	16.00	157.50	2178	9.82	17.04	156.46	2164	10.42	18.08	155.42	2149	11.02	19.12	154.38	2135
174	9.17	15.96	158.04	2186	9.77	17.00	157.00	2171	10.37	18.04	155.96	2157	10.96	19.07	154.93	2143
174.5	9.12	15.92	158.58	2193	9.72	16.96	157.54	2179	10.31	18.00	156.50	2164	10.91	19.03	155.47	2150
175	9.07	15.88	159.12	2201	9.67	16.92	158.08	2186	10.26	17.96	157.05	2172	10.85	18.99	156.01	2158
175.5	9.03	15.84	159.66	2208	9.62	16.88	158.62	2194	10.21	17.91	157.59	2179	10.80	18.95	156.55	2165
176	8.98	15.80	160.20	2216	9.57	16.84	159.16	2201	10.16	17.87	158.13	2187	10.74	18.91	157.09	2173
176.5	8.93	15.76	160.74	2223	9.52	16.79	159.71	2209	10.10	17.83	158.67	2194	10.69	18.87	157.63	2180
177	8.88	15.72	161.28	2231	9.47	16.75	160.25	2216	10.05	17.79	159.21	2202	10.64	18.83	158.17	2188
177.5	8.83	15.68	161.83	2238	9.42	16.71	160.79	2224	10.00	17.75	159.75	2209	10.58	18.79	158.71	2195
178	8.78	15.63	162.37	2246	9.37	16.67	161.33	2231	9.95	17.71	160.29	2217	10.53	18.75	159.25	2202
178.5	8.74	15.59	162.91	2253	9.32	16.63	161.87	2239	9.90	17.67	160.83	2224	10.48	18.71	159.79	2210
179	8.69	15.55	163.45	2260	9.27	16.59	162.41	2246	9.85	17.63	161.37	2232	10.43	18.66	160.34	2217
179.5	8.64	15.51	163.99	2268	9.22	16.55	162.95	2254	9.80	17.59	161.91	2239	10.38	18.62	160.88	2225
180	8.59	15.47	164.53	2275	9.17	16.51	163.49	2261	9.75	17.55	162.46	2247	10.32	18.58	161.42	2232
180.5	8.55	15.43	165.07	2283	9.12	16.47	164.03	2269	9.70	17.50	163.00	2254	10.27	18.54	161.96	2240
181	8.50	15.39	165.61	2290	9.07	16.43	164.57	2276	9.65	17.46	163.54	2262	10.22	18.50	162.50	2247
181.5	8.46	15.35	166.15	2298	9.03	16.38	165.12	2284	9.60	17.42	164.08	2269	10.17	18.46	163.04	2255
182	8.41	15.31	166.69	2305	8.98	16.34	165.66	2291	9.55	17.38	164.62	2277	10.12	18.42	163.58	2262
182.5	8.36	15.27	167.24	2313	8.93	16.30	166.20	2299	9.50	17.34	165.16	2284	10.07	18.38	164.12	2270
183	8.32	15.22	167.78	2320	8.89	16.26	166.74	2306	9.45	17.30	165.70	2292	10.02	18.34	164.66	2277
183.5	8.27	15.18	168.32	2328	8.84	16.22	167.28	2313	9.40	17.26	166.24	2299	9.97	18.30	165.20	2285

Body Composition   MALE   152-183.5 Lb.

Waist:	32 inches				32.25 inches				32.5 inches				32.75 inches			
Weight: Lb.	Fat: %	Fat: Lb.	LBM: Lb.	RMR: Cal.	Fat: %	Fat: Lb.	LBM: Lb.	RMR: Cal.	Fat: %	Fat: Lb.	LBM: Lb.	RMR: Cal.	Fat: %	Fat: Lb.	LBM: Lb.	RMR: Cal.
152	14.42	21.92	130.08	1799	15.10	22.95	129.05	1785	15.78	23.99	128.01	1770	16.47	25.03	126.97	1756
152.5	14.34	21.88	130.63	1807	15.02	22.91	129.59	1792	15.70	23.95	128.55	1778	16.39	24.99	127.51	1763
153	14.27	21.83	131.17	1814	14.95	22.87	130.13	1800	15.63	23.91	129.09	1785	16.30	24.95	128.05	1771
153.5	14.20	21.79	131.71	1822	14.87	22.83	130.67	1807	15.55	23.87	129.63	1793	16.23	24.91	128.59	1778
154	14.12	21.75	132.25	1829	14.80	22.79	131.21	1815	15.47	23.83	130.17	1800	16.15	24.86	129.14	1786
154.5	14.05	21.71	132.79	1836	14.72	22.75	131.75	1822	15.40	23.79	130.71	1808	16.07	24.82	129.68	1793
155	13.98	21.67	133.33	1844	14.65	22.71	132.29	1830	15.32	23.75	131.26	1815	15.99	24.78	130.22	1801
155.5	13.91	21.63	133.87	1851	14.58	22.67	132.83	1837	15.24	23.70	131.80	1823	15.91	24.74	130.76	1808
156	13.84	21.59	134.41	1859	14.50	22.63	133.37	1845	15.17	23.66	132.34	1830	15.83	24.70	131.30	1816
156.5	13.77	21.55	134.95	1866	14.43	22.58	133.92	1852	15.09	23.62	132.88	1838	15.76	24.66	131.84	1823
157	13.70	21.51	135.49	1874	14.36	22.54	134.46	1860	15.02	23.58	133.42	1845	15.68	24.62	132.38	1831
157.5	13.63	21.47	136.04	1881	14.29	22.50	135.00	1867	14.95	23.54	133.96	1853	15.60	24.58	132.92	1838
158	13.56	21.42	136.58	1889	14.22	22.46	135.54	1874	14.87	23.50	134.50	1860	15.53	24.54	133.46	1846
158.5	13.49	21.38	137.12	1896	14.15	22.42	136.08	1882	14.80	23.46	135.04	1868	15.45	24.50	134.00	1853
159	13.42	21.34	137.66	1904	14.08	22.38	136.62	1889	14.73	23.42	135.58	1875	15.38	24.45	134.55	1861
159.5	13.35	21.30	138.20	1911	14.01	22.34	137.16	1897	14.66	23.38	136.12	1883	15.31	24.41	135.09	1868
160	13.29	21.26	138.74	1919	13.94	22.30	137.70	1904	14.58	23.34	136.67	1890	15.23	24.37	135.63	1876
160.5	13.22	21.22	139.28	1926	13.87	22.26	138.24	1912	14.51	23.29	137.21	1898	15.16	24.33	136.17	1883
161	13.15	21.18	139.82	1934	13.80	22.22	138.78	1919	14.44	23.25	137.75	1905	15.09	24.29	136.71	1891
161.5	13.09	21.14	140.36	1941	13.73	22.17	139.33	1927	14.37	23.21	138.29	1913	15.02	24.25	137.25	1898
162	13.02	21.10	140.90	1949	13.66	22.13	139.87	1934	14.30	23.17	138.83	1920	14.94	24.21	137.79	1906
162.5	12.96	21.06	141.45	1956	13.60	22.09	140.41	1942	14.23	23.13	139.37	1927	14.87	24.17	138.33	1913
163	12.89	21.01	141.99	1964	13.53	22.05	140.95	1949	14.17	23.09	139.91	1935	14.80	24.13	138.87	1921
163.5	12.83	20.97	142.53	1971	13.46	22.01	141.49	1957	14.10	23.05	140.45	1942	14.73	24.09	139.41	1928
164	12.76	20.93	143.07	1979	13.40	21.97	142.03	1964	14.03	23.01	140.99	1950	14.66	24.04	139.96	1936
164.5	12.70	20.89	143.61	1986	13.33	21.93	142.57	1972	13.96	22.97	141.53	1957	14.59	24.00	140.50	1943
165	12.64	20.85	144.15	1994	13.27	21.89	143.11	1979	13.89	22.93	142.08	1965	14.52	23.96	141.04	1951
165.5	12.57	20.81	144.69	2001	13.20	21.85	143.65	1987	13.83	22.88	142.62	1972	14.45	23.92	141.58	1958
166	12.51	20.77	145.23	2009	13.14	21.81	144.19	1994	13.76	22.84	143.16	1980	14.39	23.88	142.12	1966
166.5	12.45	20.73	145.77	2016	13.07	21.76	144.74	2002	13.69	22.80	143.70	1987	14.32	23.84	142.66	1973
167	12.39	20.69	146.31	2024	13.01	21.72	145.28	2009	13.63	22.76	144.24	1995	14.25	23.80	143.20	1980
167.5	12.33	20.65	146.86	2031	12.94	21.68	145.82	2017	13.56	22.72	144.78	2002	14.18	23.76	143.74	1988
168	12.26	20.60	147.40	2038	12.88	21.64	146.36	2024	13.50	22.68	145.32	2010	14.12	23.72	144.28	1995
168.5	12.20	20.56	147.94	2046	12.82	21.60	146.90	2032	13.44	22.64	145.86	2017	14.05	23.68	144.82	2003
169	12.14	20.52	148.48	2053	12.76	21.56	147.44	2039	13.37	22.60	146.40	2025	13.98	23.63	145.37	2010
169.5	12.08	20.48	149.02	2061	12.70	21.52	147.98	2047	13.31	22.56	146.94	2032	13.92	23.59	145.91	2018
170	12.02	20.44	149.56	2068	12.63	21.48	148.52	2054	13.24	22.52	147.49	2040	13.85	23.55	146.45	2025
170.5	11.96	20.40	150.10	2076	12.57	21.44	149.06	2062	13.18	22.47	148.03	2047	13.79	23.51	146.99	2033
171	11.91	20.36	150.64	2083	12.51	21.40	149.60	2069	13.12	22.43	148.57	2055	13.73	23.47	147.53	2040
171.5	11.85	20.32	151.18	2091	12.45	21.35	150.15	2077	13.06	22.39	149.11	2062	13.66	23.43	148.07	2048
172	11.79	20.28	151.72	2098	12.39	21.31	150.69	2084	12.99	22.35	149.65	2070	13.60	23.39	148.61	2055
172.5	11.73	20.24	152.27	2106	12.33	21.27	151.23	2091	12.93	22.31	150.19	2077	13.53	23.35	149.15	2063
173	11.67	20.19	152.81	2113	12.27	21.23	151.77	2099	12.87	22.27	150.73	2085	13.47	23.31	149.69	2070
173.5	11.62	20.15	153.35	2121	12.21	21.19	152.31	2106	12.81	22.23	151.27	2092	13.41	23.27	150.23	2078
174	11.56	20.11	153.89	2128	12.15	21.15	152.85	2114	12.75	22.19	151.81	2100	13.35	23.22	150.78	2085
174.5	11.50	20.07	154.43	2136	12.10	21.11	153.39	2121	12.69	22.15	152.35	2107	13.29	23.18	151.32	2093
175	11.45	20.03	154.97	2143	12.04	21.07	153.93	2129	12.63	22.11	152.90	2115	13.22	23.14	151.86	2100
175.5	11.39	19.99	155.51	2151	11.98	21.03	154.47	2136	12.57	22.06	153.44	2122	13.16	23.10	152.40	2108
176	11.33	19.95	156.05	2158	11.92	20.99	155.01	2144	12.51	22.02	153.98	2130	13.10	23.06	152.94	2115
176.5	11.28	19.91	156.59	2166	11.87	20.94	155.56	2151	12.45	21.98	154.52	2137	13.04	23.02	153.48	2123
177	11.22	19.87	157.13	2173	11.81	20.90	156.10	2159	12.40	21.94	155.06	2144	12.98	22.98	154.02	2130
177.5	11.17	19.83	157.68	2181	11.75	20.86	156.64	2166	12.34	21.90	155.60	2152	12.92	22.94	154.56	2138
178	11.11	19.78	158.22	2188	11.70	20.82	157.18	2174	12.28	21.86	156.14	2159	12.86	22.90	155.10	2145
178.5	11.06	19.74	158.76	2196	11.64	20.78	157.72	2181	12.22	21.82	156.68	2167	12.80	22.86	155.64	2153
179	11.01	19.70	159.30	2203	11.59	20.74	158.26	2189	12.17	21.78	157.22	2174	12.75	22.81	156.19	2160
179.5	10.95	19.66	159.84	2211	11.53	20.70	158.80	2196	12.11	21.74	157.76	2182	12.69	22.77	156.73	2168
180	10.90	19.62	160.38	2218	11.48	20.66	159.34	2204	12.05	21.70	158.31	2189	12.63	22.73	157.27	2175
180.5	10.85	19.58	160.92	2226	11.42	20.62	159.88	2211	12.00	21.65	158.85	2197	12.57	22.69	157.81	2182
181	10.79	19.54	161.46	2233	11.37	20.58	160.42	2219	11.94	21.61	159.39	2204	12.51	22.65	158.35	2190
181.5	10.74	19.50	162.00	2241	11.31	20.53	160.97	2226	11.89	21.57	159.93	2212	12.46	22.61	158.89	2197
182	10.69	19.46	162.54	2248	11.26	20.49	161.51	2234	11.83	21.53	160.47	2219	12.40	22.57	159.43	2205
182.5	10.64	19.42	163.09	2255	11.21	20.45	162.05	2241	11.78	21.49	161.01	2227	12.34	22.53	159.97	2212
183	10.59	19.37	163.63	2263	11.15	20.41	162.59	2249	11.72	21.45	161.55	2234	12.29	22.49	160.51	2220
183.5	10.54	19.33	164.17	2270	11.10	20.37	163.13	2256	11.67	21.41	162.09	2242	12.23	22.45	161.05	2227

Body Composition MALE 152-183.5 Lb.

Weight: Lb.	Waist: 33 inches				33.25 inches				33.5 inches				33.75 inches			
	Fat: %	Fat: Lb.	LBM: Lb.	RMR: Cal.	Fat: %	Fat: Lb.	LBM: Lb.	RMR: Cal.	Fat: %	Fat: Lb.	LBM: Lb.	RMR: Cal.	Fat: %	Fat: Lb.	LBM: Lb.	RMR: Cal.
152	17.15	26.07	125.93	1742	17.83	27.10	124.90	1727	18.51	28.14	123.86	1713	19.20	29.18	122.82	1699
152.5	17.07	26.03	126.48	1749	17.75	27.06	125.44	1735	18.43	28.10	124.40	1720	19.11	29.14	123.36	1706
153	16.98	25.98	127.02	1757	17.66	27.02	125.98	1742	18.34	28.06	124.94	1728	19.02	29.10	123.90	1714
153.5	16.90	25.94	127.56	1764	17.58	26.98	126.52	1750	18.25	28.02	125.48	1735	18.93	29.06	124.44	1721
154	16.82	25.90	128.10	1772	17.49	26.94	127.06	1757	18.17	27.98	126.02	1743	18.84	29.01	124.99	1729
154.5	16.74	25.86	128.64	1779	17.41	26.90	127.60	1765	18.08	27.94	126.56	1750	18.75	28.97	125.53	1736
155	16.66	25.82	129.18	1787	17.33	26.86	128.14	1772	18.00	27.90	127.11	1758	18.67	28.93	126.07	1744
155.5	16.58	25.78	129.72	1794	17.25	26.82	128.68	1780	17.91	27.85	127.65	1765	18.58	28.89	126.61	1751
156	16.50	25.74	130.26	1802	17.16	26.78	129.22	1787	17.83	27.81	128.19	1773	18.49	28.85	127.15	1758
156.5	16.42	25.70	130.80	1809	17.08	26.73	129.77	1795	17.75	27.77	128.73	1780	18.41	28.81	127.69	1766
157	16.34	25.66	131.34	1816	17.00	26.69	130.31	1802	17.66	27.73	129.27	1788	18.32	28.77	128.23	1773
157.5	16.26	25.62	131.89	1824	16.92	26.65	130.85	1810	17.58	27.69	129.81	1795	18.24	28.73	128.77	1781
158	16.19	25.57	132.43	1831	16.84	26.61	131.39	1817	17.50	27.65	130.35	1803	18.16	28.69	129.31	1788
158.5	16.11	25.53	132.97	1839	16.76	26.57	131.93	1825	17.42	27.61	130.89	1810	18.07	28.65	129.85	1796
159	16.03	25.49	133.51	1846	16.69	26.53	132.47	1832	17.34	27.57	131.43	1818	17.99	28.60	130.40	1803
159.5	15.96	25.45	134.05	1854	16.61	26.49	133.01	1840	17.26	27.53	131.97	1825	17.91	28.56	130.94	1811
160	15.88	25.41	134.59	1861	16.53	26.45	133.55	1847	17.18	27.49	132.52	1833	17.83	28.52	131.48	1818
160.5	15.81	25.37	135.13	1869	16.45	26.41	134.09	1855	17.10	27.44	133.06	1840	17.75	28.48	132.02	1826
161	15.73	25.33	135.67	1876	16.38	26.37	134.63	1862	17.02	27.40	133.60	1848	17.66	28.44	132.56	1833
161.5	15.66	25.29	136.21	1884	16.30	26.32	135.18	1869	16.94	27.36	134.14	1855	17.58	28.40	133.10	1841
162	15.58	25.25	136.75	1891	16.22	26.28	135.72	1877	16.86	27.32	134.68	1863	17.51	28.36	133.64	1848
162.5	15.51	25.21	137.30	1899	16.15	26.24	136.26	1884	16.79	27.28	135.22	1870	17.43	28.32	134.18	1856
163	15.44	25.16	137.84	1906	16.07	26.20	136.80	1892	16.71	27.24	135.76	1878	17.35	28.28	134.72	1863
163.5	15.37	25.12	138.38	1914	16.00	26.16	137.34	1899	16.63	27.20	136.30	1885	17.27	28.24	135.26	1871
164	15.29	25.08	138.92	1921	15.93	26.12	137.88	1907	16.56	27.16	136.84	1893	17.19	28.19	135.81	1878
164.5	15.22	25.04	139.46	1929	15.85	26.08	138.42	1914	16.48	27.12	137.38	1900	17.11	28.15	136.35	1886
165	15.15	25.00	140.00	1936	15.78	26.04	138.96	1922	16.41	27.08	137.93	1908	17.04	28.11	136.89	1893
165.5	15.08	24.96	140.54	1944	15.71	26.00	139.50	1929	16.33	27.03	138.47	1915	16.96	28.07	137.43	1901
166	15.01	24.92	141.08	1951	15.64	25.96	140.04	1937	16.26	26.99	139.01	1922	16.89	28.03	137.97	1908
166.5	14.94	24.88	141.62	1959	15.56	25.91	140.59	1944	16.19	26.95	139.55	1930	16.81	27.99	138.51	1916
167	14.87	24.84	142.16	1966	15.49	25.87	141.13	1952	16.11	26.91	140.09	1937	16.74	27.95	139.05	1923
167.5	14.80	24.80	142.71	1974	15.42	25.83	141.67	1959	16.04	26.87	140.63	1945	16.66	27.91	139.59	1931
168	14.73	24.75	143.25	1981	15.35	25.79	142.21	1967	15.97	26.83	141.17	1952	16.59	27.87	140.13	1938
168.5	14.67	24.71	143.79	1989	15.28	25.75	142.75	1974	15.90	26.79	141.71	1960	16.51	27.83	140.67	1946
169	14.60	24.67	144.33	1996	15.21	25.71	143.29	1982	15.83	26.75	142.25	1967	16.44	27.78	141.22	1953
169.5	14.53	24.63	144.87	2004	15.14	25.67	143.83	1989	15.76	26.71	142.79	1975	16.37	27.74	141.76	1960
170	14.46	24.59	145.41	2011	15.08	25.63	144.37	1997	15.69	26.67	143.34	1982	16.30	27.70	142.30	1968
170.5	14.40	24.55	145.95	2019	15.01	25.59	144.91	2004	15.62	26.62	143.88	1990	16.22	27.66	142.84	1975
171	14.33	24.51	146.49	2026	14.94	25.55	145.45	2012	15.55	26.58	144.42	1997	16.15	27.62	143.38	1983
171.5	14.27	24.47	147.03	2033	14.87	25.50	146.00	2019	15.48	26.54	144.96	2005	16.08	27.58	143.92	1990
172	14.20	24.43	147.57	2041	14.80	25.46	146.54	2027	15.41	26.50	145.50	2012	16.01	27.54	144.46	1998
172.5	14.14	24.39	148.12	2048	14.74	25.42	147.08	2034	15.34	26.46	146.04	2020	15.94	27.50	145.00	2005
173	14.07	24.34	148.66	2056	14.67	25.38	147.62	2042	15.27	26.42	146.58	2027	15.87	27.46	145.54	2013
173.5	14.01	24.30	149.20	2063	14.61	25.34	148.16	2049	15.20	26.38	147.12	2035	15.80	27.42	146.08	2020
174	13.94	24.26	149.74	2071	14.54	25.30	148.70	2057	15.14	26.34	147.66	2042	15.73	27.37	146.63	2028
174.5	13.88	24.22	150.28	2078	14.47	25.26	149.24	2064	15.07	26.30	148.20	2050	15.66	27.33	147.17	2035
175	13.82	24.18	150.82	2086	14.41	25.22	149.78	2071	15.00	26.26	148.75	2057	15.60	27.29	147.71	2043
175.5	13.75	24.14	151.36	2093	14.35	25.18	150.32	2079	14.94	26.21	149.29	2065	15.53	27.25	148.25	2050
176	13.69	24.10	151.90	2101	14.28	25.14	150.86	2086	14.87	26.17	149.83	2072	15.46	27.21	148.79	2058
176.5	13.63	24.06	152.44	2108	14.22	25.09	151.41	2094	14.81	26.13	150.37	2080	15.39	27.17	149.33	2065
177	13.57	24.02	152.98	2116	14.15	25.05	151.95	2101	14.74	26.09	150.91	2087	15.33	27.13	149.87	2073
177.5	13.51	23.98	153.53	2123	14.09	25.01	152.49	2109	14.68	26.05	151.45	2095	15.26	27.09	150.41	2080
178	13.45	23.93	154.07	2131	14.03	24.97	153.03	2116	14.61	26.01	151.99	2102	15.19	27.05	150.95	2088
178.5	13.39	23.89	154.61	2138	13.97	24.93	153.57	2124	14.55	25.97	152.53	2110	15.13	27.01	151.49	2095
179	13.33	23.85	155.15	2146	13.90	24.89	154.11	2131	14.48	25.93	153.07	2117	15.06	26.96	152.04	2103
179.5	13.27	23.81	155.69	2153	13.84	24.85	154.65	2139	14.42	25.89	153.61	2124	15.00	26.92	152.58	2110
180	13.21	23.77	156.23	2161	13.78	24.81	155.19	2146	14.36	25.85	154.16	2132	14.93	26.88	153.12	2118
180.5	13.15	23.73	156.77	2168	13.72	24.77	155.73	2154	14.30	25.80	154.70	2139	14.87	26.84	153.66	2125
181	13.09	23.69	157.31	2176	13.66	24.73	156.27	2161	14.23	25.76	155.24	2147	14.81	26.80	154.20	2133
181.5	13.03	23.65	157.85	2183	13.60	24.68	156.82	2169	14.17	25.72	155.78	2154	14.74	26.76	154.74	2140
182	12.97	23.61	158.39	2191	13.54	24.64	157.36	2176	14.11	25.68	156.32	2162	14.68	26.72	155.28	2148
182.5	12.91	23.57	158.94	2198	13.48	24.60	157.90	2184	14.05	25.64	156.86	2169	14.62	26.68	155.82	2155
183	12.85	23.52	159.48	2206	13.42	24.56	158.44	2191	13.99	25.60	157.40	2177	14.56	26.64	156.36	2163
183.5	12.80	23.48	160.02	2213	13.36	24.52	158.98	2199	13.93	25.56	157.94	2184	14.49	26.60	156.90	2170

Body Composition MALE 152-183.5 Lb.

Weight: Lb.	Waist: 34 inches Fat: %	Fat: Lb.	LBM: Lb.	RMR: Cal.	34.25 inches Fat: %	Fat: Lb.	LBM: Lb.	RMR: Cal.	34.5 inches Fat: %	Fat: Lb.	LBM: Lb.	RMR: Cal.	34.75 inches Fat: %	Fat: Lb.	LBM: Lb.	RMR: Cal.
152	19.88	30.22	121.78	1684	20.56	31.25	120.75	1670	21.24	32.29	119.71	1656	21.93	33.33	118.67	1641
152.5	19.79	30.18	122.33	1692	20.47	31.21	121.29	1677	21.15	32.25	120.25	1663	21.83	33.29	119.21	1649
153	19.70	30.13	122.87	1699	20.37	31.17	121.83	1685	21.05	32.21	120.79	1671	21.73	33.25	119.75	1656
153.5	19.60	30.09	123.41	1707	20.28	31.13	122.37	1692	20.96	32.17	121.33	1678	21.63	33.21	120.29	1664
154	19.51	30.05	123.95	1714	20.19	31.09	122.91	1700	20.86	32.13	121.87	1686	21.54	33.16	120.84	1671
154.5	19.42	30.01	124.49	1722	20.10	31.05	123.45	1707	20.77	32.09	122.41	1693	21.44	33.12	121.38	1679
155	19.34	29.97	125.03	1729	20.00	31.01	123.99	1715	20.67	32.05	122.96	1700	21.34	33.08	121.92	1686
155.5	19.25	29.93	125.57	1737	19.91	30.97	124.53	1722	20.58	32.00	123.50	1708	21.25	33.04	122.46	1694
156	19.16	29.89	126.11	1744	19.82	30.93	125.07	1730	20.49	31.96	124.04	1715	21.15	33.00	123.00	1701
156.5	19.07	29.85	126.65	1752	19.73	30.88	125.62	1737	20.40	31.92	124.58	1723	21.06	32.96	123.54	1709
157	18.98	29.81	127.19	1759	19.65	30.84	126.16	1745	20.31	31.88	125.12	1730	20.97	32.92	124.08	1716
157.5	18.90	29.77	127.74	1767	19.56	30.80	126.70	1752	20.22	31.84	125.66	1738	20.87	32.88	124.62	1724
158	18.81	29.72	128.28	1774	19.47	30.76	127.24	1760	20.13	31.80	126.20	1745	20.78	32.84	125.16	1731
158.5	18.73	29.68	128.82	1782	19.38	30.72	127.78	1767	20.04	31.76	126.74	1753	20.69	32.80	125.70	1738
159	18.64	29.64	129.36	1789	19.30	30.68	128.32	1775	19.95	31.72	127.28	1760	20.60	32.75	126.25	1746
159.5	18.56	29.60	129.90	1797	19.21	30.64	128.86	1782	19.86	31.68	127.82	1768	20.51	32.71	126.79	1753
160	18.48	29.56	130.44	1804	19.12	30.60	129.40	1790	19.77	31.64	128.37	1775	20.42	32.67	127.33	1761
160.5	18.39	29.52	130.98	1811	19.04	30.56	129.94	1797	19.68	31.59	128.91	1783	20.33	32.63	127.87	1768
161	18.31	29.48	131.52	1819	18.95	30.52	130.48	1805	19.60	31.55	129.45	1790	20.24	32.59	128.41	1776
161.5	18.23	29.44	132.06	1826	18.87	30.47	131.03	1812	19.51	31.51	129.99	1798	20.15	32.55	128.95	1783
162	18.15	29.40	132.60	1834	18.79	30.43	131.57	1820	19.43	31.47	130.53	1805	20.07	32.51	129.49	1791
162.5	18.06	29.36	133.15	1841	18.70	30.39	132.11	1827	19.34	31.43	131.07	1813	19.98	32.47	130.03	1798
163	17.98	29.31	133.69	1849	18.62	30.35	132.65	1835	19.26	31.39	131.61	1820	19.89	32.43	130.57	1806
163.5	17.90	29.27	134.23	1856	18.54	30.31	133.19	1842	19.17	31.35	132.15	1828	19.81	32.39	131.11	1813
164	17.82	29.23	134.77	1864	18.46	30.27	133.73	1849	19.09	31.31	132.69	1835	19.72	32.34	131.66	1821
164.5	17.75	29.19	135.31	1871	18.38	30.23	134.27	1857	19.01	31.27	133.23	1843	19.64	32.30	132.20	1828
165	17.67	29.15	135.85	1879	18.30	30.19	134.81	1864	18.92	31.23	133.78	1850	19.55	32.26	132.74	1836
165.5	17.59	29.11	136.39	1886	18.22	30.15	135.35	1872	18.84	31.18	134.32	1858	19.47	32.22	133.28	1843
166	17.51	29.07	136.93	1894	18.14	30.11	135.89	1879	18.76	31.14	134.86	1865	19.39	32.18	133.82	1851
166.5	17.43	29.03	137.47	1901	18.06	30.06	136.44	1887	18.68	31.10	135.40	1873	19.30	32.14	134.36	1858
167	17.36	28.99	138.01	1909	17.98	30.02	136.98	1894	18.60	31.06	135.94	1880	19.22	32.10	134.90	1866
167.5	17.28	28.95	138.56	1916	17.90	29.98	137.52	1902	18.52	31.02	136.48	1888	19.14	32.06	135.44	1873
168	17.20	28.90	139.10	1924	17.82	29.94	138.06	1909	18.44	30.98	137.02	1895	19.06	32.02	135.98	1881
168.5	17.13	28.86	139.64	1931	17.75	29.90	138.60	1917	18.36	30.94	137.56	1902	18.98	31.98	136.52	1888
169	17.05	28.82	140.18	1939	17.67	29.86	139.14	1924	18.28	30.90	138.10	1910	18.90	31.93	137.07	1896
169.5	16.98	28.78	140.72	1946	17.59	29.82	139.68	1932	18.20	30.86	138.64	1917	18.82	31.89	137.61	1903
170	16.91	28.74	141.26	1954	17.52	29.78	140.22	1939	18.13	30.82	139.19	1925	18.74	31.85	138.15	1911
170.5	16.83	28.70	141.80	1961	17.44	29.74	140.76	1947	18.05	30.77	139.73	1932	18.66	31.81	138.69	1918
171	16.76	28.66	142.34	1969	17.37	29.70	141.30	1954	17.97	30.73	140.27	1940	18.58	31.77	139.23	1926
171.5	16.69	28.62	142.88	1976	17.29	29.65	141.85	1962	17.90	30.69	140.81	1947	18.50	31.73	139.77	1933
172	16.61	28.58	143.42	1984	17.22	29.61	142.39	1969	17.82	30.65	141.35	1955	18.42	31.69	140.31	1941
172.5	16.54	28.54	143.97	1991	17.14	29.57	142.93	1977	17.74	30.61	141.89	1962	18.35	31.65	140.85	1948
173	16.47	28.49	144.51	1999	17.07	29.53	143.47	1984	17.67	30.57	142.43	1970	18.27	31.61	141.39	1955
173.5	16.40	28.45	145.05	2006	17.00	29.49	144.01	1992	17.60	30.53	142.97	1977	18.19	31.57	141.93	1963
174	16.33	28.41	145.59	2013	16.93	29.45	144.55	1999	17.52	30.49	143.51	1985	18.12	31.52	142.48	1970
174.5	16.26	28.37	146.13	2021	16.85	29.41	145.09	2007	17.45	30.45	144.05	1992	18.04	31.48	143.02	1978
175	16.19	28.33	146.67	2028	16.78	29.37	145.63	2014	17.37	30.41	144.60	2000	17.97	31.44	143.56	1985
175.5	16.12	28.29	147.21	2036	16.71	29.33	146.17	2022	17.30	30.36	145.14	2007	17.89	31.40	144.10	1993
176	16.05	28.25	147.75	2043	16.64	29.29	146.71	2029	17.23	30.32	145.68	2015	17.82	31.36	144.64	2000
176.5	15.98	28.21	148.29	2051	16.57	29.24	147.26	2037	17.16	30.28	146.22	2022	17.74	31.32	145.18	2008
177	15.91	28.17	148.83	2058	16.50	29.20	147.80	2044	17.09	30.24	146.76	2030	17.67	31.28	145.72	2015
177.5	15.85	28.13	149.38	2066	16.43	29.16	148.34	2052	17.01	30.20	147.30	2037	17.60	31.24	146.26	2023
178	15.78	28.08	149.92	2073	16.36	29.12	148.88	2059	16.94	30.16	147.84	2045	17.53	31.20	146.80	2030
178.5	15.71	28.04	150.46	2081	16.29	29.08	149.42	2066	16.87	30.12	148.38	2052	17.45	31.16	147.34	2038
179	15.64	28.00	151.00	2088	16.22	29.04	149.96	2074	16.80	30.08	148.92	2060	17.38	31.11	147.89	2045
179.5	15.58	27.96	151.54	2096	16.16	29.00	150.50	2081	16.73	30.04	149.46	2067	17.31	31.07	148.43	2053
180	15.51	27.92	152.08	2103	16.09	28.96	151.04	2089	16.66	30.00	150.01	2075	17.24	31.03	148.97	2060
180.5	15.45	27.88	152.62	2111	16.02	28.92	151.58	2096	16.60	29.95	150.55	2082	17.17	30.99	149.51	2068
181	15.38	27.84	153.16	2118	15.95	28.88	152.12	2104	16.53	29.91	151.09	2090	17.10	30.95	150.05	2075
181.5	15.32	27.80	153.70	2126	15.89	28.83	152.67	2111	16.46	29.87	151.63	2097	17.03	30.91	150.59	2083
182	15.25	27.76	154.24	2133	15.82	28.79	153.21	2119	16.39	29.83	152.17	2104	16.96	30.87	151.13	2090
182.5	15.19	27.72	154.79	2141	15.75	28.75	153.75	2126	16.32	29.79	152.71	2112	16.89	30.83	151.67	2098
183	15.12	27.67	155.33	2148	15.69	28.71	154.29	2134	16.26	29.75	153.25	2119	16.82	30.79	152.21	2105
183.5	15.06	27.63	155.87	2156	15.62	28.67	154.83	2141	16.19	29.71	153.79	2127	16.76	30.75	152.75	2113

Body Composition MALE 152-183.5 Lb.

Weight: Lb.	Waist: 35 inches				35.25 inches				35.5 inches				35.75 inches			
	Fat: %	Fat: Lb.	LBM: Lb.	RMR: Cal.	Fat: %	Fat: Lb.	LBM: Lb.	RMR: Cal.	Fat: %	Fat: Lb.	LBM: Lb.	RMR: Cal.	Fat: %	Fat: Lb.	LBM: Lb.	RMR: Cal.
152	22.61	34.37	117.63	1627	23.29	35.40	116.60	1613	23.97	36.44	115.56	1598	24.66	37.48	114.52	1584
152.5	22.51	34.33	118.18	1634	23.19	35.36	117.14	1620	23.87	36.40	116.10	1606	24.55	37.44	115.06	1591
153	22.41	34.28	118.72	1642	23.09	35.32	117.68	1627	23.76	36.36	116.64	1613	24.44	37.40	115.60	1599
153.5	22.31	34.24	119.26	1649	22.98	35.28	118.22	1635	23.66	36.32	117.18	1621	24.34	37.36	116.14	1606
154	22.21	34.20	119.80	1657	22.88	35.24	118.76	1642	23.56	36.28	117.72	1628	24.23	37.31	116.69	1614
154.5	22.11	34.16	120.34	1664	22.78	35.20	119.30	1650	23.45	36.24	118.26	1636	24.13	37.27	117.23	1621
155	22.01	34.12	120.88	1672	22.68	35.16	119.84	1657	23.35	36.20	118.81	1643	24.02	37.23	117.77	1629
155.5	21.92	34.08	121.42	1679	22.58	35.12	120.38	1665	23.25	36.15	119.35	1651	23.92	37.19	118.31	1636
156	21.82	34.04	121.96	1687	22.48	35.08	120.92	1672	23.15	36.11	119.89	1658	23.81	37.15	118.85	1644
156.5	21.72	34.00	122.50	1694	22.39	35.03	121.47	1680	23.05	36.07	120.43	1666	23.71	37.11	119.39	1651
157	21.63	33.96	123.04	1702	22.29	34.99	122.01	1687	22.95	36.03	120.97	1673	23.61	37.07	119.93	1659
157.5	21.53	33.92	123.59	1709	22.19	34.95	122.55	1695	22.85	35.99	121.51	1680	23.51	37.03	120.47	1666
158	21.44	33.87	124.13	1717	22.10	34.91	123.09	1702	22.75	35.95	122.05	1688	23.41	36.99	121.01	1674
158.5	21.35	33.83	124.67	1724	22.00	34.87	123.63	1710	22.65	35.91	122.59	1695	23.31	36.95	121.55	1681
159	21.25	33.79	125.21	1732	21.91	34.83	124.17	1717	22.56	35.87	123.13	1703	23.21	36.90	122.10	1689
159.5	21.16	33.75	125.75	1739	21.81	34.79	124.71	1725	22.46	35.83	123.67	1710	23.11	36.86	122.64	1696
160	21.07	33.71	126.29	1747	21.72	34.75	125.25	1732	22.37	35.79	124.22	1718	23.01	36.82	123.18	1704
160.5	20.98	33.67	126.83	1754	21.62	34.71	125.79	1740	22.27	35.74	124.76	1725	22.92	36.78	123.72	1711
161	20.89	33.63	127.37	1762	21.53	34.67	126.33	1747	22.18	35.70	125.30	1733	22.82	36.74	124.26	1719
161.5	20.80	33.59	127.91	1769	21.44	34.62	126.88	1755	22.08	35.66	125.84	1740	22.72	36.70	124.80	1726
162	20.71	33.55	128.45	1777	21.35	34.58	127.42	1762	21.99	35.62	126.38	1748	22.63	36.66	125.34	1733
162.5	20.62	33.51	129.00	1784	21.26	34.54	127.96	1770	21.90	35.58	126.92	1755	22.53	36.62	125.88	1741
163	20.53	33.46	129.54	1791	21.17	34.50	128.50	1777	21.80	35.54	127.46	1763	22.44	36.58	126.42	1748
163.5	20.44	33.42	130.08	1799	21.08	34.46	129.04	1785	21.71	35.50	128.00	1770	22.35	36.54	126.96	1756
164	20.35	33.38	130.62	1806	20.99	34.42	129.58	1792	21.62	35.46	128.54	1778	22.25	36.49	127.51	1763
164.5	20.27	33.34	131.16	1814	20.90	34.38	130.12	1800	21.53	35.42	129.08	1785	22.16	36.45	128.05	1771
165	20.18	33.30	131.70	1821	20.81	34.34	130.66	1807	21.44	35.38	129.63	1793	22.07	36.41	128.59	1778
165.5	20.10	33.26	132.24	1829	20.72	34.30	131.20	1815	21.35	35.33	130.17	1800	21.98	36.37	129.13	1786
166	20.01	33.22	132.78	1836	20.64	34.26	131.74	1822	21.26	35.29	130.71	1808	21.89	36.33	129.67	1793
166.5	19.93	33.18	133.32	1844	20.55	34.21	132.29	1830	21.17	35.25	131.25	1815	21.80	36.29	130.21	1801
167	19.84	33.14	133.86	1851	20.46	34.17	132.83	1837	21.08	35.21	131.79	1823	21.71	36.25	130.75	1808
167.5	19.76	33.10	134.41	1859	20.38	34.13	133.37	1844	21.00	35.17	132.33	1830	21.62	36.21	131.29	1816
168	19.68	33.05	134.95	1866	20.29	34.09	133.91	1852	20.91	35.13	132.87	1838	21.53	36.17	131.83	1823
168.5	19.59	33.01	135.49	1874	20.21	34.05	134.45	1859	20.82	35.09	133.41	1845	21.44	36.13	132.37	1831
169	19.51	32.97	136.03	1881	20.12	34.01	134.99	1867	20.74	35.05	133.95	1853	21.35	36.08	132.92	1838
169.5	19.43	32.93	136.57	1889	20.04	33.97	135.53	1874	20.65	35.01	134.49	1860	21.26	36.04	133.46	1846
170	19.35	32.89	137.11	1896	19.96	33.93	136.07	1882	20.57	34.97	135.04	1868	21.18	36.00	134.00	1853
170.5	19.27	32.85	137.65	1904	19.87	33.89	136.61	1889	20.48	34.92	135.58	1875	21.09	35.96	134.54	1861
171	19.19	32.81	138.19	1911	19.79	33.85	137.15	1897	20.40	34.88	136.12	1882	21.01	35.92	135.08	1868
171.5	19.11	32.77	138.73	1919	19.71	33.80	137.70	1904	20.32	34.84	136.66	1890	20.92	35.88	135.62	1876
172	19.03	32.73	139.27	1926	19.63	33.76	138.24	1912	20.23	34.80	137.20	1897	20.84	35.84	136.16	1883
172.5	18.95	32.69	139.82	1934	19.55	33.72	138.78	1919	20.15	34.76	137.74	1905	20.75	35.80	136.70	1891
173	18.87	32.64	140.36	1941	19.47	33.68	139.32	1927	20.07	34.72	138.28	1912	20.67	35.76	137.24	1898
173.5	18.79	32.60	140.90	1949	19.39	33.64	139.86	1934	19.99	34.68	138.82	1920	20.59	35.72	137.78	1906
174	18.71	32.56	141.44	1956	19.31	33.60	140.40	1942	19.91	34.64	139.36	1927	20.50	35.67	138.33	1913
174.5	18.64	32.52	141.98	1964	19.23	33.56	140.94	1949	19.83	34.60	139.90	1935	20.42	35.63	138.87	1921
175	18.56	32.48	142.52	1971	19.15	33.52	141.48	1957	19.75	34.56	140.45	1942	20.34	35.59	139.41	1928
175.5	18.48	32.44	143.06	1979	19.07	33.48	142.02	1964	19.67	34.51	140.99	1950	20.26	35.55	139.95	1935
176	18.41	32.40	143.60	1986	19.00	33.44	142.56	1972	19.59	34.47	141.53	1957	20.18	35.51	140.49	1943
176.5	18.33	32.36	144.14	1993	18.92	33.39	143.11	1979	19.51	34.43	142.07	1965	20.10	35.47	141.03	1950
177	18.26	32.32	144.68	2001	18.84	33.35	143.65	1987	19.43	34.39	142.61	1972	20.02	35.43	141.57	1958
177.5	18.18	32.28	145.23	2008	18.77	33.31	144.19	1994	19.35	34.35	143.15	1980	19.94	35.39	142.11	1965
178	18.11	32.23	145.77	2016	18.69	33.27	144.73	2002	19.27	34.31	143.69	1987	19.86	35.35	142.65	1973
178.5	18.04	32.19	146.31	2023	18.62	33.23	145.27	2009	19.20	34.27	144.23	1995	19.78	35.31	143.19	1980
179	17.96	32.15	146.85	2031	18.54	33.19	145.81	2017	19.12	34.23	144.77	2002	19.70	35.26	143.74	1988
179.5	17.89	32.11	147.39	2038	18.47	33.15	146.35	2024	19.05	34.19	145.31	2010	19.62	35.22	144.28	1995
180	17.82	32.07	147.93	2046	18.39	33.11	146.89	2032	18.97	34.15	145.86	2017	19.55	35.18	144.82	2003
180.5	17.74	32.03	148.47	2053	18.32	33.07	147.43	2039	18.89	34.10	146.40	2025	19.47	35.14	145.36	2010
181	17.67	31.99	149.01	2061	18.25	33.03	147.97	2046	18.82	34.06	146.94	2032	19.39	35.10	145.90	2018
181.5	17.60	31.95	149.55	2068	18.17	32.98	148.52	2054	18.74	34.02	147.48	2040	19.32	35.06	146.44	2025
182	17.53	31.91	150.09	2076	18.10	32.94	149.06	2061	18.67	33.98	148.02	2047	19.24	35.02	146.98	2033
182.5	17.46	31.87	150.64	2083	18.03	32.90	149.60	2069	18.60	33.94	148.56	2055	19.17	34.98	147.52	2040
183	17.39	31.82	151.18	2091	17.96	32.86	150.14	2076	18.52	33.90	149.10	2062	19.09	34.94	148.06	2048
183.5	17.32	31.78	151.72	2098	17.89	32.82	150.68	2084	18.45	33.86	149.64	2070	19.02	34.90	148.60	2055

Body Composition   MALE   152-183.5 Lb.

Weight: Lb.	Waist: 36 inches				36.25 inches				36.5 inches				36.75 inches			
	Fat: %	Fat: Lb.	LBM: Lb.	RMR: Cal.	Fat: %	Fat: Lb.	LBM: Lb.	RMR: Cal.	Fat: %	Fat: Lb.	LBM: Lb.	RMR: Cal.	Fat: %	Fat: Lb.	LBM: Lb.	RMR: Cal.
152	25.34	38.52	113.48	1569	26.02	39.55	112.45	1555	26.70	40.59	111.41	1541	27.39	41.63	110.37	1526
152.5	25.23	38.48	114.03	1577	25.91	39.51	112.99	1563	26.59	40.55	111.95	1548	27.27	41.59	110.91	1534
153	25.12	38.43	114.57	1584	25.80	39.47	113.53	1570	26.48	40.51	112.49	1556	27.15	41.55	111.45	1541
153.5	25.01	38.39	115.11	1592	25.69	39.43	114.07	1578	26.36	40.47	113.03	1563	27.04	41.51	111.99	1549
154	24.90	38.35	115.65	1599	25.58	39.39	114.61	1585	26.25	40.43	113.57	1571	26.93	41.46	112.54	1556
154.5	24.80	38.31	116.19	1607	25.47	39.35	115.15	1593	26.14	40.39	114.11	1578	26.81	41.42	113.08	1564
155	24.69	38.27	116.73	1614	25.36	39.31	115.69	1600	26.03	40.35	114.66	1586	26.70	41.38	113.62	1571
155.5	24.58	38.23	117.27	1622	25.25	39.27	116.23	1608	25.92	40.30	115.20	1593	26.59	41.34	114.16	1579
156	24.48	38.19	117.81	1629	25.14	39.23	116.77	1615	25.81	40.26	115.74	1601	26.47	41.30	114.70	1586
156.5	24.38	38.15	118.35	1637	25.04	39.18	117.32	1622	25.70	40.22	116.28	1608	26.36	41.26	115.24	1594
157	24.27	38.11	118.89	1644	24.93	39.14	117.86	1630	25.59	40.18	116.82	1616	26.25	41.22	115.78	1601
157.5	24.17	38.07	119.44	1652	24.83	39.10	118.40	1637	25.49	40.14	117.36	1623	26.14	41.18	116.32	1609
158	24.07	38.02	119.98	1659	24.72	39.06	118.94	1645	25.38	40.10	117.90	1631	26.04	41.14	116.86	1616
158.5	23.96	37.98	120.52	1667	24.62	39.02	119.48	1652	25.27	40.06	118.44	1638	25.93	41.10	117.40	1624
159	23.86	37.94	121.06	1674	24.52	38.98	120.02	1660	25.17	40.02	118.98	1646	25.82	41.05	117.95	1631
159.5	23.76	37.90	121.60	1682	24.41	38.94	120.56	1667	25.06	39.98	119.52	1653	25.71	41.01	118.49	1639
160	23.66	37.86	122.14	1689	24.31	38.90	121.10	1675	24.96	39.94	120.07	1660	25.61	40.97	119.03	1646
160.5	23.56	37.82	122.68	1697	24.21	38.86	121.64	1682	24.86	39.89	120.61	1668	25.50	40.93	119.57	1654
161	23.46	37.78	123.22	1704	24.11	38.82	122.18	1690	24.75	39.85	121.15	1675	25.40	40.89	120.11	1661
161.5	23.37	37.74	123.76	1712	24.01	38.77	122.73	1697	24.65	39.81	121.69	1683	25.29	40.85	120.65	1669
162	23.27	37.70	124.30	1719	23.91	38.73	123.27	1705	24.55	39.77	122.23	1690	25.19	40.81	121.19	1676
162.5	23.17	37.66	124.85	1727	23.81	38.69	123.81	1712	24.45	39.73	122.77	1698	25.09	40.77	121.73	1684
163	23.08	37.61	125.39	1734	23.71	38.65	124.35	1720	24.35	39.69	123.31	1705	24.99	40.73	122.27	1691
163.5	22.98	37.57	125.93	1742	23.61	38.61	124.89	1727	24.25	39.65	123.85	1713	24.88	40.69	122.81	1699
164	22.89	37.53	126.47	1749	23.52	38.57	125.43	1735	24.15	39.61	124.39	1720	24.78	40.64	123.36	1706
164.5	22.79	37.49	127.01	1757	23.42	38.53	125.97	1742	24.05	39.57	124.93	1728	24.68	40.60	123.90	1713
165	22.70	37.45	127.55	1764	23.33	38.49	126.51	1750	23.95	39.53	125.48	1735	24.58	40.56	124.44	1721
165.5	22.60	37.41	128.09	1771	23.23	38.45	127.05	1757	23.86	39.48	126.02	1743	24.48	40.52	124.98	1728
166	22.51	37.37	128.63	1779	23.14	38.41	127.59	1765	23.76	39.44	126.56	1750	24.39	40.48	125.52	1736
166.5	22.42	37.33	129.17	1786	23.04	38.36	128.14	1772	23.66	39.40	127.10	1758	24.29	40.44	126.06	1743
167	22.33	37.29	129.71	1794	22.95	38.32	128.68	1780	23.57	39.36	127.64	1765	24.19	40.40	126.60	1751
167.5	22.24	37.25	130.26	1801	22.86	38.28	129.22	1787	23.47	39.32	128.18	1773	24.09	40.36	127.14	1758
168	22.15	37.20	130.80	1809	22.76	38.24	129.76	1795	23.38	39.28	128.72	1780	24.00	40.32	127.68	1766
168.5	22.06	37.16	131.34	1816	22.67	38.20	130.30	1802	23.29	39.24	129.26	1788	23.90	40.28	128.22	1773
169	21.97	37.12	131.88	1824	22.58	38.16	130.84	1810	23.19	39.20	129.80	1795	23.81	40.23	128.77	1781
169.5	21.88	37.08	132.42	1831	22.49	38.12	131.38	1817	23.10	39.16	130.34	1803	23.71	40.19	129.31	1788
170	21.79	37.04	132.96	1839	22.40	38.08	131.92	1824	23.01	39.12	130.89	1810	23.62	40.15	129.85	1796
170.5	21.70	37.00	133.50	1846	22.31	38.04	132.46	1832	22.92	39.07	131.43	1818	23.53	40.11	130.39	1803
171	21.61	36.96	134.04	1854	22.22	38.00	133.00	1839	22.83	39.03	131.97	1825	23.43	40.07	130.93	1811
171.5	21.53	36.92	134.58	1861	22.13	37.95	133.55	1847	22.74	38.99	132.51	1833	23.34	40.03	131.47	1818
172	21.44	36.88	135.12	1869	22.04	37.91	134.09	1854	22.65	38.95	133.05	1840	23.25	39.99	132.01	1826
172.5	21.35	36.84	135.67	1876	21.96	37.87	134.63	1862	22.56	38.91	133.59	1848	23.16	39.95	132.55	1833
173	21.27	36.79	136.21	1884	21.87	37.83	135.17	1869	22.47	38.87	134.13	1855	23.07	39.91	133.09	1841
173.5	21.18	36.75	136.75	1891	21.78	37.79	135.71	1877	22.38	38.83	134.67	1863	22.98	39.87	133.63	1848
174	21.10	36.71	137.29	1899	21.70	37.75	136.25	1884	22.29	38.79	135.21	1870	22.89	39.82	134.18	1856
174.5	21.01	36.67	137.83	1906	21.61	37.71	136.79	1892	22.20	38.75	135.75	1877	22.80	39.78	134.72	1863
175	20.93	36.63	138.37	1914	21.52	37.67	137.33	1899	22.12	38.71	136.30	1885	22.71	39.74	135.26	1871
175.5	20.85	36.59	138.91	1921	21.44	37.63	137.87	1907	22.03	38.66	136.84	1892	22.62	39.70	135.80	1878
176	20.77	36.55	139.45	1929	21.36	37.59	138.41	1914	21.94	38.62	137.38	1900	22.53	39.66	136.34	1886
176.5	20.68	36.51	139.99	1936	21.27	37.54	138.96	1922	21.86	38.58	137.92	1907	22.45	39.62	136.88	1893
177	20.60	36.47	140.53	1944	21.19	37.50	139.50	1929	21.77	38.54	138.46	1915	22.36	39.58	137.42	1901
177.5	20.52	36.43	141.08	1951	21.11	37.46	140.04	1937	21.69	38.50	139.00	1922	22.27	39.54	137.96	1908
178	20.44	36.38	141.62	1959	21.02	37.42	140.58	1944	21.61	38.46	139.54	1930	22.19	39.50	138.50	1916
178.5	20.36	36.34	142.16	1966	20.94	37.38	141.12	1952	21.52	38.42	140.08	1937	22.10	39.46	139.04	1923
179	20.28	36.30	142.70	1974	20.86	37.34	141.66	1959	21.44	38.38	140.62	1945	22.02	39.41	139.59	1930
179.5	20.20	36.26	143.24	1981	20.78	37.30	142.20	1967	21.36	38.34	141.16	1952	21.94	39.37	140.13	1938
180	20.12	36.22	143.78	1988	20.70	37.26	142.74	1974	21.28	38.30	141.71	1960	21.85	39.33	140.67	1945
180.5	20.04	36.18	144.32	1996	20.62	37.22	143.28	1982	21.19	38.25	142.25	1967	21.77	39.29	141.21	1953
181	19.97	36.14	144.86	2003	20.54	37.18	143.82	1989	21.11	38.21	142.79	1975	21.69	39.25	141.75	1960
181.5	19.89	36.10	145.40	2011	20.46	37.13	144.37	1997	21.03	38.17	143.33	1982	21.60	39.21	142.29	1968
182	19.81	36.06	145.94	2018	20.38	37.09	144.91	2004	20.95	38.13	143.87	1990	21.52	39.17	142.83	1975
182.5	19.73	36.02	146.49	2026	20.30	37.05	145.45	2012	20.87	38.09	144.41	1997	21.44	39.13	143.37	1983
183	19.66	35.97	147.03	2033	20.22	37.01	145.99	2019	20.79	38.05	144.95	2005	21.36	39.09	143.91	1990
183.5	19.58	35.93	147.57	2041	20.15	36.97	146.53	2027	20.71	38.01	145.49	2012	21.28	39.05	144.45	1998

Body Composition MALE 152-183.5 Lb.

Weight: Lb.	Waist: 37 inches Fat: %	Fat: Lb.	LBM: Lb.	RMR: Cal.	37.25 inches Fat: %	Fat: Lb.	LBM: Lb.	RMR: Cal.	37.5 inches Fat: %	Fat: Lb.	LBM: Lb.	RMR: Cal.	37.75 inches Fat: %	Fat: Lb.	LBM: Lb.	RMR: Cal.
152	28.07	42.67	109.33	1512	28.75	43.70	108.30	1498	29.43	44.74	107.26	1483	30.12	45.78	106.22	1469
152.5	27.95	42.63	109.88	1520	28.63	43.66	108.84	1505	29.31	44.70	107.80	1491	29.99	45.74	106.76	1477
153	27.83	42.58	110.42	1527	28.51	43.62	109.38	1513	29.19	44.66	108.34	1498	29.87	45.70	107.30	1484
153.5	27.72	42.54	110.96	1535	28.39	43.58	109.92	1520	29.07	44.62	108.88	1506	29.74	45.66	107.84	1491
154	27.60	42.50	111.50	1542	28.27	43.54	110.46	1528	28.95	44.58	109.42	1513	29.62	45.61	108.39	1499
154.5	27.48	42.46	112.04	1549	28.15	43.50	111.00	1535	28.83	44.54	109.96	1521	29.50	45.57	108.93	1506
155	27.37	42.42	112.58	1557	28.04	43.46	111.54	1543	28.71	44.50	110.51	1528	29.38	45.53	109.47	1514
155.5	27.25	42.38	113.12	1564	27.92	43.42	112.08	1550	28.59	44.45	111.05	1536	29.25	45.49	110.01	1521
156	27.14	42.34	113.66	1572	27.80	43.38	112.62	1558	28.47	44.41	111.59	1543	29.13	45.45	110.55	1529
156.5	27.03	42.30	114.20	1579	27.69	43.33	113.17	1565	28.35	44.37	112.13	1551	29.02	45.41	111.09	1536
157	26.91	42.26	114.74	1587	27.58	43.29	113.71	1573	28.24	44.33	112.67	1558	28.90	45.37	111.63	1544
157.5	26.80	42.22	115.29	1594	27.46	43.25	114.25	1580	28.12	44.29	113.21	1566	28.78	45.33	112.17	1551
158	26.69	42.17	115.83	1602	27.35	43.21	114.79	1588	28.01	44.25	113.75	1573	28.66	45.29	112.71	1559
158.5	26.58	42.13	116.37	1609	27.24	43.17	115.33	1595	27.89	44.21	114.29	1581	28.55	45.25	113.25	1566
159	26.47	42.09	116.91	1617	27.13	43.13	115.87	1602	27.78	44.17	114.83	1588	28.43	45.20	113.80	1574
159.5	26.36	42.05	117.45	1624	27.01	43.09	116.41	1610	27.67	44.13	115.37	1596	28.32	45.16	114.34	1581
160	26.26	42.01	117.99	1632	26.90	43.05	116.95	1617	27.55	44.09	115.92	1603	28.20	45.12	114.88	1589
160.5	26.15	41.97	118.53	1639	26.80	43.01	117.49	1625	27.44	44.04	116.46	1611	28.09	45.08	115.42	1596
161	26.04	41.93	119.07	1647	26.69	42.97	118.03	1632	27.33	44.00	117.00	1618	27.98	45.04	115.96	1604
161.5	25.94	41.89	119.61	1654	26.58	42.92	118.58	1640	27.22	43.96	117.54	1626	27.86	45.00	116.50	1611
162	25.83	41.85	120.15	1662	26.47	42.88	119.12	1647	27.11	43.92	118.08	1633	27.75	44.96	117.04	1619
162.5	25.73	41.81	120.70	1669	26.36	42.84	119.66	1655	27.00	43.88	118.62	1641	27.64	44.92	117.58	1626
163	25.62	41.76	121.24	1677	26.26	42.80	120.20	1662	26.90	43.84	119.16	1648	27.53	44.88	118.12	1634
163.5	25.52	41.72	121.78	1684	26.15	42.76	120.74	1670	26.79	43.80	119.70	1655	27.42	44.84	118.66	1641
164	25.42	41.68	122.32	1692	26.05	42.72	121.28	1677	26.68	43.76	120.24	1663	27.31	44.79	119.21	1649
164.5	25.31	41.64	122.86	1699	25.94	42.68	121.82	1685	26.58	43.72	120.78	1670	27.21	44.75	119.75	1656
165	25.21	41.60	123.40	1707	25.84	42.64	122.36	1692	26.47	43.68	121.33	1678	27.10	44.71	120.29	1664
165.5	25.11	41.56	123.94	1714	25.74	42.60	122.90	1700	26.36	43.63	121.87	1685	26.99	44.67	120.83	1671
166	25.01	41.52	124.48	1722	25.64	42.56	123.44	1707	26.26	43.59	122.41	1693	26.89	44.63	121.37	1679
166.5	24.91	41.48	125.02	1729	25.53	42.51	123.99	1715	26.16	43.55	122.95	1700	26.78	44.59	121.91	1686
167	24.81	41.44	125.56	1737	25.43	42.47	124.53	1722	26.05	43.51	123.49	1708	26.68	44.55	122.45	1694
167.5	24.71	41.40	126.11	1744	25.33	42.43	125.07	1730	25.95	43.47	124.03	1715	26.57	44.51	122.99	1701
168	24.62	41.35	126.65	1752	25.23	42.39	125.61	1737	25.85	43.43	124.57	1723	26.47	44.47	123.53	1708
168.5	24.52	41.31	127.19	1759	25.13	42.35	126.15	1745	25.75	43.39	125.11	1730	26.37	44.43	124.07	1716
169	24.42	41.27	127.73	1766	25.04	42.31	126.69	1752	25.65	43.35	125.65	1738	26.26	44.38	124.62	1723
169.5	24.33	41.23	128.27	1774	24.94	42.27	127.23	1760	25.55	43.31	126.19	1745	26.16	44.34	125.16	1731
170	24.23	41.19	128.81	1781	24.84	42.23	127.77	1767	25.45	43.27	126.74	1753	26.06	44.30	125.70	1738
170.5	24.13	41.15	129.35	1789	24.74	42.19	128.31	1775	25.35	43.22	127.28	1760	25.96	44.26	126.24	1746
171	24.04	41.11	129.89	1796	24.65	42.15	128.85	1782	25.25	43.18	127.82	1768	25.86	44.22	126.78	1753
171.5	23.95	41.07	130.43	1804	24.55	42.10	129.40	1790	25.16	43.14	128.36	1775	25.76	44.18	127.32	1761
172	23.85	41.03	130.97	1811	24.46	42.06	129.94	1797	25.06	43.10	128.90	1783	25.66	44.14	127.86	1768
172.5	23.76	40.99	131.52	1819	24.36	42.02	130.48	1805	24.96	43.06	129.44	1790	25.56	44.10	128.40	1776
173	23.67	40.94	132.06	1826	24.27	41.98	131.02	1812	24.87	43.02	129.98	1798	25.47	44.06	128.94	1783
173.5	23.58	40.90	132.60	1834	24.17	41.94	131.56	1819	24.77	42.98	130.52	1805	25.37	44.02	129.48	1791
174	23.48	40.86	133.14	1841	24.08	41.90	132.10	1827	24.68	42.94	131.06	1813	25.27	43.97	130.03	1798
174.5	23.39	40.82	133.68	1849	23.99	41.86	132.64	1834	24.58	42.90	131.60	1820	25.18	43.93	130.57	1806
175	23.30	40.78	134.22	1856	23.90	41.82	133.18	1842	24.49	42.86	132.15	1828	25.08	43.89	131.11	1813
175.5	23.21	40.74	134.76	1864	23.80	41.78	133.72	1849	24.40	42.81	132.69	1835	24.99	43.85	131.65	1821
176	23.12	40.70	135.30	1871	23.71	41.74	134.26	1857	24.30	42.77	133.23	1843	24.89	43.81	132.19	1828
176.5	23.04	40.66	135.84	1879	23.62	41.69	134.81	1864	24.21	42.73	133.77	1850	24.80	43.77	132.73	1836
177	22.95	40.62	136.38	1886	23.53	41.65	135.35	1872	24.12	42.69	134.31	1857	24.71	43.73	133.27	1843
177.5	22.86	40.58	136.93	1894	23.44	41.61	135.89	1879	24.03	42.65	134.85	1865	24.61	43.69	133.81	1851
178	22.77	40.53	137.47	1901	23.35	41.57	136.43	1887	23.94	42.61	135.39	1872	24.52	43.65	134.35	1858
178.5	22.69	40.49	138.01	1909	23.27	41.53	136.97	1894	23.85	42.57	135.93	1880	24.43	43.61	134.89	1866
179	22.60	40.45	138.55	1916	23.18	41.49	137.51	1902	23.76	42.53	136.47	1887	24.34	43.56	135.44	1873
179.5	22.51	40.41	139.09	1924	23.09	41.45	138.05	1909	23.67	42.49	137.01	1895	24.25	43.52	135.98	1881
180	22.43	40.37	139.63	1931	23.00	41.41	138.59	1917	23.58	42.45	137.56	1902	24.16	43.48	136.52	1888
180.5	22.34	40.33	140.17	1939	22.92	41.37	139.13	1924	23.49	42.40	138.10	1910	24.07	43.44	137.06	1896
181	22.26	40.29	140.71	1946	22.83	41.33	139.67	1932	23.40	42.36	138.64	1917	23.98	43.40	137.60	1903
181.5	22.17	40.25	141.25	1954	22.75	41.28	140.22	1939	23.32	42.32	139.18	1925	23.89	43.36	138.14	1910
182	22.09	40.21	141.79	1961	22.66	41.24	140.76	1947	23.23	42.28	139.72	1932	23.80	43.32	138.68	1918
182.5	22.01	40.17	142.34	1968	22.58	41.20	141.30	1954	23.15	42.24	140.26	1940	23.71	43.28	139.22	1925
183	21.93	40.12	142.88	1976	22.49	41.16	141.84	1962	23.06	42.20	140.80	1947	23.63	43.24	139.76	1933
183.5	21.84	40.08	143.42	1983	22.41	41.12	142.38	1969	22.97	42.16	141.34	1955	23.54	43.20	140.30	1940

Body Composition MALE 152-183.5 Lb.

Weight: Lb.	Waist: 38 inches				38.25 inches				38.5 inches				38.75 inches			
	Fat: %	Fat: Lb.	LBM: Lb.	RMR: Cal.	Fat: %	Fat: Lb.	LBM: Lb.	RMR: Cal.	Fat: %	Fat: Lb.	LBM: Lb.	RMR: Cal.	Fat: %	Fat: Lb.	LBM: Lb.	RMR: Cal.
152	30.80	46.82	105.18	1455	31.48	47.85	104.15	1440	32.17	48.89	103.11	1426	32.85	49.93	102.07	1412
152.5	30.67	46.78	105.73	1462	31.35	47.81	104.69	1448	32.03	48.85	103.65	1433	32.71	49.89	102.61	1419
153	30.55	46.73	106.27	1470	31.22	47.77	105.23	1455	31.90	48.81	104.19	1441	32.58	49.85	103.15	1427
153.5	30.42	46.69	106.81	1477	31.09	47.73	105.77	1463	31.77	48.77	104.73	1448	32.45	49.81	103.69	1434
154	30.29	46.65	107.35	1485	30.97	47.69	106.31	1470	31.64	48.73	105.27	1456	32.31	49.76	104.24	1442
154.5	30.17	46.61	107.89	1492	30.84	47.65	106.85	1478	31.51	48.69	105.81	1463	32.18	49.72	104.78	1449
155	30.05	46.57	108.43	1500	30.71	47.61	107.39	1485	31.38	48.65	106.36	1471	32.05	49.68	105.32	1457
155.5	29.92	46.53	108.97	1507	30.59	47.57	107.93	1493	31.26	48.60	106.90	1478	31.92	49.64	105.86	1464
156	29.80	46.49	109.51	1515	30.47	47.53	108.47	1500	31.13	48.56	107.44	1486	31.80	49.60	106.40	1472
156.5	29.68	46.45	110.05	1522	30.34	47.48	109.02	1508	31.00	48.52	107.98	1493	31.67	49.56	106.94	1479
157	29.56	46.41	110.59	1530	30.22	47.44	109.56	1515	30.88	48.48	108.52	1501	31.54	49.52	107.48	1486
157.5	29.44	46.37	111.14	1537	30.10	47.40	110.10	1523	30.76	48.44	109.06	1508	31.41	49.48	108.02	1494
158	29.32	46.32	111.68	1544	29.98	47.36	110.64	1530	30.63	48.40	109.60	1516	31.29	49.44	108.56	1501
158.5	29.20	46.28	112.22	1552	29.86	47.32	111.18	1538	30.51	48.36	110.14	1523	31.16	49.40	109.10	1509
159	29.08	46.24	112.76	1559	29.74	47.28	111.72	1545	30.39	48.32	110.68	1531	31.04	49.35	109.65	1516
159.5	28.97	46.20	113.30	1567	29.62	47.24	112.26	1553	30.27	48.28	111.22	1538	30.92	49.31	110.19	1524
160	28.85	46.16	113.84	1574	29.50	47.20	112.80	1560	30.15	48.24	111.77	1546	30.80	49.27	110.73	1531
160.5	28.73	46.12	114.38	1582	29.38	47.16	113.34	1568	30.03	48.19	112.31	1553	30.67	49.23	111.27	1539
161	28.62	46.08	114.92	1589	29.26	47.12	113.88	1575	29.91	48.15	112.85	1561	30.55	49.19	111.81	1546
161.5	28.51	46.04	115.46	1597	29.15	47.07	114.43	1583	29.79	48.11	113.39	1568	30.43	49.15	112.35	1554
162	28.39	46.00	116.00	1604	29.03	47.03	114.97	1590	29.67	48.07	113.93	1576	30.31	49.11	112.89	1561
162.5	28.28	45.96	116.55	1612	28.92	46.99	115.51	1597	29.56	48.03	114.47	1583	30.20	49.07	113.43	1569
163	28.17	45.91	117.09	1619	28.80	46.95	116.05	1605	29.44	47.99	115.01	1591	30.08	49.03	113.97	1576
163.5	28.06	45.87	117.63	1627	28.69	46.91	116.59	1612	29.33	47.95	115.55	1598	29.96	48.99	114.51	1584
164	27.95	45.83	118.17	1634	28.58	46.87	117.13	1620	29.21	47.91	116.09	1606	29.84	48.94	115.06	1591
164.5	27.84	45.79	118.71	1642	28.47	46.83	117.67	1627	29.10	47.87	116.63	1613	29.73	48.90	115.60	1599
165	27.73	45.75	119.25	1649	28.36	46.79	118.21	1635	28.98	47.83	117.18	1621	29.61	48.86	116.14	1606
165.5	27.62	45.71	119.79	1657	28.25	46.75	118.75	1642	28.87	47.78	117.72	1628	29.50	48.82	116.68	1614
166	27.51	45.67	120.33	1664	28.14	46.71	119.29	1650	28.76	47.74	118.26	1635	29.39	48.78	117.22	1621
166.5	27.40	45.63	120.87	1672	28.03	46.66	119.84	1657	28.65	47.70	118.80	1643	29.27	48.74	117.76	1629
167	27.30	45.59	121.41	1679	27.92	46.62	120.38	1665	28.54	47.66	119.34	1650	29.16	48.70	118.30	1636
167.5	27.19	45.55	121.96	1687	27.81	46.58	120.92	1672	28.43	47.62	119.88	1658	29.05	48.66	118.84	1644
168	27.09	45.50	122.50	1694	27.70	46.54	121.46	1680	28.32	47.58	120.42	1665	28.94	48.62	119.38	1651
168.5	26.98	45.46	123.04	1702	27.60	46.50	122.00	1687	28.21	47.54	120.96	1673	28.83	48.58	119.92	1659
169	26.88	45.42	123.58	1709	27.49	46.46	122.54	1695	28.10	47.50	121.50	1680	28.72	48.53	120.47	1666
169.5	26.77	45.38	124.12	1717	27.39	46.42	123.08	1702	28.00	47.46	122.04	1688	28.61	48.49	121.01	1674
170	26.67	45.34	124.66	1724	27.28	46.38	123.62	1710	27.89	47.42	122.59	1695	28.50	48.45	121.55	1681
170.5	26.57	45.30	125.20	1732	27.18	46.34	124.16	1717	27.79	47.37	123.13	1703	28.39	48.41	122.09	1688
171	26.47	45.26	125.74	1739	27.07	46.30	124.70	1725	27.68	47.33	123.67	1710	28.29	48.37	122.63	1696
171.5	26.37	45.22	126.28	1746	26.97	46.25	125.25	1732	27.58	47.29	124.21	1718	28.18	48.33	123.17	1703
172	26.27	45.18	126.82	1754	26.87	46.21	125.79	1740	27.47	47.25	124.75	1725	28.07	48.29	123.71	1711
172.5	26.17	45.14	127.37	1761	26.77	46.17	126.33	1747	27.37	47.21	125.29	1733	27.97	48.25	124.25	1718
173	26.07	45.09	127.91	1769	26.67	46.13	126.87	1755	27.27	47.17	125.83	1740	27.87	48.21	124.79	1726
173.5	25.97	45.05	128.45	1776	26.57	46.09	127.41	1762	27.16	47.13	126.37	1748	27.76	48.17	125.33	1733
174	25.87	45.01	128.99	1784	26.47	46.05	127.95	1770	27.06	47.09	126.91	1755	27.66	48.12	125.88	1741
174.5	25.77	44.97	129.53	1791	26.37	46.01	128.49	1777	26.96	47.05	127.45	1763	27.56	48.08	126.42	1748
175	25.67	44.93	130.07	1799	26.27	45.97	129.03	1785	26.86	47.01	128.00	1770	27.45	48.04	126.96	1756
175.5	25.58	44.89	130.61	1806	26.17	45.93	129.57	1792	26.76	46.96	128.54	1778	27.35	48.00	127.50	1763
176	25.48	44.85	131.15	1814	26.07	45.89	130.11	1799	26.66	46.92	129.08	1785	27.25	47.96	128.04	1771
176.5	25.39	44.81	131.69	1821	25.97	45.84	130.66	1807	26.56	46.88	129.62	1793	27.15	47.92	128.58	1778
177	25.29	44.77	132.23	1829	25.88	45.80	131.20	1814	26.46	46.84	130.16	1800	27.05	47.88	129.12	1786
177.5	25.20	44.73	132.78	1836	25.78	45.76	131.74	1822	26.37	46.80	130.70	1808	26.95	47.84	129.66	1793
178	25.10	44.68	133.32	1844	25.69	45.72	132.28	1829	26.27	46.76	131.24	1815	26.85	47.80	130.20	1801
178.5	25.01	44.64	133.86	1851	25.59	45.68	132.82	1837	26.17	46.72	131.78	1823	26.75	47.76	130.74	1808
179	24.92	44.60	134.40	1859	25.50	45.64	133.36	1844	26.08	46.68	132.32	1830	26.66	47.71	131.29	1816
179.5	24.83	44.56	134.94	1866	25.40	45.60	133.90	1852	25.98	46.64	132.86	1838	26.56	47.67	131.83	1823
180	24.73	44.52	135.48	1874	25.31	45.56	134.44	1859	25.89	46.60	133.41	1845	26.46	47.63	132.37	1831
180.5	24.64	44.48	136.02	1881	25.22	45.52	134.98	1867	25.79	46.55	133.95	1852	26.37	47.59	132.91	1838
181	24.55	44.44	136.56	1889	25.12	45.48	135.52	1874	25.70	46.51	134.49	1860	26.27	47.55	133.45	1846
181.5	24.46	44.40	137.10	1896	25.03	45.43	136.07	1882	25.60	46.47	135.03	1867	26.18	47.51	133.99	1853
182	24.37	44.36	137.64	1904	24.94	45.39	136.61	1889	25.51	46.43	135.57	1875	26.08	47.47	134.53	1861
182.5	24.28	44.32	138.19	1911	24.85	45.35	137.15	1897	25.42	46.39	136.11	1882	25.99	47.43	135.07	1868
183	24.19	44.27	138.73	1919	24.76	45.31	137.69	1904	25.33	46.35	136.65	1890	25.89	47.39	135.61	1876
183.5	24.11	44.23	139.27	1926	24.67	45.27	138.23	1912	25.24	46.31	137.19	1897	25.80	47.35	136.15	1883

Body Composition   MALE   152-183.5 Lb.

Weight: Lb.	Waist: 39 inches Fat: %	Fat: Lb.	LBM: Lb.	RMR: Cal.	39.25 inches Fat: %	Fat: Lb.	LBM: Lb.	RMR: Cal.	39.5 inches Fat: %	Fat: Lb.	LBM: Lb.	RMR: Cal.	39.75 inches Fat: %	Fat: Lb.	LBM: Lb.	RMR: Cal.
152	33.53	50.97	101.03	1397	34.21	52.00	100.00	1383	34.90	53.04	98.96	1369	35.58	54.08	97.92	1354
152.5	33.39	50.93	101.58	1405	34.07	51.96	100.54	1390	34.75	53.00	99.50	1376	35.43	54.04	98.46	1362
153	33.26	50.88	102.12	1412	33.94	51.92	101.08	1398	34.61	52.96	100.04	1384	35.29	54.00	99.00	1369
153.5	33.12	50.84	102.66	1420	33.80	51.88	101.62	1405	34.47	52.92	100.58	1391	35.15	53.96	99.54	1377
154	32.99	50.80	103.20	1427	33.66	51.84	102.16	1413	34.34	52.88	101.12	1399	35.01	53.91	100.09	1384
154.5	32.86	50.76	103.74	1435	33.53	51.80	102.70	1420	34.20	52.84	101.66	1406	34.87	53.87	100.63	1392
155	32.72	50.72	104.28	1442	33.39	51.76	103.24	1428	34.06	52.80	102.21	1413	34.73	53.83	101.17	1399
155.5	32.59	50.68	104.82	1450	33.26	51.72	103.78	1435	33.93	52.75	102.75	1421	34.59	53.79	101.71	1407
156	32.46	50.64	105.36	1457	33.13	51.68	104.32	1443	33.79	52.71	103.29	1428	34.46	53.75	102.25	1414
156.5	32.33	50.60	105.90	1465	32.99	51.63	104.87	1450	33.66	52.67	103.83	1436	34.32	53.71	102.79	1422
157	32.20	50.56	106.44	1472	32.86	51.59	105.41	1458	33.52	52.63	104.37	1443	34.18	53.67	103.33	1429
157.5	32.07	50.52	106.99	1480	32.73	51.55	105.95	1465	33.39	52.59	104.91	1451	34.05	53.63	103.87	1437
158	31.95	50.47	107.53	1487	32.60	51.51	106.49	1473	33.26	52.55	105.45	1458	33.92	53.59	104.41	1444
158.5	31.82	50.43	108.07	1495	32.47	51.47	107.03	1480	33.13	52.51	105.99	1466	33.78	53.55	104.95	1452
159	31.69	50.39	108.61	1502	32.35	51.43	107.57	1488	33.00	52.47	106.53	1473	33.65	53.50	105.50	1459
159.5	31.57	50.35	109.15	1510	32.22	51.39	108.11	1495	32.87	52.43	107.07	1481	33.52	53.46	106.04	1466
160	31.44	50.31	109.69	1517	32.09	51.35	108.65	1503	32.74	52.39	107.62	1488	33.39	53.42	106.58	1474
160.5	31.32	50.27	110.23	1524	31.97	51.31	109.19	1510	32.61	52.34	108.16	1496	33.26	53.38	107.12	1481
161	31.20	50.23	110.77	1532	31.84	51.27	109.73	1518	32.49	52.30	108.70	1503	33.13	53.34	107.66	1489
161.5	31.08	50.19	111.31	1539	31.72	51.22	110.28	1525	32.36	52.26	109.24	1511	33.00	53.30	108.20	1496
162	30.95	50.15	111.85	1547	31.59	51.18	110.82	1533	32.24	52.22	109.78	1518	32.88	53.26	108.74	1504
162.5	30.83	50.11	112.40	1554	31.47	51.14	111.36	1540	32.11	52.18	110.32	1526	32.75	53.22	109.28	1511
163	30.71	50.06	112.94	1562	31.35	51.10	111.90	1548	31.99	52.14	110.86	1533	32.62	53.18	109.82	1519
163.5	30.60	50.02	113.48	1569	31.23	51.06	112.44	1555	31.86	52.10	111.40	1541	32.50	53.14	110.36	1526
164	30.48	49.98	114.02	1577	31.11	51.02	112.98	1563	31.74	52.06	111.94	1548	32.37	53.09	110.91	1534
164.5	30.36	49.94	114.56	1584	30.99	50.98	113.52	1570	31.62	52.02	112.48	1556	32.25	53.05	111.45	1541
165	30.24	49.90	115.10	1592	30.87	50.94	114.06	1577	31.50	51.98	113.03	1563	32.13	53.01	111.99	1549
165.5	30.13	49.86	115.64	1599	30.75	50.90	114.60	1585	31.38	51.93	113.57	1571	32.01	52.97	112.53	1556
166	30.01	49.82	116.18	1607	30.64	50.86	115.14	1592	31.26	51.89	114.11	1578	31.89	52.93	113.07	1564
166.5	29.90	49.78	116.72	1614	30.52	50.81	115.69	1600	31.14	51.85	114.65	1586	31.77	52.89	113.61	1571
167	29.78	49.74	117.26	1622	30.40	50.77	116.23	1607	31.02	51.81	115.19	1593	31.65	52.85	114.15	1579
167.5	29.67	49.70	117.81	1629	30.29	50.73	116.77	1615	30.91	51.77	115.73	1601	31.53	52.81	114.69	1586
168	29.56	49.65	118.35	1637	30.17	50.69	117.31	1622	30.79	51.73	116.27	1608	31.41	52.77	115.23	1594
168.5	29.44	49.61	118.89	1644	30.06	50.65	117.85	1630	30.68	51.69	116.81	1616	31.29	52.73	115.77	1601
169	29.33	49.57	119.43	1652	29.95	50.61	118.39	1637	30.56	51.65	117.35	1623	31.17	52.69	116.32	1609
169.5	29.22	49.53	119.97	1659	29.83	50.57	118.93	1645	30.45	51.61	117.89	1630	31.06	52.64	116.86	1616
170	29.11	49.49	120.51	1667	29.72	50.53	119.47	1652	30.33	51.57	118.44	1638	30.94	52.60	117.40	1624
170.5	29.00	49.45	121.05	1674	29.61	50.49	120.01	1660	30.22	51.52	118.98	1645	30.83	52.56	117.94	1631
171	28.89	49.41	121.59	1682	29.50	50.45	120.55	1667	30.11	51.48	119.52	1653	30.71	52.52	118.48	1639
171.5	28.79	49.37	122.13	1689	29.39	50.40	121.10	1675	30.00	51.44	120.06	1660	30.60	52.48	119.02	1646
172	28.68	49.33	122.67	1697	29.28	50.36	121.64	1682	29.88	51.40	120.60	1668	30.49	52.44	119.56	1654
172.5	28.57	49.29	123.22	1704	29.17	50.32	122.18	1690	29.77	51.36	121.14	1675	30.38	52.40	120.10	1661
173	28.46	49.24	123.76	1712	29.06	50.28	122.72	1697	29.66	51.32	121.68	1683	30.26	52.36	120.64	1668
173.5	28.36	49.20	124.30	1719	28.96	50.24	123.26	1705	29.56	51.28	122.22	1690	30.15	52.32	121.18	1676
174	28.25	49.16	124.84	1727	28.85	50.20	123.80	1712	29.45	51.24	122.76	1698	30.04	52.27	121.73	1683
174.5	28.15	49.12	125.38	1734	28.74	50.16	124.34	1720	29.34	51.20	123.30	1705	29.93	52.23	122.27	1691
175	28.05	49.08	125.92	1741	28.64	50.12	124.88	1727	29.23	51.16	123.85	1713	29.82	52.19	122.81	1698
175.5	27.94	49.04	126.46	1749	28.53	50.08	125.42	1735	29.12	51.11	124.39	1720	29.72	52.15	123.35	1706
176	27.84	49.00	127.00	1756	28.43	50.04	125.96	1742	29.02	51.07	124.93	1728	29.61	52.11	123.89	1713
176.5	27.74	48.96	127.54	1764	28.33	49.99	126.51	1750	28.91	51.03	125.47	1735	29.50	52.07	124.43	1721
177	27.64	48.92	128.08	1771	28.22	49.95	127.05	1757	28.81	50.99	126.01	1743	29.39	52.03	124.97	1728
177.5	27.54	48.88	128.63	1779	28.12	49.91	127.59	1765	28.70	50.95	126.55	1750	29.29	51.99	125.51	1736
178	27.43	48.83	129.17	1786	28.02	49.87	128.13	1772	28.60	50.91	127.09	1758	29.18	51.95	126.05	1743
178.5	27.34	48.79	129.71	1794	27.92	49.83	128.67	1779	28.50	50.87	127.63	1765	29.08	51.91	126.59	1751
179	27.24	48.75	130.25	1801	27.82	49.79	129.21	1787	28.39	50.83	128.17	1773	28.97	51.86	127.14	1758
179.5	27.14	48.71	130.79	1809	27.72	49.75	129.75	1794	28.29	50.79	128.71	1780	28.87	51.82	127.68	1766
180	27.04	48.67	131.33	1816	27.62	49.71	130.29	1802	28.19	50.75	129.26	1788	28.77	51.78	128.22	1773
180.5	26.94	48.63	131.87	1824	27.52	49.67	130.83	1809	28.09	50.70	129.80	1795	28.67	51.74	128.76	1781
181	26.84	48.59	132.41	1831	27.42	49.63	131.37	1817	27.99	50.66	130.34	1803	28.56	51.70	129.30	1788
181.5	26.75	48.55	132.95	1839	27.32	49.58	131.92	1824	27.89	50.62	130.88	1810	28.46	51.66	129.84	1796
182	26.65	48.51	133.49	1846	27.22	49.54	132.46	1832	27.79	50.58	131.42	1818	28.36	51.62	130.38	1803
182.5	26.56	48.47	134.04	1854	27.12	49.50	133.00	1839	27.69	50.54	131.96	1825	28.26	51.58	130.92	1811
183	26.46	48.42	134.58	1861	27.03	49.46	133.54	1847	27.60	50.50	132.50	1832	28.16	51.54	131.46	1818
183.5	26.37	48.38	135.12	1869	26.93	49.42	134.08	1854	27.50	50.46	133.04	1840	28.06	51.50	132.00	1826

Body Composition MALE 152-183.5 Lb.

Weight: Lb.	Waist: 40 inches				40.25 inches				40.5 inches				40.75 inches			
	Fat: %	Fat: Lb.	LBM: Lb.	RMR: Cal.	Fat: %	Fat: Lb.	LBM: Lb.	RMR: Cal.	Fat: %	Fat: Lb.	LBM: Lb.	RMR: Cal.	Fat: %	Fat: Lb.	LBM: Lb.	RMR: Cal.
152	36.26	55.12	96.88	1340	36.94	56.15	95.85	1326	37.63	57.19	94.81	1311	38.31	58.23	93.77	1297
152.5	36.11	55.08	97.43	1347	36.80	56.11	96.39	1333	37.48	57.15	95.35	1319	38.16	58.19	94.31	1304
153	35.97	55.03	97.97	1355	36.65	56.07	96.93	1341	37.33	57.11	95.89	1326	38.00	58.15	94.85	1312
153.5	35.83	54.99	98.51	1362	36.50	56.03	97.47	1348	37.18	57.07	96.43	1334	37.85	58.11	95.39	1319
154	35.68	54.95	99.05	1370	36.36	55.99	98.01	1355	37.03	57.03	96.97	1341	37.70	58.06	95.94	1327
154.5	35.54	54.91	99.59	1377	36.21	55.95	98.55	1363	36.88	56.99	97.51	1349	37.56	58.02	96.48	1334
155	35.40	54.87	100.13	1385	36.07	55.91	99.09	1370	36.74	56.95	98.06	1356	37.41	57.98	97.02	1342
155.5	35.26	54.83	100.67	1392	35.93	55.87	99.63	1378	36.59	56.90	98.60	1364	37.26	57.94	97.56	1349
156	35.12	54.79	101.21	1400	35.79	55.83	100.17	1385	36.45	56.86	99.14	1371	37.12	57.90	98.10	1357
156.5	34.98	54.75	101.75	1407	35.65	55.78	100.72	1393	36.31	56.82	99.68	1379	36.97	57.86	98.64	1364
157	34.84	54.71	102.29	1415	35.51	55.74	101.26	1400	36.17	56.78	100.22	1386	36.83	57.82	99.18	1372
157.5	34.71	54.67	102.84	1422	35.37	55.70	101.80	1408	36.03	56.74	100.76	1394	36.68	57.78	99.72	1379
158	34.57	54.62	103.38	1430	35.23	55.66	102.34	1415	35.89	56.70	101.30	1401	36.54	57.74	100.26	1387
158.5	34.44	54.58	103.92	1437	35.09	55.62	102.88	1423	35.75	56.66	101.84	1408	36.40	57.70	100.80	1394
159	34.30	54.54	104.46	1445	34.96	55.58	103.42	1430	35.61	56.62	102.38	1416	36.26	57.65	101.35	1402
159.5	34.17	54.50	105.00	1452	34.82	55.54	103.96	1438	35.47	56.58	102.92	1423	36.12	57.61	101.89	1409
160	34.04	54.46	105.54	1460	34.69	55.50	104.50	1445	35.33	56.54	103.47	1431	35.98	57.57	102.43	1417
160.5	33.91	54.42	106.08	1467	34.55	55.46	105.04	1453	35.20	56.49	104.01	1438	35.85	57.53	102.97	1424
161	33.78	54.38	106.62	1475	34.42	55.42	105.58	1460	35.06	56.45	104.55	1446	35.71	57.49	103.51	1432
161.5	33.65	54.34	107.16	1482	34.29	55.37	106.13	1468	34.93	56.41	105.09	1453	35.57	57.45	104.05	1439
162	33.52	54.30	107.70	1490	34.16	55.33	106.67	1475	34.80	56.37	105.63	1461	35.44	57.41	104.59	1447
162.5	33.39	54.26	108.25	1497	34.03	55.29	107.21	1483	34.66	56.33	106.17	1468	35.30	57.37	105.13	1454
163	33.26	54.21	108.79	1505	33.90	55.25	107.75	1490	34.53	56.29	106.71	1476	35.17	57.33	105.67	1461
163.5	33.13	54.17	109.33	1512	33.77	55.21	108.29	1498	34.40	56.25	107.25	1483	35.04	57.29	106.21	1469
164	33.01	54.13	109.87	1519	33.64	55.17	108.83	1505	34.27	56.21	107.79	1491	34.91	57.24	106.76	1476
164.5	32.88	54.09	110.41	1527	33.51	55.13	109.37	1513	34.14	56.17	108.33	1498	34.77	57.20	107.30	1484
165	32.76	54.05	110.95	1534	33.39	55.09	109.91	1520	34.02	56.13	108.88	1506	34.64	57.16	107.84	1491
165.5	32.63	54.01	111.49	1542	33.26	55.05	110.45	1528	33.89	56.08	109.42	1513	34.51	57.12	108.38	1499
166	32.51	53.97	112.03	1549	33.14	55.01	110.99	1535	33.76	56.04	109.96	1521	34.39	57.08	108.92	1506
166.5	32.39	53.93	112.57	1557	33.01	54.96	111.54	1543	33.63	56.00	110.50	1528	34.26	57.04	109.46	1514
167	32.27	53.89	113.11	1564	32.89	54.92	112.08	1550	33.51	55.96	111.04	1536	34.13	57.00	110.00	1521
167.5	32.15	53.85	113.66	1572	32.77	54.88	112.62	1558	33.39	55.92	111.58	1543	34.00	56.96	110.54	1529
168	32.03	53.80	114.20	1579	32.64	54.84	113.16	1565	33.26	55.88	112.12	1551	33.88	56.92	111.08	1536
168.5	31.91	53.76	114.74	1587	32.52	54.80	113.70	1572	33.14	55.84	112.66	1558	33.75	56.88	111.62	1544
169	31.79	53.72	115.28	1594	32.40	54.76	114.24	1580	33.02	55.80	113.20	1566	33.63	56.83	112.17	1551
169.5	31.67	53.68	115.82	1602	32.28	54.72	114.78	1587	32.89	55.76	113.74	1573	33.51	56.79	112.71	1559
170	31.55	53.64	116.36	1609	32.16	54.68	115.32	1595	32.77	55.72	114.29	1581	33.38	56.75	113.25	1566
170.5	31.44	53.60	116.90	1617	32.04	54.64	115.86	1602	32.65	55.67	114.83	1588	33.26	56.71	113.79	1574
171	31.32	53.56	117.44	1624	31.93	54.60	116.40	1610	32.53	55.63	115.37	1596	33.14	56.67	114.33	1581
171.5	31.21	53.52	117.98	1632	31.81	54.55	116.95	1617	32.42	55.59	115.91	1603	33.02	56.63	114.87	1589
172	31.09	53.48	118.52	1639	31.69	54.51	117.49	1625	32.30	55.55	116.45	1610	32.90	56.59	115.41	1596
172.5	30.98	53.44	119.07	1647	31.58	54.47	118.03	1632	32.18	55.51	116.99	1618	32.78	56.55	115.95	1604
173	30.86	53.39	119.61	1654	31.46	54.43	118.57	1640	32.06	55.47	117.53	1625	32.66	56.51	116.49	1611
173.5	30.75	53.35	120.15	1662	31.35	54.39	119.11	1647	31.95	55.43	118.07	1633	32.54	56.47	117.03	1619
174	30.64	53.31	120.69	1669	31.24	54.35	119.65	1655	31.83	55.39	118.61	1640	32.43	56.42	117.58	1626
174.5	30.53	53.27	121.23	1677	31.12	54.31	120.19	1662	31.72	55.35	119.15	1648	32.31	56.38	118.12	1634
175	30.42	53.23	121.77	1684	31.01	54.27	120.73	1670	31.60	55.31	119.70	1655	32.20	56.34	118.66	1641
175.5	30.31	53.19	122.31	1692	30.90	54.23	121.27	1677	31.49	55.26	120.24	1663	32.08	56.30	119.20	1649
176	30.20	53.15	122.85	1699	30.79	54.19	121.81	1685	31.38	55.22	120.78	1670	31.97	56.26	119.74	1656
176.5	30.09	53.11	123.39	1707	30.68	54.14	122.36	1692	31.26	55.18	121.32	1678	31.85	56.22	120.28	1663
177	29.98	53.07	123.93	1714	30.57	54.10	122.90	1700	31.15	55.14	121.86	1685	31.74	56.18	120.82	1671
177.5	29.87	53.03	124.48	1721	30.46	54.06	123.44	1707	31.04	55.10	122.40	1693	31.63	56.14	121.36	1678
178	29.77	52.98	125.02	1729	30.35	54.02	123.98	1715	30.93	55.06	122.94	1700	31.51	56.10	121.90	1686
178.5	29.66	52.94	125.56	1736	30.24	53.98	124.52	1722	30.82	55.02	123.48	1708	31.40	56.06	122.44	1693
179	29.55	52.90	126.10	1744	30.13	53.94	125.06	1730	30.71	54.98	124.02	1715	31.29	56.01	122.99	1701
179.5	29.45	52.86	126.64	1751	30.03	53.90	125.60	1737	30.61	54.94	124.56	1723	31.18	55.97	123.53	1708
180	29.34	52.82	127.18	1759	29.92	53.86	126.14	1745	30.50	54.90	125.11	1730	31.07	55.93	124.07	1716
180.5	29.24	52.78	127.72	1766	29.82	53.82	126.68	1752	30.39	54.85	125.65	1738	30.96	55.89	124.61	1723
181	29.14	52.74	128.26	1774	29.71	53.78	127.22	1760	30.28	54.81	126.19	1745	30.86	55.85	125.15	1731
181.5	29.03	52.70	128.80	1781	29.61	53.73	127.77	1767	30.18	54.77	126.73	1753	30.75	55.81	125.69	1738
182	28.93	52.66	129.34	1789	29.50	53.69	128.31	1774	30.07	54.73	127.27	1760	30.64	55.77	126.23	1746
182.5	28.83	52.62	129.89	1796	29.40	53.65	128.85	1782	29.97	54.69	127.81	1768	30.54	55.73	126.77	1753
183	28.73	52.57	130.43	1804	29.30	53.61	129.39	1789	29.86	54.65	128.35	1775	30.43	55.69	127.31	1761
183.5	28.63	52.53	130.97	1811	29.19	53.57	129.93	1797	29.76	54.61	128.89	1783	30.32	55.65	127.85	1768

Body Composition   MALE   152-183.5 Lb.

Weight: Lb.	Waist: 41 inches Fat: %	Fat: Lb.	LBM: Lb.	RMR: Cal.	41.25 inches Fat: %	Fat: Lb.	LBM: Lb.	RMR: Cal.	41.5 inches Fat: %	Fat: Lb.	LBM: Lb.	RMR: Cal.	41.75 inches Fat: %	Fat: Lb.	LBM: Lb.	RMR: Cal.
152	38.99	59.27	92.73	1283	39.67	60.30	91.70	1268	40.36	61.34	90.66	1254	41.04	62.38	89.62	1239
152.5	38.84	59.23	93.28	1290	39.52	60.26	92.24	1276	40.20	61.30	91.20	1261	40.88	62.34	90.16	1247
153	38.68	59.18	93.82	1297	39.36	60.22	92.78	1283	40.04	61.26	91.74	1269	40.72	62.30	90.70	1254
153.5	38.53	59.14	94.36	1305	39.21	60.18	93.32	1291	39.88	61.22	92.28	1276	40.56	62.26	91.24	1262
154	38.38	59.10	94.90	1312	39.05	60.14	93.86	1298	39.73	61.18	92.82	1284	40.40	62.21	91.79	1269
154.5	38.23	59.06	95.44	1320	38.90	60.10	94.40	1306	39.57	61.14	93.36	1291	40.24	62.17	92.33	1277
155	38.08	59.02	95.98	1327	38.75	60.06	94.94	1313	39.42	61.10	93.91	1299	40.09	62.13	92.87	1284
155.5	37.93	58.98	96.52	1335	38.60	60.02	95.48	1321	39.26	61.05	94.45	1306	39.93	62.09	93.41	1292
156	37.78	58.94	97.06	1342	38.45	59.98	96.02	1328	39.11	61.01	94.99	1314	39.78	62.05	93.95	1299
156.5	37.63	58.90	97.60	1350	38.30	59.93	96.57	1336	38.96	60.97	95.53	1321	39.62	62.01	94.49	1307
157	37.49	58.86	98.14	1357	38.15	59.89	97.11	1343	38.81	60.93	96.07	1329	39.47	61.97	95.03	1314
157.5	37.34	58.82	98.69	1365	38.00	59.85	97.65	1350	38.66	60.89	96.61	1336	39.32	61.93	95.57	1322
158	37.20	58.77	99.23	1372	37.86	59.81	98.19	1358	38.51	60.85	97.15	1344	39.17	61.89	96.11	1329
158.5	37.06	58.73	99.77	1380	37.71	59.77	98.73	1365	38.36	60.81	97.69	1351	39.02	61.85	96.65	1337
159	36.91	58.69	100.31	1387	37.57	59.73	99.27	1373	38.22	60.77	98.23	1359	38.87	61.80	97.20	1344
159.5	36.77	58.65	100.85	1395	37.42	59.69	99.81	1380	38.07	60.73	98.77	1366	38.72	61.76	97.74	1352
160	36.63	58.61	101.39	1402	37.28	59.65	100.35	1388	37.93	60.69	99.32	1374	38.58	61.72	98.28	1359
160.5	36.49	58.57	101.93	1410	37.14	59.61	100.89	1395	37.78	60.64	99.86	1381	38.43	61.68	98.82	1367
161	36.35	58.53	102.47	1417	37.00	59.57	101.43	1403	37.64	60.60	100.40	1388	38.29	61.64	99.36	1374
161.5	36.21	58.49	103.01	1425	36.86	59.52	101.98	1410	37.50	60.56	100.94	1396	38.14	61.60	99.90	1382
162	36.08	58.45	103.55	1432	36.72	59.48	102.52	1418	37.36	60.52	101.48	1403	38.00	61.56	100.44	1389
162.5	35.94	58.41	104.10	1440	36.58	59.44	103.06	1425	37.22	60.48	102.02	1411	37.86	61.52	100.98	1397
163	35.81	58.36	104.64	1447	36.44	59.40	103.60	1433	37.08	60.44	102.56	1418	37.72	61.48	101.52	1404
163.5	35.67	58.32	105.18	1455	36.31	59.36	104.14	1440	36.94	60.40	103.10	1426	37.58	61.44	102.06	1412
164	35.54	58.28	105.72	1462	36.17	59.32	104.68	1448	36.80	60.36	103.64	1433	37.44	61.39	102.61	1419
164.5	35.40	58.24	106.26	1470	36.04	59.28	105.22	1455	36.67	60.32	104.18	1441	37.30	61.35	103.15	1427
165	35.27	58.20	106.80	1477	35.90	59.24	105.76	1463	36.53	60.28	104.73	1448	37.16	61.31	103.69	1434
165.5	35.14	58.16	107.34	1485	35.77	59.20	106.30	1470	36.40	60.23	105.27	1456	37.02	61.27	104.23	1441
166	35.01	58.12	107.88	1492	35.64	59.16	106.84	1478	36.26	60.19	105.81	1463	36.89	61.23	104.77	1449
166.5	34.88	58.08	108.42	1499	35.50	59.11	107.39	1485	36.13	60.15	106.35	1471	36.75	61.19	105.31	1456
167	34.75	58.04	108.96	1507	35.37	59.07	107.93	1493	35.99	60.11	106.89	1478	36.62	61.15	105.85	1464
167.5	34.62	58.00	109.51	1514	35.24	59.03	108.47	1500	35.86	60.07	107.43	1486	36.48	61.11	106.39	1471
168	34.50	57.95	110.05	1522	35.11	58.99	109.01	1508	35.73	60.03	107.97	1493	36.35	61.07	106.93	1479
168.5	34.37	57.91	110.59	1529	34.99	58.95	109.55	1515	35.60	59.99	108.51	1501	36.22	61.03	107.47	1486
169	34.24	57.87	111.13	1537	34.86	58.91	110.09	1523	35.47	59.95	109.05	1508	36.09	60.98	108.02	1494
169.5	34.12	57.83	111.67	1544	34.73	58.87	110.63	1530	35.34	59.91	109.59	1516	35.95	60.94	108.56	1501
170	33.99	57.79	112.21	1552	34.60	58.83	111.17	1538	35.21	59.87	110.14	1523	35.83	60.90	109.10	1509
170.5	33.87	57.75	112.75	1559	34.48	58.79	111.71	1545	35.09	59.82	110.68	1531	35.70	60.86	109.64	1516
171	33.75	57.71	113.29	1567	34.35	58.75	112.25	1552	34.96	59.78	111.22	1538	35.57	60.82	110.18	1524
171.5	33.63	57.67	113.83	1574	34.23	58.70	112.80	1560	34.83	59.74	111.76	1546	35.44	60.78	110.72	1531
172	33.50	57.63	114.37	1582	34.11	58.66	113.34	1567	34.71	59.70	112.30	1553	35.31	60.74	111.26	1539
172.5	33.38	57.59	114.92	1589	33.98	58.62	113.88	1575	34.59	59.66	112.84	1561	35.19	60.70	111.80	1546
173	33.26	57.54	115.46	1597	33.86	58.58	114.42	1582	34.46	59.62	113.38	1568	35.06	60.66	112.34	1554
173.5	33.14	57.50	116.00	1604	33.74	58.54	114.96	1590	34.34	59.58	113.92	1576	34.94	60.62	112.88	1561
174	33.02	57.46	116.54	1612	33.62	58.50	115.50	1597	34.22	59.54	114.46	1583	34.81	60.57	113.43	1569
174.5	32.91	57.42	117.08	1619	33.50	58.46	116.04	1605	34.10	59.50	115.00	1591	34.69	60.53	113.97	1576
175	32.79	57.38	117.62	1627	33.38	58.42	116.58	1612	33.97	59.46	115.55	1598	34.57	60.49	114.51	1584
175.5	32.67	57.34	118.16	1634	33.26	58.38	117.12	1620	33.85	59.41	116.09	1605	34.45	60.45	115.05	1591
176	32.56	57.30	118.70	1642	33.15	58.34	117.66	1627	33.73	59.37	116.63	1613	34.32	60.41	115.59	1599
176.5	32.44	57.26	119.24	1649	33.03	58.29	118.21	1635	33.62	59.33	117.17	1620	34.20	60.37	116.13	1606
177	32.33	57.22	119.78	1657	32.91	58.25	118.75	1642	33.50	59.29	117.71	1628	34.08	60.33	116.67	1614
177.5	32.21	57.18	120.33	1664	32.80	58.21	119.29	1650	33.38	59.25	118.25	1635	33.96	60.29	117.21	1621
178	32.10	57.13	120.87	1672	32.68	58.17	119.83	1657	33.26	59.21	118.79	1643	33.85	60.25	117.75	1629
178.5	31.98	57.09	121.41	1679	32.57	58.13	120.37	1665	33.15	59.17	119.33	1650	33.73	60.21	118.29	1636
179	31.87	57.05	121.95	1687	32.45	58.09	120.91	1672	33.03	59.13	119.87	1658	33.61	60.16	118.84	1643
179.5	31.76	57.01	122.49	1694	32.34	58.05	121.45	1680	32.92	59.09	120.41	1665	33.49	60.12	119.38	1651
180	31.65	56.97	123.03	1702	32.23	58.01	121.99	1687	32.80	59.05	120.96	1673	33.38	60.08	119.92	1658
180.5	31.54	56.93	123.57	1709	32.11	57.97	122.53	1695	32.69	59.00	121.50	1680	33.26	60.04	120.46	1666
181	31.43	56.89	124.11	1716	32.00	57.93	123.07	1702	32.58	58.96	122.04	1688	33.15	60.00	121.00	1673
181.5	31.32	56.85	124.65	1724	31.89	57.88	123.62	1710	32.46	58.92	122.58	1695	33.04	59.96	121.54	1681
182	31.21	56.81	125.19	1731	31.78	57.84	124.16	1717	32.35	58.88	123.12	1703	32.92	59.92	122.08	1688
182.5	31.10	56.77	125.74	1739	31.67	57.80	124.70	1725	32.24	58.84	123.66	1710	32.81	59.88	122.62	1696
183	31.00	56.72	126.28	1746	31.56	57.76	125.24	1732	32.13	58.80	124.20	1718	32.70	59.84	123.16	1703
183.5	30.89	56.68	126.82	1754	31.46	57.72	125.78	1740	32.02	58.76	124.74	1725	32.59	59.80	123.70	1711

Body Composition MALE 152-183.5 Lb.

Weight: Lb.	Waist: 42 inches Fat: %	Fat: Lb.	LBM: Lb.	RMR: Cal.	42.25 inches Fat: %	Fat: Lb.	LBM: Lb.	RMR: Cal.	42.5 inches Fat: %	Fat: Lb.	LBM: Lb.	RMR: Cal.	42.75 inches Fat: %	Fat: Lb.	LBM: Lb.	RMR: Cal.
152	41.72	63.42	88.58	1225	42.40	64.45	87.55	1211	43.09	65.49	86.51	1196	43.77	66.53	85.47	1182
152.5	41.56	63.38	89.13	1233	42.24	64.41	88.09	1218	42.92	65.45	87.05	1204	43.60	66.49	86.01	1190
153	41.39	63.33	89.67	1240	42.07	64.37	88.63	1226	42.75	65.41	87.59	1211	43.43	66.45	86.55	1197
153.5	41.23	63.29	90.21	1248	41.91	64.33	89.17	1233	42.59	65.37	88.13	1219	43.26	66.41	87.09	1205
154	41.07	63.25	90.75	1255	41.75	64.29	89.71	1241	42.42	65.33	88.67	1226	43.09	66.36	87.64	1212
154.5	40.91	63.21	91.29	1263	41.58	64.25	90.25	1248	42.26	65.29	89.21	1234	42.93	66.32	88.18	1219
155	40.75	63.17	91.83	1270	41.42	64.21	90.79	1256	42.09	65.25	89.76	1241	42.76	66.28	88.72	1227
155.5	40.60	63.13	92.37	1277	41.26	64.17	91.33	1263	41.93	65.20	90.30	1249	42.60	66.24	89.26	1234
156	40.44	63.09	92.91	1285	41.11	64.13	91.87	1271	41.77	65.16	90.84	1256	42.44	66.20	89.80	1242
156.5	40.29	63.05	93.45	1292	40.95	64.08	92.42	1278	41.61	65.12	91.38	1264	42.27	66.16	90.34	1249
157	40.13	63.01	93.99	1300	40.79	64.04	92.96	1286	41.45	65.08	91.92	1271	42.11	66.12	90.88	1257
157.5	39.98	62.97	94.54	1307	40.64	64.00	93.50	1293	41.30	65.04	92.46	1279	41.95	66.08	91.42	1264
158	39.83	62.92	95.08	1315	40.48	63.96	94.04	1301	41.14	65.00	93.00	1286	41.80	66.04	91.96	1272
158.5	39.67	62.88	95.62	1322	40.33	63.92	94.58	1308	40.98	64.96	93.54	1294	41.64	66.00	92.50	1279
159	39.52	62.84	96.16	1330	40.18	63.88	95.12	1316	40.83	64.92	94.08	1301	41.48	65.95	93.05	1287
159.5	39.37	62.80	96.70	1337	40.02	63.84	95.66	1323	40.67	64.88	94.62	1309	41.33	65.91	93.59	1294
160	39.23	62.76	97.24	1345	39.87	63.80	96.20	1330	40.52	64.84	95.17	1316	41.17	65.87	94.13	1302
160.5	39.08	62.72	97.78	1352	39.72	63.76	96.74	1338	40.37	64.79	95.71	1324	41.02	65.83	94.67	1309
161	38.93	62.68	98.32	1360	39.57	63.72	97.28	1345	40.22	64.75	96.25	1331	40.86	65.79	95.21	1317
161.5	38.78	62.64	98.86	1367	39.43	63.67	97.83	1353	40.07	64.71	96.79	1339	40.71	65.75	95.75	1324
162	38.64	62.60	99.40	1375	39.28	63.63	98.37	1360	39.92	64.67	97.33	1346	40.56	65.71	96.29	1332
162.5	38.50	62.56	99.95	1382	39.13	63.59	98.91	1368	39.77	64.63	97.87	1354	40.41	65.67	96.83	1339
163	38.35	62.51	100.49	1390	38.99	63.55	99.45	1375	39.63	64.59	98.41	1361	40.26	65.63	97.37	1347
163.5	38.21	62.47	101.03	1397	38.84	63.51	99.99	1383	39.48	64.55	98.95	1369	40.11	65.59	97.91	1354
164	38.07	62.43	101.57	1405	38.70	63.47	100.53	1390	39.33	64.51	99.49	1376	39.97	65.54	98.46	1362
164.5	37.93	62.39	102.11	1412	38.56	63.43	101.07	1398	39.19	64.47	100.03	1383	39.82	65.50	99.00	1369
165	37.79	62.35	102.65	1420	38.42	63.39	101.61	1405	39.05	64.43	100.58	1391	39.67	65.46	99.54	1377
165.5	37.65	62.31	103.19	1427	38.28	63.35	102.15	1413	38.90	64.38	101.12	1398	39.53	65.42	100.08	1384
166	37.51	62.27	103.73	1435	38.14	63.31	102.69	1420	38.76	64.34	101.66	1406	39.39	65.38	100.62	1392
166.5	37.37	62.23	104.27	1442	38.00	63.26	103.24	1428	38.62	64.30	102.20	1413	39.24	65.34	101.16	1399
167	37.24	62.19	104.81	1450	37.86	63.22	103.78	1435	38.48	64.26	102.74	1421	39.10	65.30	101.70	1407
167.5	37.10	62.15	105.36	1457	37.72	63.18	104.32	1443	38.34	64.22	103.28	1428	38.96	65.26	102.24	1414
168	36.97	62.10	105.90	1465	37.58	63.14	104.86	1450	38.20	64.18	103.82	1436	38.82	65.22	102.78	1421
168.5	36.83	62.06	106.44	1472	37.45	63.10	105.40	1458	38.06	64.14	104.36	1443	38.68	65.18	103.32	1429
169	36.70	62.02	106.98	1480	37.31	63.06	105.94	1465	37.93	64.10	104.90	1451	38.54	65.13	103.87	1436
169.5	36.57	61.98	107.52	1487	37.18	63.02	106.48	1473	37.79	64.06	105.44	1458	38.40	65.09	104.41	1444
170	36.44	61.94	108.06	1494	37.05	62.98	107.02	1480	37.66	64.02	105.99	1466	38.27	65.05	104.95	1451
170.5	36.30	61.90	108.60	1502	36.91	62.94	107.56	1488	37.52	63.97	106.53	1473	38.13	65.01	105.49	1459
171	36.17	61.86	109.14	1509	36.78	62.90	108.10	1495	37.39	63.93	107.07	1481	37.99	64.97	106.03	1466
171.5	36.04	61.82	109.68	1517	36.65	62.85	108.65	1503	37.25	63.89	107.61	1488	37.86	64.93	106.57	1474
172	35.92	61.78	110.22	1524	36.52	62.81	109.19	1510	37.12	63.85	108.15	1496	37.73	64.89	107.11	1481
172.5	35.79	61.74	110.77	1532	36.39	62.77	109.73	1518	36.99	63.81	108.69	1503	37.59	64.85	107.65	1489
173	35.66	61.69	111.31	1539	36.26	62.73	110.27	1525	36.86	63.77	109.23	1511	37.46	64.81	108.19	1496
173.5	35.53	61.65	111.85	1547	36.13	62.69	110.81	1532	36.73	63.73	109.77	1518	37.33	64.77	108.73	1504
174	35.41	61.61	112.39	1554	36.01	62.65	111.35	1540	36.60	63.69	110.31	1526	37.20	64.72	109.28	1511
174.5	35.28	61.57	112.93	1562	35.88	62.61	111.89	1547	36.47	63.65	110.85	1533	37.07	64.68	109.82	1519
175	35.16	61.53	113.47	1569	35.75	62.57	112.43	1555	36.35	63.61	111.40	1541	36.94	64.64	110.36	1526
175.5	35.04	61.49	114.01	1577	35.63	62.53	112.97	1562	36.22	63.56	111.94	1548	36.81	64.60	110.90	1534
176	34.91	61.45	114.55	1584	35.50	62.49	113.51	1570	36.09	63.52	112.48	1556	36.68	64.56	111.44	1541
176.5	34.79	61.41	115.09	1592	35.38	62.44	114.06	1577	35.97	63.48	113.02	1563	36.55	64.52	111.98	1549
177	34.67	61.37	115.63	1599	35.26	62.40	114.60	1585	35.84	63.44	113.56	1571	36.43	64.48	112.52	1556
177.5	34.55	61.33	116.18	1607	35.13	62.36	115.14	1592	35.72	63.40	114.10	1578	36.30	64.44	113.06	1564
178	34.43	61.28	116.72	1614	35.01	62.32	115.68	1600	35.59	63.36	114.64	1585	36.18	64.40	113.60	1571
178.5	34.31	61.24	117.26	1622	34.89	62.28	116.22	1607	35.47	63.32	115.18	1593	36.05	64.36	114.14	1579
179	34.19	61.20	117.80	1629	34.77	62.24	116.76	1615	35.35	63.28	115.72	1600	35.93	64.31	114.69	1586
179.5	34.07	61.16	118.34	1637	34.65	62.20	117.30	1622	35.23	63.24	116.26	1608	35.81	64.27	115.23	1594
180	33.96	61.12	118.88	1644	34.53	62.16	117.84	1630	35.11	63.20	116.81	1615	35.68	64.23	115.77	1601
180.5	33.84	61.08	119.42	1652	34.41	62.12	118.38	1637	34.99	63.15	117.35	1623	35.56	64.19	116.31	1609
181	33.72	61.04	119.96	1659	34.30	62.08	118.92	1645	34.87	63.11	117.89	1630	35.44	64.15	116.85	1616
181.5	33.61	61.00	120.50	1667	34.18	62.03	119.47	1652	34.75	63.07	118.43	1638	35.32	64.11	117.39	1624
182	33.49	60.96	121.04	1674	34.06	61.99	120.01	1660	34.63	63.03	118.97	1645	35.20	64.07	117.93	1631
182.5	33.38	60.92	121.59	1682	33.95	61.95	120.55	1667	34.52	62.99	119.51	1653	35.08	64.03	118.47	1638
183	33.26	60.87	122.13	1689	33.83	61.91	121.09	1675	34.40	62.95	120.05	1660	34.97	63.99	119.01	1646
183.5	33.15	60.83	122.67	1696	33.72	61.87	121.63	1682	34.28	62.91	120.59	1668	34.85	63.95	119.55	1653

Body Composition MALE 184-215.5 Lb.

Weight: Lb.	Waist: 29 inches				29.25 inches				29.5 inches				29.75 inches			
	Fat: %	Fat: Lb.	LBM: Lb.	RMR: Cal.	Fat: %	Fat: Lb.	LBM: Lb.	RMR: Cal.	Fat: %	Fat: Lb.	LBM: Lb.	RMR: Cal.	Fat: %	Fat: Lb.	LBM: Lb.	RMR: Cal.
184	3.72	6.84	177.16	2450	4.28	7.88	176.12	2436	4.85	8.92	175.08	2421	5.41	9.95	174.05	2407
184.5	3.69	6.80	177.70	2458	4.25	7.84	176.66	2443	4.81	8.88	175.62	2429	5.37	9.91	174.59	2415
185	3.65	6.76	178.24	2465	4.21	7.80	177.20	2451	4.78	8.83	176.17	2436	5.34	9.87	175.13	2422
185.5	3.62	6.72	178.78	2473	4.18	7.76	177.74	2458	4.74	8.79	176.71	2444	5.30	9.83	175.67	2429
186	3.59	6.68	179.32	2480	4.15	7.72	178.28	2466	4.71	8.75	177.25	2451	5.26	9.79	176.21	2437
186.5	3.56	6.64	179.86	2488	4.12	7.67	178.83	2473	4.67	8.71	177.79	2459	5.23	9.75	176.75	2444
187	3.53	6.60	180.40	2495	4.08	7.63	179.37	2481	4.64	8.67	178.33	2466	5.19	9.71	177.29	2452
187.5	3.50	6.56	180.95	2502	4.05	7.59	179.91	2488	4.60	8.63	178.87	2474	5.16	9.67	177.83	2459
188	3.46	6.51	181.49	2510	4.02	7.55	180.45	2496	4.57	8.59	179.41	2481	5.12	9.63	178.37	2467
188.5	3.43	6.47	182.03	2517	3.98	7.51	180.99	2503	4.53	8.55	179.95	2489	5.09	9.59	178.91	2474
189	3.40	6.43	182.57	2525	3.95	7.47	181.53	2511	4.50	8.51	180.49	2496	5.05	9.54	179.46	2482
189.5	3.37	6.39	183.11	2532	3.92	7.43	182.07	2518	4.47	8.47	181.03	2504	5.02	9.50	180.00	2489
190	3.34	6.35	183.65	2540	3.89	7.39	182.61	2526	4.43	8.43	181.58	2511	4.98	9.46	180.54	2497
190.5	3.31	6.31	184.19	2547	3.86	7.35	183.15	2533	4.40	8.38	182.12	2519	4.95	9.42	181.08	2504
191	3.28	6.27	184.73	2555	3.82	7.31	183.69	2540	4.37	8.34	182.66	2526	4.91	9.38	181.62	2512
191.5	3.25	6.23	185.27	2562	3.79	7.26	184.24	2548	4.34	8.30	183.20	2534	4.88	9.34	182.16	2519
192	3.22	6.19	185.81	2570	3.76	7.22	184.78	2555	4.30	8.26	183.74	2541	4.84	9.30	182.70	2527
192.5	3.19	6.14	186.36	2577	3.73	7.18	185.32	2563	4.27	8.22	184.28	2549	4.81	9.26	183.24	2534
193	3.16	6.10	186.90	2585	3.70	7.14	185.86	2570	4.24	8.18	184.82	2556	4.78	9.22	183.78	2542
193.5	3.13	6.06	187.44	2592	3.67	7.10	186.40	2578	4.21	8.14	185.36	2564	4.74	9.18	184.32	2549
194	3.10	6.02	187.98	2600	3.64	7.06	186.94	2585	4.17	8.10	185.90	2571	4.71	9.13	184.87	2557
194.5	3.08	5.98	188.52	2607	3.61	7.02	187.48	2593	4.14	8.06	186.44	2579	4.68	9.09	185.41	2564
195	3.05	5.94	189.06	2615	3.58	6.98	188.02	2600	4.11	8.01	186.99	2586	4.64	9.05	185.95	2572
195.5	3.02	5.90	189.60	2622	3.55	6.94	188.56	2608	4.08	7.97	187.53	2593	4.61	9.01	186.49	2579
196	2.99	5.86	190.14	2630	3.52	6.90	189.10	2615	4.05	7.93	188.07	2601	4.58	8.97	187.03	2587
196.5	2.96	5.82	190.68	2637	3.49	6.85	189.65	2623	4.02	7.89	188.61	2608	4.54	8.93	187.57	2594
197	2.93	5.78	191.22	2645	3.46	6.81	190.19	2630	3.99	7.85	189.15	2616	4.51	8.89	188.11	2602
197.5	2.90	5.73	191.77	2652	3.43	6.77	190.73	2638	3.95	7.81	189.69	2623	4.48	8.85	188.65	2609
198	2.88	5.69	192.31	2660	3.40	6.73	191.27	2645	3.92	7.77	190.23	2631	4.45	8.81	189.19	2617
198.5	2.85	5.65	192.85	2667	3.37	6.69	191.81	2653	3.89	7.73	190.77	2638	4.42	8.77	189.73	2624
199	2.82	5.61	193.39	2675	3.34	6.65	192.35	2660	3.86	7.69	191.31	2646	4.38	8.72	190.28	2632
199.5	2.79	5.57	193.93	2682	3.31	6.61	192.89	2668	3.83	7.65	191.85	2653	4.35	8.68	190.82	2639
200	2.77	5.53	194.47	2690	3.28	6.57	193.43	2675	3.80	7.61	192.40	2661	4.32	8.64	191.36	2646
200.5	2.74	5.49	195.01	2697	3.26	6.53	193.97	2683	3.77	7.56	192.94	2668	4.29	8.60	191.90	2654
201	2.71	5.45	195.55	2704	3.23	6.49	194.51	2690	3.74	7.52	193.48	2676	4.26	8.56	192.44	2661
201.5	2.68	5.41	196.09	2712	3.20	6.44	195.06	2698	3.71	7.48	194.02	2683	4.23	8.52	192.98	2669
202	2.66	5.37	196.63	2719	3.17	6.40	195.60	2705	3.68	7.44	194.56	2691	4.20	8.48	193.52	2676
202.5	2.63	5.32	197.18	2727	3.14	6.36	196.14	2713	3.65	7.40	195.10	2698	4.17	8.44	194.06	2684
203	2.60	5.28	197.72	2734	3.11	6.32	196.68	2720	3.63	7.36	195.64	2706	4.14	8.40	194.60	2691
203.5	2.58	5.24	198.26	2742	3.09	6.28	197.22	2728	3.60	7.32	196.18	2713	4.11	8.36	195.14	2699
204	2.55	5.20	198.80	2749	3.06	6.24	197.76	2735	3.57	7.28	196.72	2721	4.08	8.31	195.69	2706
204.5	2.52	5.16	199.34	2757	3.03	6.20	198.30	2743	3.54	7.24	197.26	2728	4.05	8.27	196.23	2714
205	2.50	5.12	199.88	2764	3.00	6.16	198.84	2750	3.51	7.19	197.81	2736	4.02	8.23	196.77	2721
205.5	2.47	5.08	200.42	2772	2.98	6.12	199.38	2757	3.48	7.15	198.35	2743	3.99	8.19	197.31	2729
206	2.45	5.04	200.96	2779	2.95	6.08	199.92	2765	3.45	7.11	198.89	2751	3.96	8.15	197.85	2736
206.5	2.42	5.00	201.50	2787	2.92	6.03	200.47	2772	3.42	7.07	199.43	2758	3.93	8.11	198.39	2744
207	2.39	4.96	202.04	2794	2.90	5.99	201.01	2780	3.40	7.03	199.97	2766	3.90	8.07	198.93	2751
207.5	2.37	4.91	202.59	2802	2.87	5.95	201.55	2787	3.37	6.99	200.51	2773	3.87	8.03	199.47	2759
208	2.34	4.87	203.13	2809	2.84	5.91	202.09	2795	3.34	6.95	201.05	2781	3.84	7.99	200.01	2766
208.5	2.32	4.83	203.67	2817	2.82	5.87	202.63	2802	3.31	6.91	201.59	2788	3.81	7.95	200.55	2774
209	2.29	4.79	204.21	2824	2.79	5.83	203.17	2810	3.29	6.87	202.13	2795	3.78	7.90	201.10	2781
209.5	2.27	4.75	204.75	2832	2.76	5.79	203.71	2817	3.26	6.83	202.67	2803	3.75	7.86	201.64	2789
210	2.24	4.71	205.29	2839	2.74	5.75	204.25	2825	3.23	6.78	203.22	2810	3.73	7.82	202.18	2796
210.5	2.22	4.67	205.83	2847	2.71	5.71	204.79	2832	3.20	6.74	203.76	2818	3.70	7.78	202.72	2804
211	2.19	4.63	206.37	2854	2.69	5.67	205.33	2840	3.18	6.70	204.30	2825	3.67	7.74	203.26	2811
211.5	2.17	4.59	206.91	2862	2.66	5.62	205.88	2847	3.15	6.66	204.84	2833	3.64	7.70	203.80	2819
212	2.14	4.55	207.45	2869	2.63	5.58	206.42	2855	3.12	6.62	205.38	2840	3.61	7.66	204.34	2826
212.5	2.12	4.51	208.00	2877	2.61	5.54	206.96	2862	3.10	6.58	205.92	2848	3.58	7.62	204.88	2834
213	2.10	4.46	208.54	2884	2.58	5.50	207.50	2870	3.07	6.54	206.46	2855	3.56	7.58	205.42	2841
213.5	2.07	4.42	209.08	2892	2.56	5.46	208.04	2877	3.04	6.50	207.00	2863	3.53	7.54	205.96	2848
214	2.05	4.38	209.62	2899	2.53	5.42	208.58	2885	3.02	6.46	207.54	2870	3.50	7.49	206.51	2856
214.5	2.02	4.34	210.16	2906	2.51	5.38	209.12	2892	2.99	6.42	208.08	2878	3.47	7.45	207.05	2863
215	2.00	4.30	210.70	2914	2.48	5.34	209.66	2900	2.97	6.38	208.63	2885	3.45	7.41	207.59	2871
215.5	1.98	4.26	211.24	2921	2.46	5.30	210.20	2907	2.94	6.33	209.17	2893	3.42	7.37	208.13	2878

Body Composition MALE 184-215.5 Lb.

Weight: Lb.	Waist: 30 inches				30.25 inches				30.5 inches				30.75 inches			
	Fat: %	Fat: Lb.	LBM: Lb.	RMR: Cal.	Fat: %	Fat: Lb.	LBM: Lb.	RMR: Cal.	Fat: %	Fat: Lb.	LBM: Lb.	RMR: Cal.	Fat: %	Fat: Lb.	LBM: Lb.	RMR: Cal.
184	5.97	10.99	173.01	2393	6.54	12.03	171.97	2378	7.10	13.07	170.93	2364	7.67	14.10	169.90	2350
184.5	5.94	10.95	173.55	2400	6.50	11.99	172.51	2386	7.06	13.03	171.47	2371	7.62	14.06	170.44	2357
185	5.90	10.91	174.09	2408	6.46	11.95	173.05	2393	7.02	12.99	172.02	2379	7.58	14.02	170.98	2365
185.5	5.86	10.87	174.63	2415	6.42	11.91	173.59	2401	6.98	12.94	172.56	2386	7.54	13.98	171.52	2372
186	5.82	10.83	175.17	2423	6.38	11.87	174.13	2408	6.94	12.90	173.10	2394	7.49	13.94	172.06	2380
186.5	5.78	10.79	175.71	2430	6.34	11.82	174.68	2416	6.90	12.86	173.64	2401	7.45	13.90	172.60	2387
187	5.75	10.75	176.25	2438	6.30	11.78	175.22	2423	6.86	12.82	174.18	2409	7.41	13.86	173.14	2395
187.5	5.71	10.71	176.80	2445	6.26	11.74	175.76	2431	6.82	12.78	174.72	2416	7.37	13.82	173.68	2402
188	5.67	10.66	177.34	2453	6.22	11.70	176.30	2438	6.78	12.74	175.26	2424	7.33	13.78	174.22	2410
188.5	5.64	10.62	177.88	2460	6.19	11.66	176.84	2446	6.74	12.70	175.80	2431	7.29	13.74	174.76	2417
189	5.60	10.58	178.42	2468	6.15	11.62	177.38	2453	6.70	12.66	176.34	2439	7.25	13.69	175.31	2424
189.5	5.56	10.54	178.96	2475	6.11	11.58	177.92	2461	6.66	12.62	176.88	2446	7.21	13.65	175.85	2432
190	5.53	10.50	179.50	2482	6.07	11.54	178.46	2468	6.62	12.58	177.43	2454	7.16	13.61	176.39	2439
190.5	5.49	10.46	180.04	2490	6.03	11.50	179.00	2476	6.58	12.53	177.97	2461	7.12	13.57	176.93	2447
191	5.45	10.42	180.58	2497	6.00	11.46	179.54	2483	6.54	12.49	178.51	2469	7.08	13.53	177.47	2454
191.5	5.42	10.38	181.12	2505	5.96	11.41	180.09	2491	6.50	12.45	179.05	2476	7.04	13.49	178.01	2462
192	5.38	10.34	181.66	2512	5.92	11.37	180.63	2498	6.46	12.41	179.59	2484	7.00	13.45	178.55	2469
192.5	5.35	10.30	182.21	2520	5.89	11.33	181.17	2506	6.43	12.37	180.13	2491	6.96	13.41	179.09	2477
193	5.31	10.25	182.75	2527	5.85	11.29	181.71	2513	6.39	12.33	180.67	2499	6.93	13.37	179.63	2484
193.5	5.28	10.21	183.29	2535	5.81	11.25	182.25	2521	6.35	12.29	181.21	2506	6.89	13.33	180.17	2492
194	5.24	10.17	183.83	2542	5.78	11.21	182.79	2528	6.31	12.25	181.75	2514	6.85	13.28	180.72	2499
194.5	5.21	10.13	184.37	2550	5.74	11.17	183.33	2535	6.28	12.21	182.29	2521	6.81	13.24	181.26	2507
195	5.17	10.09	184.91	2557	5.71	11.13	183.87	2543	6.24	12.17	182.84	2529	6.77	13.20	181.80	2514
195.5	5.14	10.05	185.45	2565	5.67	11.09	184.41	2550	6.20	12.12	183.38	2536	6.73	13.16	182.34	2522
196	5.11	10.01	185.99	2572	5.64	11.05	184.95	2558	6.16	12.08	183.92	2544	6.69	13.12	182.88	2529
196.5	5.07	9.97	186.53	2580	5.60	11.00	185.50	2565	6.13	12.04	184.46	2551	6.66	13.08	183.42	2537
197	5.04	9.93	187.07	2587	5.57	10.96	186.04	2573	6.09	12.00	185.00	2559	6.62	13.04	183.96	2544
197.5	5.01	9.88	187.62	2595	5.53	10.92	186.58	2580	6.06	11.96	185.54	2566	6.58	13.00	184.50	2552
198	4.97	9.84	188.16	2602	5.50	10.88	187.12	2588	6.02	11.92	186.08	2574	6.54	12.96	185.04	2559
198.5	4.94	9.80	188.70	2610	5.46	10.84	187.66	2595	5.98	11.88	186.62	2581	6.51	12.92	185.58	2567
199	4.91	9.76	189.24	2617	5.43	10.80	188.20	2603	5.95	11.84	187.16	2588	6.47	12.87	186.13	2574
199.5	4.87	9.72	189.78	2625	5.39	10.76	188.74	2610	5.91	11.80	187.70	2596	6.43	12.83	186.67	2582
200	4.84	9.68	190.32	2632	5.36	10.72	189.28	2618	5.88	11.76	188.25	2603	6.40	12.79	187.21	2589
200.5	4.81	9.64	190.86	2640	5.32	10.68	189.82	2625	5.84	11.71	188.79	2611	6.36	12.75	187.75	2597
201	4.78	9.60	191.40	2647	5.29	10.64	190.36	2633	5.81	11.67	189.33	2618	6.32	12.71	188.29	2604
201.5	4.74	9.56	191.94	2655	5.26	10.59	190.91	2640	5.77	11.63	189.87	2626	6.29	12.67	188.83	2612
202	4.71	9.52	192.48	2662	5.22	10.55	191.45	2648	5.74	11.59	190.41	2633	6.25	12.63	189.37	2619
202.5	4.68	9.47	193.03	2670	5.19	10.51	191.99	2655	5.70	11.55	190.95	2641	6.22	12.59	189.91	2626
203	4.65	9.43	193.57	2677	5.16	10.47	192.53	2663	5.67	11.51	191.49	2648	6.18	12.55	190.45	2634
203.5	4.62	9.39	194.11	2684	5.13	10.43	193.07	2670	5.64	11.47	192.03	2656	6.15	12.51	190.99	2641
204	4.58	9.35	194.65	2692	5.09	10.39	193.61	2678	5.60	11.43	192.57	2663	6.11	12.46	191.54	2649
204.5	4.55	9.31	195.19	2699	5.06	10.35	194.15	2685	5.57	11.39	193.11	2671	6.08	12.42	192.08	2656
205	4.52	9.27	195.73	2707	5.03	10.31	194.69	2693	5.53	11.35	193.66	2678	6.04	12.38	192.62	2664
205.5	4.49	9.23	196.27	2714	5.00	10.27	195.23	2700	5.50	11.30	194.20	2686	6.01	12.34	193.16	2671
206	4.46	9.19	196.81	2722	4.96	10.23	195.77	2708	5.47	11.26	194.74	2693	5.97	12.30	193.70	2679
206.5	4.43	9.15	197.35	2729	4.93	10.18	196.32	2715	5.43	11.22	195.28	2701	5.94	12.26	194.24	2686
207	4.40	9.11	197.89	2737	4.90	10.14	196.86	2723	5.40	11.18	195.82	2708	5.90	12.22	194.78	2694
207.5	4.37	9.07	198.44	2744	4.87	10.10	197.40	2730	5.37	11.14	196.36	2716	5.87	12.18	195.32	2701
208	4.34	9.02	198.98	2752	4.84	10.06	197.94	2737	5.34	11.10	196.90	2723	5.83	12.14	195.86	2709
208.5	4.31	8.98	199.52	2759	4.81	10.02	198.48	2745	5.30	11.06	197.44	2731	5.80	12.10	196.40	2716
209	4.28	8.94	200.06	2767	4.77	9.98	199.02	2752	5.27	11.02	197.98	2738	5.77	12.05	196.95	2724
209.5	4.25	8.90	200.60	2774	4.74	9.94	199.56	2760	5.24	10.98	198.52	2746	5.73	12.01	197.49	2731
210	4.22	8.86	201.14	2782	4.71	9.90	200.10	2767	5.21	10.94	199.07	2753	5.70	11.97	198.03	2739
210.5	4.19	8.82	201.68	2789	4.68	9.86	200.64	2775	5.18	10.89	199.61	2761	5.67	11.93	198.57	2746
211	4.16	8.78	202.22	2797	4.65	9.82	201.18	2782	5.14	10.85	200.15	2768	5.64	11.89	199.11	2754
211.5	4.13	8.74	202.76	2804	4.62	9.77	201.73	2790	5.11	10.81	200.69	2776	5.60	11.85	199.65	2761
212	4.10	8.70	203.30	2812	4.59	9.73	202.27	2797	5.08	10.77	201.23	2783	5.57	11.81	200.19	2769
212.5	4.07	8.66	203.85	2819	4.56	9.69	202.81	2805	5.05	10.73	201.77	2790	5.54	11.77	200.73	2776
213	4.04	8.61	204.39	2827	4.53	9.65	203.35	2812	5.02	10.69	202.31	2798	5.51	11.73	201.27	2784
213.5	4.02	8.57	204.93	2834	4.50	9.61	203.89	2820	4.99	10.65	202.85	2805	5.47	11.69	201.81	2791
214	3.99	8.53	205.47	2842	4.47	9.57	204.43	2827	4.96	10.61	203.39	2813	5.44	11.64	202.36	2799
214.5	3.96	8.49	206.01	2849	4.44	9.53	204.97	2835	4.93	10.57	203.93	2820	5.41	11.60	202.90	2806
215	3.93	8.45	206.55	2857	4.41	9.49	205.51	2842	4.90	10.53	204.48	2828	5.38	11.56	203.44	2814
215.5	3.90	8.41	207.09	2864	4.38	9.45	206.05	2850	4.86	10.48	205.02	2835	5.35	11.52	203.98	2821

Body Composition MALE 184-215.5 Lb.

Weight: Lb.	Waist: 31 inches				31.25 inches				31.5 inches				31.75 inches			
	Fat: %	Fat: Lb.	LBM: Lb.	RMR: Cal.	Fat: %	Fat: Lb.	LBM: Lb.	RMR: Cal.	Fat: %	Fat: Lb.	LBM: Lb.	RMR: Cal.	Fat: %	Fat: Lb.	LBM: Lb.	RMR: Cal.
184	8.23	15.14	168.86	2335	8.79	16.18	167.82	2321	9.36	17.22	166.78	2307	9.92	18.25	165.75	2292
184.5	8.18	15.10	169.40	2343	8.75	16.14	168.36	2328	9.31	17.18	167.32	2314	9.87	18.21	166.29	2300
185	8.14	15.06	169.94	2350	8.70	16.10	168.90	2336	9.26	17.14	167.87	2322	9.82	18.17	166.83	2307
185.5	8.10	15.02	170.48	2358	8.66	16.06	169.44	2343	9.22	17.09	168.41	2329	9.77	18.13	167.37	2315
186	8.05	14.98	171.02	2365	8.61	16.02	169.98	2351	9.17	17.05	168.95	2337	9.73	18.09	167.91	2322
186.5	8.01	14.94	171.56	2373	8.57	15.97	170.53	2358	9.12	17.01	169.49	2344	9.68	18.05	168.45	2330
187	7.97	14.90	172.10	2380	8.52	15.93	171.07	2366	9.08	16.97	170.03	2352	9.63	18.01	168.99	2337
187.5	7.92	14.86	172.65	2388	8.48	15.89	171.61	2373	9.03	16.93	170.57	2359	9.58	17.97	169.53	2345
188	7.88	14.81	173.19	2395	8.43	15.85	172.15	2381	8.98	16.89	171.11	2366	9.54	17.93	170.07	2352
188.5	7.84	14.77	173.73	2403	8.39	15.81	172.69	2388	8.94	16.85	171.65	2374	9.49	17.89	170.61	2360
189	7.79	14.73	174.27	2410	8.34	15.77	173.23	2396	8.89	16.81	172.19	2381	9.44	17.84	171.16	2367
189.5	7.75	14.69	174.81	2418	8.30	15.73	173.77	2403	8.85	16.77	172.73	2389	9.39	17.80	171.70	2375
190	7.71	14.65	175.35	2425	8.26	15.69	174.31	2411	8.80	16.73	173.28	2396	9.35	17.76	172.24	2382
190.5	7.67	14.61	175.89	2433	8.21	15.65	174.85	2418	8.76	16.68	173.82	2404	9.30	17.72	172.78	2390
191	7.63	14.57	176.43	2440	8.17	15.61	175.39	2426	8.71	16.64	174.36	2411	9.26	17.68	173.32	2397
191.5	7.59	14.53	176.97	2448	8.13	15.56	175.94	2433	8.67	16.60	174.90	2419	9.21	17.64	173.86	2404
192	7.54	14.49	177.51	2455	8.09	15.52	176.48	2441	8.63	16.56	175.44	2426	9.17	17.60	174.40	2412
192.5	7.50	14.45	178.06	2463	8.04	15.48	177.02	2448	8.58	16.52	175.98	2434	9.12	17.56	174.94	2419
193	7.46	14.40	178.60	2470	8.00	15.44	177.56	2456	8.54	16.48	176.52	2441	9.08	17.52	175.48	2427
193.5	7.42	14.36	179.14	2477	7.96	15.40	178.10	2463	8.50	16.44	177.06	2449	9.03	17.48	176.02	2434
194	7.38	14.32	179.68	2485	7.92	15.36	178.64	2471	8.45	16.40	177.60	2456	8.99	17.43	176.57	2442
194.5	7.34	14.28	180.22	2492	7.88	15.32	179.18	2478	8.41	16.36	178.14	2464	8.94	17.39	177.11	2449
195	7.30	14.24	180.76	2500	7.83	15.28	179.72	2486	8.37	16.32	178.69	2471	8.90	17.35	177.65	2457
195.5	7.26	14.20	181.30	2507	7.79	15.24	180.26	2493	8.32	16.27	179.23	2479	8.85	17.31	178.19	2464
196	7.22	14.16	181.84	2515	7.75	15.20	180.80	2501	8.28	16.23	179.77	2486	8.81	17.27	178.73	2472
196.5	7.18	14.12	182.38	2522	7.71	15.15	181.35	2508	8.24	16.19	180.31	2494	8.77	17.23	179.27	2479
197	7.15	14.08	182.92	2530	7.67	15.11	181.89	2515	8.20	16.15	180.85	2501	8.73	17.19	179.81	2487
197.5	7.11	14.04	183.47	2537	7.63	15.07	182.43	2523	8.16	16.11	181.39	2509	8.68	17.15	180.35	2494
198	7.07	13.99	184.01	2545	7.59	15.03	182.97	2530	8.12	16.07	181.93	2516	8.64	17.11	180.89	2502
198.5	7.03	13.95	184.55	2552	7.55	14.99	183.51	2538	8.07	16.03	182.47	2524	8.60	17.07	181.43	2509
199	6.99	13.91	185.09	2560	7.51	14.95	184.05	2545	8.03	15.99	183.01	2531	8.56	17.02	181.98	2517
199.5	6.95	13.87	185.63	2567	7.47	14.91	184.59	2553	7.99	15.95	183.55	2539	8.51	16.98	182.52	2524
200	6.91	13.83	186.17	2575	7.43	14.87	185.13	2560	7.95	15.91	184.10	2546	8.47	16.94	183.06	2532
200.5	6.88	13.79	186.71	2582	7.39	14.83	185.67	2568	7.91	15.86	184.64	2554	8.43	16.90	183.60	2539
201	6.84	13.75	187.25	2590	7.36	14.79	186.21	2575	7.87	15.82	185.18	2561	8.39	16.86	184.14	2547
201.5	6.80	13.71	187.79	2597	7.32	14.74	186.76	2583	7.83	15.78	185.72	2568	8.35	16.82	184.68	2554
202	6.77	13.67	188.33	2605	7.28	14.70	187.30	2590	7.79	15.74	186.26	2576	8.31	16.78	185.22	2562
202.5	6.73	13.63	188.88	2612	7.24	14.66	187.84	2598	7.75	15.70	186.80	2583	8.27	16.74	185.76	2569
203	6.69	13.58	189.42	2620	7.20	14.62	188.38	2605	7.71	15.66	187.34	2591	8.22	16.70	186.30	2577
203.5	6.66	13.54	189.96	2627	7.16	14.58	188.92	2613	7.67	15.62	187.88	2598	8.18	16.66	186.84	2584
204	6.62	13.50	190.50	2635	7.13	14.54	189.46	2620	7.64	15.58	188.42	2606	8.14	16.61	187.39	2592
204.5	6.58	13.46	191.04	2642	7.09	14.50	190.00	2628	7.60	15.54	188.96	2613	8.10	16.57	187.93	2599
205	6.55	13.42	191.58	2650	7.05	14.46	190.54	2635	7.56	15.50	189.51	2621	8.06	16.53	188.47	2607
205.5	6.51	13.38	192.12	2657	7.02	14.42	191.08	2643	7.52	15.45	190.05	2628	8.03	16.49	189.01	2614
206	6.47	13.34	192.66	2665	6.98	14.38	191.62	2650	7.48	15.41	190.59	2636	7.99	16.45	189.55	2621
206.5	6.44	13.30	193.20	2672	6.94	14.33	192.17	2658	7.44	15.37	191.13	2643	7.95	16.41	190.09	2629
207	6.40	13.26	193.74	2679	6.91	14.29	192.71	2665	7.41	15.33	191.67	2651	7.91	16.37	190.63	2636
207.5	6.37	13.22	194.29	2687	6.87	14.25	193.25	2673	7.37	15.29	192.21	2658	7.87	16.33	191.17	2644
208	6.33	13.17	194.83	2694	6.83	14.21	193.79	2680	7.33	15.25	192.75	2666	7.83	16.29	191.71	2651
208.5	6.30	13.13	195.37	2702	6.80	14.17	194.33	2688	7.29	15.21	193.29	2673	7.79	16.25	192.25	2659
209	6.26	13.09	195.91	2709	6.76	14.13	194.87	2695	7.26	15.17	193.83	2681	7.75	16.20	192.80	2666
209.5	6.23	13.05	196.45	2717	6.72	14.09	195.41	2703	7.22	15.13	194.37	2688	7.72	16.16	193.34	2674
210	6.20	13.01	196.99	2724	6.69	14.05	195.95	2710	7.18	15.09	194.92	2696	7.68	16.12	193.88	2681
210.5	6.16	12.97	197.53	2732	6.65	14.01	196.49	2718	7.15	15.04	195.46	2703	7.64	16.08	194.42	2689
211	6.13	12.93	198.07	2739	6.62	13.97	197.03	2725	7.11	15.00	196.00	2711	7.60	16.04	194.96	2696
211.5	6.09	12.89	198.61	2747	6.58	13.92	197.58	2732	7.07	14.96	196.54	2718	7.56	16.00	195.50	2704
212	6.06	12.85	199.15	2754	6.55	13.88	198.12	2740	7.04	14.92	197.08	2726	7.53	15.96	196.04	2711
212.5	6.03	12.81	199.70	2762	6.51	13.84	198.66	2747	7.00	14.88	197.62	2733	7.49	15.92	196.58	2719
213	5.99	12.76	200.24	2769	6.48	13.80	199.20	2755	6.97	14.84	198.16	2741	7.45	15.88	197.12	2726
213.5	5.96	12.72	200.78	2777	6.45	13.76	199.74	2762	6.93	14.80	198.70	2748	7.42	15.84	197.66	2734
214	5.93	12.68	201.32	2784	6.41	13.72	200.28	2770	6.90	14.76	199.24	2756	7.38	15.79	198.21	2741
214.5	5.89	12.64	201.86	2792	6.38	13.68	200.82	2777	6.86	14.72	199.78	2763	7.34	15.75	198.75	2749
215	5.86	12.60	202.40	2799	6.34	13.64	201.36	2785	6.83	14.68	200.33	2770	7.31	15.71	199.29	2756
215.5	5.83	12.56	202.94	2807	6.31	13.60	201.90	2792	6.79	14.63	200.87	2778	7.27	15.67	199.83	2764

Body Composition　MALE　184-215.5 Lb.

Weight: Lb.	Waist: 32 inches Fat: %	Fat: Lb.	LBM: Lb.	RMR: Cal.	32.25 inches Fat: %	Fat: Lb.	LBM: Lb.	RMR: Cal.	32.5 inches Fat: %	Fat: Lb.	LBM: Lb.	RMR: Cal.	32.75 inches Fat: %	Fat: Lb.	LBM: Lb.	RMR: Cal.
184	10.48	19.29	164.71	2278	11.05	20.33	163.67	2264	11.61	21.37	162.63	2249	12.18	22.40	161.60	2235
184.5	10.43	19.25	165.25	2285	11.00	20.29	164.21	2271	11.56	21.33	163.17	2257	12.12	22.36	162.14	2242
185	10.38	19.21	165.79	2293	10.94	20.25	164.75	2279	11.51	21.29	163.72	2264	12.07	22.32	162.68	2250
185.5	10.33	19.17	166.33	2300	10.89	20.21	165.29	2286	11.45	21.24	164.26	2272	12.01	22.28	163.22	2257
186	10.28	19.13	166.87	2308	10.84	20.17	165.83	2293	11.40	21.20	164.80	2279	11.96	22.24	163.76	2265
186.5	10.23	19.09	167.41	2315	10.79	20.12	166.38	2301	11.35	21.16	165.34	2287	11.90	22.20	164.30	2272
187	10.19	19.05	167.95	2323	10.74	20.08	166.92	2308	11.29	21.12	165.88	2294	11.85	22.16	164.84	2280
187.5	10.14	19.01	168.50	2330	10.69	20.04	167.46	2316	11.24	21.08	166.42	2302	11.80	22.12	165.38	2287
188	10.09	18.96	169.04	2338	10.64	20.00	168.00	2323	11.19	21.04	166.96	2309	11.74	22.08	165.92	2295
188.5	10.04	18.92	169.58	2345	10.59	19.96	168.54	2331	11.14	21.00	167.50	2317	11.69	22.04	166.46	2302
189	9.99	18.88	170.12	2353	10.54	19.92	169.08	2338	11.09	20.96	168.04	2324	11.64	21.99	167.01	2310
189.5	9.94	18.84	170.66	2360	10.49	19.88	169.62	2346	11.04	20.92	168.58	2332	11.58	21.95	167.55	2317
190	9.89	18.80	171.20	2368	10.44	19.84	170.16	2353	10.99	20.88	169.13	2339	11.53	21.91	168.09	2325
190.5	9.85	18.76	171.74	2375	10.39	19.80	170.70	2361	10.94	20.83	169.67	2346	11.48	21.87	168.63	2332
191	9.80	18.72	172.28	2383	10.34	19.76	171.24	2368	10.89	20.79	170.21	2354	11.43	21.83	169.17	2340
191.5	9.75	18.68	172.82	2390	10.29	19.71	171.79	2376	10.84	20.75	170.75	2361	11.38	21.79	169.71	2347
192	9.71	18.64	173.36	2398	10.25	19.67	172.33	2383	10.79	20.71	171.29	2369	11.33	21.75	170.25	2355
192.5	9.66	18.60	173.91	2405	10.20	19.63	172.87	2391	10.74	20.67	171.83	2376	11.28	21.71	170.79	2362
193	9.61	18.55	174.45	2413	10.15	19.59	173.41	2398	10.69	20.63	172.37	2384	11.23	21.67	171.33	2370
193.5	9.57	18.51	174.99	2420	10.10	19.55	173.95	2406	10.64	20.59	172.91	2391	11.18	21.63	171.87	2377
194	9.52	18.47	175.53	2428	10.06	19.51	174.49	2413	10.59	20.55	173.45	2399	11.13	21.58	172.42	2385
194.5	9.48	18.43	176.07	2435	10.01	19.47	175.03	2421	10.54	20.51	173.99	2406	11.08	21.54	172.96	2392
195	9.43	18.39	176.61	2443	9.96	19.43	175.57	2428	10.49	20.47	174.54	2414	11.03	21.50	173.50	2399
195.5	9.39	18.35	177.15	2450	9.92	19.39	176.11	2436	10.45	20.42	175.08	2421	10.98	21.46	174.04	2407
196	9.34	18.31	177.69	2457	9.87	19.35	176.65	2443	10.40	20.38	175.62	2429	10.93	21.42	174.58	2414
196.5	9.30	18.27	178.23	2465	9.82	19.30	177.20	2451	10.35	20.34	176.16	2436	10.88	21.38	175.12	2422
197	9.25	18.23	178.77	2472	9.78	19.26	177.74	2458	10.31	20.30	176.70	2444	10.83	21.34	175.66	2429
197.5	9.21	18.19	179.32	2480	9.73	19.22	178.28	2466	10.26	20.26	177.24	2451	10.78	21.30	176.20	2437
198	9.16	18.14	179.86	2487	9.69	19.18	178.82	2473	10.21	20.22	177.78	2459	10.74	21.26	176.74	2444
198.5	9.12	18.10	180.40	2495	9.64	19.14	179.36	2481	10.17	20.18	178.32	2466	10.69	21.22	177.28	2452
199	9.08	18.06	180.94	2502	9.60	19.10	179.90	2488	10.12	20.14	178.86	2474	10.64	21.17	177.83	2459
199.5	9.03	18.02	181.48	2510	9.55	19.06	180.44	2496	10.07	20.10	179.40	2481	10.59	21.13	178.37	2467
200	8.99	17.98	182.02	2517	9.51	19.02	180.98	2503	10.03	20.06	179.95	2489	10.55	21.09	178.91	2474
200.5	8.95	17.94	182.56	2525	9.46	18.98	181.52	2510	9.98	20.01	180.49	2496	10.50	21.05	179.45	2482
201	8.90	17.90	183.10	2532	9.42	18.94	182.06	2518	9.94	19.97	181.03	2504	10.45	21.01	179.99	2489
201.5	8.86	17.86	183.64	2540	9.38	18.89	182.61	2525	9.89	19.93	181.57	2511	10.41	20.97	180.53	2497
202	8.82	17.82	184.18	2547	9.33	18.85	183.15	2533	9.85	19.89	182.11	2519	10.36	20.93	181.07	2504
202.5	8.78	17.78	184.73	2555	9.29	18.81	183.69	2540	9.80	19.85	182.65	2526	10.31	20.89	181.61	2512
203	8.74	17.73	185.27	2562	9.25	18.77	184.23	2548	9.76	19.81	183.19	2534	10.27	20.85	182.15	2519
203.5	8.69	17.69	185.81	2570	9.20	18.73	184.77	2555	9.71	19.77	183.73	2541	10.22	20.81	182.69	2527
204	8.65	17.65	186.35	2577	9.16	18.69	185.31	2563	9.67	19.73	184.27	2548	10.18	20.76	183.24	2534
204.5	8.61	17.61	186.89	2585	9.12	18.65	185.85	2570	9.63	19.69	184.81	2556	10.13	20.72	183.78	2542
205	8.57	17.57	187.43	2592	9.08	18.61	186.39	2578	9.58	19.65	185.36	2563	10.09	20.68	184.32	2549
205.5	8.53	17.53	187.97	2600	9.03	18.57	186.93	2585	9.54	19.60	185.90	2571	10.04	20.64	184.86	2557
206	8.49	17.49	188.51	2607	8.99	18.53	187.47	2593	9.50	19.56	186.44	2578	10.00	20.60	185.40	2564
206.5	8.45	17.45	189.05	2615	8.95	18.48	188.02	2600	9.45	19.52	186.98	2586	9.96	20.56	185.94	2572
207	8.41	17.41	189.59	2622	8.91	18.44	188.56	2608	9.41	19.48	187.52	2593	9.91	20.52	186.48	2579
207.5	8.37	17.37	190.14	2630	8.87	18.40	189.10	2615	9.37	19.44	188.06	2601	9.87	20.48	187.02	2587
208	8.33	17.32	190.68	2637	8.83	18.36	189.64	2623	9.33	19.40	188.60	2608	9.83	20.44	187.56	2594
208.5	8.29	17.28	191.22	2645	8.79	18.32	190.18	2630	9.28	19.36	189.14	2616	9.78	20.40	188.10	2601
209	8.25	17.24	191.76	2652	8.75	18.28	190.72	2638	9.24	19.32	189.68	2623	9.74	20.35	188.65	2609
209.5	8.21	17.20	192.30	2659	8.71	18.24	191.26	2645	9.20	19.28	190.22	2631	9.70	20.31	189.19	2616
210	8.17	17.16	192.84	2667	8.67	18.20	191.80	2653	9.16	19.24	190.77	2638	9.65	20.27	189.73	2624
210.5	8.13	17.12	193.38	2674	8.63	18.16	192.34	2660	9.12	19.19	191.31	2646	9.61	20.23	190.27	2631
211	8.09	17.08	193.92	2682	8.59	18.12	192.88	2668	9.08	19.15	191.85	2653	9.57	20.19	190.81	2639
211.5	8.06	17.04	194.46	2689	8.55	18.07	193.43	2675	9.04	19.11	192.39	2661	9.53	20.15	191.35	2646
212	8.02	17.00	195.00	2697	8.51	18.03	193.97	2683	9.00	19.07	192.93	2668	9.49	20.11	191.89	2654
212.5	7.98	16.96	195.55	2704	8.47	17.99	194.51	2690	8.96	19.03	193.47	2676	9.44	20.07	192.43	2661
213	7.94	16.91	196.09	2712	8.43	17.95	195.05	2698	8.92	18.99	194.01	2683	9.40	20.03	192.97	2669
213.5	7.90	16.87	196.63	2719	8.39	17.91	195.59	2705	8.87	18.95	194.55	2691	9.36	19.99	193.51	2676
214	7.87	16.83	197.17	2727	8.35	17.87	196.13	2712	8.84	18.91	195.09	2698	9.32	19.94	194.06	2684
214.5	7.83	16.79	197.71	2734	8.31	17.83	196.67	2720	8.80	18.87	195.63	2706	9.28	19.90	194.60	2691
215	7.79	16.75	198.25	2742	8.27	17.79	197.21	2727	8.76	18.83	196.18	2713	9.24	19.86	195.14	2699
215.5	7.75	16.71	198.79	2749	8.24	17.75	197.75	2735	8.72	18.78	196.72	2721	9.20	19.82	195.68	2706

Body Composition MALE 184-215.5 Lb.

Weight: Lb.	Waist: 33 inches				33.25 inches				33.5 inches				33.75 inches			
	Fat: %	Fat: Lb.	LBM: Lb.	RMR: Cal.	Fat: %	Fat: Lb.	LBM: Lb.	RMR: Cal.	Fat: %	Fat: Lb.	LBM: Lb.	RMR: Cal.	Fat: %	Fat: Lb.	LBM: Lb.	RMR: Cal.
184	12.74	23.44	160.56	2221	13.30	24.48	159.52	2206	13.87	25.52	158.48	2192	14.43	26.55	157.45	2177
184.5	12.68	23.40	161.10	2228	13.25	24.44	160.06	2214	13.81	25.48	159.02	2199	14.37	26.51	157.99	2185
185	12.63	23.36	161.64	2235	13.19	24.40	160.60	2221	13.75	25.44	159.57	2207	14.31	26.47	158.53	2192
185.5	12.57	23.32	162.18	2243	13.13	24.36	161.14	2229	13.69	25.39	160.11	2214	14.25	26.43	159.07	2200
186	12.52	23.28	162.72	2250	13.07	24.32	161.68	2236	13.63	25.35	160.65	2222	14.19	26.39	159.61	2207
186.5	12.46	23.24	163.26	2258	13.02	24.27	162.23	2244	13.57	25.31	161.19	2229	14.13	26.35	160.15	2215
187	12.40	23.20	163.80	2265	12.96	24.23	162.77	2251	13.51	25.27	161.73	2237	14.07	26.31	160.69	2222
187.5	12.35	23.16	164.35	2273	12.90	24.19	163.31	2259	13.46	25.23	162.27	2244	14.01	26.27	161.23	2230
188	12.29	23.11	164.89	2280	12.85	24.15	163.85	2266	13.40	25.19	162.81	2252	13.95	26.23	161.77	2237
188.5	12.24	23.07	165.43	2288	12.79	24.11	164.39	2274	13.34	25.15	163.35	2259	13.89	26.19	162.31	2245
189	12.19	23.03	165.97	2295	12.74	24.07	164.93	2281	13.28	25.11	163.89	2267	13.83	26.14	162.86	2252
189.5	12.13	22.99	166.51	2303	12.68	24.03	165.47	2288	13.23	25.07	164.43	2274	13.77	26.10	163.40	2260
190	12.08	22.95	167.05	2310	12.63	23.99	166.01	2296	13.17	25.03	164.98	2282	13.72	26.06	163.94	2267
190.5	12.03	22.91	167.59	2318	12.57	23.95	166.55	2303	13.11	24.98	165.52	2289	13.66	26.02	164.48	2275
191	11.97	22.87	168.13	2325	12.52	23.91	167.09	2311	13.06	24.94	166.06	2297	13.60	25.98	165.02	2282
191.5	11.92	22.83	168.67	2333	12.46	23.86	167.64	2318	13.00	24.90	166.60	2304	13.55	25.94	165.56	2290
192	11.87	22.79	169.21	2340	12.41	23.82	168.18	2326	12.95	24.86	167.14	2312	13.49	25.90	166.10	2297
192.5	11.82	22.75	169.76	2348	12.35	23.78	168.72	2333	12.89	24.82	167.68	2319	13.43	25.86	166.64	2305
193	11.76	22.70	170.30	2355	12.30	23.74	169.26	2341	12.84	24.78	168.22	2326	13.38	25.82	167.18	2312
193.5	11.71	22.66	170.84	2363	12.25	23.70	169.80	2348	12.78	24.74	168.76	2334	13.32	25.78	167.72	2320
194	11.66	22.62	171.38	2370	12.20	23.66	170.34	2356	12.73	24.70	169.30	2341	13.27	25.73	168.27	2327
194.5	11.61	22.58	171.92	2378	12.14	23.62	170.88	2363	12.68	24.66	169.84	2349	13.21	25.69	168.81	2335
195	11.56	22.54	172.46	2385	12.09	23.58	171.42	2371	12.62	24.62	170.39	2356	13.16	25.65	169.35	2342
195.5	11.51	22.50	173.00	2393	12.04	23.54	171.96	2378	12.57	24.57	170.93	2364	13.10	25.61	169.89	2350
196	11.46	22.46	173.54	2400	11.99	23.50	172.50	2386	12.52	24.53	171.47	2371	13.05	25.57	170.43	2357
196.5	11.41	22.42	174.08	2408	11.94	23.45	173.05	2393	12.46	24.49	172.01	2379	12.99	25.53	170.97	2365
197	11.36	22.38	174.62	2415	11.89	23.41	173.59	2401	12.41	24.45	172.55	2386	12.94	25.49	171.51	2372
197.5	11.31	22.34	175.17	2423	11.83	23.37	174.13	2408	12.36	24.41	173.09	2394	12.88	25.45	172.05	2379
198	11.26	22.29	175.71	2430	11.78	23.33	174.67	2416	12.31	24.37	173.63	2401	12.83	25.41	172.59	2387
198.5	11.21	22.25	176.25	2437	11.73	23.29	175.21	2423	12.26	24.33	174.17	2409	12.78	25.37	173.13	2394
199	11.16	22.21	176.79	2445	11.68	23.25	175.75	2431	12.20	24.29	174.71	2416	12.73	25.32	173.68	2402
199.5	11.11	22.17	177.33	2452	11.63	23.21	176.29	2438	12.15	24.25	175.25	2424	12.67	25.28	174.22	2409
200	11.07	22.13	177.87	2460	11.58	23.17	176.83	2446	12.10	24.21	175.80	2431	12.62	25.24	174.76	2417
200.5	11.02	22.09	178.41	2467	11.53	23.13	177.37	2453	12.05	24.16	176.34	2439	12.57	25.20	175.30	2424
201	10.97	22.05	178.95	2475	11.49	23.09	177.91	2461	12.00	24.12	176.88	2446	12.52	25.16	175.84	2432
201.5	10.92	22.01	179.49	2482	11.44	23.04	178.46	2468	11.95	24.08	177.42	2454	12.47	25.12	176.38	2439
202	10.87	21.97	180.03	2490	11.39	23.00	179.00	2476	11.90	24.04	177.96	2461	12.42	25.08	176.92	2447
202.5	10.83	21.93	180.58	2497	11.34	22.96	179.54	2483	11.85	24.00	178.50	2469	12.36	25.04	177.46	2454
203	10.78	21.88	181.12	2505	11.29	22.92	180.08	2490	11.80	23.96	179.04	2476	12.31	25.00	178.00	2462
203.5	10.73	21.84	181.66	2512	11.24	22.88	180.62	2498	11.75	23.92	179.58	2484	12.26	24.96	178.54	2469
204	10.69	21.80	182.20	2520	11.20	22.84	181.16	2505	11.70	23.88	180.12	2491	12.21	24.91	179.09	2477
204.5	10.64	21.76	182.74	2527	11.15	22.80	181.70	2513	11.66	23.84	180.66	2499	12.16	24.87	179.63	2484
205	10.60	21.72	183.28	2535	11.10	22.76	182.24	2520	11.61	23.80	181.21	2506	12.11	24.83	180.17	2492
205.5	10.55	21.68	183.82	2542	11.05	22.72	182.78	2528	11.56	23.75	181.75	2514	12.06	24.79	180.71	2499
206	10.50	21.64	184.36	2550	11.01	22.68	183.32	2535	11.51	23.71	182.29	2521	12.01	24.75	181.25	2507
206.5	10.46	21.60	184.90	2557	10.96	22.63	183.87	2543	11.46	23.67	182.83	2529	11.97	24.71	181.79	2514
207	10.41	21.56	185.44	2565	10.91	22.59	184.41	2550	11.42	23.63	183.37	2536	11.92	24.67	182.33	2522
207.5	10.37	21.52	185.99	2572	10.87	22.55	184.95	2558	11.37	23.59	183.91	2543	11.87	24.63	182.87	2529
208	10.32	21.47	186.53	2580	10.82	22.51	185.49	2565	11.32	23.55	184.45	2551	11.82	24.59	183.41	2537
208.5	10.28	21.43	187.07	2587	10.78	22.47	186.03	2573	11.27	23.51	184.99	2558	11.77	24.55	183.95	2544
209	10.24	21.39	187.61	2595	10.73	22.43	186.57	2580	11.23	23.47	185.53	2566	11.72	24.50	184.50	2552
209.5	10.19	21.35	188.15	2602	10.69	22.39	187.11	2588	11.18	23.43	186.07	2573	11.68	24.46	185.04	2559
210	10.15	21.31	188.69	2610	10.64	22.35	187.65	2595	11.14	23.39	186.62	2581	11.63	24.42	185.58	2567
210.5	10.10	21.27	189.23	2617	10.60	22.31	188.19	2603	11.09	23.34	187.16	2588	11.58	24.38	186.12	2574
211	10.06	21.23	189.77	2625	10.55	22.27	188.73	2610	11.04	23.30	187.70	2596	11.54	24.34	186.66	2582
211.5	10.02	21.19	190.31	2632	10.51	22.22	189.28	2618	11.00	23.26	188.24	2603	11.49	24.30	187.20	2589
212	9.97	21.15	190.85	2640	10.46	22.18	189.82	2625	10.95	23.22	188.78	2611	11.44	24.26	187.74	2596
212.5	9.93	21.11	191.40	2647	10.42	22.14	190.36	2633	10.91	23.18	189.32	2618	11.40	24.22	188.28	2604
213	9.89	21.06	191.94	2654	10.38	22.10	190.90	2640	10.86	23.14	189.86	2626	11.35	24.18	188.82	2611
213.5	9.85	21.02	192.48	2662	10.33	22.06	191.44	2648	10.82	23.10	190.40	2633	11.30	24.14	189.36	2619
214	9.80	20.98	193.02	2669	10.29	22.02	191.98	2655	10.77	23.06	190.94	2641	11.26	24.09	189.91	2626
214.5	9.76	20.94	193.56	2677	10.25	21.98	192.52	2663	10.73	23.02	191.48	2648	11.21	24.05	190.45	2634
215	9.72	20.90	194.10	2684	10.20	21.94	193.06	2670	10.69	22.98	192.03	2656	11.17	24.01	190.99	2641
215.5	9.68	20.86	194.64	2692	10.16	21.90	193.60	2678	10.64	22.93	192.57	2663	11.12	23.97	191.53	2649

Body Composition   MALE   184-215.5 Lb.

Weight: Lb.	Waist: 34 inches Fat: %	Fat: Lb.	LBM: Lb.	RMR: Cal.	34.25 inches Fat: %	Fat: Lb.	LBM: Lb.	RMR: Cal.	34.5 inches Fat: %	Fat: Lb.	LBM: Lb.	RMR: Cal.	34.75 inches Fat: %	Fat: Lb.	LBM: Lb.	RMR: Cal.
184	15.00	27.59	156.41	2163	15.56	28.63	155.37	2149	16.12	29.67	154.33	2134	16.69	30.70	153.30	2120
184.5	14.93	27.55	156.95	2171	15.50	28.59	155.91	2156	16.06	29.63	154.87	2142	16.62	30.66	153.84	2128
185	14.87	27.51	157.49	2178	15.43	28.55	156.45	2164	15.99	29.59	155.42	2149	16.55	30.62	154.38	2135
185.5	14.81	27.47	158.03	2186	15.37	28.51	156.99	2171	15.93	29.54	155.96	2157	16.49	30.58	154.92	2143
186	14.75	27.43	158.57	2193	15.30	28.47	157.53	2179	15.86	29.50	156.50	2164	16.42	30.54	155.46	2150
186.5	14.68	27.39	159.11	2201	15.24	28.42	158.08	2186	15.80	29.46	157.04	2172	16.35	30.50	156.00	2157
187	14.62	27.35	159.65	2208	15.18	28.38	158.62	2194	15.73	29.42	157.58	2179	16.29	30.46	156.54	2165
187.5	14.56	27.31	160.20	2215	15.12	28.34	159.16	2201	15.67	29.38	158.12	2187	16.22	30.42	157.08	2172
188	14.50	27.26	160.74	2223	15.05	28.30	159.70	2209	15.61	29.34	158.66	2194	16.16	30.38	157.62	2180
188.5	14.44	27.22	161.28	2230	14.99	28.26	160.24	2216	15.54	29.30	159.20	2202	16.09	30.34	158.16	2187
189	14.38	27.18	161.82	2238	14.93	28.22	160.78	2224	15.48	29.26	159.74	2209	16.03	30.29	158.71	2195
189.5	14.32	27.14	162.36	2245	14.87	28.18	161.32	2231	15.42	29.22	160.28	2217	15.96	30.25	159.25	2202
190	14.26	27.10	162.90	2253	14.81	28.14	161.86	2239	15.36	29.18	160.83	2224	15.90	30.21	159.79	2210
190.5	14.20	27.06	163.44	2260	14.75	28.10	162.40	2246	15.29	29.13	161.37	2232	15.84	30.17	160.33	2217
191	14.15	27.02	163.98	2268	14.69	28.06	162.94	2254	15.23	29.09	161.91	2239	15.78	30.13	160.87	2225
191.5	14.09	26.98	164.52	2275	14.63	28.01	163.49	2261	15.17	29.05	162.45	2247	15.71	30.09	161.41	2232
192	14.03	26.94	165.06	2283	14.57	27.97	164.03	2268	15.11	29.01	162.99	2254	15.65	30.05	161.95	2240
192.5	13.97	26.90	165.61	2290	14.51	27.93	164.57	2276	15.05	28.97	163.53	2262	15.59	30.01	162.49	2247
193	13.91	26.85	166.15	2298	14.45	27.89	165.11	2283	14.99	28.93	164.07	2269	15.53	29.97	163.03	2255
193.5	13.86	26.81	166.69	2305	14.39	27.85	165.65	2291	14.93	28.89	164.61	2277	15.47	29.93	163.57	2262
194	13.80	26.77	167.23	2313	14.33	27.81	166.19	2298	14.87	28.85	165.15	2284	15.40	29.88	164.12	2270
194.5	13.74	26.73	167.77	2320	14.28	27.77	166.73	2306	14.81	28.81	165.69	2292	15.34	29.84	164.66	2277
195	13.69	26.69	168.31	2328	14.22	27.73	167.27	2313	14.75	28.77	166.24	2299	15.28	29.80	165.20	2285
195.5	13.63	26.65	168.85	2335	14.16	27.69	167.81	2321	14.69	28.72	166.78	2307	15.22	29.76	165.74	2292
196	13.58	26.61	169.39	2343	14.10	27.65	168.35	2328	14.63	28.68	167.32	2314	15.16	29.72	166.28	2300
196.5	13.52	26.57	169.93	2350	14.05	27.60	168.90	2336	14.58	28.64	167.86	2321	15.10	29.68	166.82	2307
197	13.46	26.53	170.47	2358	13.99	27.56	169.44	2343	14.52	28.60	168.40	2329	15.04	29.64	167.36	2315
197.5	13.41	26.49	171.02	2365	13.94	27.52	169.98	2351	14.46	28.56	168.94	2336	14.99	29.60	167.90	2322
198	13.36	26.44	171.56	2373	13.88	27.48	170.52	2358	14.40	28.52	169.48	2344	14.93	29.56	168.44	2330
198.5	13.30	26.40	172.10	2380	13.82	27.44	171.06	2366	14.35	28.48	170.02	2351	14.87	29.52	168.98	2337
199	13.25	26.36	172.64	2388	13.77	27.40	171.60	2373	14.29	28.44	170.56	2359	14.81	29.47	169.53	2345
199.5	13.19	26.32	173.18	2395	13.71	27.36	172.14	2381	14.23	28.40	171.10	2366	14.75	29.43	170.07	2352
200	13.14	26.28	173.72	2403	13.66	27.32	172.68	2388	14.18	28.36	171.65	2374	14.70	29.39	170.61	2360
200.5	13.09	26.24	174.26	2410	13.60	27.28	173.22	2396	14.12	28.31	172.19	2381	14.64	29.35	171.15	2367
201	13.03	26.20	174.80	2418	13.55	27.24	173.76	2403	14.07	28.27	172.73	2389	14.58	29.31	171.69	2374
201.5	12.98	26.16	175.34	2425	13.50	27.19	174.31	2411	14.01	28.23	173.27	2396	14.53	29.27	172.23	2382
202	12.93	26.12	175.88	2432	13.44	27.15	174.85	2418	13.96	28.19	173.81	2404	14.47	29.23	172.77	2389
202.5	12.88	26.08	176.43	2440	13.39	27.11	175.39	2426	13.90	28.15	174.35	2411	14.41	29.19	173.31	2397
203	12.82	26.03	176.97	2447	13.34	27.07	175.93	2433	13.85	28.11	174.89	2419	14.36	29.15	173.85	2404
203.5	12.77	25.99	177.51	2455	13.28	27.03	176.47	2441	13.79	28.07	175.43	2426	14.30	29.11	174.39	2412
204	12.72	25.95	178.05	2462	13.23	26.99	177.01	2448	13.74	28.03	175.97	2434	14.25	29.06	174.94	2419
204.5	12.67	25.91	178.59	2470	13.18	26.95	177.55	2456	13.69	27.99	176.51	2441	14.19	29.02	175.48	2427
205	12.62	25.87	179.13	2477	13.13	26.91	178.09	2463	13.63	27.95	177.06	2449	14.14	28.98	176.02	2434
205.5	12.57	25.83	179.67	2485	13.07	26.87	178.63	2471	13.58	27.90	177.60	2456	14.08	28.94	176.56	2442
206	12.52	25.79	180.21	2492	13.02	26.83	179.17	2478	13.53	27.86	178.14	2464	14.03	28.90	177.10	2449
206.5	12.47	25.75	180.75	2500	12.97	26.78	179.72	2485	13.47	27.82	178.68	2471	13.98	28.86	177.64	2457
207	12.42	25.71	181.29	2507	12.92	26.74	180.26	2493	13.42	27.78	179.22	2479	13.92	28.82	178.18	2464
207.5	12.37	25.67	181.84	2515	12.87	26.70	180.80	2500	13.37	27.74	179.76	2486	13.87	28.78	178.72	2472
208	12.32	25.62	182.38	2522	12.82	26.66	181.34	2508	13.32	27.70	180.30	2494	13.82	28.74	179.26	2479
208.5	12.27	25.58	182.92	2530	12.77	26.62	181.88	2515	13.27	27.66	180.84	2501	13.76	28.70	179.80	2487
209	12.22	25.54	183.46	2537	12.72	26.58	182.42	2523	13.21	27.62	181.38	2509	13.71	28.65	180.35	2494
209.5	12.17	25.50	184.00	2545	12.67	26.54	182.96	2530	13.16	27.58	181.92	2516	13.66	28.61	180.89	2502
210	12.12	25.46	184.54	2552	12.62	26.50	183.50	2538	13.11	27.54	182.47	2523	13.61	28.57	181.43	2509
210.5	12.08	25.42	185.08	2560	12.57	26.46	184.04	2545	13.06	27.49	183.01	2531	13.55	28.53	181.97	2517
211	12.03	25.38	185.62	2567	12.52	26.42	184.58	2553	13.01	27.45	183.55	2538	13.50	28.49	182.51	2524
211.5	11.98	25.34	186.16	2575	12.47	26.37	185.13	2560	12.96	27.41	184.09	2546	13.45	28.45	183.05	2532
212	11.93	25.30	186.70	2582	12.42	26.33	185.67	2568	12.91	27.37	184.63	2553	13.40	28.41	183.59	2539
212.5	11.88	25.26	187.25	2590	12.37	26.29	186.21	2575	12.86	27.33	185.17	2561	13.35	28.37	184.13	2547
213	11.84	25.21	187.79	2597	12.32	26.25	186.75	2583	12.81	27.29	185.71	2568	13.30	28.33	184.67	2554
213.5	11.79	25.17	188.33	2605	12.28	26.21	187.29	2590	12.76	27.25	186.25	2576	13.25	28.29	185.21	2562
214	11.74	25.13	188.87	2612	12.23	26.17	187.83	2598	12.71	27.21	186.79	2583	13.20	28.24	185.76	2569
214.5	11.70	25.09	189.41	2620	12.18	26.13	188.37	2605	12.66	27.17	187.33	2591	13.15	28.20	186.30	2576
215	11.65	25.05	189.95	2627	12.13	26.09	188.91	2613	12.62	27.13	187.88	2598	13.10	28.16	186.84	2584
215.5	11.61	25.01	190.49	2634	12.09	26.05	189.45	2620	12.57	27.08	188.42	2606	13.05	28.12	187.38	2591

Body Composition MALE 184-215.5 Lb.

Weight: Lb.	Waist: 35 inches				35.25 inches				35.5 inches				35.75 inches			
	Fat: %	Fat: Lb.	LBM: Lb.	RMR: Cal.	Fat: %	Fat: Lb.	LBM: Lb.	RMR: Cal.	Fat: %	Fat: Lb.	LBM: Lb.	RMR: Cal.	Fat: %	Fat: Lb.	LBM: Lb.	RMR: Cal.
184	17.25	31.74	152.26	2106	17.81	32.78	151.22	2091	18.38	33.82	150.18	2077	18.94	34.85	149.15	2063
184.5	17.18	31.70	152.80	2113	17.74	32.74	151.76	2099	18.31	33.78	150.72	2085	18.87	34.81	149.69	2070
185	17.11	31.66	153.34	2121	17.67	32.70	152.30	2106	18.24	33.74	151.27	2092	18.80	34.77	150.23	2078
185.5	17.05	31.62	153.88	2128	17.60	32.66	152.84	2114	18.16	33.69	151.81	2099	18.72	34.73	150.77	2085
186	16.98	31.58	154.42	2136	17.54	32.62	153.38	2121	18.09	33.65	152.35	2107	18.65	34.69	151.31	2093
186.5	16.91	31.54	154.96	2143	17.47	32.57	153.93	2129	18.02	33.61	152.89	2114	18.58	34.65	151.85	2100
187	16.84	31.50	155.50	2151	17.40	32.53	154.47	2136	17.95	33.57	153.43	2122	18.51	34.61	152.39	2108
187.5	16.78	31.46	156.05	2158	17.33	32.49	155.01	2144	17.88	33.53	153.97	2129	18.44	34.57	152.93	2115
188	16.71	31.41	156.59	2166	17.26	32.45	155.55	2151	17.81	33.49	154.51	2137	18.37	34.53	153.47	2123
188.5	16.64	31.37	157.13	2173	17.19	32.41	156.09	2159	17.74	33.45	155.05	2144	18.29	34.49	154.01	2130
189	16.58	31.33	157.67	2181	17.13	32.37	156.63	2166	17.68	33.41	155.59	2152	18.22	34.44	154.56	2138
189.5	16.51	31.29	158.21	2188	17.06	32.33	157.17	2174	17.61	33.37	156.13	2159	18.15	34.40	155.10	2145
190	16.45	31.25	158.75	2196	16.99	32.29	157.71	2181	17.54	33.33	156.68	2167	18.09	34.36	155.64	2152
190.5	16.38	31.21	159.29	2203	16.93	32.25	158.25	2189	17.47	33.28	157.22	2174	18.02	34.32	156.18	2160
191	16.32	31.17	159.83	2210	16.86	32.21	158.79	2196	17.40	33.24	157.76	2182	17.95	34.28	156.72	2167
191.5	16.25	31.13	160.37	2218	16.80	32.16	159.34	2204	17.34	33.20	158.30	2189	17.88	34.24	157.26	2175
192	16.19	31.09	160.91	2225	16.73	32.12	159.88	2211	17.27	33.16	158.84	2197	17.81	34.20	157.80	2182
192.5	16.13	31.05	161.46	2233	16.67	32.08	160.42	2219	17.21	33.12	159.38	2204	17.74	34.16	158.34	2190
193	16.06	31.00	162.00	2240	16.60	32.04	160.96	2226	17.14	33.08	159.92	2212	17.68	34.12	158.88	2197
193.5	16.00	30.96	162.54	2248	16.54	32.00	161.50	2234	17.07	33.04	160.46	2219	17.61	34.08	159.42	2205
194	15.94	30.92	163.08	2255	16.47	31.96	162.04	2241	17.01	33.00	161.00	2227	17.54	34.03	159.97	2212
194.5	15.88	30.88	163.62	2263	16.41	31.92	162.58	2249	16.94	32.96	161.54	2234	17.48	33.99	160.51	2220
195	15.82	30.84	164.16	2270	16.35	31.88	163.12	2256	16.88	32.92	162.09	2242	17.41	33.95	161.05	2227
195.5	15.75	30.80	164.70	2278	16.28	31.84	163.66	2263	16.82	32.87	162.63	2249	17.35	33.91	161.59	2235
196	15.69	30.76	165.24	2285	16.22	31.80	164.20	2271	16.75	32.83	163.17	2257	17.28	33.87	162.13	2242
196.5	15.63	30.72	165.78	2293	16.16	31.75	164.75	2278	16.69	32.79	163.71	2264	17.22	33.83	162.67	2250
197	15.57	30.68	166.32	2300	16.10	31.71	165.29	2286	16.62	32.75	164.25	2272	17.15	33.79	163.21	2257
197.5	15.51	30.64	166.87	2308	16.04	31.67	165.83	2293	16.56	32.71	164.79	2279	17.09	33.75	163.75	2265
198	15.45	30.59	167.41	2315	15.98	31.63	166.37	2301	16.50	32.67	165.33	2287	17.02	33.71	164.29	2272
198.5	15.39	30.55	167.95	2323	15.91	31.59	166.91	2308	16.44	32.63	165.87	2294	16.96	33.67	164.83	2280
199	15.33	30.51	168.49	2330	15.85	31.55	167.45	2316	16.38	32.59	166.41	2301	16.90	33.62	165.38	2287
199.5	15.27	30.47	169.03	2338	15.79	31.51	167.99	2323	16.31	32.55	166.95	2309	16.83	33.58	165.92	2295
200	15.22	30.43	169.57	2345	15.73	31.47	168.53	2331	16.25	32.51	167.50	2316	16.77	33.54	166.46	2302
200.5	15.16	30.39	170.11	2353	15.67	31.43	169.07	2338	16.19	32.46	168.04	2324	16.71	33.50	167.00	2310
201	15.10	30.35	170.65	2360	15.61	31.39	169.61	2346	16.13	32.42	168.58	2331	16.65	33.46	167.54	2317
201.5	15.04	30.31	171.19	2368	15.56	31.34	170.16	2353	16.07	32.38	169.12	2339	16.59	33.42	168.08	2325
202	14.98	30.27	171.73	2375	15.50	31.30	170.70	2361	16.01	32.34	169.66	2346	16.52	33.38	168.62	2332
202.5	14.93	30.23	172.28	2383	15.44	31.26	171.24	2368	15.95	32.30	170.20	2354	16.46	33.34	169.16	2340
203	14.87	30.18	172.82	2390	15.38	31.22	171.78	2376	15.89	32.26	170.74	2361	16.40	33.30	169.70	2347
203.5	14.81	30.14	173.36	2398	15.32	31.18	172.32	2383	15.83	32.22	171.28	2369	16.34	33.26	170.24	2354
204	14.76	30.10	173.90	2405	15.26	31.14	172.86	2391	15.77	32.18	171.82	2376	16.28	33.21	170.79	2362
204.5	14.70	30.06	174.44	2412	15.21	31.10	173.40	2398	15.71	32.14	172.36	2384	16.22	33.17	171.33	2369
205	14.64	30.02	174.98	2420	15.15	31.06	173.94	2406	15.66	32.10	172.91	2391	16.16	33.13	171.87	2377
205.5	14.59	29.98	175.52	2427	15.09	31.02	174.48	2413	15.60	32.05	173.45	2399	16.10	33.09	172.41	2384
206	14.53	29.94	176.06	2435	15.04	30.98	175.02	2421	15.54	32.01	173.99	2406	16.04	33.05	172.95	2392
206.5	14.48	29.90	176.60	2442	14.98	30.93	175.57	2428	15.48	31.97	174.53	2414	15.99	33.01	173.49	2399
207	14.42	29.86	177.14	2450	14.92	30.89	176.11	2436	15.43	31.93	175.07	2421	15.93	32.97	174.03	2407
207.5	14.37	29.82	177.69	2457	14.87	30.85	176.65	2443	15.37	31.89	175.61	2429	15.87	32.93	174.57	2414
208	14.31	29.77	178.23	2465	14.81	30.81	177.19	2451	15.31	31.85	176.15	2436	15.81	32.89	175.11	2422
208.5	14.26	29.73	178.77	2472	14.76	30.77	177.73	2458	15.26	31.81	176.69	2444	15.75	32.85	175.65	2429
209	14.21	29.69	179.31	2480	14.70	30.73	178.27	2465	15.20	31.77	177.23	2451	15.70	32.80	176.20	2437
209.5	14.15	29.65	179.85	2487	14.65	30.69	178.81	2473	15.14	31.73	177.77	2459	15.64	32.76	176.74	2444
210	14.10	29.61	180.39	2495	14.59	30.65	179.35	2480	15.09	31.69	178.32	2466	15.58	32.72	177.28	2452
210.5	14.05	29.57	180.93	2502	14.54	30.61	179.89	2488	15.03	31.64	178.86	2474	15.53	32.68	177.82	2459
211	13.99	29.53	181.47	2510	14.49	30.57	180.43	2495	14.98	31.60	179.40	2481	15.47	32.64	178.36	2467
211.5	13.94	29.49	182.01	2517	14.43	30.52	180.98	2503	14.92	31.56	179.94	2489	15.41	32.60	178.90	2474
212	13.89	29.45	182.55	2525	14.38	30.48	181.52	2510	14.87	31.52	180.48	2496	15.36	32.56	179.44	2482
212.5	13.84	29.41	183.10	2532	14.33	30.44	182.06	2518	14.81	31.48	181.02	2504	15.30	32.52	179.98	2489
213	13.79	29.36	183.64	2540	14.27	30.40	182.60	2525	14.76	31.44	181.56	2511	15.25	32.48	180.52	2497
213.5	13.73	29.32	184.18	2547	14.22	30.36	183.14	2533	14.71	31.40	182.10	2518	15.19	32.44	181.06	2504
214	13.68	29.28	184.72	2555	14.17	30.32	183.68	2540	14.65	31.36	182.64	2526	15.14	32.39	181.61	2512
214.5	13.63	29.24	185.26	2562	14.12	30.28	184.22	2548	14.60	31.32	183.18	2533	15.08	32.35	182.15	2519
215	13.58	29.20	185.80	2570	14.06	30.24	184.76	2555	14.55	31.28	183.73	2541	15.03	32.31	182.69	2527
215.5	13.53	29.16	186.34	2577	14.01	30.20	185.30	2563	14.49	31.23	184.27	2548	14.98	32.27	183.23	2534

Body Composition MALE 184-215.5 Lb.

Weight: Lb.	Waist: 36 inches Fat: %	Fat: Lb.	LBM: Lb.	RMR: Cal.	36.25 inches Fat: %	Fat: Lb.	LBM: Lb.	RMR: Cal.	36.5 inches Fat: %	Fat: Lb.	LBM: Lb.	RMR: Cal.	36.75 inches Fat: %	Fat: Lb.	LBM: Lb.	RMR: Cal.
184	19.51	35.89	148.11	2048	20.07	36.93	147.07	2034	20.63	37.97	146.03	2020	21.20	39.00	145.00	2005
184.5	19.43	35.85	148.65	2056	19.99	36.89	147.61	2041	20.56	37.93	146.57	2027	21.12	38.96	145.54	2013
185	19.36	35.81	149.19	2063	19.92	36.85	148.15	2049	20.48	37.89	147.12	2035	21.04	38.92	146.08	2020
185.5	19.28	35.77	149.73	2071	19.84	36.81	148.69	2056	20.40	37.84	147.66	2042	20.96	38.88	146.62	2028
186	19.21	35.73	150.27	2078	19.77	36.77	149.23	2064	20.32	37.80	148.20	2050	20.88	38.84	147.16	2035
186.5	19.14	35.69	150.81	2086	19.69	36.72	149.78	2071	20.25	37.76	148.74	2057	20.80	38.80	147.70	2043
187	19.06	35.65	151.35	2093	19.62	36.68	150.32	2079	20.17	37.72	149.28	2065	20.73	38.76	148.24	2050
187.5	18.99	35.61	151.90	2101	19.54	36.64	150.86	2086	20.10	37.68	149.82	2072	20.65	38.72	148.78	2058
188	18.92	35.56	152.44	2108	19.47	36.60	151.40	2094	20.02	37.64	150.36	2079	20.57	38.68	149.32	2065
188.5	18.85	35.52	152.98	2116	19.40	36.56	151.94	2101	19.95	37.60	150.90	2087	20.50	38.64	149.86	2073
189	18.77	35.48	153.52	2123	19.32	36.52	152.48	2109	19.87	37.56	151.44	2094	20.42	38.59	150.41	2080
189.5	18.70	35.44	154.06	2131	19.25	36.48	153.02	2116	19.80	37.52	151.98	2102	20.34	38.55	150.95	2088
190	18.63	35.40	154.60	2138	19.18	36.44	153.56	2124	19.72	37.48	152.53	2109	20.27	38.51	151.49	2095
190.5	18.56	35.36	155.14	2146	19.11	36.40	154.10	2131	19.65	37.43	153.07	2117	20.20	38.47	152.03	2103
191	18.49	35.32	155.68	2153	19.03	36.36	154.64	2139	19.58	37.39	153.61	2124	20.12	38.43	152.57	2110
191.5	18.42	35.28	156.22	2161	18.96	36.31	155.19	2146	19.50	37.35	154.15	2132	20.05	38.39	153.11	2118
192	18.35	35.24	156.76	2168	18.89	36.27	155.73	2154	19.43	37.31	154.69	2139	19.97	38.35	153.65	2125
192.5	18.28	35.20	157.31	2176	18.82	36.23	156.27	2161	19.36	37.27	155.23	2147	19.90	38.31	154.19	2132
193	18.21	35.15	157.85	2183	18.75	36.19	156.81	2169	19.29	37.23	155.77	2154	19.83	38.27	154.73	2140
193.5	18.15	35.11	158.39	2190	18.68	36.15	157.35	2176	19.22	37.19	156.31	2162	19.75	38.23	155.27	2147
194	18.08	35.07	158.93	2198	18.61	36.11	157.89	2184	19.15	37.15	156.85	2169	19.68	38.18	155.82	2155
194.5	18.01	35.03	159.47	2205	18.54	36.07	158.43	2191	19.08	37.11	157.39	2177	19.61	38.14	156.36	2162
195	17.94	34.99	160.01	2213	18.48	36.03	158.97	2199	19.01	37.07	157.94	2184	19.54	38.10	156.90	2170
195.5	17.88	34.95	160.55	2220	18.41	35.99	159.51	2206	18.94	37.02	158.48	2192	19.47	38.06	157.44	2177
196	17.81	34.91	161.09	2228	18.34	35.95	160.05	2214	18.87	36.98	159.02	2199	19.40	38.02	157.98	2185
196.5	17.74	34.87	161.63	2235	18.27	35.90	160.60	2221	18.80	36.94	159.56	2207	19.33	37.98	158.52	2192
197	17.68	34.83	162.17	2243	18.20	35.86	161.14	2229	18.73	36.90	160.10	2214	19.26	37.94	159.06	2200
197.5	17.61	34.79	162.72	2250	18.14	35.82	161.68	2236	18.66	36.86	160.64	2222	19.19	37.90	159.60	2207
198	17.55	34.74	163.26	2258	18.07	35.78	162.22	2243	18.60	36.82	161.18	2229	19.12	37.86	160.14	2215
198.5	17.48	34.70	163.80	2265	18.01	35.74	162.76	2251	18.53	36.78	161.72	2237	19.05	37.82	160.68	2222
199	17.42	34.66	164.34	2273	17.94	35.70	163.30	2258	18.46	36.74	162.26	2244	18.98	37.77	161.23	2230
199.5	17.35	34.62	164.88	2280	17.87	35.66	163.84	2266	18.39	36.70	162.80	2252	18.91	37.73	161.77	2237
200	17.29	34.58	165.42	2288	17.81	35.62	164.38	2273	18.33	36.66	163.35	2259	18.85	37.69	162.31	2245
200.5	17.23	34.54	165.96	2295	17.74	35.58	164.92	2281	18.26	36.61	163.89	2267	18.78	37.65	162.85	2252
201	17.16	34.50	166.50	2303	17.68	35.54	165.46	2288	18.20	36.57	164.43	2274	18.71	37.61	163.39	2260
201.5	17.10	34.46	167.04	2310	17.62	35.49	166.01	2296	18.13	36.53	164.97	2282	18.64	37.57	163.93	2267
202	17.04	34.42	167.58	2318	17.55	35.45	166.55	2303	18.06	36.49	165.51	2289	18.58	37.53	164.47	2275
202.5	16.98	34.38	168.13	2325	17.49	35.41	167.09	2311	18.00	36.45	166.05	2296	18.51	37.49	165.01	2282
203	16.91	34.33	168.67	2333	17.42	35.37	167.63	2318	17.94	36.41	166.59	2304	18.45	37.45	165.55	2290
203.5	16.85	34.29	169.21	2340	17.36	35.33	168.17	2326	17.87	36.37	167.13	2311	18.38	37.41	166.09	2297
204	16.79	34.25	169.75	2348	17.30	35.29	168.71	2333	17.81	36.33	167.67	2319	18.32	37.36	166.64	2305
204.5	16.73	34.21	170.29	2355	17.24	35.25	169.25	2341	17.74	36.29	168.21	2326	18.25	37.32	167.18	2312
205	16.67	34.17	170.83	2363	17.17	35.21	169.79	2348	17.68	36.25	168.76	2334	18.19	37.28	167.72	2320
205.5	16.61	34.13	171.37	2370	17.11	35.17	170.33	2356	17.62	36.20	169.30	2341	18.12	37.24	168.26	2327
206	16.55	34.09	171.91	2378	17.05	35.13	170.87	2363	17.55	36.16	169.84	2349	18.06	37.20	168.80	2334
206.5	16.49	34.05	172.45	2385	16.99	35.08	171.42	2371	17.49	36.12	170.38	2356	17.99	37.16	169.34	2342
207	16.43	34.01	172.99	2393	16.93	35.04	171.96	2378	17.43	36.08	170.92	2364	17.93	37.12	169.88	2349
207.5	16.37	33.97	173.54	2400	16.87	35.00	172.50	2386	17.37	36.04	171.46	2371	17.87	37.08	170.42	2357
208	16.31	33.92	174.08	2407	16.81	34.96	173.04	2393	17.31	36.00	172.00	2379	17.81	37.04	170.96	2364
208.5	16.25	33.88	174.62	2415	16.75	34.92	173.58	2401	17.25	35.96	172.54	2386	17.74	37.00	171.50	2372
209	16.19	33.84	175.16	2422	16.69	34.88	174.12	2408	17.19	35.92	173.08	2394	17.68	36.95	172.05	2379
209.5	16.13	33.80	175.70	2430	16.63	34.84	174.66	2416	17.12	35.88	173.62	2401	17.62	36.91	172.59	2387
210	16.08	33.76	176.24	2437	16.57	34.80	175.20	2423	17.06	35.84	174.17	2409	17.56	36.87	173.13	2394
210.5	16.02	33.72	176.78	2445	16.51	34.76	175.74	2431	17.00	35.79	174.71	2416	17.50	36.83	173.67	2402
211	15.96	33.68	177.32	2452	16.45	34.72	176.28	2438	16.94	35.75	175.25	2424	17.44	36.79	174.21	2409
211.5	15.90	33.64	177.86	2460	16.39	34.67	176.83	2445	16.89	35.71	175.79	2431	17.38	36.75	174.75	2417
212	15.85	33.60	178.40	2467	16.34	34.63	177.37	2453	16.83	35.67	176.33	2439	17.32	36.71	175.29	2424
212.5	15.79	33.56	178.95	2475	16.28	34.59	177.91	2460	16.77	35.63	176.87	2446	17.26	36.67	175.83	2432
213	15.73	33.51	179.49	2482	16.22	34.55	178.45	2468	16.71	35.59	177.41	2454	17.20	36.63	176.37	2439
213.5	15.68	33.47	180.03	2490	16.16	34.51	178.99	2475	16.65	35.55	177.95	2461	17.14	36.59	176.91	2447
214	15.62	33.43	180.57	2497	16.11	34.47	179.53	2483	16.59	35.51	178.49	2469	17.08	36.54	177.46	2454
214.5	15.57	33.39	181.11	2505	16.05	34.43	180.07	2490	16.53	35.47	179.03	2476	17.02	36.50	178.00	2462
215	15.51	33.35	181.65	2512	15.99	34.39	180.61	2498	16.48	35.43	179.58	2484	16.96	36.46	178.54	2469
215.5	15.46	33.31	182.19	2520	15.94	34.35	181.15	2505	16.42	35.38	180.12	2491	16.90	36.42	179.08	2477

Body Composition   MALE   184-215.5 Lb.

Weight: Lb.	Waist: 37 inches				37.25 inches				37.5 inches				37.75 inches			
	Fat: %	Fat: Lb.	LBM: Lb.	RMR: Cal.	Fat: %	Fat: Lb.	LBM: Lb.	RMR: Cal.	Fat: %	Fat: Lb.	LBM: Lb.	RMR: Cal.	Fat: %	Fat: Lb.	LBM: Lb.	RMR: Cal.
184	21.76	40.04	143.96	1991	22.33	41.08	142.92	1977	22.89	42.12	141.88	1962	23.45	43.15	140.85	1948
184.5	21.68	40.00	144.50	1998	22.24	41.04	143.46	1984	22.81	42.08	142.42	1970	23.37	43.11	141.39	1955
185	21.60	39.96	145.04	2006	22.16	41.00	144.00	1992	22.72	42.04	142.97	1977	23.28	43.07	141.93	1963
185.5	21.52	39.92	145.58	2013	22.08	40.96	144.54	1999	22.64	41.99	143.51	1985	23.20	43.03	142.47	1970
186	21.44	39.88	146.12	2021	22.00	40.92	145.08	2007	22.56	41.95	144.05	1992	23.11	42.99	143.01	1978
186.5	21.36	39.84	146.66	2028	21.92	40.87	145.63	2014	22.47	41.91	144.59	2000	23.03	42.95	143.55	1985
187	21.28	39.80	147.20	2036	21.84	40.83	146.17	2021	22.39	41.87	145.13	2007	22.95	42.91	144.09	1993
187.5	21.20	39.76	147.75	2043	21.76	40.79	146.71	2029	22.31	41.83	145.67	2015	22.86	42.87	144.63	2000
188	21.12	39.71	148.29	2051	21.68	40.75	147.25	2036	22.23	41.79	146.21	2022	22.78	42.83	145.17	2008
188.5	21.05	39.67	148.83	2058	21.60	40.71	147.79	2044	22.15	41.75	146.75	2030	22.70	42.79	145.71	2015
189	20.97	39.63	149.37	2066	21.52	40.67	148.33	2051	22.07	41.71	147.29	2037	22.62	42.74	146.26	2023
189.5	20.89	39.59	149.91	2073	21.44	40.63	148.87	2059	21.99	41.67	147.83	2045	22.53	42.70	146.80	2030
190	20.82	39.55	150.45	2081	21.36	40.59	149.41	2066	21.91	41.63	148.38	2052	22.45	42.66	147.34	2038
190.5	20.74	39.51	150.99	2088	21.28	40.55	149.95	2074	21.83	41.58	148.92	2060	22.37	42.62	147.88	2045
191	20.66	39.47	151.53	2096	21.21	40.51	150.49	2081	21.75	41.54	149.46	2067	22.29	42.58	148.42	2053
191.5	20.59	39.43	152.07	2103	21.13	40.46	151.04	2089	21.67	41.50	150.00	2074	22.21	42.54	148.96	2060
192	20.51	39.39	152.61	2111	21.05	40.42	151.58	2096	21.59	41.46	150.54	2082	22.13	42.50	149.50	2068
192.5	20.44	39.35	153.16	2118	20.98	40.38	152.12	2104	21.52	41.42	151.08	2089	22.06	42.46	150.04	2075
193	20.36	39.30	153.70	2126	20.90	40.34	152.66	2111	21.44	41.38	151.62	2097	21.98	42.42	150.58	2083
193.5	20.29	39.26	154.24	2133	20.83	40.30	153.20	2119	21.36	41.34	152.16	2104	21.90	42.38	151.12	2090
194	20.22	39.22	154.78	2141	20.75	40.26	153.74	2126	21.29	41.30	152.70	2112	21.82	42.33	151.67	2098
194.5	20.14	39.18	155.32	2148	20.68	40.22	154.28	2134	21.21	41.26	153.24	2119	21.74	42.29	152.21	2105
195	20.07	39.14	155.86	2156	20.60	40.18	154.82	2141	21.14	41.22	153.79	2127	21.67	42.25	152.75	2112
195.5	20.00	39.10	156.40	2163	20.53	40.14	155.36	2149	21.06	41.17	154.33	2134	21.59	42.21	153.29	2120
196	19.93	39.06	156.94	2171	20.46	40.10	155.90	2156	20.99	41.13	154.87	2142	21.52	42.17	153.83	2127
196.5	19.86	39.02	157.48	2178	20.38	40.05	156.45	2164	20.91	41.09	155.41	2149	21.44	42.13	154.37	2135
197	19.78	38.98	158.02	2185	20.31	40.01	156.99	2171	20.84	41.05	155.95	2157	21.36	42.09	154.91	2142
197.5	19.71	38.94	158.57	2193	20.24	39.97	157.53	2179	20.76	41.01	156.49	2164	21.29	42.05	155.45	2150
198	19.64	38.89	159.11	2200	20.17	39.93	158.07	2186	20.69	40.97	157.03	2172	21.22	42.01	155.99	2157
198.5	19.57	38.85	159.65	2208	20.10	39.89	158.61	2194	20.62	40.93	157.57	2179	21.14	41.97	156.53	2165
199	19.50	38.81	160.19	2215	20.02	39.85	159.15	2201	20.55	40.89	158.11	2187	21.07	41.92	157.08	2172
199.5	19.43	38.77	160.73	2223	19.95	39.81	159.69	2209	20.47	40.85	158.65	2194	20.99	41.88	157.62	2180
200	19.37	38.73	161.27	2230	19.88	39.77	160.23	2216	20.40	40.81	159.20	2202	20.92	41.84	158.16	2187
200.5	19.30	38.69	161.81	2238	19.81	39.73	160.77	2223	20.33	40.76	159.74	2209	20.85	41.80	158.70	2195
201	19.23	38.65	162.35	2245	19.74	39.69	161.31	2231	20.26	40.72	160.28	2217	20.78	41.76	159.24	2202
201.5	19.16	38.61	162.89	2253	19.67	39.64	161.86	2238	20.19	40.68	160.82	2224	20.70	41.72	159.78	2210
202	19.09	38.57	163.43	2260	19.61	39.60	162.40	2246	20.12	40.64	161.36	2232	20.63	41.68	160.32	2217
202.5	19.02	38.53	163.98	2268	19.54	39.56	162.94	2253	20.05	40.60	161.90	2239	20.56	41.64	160.86	2225
203	18.96	38.48	164.52	2275	19.47	39.52	163.48	2261	19.98	40.56	162.44	2247	20.49	41.60	161.40	2232
203.5	18.89	38.44	165.06	2283	19.40	39.48	164.02	2268	19.91	40.52	162.98	2254	20.42	41.56	161.94	2240
204	18.82	38.40	165.60	2290	19.33	39.44	164.56	2276	19.84	40.48	163.52	2262	20.35	41.51	162.49	2247
204.5	18.76	38.36	166.14	2298	19.27	39.40	165.10	2283	19.77	40.44	164.06	2269	20.28	41.47	163.03	2255
205	18.69	38.32	166.68	2305	19.20	39.36	165.64	2291	19.70	40.40	164.61	2276	20.21	41.43	163.57	2262
205.5	18.63	38.28	167.22	2313	19.13	39.32	166.18	2298	19.64	40.35	165.15	2284	20.14	41.39	164.11	2270
206	18.56	38.24	167.76	2320	19.07	39.28	166.72	2306	19.57	40.31	165.69	2291	20.07	41.35	164.65	2277
206.5	18.50	38.20	168.30	2328	19.00	39.23	167.27	2313	19.50	40.27	166.23	2299	20.00	41.31	165.19	2285
207	18.43	38.16	168.84	2335	18.93	39.19	167.81	2321	19.44	40.23	166.77	2306	19.94	41.27	165.73	2292
207.5	18.37	38.12	169.39	2343	18.87	39.15	168.35	2328	19.37	40.19	167.31	2314	19.87	41.23	166.27	2300
208	18.30	38.07	169.93	2350	18.80	39.11	168.89	2336	19.30	40.15	167.85	2321	19.80	41.19	166.81	2307
208.5	18.24	38.03	170.47	2358	18.74	39.07	169.43	2343	19.24	40.11	168.39	2329	19.73	41.15	167.35	2315
209	18.18	37.99	171.01	2365	18.67	39.03	169.97	2351	19.17	40.07	168.93	2336	19.67	41.10	167.90	2322
209.5	18.12	37.95	171.55	2373	18.61	38.99	170.51	2358	19.11	40.03	169.47	2344	19.60	41.06	168.44	2329
210	18.05	37.91	172.09	2380	18.55	38.95	171.05	2366	19.04	39.99	170.02	2351	19.53	41.02	168.98	2337
210.5	17.99	37.87	172.63	2387	18.48	38.91	171.59	2373	18.98	39.94	170.56	2359	19.47	40.98	169.52	2344
211	17.93	37.83	173.17	2395	18.42	38.87	172.13	2381	18.91	39.90	171.10	2366	19.40	40.94	170.06	2352
211.5	17.87	37.79	173.71	2402	18.36	38.82	172.68	2388	18.85	39.86	171.64	2374	19.34	40.90	170.60	2359
212	17.80	37.75	174.25	2410	18.29	38.78	173.22	2396	18.78	39.82	172.18	2381	19.27	40.86	171.14	2367
212.5	17.74	37.71	174.80	2417	18.23	38.74	173.76	2403	18.72	39.78	172.72	2389	19.21	40.82	171.68	2374
213	17.68	37.66	175.34	2425	18.17	38.70	174.30	2411	18.66	39.74	173.26	2396	19.14	40.78	172.22	2382
213.5	17.62	37.62	175.88	2432	18.11	38.66	174.84	2418	18.59	39.70	173.80	2404	19.08	40.74	172.76	2389
214	17.56	37.58	176.42	2440	18.05	38.62	175.38	2426	18.53	39.66	174.34	2411	19.02	40.69	173.31	2397
214.5	17.50	37.54	176.96	2447	17.99	38.58	175.92	2433	18.47	39.62	174.88	2419	18.95	40.65	173.85	2404
215	17.44	37.50	177.50	2455	17.92	38.54	176.46	2440	18.41	39.58	175.43	2426	18.89	40.61	174.39	2412
215.5	17.38	37.46	178.04	2462	17.86	38.50	177.00	2448	18.35	39.53	175.97	2434	18.83	40.57	174.93	2419

Body Composition   MALE   184-215.5 Lb.

Weight: Lb.	Waist: 38 inches Fat: %	Fat: Lb.	LBM: Lb.	RMR: Cal.	38.25 inches Fat: %	Fat: Lb.	LBM: Lb.	RMR: Cal.	38.5 inches Fat: %	Fat: Lb.	LBM: Lb.	RMR: Cal.	38.75 inches Fat: %	Fat: Lb.	LBM: Lb.	RMR: Cal.
184	24.02	44.19	139.81	1934	24.58	45.23	138.77	1919	25.15	46.27	137.73	1905	25.71	47.30	136.70	1890
184.5	23.93	44.15	140.35	1941	24.49	45.19	139.31	1927	25.05	46.23	138.27	1912	25.62	47.26	137.24	1898
185	23.84	44.11	140.89	1949	24.40	45.15	139.85	1934	24.96	46.19	138.82	1920	25.53	47.22	137.78	1905
185.5	23.76	44.07	141.43	1956	24.32	45.11	140.39	1942	24.88	46.14	139.36	1927	25.43	47.18	138.32	1913
186	23.67	44.03	141.97	1963	24.23	45.07	140.93	1949	24.79	46.10	139.90	1935	25.34	47.14	138.86	1920
186.5	23.59	43.99	142.51	1971	24.14	45.02	141.48	1957	24.70	46.06	140.44	1942	25.25	47.10	139.40	1928
187	23.50	43.95	143.05	1978	24.06	44.98	142.02	1964	24.61	46.02	140.98	1950	25.16	47.06	139.94	1935
187.5	23.42	43.91	143.60	1986	23.97	44.94	142.56	1972	24.52	45.98	141.52	1957	25.08	47.02	140.48	1943
188	23.33	43.86	144.14	1993	23.88	44.90	143.10	1979	24.44	45.94	142.06	1965	24.99	46.98	141.02	1950
188.5	23.25	43.82	144.68	2001	23.80	44.86	143.64	1987	24.35	45.90	142.60	1972	24.90	46.94	141.56	1958
189	23.17	43.78	145.22	2008	23.71	44.82	144.18	1994	24.26	45.86	143.14	1980	24.81	46.89	142.11	1965
189.5	23.08	43.74	145.76	2016	23.63	44.78	144.72	2001	24.18	45.82	143.68	1987	24.72	46.85	142.65	1973
190	23.00	43.70	146.30	2023	23.55	44.74	145.26	2009	24.09	45.78	144.23	1995	24.64	46.81	143.19	1980
190.5	22.92	43.66	146.84	2031	23.46	44.70	145.80	2016	24.01	45.73	144.77	2002	24.55	46.77	143.73	1988
191	22.84	43.62	147.38	2038	23.38	44.66	146.34	2024	23.92	45.69	145.31	2010	24.47	46.73	144.27	1995
191.5	22.76	43.58	147.92	2046	23.30	44.61	146.89	2031	23.84	45.65	145.85	2017	24.38	46.69	144.81	2003
192	22.68	43.54	148.46	2053	23.22	44.57	147.43	2039	23.76	45.61	146.39	2025	24.30	46.65	145.35	2010
192.5	22.59	43.50	149.01	2061	23.13	44.53	147.97	2046	23.67	45.57	146.93	2032	24.21	46.61	145.89	2018
193	22.52	43.45	149.55	2068	23.05	44.49	148.51	2054	23.59	45.53	147.47	2040	24.13	46.57	146.43	2025
193.5	22.44	43.41	150.09	2076	22.97	44.45	149.05	2061	23.51	45.49	148.01	2047	24.04	46.53	146.97	2033
194	22.36	43.37	150.63	2083	22.89	44.41	149.59	2069	23.43	45.45	148.55	2054	23.96	46.48	147.52	2040
194.5	22.28	43.33	151.17	2091	22.81	44.37	150.13	2076	23.34	45.41	149.09	2062	23.88	46.44	148.06	2048
195	22.20	43.29	151.71	2098	22.73	44.33	150.67	2084	23.26	45.37	149.64	2069	23.80	46.40	148.60	2055
195.5	22.12	43.25	152.25	2106	22.65	44.29	151.21	2091	23.18	45.32	150.18	2077	23.71	46.36	149.14	2063
196	22.04	43.21	152.79	2113	22.57	44.25	151.75	2099	23.10	45.28	150.72	2084	23.63	46.32	149.68	2070
196.5	21.97	43.17	153.33	2121	22.50	44.20	152.30	2106	23.02	45.24	151.26	2092	23.55	46.28	150.22	2078
197	21.89	43.13	153.87	2128	22.42	44.16	152.84	2114	22.94	45.20	151.80	2099	23.47	46.24	150.76	2085
197.5	21.82	43.09	154.42	2136	22.34	44.12	153.38	2121	22.87	45.16	152.34	2107	23.39	46.20	151.30	2093
198	21.74	43.04	154.96	2143	22.26	44.08	153.92	2129	22.79	45.12	152.88	2114	23.31	46.16	151.84	2100
198.5	21.66	43.00	155.50	2151	22.19	44.04	154.46	2136	22.71	45.08	153.42	2122	23.23	46.12	152.38	2107
199	21.59	42.96	156.04	2158	22.11	44.00	155.00	2144	22.63	45.04	153.96	2129	23.15	46.07	152.93	2115
199.5	21.51	42.92	156.58	2165	22.03	43.96	155.54	2151	22.55	45.00	154.50	2137	23.07	46.03	153.47	2122
200	21.44	42.88	157.12	2173	21.96	43.92	156.08	2159	22.48	44.96	155.05	2144	23.00	45.99	154.01	2130
200.5	21.37	42.84	157.66	2180	21.88	43.88	156.62	2166	22.40	44.91	155.59	2152	22.92	45.95	154.55	2137
201	21.29	42.80	158.20	2188	21.81	43.84	157.16	2174	22.32	44.87	156.13	2159	22.84	45.91	155.09	2145
201.5	21.22	42.76	158.74	2195	21.73	43.79	157.71	2181	22.25	44.83	156.67	2167	22.76	45.87	155.63	2152
202	21.15	42.72	159.28	2203	21.66	43.75	158.25	2189	22.17	44.79	157.21	2174	22.69	45.83	156.17	2160
202.5	21.07	42.68	159.83	2210	21.59	43.71	158.79	2196	22.10	44.75	157.75	2182	22.61	45.79	156.71	2167
203	21.00	42.63	160.37	2218	21.51	43.67	159.33	2204	22.02	44.71	158.29	2189	22.54	45.75	157.25	2175
203.5	20.93	42.59	160.91	2225	21.44	43.63	159.87	2211	21.95	44.67	158.83	2197	22.46	45.71	157.79	2182
204	20.86	42.55	161.45	2233	21.37	43.59	160.41	2218	21.88	44.63	159.37	2204	22.38	45.66	158.34	2190
204.5	20.79	42.51	161.99	2240	21.30	43.55	160.95	2226	21.80	44.59	159.91	2212	22.31	45.62	158.88	2197
205	20.72	42.47	162.53	2248	21.22	43.51	161.49	2233	21.73	44.55	160.46	2219	22.24	45.58	159.42	2205
205.5	20.65	42.43	163.07	2255	21.15	43.47	162.03	2241	21.66	44.51	161.00	2227	22.16	45.54	159.96	2212
206	20.58	42.39	163.61	2263	21.08	43.43	162.57	2248	21.58	44.46	161.54	2234	22.09	45.50	160.50	2220
206.5	20.51	42.35	164.15	2270	21.01	43.38	163.12	2256	21.51	44.42	162.08	2242	22.01	45.46	161.04	2227
207	20.44	42.31	164.69	2278	20.94	43.34	163.66	2263	21.44	44.38	162.62	2249	21.94	45.42	161.58	2235
207.5	20.37	42.27	165.24	2285	20.87	43.30	164.20	2271	21.37	44.34	163.16	2257	21.87	45.38	162.12	2242
208	20.30	42.22	165.78	2293	20.80	43.26	164.74	2278	21.30	44.30	163.70	2264	21.80	45.34	162.66	2250
208.5	20.23	42.18	166.32	2300	20.73	43.22	165.28	2286	21.23	44.26	164.24	2271	21.72	45.30	163.20	2257
209	20.16	42.14	166.86	2308	20.66	43.18	165.82	2293	21.16	44.22	164.78	2279	21.65	45.25	163.75	2265
209.5	20.10	42.10	167.40	2315	20.59	43.14	166.36	2301	21.09	44.18	165.32	2286	21.58	45.21	164.29	2272
210	20.03	42.06	167.94	2323	20.52	43.10	166.90	2308	21.02	44.14	165.87	2294	21.51	45.17	164.83	2280
210.5	19.96	42.02	168.48	2330	20.45	43.06	167.44	2316	20.95	44.09	166.41	2301	21.44	45.13	165.37	2287
211	19.89	41.98	169.02	2338	20.39	43.02	167.98	2323	20.88	44.05	166.95	2309	21.37	45.09	165.91	2295
211.5	19.83	41.94	169.56	2345	20.32	42.97	168.53	2331	20.81	44.01	167.49	2316	21.30	45.05	166.45	2302
212	19.76	41.90	170.10	2353	20.25	42.93	169.07	2338	20.74	43.97	168.03	2324	21.23	45.01	166.99	2309
212.5	19.70	41.86	170.65	2360	20.18	42.89	169.61	2346	20.67	43.93	168.57	2331	21.16	44.97	167.53	2317
213	19.63	41.81	171.19	2368	20.12	42.85	170.15	2353	20.61	43.89	169.11	2339	21.09	44.93	168.07	2324
213.5	19.57	41.77	171.73	2375	20.05	42.81	170.69	2361	20.54	43.85	169.65	2346	21.02	44.89	168.61	2332
214	19.50	41.73	172.27	2382	19.99	42.77	171.23	2368	20.47	43.81	170.19	2354	20.96	44.84	169.16	2339
214.5	19.44	41.69	172.81	2390	19.92	42.73	171.77	2376	20.40	43.77	170.73	2361	20.89	44.80	169.70	2347
215	19.37	41.65	173.35	2397	19.85	42.69	172.31	2383	20.34	43.73	171.28	2369	20.82	44.76	170.24	2354
215.5	19.31	41.61	173.89	2405	19.79	42.65	172.85	2391	20.27	43.68	171.82	2376	20.75	44.72	170.78	2362

Body Composition MALE 184-215.5 Lb.

Weight: Lb.	Waist: 39 inches Fat: %	Fat: Lb.	LBM: Lb.	RMR: Cal.	39.25 inches Fat: %	Fat: Lb.	LBM: Lb.	RMR: Cal.	39.5 inches Fat: %	Fat: Lb.	LBM: Lb.	RMR: Cal.	39.75 inches Fat: %	Fat: Lb.	LBM: Lb.	RMR: Cal.
184	26.27	48.34	135.66	1876	26.84	49.38	134.62	1862	27.40	50.42	133.58	1847	27.96	51.45	132.55	1833
184.5	26.18	48.30	136.20	1884	26.74	49.34	135.16	1869	27.30	50.38	134.12	1855	27.87	51.41	133.09	1841
185	26.09	48.26	136.74	1891	26.65	49.30	135.70	1877	27.21	50.34	134.67	1862	27.77	51.37	133.63	1848
185.5	25.99	48.22	137.28	1899	26.55	49.26	136.24	1884	27.11	50.29	135.21	1870	27.67	51.33	134.17	1856
186	25.90	48.18	137.82	1906	26.46	49.22	136.78	1892	27.02	50.25	135.75	1877	27.58	51.29	134.71	1863
186.5	25.81	48.14	138.36	1914	26.37	49.17	137.33	1899	26.92	50.21	136.29	1885	27.48	51.25	135.25	1871
187	25.72	48.10	138.90	1921	26.27	49.13	137.87	1907	26.83	50.17	136.83	1892	27.38	51.21	135.79	1878
187.5	25.63	48.06	139.45	1929	26.18	49.09	138.41	1914	26.74	50.13	137.37	1900	27.29	51.17	136.33	1885
188	25.54	48.01	139.99	1936	26.09	49.05	138.95	1922	26.64	50.09	137.91	1907	27.19	51.13	136.87	1893
188.5	25.45	47.97	140.53	1943	26.00	49.01	139.49	1929	26.55	50.05	138.45	1915	27.10	51.09	137.41	1900
189	25.36	47.93	141.07	1951	25.91	48.97	140.03	1937	26.46	50.01	138.99	1922	27.01	51.04	137.96	1908
189.5	25.27	47.89	141.61	1958	25.82	48.93	140.57	1944	26.37	49.97	139.53	1930	26.91	51.00	138.50	1915
190	25.18	47.85	142.15	1966	25.73	48.89	141.11	1952	26.28	49.93	140.08	1937	26.82	50.96	139.04	1923
190.5	25.10	47.81	142.69	1973	25.64	48.85	141.65	1959	26.19	49.88	140.62	1945	26.73	50.92	139.58	1930
191	25.01	47.77	143.23	1981	25.55	48.81	142.19	1967	26.10	49.84	141.16	1952	26.64	50.88	140.12	1938
191.5	24.92	47.73	143.77	1988	25.46	48.76	142.74	1974	26.01	49.80	141.70	1960	26.55	50.84	140.66	1945
192	24.84	47.69	144.31	1996	25.38	48.72	143.28	1982	25.92	49.76	142.24	1967	26.46	50.80	141.20	1953
192.5	24.75	47.65	144.86	2003	25.29	48.68	143.82	1989	25.83	49.72	142.78	1975	26.37	50.76	141.74	1960
193	24.67	47.60	145.40	2011	25.20	48.64	144.36	1996	25.74	49.68	143.32	1982	26.28	50.72	142.28	1968
193.5	24.58	47.56	145.94	2018	25.12	48.60	144.90	2004	25.65	49.64	143.86	1990	26.19	50.68	142.82	1975
194	24.50	47.52	146.48	2026	25.03	48.56	145.44	2011	25.57	49.60	144.40	1997	26.10	50.63	143.37	1983
194.5	24.41	47.48	147.02	2033	24.95	48.52	145.98	2019	25.48	49.56	144.94	2005	26.01	50.59	143.91	1990
195	24.33	47.44	147.56	2041	24.86	48.48	146.52	2026	25.39	49.52	145.49	2012	25.92	50.55	144.45	1998
195.5	24.25	47.40	148.10	2048	24.78	48.44	147.06	2034	25.31	49.47	146.03	2020	25.84	50.51	144.99	2005
196	24.16	47.36	148.64	2056	24.69	48.40	147.60	2041	25.22	49.43	146.57	2027	25.75	50.47	145.53	2013
196.5	24.08	47.32	149.18	2063	24.61	48.35	148.15	2049	25.14	49.39	147.11	2035	25.66	50.43	146.07	2020
197	24.00	47.28	149.72	2071	24.52	48.31	148.69	2056	25.05	49.35	147.65	2042	25.58	50.39	146.61	2028
197.5	23.92	47.24	150.27	2078	24.44	48.27	149.23	2064	24.97	49.31	148.19	2049	25.49	50.35	147.15	2035
198	23.84	47.19	150.81	2086	24.36	48.23	149.77	2071	24.88	49.27	148.73	2057	25.41	50.31	147.69	2043
198.5	23.75	47.15	151.35	2093	24.28	48.19	150.31	2079	24.80	49.23	149.27	2064	25.32	50.27	148.23	2050
199	23.67	47.11	151.89	2101	24.20	48.15	150.85	2086	24.72	49.19	149.81	2072	25.24	50.22	148.78	2058
199.5	23.59	47.07	152.43	2108	24.11	48.11	151.39	2094	24.63	49.15	150.35	2079	25.15	50.18	149.32	2065
200	23.52	47.03	152.97	2116	24.03	48.07	151.93	2101	24.55	49.11	150.90	2087	25.07	50.14	149.86	2073
200.5	23.44	46.99	153.51	2123	23.95	48.03	152.47	2109	24.47	49.06	151.44	2094	24.99	50.10	150.40	2080
201	23.36	46.95	154.05	2131	23.87	47.99	153.01	2116	24.39	49.02	151.98	2102	24.91	50.06	150.94	2087
201.5	23.28	46.91	154.59	2138	23.79	47.94	153.56	2124	24.31	48.98	152.52	2109	24.82	50.02	151.48	2095
202	23.20	46.87	155.13	2146	23.71	47.90	154.10	2131	24.23	48.94	153.06	2117	24.74	49.98	152.02	2102
202.5	23.12	46.83	155.68	2153	23.64	47.86	154.64	2139	24.15	48.90	153.60	2124	24.66	49.94	152.56	2110
203	23.05	46.78	156.22	2160	23.56	47.82	155.18	2146	24.07	48.86	154.14	2132	24.58	49.90	153.10	2117
203.5	22.97	46.74	156.76	2168	23.48	47.78	155.72	2154	23.99	48.82	154.68	2139	24.50	49.86	153.64	2125
204	22.89	46.70	157.30	2175	23.40	47.74	156.26	2161	23.91	48.78	155.22	2147	24.42	49.81	154.19	2132
204.5	22.82	46.66	157.84	2183	23.32	47.70	156.80	2169	23.83	48.74	155.76	2154	24.34	49.77	154.73	2140
205	22.74	46.62	158.38	2190	23.25	47.66	157.34	2176	23.75	48.70	156.31	2162	24.26	49.73	155.27	2147
205.5	22.67	46.58	158.92	2198	23.17	47.62	157.88	2184	23.68	48.65	156.85	2169	24.18	49.69	155.81	2155
206	22.59	46.54	159.46	2205	23.09	47.58	158.42	2191	23.60	48.61	157.39	2177	24.10	49.65	156.35	2162
206.5	22.52	46.50	160.00	2213	23.02	47.53	158.97	2198	23.52	48.57	157.93	2184	24.02	49.61	156.89	2170
207	22.44	46.46	160.54	2220	22.94	47.49	159.51	2206	23.44	48.53	158.47	2192	23.95	49.57	157.43	2177
207.5	22.37	46.42	161.09	2228	22.87	47.45	160.05	2213	23.37	48.49	159.01	2199	23.87	49.53	157.97	2185
208	22.30	46.37	161.63	2235	22.79	47.41	160.59	2221	23.29	48.45	159.55	2207	23.79	49.49	158.51	2192
208.5	22.22	46.33	162.17	2243	22.72	47.37	161.13	2228	23.22	48.41	160.09	2214	23.71	49.45	159.05	2200
209	22.15	46.29	162.71	2250	22.65	47.33	161.67	2236	23.14	48.37	160.63	2222	23.64	49.40	159.60	2207
209.5	22.08	46.25	163.25	2258	22.57	47.29	162.21	2243	23.07	48.33	161.17	2229	23.56	49.36	160.14	2215
210	22.00	46.21	163.79	2265	22.50	47.25	162.75	2251	22.99	48.29	161.72	2237	23.49	49.32	160.68	2222
210.5	21.93	46.17	164.33	2273	22.43	47.21	163.29	2258	22.92	48.24	162.26	2244	23.41	49.28	161.22	2230
211	21.86	46.13	164.87	2280	22.35	47.17	163.83	2266	22.85	48.20	162.80	2251	23.34	49.24	161.76	2237
211.5	21.79	46.09	165.41	2288	22.28	47.12	164.38	2273	22.77	48.16	163.34	2259	23.26	49.20	162.30	2245
212	21.72	46.05	165.95	2295	22.21	47.08	164.92	2281	22.70	48.12	163.88	2266	23.19	49.16	162.84	2252
212.5	21.65	46.01	166.50	2303	22.14	47.04	165.46	2288	22.63	48.08	164.42	2274	23.11	49.12	163.38	2260
213	21.58	45.96	167.04	2310	22.07	47.00	166.00	2296	22.55	48.04	164.96	2281	23.04	49.08	163.92	2267
213.5	21.51	45.92	167.58	2318	22.00	46.96	166.54	2303	22.48	48.00	165.50	2289	22.97	49.04	164.46	2275
214	21.44	45.88	168.12	2325	21.93	46.92	167.08	2311	22.41	47.96	166.04	2296	22.89	48.99	165.01	2282
214.5	21.37	45.84	168.66	2333	21.85	46.88	167.62	2318	22.34	47.92	166.58	2304	22.82	48.95	165.55	2290
215	21.30	45.80	169.20	2340	21.78	46.84	168.16	2326	22.27	47.88	167.13	2311	22.75	48.91	166.09	2297
215.5	21.23	45.76	169.74	2348	21.72	46.80	168.70	2333	22.20	47.83	167.67	2319	22.68	48.87	166.63	2304

Body Composition MALE 184-215.5 Lb.

Weight: Lb.	Waist: 40 inches Fat: %	Fat: Lb.	LBM: Lb.	RMR: Cal.	40.25 inches Fat: %	Fat: Lb.	LBM: Lb.	RMR: Cal.	40.5 inches Fat: %	Fat: Lb.	LBM: Lb.	RMR: Cal.	40.75 inches Fat: %	Fat: Lb.	LBM: Lb.	RMR: Cal.
184	28.53	52.49	131.51	1819	29.09	53.53	130.47	1804	29.66	54.57	129.43	1790	30.22	55.60	128.40	1776
184.5	28.43	52.45	132.05	1826	28.99	53.49	131.01	1812	29.55	54.53	129.97	1798	30.12	55.56	128.94	1783
185	28.33	52.41	132.59	1834	28.89	53.45	131.55	1819	29.45	54.49	130.52	1805	30.01	55.52	129.48	1791
185.5	28.23	52.37	133.13	1841	28.79	53.41	132.09	1827	29.35	54.44	131.06	1813	29.91	55.48	130.02	1798
186	28.13	52.33	133.67	1849	28.69	53.37	132.63	1834	29.25	54.40	131.60	1820	29.81	55.44	130.56	1806
186.5	28.04	52.29	134.21	1856	28.59	53.32	133.18	1842	29.15	54.36	132.14	1827	29.70	55.40	131.10	1813
187	27.94	52.25	134.75	1864	28.49	53.28	133.72	1849	29.05	54.32	132.68	1835	29.60	55.36	131.64	1821
187.5	27.84	52.21	135.30	1871	28.40	53.24	134.26	1857	28.95	54.28	133.22	1842	29.50	55.32	132.18	1828
188	27.75	52.16	135.84	1879	28.30	53.20	134.80	1864	28.85	54.24	133.76	1850	29.40	55.28	132.72	1836
188.5	27.65	52.12	136.38	1886	28.20	53.16	135.34	1872	28.75	54.20	134.30	1857	29.30	55.24	133.26	1843
189	27.56	52.08	136.92	1894	28.11	53.12	135.88	1879	28.65	54.16	134.84	1865	29.20	55.19	133.81	1851
189.5	27.46	52.04	137.46	1901	28.01	53.08	136.42	1887	28.56	54.12	135.38	1872	29.10	55.15	134.35	1858
190	27.37	52.00	138.00	1909	27.91	53.04	136.96	1894	28.46	54.08	135.93	1880	29.01	55.11	134.89	1865
190.5	27.28	51.96	138.54	1916	27.82	53.00	137.50	1902	28.36	54.03	136.47	1887	28.91	55.07	135.43	1873
191	27.18	51.92	139.08	1924	27.73	52.96	138.04	1909	28.27	53.99	137.01	1895	28.81	55.03	135.97	1880
191.5	27.09	51.88	139.62	1931	27.63	52.91	138.59	1917	28.17	53.95	137.55	1902	28.72	54.99	136.51	1888
192	27.00	51.84	140.16	1938	27.54	52.87	139.13	1924	28.08	53.91	138.09	1910	28.62	54.95	137.05	1895
192.5	26.91	51.80	140.71	1946	27.45	52.83	139.67	1932	27.98	53.87	138.63	1917	28.52	54.91	137.59	1903
193	26.82	51.75	141.25	1953	27.35	52.79	140.21	1939	27.89	53.83	139.17	1925	28.43	54.87	138.13	1910
193.5	26.73	51.71	141.79	1961	27.26	52.75	140.75	1947	27.80	53.79	139.71	1932	28.33	54.83	138.67	1918
194	26.64	51.67	142.33	1968	27.17	52.71	141.29	1954	27.70	53.75	140.25	1940	28.24	54.78	139.22	1925
194.5	26.55	51.63	142.87	1976	27.08	52.67	141.83	1962	27.61	53.71	140.79	1947	28.15	54.74	139.76	1933
195	26.46	51.59	143.41	1983	26.99	52.63	142.37	1969	27.52	53.67	141.34	1955	28.05	54.70	140.30	1940
195.5	26.37	51.55	143.95	1991	26.90	52.59	142.91	1976	27.43	53.62	141.88	1962	27.96	54.66	140.84	1948
196	26.28	51.51	144.49	1998	26.81	52.55	143.45	1984	27.34	53.58	142.42	1970	27.87	54.62	141.38	1955
196.5	26.19	51.47	145.03	2006	26.72	52.50	144.00	1991	27.25	53.54	142.96	1977	27.78	54.58	141.92	1963
197	26.10	51.43	145.57	2013	26.63	52.46	144.54	1999	27.16	53.50	143.50	1985	27.68	54.54	142.46	1970
197.5	26.02	51.39	146.12	2021	26.54	52.42	145.08	2006	27.07	53.46	144.04	1992	27.59	54.50	143.00	1978
198	25.93	51.34	146.66	2028	26.46	52.38	145.62	2014	26.98	53.42	144.58	2000	27.50	54.46	143.54	1985
198.5	25.85	51.30	147.20	2036	26.37	52.34	146.16	2021	26.89	53.38	145.12	2007	27.41	54.42	144.08	1993
199	25.76	51.26	147.74	2043	26.28	52.30	146.70	2029	26.80	53.34	145.66	2015	27.32	54.37	144.63	2000
199.5	25.67	51.22	148.28	2051	26.19	52.26	147.24	2036	26.71	53.30	146.20	2022	27.23	54.33	145.17	2008
200	25.59	51.18	148.82	2058	26.11	52.22	147.78	2044	26.63	53.26	146.75	2029	27.15	54.29	145.71	2015
200.5	25.51	51.14	149.36	2066	26.02	52.18	148.32	2051	26.54	53.21	147.29	2037	27.06	54.25	146.25	2023
201	25.42	51.10	149.90	2073	25.94	52.14	148.86	2059	26.45	53.17	147.83	2044	26.97	54.21	146.79	2030
201.5	25.34	51.06	150.44	2081	25.85	52.09	149.41	2066	26.37	53.13	148.37	2052	26.88	54.17	147.33	2038
202	25.26	51.02	150.98	2088	25.77	52.05	149.95	2074	26.28	53.09	148.91	2059	26.80	54.13	147.87	2045
202.5	25.17	50.98	151.53	2096	25.69	52.01	150.49	2081	26.20	53.05	149.45	2067	26.71	54.09	148.41	2053
203	25.09	50.93	152.07	2103	25.60	51.97	151.03	2089	26.11	53.01	149.99	2074	26.62	54.05	148.95	2060
203.5	25.01	50.89	152.61	2111	25.52	51.93	151.57	2096	26.03	52.97	150.53	2082	26.54	54.01	149.49	2068
204	24.93	50.85	153.15	2118	25.44	51.89	152.11	2104	25.94	52.93	151.07	2089	26.45	53.96	150.04	2075
204.5	24.85	50.81	153.69	2126	25.35	51.85	152.65	2111	25.86	52.89	151.61	2097	26.37	53.92	150.58	2082
205	24.77	50.77	154.23	2133	25.27	51.81	153.19	2119	25.78	52.85	152.16	2104	26.28	53.88	151.12	2090
205.5	24.69	50.73	154.77	2140	25.19	51.77	153.73	2126	25.70	52.80	152.70	2112	26.20	53.84	151.66	2097
206	24.61	50.69	155.31	2148	25.11	51.73	154.27	2134	25.61	52.76	153.24	2119	26.12	53.80	152.20	2105
206.5	24.53	50.65	155.85	2155	25.03	51.68	154.82	2141	25.53	52.72	153.78	2127	26.03	53.76	152.74	2112
207	24.45	50.61	156.39	2163	24.95	51.64	155.36	2149	25.45	52.68	154.32	2134	25.95	53.72	153.28	2120
207.5	24.37	50.57	156.94	2170	24.87	51.60	155.90	2156	25.37	52.64	154.86	2142	25.87	53.68	153.82	2127
208	24.29	50.52	157.48	2178	24.79	51.56	156.44	2164	25.29	52.60	155.40	2149	25.79	53.64	154.36	2135
208.5	24.21	50.48	158.02	2185	24.71	51.52	156.98	2171	25.21	52.56	155.94	2157	25.71	53.60	154.90	2142
209	24.13	50.44	158.56	2193	24.63	51.48	157.52	2179	25.13	52.52	156.48	2164	25.62	53.55	155.45	2150
209.5	24.06	50.40	159.10	2200	24.55	51.44	158.06	2186	25.05	52.48	157.02	2172	25.54	53.51	155.99	2157
210	23.98	50.36	159.64	2208	24.48	51.40	158.60	2193	24.97	52.44	157.57	2179	25.46	53.47	156.53	2165
210.5	23.90	50.32	160.18	2215	24.40	51.36	159.14	2201	24.89	52.39	158.11	2187	25.38	53.43	157.07	2172
211	23.83	50.28	160.72	2223	24.32	51.32	159.68	2208	24.81	52.35	158.65	2194	25.30	53.39	157.61	2180
211.5	23.75	50.24	161.26	2230	24.24	51.27	160.23	2216	24.73	52.31	159.19	2202	25.22	53.35	158.15	2187
212	23.68	50.20	161.80	2238	24.17	51.23	160.77	2223	24.66	52.27	159.73	2209	25.15	53.31	158.69	2195
212.5	23.60	50.16	162.35	2245	24.09	51.19	161.31	2231	24.58	52.23	160.27	2217	25.07	53.27	159.23	2202
213	23.53	50.11	162.89	2253	24.01	51.15	161.85	2238	24.50	52.19	160.81	2224	24.99	53.23	159.77	2210
213.5	23.45	50.07	163.43	2260	23.94	51.11	162.39	2246	24.43	52.15	161.35	2231	24.91	53.19	160.31	2217
214	23.38	50.03	163.97	2268	23.86	51.07	162.93	2253	24.35	52.11	161.89	2239	24.83	53.14	160.86	2225
214.5	23.31	49.99	164.51	2275	23.79	51.03	163.47	2261	24.27	52.07	162.43	2246	24.76	53.10	161.40	2232
215	23.23	49.95	165.05	2283	23.72	50.99	164.01	2268	24.20	52.03	162.98	2254	24.68	53.06	161.94	2240
215.5	23.16	49.91	165.59	2290	23.64	50.95	164.55	2276	24.12	51.98	163.52	2261	24.60	53.02	162.48	2247

Body Composition　MALE　184-215.5 Lb.

Weight: Lb.	Waist: 41 inches				41.25 inches				41.5 inches				41.75 inches			
	Fat: %	Fat: Lb.	LBM: Lb.	RMR: Cal.	Fat: %	Fat: Lb.	LBM: Lb.	RMR: Cal.	Fat: %	Fat: Lb.	LBM: Lb.	RMR: Cal.	Fat: %	Fat: Lb.	LBM: Lb.	RMR: Cal.
184	30.78	56.64	127.36	1761	31.35	57.68	126.32	1747	31.91	58.72	125.28	1733	32.48	59.75	124.25	1718
184.5	30.68	56.60	127.90	1769	31.24	57.64	126.86	1754	31.80	58.68	125.82	1740	32.37	59.71	124.79	1726
185	30.57	56.56	128.44	1776	31.13	57.60	127.40	1762	31.69	58.64	126.37	1748	32.26	59.67	125.33	1733
185.5	30.47	56.52	128.98	1784	31.03	57.56	127.94	1769	31.59	58.59	126.91	1755	32.15	59.63	125.87	1741
186	30.36	56.48	129.52	1791	30.92	57.52	128.48	1777	31.48	58.55	127.45	1763	32.04	59.59	126.41	1748
186.5	30.26	56.44	130.06	1799	30.82	57.47	129.03	1784	31.37	58.51	127.99	1770	31.93	59.55	126.95	1756
187	30.16	56.40	130.60	1806	30.71	57.43	129.57	1792	31.27	58.47	128.53	1778	31.82	59.51	127.49	1763
187.5	30.06	56.36	131.15	1814	30.61	57.39	130.11	1799	31.16	58.43	129.07	1785	31.72	59.47	128.03	1771
188	29.95	56.31	131.69	1821	30.51	57.35	130.65	1807	31.06	58.39	129.61	1793	31.61	59.43	128.57	1778
188.5	29.85	56.27	132.23	1829	30.40	57.31	131.19	1814	30.95	58.35	130.15	1800	31.50	59.39	129.11	1786
189	29.75	56.23	132.77	1836	30.30	57.27	131.73	1822	30.85	58.31	130.69	1807	31.40	59.34	129.66	1793
189.5	29.65	56.19	133.31	1844	30.20	57.23	132.27	1829	30.75	58.27	131.23	1815	31.29	59.30	130.20	1801
190	29.55	56.15	133.85	1851	30.10	57.19	132.81	1837	30.64	58.23	131.78	1822	31.19	59.26	130.74	1808
190.5	29.45	56.11	134.39	1859	30.00	57.15	133.35	1844	30.54	58.18	132.32	1830	31.09	59.22	131.28	1816
191	29.35	56.07	134.93	1866	29.90	57.11	133.89	1852	30.44	58.14	132.86	1837	30.98	59.18	131.82	1823
191.5	29.26	56.03	135.47	1874	29.80	57.06	134.44	1859	30.34	58.10	133.40	1845	30.88	59.14	132.36	1831
192	29.16	55.99	136.01	1881	29.70	57.02	134.98	1867	30.24	58.06	133.94	1852	30.78	59.10	132.90	1838
192.5	29.06	55.95	136.56	1889	29.60	56.98	135.52	1874	30.14	58.02	134.48	1860	30.68	59.06	133.44	1846
193	28.97	55.90	137.10	1896	29.50	56.94	136.06	1882	30.04	57.98	135.02	1867	30.58	59.02	133.98	1853
193.5	28.87	55.86	137.64	1904	29.41	56.90	136.60	1889	29.94	57.94	135.56	1875	30.48	58.98	134.52	1860
194	28.77	55.82	138.18	1911	29.31	56.86	137.14	1897	29.84	57.90	136.10	1882	30.38	58.93	135.07	1868
194.5	28.68	55.78	138.72	1918	29.21	56.82	137.68	1904	29.75	57.86	136.64	1890	30.28	58.89	135.61	1875
195	28.58	55.74	139.26	1926	29.12	56.78	138.22	1912	29.65	57.82	137.19	1897	30.18	58.85	136.15	1883
195.5	28.49	55.70	139.80	1933	29.02	56.74	138.76	1919	29.55	57.77	137.73	1905	30.08	58.81	136.69	1890
196	28.40	55.66	140.34	1941	28.93	56.70	139.30	1927	29.46	57.73	138.27	1912	29.98	58.77	137.23	1898
196.5	28.30	55.62	140.88	1948	28.83	56.65	139.85	1934	29.36	57.69	138.81	1920	29.89	58.73	137.77	1905
197	28.21	55.58	141.42	1956	28.74	56.61	140.39	1942	29.26	57.65	139.35	1927	29.79	58.69	138.31	1913
197.5	28.12	55.54	141.97	1963	28.64	56.57	140.93	1949	29.17	57.61	139.89	1935	29.69	58.65	138.85	1920
198	28.03	55.49	142.51	1971	28.55	56.53	141.47	1957	29.08	57.57	140.43	1942	29.60	58.61	139.39	1928
198.5	27.94	55.45	143.05	1978	28.46	56.49	142.01	1964	28.98	57.53	140.97	1950	29.50	58.57	139.93	1935
199	27.85	55.41	143.59	1986	28.37	56.45	142.55	1971	28.89	57.49	141.51	1957	29.41	58.52	140.48	1943
199.5	27.75	55.37	144.13	1993	28.27	56.41	143.09	1979	28.79	57.45	142.05	1965	29.32	58.48	141.02	1950
200	27.67	55.33	144.67	2001	28.18	56.37	143.63	1986	28.70	57.41	142.60	1972	29.22	58.44	141.56	1958
200.5	27.58	55.29	145.21	2008	28.09	56.33	144.17	1994	28.61	57.36	143.14	1980	29.13	58.40	142.10	1965
201	27.49	55.25	145.75	2016	28.00	56.29	144.71	2001	28.52	57.32	143.68	1987	29.04	58.36	142.64	1973
201.5	27.40	55.21	146.29	2023	27.91	56.24	145.26	2009	28.43	57.28	144.22	1995	28.94	58.32	143.18	1980
202	27.31	55.17	146.83	2031	27.82	56.20	145.80	2016	28.34	57.24	144.76	2002	28.85	58.28	143.72	1988
202.5	27.22	55.13	147.38	2038	27.73	56.16	146.34	2024	28.25	57.20	145.30	2009	28.76	58.24	144.26	1995
203	27.13	55.08	147.92	2046	27.65	56.12	146.88	2031	28.16	57.16	145.84	2017	28.67	58.20	144.80	2003
203.5	27.05	55.04	148.46	2053	27.56	56.08	147.42	2039	28.07	57.12	146.38	2024	28.58	58.16	145.34	2010
204	26.96	55.00	149.00	2061	27.47	56.04	147.96	2046	27.98	57.08	146.92	2032	28.49	58.11	145.89	2018
204.5	26.88	54.96	149.54	2068	27.38	56.00	148.50	2054	27.89	57.04	147.46	2039	28.40	58.07	146.43	2025
205	26.79	54.92	150.08	2076	27.30	55.96	149.04	2061	27.80	57.00	148.01	2047	28.31	58.03	146.97	2033
205.5	26.71	54.88	150.62	2083	27.21	55.92	149.58	2069	27.71	56.95	148.55	2054	28.22	57.99	147.51	2040
206	26.62	54.84	151.16	2091	27.12	55.88	150.12	2076	27.63	56.91	149.09	2062	28.13	57.95	148.05	2048
206.5	26.54	54.80	151.70	2098	27.04	55.83	150.67	2084	27.54	56.87	149.63	2069	28.04	57.91	148.59	2055
207	26.45	54.76	152.24	2106	26.95	55.79	151.21	2091	27.45	56.83	150.17	2077	27.96	57.87	149.13	2062
207.5	26.37	54.72	152.79	2113	26.87	55.75	151.75	2099	27.37	56.79	150.71	2084	27.87	57.83	149.67	2070
208	26.29	54.67	153.33	2120	26.78	55.71	152.29	2106	27.28	56.75	151.25	2092	27.78	57.79	150.21	2077
208.5	26.20	54.63	153.87	2128	26.70	55.67	152.83	2114	27.20	56.71	151.79	2099	27.70	57.75	150.75	2085
209	26.12	54.59	154.41	2135	26.62	55.63	153.37	2121	27.11	56.67	152.33	2107	27.61	57.70	151.30	2092
209.5	26.04	54.55	154.95	2143	26.53	55.59	153.91	2129	27.03	56.63	152.87	2114	27.52	57.66	151.84	2100
210	25.96	54.51	155.49	2150	26.45	55.55	154.45	2136	26.95	56.59	153.42	2122	27.44	57.62	152.38	2107
210.5	25.88	54.47	156.03	2158	26.37	55.51	154.99	2144	26.86	56.54	153.96	2129	27.35	57.58	152.92	2115
211	25.80	54.43	156.57	2165	26.29	55.47	155.53	2151	26.78	56.50	154.50	2137	27.27	57.54	153.46	2122
211.5	25.71	54.39	157.11	2173	26.21	55.42	156.08	2159	26.70	56.46	155.04	2144	27.19	57.50	154.00	2130
212	25.63	54.35	157.65	2180	26.12	55.38	156.62	2166	26.61	56.42	155.58	2152	27.10	57.46	154.54	2137
212.5	25.56	54.31	158.20	2188	26.04	55.34	157.16	2173	26.53	56.38	156.12	2159	27.02	57.42	155.08	2145
213	25.48	54.26	158.74	2195	25.96	55.30	157.70	2181	26.45	56.34	156.66	2167	26.94	57.38	155.62	2152
213.5	25.40	54.22	159.28	2203	25.88	55.26	158.24	2188	26.37	56.30	157.20	2174	26.86	57.34	156.16	2160
214	25.32	54.18	159.82	2210	25.80	55.22	158.78	2196	26.29	56.26	157.74	2182	26.77	57.29	156.71	2167
214.5	25.24	54.14	160.36	2218	25.72	55.18	159.32	2203	26.21	56.22	158.28	2189	26.69	57.25	157.25	2175
215	25.16	54.10	160.90	2225	25.65	55.14	159.86	2211	26.13	56.18	158.83	2197	26.61	57.21	157.79	2182
215.5	25.09	54.06	161.44	2233	25.57	55.10	160.40	2218	26.05	56.13	159.37	2204	26.53	57.17	158.33	2190

Body Composition MALE 184-215.5 Lb.

Weight: Lb.	Waist: 42 inches				42.25 inches				42.5 inches				42.75 inches			
	Fat: %	Fat: Lb.	LBM: Lb.	RMR: Cal.	Fat: %	Fat: Lb.	LBM: Lb.	RMR: Cal.	Fat: %	Fat: Lb.	LBM: Lb.	RMR: Cal.	Fat: %	Fat: Lb.	LBM: Lb.	RMR: Cal.
184	33.04	60.79	123.21	1704	33.60	61.83	122.17	1690	34.17	62.87	121.13	1675	34.73	63.90	120.10	1661
184.5	32.93	60.75	123.75	1711	33.49	61.79	122.71	1697	34.05	62.83	121.67	1683	34.61	63.86	120.64	1668
185	32.82	60.71	124.29	1719	33.38	61.75	123.25	1705	33.94	62.79	122.22	1690	34.50	63.82	121.18	1676
185.5	32.71	60.67	124.83	1726	33.26	61.71	123.79	1712	33.82	62.74	122.76	1698	34.38	63.78	121.72	1683
186	32.60	60.63	125.37	1734	33.15	61.67	124.33	1720	33.71	62.70	123.30	1705	34.27	63.74	122.26	1691
186.5	32.49	60.59	125.91	1741	33.04	61.62	124.88	1727	33.60	62.66	123.84	1713	34.16	63.70	122.80	1698
187	32.38	60.55	126.45	1749	32.93	61.58	125.42	1735	33.49	62.62	124.38	1720	34.04	63.66	123.34	1706
187.5	32.27	60.51	127.00	1756	32.82	61.54	125.96	1742	33.38	62.58	124.92	1728	33.93	63.62	123.88	1713
188	32.16	60.46	127.54	1764	32.71	61.50	126.50	1749	33.27	62.54	125.46	1735	33.82	63.58	124.42	1721
188.5	32.05	60.42	128.08	1771	32.61	61.46	127.04	1757	33.16	62.50	126.00	1743	33.71	63.54	124.96	1728
189	31.95	60.38	128.62	1779	32.50	61.42	127.58	1764	33.05	62.46	126.54	1750	33.59	63.49	125.51	1736
189.5	31.84	60.34	129.16	1786	32.39	61.38	128.12	1772	32.94	62.42	127.08	1758	33.48	63.45	126.05	1743
190	31.74	60.30	129.70	1794	32.28	61.34	128.66	1779	32.83	62.38	127.63	1765	33.38	63.41	126.59	1751
190.5	31.63	60.26	130.24	1801	32.18	61.30	129.20	1787	32.72	62.33	128.17	1773	33.27	63.37	127.13	1758
191	31.53	60.22	130.78	1809	32.07	61.26	129.74	1794	32.61	62.29	128.71	1780	33.16	63.33	127.67	1766
191.5	31.42	60.18	131.32	1816	31.97	61.21	130.29	1802	32.51	62.25	129.25	1787	33.05	63.29	128.21	1773
192	31.32	60.14	131.86	1824	31.86	61.17	130.83	1809	32.40	62.21	129.79	1795	32.94	63.25	128.75	1781
192.5	31.22	60.10	132.41	1831	31.76	61.13	131.37	1817	32.30	62.17	130.33	1802	32.84	63.21	129.29	1788
193	31.12	60.05	132.95	1839	31.65	61.09	131.91	1824	32.19	62.13	130.87	1810	32.73	63.17	129.83	1796
193.5	31.01	60.01	133.49	1846	31.55	61.05	132.45	1832	32.09	62.09	131.41	1817	32.62	63.13	130.37	1803
194	30.91	59.97	134.03	1854	31.45	61.01	132.99	1839	31.98	62.05	131.95	1825	32.52	63.08	130.92	1811
194.5	30.81	59.93	134.57	1861	31.35	60.97	133.53	1847	31.88	62.01	132.49	1832	32.41	63.04	131.46	1818
195	30.71	59.89	135.11	1869	31.24	60.93	134.07	1854	31.78	61.97	133.04	1840	32.31	63.00	132.00	1826
195.5	30.61	59.85	135.65	1876	31.14	60.89	134.61	1862	31.67	61.92	133.58	1847	32.21	62.96	132.54	1833
196	30.51	59.81	136.19	1884	31.04	60.85	135.15	1869	31.57	61.88	134.12	1855	32.10	62.92	133.08	1840
196.5	30.42	59.77	136.73	1891	30.94	60.80	135.70	1877	31.47	61.84	134.66	1862	32.00	62.88	133.62	1848
197	30.32	59.73	137.27	1898	30.84	60.76	136.24	1884	31.37	61.80	135.20	1870	31.90	62.84	134.16	1855
197.5	30.22	59.69	137.82	1906	30.75	60.72	136.78	1892	31.27	61.76	135.74	1877	31.80	62.80	134.70	1863
198	30.12	59.64	138.36	1913	30.65	60.68	137.32	1899	31.17	61.72	136.28	1885	31.70	62.76	135.24	1870
198.5	30.03	59.60	138.90	1921	30.55	60.64	137.86	1907	31.07	61.68	136.82	1892	31.59	62.72	135.78	1878
199	29.93	59.56	139.44	1928	30.45	60.60	138.40	1914	30.97	61.64	137.36	1900	31.49	62.67	136.33	1885
199.5	29.84	59.52	139.98	1936	30.36	60.56	138.94	1922	30.88	61.60	137.90	1907	31.40	62.63	136.87	1893
200	29.74	59.48	140.52	1943	30.26	60.52	139.48	1929	30.78	61.56	138.45	1915	31.30	62.59	137.41	1900
200.5	29.65	59.44	141.06	1951	30.16	60.48	140.02	1937	30.68	61.51	138.99	1922	31.20	62.55	137.95	1908
201	29.55	59.40	141.60	1958	30.07	60.44	140.56	1944	30.58	61.47	139.53	1930	31.10	62.51	138.49	1915
201.5	29.46	59.36	142.14	1966	29.97	60.39	141.11	1951	30.49	61.43	140.07	1937	31.00	62.47	139.03	1923
202	29.36	59.32	142.68	1973	29.88	60.35	141.65	1959	30.39	61.39	140.61	1945	30.91	62.43	139.57	1930
202.5	29.27	59.28	143.23	1981	29.78	60.31	142.19	1966	30.30	61.35	141.15	1952	30.81	62.39	140.11	1938
203	29.18	59.23	143.77	1988	29.69	60.27	142.73	1974	30.20	61.31	141.69	1960	30.71	62.35	140.65	1945
203.5	29.09	59.19	144.31	1996	29.60	60.23	143.27	1981	30.11	61.27	142.23	1967	30.62	62.31	141.19	1953
204	29.00	59.15	144.85	2003	29.50	60.19	143.81	1989	30.01	61.23	142.77	1975	30.52	62.26	141.74	1960
204.5	28.91	59.11	145.39	2011	29.41	60.15	144.35	1996	29.92	61.19	143.31	1982	30.43	62.22	142.28	1968
205	28.81	59.07	145.93	2018	29.32	60.11	144.89	2004	29.83	61.15	143.86	1990	30.33	62.18	142.82	1975
205.5	28.72	59.03	146.47	2026	29.23	60.07	145.43	2011	29.73	61.10	144.40	1997	30.24	62.14	143.36	1983
206	28.63	58.99	147.01	2033	29.14	60.03	145.97	2019	29.64	61.06	144.94	2004	30.15	62.10	143.90	1990
206.5	28.55	58.95	147.55	2041	29.05	59.98	146.52	2026	29.55	61.02	145.48	2012	30.05	62.06	144.44	1998
207	28.46	58.91	148.09	2048	28.96	59.94	147.06	2034	29.46	60.98	146.02	2019	29.96	62.02	144.98	2005
207.5	28.37	58.87	148.64	2056	28.87	59.90	147.60	2041	29.37	60.94	146.56	2027	29.87	61.98	145.52	2013
208	28.28	58.82	149.18	2063	28.78	59.86	148.14	2049	29.28	60.90	147.10	2034	29.78	61.94	146.06	2020
208.5	28.19	58.78	149.72	2071	28.69	59.82	148.68	2056	29.19	60.86	147.64	2042	29.69	61.90	146.60	2028
209	28.11	58.74	150.26	2078	28.60	59.78	149.22	2064	29.10	60.82	148.18	2049	29.60	61.85	147.15	2035
209.5	28.02	58.70	150.80	2086	28.51	59.74	149.76	2071	29.01	60.78	148.72	2057	29.51	61.81	147.69	2043
210	27.93	58.66	151.34	2093	28.43	59.70	150.30	2079	28.92	60.74	149.27	2064	29.42	61.77	148.23	2050
210.5	27.85	58.62	151.88	2101	28.34	59.66	150.84	2086	28.83	60.69	149.81	2072	29.33	61.73	148.77	2057
211	27.76	58.58	152.42	2108	28.25	59.62	151.38	2094	28.75	60.65	150.35	2079	29.24	61.69	149.31	2065
211.5	27.68	58.54	152.96	2115	28.17	59.57	151.93	2101	28.66	60.61	150.89	2087	29.15	61.65	149.85	2072
212	27.59	58.50	153.50	2123	28.08	59.53	152.47	2109	28.57	60.57	151.43	2094	29.06	61.61	150.39	2080
212.5	27.51	58.46	154.05	2130	28.00	59.49	153.01	2116	28.48	60.53	151.97	2102	28.97	61.57	150.93	2087
213	27.42	58.41	154.59	2138	27.91	59.45	153.55	2124	28.40	60.49	152.51	2109	28.89	61.53	151.47	2095
213.5	27.34	58.37	155.13	2145	27.83	59.41	154.09	2131	28.31	60.45	153.05	2117	28.80	61.49	152.01	2102
214	27.26	58.33	155.67	2153	27.74	59.37	154.63	2139	28.23	60.41	153.59	2124	28.71	61.44	152.56	2110
214.5	27.18	58.29	156.21	2160	27.66	59.33	155.17	2146	28.14	60.37	154.13	2132	28.63	61.40	153.10	2117
215	27.09	58.25	156.75	2168	27.58	59.29	155.71	2154	28.06	60.33	154.68	2139	28.54	61.36	153.64	2125
215.5	27.01	58.21	157.29	2175	27.49	59.25	156.25	2161	27.97	60.28	155.22	2147	28.46	61.32	154.18	2132

Body Composition   MALE   184-215.5 Lb.

Weight: Lb.	Waist: 43 inches				43.25 inches				43.5 inches				43.75 inches			
	Fat: %	Fat: Lb.	LBM: Lb.	RMR: Cal.	Fat: %	Fat: Lb.	LBM: Lb.	RMR: Cal.	Fat: %	Fat: Lb.	LBM: Lb.	RMR: Cal.	Fat: %	Fat: Lb.	LBM: Lb.	RMR: Cal.
184	35.29	64.94	119.06	1647	35.86	65.98	118.02	1632	36.42	67.02	116.98	1618	36.99	68.05	115.95	1604
184.5	35.18	64.90	119.60	1654	35.74	65.94	118.56	1640	36.30	66.98	117.52	1625	36.86	68.01	116.49	1611
185	35.06	64.86	120.14	1662	35.62	65.90	119.10	1647	36.18	66.94	118.07	1633	36.74	67.97	117.03	1618
185.5	34.94	64.82	120.68	1669	35.50	65.86	119.64	1655	36.06	66.89	118.61	1640	36.62	67.93	117.57	1626
186	34.83	64.78	121.22	1677	35.38	65.82	120.18	1662	35.94	66.85	119.15	1648	36.50	67.89	118.11	1633
186.5	34.71	64.74	121.76	1684	35.27	65.77	120.73	1670	35.82	66.81	119.69	1655	36.38	67.85	118.65	1641
187	34.60	64.70	122.30	1691	35.15	65.73	121.27	1677	35.71	66.77	120.23	1663	36.26	67.81	119.19	1648
187.5	34.48	64.66	122.85	1699	35.04	65.69	121.81	1685	35.59	66.73	120.77	1670	36.14	67.77	119.73	1656
188	34.37	64.61	123.39	1706	34.92	65.65	122.35	1692	35.47	66.69	121.31	1678	36.02	67.73	120.27	1663
188.5	34.26	64.57	123.93	1714	34.81	65.61	122.89	1700	35.36	66.65	121.85	1685	35.91	67.69	120.81	1671
189	34.14	64.53	124.47	1721	34.69	65.57	123.43	1707	35.24	66.61	122.39	1693	35.79	67.64	121.36	1678
189.5	34.03	64.49	125.01	1729	34.58	65.53	123.97	1715	35.13	66.57	122.93	1700	35.67	67.60	121.90	1686
190	33.92	64.45	125.55	1736	34.47	65.49	124.51	1722	35.01	66.53	123.48	1708	35.56	67.56	122.44	1693
190.5	33.81	64.41	126.09	1744	34.36	65.45	125.05	1729	34.90	66.48	124.02	1715	35.44	67.52	122.98	1701
191	33.70	64.37	126.63	1751	34.24	65.41	125.59	1737	34.79	66.44	124.56	1723	35.33	67.48	123.52	1708
191.5	33.59	64.33	127.17	1759	34.13	65.36	126.14	1744	34.67	66.40	125.10	1730	35.22	67.44	124.06	1716
192	33.48	64.29	127.71	1766	34.02	65.32	126.68	1752	34.56	66.36	125.64	1738	35.10	67.40	124.60	1723
192.5	33.37	64.25	128.26	1774	33.91	65.28	127.22	1759	34.45	66.32	126.18	1745	34.99	67.36	125.14	1731
193	33.27	64.20	128.80	1781	33.80	65.24	127.76	1767	34.34	66.28	126.72	1753	34.88	67.32	125.68	1738
193.5	33.16	64.16	129.34	1789	33.70	65.20	128.30	1774	34.23	66.24	127.26	1760	34.77	67.28	126.22	1746
194	33.05	64.12	129.88	1796	33.59	65.16	128.84	1782	34.12	66.20	127.80	1768	34.66	67.23	126.77	1753
194.5	32.95	64.08	130.42	1804	33.48	65.12	129.38	1789	34.01	66.16	128.34	1775	34.55	67.19	127.31	1761
195	32.84	64.04	130.96	1811	33.37	65.08	129.92	1797	33.91	66.12	128.89	1782	34.44	67.15	127.85	1768
195.5	32.74	64.00	131.50	1819	33.27	65.04	130.46	1804	33.80	66.07	129.43	1790	34.33	67.11	128.39	1776
196	32.63	63.96	132.04	1826	33.16	65.00	131.00	1812	33.69	66.03	129.97	1797	34.22	67.07	128.93	1783
196.5	32.53	63.92	132.58	1834	33.06	64.95	131.55	1819	33.58	65.99	130.51	1805	34.11	67.03	129.47	1791
197	32.42	63.88	133.12	1841	32.95	64.91	132.09	1827	33.48	65.95	131.05	1812	34.00	66.99	130.01	1798
197.5	32.32	63.84	133.67	1849	32.85	64.87	132.63	1834	33.37	65.91	131.59	1820	33.90	66.95	130.55	1806
198	32.22	63.79	134.21	1856	32.74	64.83	133.17	1842	33.27	65.87	132.13	1827	33.79	66.91	131.09	1813
198.5	32.12	63.75	134.75	1864	32.64	64.79	133.71	1849	33.16	65.83	132.67	1835	33.69	66.87	131.63	1821
199	32.02	63.71	135.29	1871	32.54	64.75	134.25	1857	33.06	65.79	133.21	1842	33.58	66.82	132.18	1828
199.5	31.92	63.67	135.83	1879	32.44	64.71	134.79	1864	32.96	65.75	133.75	1850	33.48	66.78	132.72	1835
200	31.82	63.63	136.37	1886	32.33	64.67	135.33	1872	32.85	65.71	134.30	1857	33.37	66.74	133.26	1843
200.5	31.72	63.59	136.91	1893	32.23	64.63	135.87	1879	32.75	65.66	134.84	1865	33.27	66.70	133.80	1850
201	31.62	63.55	137.45	1901	32.13	64.59	136.41	1887	32.65	65.62	135.38	1872	33.16	66.66	134.34	1858
201.5	31.52	63.51	137.99	1908	32.03	64.54	136.96	1894	32.55	65.58	135.92	1880	33.06	66.62	134.88	1865
202	31.42	63.47	138.53	1916	31.93	64.50	137.50	1902	32.45	65.54	136.46	1887	32.96	66.58	135.42	1873
202.5	31.32	63.43	139.08	1923	31.83	64.46	138.04	1909	32.35	65.50	137.00	1895	32.86	66.54	135.96	1880
203	31.22	63.38	139.62	1931	31.73	64.42	138.58	1917	32.25	65.46	137.54	1902	32.76	66.50	136.50	1888
203.5	31.13	63.34	140.16	1938	31.64	64.38	139.12	1924	32.15	65.42	138.08	1910	32.66	66.46	137.04	1895
204	31.03	63.30	140.70	1946	31.54	64.34	139.66	1932	32.05	65.38	138.62	1917	32.56	66.41	137.59	1903
204.5	30.93	63.26	141.24	1953	31.44	64.30	140.20	1939	31.95	65.34	139.16	1925	32.46	66.37	138.13	1910
205	30.84	63.22	141.78	1961	31.35	64.26	140.74	1946	31.85	65.30	139.71	1932	32.36	66.33	138.67	1918
205.5	30.74	63.18	142.32	1968	31.25	64.22	141.28	1954	31.75	65.25	140.25	1940	32.26	66.29	139.21	1925
206	30.65	63.14	142.86	1976	31.15	64.18	141.82	1961	31.66	65.21	140.79	1947	32.16	66.25	139.75	1933
206.5	30.56	63.10	143.40	1983	31.06	64.13	142.37	1969	31.56	65.17	141.33	1955	32.06	66.21	140.29	1940
207	30.46	63.06	143.94	1991	30.96	64.09	142.91	1976	31.46	65.13	141.87	1962	31.97	66.17	140.83	1948
207.5	30.37	63.02	144.49	1998	30.87	64.05	143.45	1984	31.37	65.09	142.41	1970	31.87	66.13	141.37	1955
208	30.28	62.97	145.03	2006	30.77	64.01	143.99	1991	31.27	65.05	142.95	1977	31.77	66.09	141.91	1963
208.5	30.18	62.93	145.57	2013	30.68	63.97	144.53	1999	31.18	65.01	143.49	1984	31.68	66.05	142.45	1970
209	30.09	62.89	146.11	2021	30.59	63.93	145.07	2006	31.08	64.97	144.03	1992	31.58	66.00	143.00	1978
209.5	30.00	62.85	146.65	2028	30.50	63.89	145.61	2014	30.99	64.93	144.57	1999	31.49	65.96	143.54	1985
210	29.91	62.81	147.19	2036	30.40	63.85	146.15	2021	30.90	64.89	145.12	2007	31.39	65.92	144.08	1993
210.5	29.82	62.77	147.73	2043	30.31	63.81	146.69	2029	30.80	64.84	145.66	2014	31.30	65.88	144.62	2000
211	29.73	62.73	148.27	2051	30.22	63.77	147.23	2036	30.71	64.80	146.20	2022	31.20	65.84	145.16	2008
211.5	29.64	62.69	148.81	2058	30.13	63.72	147.78	2044	30.62	64.76	146.74	2029	31.11	65.80	145.70	2015
212	29.55	62.65	149.35	2066	30.04	63.68	148.32	2051	30.53	64.72	147.28	2037	31.02	65.76	146.24	2023
212.5	29.46	62.61	149.90	2073	29.95	63.64	148.86	2059	30.44	64.68	147.82	2044	30.93	65.72	146.78	2030
213	29.37	62.56	150.44	2081	29.86	63.60	149.40	2066	30.35	64.64	148.36	2052	30.83	65.68	147.32	2037
213.5	29.28	62.52	150.98	2088	29.77	63.56	149.94	2074	30.26	64.60	148.90	2059	30.74	65.64	147.86	2045
214	29.20	62.48	151.52	2095	29.68	63.52	150.48	2081	30.17	64.56	149.44	2067	30.65	65.59	148.41	2052
214.5	29.11	62.44	152.06	2103	29.59	63.48	151.02	2089	30.08	64.52	149.98	2074	30.56	65.55	148.95	2060
215	29.02	62.40	152.60	2110	29.51	63.44	151.56	2096	29.99	64.48	150.53	2082	30.47	65.51	149.49	2067
215.5	28.94	62.36	153.14	2118	29.42	63.40	152.10	2104	29.90	64.43	151.07	2089	30.38	65.47	150.03	2075

Body Composition   MALE   184-215.5 Lb.

Weight: Lb.	Waist: 44 inches Fat: %	Fat: Lb.	LBM: Lb.	RMR: Cal.	44.25 inches Fat: %	Fat: Lb.	LBM: Lb.	RMR: Cal.	44.5 inches Fat: %	Fat: Lb.	LBM: Lb.	RMR: Cal.	44.75 inches Fat: %	Fat: Lb.	LBM: Lb.	RMR: Cal.
184	37.55	69.09	114.91	1589	38.11	70.13	113.87	1575	38.68	71.17	112.83	1560	39.24	72.20	111.80	1546
184.5	37.43	69.05	115.45	1597	37.99	70.09	114.41	1582	38.55	71.13	113.37	1568	39.11	72.16	112.34	1554
185	37.30	69.01	115.99	1604	37.86	70.05	114.95	1590	38.42	71.09	113.92	1575	38.99	72.12	112.88	1561
185.5	37.18	68.97	116.53	1612	37.74	70.01	115.49	1597	38.30	71.04	114.46	1583	38.86	72.08	113.42	1569
186	37.06	68.93	117.07	1619	37.62	69.97	116.03	1605	38.17	71.00	115.00	1590	38.73	72.04	113.96	1576
186.5	36.94	68.89	117.61	1627	37.49	69.92	116.58	1612	38.05	70.96	115.54	1598	38.61	72.00	114.50	1584
187	36.82	68.85	118.15	1634	37.37	69.88	117.12	1620	37.93	70.92	116.08	1605	38.48	71.96	115.04	1591
187.5	36.70	68.81	118.70	1642	37.25	69.84	117.66	1627	37.80	70.88	116.62	1613	38.36	71.92	115.58	1599
188	36.58	68.76	119.24	1649	37.13	69.80	118.20	1635	37.68	70.84	117.16	1620	38.23	71.88	116.12	1606
188.5	36.46	68.72	119.78	1657	37.01	69.76	118.74	1642	37.56	70.80	117.70	1628	38.11	71.84	116.66	1613
189	36.34	68.68	120.32	1664	36.89	69.72	119.28	1650	37.44	70.76	118.24	1635	37.99	71.79	117.21	1621
189.5	36.22	68.64	120.86	1671	36.77	69.68	119.82	1657	37.32	70.72	118.78	1643	37.86	71.75	117.75	1628
190	36.11	68.60	121.40	1679	36.65	69.64	120.36	1665	37.20	70.68	119.33	1650	37.74	71.71	118.29	1636
190.5	35.99	68.56	121.94	1686	36.53	69.60	120.90	1672	37.08	70.63	119.87	1658	37.62	71.67	118.83	1643
191	35.87	68.52	122.48	1694	36.42	69.56	121.44	1680	36.96	70.59	120.41	1665	37.50	71.63	119.37	1651
191.5	35.76	68.48	123.02	1701	36.30	69.51	121.99	1687	36.84	70.55	120.95	1673	37.38	71.59	119.91	1658
192	35.64	68.44	123.56	1709	36.18	69.47	122.53	1695	36.72	70.51	121.49	1680	37.26	71.55	120.45	1666
192.5	35.53	68.40	124.11	1716	36.07	69.43	123.07	1702	36.61	70.47	122.03	1688	37.15	71.51	120.99	1673
193	35.42	68.35	124.65	1724	35.95	69.39	123.61	1710	36.49	70.43	122.57	1695	37.03	71.47	121.53	1681
193.5	35.30	68.31	125.19	1731	35.84	69.35	124.15	1717	36.38	70.39	123.11	1703	36.91	71.43	122.07	1688
194	35.19	68.27	125.73	1739	35.73	69.31	124.69	1724	36.26	70.35	123.65	1710	36.80	71.38	122.62	1696
194.5	35.08	68.23	126.27	1746	35.61	69.27	125.23	1732	36.15	70.31	124.19	1718	36.68	71.34	123.16	1703
195	34.97	68.19	126.81	1754	35.50	69.23	125.77	1739	36.03	70.27	124.74	1725	36.57	71.30	123.70	1711
195.5	34.86	68.15	127.35	1761	35.39	69.19	126.31	1747	35.92	70.22	125.28	1733	36.45	71.26	124.24	1718
196	34.75	68.11	127.89	1769	35.28	69.15	126.85	1754	35.81	70.18	125.82	1740	36.34	71.22	124.78	1726
196.5	34.64	68.07	128.43	1776	35.17	69.10	127.40	1762	35.70	70.14	126.36	1748	36.22	71.18	125.32	1733
197	34.53	68.03	128.97	1784	35.06	69.06	127.94	1769	35.58	70.10	126.90	1755	36.11	71.14	125.86	1741
197.5	34.42	67.99	129.52	1791	34.95	69.02	128.48	1777	35.47	70.06	127.44	1762	36.00	71.10	126.40	1748
198	34.32	67.94	130.06	1799	34.84	68.98	129.02	1784	35.36	70.02	127.98	1770	35.89	71.06	126.94	1756
198.5	34.21	67.90	130.60	1806	34.73	68.94	129.56	1792	35.25	69.98	128.52	1777	35.78	71.02	127.48	1763
199	34.10	67.86	131.14	1814	34.62	68.90	130.10	1799	35.14	69.94	129.06	1785	35.67	70.97	128.03	1771
199.5	34.00	67.82	131.68	1821	34.52	68.86	130.64	1807	35.04	69.90	129.60	1792	35.56	70.93	128.57	1778
200	33.89	67.78	132.22	1829	34.41	68.82	131.18	1814	34.93	69.86	130.15	1800	35.45	70.89	129.11	1786
200.5	33.79	67.74	132.76	1836	34.30	68.78	131.72	1822	34.82	69.81	130.69	1807	35.34	70.85	129.65	1793
201	33.68	67.70	133.30	1844	34.20	68.74	132.26	1829	34.71	69.77	131.23	1815	35.23	70.81	130.19	1801
201.5	33.58	67.66	133.84	1851	34.09	68.69	132.81	1837	34.61	69.73	131.77	1822	35.12	70.77	130.73	1808
202	33.47	67.62	134.38	1859	33.99	68.65	133.35	1844	34.50	69.69	132.31	1830	35.01	70.73	131.27	1815
202.5	33.37	67.58	134.93	1866	33.88	68.61	133.89	1852	34.40	69.65	132.85	1837	34.91	70.69	131.81	1823
203	33.27	67.53	135.47	1873	33.78	68.57	134.43	1859	34.29	69.61	133.39	1845	34.80	70.65	132.35	1830
203.5	33.17	67.49	136.01	1881	33.68	68.53	134.97	1867	34.19	69.57	133.93	1852	34.70	70.61	132.89	1838
204	33.06	67.45	136.55	1888	33.57	68.49	135.51	1874	34.08	69.53	134.47	1860	34.59	70.56	133.44	1845
204.5	32.96	67.41	137.09	1896	33.47	68.45	136.05	1882	33.98	69.49	135.01	1867	34.49	70.52	133.98	1853
205	32.86	67.37	137.63	1903	33.37	68.41	136.59	1889	33.88	69.45	135.56	1875	34.38	70.48	134.52	1860
205.5	32.76	67.33	138.17	1911	33.27	68.37	137.13	1897	33.77	69.40	136.10	1882	34.28	70.44	135.06	1868
206	32.66	67.29	138.71	1918	33.17	68.33	137.67	1904	33.67	69.36	136.64	1890	34.18	70.40	135.60	1875
206.5	32.57	67.25	139.25	1926	33.07	68.28	138.22	1912	33.57	69.32	137.18	1897	34.07	70.36	136.14	1883
207	32.47	67.21	139.79	1933	32.97	68.24	138.76	1919	33.47	69.28	137.72	1905	33.97	70.32	136.68	1890
207.5	32.37	67.17	140.34	1941	32.87	68.20	139.30	1926	33.37	69.24	138.26	1912	33.87	70.28	137.22	1898
208	32.27	67.12	140.88	1948	32.77	68.16	139.84	1934	33.27	69.20	138.80	1920	33.77	70.24	137.76	1905
208.5	32.17	67.08	141.42	1956	32.67	68.12	140.38	1941	33.17	69.16	139.34	1927	33.67	70.20	138.30	1913
209	32.08	67.04	141.96	1963	32.57	68.08	140.92	1949	33.07	69.12	139.88	1935	33.57	70.15	138.85	1920
209.5	31.98	67.00	142.50	1971	32.48	68.04	141.46	1956	32.97	69.08	140.42	1942	33.47	70.11	139.39	1928
210	31.89	66.96	143.04	1978	32.38	68.00	142.00	1964	32.87	69.04	140.97	1950	33.37	70.07	139.93	1935
210.5	31.79	66.92	143.58	1986	32.28	67.96	142.54	1971	32.78	68.99	141.51	1957	33.27	70.03	140.47	1943
211	31.70	66.88	144.12	1993	32.19	67.92	143.08	1979	32.68	68.95	142.05	1965	33.17	69.99	141.01	1950
211.5	31.60	66.84	144.66	2001	32.09	67.87	143.63	1986	32.58	68.91	142.59	1972	33.07	69.95	141.55	1958
212	31.51	66.80	145.20	2008	32.00	67.83	144.17	1994	32.49	68.87	143.13	1979	32.98	69.91	142.09	1965
212.5	31.41	66.76	145.75	2016	31.90	67.79	144.71	2001	32.39	68.83	143.67	1987	32.88	69.87	142.63	1973
213	31.32	66.71	146.29	2023	31.81	67.75	145.25	2009	32.30	68.79	144.21	1994	32.78	69.83	143.17	1980
213.5	31.23	66.67	146.83	2031	31.71	67.71	145.79	2016	32.20	68.75	144.75	2002	32.69	69.79	143.71	1988
214	31.14	66.63	147.37	2038	31.62	67.67	146.33	2024	32.11	68.71	145.29	2009	32.59	69.74	144.26	1995
214.5	31.04	66.59	147.91	2046	31.53	67.63	146.87	2031	32.01	68.67	145.83	2017	32.50	69.70	144.80	2003
215	30.95	66.55	148.45	2053	31.44	67.59	147.41	2039	31.92	68.63	146.38	2024	32.40	69.66	145.34	2010
215.5	30.86	66.51	148.99	2061	31.34	67.55	147.95	2046	31.83	68.58	146.92	2032	32.31	69.62	145.88	2017

Body Composition   MALE   184-215.5 Lb.

Weight: Lb.	Waist: 45 inches Fat: %	Fat: Lb.	LBM: Lb.	RMR: Cal.	45.25 inches Fat: %	Fat: Lb.	LBM: Lb.	RMR: Cal.	45.5 inches Fat: %	Fat: Lb.	LBM: Lb.	RMR: Cal.	45.75 inches Fat: %	Fat: Lb.	LBM: Lb.	RMR: Cal.
184	39.81	73.24	110.76	1532	40.37	74.28	109.72	1517	40.93	75.32	108.68	1503	41.50	76.35	107.65	1489
184.5	39.68	73.20	111.30	1539	40.24	74.24	110.26	1525	40.80	75.28	109.22	1511	41.36	76.31	108.19	1496
185	39.55	73.16	111.84	1547	40.11	74.20	110.80	1532	40.67	75.24	109.77	1518	41.23	76.27	108.73	1504
185.5	39.42	73.12	112.38	1554	39.98	74.16	111.34	1540	40.54	75.19	110.31	1526	41.10	76.23	109.27	1511
186	39.29	73.08	112.92	1562	39.85	74.12	111.88	1547	40.40	75.15	110.85	1533	40.96	76.19	109.81	1519
186.5	39.16	73.04	113.46	1569	39.72	74.07	112.43	1555	40.27	75.11	111.39	1540	40.83	76.15	110.35	1526
187	39.04	73.00	114.00	1577	39.59	74.03	112.97	1562	40.14	75.07	111.93	1548	40.70	76.11	110.89	1534
187.5	38.91	72.96	114.55	1584	39.46	73.99	113.51	1570	40.02	75.03	112.47	1555	40.57	76.07	111.43	1541
188	38.78	72.91	115.09	1592	39.34	73.95	114.05	1577	39.89	74.99	113.01	1563	40.44	76.03	111.97	1549
188.5	38.66	72.87	115.63	1599	39.21	73.91	114.59	1585	39.76	74.95	113.55	1570	40.31	75.99	112.51	1556
189	38.54	72.83	116.17	1607	39.08	73.87	115.13	1592	39.63	74.91	114.09	1578	40.18	75.94	113.06	1564
189.5	38.41	72.79	116.71	1614	38.96	73.83	115.67	1600	39.51	74.87	114.63	1585	40.05	75.90	113.60	1571
190	38.29	72.75	117.25	1622	38.84	73.79	116.21	1607	39.38	74.83	115.18	1593	39.93	75.86	114.14	1579
190.5	38.17	72.71	117.79	1629	38.71	73.75	116.75	1615	39.26	74.78	115.72	1600	39.80	75.82	114.68	1586
191	38.05	72.67	118.33	1637	38.59	73.71	117.29	1622	39.13	74.74	116.26	1608	39.68	75.78	115.22	1593
191.5	37.93	72.63	118.87	1644	38.47	73.66	117.84	1630	39.01	74.70	116.80	1615	39.55	75.74	115.76	1601
192	37.81	72.59	119.41	1651	38.35	73.62	118.38	1637	38.89	74.66	117.34	1623	39.43	75.70	116.30	1608
192.5	37.69	72.55	119.96	1659	38.22	73.58	118.92	1645	38.76	74.62	117.88	1630	39.30	75.66	116.84	1616
193	37.57	72.50	120.50	1666	38.10	73.54	119.46	1652	38.64	74.58	118.42	1638	39.18	75.62	117.38	1623
193.5	37.45	72.46	121.04	1674	37.98	73.50	120.00	1660	38.52	74.54	118.96	1645	39.06	75.58	117.92	1631
194	37.33	72.42	121.58	1681	37.87	73.46	120.54	1667	38.40	74.50	119.50	1653	38.94	75.53	118.47	1638
194.5	37.21	72.38	122.12	1689	37.75	73.42	121.08	1675	38.28	74.46	120.04	1660	38.81	75.49	119.01	1646
195	37.10	72.34	122.66	1696	37.63	73.38	121.62	1682	38.16	74.42	120.59	1668	38.69	75.45	119.55	1653
195.5	36.98	72.30	123.20	1704	37.51	73.34	122.16	1690	38.04	74.37	121.13	1675	38.57	75.41	120.09	1661
196	36.87	72.26	123.74	1711	37.40	73.30	122.70	1697	37.93	74.33	121.67	1683	38.45	75.37	120.63	1668
196.5	36.75	72.22	124.28	1719	37.28	73.25	123.25	1704	37.81	74.29	122.21	1690	38.34	75.33	121.17	1676
197	36.64	72.18	124.82	1726	37.16	73.21	123.79	1712	37.69	74.25	122.75	1698	38.22	75.29	121.71	1683
197.5	36.52	72.14	125.37	1734	37.05	73.17	124.33	1719	37.57	74.21	123.29	1705	38.10	75.25	122.25	1691
198	36.41	72.09	125.91	1741	36.94	73.13	124.87	1727	37.46	74.17	123.83	1713	37.98	75.21	122.79	1698
198.5	36.30	72.05	126.45	1749	36.82	73.09	125.41	1734	37.34	74.13	124.37	1720	37.87	75.17	123.33	1706
199	36.19	72.01	126.99	1756	36.71	73.05	125.95	1742	37.23	74.09	124.91	1728	37.75	75.12	123.88	1713
199.5	36.08	71.97	127.53	1764	36.60	73.01	126.49	1749	37.12	74.05	125.45	1735	37.64	75.08	124.42	1721
200	35.97	71.93	128.07	1771	36.48	72.97	127.03	1757	37.00	74.01	126.00	1743	37.52	75.04	124.96	1728
200.5	35.85	71.89	128.61	1779	36.37	72.93	127.57	1764	36.89	73.96	126.54	1750	37.41	75.00	125.50	1736
201	35.75	71.85	129.15	1786	36.26	72.89	128.11	1772	36.78	73.92	127.08	1757	37.29	74.96	126.04	1743
201.5	35.64	71.81	129.69	1794	36.15	72.84	128.66	1779	36.67	73.88	127.62	1765	37.18	74.92	126.58	1751
202	35.53	71.77	130.23	1801	36.04	72.80	129.20	1787	36.55	73.84	128.16	1772	37.07	74.88	127.12	1758
202.5	35.42	71.73	130.78	1809	35.93	72.76	129.74	1794	36.44	73.80	128.70	1780	36.96	74.84	127.66	1766
203	35.31	71.68	131.32	1816	35.82	72.72	130.28	1802	36.33	73.76	129.24	1787	36.85	74.80	128.20	1773
203.5	35.21	71.64	131.86	1824	35.72	72.68	130.82	1809	36.23	73.72	129.78	1795	36.73	74.76	128.74	1781
204	35.10	71.60	132.40	1831	35.61	72.64	131.36	1817	36.12	73.68	130.32	1802	36.62	74.71	129.29	1788
204.5	34.99	71.56	132.94	1839	35.50	72.60	131.90	1824	36.01	73.64	130.86	1810	36.52	74.67	129.83	1796
205	34.89	71.52	133.48	1846	35.39	72.56	132.44	1832	35.90	73.60	131.41	1817	36.41	74.63	130.37	1803
205.5	34.78	71.48	134.02	1854	35.29	72.52	132.98	1839	35.79	73.55	131.95	1825	36.30	74.59	130.91	1810
206	34.68	71.44	134.56	1861	35.18	72.48	133.52	1847	35.69	73.51	132.49	1832	36.19	74.55	131.45	1818
206.5	34.57	71.40	135.10	1868	35.08	72.43	134.07	1854	35.58	73.47	133.03	1840	36.08	74.51	131.99	1825
207	34.47	71.36	135.64	1876	34.97	72.39	134.61	1862	35.47	73.43	133.57	1847	35.98	74.47	132.53	1833
207.5	34.37	71.32	136.19	1883	34.87	72.35	135.15	1869	35.37	73.39	134.11	1855	35.87	74.43	133.07	1840
208	34.27	71.27	136.73	1891	34.77	72.31	135.69	1877	35.26	73.35	134.65	1862	35.76	74.39	133.61	1848
208.5	34.16	71.23	137.27	1898	34.66	72.27	136.23	1884	35.16	73.31	135.19	1870	35.66	74.35	134.15	1855
209	34.06	71.19	137.81	1906	34.56	72.23	136.77	1892	35.06	73.27	135.73	1877	35.55	74.30	134.70	1863
209.5	33.96	71.15	138.35	1913	34.46	72.19	137.31	1899	34.95	73.23	136.27	1885	35.45	74.26	135.24	1870
210	33.86	71.11	138.89	1921	34.36	72.15	137.85	1907	34.85	73.19	136.82	1892	35.34	74.22	135.78	1878
210.5	33.76	71.07	139.43	1928	34.25	72.11	138.39	1914	34.75	73.14	137.36	1900	35.24	74.18	136.32	1885
211	33.66	71.03	139.97	1936	34.15	72.07	138.93	1921	34.65	73.10	137.90	1907	35.14	74.14	136.86	1893
211.5	33.56	70.99	140.51	1943	34.05	72.02	139.48	1929	34.54	73.06	138.44	1915	35.04	74.10	137.40	1900
212	33.47	70.95	141.05	1951	33.95	71.98	140.02	1936	34.44	73.02	138.98	1922	34.93	74.06	137.94	1908
212.5	33.37	70.91	141.60	1958	33.86	71.94	140.56	1944	34.34	72.98	139.52	1930	34.83	74.02	138.48	1915
213	33.27	70.86	142.14	1966	33.76	71.90	141.10	1951	34.24	72.94	140.06	1937	34.73	73.98	139.02	1923
213.5	33.17	70.82	142.68	1973	33.66	71.86	141.64	1959	34.14	72.90	140.60	1945	34.63	73.94	139.56	1930
214	33.08	70.78	143.22	1981	33.56	71.82	142.18	1966	34.05	72.86	141.14	1952	34.53	73.89	140.11	1938
214.5	32.98	70.74	143.76	1988	33.46	71.78	142.72	1974	33.95	72.82	141.68	1959	34.43	73.85	140.65	1945
215	32.88	70.70	144.30	1996	33.37	71.74	143.26	1981	33.85	72.78	142.23	1967	34.33	73.81	141.19	1953
215.5	32.79	70.66	144.84	2003	33.27	71.70	143.80	1989	33.75	72.73	142.77	1974	34.23	73.77	141.73	1960

Body Composition   MALE   184-215.5 Lb.

Weight: Lb.	Waist: 46 inches				46.25 inches				46.5 inches				46.75 inches			
	Fat: %	Fat: Lb.	LBM: Lb.	RMR: Cal.	Fat: %	Fat: Lb.	LBM: Lb.	RMR: Cal.	Fat: %	Fat: Lb.	LBM: Lb.	RMR: Cal.	Fat: %	Fat: Lb.	LBM: Lb.	RMR: Cal.
184	42.06	77.39	106.61	1474	42.62	78.43	105.57	1460	43.19	79.47	104.53	1446	43.75	80.50	103.50	1431
184.5	41.92	77.35	107.15	1482	42.49	78.39	106.11	1468	43.05	79.43	105.07	1453	43.61	80.46	104.04	1439
185	41.79	77.31	107.69	1489	42.35	78.35	106.65	1475	42.91	79.39	105.62	1461	43.47	80.42	104.58	1446
185.5	41.65	77.27	108.23	1497	42.21	78.31	107.19	1482	42.77	79.34	106.16	1468	43.33	80.38	105.12	1454
186	41.52	77.23	108.77	1504	42.08	78.27	107.73	1490	42.64	79.30	106.70	1476	43.19	80.34	105.66	1461
186.5	41.39	77.19	109.31	1512	41.94	78.22	108.28	1497	42.50	79.26	107.24	1483	43.06	80.30	106.20	1469
187	41.25	77.15	109.85	1519	41.81	78.18	108.82	1505	42.36	79.22	107.78	1491	42.92	80.26	106.74	1476
187.5	41.12	77.11	110.40	1527	41.68	78.14	109.36	1512	42.23	79.18	108.32	1498	42.78	80.22	107.28	1484
188	40.99	77.06	110.94	1534	41.54	78.10	109.90	1520	42.10	79.14	108.86	1506	42.65	80.18	107.82	1491
188.5	40.86	77.02	111.48	1542	41.41	78.06	110.44	1527	41.96	79.10	109.40	1513	42.51	80.14	108.36	1499
189	40.73	76.98	112.02	1549	41.28	78.02	110.98	1535	41.83	79.06	109.94	1521	42.38	80.09	108.91	1506
189.5	40.60	76.94	112.56	1557	41.15	77.98	111.52	1542	41.70	79.02	110.48	1528	42.24	80.05	109.45	1514
190	40.47	76.90	113.10	1564	41.02	77.94	112.06	1550	41.57	78.98	111.03	1535	42.11	80.01	109.99	1521
190.5	40.35	76.86	113.64	1572	40.89	77.90	112.60	1557	41.44	78.93	111.57	1543	41.98	79.97	110.53	1529
191	40.22	76.82	114.18	1579	40.76	77.86	113.14	1565	41.31	78.89	112.11	1550	41.85	79.93	111.07	1536
191.5	40.09	76.78	114.72	1587	40.63	77.81	113.69	1572	41.18	78.85	112.65	1558	41.72	79.89	111.61	1544
192	39.97	76.74	115.26	1594	40.51	77.77	114.23	1580	41.05	78.81	113.19	1565	41.59	79.85	112.15	1551
192.5	39.84	76.70	115.81	1602	40.38	77.73	114.77	1587	40.92	78.77	113.73	1573	41.46	79.81	112.69	1559
193	39.72	76.65	116.35	1609	40.25	77.69	115.31	1595	40.79	78.73	114.27	1580	41.33	79.77	113.23	1566
193.5	39.59	76.61	116.89	1617	40.13	77.65	115.85	1602	40.67	78.69	114.81	1588	41.20	79.73	113.77	1574
194	39.47	76.57	117.43	1624	40.00	77.61	116.39	1610	40.54	78.65	115.35	1595	41.07	79.68	114.32	1581
194.5	39.35	76.53	117.97	1632	39.88	77.57	116.93	1617	40.41	78.61	115.89	1603	40.95	79.64	114.86	1588
195	39.23	76.49	118.51	1639	39.76	77.53	117.47	1625	40.29	78.57	116.44	1610	40.82	79.60	115.40	1596
195.5	39.10	76.45	119.05	1646	39.64	77.49	118.01	1632	40.17	78.52	116.98	1618	40.70	79.56	115.94	1603
196	38.98	76.41	119.59	1654	39.51	77.45	118.55	1640	40.04	78.48	117.52	1625	40.57	79.52	116.48	1611
196.5	38.86	76.37	120.13	1661	39.39	77.40	119.10	1647	39.92	78.44	118.06	1633	40.45	79.48	117.02	1618
197	38.74	76.33	120.67	1669	39.27	77.36	119.64	1655	39.80	78.40	118.60	1640	40.32	79.44	117.56	1626
197.5	38.63	76.29	121.22	1676	39.15	77.32	120.18	1662	39.68	78.36	119.14	1648	40.20	79.40	118.10	1633
198	38.51	76.24	121.76	1684	39.03	77.28	120.72	1670	39.56	78.32	119.68	1655	40.08	79.36	118.64	1641
198.5	38.39	76.20	122.30	1691	38.91	77.24	121.26	1677	39.43	78.28	120.22	1663	39.96	79.32	119.18	1648
199	38.27	76.16	122.84	1699	38.79	77.20	121.80	1685	39.32	78.24	120.76	1670	39.84	79.27	119.73	1656
199.5	38.16	76.12	123.38	1706	38.68	77.16	122.34	1692	39.20	78.20	121.30	1678	39.72	79.23	120.27	1663
200	38.04	76.08	123.92	1714	38.56	77.12	122.88	1699	39.08	78.16	121.85	1685	39.60	79.19	120.81	1671
200.5	37.92	76.04	124.46	1721	38.44	77.08	123.42	1707	38.96	78.11	122.39	1693	39.48	79.15	121.35	1678
201	37.81	76.00	125.00	1729	38.33	77.04	123.96	1714	38.84	78.07	122.93	1700	39.36	79.11	121.89	1686
201.5	37.70	75.96	125.54	1736	38.21	76.99	124.51	1722	38.73	78.03	123.47	1708	39.24	79.07	122.43	1693
202	37.58	75.92	126.08	1744	38.10	76.95	125.05	1729	38.61	77.99	124.01	1715	39.12	79.03	122.97	1701
202.5	37.47	75.88	126.63	1751	37.98	76.91	125.59	1737	38.49	77.95	124.55	1723	39.01	78.99	123.51	1708
203	37.36	75.83	127.17	1759	37.87	76.87	126.13	1744	38.38	77.91	125.09	1730	38.89	78.95	124.05	1716
203.5	37.24	75.79	127.71	1766	37.75	76.83	126.67	1752	38.26	77.87	125.63	1737	38.77	78.91	124.59	1723
204	37.13	75.75	128.25	1774	37.64	76.79	127.21	1759	38.15	77.83	126.17	1745	38.66	78.86	125.14	1731
204.5	37.02	75.71	128.79	1781	37.53	76.75	127.75	1767	38.04	77.79	126.71	1752	38.54	78.82	125.68	1738
205	36.91	75.67	129.33	1789	37.42	76.71	128.29	1774	37.92	77.75	127.26	1760	38.43	78.78	126.22	1746
205.5	36.80	75.63	129.87	1796	37.31	76.67	128.83	1782	37.81	77.70	127.80	1767	38.32	78.74	126.76	1753
206	36.69	75.59	130.41	1804	37.20	76.63	129.37	1789	37.70	77.66	128.34	1775	38.20	78.70	127.30	1761
206.5	36.58	75.55	130.95	1811	37.09	76.58	129.92	1797	37.59	77.62	128.88	1782	38.09	78.66	127.84	1768
207	36.48	75.51	131.49	1819	36.98	76.54	130.46	1804	37.48	77.58	129.42	1790	37.98	78.62	128.38	1776
207.5	36.37	75.47	132.04	1826	36.87	76.50	131.00	1812	37.37	77.54	129.96	1797	37.87	78.58	128.92	1783
208	36.26	75.42	132.58	1834	36.76	76.46	131.54	1819	37.26	77.50	130.50	1805	37.76	78.54	129.46	1790
208.5	36.15	75.38	133.12	1841	36.65	76.42	132.08	1827	37.15	77.46	131.04	1812	37.65	78.50	130.00	1798
209	36.05	75.34	133.66	1848	36.55	76.38	132.62	1834	37.04	77.42	131.58	1820	37.54	78.45	130.55	1805
209.5	35.94	75.30	134.20	1856	36.44	76.34	133.16	1842	36.93	77.38	132.12	1827	37.43	78.41	131.09	1813
210	35.84	75.26	134.74	1863	36.33	76.30	133.70	1849	36.83	77.34	132.67	1835	37.32	78.37	131.63	1820
210.5	35.73	75.22	135.28	1871	36.23	76.26	134.24	1857	36.72	77.29	133.21	1842	37.21	78.33	132.17	1828
211	35.63	75.18	135.82	1878	36.12	76.22	134.78	1864	36.61	77.25	133.75	1850	37.10	78.29	132.71	1835
211.5	35.53	75.14	136.36	1886	36.02	76.17	135.33	1872	36.51	77.21	134.29	1857	37.00	78.25	133.25	1843
212	35.42	75.10	136.90	1893	35.91	76.13	135.87	1879	36.40	77.17	134.83	1865	36.89	78.21	133.79	1850
212.5	35.32	75.06	137.45	1901	35.81	76.09	136.41	1887	36.30	77.13	135.37	1872	36.78	78.17	134.33	1858
213	35.22	75.01	137.99	1908	35.70	76.05	136.95	1894	36.19	77.09	135.91	1880	36.68	78.13	134.87	1865
213.5	35.12	74.97	138.53	1916	35.60	76.01	137.49	1901	36.09	77.05	136.45	1887	36.57	78.09	135.41	1873
214	35.01	74.93	139.07	1923	35.50	75.97	138.03	1909	35.98	77.01	136.99	1895	36.47	78.04	135.96	1880
214.5	34.91	74.89	139.61	1931	35.40	75.93	138.57	1916	35.88	76.97	137.53	1902	36.37	78.00	136.50	1888
215	34.81	74.85	140.15	1938	35.30	75.89	139.11	1924	35.78	76.93	138.08	1910	36.26	77.96	137.04	1895
215.5	34.71	74.81	140.69	1946	35.20	75.85	139.65	1931	35.68	76.88	138.62	1917	36.16	77.92	137.58	1903

Body Composition MALE 184-215.5 Lb.

Weight: Lb.	Waist: 47 inches				47.25 inches				47.5 inches				47.75 inches			
	Fat: %	Fat: Lb.	LBM: Lb.	RMR: Cal.	Fat: %	Fat: Lb.	LBM: Lb.	RMR: Cal.	Fat: %	Fat: Lb.	LBM: Lb.	RMR: Cal.	Fat: %	Fat: Lb.	LBM: Lb.	RMR: Cal.
184	44.32	81.54	102.46	1417	44.88	82.58	101.42	1403	45.44	83.62	100.38	1388	46.01	84.65	99.35	1374
184.5	44.17	81.50	103.00	1424	44.74	82.54	101.96	1410	45.30	83.58	100.92	1396	45.86	84.61	99.89	1381
185	44.03	81.46	103.54	1432	44.59	82.50	102.50	1418	45.15	83.54	101.47	1403	45.71	84.57	100.43	1389
185.5	43.89	81.42	104.08	1439	44.45	82.46	103.04	1425	45.01	83.49	102.01	1411	45.57	84.53	100.97	1396
186	43.75	81.38	104.62	1447	44.31	82.42	103.58	1433	44.87	83.45	102.55	1418	45.43	84.49	101.51	1404
186.5	43.61	81.34	105.16	1454	44.17	82.37	104.13	1440	44.72	83.41	103.09	1426	45.28	84.45	102.05	1411
187	43.47	81.30	105.70	1462	44.03	82.33	104.67	1448	44.58	83.37	103.63	1433	45.14	84.41	102.59	1419
187.5	43.34	81.26	106.25	1469	43.89	82.29	105.21	1455	44.44	83.33	104.17	1441	45.00	84.37	103.13	1426
188	43.20	81.21	106.79	1477	43.75	82.25	105.75	1463	44.30	83.29	104.71	1448	44.85	84.33	103.67	1434
188.5	43.06	81.17	107.33	1484	43.61	82.21	106.29	1470	44.16	83.25	105.25	1456	44.71	84.29	104.21	1441
189	42.93	81.13	107.87	1492	43.48	82.17	106.83	1477	44.02	83.21	105.79	1463	44.57	84.24	104.76	1449
189.5	42.79	81.09	108.41	1499	43.34	82.13	107.37	1485	43.89	83.17	106.33	1471	44.43	84.20	105.30	1456
190	42.66	81.05	108.95	1507	43.20	82.09	107.91	1492	43.75	83.13	106.88	1478	44.30	84.16	105.84	1464
190.5	42.52	81.01	109.49	1514	43.07	82.05	108.45	1500	43.61	83.08	107.42	1486	44.16	84.12	106.38	1471
191	42.39	80.97	110.03	1522	42.93	82.01	108.99	1507	43.48	83.04	107.96	1493	44.02	84.08	106.92	1479
191.5	42.26	80.93	110.57	1529	42.80	81.96	109.54	1515	43.34	83.00	108.50	1501	43.88	84.04	107.46	1486
192	42.13	80.89	111.11	1537	42.67	81.92	110.08	1522	43.21	82.96	109.04	1508	43.75	84.00	108.00	1494
192.5	42.00	80.85	111.66	1544	42.54	81.88	110.62	1530	43.08	82.92	109.58	1515	43.61	83.96	108.54	1501
193	41.87	80.80	112.20	1552	42.40	81.84	111.16	1537	42.94	82.88	110.12	1523	43.48	83.92	109.08	1509
193.5	41.74	80.76	112.74	1559	42.27	81.80	111.70	1545	42.81	82.84	110.66	1530	43.35	83.88	109.62	1516
194	41.61	80.72	113.28	1567	42.14	81.76	112.24	1552	42.68	82.80	111.20	1538	43.21	83.83	110.17	1524
194.5	41.48	80.68	113.82	1574	42.01	81.72	112.78	1560	42.55	82.76	111.74	1545	43.08	83.79	110.71	1531
195	41.35	80.64	114.36	1582	41.89	81.68	113.32	1567	42.42	82.72	112.29	1553	42.95	83.75	111.25	1539
195.5	41.23	80.60	114.90	1589	41.76	81.64	113.86	1575	42.29	82.67	112.83	1560	42.82	83.71	111.79	1546
196	41.10	80.56	115.44	1597	41.63	81.60	114.40	1582	42.16	82.63	113.37	1568	42.69	83.67	112.33	1554
196.5	40.98	80.52	115.98	1604	41.50	81.55	114.95	1590	42.03	82.59	113.91	1575	42.56	83.63	112.87	1561
197	40.85	80.48	116.52	1612	41.38	81.51	115.49	1597	41.90	82.55	114.45	1583	42.43	83.59	113.41	1568
197.5	40.73	80.44	117.07	1619	41.25	81.47	116.03	1605	41.78	82.51	114.99	1590	42.30	83.55	113.95	1576
198	40.60	80.39	117.61	1626	41.13	81.43	116.57	1612	41.65	82.47	115.53	1598	42.18	83.51	114.49	1583
198.5	40.48	80.35	118.15	1634	41.00	81.39	117.11	1620	41.53	82.43	116.07	1605	42.05	83.47	115.03	1591
199	40.36	80.31	118.69	1641	40.88	81.35	117.65	1627	41.40	82.39	116.61	1613	41.92	83.42	115.58	1598
199.5	40.24	80.27	119.23	1649	40.76	81.31	118.19	1635	41.28	82.35	117.15	1620	41.80	83.38	116.12	1606
200	40.12	80.23	119.77	1656	40.63	81.27	118.73	1642	41.15	82.31	117.70	1628	41.67	83.34	116.66	1613
200.5	39.99	80.19	120.31	1664	40.51	81.23	119.27	1650	41.03	82.26	118.24	1635	41.55	83.30	117.20	1621
201	39.87	80.15	120.85	1671	40.39	81.19	119.81	1657	40.91	82.22	118.78	1643	41.42	83.26	117.74	1628
201.5	39.76	80.11	121.39	1679	40.27	81.14	120.36	1665	40.79	82.18	119.32	1650	41.30	83.22	118.28	1636
202	39.64	80.07	121.93	1686	40.15	81.10	120.90	1672	40.66	82.14	119.86	1658	41.18	83.18	118.82	1643
202.5	39.52	80.03	122.48	1694	40.03	81.06	121.44	1679	40.54	82.10	120.40	1665	41.06	83.14	119.36	1651
203	39.40	79.98	123.02	1701	39.91	81.02	121.98	1687	40.42	82.06	120.94	1673	40.93	83.10	119.90	1658
203.5	39.28	79.94	123.56	1709	39.79	80.98	122.52	1694	40.30	82.02	121.48	1680	40.81	83.06	120.44	1666
204	39.17	79.90	124.10	1716	39.68	80.94	123.06	1702	40.18	81.98	122.02	1688	40.69	83.01	120.99	1673
204.5	39.05	79.86	124.64	1724	39.56	80.90	123.60	1709	40.07	81.94	122.56	1695	40.57	82.97	121.53	1681
205	38.94	79.82	125.18	1731	39.44	80.86	124.14	1717	39.95	81.90	123.11	1703	40.45	82.93	122.07	1688
205.5	38.82	79.78	125.72	1739	39.33	80.82	124.68	1724	39.83	81.85	123.65	1710	40.34	82.89	122.61	1696
206	38.71	79.74	126.26	1746	39.21	80.78	125.22	1732	39.72	81.81	124.19	1718	40.22	82.85	123.15	1703
206.5	38.59	79.70	126.80	1754	39.10	80.73	125.77	1739	39.60	81.77	124.73	1725	40.10	82.81	123.69	1711
207	38.48	79.66	127.34	1761	38.98	80.69	126.31	1747	39.48	81.73	125.27	1732	39.98	82.77	124.23	1718
207.5	38.37	79.62	127.89	1769	38.87	80.65	126.85	1754	39.37	81.69	125.81	1740	39.87	82.73	124.77	1726
208	38.26	79.57	128.43	1776	38.76	80.61	127.39	1762	39.25	81.65	126.35	1747	39.75	82.69	125.31	1733
208.5	38.15	79.53	128.97	1784	38.64	80.57	127.93	1769	39.14	81.61	126.89	1755	39.64	82.65	125.85	1741
209	38.03	79.49	129.51	1791	38.53	80.53	128.47	1777	39.03	81.57	127.43	1762	39.52	82.60	126.40	1748
209.5	37.92	79.45	130.05	1799	38.42	80.49	129.01	1784	38.91	81.53	127.97	1770	39.41	82.56	126.94	1756
210	37.81	79.41	130.59	1806	38.31	80.45	129.55	1792	38.80	81.49	128.52	1777	39.30	82.52	127.48	1763
210.5	37.70	79.37	131.13	1814	38.20	80.41	130.09	1799	38.69	81.44	129.06	1785	39.18	82.48	128.02	1770
211	37.60	79.33	131.67	1821	38.09	80.37	130.63	1807	38.58	81.40	129.60	1792	39.07	82.44	128.56	1778
211.5	37.49	79.29	132.21	1829	37.98	80.32	131.18	1814	38.47	81.36	130.14	1800	38.96	82.40	129.10	1785
212	37.38	79.25	132.75	1836	37.87	80.28	131.72	1822	38.36	81.32	130.68	1807	38.85	82.36	129.64	1793
212.5	37.27	79.21	133.30	1843	37.76	80.24	132.26	1829	38.25	81.28	131.22	1815	38.74	82.32	130.18	1800
213	37.17	79.16	133.84	1851	37.65	80.20	132.80	1837	38.14	81.24	131.76	1822	38.63	82.28	130.72	1808
213.5	37.06	79.12	134.38	1858	37.55	80.16	133.34	1844	38.03	81.20	132.30	1830	38.52	82.24	131.26	1815
214	36.95	79.08	134.92	1866	37.44	80.12	133.88	1852	37.92	81.16	132.84	1837	38.41	82.19	131.81	1823
214.5	36.85	79.04	135.46	1873	37.33	80.08	134.42	1859	37.82	81.12	133.38	1845	38.30	82.15	132.35	1830
215	36.74	79.00	136.00	1881	37.23	80.04	134.96	1867	37.71	81.08	133.93	1852	38.19	82.11	132.89	1838
215.5	36.64	78.96	136.54	1888	37.12	80.00	135.50	1874	37.60	81.03	134.47	1860	38.08	82.07	133.43	1845

Body Composition MALE 184-215.5 Lb.

Weight: Lb.	Waist: 48 inches Fat: %	Fat: Lb.	LBM: Lb.	RMR: Cal.	48.25 inches Fat: %	Fat: Lb.	LBM: Lb.	RMR: Cal.	48.5 inches Fat: %	Fat: Lb.	LBM: Lb.	RMR: Cal.	48.75 inches Fat: %	Fat: Lb.	LBM: Lb.	RMR: Cal.
184	46.57	85.69	98.31	1360	47.14	86.73	97.27	1345	47.70	87.77	96.23	1331	48.26	88.80	95.20	1317
184.5	46.42	85.65	98.85	1367	46.99	86.69	97.81	1353	47.55	87.73	96.77	1338	48.11	88.76	95.74	1324
185	46.28	85.61	99.39	1375	46.84	86.65	98.35	1360	47.40	87.69	97.32	1346	47.96	88.72	96.28	1332
185.5	46.13	85.57	99.93	1382	46.69	86.61	98.89	1368	47.25	87.64	97.86	1353	47.81	88.68	96.82	1339
186	45.98	85.53	100.47	1390	46.54	86.57	99.43	1375	47.10	87.60	98.40	1361	47.66	88.64	97.36	1346
186.5	45.84	85.49	101.01	1397	46.39	86.52	99.98	1383	46.95	87.56	98.94	1368	47.51	88.60	97.90	1354
187	45.69	85.45	101.55	1404	46.25	86.48	100.52	1390	46.80	87.52	99.48	1376	47.36	88.56	98.44	1361
187.5	45.55	85.41	102.10	1412	46.10	86.44	101.06	1398	46.66	87.48	100.02	1383	47.21	88.52	98.98	1369
188	45.41	85.36	102.64	1419	45.96	86.40	101.60	1405	46.51	87.44	100.56	1391	47.06	88.48	99.52	1376
188.5	45.26	85.32	103.18	1427	45.81	86.36	102.14	1413	46.36	87.40	101.10	1398	46.92	88.44	100.06	1384
189	45.12	85.28	103.72	1434	45.67	86.32	102.68	1420	46.22	87.36	101.64	1406	46.77	88.39	100.61	1391
189.5	44.98	85.24	104.26	1442	45.53	86.28	103.22	1428	46.08	87.32	102.18	1413	46.62	88.35	101.15	1399
190	44.84	85.20	104.80	1449	45.39	86.24	103.76	1435	45.93	87.28	102.73	1421	46.48	88.31	101.69	1406
190.5	44.70	85.16	105.34	1457	45.25	86.20	104.30	1443	45.79	87.23	103.27	1428	46.34	88.27	102.23	1414
191	44.56	85.12	105.88	1464	45.11	86.16	104.84	1450	45.65	87.19	103.81	1436	46.19	88.23	102.77	1421
191.5	44.43	85.08	106.42	1472	44.97	86.11	105.39	1457	45.51	87.15	104.35	1443	46.05	88.19	103.31	1429
192	44.29	85.04	106.96	1479	44.83	86.07	105.93	1465	45.37	87.11	104.89	1451	45.91	88.15	103.85	1436
192.5	44.15	85.00	107.51	1487	44.69	86.03	106.47	1472	45.23	87.07	105.43	1458	45.77	88.11	104.39	1444
193	44.02	84.95	108.05	1494	44.56	85.99	107.01	1480	45.09	87.03	105.97	1466	45.63	88.07	104.93	1451
193.5	43.88	84.91	108.59	1502	44.42	85.95	107.55	1487	44.96	86.99	106.51	1473	45.49	88.03	105.47	1459
194	43.75	84.87	109.13	1509	44.28	85.91	108.09	1495	44.82	86.95	107.05	1481	45.35	87.98	106.02	1466
194.5	43.61	84.83	109.67	1517	44.15	85.87	108.63	1502	44.68	86.91	107.59	1488	45.22	87.94	106.56	1474
195	43.48	84.79	110.21	1524	44.01	85.83	109.17	1510	44.55	86.87	108.14	1496	45.08	87.90	107.10	1481
195.5	43.35	84.75	110.75	1532	43.88	85.79	109.71	1517	44.41	86.82	108.68	1503	44.94	87.86	107.64	1489
196	43.22	84.71	111.29	1539	43.75	85.75	110.25	1525	44.28	86.78	109.22	1510	44.81	87.82	108.18	1496
196.5	43.09	84.67	111.83	1547	43.62	85.70	110.80	1532	44.14	86.74	109.76	1518	44.67	87.78	108.72	1504
197	42.96	84.63	112.37	1554	43.48	85.66	111.34	1540	44.01	86.70	110.30	1525	44.54	87.74	109.26	1511
197.5	42.83	84.59	112.92	1562	43.35	85.62	111.88	1547	43.88	86.66	110.84	1533	44.40	87.70	109.80	1519
198	42.70	84.54	113.46	1569	43.22	85.58	112.42	1555	43.75	86.62	111.38	1540	44.27	87.66	110.34	1526
198.5	42.57	84.50	114.00	1577	43.09	85.54	112.96	1562	43.62	86.58	111.92	1548	44.14	87.62	110.88	1534
199	42.44	84.46	114.54	1584	42.96	85.50	113.50	1570	43.49	86.54	112.46	1555	44.01	87.57	111.43	1541
199.5	42.32	84.42	115.08	1592	42.84	85.46	114.04	1577	43.36	86.50	113.00	1563	43.88	87.53	111.97	1548
200	42.19	84.38	115.62	1599	42.71	85.42	114.58	1585	43.23	86.46	113.55	1570	43.75	87.49	112.51	1556
200.5	42.06	84.34	116.16	1607	42.58	85.38	115.12	1592	43.10	86.41	114.09	1578	43.62	87.45	113.05	1563
201	41.94	84.30	116.70	1614	42.46	85.34	115.66	1600	42.97	86.37	114.63	1585	43.49	87.41	113.59	1571
201.5	41.81	84.26	117.24	1621	42.33	85.29	116.21	1607	42.84	86.33	115.17	1593	43.36	87.37	114.13	1578
202	41.69	84.22	117.78	1629	42.20	85.25	116.75	1615	42.72	86.29	115.71	1600	43.23	87.33	114.67	1586
202.5	41.57	84.18	118.33	1636	42.08	85.21	117.29	1622	42.59	86.25	116.25	1608	43.10	87.29	115.21	1593
203	41.45	84.13	118.87	1644	41.96	85.17	117.83	1630	42.47	86.21	116.79	1615	42.98	87.25	115.75	1601
203.5	41.32	84.09	119.41	1651	41.83	85.13	118.37	1637	42.34	86.17	117.33	1623	42.85	87.21	116.29	1608
204	41.20	84.05	119.95	1659	41.71	85.09	118.91	1645	42.22	86.13	117.87	1630	42.73	87.16	116.84	1616
204.5	41.08	84.01	120.49	1666	41.59	85.05	119.45	1652	42.10	86.09	118.41	1638	42.60	87.12	117.38	1623
205	40.96	83.97	121.03	1674	41.47	85.01	119.99	1659	41.97	86.05	118.96	1645	42.48	87.08	117.92	1631
205.5	40.84	83.93	121.57	1681	41.35	84.97	120.53	1667	41.85	86.00	119.50	1653	42.36	87.04	118.46	1638
206	40.72	83.89	122.11	1689	41.23	84.93	121.07	1674	41.73	85.96	120.04	1660	42.23	87.00	119.00	1646
206.5	40.60	83.85	122.65	1696	41.11	84.88	121.62	1682	41.61	85.92	120.58	1668	42.11	86.96	119.54	1653
207	40.49	83.81	123.19	1704	40.99	84.84	122.16	1689	41.49	85.88	121.12	1675	41.99	86.92	120.08	1661
207.5	40.37	83.77	123.74	1711	40.87	84.80	122.70	1697	41.37	85.84	121.66	1683	41.87	86.88	120.62	1668
208	40.25	83.72	124.28	1719	40.75	84.76	123.24	1704	41.25	85.80	122.20	1690	41.75	86.84	121.16	1676
208.5	40.14	83.68	124.82	1726	40.63	84.72	123.78	1712	41.13	85.76	122.74	1698	41.63	86.80	121.70	1683
209	40.02	83.64	125.36	1734	40.52	84.68	124.32	1719	41.01	85.72	123.28	1705	41.51	86.75	122.25	1691
209.5	39.91	83.60	125.90	1741	40.40	84.64	124.86	1727	40.90	85.68	123.82	1712	41.39	86.71	122.79	1698
210	39.79	83.56	126.44	1749	40.28	84.60	125.40	1734	40.78	85.64	124.37	1720	41.27	86.67	123.33	1706
210.5	39.68	83.52	126.98	1756	40.17	84.56	125.94	1742	40.66	85.59	124.91	1727	41.16	86.63	123.87	1713
211	39.56	83.48	127.52	1764	40.05	84.52	126.48	1749	40.55	85.55	125.45	1735	41.04	86.59	124.41	1721
211.5	39.45	83.44	128.06	1771	39.94	84.47	127.03	1757	40.43	85.51	125.99	1742	40.92	86.55	124.95	1728
212	39.34	83.40	128.60	1779	39.83	84.43	127.57	1764	40.32	85.47	126.53	1750	40.81	86.51	125.49	1736
212.5	39.23	83.36	129.15	1786	39.71	84.39	128.11	1772	40.20	85.43	127.07	1757	40.69	86.47	126.03	1743
213	39.11	83.31	129.69	1794	39.60	84.35	128.65	1779	40.09	85.39	127.61	1765	40.58	86.43	126.57	1751
213.5	39.00	83.27	130.23	1801	39.49	84.31	129.19	1787	39.98	85.35	128.15	1772	40.46	86.39	127.11	1758
214	38.89	83.23	130.77	1809	39.38	84.27	129.73	1794	39.86	85.31	128.69	1780	40.35	86.34	127.66	1765
214.5	38.78	83.19	131.31	1816	39.27	84.23	130.27	1802	39.75	85.27	129.23	1787	40.23	86.30	128.20	1773
215	38.67	83.15	131.85	1823	39.16	84.19	130.81	1809	39.64	85.23	129.78	1795	40.12	86.26	128.74	1780
215.5	38.57	83.11	132.39	1831	39.05	84.15	131.35	1817	39.53	85.18	130.32	1802	40.01	86.22	129.28	1788

Body Composition MALE 216-247.5 Lb.

Weight: Lb.	Waist: 30 inches				30.25 inches				30.5 inches				30.75 inches			
	Fat: %	Fat: Lb.	LBM: Lb.	RMR: Cal.	Fat: %	Fat: Lb.	LBM: Lb.	RMR: Cal.	Fat: %	Fat: Lb.	LBM: Lb.	RMR: Cal.	Fat: %	Fat: Lb.	LBM: Lb.	RMR: Cal.
216	3.87	8.37	207.63	2872	4.35	9.41	206.59	2857	4.83	10.44	205.56	2843	5.32	11.48	204.52	2829
216.5	3.85	8.33	208.17	2879	4.33	9.36	207.14	2865	4.80	10.40	206.10	2850	5.28	11.44	205.06	2836
217	3.82	8.29	208.71	2887	4.30	9.32	207.68	2872	4.77	10.36	206.64	2858	5.25	11.40	205.60	2843
217.5	3.79	8.25	209.26	2894	4.27	9.28	208.22	2880	4.74	10.32	207.18	2865	5.22	11.36	206.14	2851
218	3.76	8.20	209.80	2901	4.24	9.24	208.76	2887	4.72	10.28	207.72	2873	5.19	11.32	206.68	2858
218.5	3.74	8.16	210.34	2909	4.21	9.20	209.30	2895	4.69	10.24	208.26	2880	5.16	11.28	207.22	2866
219	3.71	8.12	210.88	2916	4.18	9.16	209.84	2902	4.66	10.20	208.80	2888	5.13	11.23	207.77	2873
219.5	3.68	8.08	211.42	2924	4.15	9.12	210.38	2910	4.63	10.16	209.34	2895	5.10	11.19	208.31	2881
220	3.65	8.04	211.96	2931	4.13	9.08	210.92	2917	4.60	10.12	209.89	2903	5.07	11.15	208.85	2888
220.5	3.63	8.00	212.50	2939	4.10	9.04	211.46	2925	4.57	10.07	210.43	2910	5.04	11.11	209.39	2896
221	3.60	7.96	213.04	2946	4.07	9.00	212.00	2932	4.54	10.03	210.97	2918	5.01	11.07	209.93	2903
221.5	3.57	7.92	213.58	2954	4.04	8.95	212.55	2940	4.51	9.99	211.51	2925	4.98	11.03	210.47	2911
222	3.55	7.88	214.12	2961	4.02	8.91	213.09	2947	4.48	9.95	212.05	2933	4.95	10.99	211.01	2918
222.5	3.52	7.84	214.67	2969	3.99	8.87	213.63	2954	4.45	9.91	212.59	2940	4.92	10.95	211.55	2926
223	3.50	7.79	215.21	2976	3.96	8.83	214.17	2962	4.43	9.87	213.13	2948	4.89	10.91	212.09	2933
223.5	3.47	7.75	215.75	2984	3.93	8.79	214.71	2969	4.40	9.83	213.67	2955	4.86	10.87	212.63	2941
224	3.44	7.71	216.29	2991	3.91	8.75	215.25	2977	4.37	9.79	214.21	2963	4.83	10.82	213.18	2948
224.5	3.42	7.67	216.83	2999	3.88	8.71	215.79	2984	4.34	9.75	214.75	2970	4.80	10.78	213.72	2956
225	3.39	7.63	217.37	3006	3.85	8.67	216.33	2992	4.31	9.70	215.30	2978	4.77	10.74	214.26	2963
225.5	3.37	7.59	217.91	3014	3.83	8.63	216.87	2999	4.29	9.66	215.84	2985	4.75	10.70	214.80	2971
226	3.34	7.55	218.45	3021	3.80	8.59	217.41	3007	4.26	9.62	216.38	2992	4.72	10.66	215.34	2978
226.5	3.31	7.51	218.99	3029	3.77	8.54	217.96	3014	4.23	9.58	216.92	3000	4.69	10.62	215.88	2986
227	3.29	7.47	219.53	3036	3.75	8.50	218.50	3022	4.20	9.54	217.46	3007	4.66	10.58	216.42	2993
227.5	3.26	7.42	220.08	3044	3.72	8.46	219.04	3029	4.18	9.50	218.00	3015	4.63	10.54	216.96	3001
228	3.24	7.38	220.62	3051	3.69	8.42	219.58	3037	4.15	9.46	218.54	3022	4.60	10.50	217.50	3008
228.5	3.21	7.34	221.16	3059	3.67	8.38	220.12	3044	4.12	9.42	219.08	3030	4.58	10.46	218.04	3016
229	3.19	7.30	221.70	3066	3.64	8.34	220.66	3052	4.09	9.38	219.62	3037	4.55	10.41	218.59	3023
229.5	3.16	7.26	222.24	3074	3.62	8.30	221.20	3059	4.07	9.34	220.16	3045	4.52	10.37	219.13	3031
230	3.14	7.22	222.78	3081	3.59	8.26	221.74	3067	4.04	9.30	220.71	3052	4.49	10.33	219.67	3038
230.5	3.11	7.18	223.32	3089	3.56	8.22	222.28	3074	4.01	9.25	221.25	3060	4.46	10.29	220.21	3045
231	3.09	7.14	223.86	3096	3.54	8.18	222.82	3082	3.99	9.21	221.79	3067	4.44	10.25	220.75	3053
231.5	3.07	7.10	224.40	3103	3.51	8.13	223.37	3089	3.96	9.17	222.33	3075	4.41	10.21	221.29	3060
232	3.04	7.06	224.94	3111	3.49	8.09	223.91	3097	3.94	9.13	222.87	3082	4.38	10.17	221.83	3068
232.5	3.02	7.01	225.49	3118	3.46	8.05	224.45	3104	3.91	9.09	223.41	3090	4.36	10.13	222.37	3075
233	2.99	6.97	226.03	3126	3.44	8.01	224.99	3112	3.88	9.05	223.95	3097	4.33	10.09	222.91	3083
233.5	2.97	6.93	226.57	3133	3.41	7.97	225.53	3119	3.86	9.01	224.49	3105	4.30	10.05	223.45	3090
234	2.95	6.89	227.11	3141	3.39	7.93	226.07	3127	3.83	8.97	225.03	3112	4.28	10.00	224.00	3098
234.5	2.92	6.85	227.65	3148	3.36	7.89	226.61	3134	3.81	8.93	225.57	3120	4.25	9.96	224.54	3105
235	2.90	6.81	228.19	3156	3.34	7.85	227.15	3142	3.78	8.88	226.12	3127	4.22	9.92	225.08	3113
235.5	2.87	6.77	228.73	3163	3.31	7.81	227.69	3149	3.76	8.84	226.66	3135	4.20	9.88	225.62	3120
236	2.85	6.73	229.27	3171	3.29	7.77	228.23	3156	3.73	8.80	227.20	3142	4.17	9.84	226.16	3128
236.5	2.83	6.69	229.81	3178	3.27	7.72	228.78	3164	3.70	8.76	227.74	3150	4.14	9.80	226.70	3135
237	2.80	6.65	230.35	3186	3.24	7.68	229.32	3171	3.68	8.72	228.28	3157	4.12	9.76	227.24	3143
237.5	2.78	6.60	230.90	3193	3.22	7.64	229.86	3179	3.65	8.68	228.82	3165	4.09	9.72	227.78	3150
238	2.76	6.56	231.44	3201	3.19	7.60	230.40	3186	3.63	8.64	229.36	3172	4.07	9.68	228.32	3158
238.5	2.74	6.52	231.98	3208	3.17	7.56	230.94	3194	3.61	8.60	229.90	3180	4.04	9.64	228.86	3165
239	2.71	6.48	232.52	3216	3.15	7.52	231.48	3201	3.58	8.56	230.44	3187	4.01	9.59	229.41	3173
239.5	2.69	6.44	233.06	3223	3.12	7.48	232.02	3209	3.56	8.52	230.98	3195	3.99	9.55	229.95	3180
240	2.67	6.40	233.60	3231	3.10	7.44	232.56	3216	3.53	8.48	231.53	3202	3.96	9.51	230.49	3188
240.5	2.64	6.36	234.14	3238	3.08	7.40	233.10	3224	3.51	8.43	232.07	3209	3.94	9.47	231.03	3195
241	2.62	6.32	234.68	3246	3.05	7.36	233.64	3231	3.48	8.39	232.61	3217	3.91	9.43	231.57	3203
241.5	2.60	6.28	235.22	3253	3.03	7.31	234.19	3239	3.46	8.35	233.15	3224	3.89	9.39	232.11	3210
242	2.58	6.24	235.76	3261	3.01	7.27	234.73	3246	3.43	8.31	233.69	3232	3.86	9.35	232.65	3218
242.5	2.55	6.19	236.31	3268	2.98	7.23	235.27	3254	3.41	8.27	234.23	3239	3.84	9.31	233.19	3225
243	2.53	6.15	236.85	3276	2.96	7.19	235.81	3261	3.39	8.23	234.77	3247	3.81	9.27	233.73	3233
243.5	2.51	6.11	237.39	3283	2.94	7.15	236.35	3269	3.36	8.19	235.31	3254	3.79	9.23	234.27	3240
244	2.49	6.07	237.93	3291	2.91	7.11	236.89	3276	3.34	8.15	235.85	3262	3.76	9.18	234.82	3247
244.5	2.47	6.03	238.47	3298	2.89	7.07	237.43	3284	3.32	8.11	236.39	3269	3.74	9.14	235.36	3255
245	2.44	5.99	239.01	3306	2.87	7.03	237.97	3291	3.29	8.07	236.94	3277	3.72	9.10	235.90	3262
245.5	2.42	5.95	239.55	3313	2.85	6.99	238.51	3299	3.27	8.02	237.48	3284	3.69	9.06	236.44	3270
246	2.40	5.91	240.09	3320	2.82	6.95	239.05	3306	3.25	7.98	238.02	3292	3.67	9.02	236.98	3277
246.5	2.38	5.87	240.63	3328	2.80	6.90	239.60	3314	3.22	7.94	238.56	3299	3.64	8.98	237.52	3285
247	2.36	5.83	241.17	3335	2.78	6.86	240.14	3321	3.20	7.90	239.10	3307	3.62	8.94	238.06	3292
247.5	2.34	5.78	241.72	3343	2.76	6.82	240.68	3329	3.18	7.86	239.64	3314	3.59	8.90	238.60	3300

Body Composition   MALE   216-247.5 Lb.

Weight: Lb.	Waist: 31 inches Fat: %	Fat: Lb.	LBM: Lb.	RMR: Cal.	31.25 inches Fat: %	Fat: Lb.	LBM: Lb.	RMR: Cal.	31.5 inches Fat: %	Fat: Lb.	LBM: Lb.	RMR: Cal.	31.75 inches Fat: %	Fat: Lb.	LBM: Lb.	RMR: Cal.
216	5.80	12.52	203.48	2814	6.28	13.56	202.44	2800	6.76	14.59	201.41	2785	7.24	15.63	200.37	2771
216.5	5.76	12.48	204.02	2822	6.24	13.51	202.99	2807	6.72	14.55	201.95	2793	7.20	15.59	200.91	2779
217	5.73	12.44	204.56	2829	6.21	13.47	203.53	2815	6.69	14.51	202.49	2800	7.17	15.55	201.45	2786
217.5	5.70	12.40	205.11	2837	6.18	13.43	204.07	2822	6.65	14.47	203.03	2808	7.13	15.51	201.99	2794
218	5.67	12.35	205.65	2844	6.14	13.39	204.61	2830	6.62	14.43	203.57	2815	7.09	15.47	202.53	2801
218.5	5.64	12.31	206.19	2852	6.11	13.35	205.15	2837	6.58	14.39	204.11	2823	7.06	15.43	203.07	2809
219	5.60	12.27	206.73	2859	6.08	13.31	205.69	2845	6.55	14.35	204.65	2830	7.02	15.38	203.62	2816
219.5	5.57	12.23	207.27	2867	6.04	13.27	206.23	2852	6.52	14.31	205.19	2838	6.99	15.34	204.16	2823
220	5.54	12.19	207.81	2874	6.01	13.23	206.77	2860	6.48	14.27	205.74	2845	6.96	15.30	204.70	2831
220.5	5.51	12.15	208.35	2881	5.98	13.19	207.31	2867	6.45	14.22	206.28	2853	6.92	15.26	205.24	2838
221	5.48	12.11	208.89	2889	5.95	13.15	207.85	2875	6.42	14.18	206.82	2860	6.89	15.22	205.78	2846
221.5	5.45	12.07	209.43	2896	5.92	13.10	208.40	2882	6.38	14.14	207.36	2868	6.85	15.18	206.32	2853
222	5.42	12.03	209.97	2904	5.88	13.06	208.94	2890	6.35	14.10	207.90	2875	6.82	15.14	206.86	2861
222.5	5.39	11.99	210.52	2911	5.85	13.02	209.48	2897	6.32	14.06	208.44	2883	6.79	15.10	207.40	2868
223	5.36	11.94	211.06	2919	5.82	12.98	210.02	2905	6.29	14.02	208.98	2890	6.75	15.06	207.94	2876
223.5	5.33	11.90	211.60	2926	5.79	12.94	210.56	2912	6.25	13.98	209.52	2898	6.72	15.02	208.48	2883
224	5.30	11.86	212.14	2934	5.76	12.90	211.10	2920	6.22	13.94	210.06	2905	6.69	14.97	209.03	2891
224.5	5.27	11.82	212.68	2941	5.73	12.86	211.64	2927	6.19	13.90	210.60	2913	6.65	14.93	209.57	2898
225	5.24	11.78	213.22	2949	5.70	12.82	212.18	2934	6.16	13.86	211.15	2920	6.62	14.89	210.11	2906
225.5	5.21	11.74	213.76	2956	5.67	12.78	212.72	2942	6.13	13.81	211.69	2928	6.59	14.85	210.65	2913
226	5.18	11.70	214.30	2964	5.64	12.74	213.26	2949	6.09	13.77	212.23	2935	6.55	14.81	211.19	2921
226.5	5.15	11.66	214.84	2971	5.60	12.69	213.81	2957	6.06	13.73	212.77	2943	6.52	14.77	211.73	2928
227	5.12	11.62	215.38	2979	5.57	12.65	214.35	2964	6.03	13.69	213.31	2950	6.49	14.73	212.27	2936
227.5	5.09	11.58	215.93	2986	5.54	12.61	214.89	2972	6.00	13.65	213.85	2958	6.46	14.69	212.81	2943
228	5.06	11.53	216.47	2994	5.51	12.57	215.43	2979	5.97	13.61	214.39	2965	6.42	14.65	213.35	2951
228.5	5.03	11.49	217.01	3001	5.48	12.53	215.97	2987	5.94	13.57	214.93	2973	6.39	14.61	213.89	2958
229	5.00	11.45	217.55	3009	5.45	12.49	216.51	2994	5.91	13.53	215.47	2980	6.36	14.56	214.44	2966
229.5	4.97	11.41	218.09	3016	5.42	12.45	217.05	3002	5.88	13.49	216.01	2987	6.33	14.52	214.98	2973
230	4.94	11.37	218.63	3024	5.39	12.41	217.59	3009	5.85	13.45	216.56	2995	6.30	14.48	215.52	2981
230.5	4.91	11.33	219.17	3031	5.37	12.37	218.13	3017	5.82	13.40	217.10	3002	6.27	14.44	216.06	2988
231	4.89	11.29	219.71	3039	5.34	12.33	218.67	3024	5.78	13.36	217.64	3010	6.23	14.40	216.60	2996
231.5	4.86	11.25	220.25	3046	5.31	12.28	219.22	3032	5.75	13.32	218.18	3017	6.20	14.36	217.14	3003
232	4.83	11.21	220.79	3054	5.28	12.24	219.76	3039	5.72	13.28	218.72	3025	6.17	14.32	217.68	3011
232.5	4.80	11.17	221.34	3061	5.25	12.20	220.30	3047	5.69	13.24	219.26	3032	6.14	14.28	218.22	3018
233	4.77	11.12	221.88	3069	5.22	12.16	220.84	3054	5.66	13.20	219.80	3040	6.11	14.24	218.76	3025
233.5	4.75	11.08	222.42	3076	5.19	12.12	221.38	3062	5.64	13.16	220.34	3047	6.08	14.20	219.30	3033
234	4.72	11.04	222.96	3084	5.16	12.08	221.92	3069	5.61	13.12	220.88	3055	6.05	14.15	219.85	3040
234.5	4.69	11.00	223.50	3091	5.13	12.04	222.46	3077	5.58	13.08	221.42	3062	6.02	14.11	220.39	3048
235	4.66	10.96	224.04	3098	5.11	12.00	223.00	3084	5.55	13.04	221.97	3070	5.99	14.07	220.93	3055
235.5	4.64	10.92	224.58	3106	5.08	11.96	223.54	3092	5.52	12.99	222.51	3077	5.96	14.03	221.47	3063
236	4.61	10.88	225.12	3113	5.05	11.92	224.08	3099	5.49	12.95	223.05	3085	5.93	13.99	222.01	3070
236.5	4.58	10.84	225.66	3121	5.02	11.87	224.63	3107	5.46	12.91	223.59	3092	5.90	13.95	222.55	3078
237	4.56	10.80	226.20	3128	4.99	11.83	225.17	3114	5.43	12.87	224.13	3100	5.87	13.91	223.09	3085
237.5	4.53	10.76	226.75	3136	4.97	11.79	225.71	3122	5.40	12.83	224.67	3107	5.84	13.87	223.63	3093
238	4.50	10.71	227.29	3143	4.94	11.75	226.25	3129	5.37	12.79	225.21	3115	5.81	13.83	224.17	3100
238.5	4.48	10.67	227.83	3151	4.91	11.71	226.79	3136	5.35	12.75	225.75	3122	5.78	13.79	224.71	3108
239	4.45	10.63	228.37	3158	4.88	11.67	227.33	3144	5.32	12.71	226.29	3130	5.75	13.74	225.26	3115
239.5	4.42	10.59	228.91	3166	4.86	11.63	227.87	3151	5.29	12.67	226.83	3137	5.72	13.70	225.80	3123
240	4.40	10.55	229.45	3173	4.83	11.59	228.41	3159	5.26	12.63	227.38	3145	5.69	13.66	226.34	3130
240.5	4.37	10.51	229.99	3181	4.80	11.55	228.95	3166	5.23	12.58	227.92	3152	5.66	13.62	226.88	3138
241	4.34	10.47	230.53	3188	4.77	11.51	229.49	3174	5.20	12.54	228.46	3160	5.64	13.58	227.42	3145
241.5	4.32	10.43	231.07	3196	4.75	11.46	230.04	3181	5.18	12.50	229.00	3167	5.61	13.54	227.96	3153
242	4.29	10.39	231.61	3203	4.72	11.42	230.58	3189	5.15	12.46	229.54	3175	5.58	13.50	228.50	3160
242.5	4.27	10.35	232.16	3211	4.69	11.38	231.12	3196	5.12	12.42	230.08	3182	5.55	13.46	229.04	3168
243	4.24	10.30	232.70	3218	4.67	11.34	231.66	3204	5.09	12.38	230.62	3189	5.52	13.42	229.58	3175
243.5	4.21	10.26	233.24	3226	4.64	11.30	232.20	3211	5.07	12.34	231.16	3197	5.49	13.38	230.12	3183
244	4.19	10.22	233.78	3233	4.61	11.26	232.74	3219	5.04	12.30	231.70	3204	5.46	13.33	230.67	3190
244.5	4.16	10.18	234.32	3241	4.59	11.22	233.28	3226	5.01	12.26	232.24	3212	5.44	13.29	231.21	3198
245	4.14	10.14	234.86	3248	4.56	11.18	233.82	3234	4.99	12.22	232.79	3219	5.41	13.25	231.75	3205
245.5	4.11	10.10	235.40	3256	4.54	11.14	234.36	3241	4.96	12.17	233.33	3227	5.38	13.21	232.29	3213
246	4.09	10.06	235.94	3263	4.51	11.10	234.90	3249	4.93	12.13	233.87	3234	5.35	13.17	232.83	3220
246.5	4.06	10.02	236.48	3271	4.48	11.05	235.45	3256	4.91	12.09	234.41	3242	5.33	13.13	233.37	3228
247	4.04	9.98	237.02	3278	4.46	11.01	235.99	3264	4.88	12.05	234.95	3249	5.30	13.09	233.91	3235
247.5	4.01	9.94	237.57	3286	4.43	10.97	236.53	3271	4.85	12.01	235.49	3257	5.27	13.05	234.45	3242

Body Composition MALE 216-247.5 Lb.

Weight: Lb.	Waist: 32 inches Fat: %	Fat: Lb.	LBM: Lb.	RMR: Cal.	32.25 inches Fat: %	Fat: Lb.	LBM: Lb.	RMR: Cal.	32.5 inches Fat: %	Fat: Lb.	LBM: Lb.	RMR: Cal.	32.75 inches Fat: %	Fat: Lb.	LBM: Lb.	RMR: Cal.
216	7.72	16.67	199.33	2757	8.20	17.71	198.29	2742	8.68	18.74	197.26	2728	9.16	19.78	196.22	2714
216.5	7.68	16.63	199.87	2764	8.16	17.66	198.84	2750	8.64	18.70	197.80	2736	9.12	19.74	196.76	2721
217	7.64	16.59	200.41	2772	8.12	17.62	199.38	2757	8.60	18.66	198.34	2743	9.08	19.70	197.30	2729
217.5	7.61	16.55	200.96	2779	8.08	17.58	199.92	2765	8.56	18.62	198.88	2751	9.04	19.66	197.84	2736
218	7.57	16.50	201.50	2787	8.05	17.54	200.46	2772	8.52	18.58	199.42	2758	9.00	19.62	198.38	2744
218.5	7.53	16.46	202.04	2794	8.01	17.50	201.00	2780	8.48	18.54	199.96	2765	8.96	19.58	198.92	2751
219	7.50	16.42	202.58	2802	7.97	17.46	201.54	2787	8.45	18.50	200.50	2773	8.92	19.53	199.47	2759
219.5	7.46	16.38	203.12	2809	7.94	17.42	202.08	2795	8.41	18.46	201.04	2780	8.88	19.49	200.01	2766
220	7.43	16.34	203.66	2817	7.90	17.38	202.62	2802	8.37	18.42	201.59	2788	8.84	19.45	200.55	2774
220.5	7.39	16.30	204.20	2824	7.86	17.34	203.16	2810	8.33	18.37	202.13	2795	8.80	19.41	201.09	2781
221	7.36	16.26	204.74	2832	7.83	17.30	203.70	2817	8.30	18.33	202.67	2803	8.76	19.37	201.63	2789
221.5	7.32	16.22	205.28	2839	7.79	17.25	204.25	2825	8.26	18.29	203.21	2810	8.73	19.33	202.17	2796
222	7.29	16.18	205.82	2847	7.75	17.21	204.79	2832	8.22	18.25	203.75	2818	8.69	19.29	202.71	2804
222.5	7.25	16.14	206.37	2854	7.72	17.17	205.33	2840	8.18	18.21	204.29	2825	8.65	19.25	203.25	2811
223	7.22	16.09	206.91	2862	7.68	17.13	205.87	2847	8.15	18.17	204.83	2833	8.61	19.21	203.79	2818
223.5	7.18	16.05	207.45	2869	7.65	17.09	206.41	2855	8.11	18.13	205.37	2840	8.58	19.17	204.33	2826
224	7.15	16.01	207.99	2876	7.61	17.05	206.95	2862	8.07	18.09	205.91	2848	8.54	19.12	204.88	2833
224.5	7.11	15.97	208.53	2884	7.58	17.01	207.49	2870	8.04	18.05	206.45	2855	8.50	19.08	205.42	2841
225	7.08	15.93	209.07	2891	7.54	16.97	208.03	2877	8.00	18.01	207.00	2863	8.46	19.04	205.96	2848
225.5	7.05	15.89	209.61	2899	7.51	16.93	208.57	2885	7.97	17.96	207.54	2870	8.43	19.00	206.50	2856
226	7.01	15.85	210.15	2906	7.47	16.89	209.11	2892	7.93	17.92	208.08	2878	8.39	18.96	207.04	2863
226.5	6.98	15.81	210.69	2914	7.44	16.84	209.66	2900	7.89	17.88	208.62	2885	8.35	18.92	207.58	2871
227	6.95	15.77	211.23	2921	7.40	16.80	210.20	2907	7.86	17.84	209.16	2893	8.32	18.88	208.12	2878
227.5	6.91	15.73	211.78	2929	7.37	16.76	210.74	2914	7.82	17.80	209.70	2900	8.28	18.84	208.66	2886
228	6.88	15.68	212.32	2936	7.33	16.72	211.28	2922	7.79	17.76	210.24	2908	8.24	18.80	209.20	2893
228.5	6.85	15.64	212.86	2944	7.30	16.68	211.82	2929	7.75	17.72	210.78	2915	8.21	18.76	209.74	2901
229	6.81	15.60	213.40	2951	7.27	16.64	212.36	2937	7.72	17.68	211.32	2923	8.17	18.71	210.29	2908
229.5	6.78	15.56	213.94	2959	7.23	16.60	212.90	2944	7.68	17.64	211.86	2930	8.14	18.67	210.83	2916
230	6.75	15.52	214.48	2966	7.20	16.56	213.44	2952	7.65	17.60	212.41	2938	8.10	18.63	211.37	2923
230.5	6.72	15.48	215.02	2974	7.17	16.52	213.98	2959	7.62	17.55	212.95	2945	8.07	18.59	211.91	2931
231	6.68	15.44	215.56	2981	7.13	16.48	214.52	2967	7.58	17.51	213.49	2953	8.03	18.55	212.45	2938
231.5	6.65	15.40	216.10	2989	7.10	16.43	215.07	2974	7.55	17.47	214.03	2960	8.00	18.51	212.99	2946
232	6.62	15.36	216.64	2996	7.07	16.39	215.61	2982	7.51	17.43	214.57	2967	7.96	18.47	213.53	2953
232.5	6.59	15.32	217.19	3004	7.03	16.35	216.15	2989	7.48	17.39	215.11	2975	7.93	18.43	214.07	2961
233	6.56	15.27	217.73	3011	7.00	16.31	216.69	2997	7.45	17.35	215.65	2982	7.89	18.39	214.61	2968
233.5	6.52	15.23	218.27	3019	6.97	16.27	217.23	3004	7.41	17.31	216.19	2990	7.86	18.35	215.15	2976
234	6.49	15.19	218.81	3026	6.94	16.23	217.77	3012	7.38	17.27	216.73	2997	7.82	18.30	215.70	2983
234.5	6.46	15.15	219.35	3034	6.90	16.19	218.31	3019	7.35	17.23	217.27	3005	7.79	18.26	216.24	2991
235	6.43	15.11	219.89	3041	6.87	16.15	218.85	3027	7.31	17.19	217.82	3012	7.75	18.22	216.78	2998
235.5	6.40	15.07	220.43	3049	6.84	16.11	219.39	3034	7.28	17.14	218.36	3020	7.72	18.18	217.32	3006
236	6.37	15.03	220.97	3056	6.81	16.07	219.93	3042	7.25	17.10	218.90	3027	7.69	18.14	217.86	3013
236.5	6.34	14.99	221.51	3064	6.78	16.02	220.48	3049	7.21	17.06	219.44	3035	7.65	18.10	218.40	3020
237	6.31	14.95	222.05	3071	6.74	15.98	221.02	3057	7.18	17.02	219.98	3042	7.62	18.06	218.94	3028
237.5	6.28	14.91	222.60	3078	6.71	15.94	221.56	3064	7.15	16.98	220.52	3050	7.59	18.02	219.48	3035
238	6.25	14.86	223.14	3086	6.68	15.90	222.10	3072	7.12	16.94	221.06	3057	7.55	17.98	220.02	3043
238.5	6.22	14.82	223.68	3093	6.65	15.86	222.64	3079	7.09	16.90	221.60	3065	7.52	17.94	220.56	3050
239	6.18	14.78	224.22	3101	6.62	15.82	223.18	3087	7.05	16.86	222.14	3072	7.49	17.89	221.11	3058
239.5	6.15	14.74	224.76	3108	6.59	15.78	223.72	3094	7.02	16.82	222.68	3080	7.45	17.85	221.65	3065
240	6.12	14.70	225.30	3116	6.56	15.74	224.26	3102	6.99	16.78	223.23	3087	7.42	17.81	222.19	3073
240.5	6.10	14.66	225.84	3123	6.53	15.70	224.80	3109	6.96	16.73	223.77	3095	7.39	17.77	222.73	3080
241	6.07	14.62	226.38	3131	6.50	15.66	225.34	3117	6.93	16.69	224.31	3102	7.36	17.73	223.27	3088
241.5	6.04	14.58	226.92	3138	6.47	15.61	225.89	3124	6.90	16.65	224.85	3110	7.32	17.69	223.81	3095
242	6.01	14.54	227.46	3146	6.44	15.57	226.43	3131	6.86	16.61	225.39	3117	7.29	17.65	224.35	3103
242.5	5.98	14.50	228.01	3153	6.41	15.53	226.97	3139	6.83	16.57	225.93	3125	7.26	17.61	224.89	3110
243	5.95	14.45	228.55	3161	6.38	15.49	227.51	3146	6.80	16.53	226.47	3132	7.23	17.57	225.43	3118
243.5	5.92	14.41	229.09	3168	6.35	15.45	228.05	3154	6.77	16.49	227.01	3140	7.20	17.53	225.97	3125
244	5.89	14.37	229.63	3176	6.32	15.41	228.59	3161	6.74	16.45	227.55	3147	7.17	17.48	226.52	3133
244.5	5.86	14.33	230.17	3183	6.29	15.37	229.13	3169	6.71	16.41	228.09	3155	7.13	17.44	227.06	3140
245	5.83	14.29	230.71	3191	6.26	15.33	229.67	3176	6.68	16.37	228.64	3162	7.10	17.40	227.60	3148
245.5	5.80	14.25	231.25	3198	6.23	15.29	230.21	3184	6.65	16.32	229.18	3170	7.07	17.36	228.14	3155
246	5.78	14.21	231.79	3206	6.20	15.25	230.75	3191	6.62	16.28	229.72	3177	7.04	17.32	228.68	3163
246.5	5.75	14.17	232.33	3213	6.17	15.20	231.30	3199	6.59	16.24	230.26	3184	7.01	17.28	229.22	3170
247	5.72	14.13	232.87	3221	6.14	15.16	231.84	3206	6.56	16.20	230.80	3192	6.98	17.24	229.76	3178
247.5	5.69	14.09	233.42	3228	6.11	15.12	232.38	3214	6.53	16.16	231.34	3199	6.95	17.20	230.30	3185

Body Composition MALE 216-247.5 Lb.

Weight: Lb.	Waist: 33 inches				33.25 inches				33.5 inches				33.75 inches			
	Fat: %	Fat: Lb.	LBM: Lb.	RMR: Cal.	Fat: %	Fat: Lb.	LBM: Lb.	RMR: Cal.	Fat: %	Fat: Lb.	LBM: Lb.	RMR: Cal.	Fat: %	Fat: Lb.	LBM: Lb.	RMR: Cal.
216	9.64	20.82	195.18	2699	10.12	21.86	194.14	2685	10.60	22.89	193.11	2671	11.08	23.93	192.07	2656
216.5	9.60	20.78	195.72	2707	10.08	21.81	194.69	2693	10.56	22.85	193.65	2678	11.03	23.89	192.61	2664
217	9.56	20.74	196.26	2714	10.03	21.77	195.23	2700	10.51	22.81	194.19	2686	10.99	23.85	193.15	2671
217.5	9.51	20.70	196.81	2722	9.99	21.73	195.77	2707	10.47	22.77	194.73	2693	10.95	23.81	193.69	2679
218	9.47	20.65	197.35	2729	9.95	21.69	196.31	2715	10.43	22.73	195.27	2701	10.90	23.77	194.23	2686
218.5	9.43	20.61	197.89	2737	9.91	21.65	196.85	2722	10.38	22.69	195.81	2708	10.86	23.73	194.77	2694
219	9.39	20.57	198.43	2744	9.87	21.61	197.39	2730	10.34	22.65	196.35	2716	10.81	23.68	195.32	2701
219.5	9.35	20.53	198.97	2752	9.83	21.57	197.93	2737	10.30	22.61	196.89	2723	10.77	23.64	195.86	2709
220	9.31	20.49	199.51	2759	9.79	21.53	198.47	2745	10.26	22.57	197.44	2731	10.73	23.60	196.40	2716
220.5	9.27	20.45	200.05	2767	9.74	21.49	199.01	2752	10.21	22.52	197.98	2738	10.69	23.56	196.94	2724
221	9.23	20.41	200.59	2774	9.70	21.45	199.55	2760	10.17	22.48	198.52	2745	10.64	23.52	197.48	2731
221.5	9.20	20.37	201.13	2782	9.66	21.40	200.10	2767	10.13	22.44	199.06	2753	10.60	23.48	198.02	2739
222	9.16	20.33	201.67	2789	9.62	21.36	200.64	2775	10.09	22.40	199.60	2760	10.56	23.44	198.56	2746
222.5	9.12	20.29	202.22	2797	9.58	21.32	201.18	2782	10.05	22.36	200.14	2768	10.52	23.40	199.10	2754
223	9.08	20.24	202.76	2804	9.54	21.28	201.72	2790	10.01	22.32	200.68	2775	10.47	23.36	199.64	2761
223.5	9.04	20.20	203.30	2812	9.50	21.24	202.26	2797	9.97	22.28	201.22	2783	10.43	23.32	200.18	2769
224	9.00	20.16	203.84	2819	9.46	21.20	202.80	2805	9.93	22.24	201.76	2790	10.39	23.27	200.73	2776
224.5	8.96	20.12	204.38	2827	9.42	21.16	203.34	2812	9.89	22.20	202.30	2798	10.35	23.23	201.27	2784
225	8.92	20.08	204.92	2834	9.39	21.12	203.88	2820	9.85	22.16	202.85	2805	10.31	23.19	201.81	2791
225.5	8.89	20.04	205.46	2842	9.35	21.08	204.42	2827	9.81	22.11	203.39	2813	10.27	23.15	202.35	2798
226	8.85	20.00	206.00	2849	9.31	21.04	204.96	2835	9.77	22.07	203.93	2820	10.23	23.11	202.89	2806
226.5	8.81	19.96	206.54	2856	9.27	20.99	205.51	2842	9.73	22.03	204.47	2828	10.19	23.07	203.43	2813
227	8.77	19.92	207.08	2864	9.23	20.95	206.05	2850	9.69	21.99	205.01	2835	10.14	23.03	203.97	2821
227.5	8.74	19.88	207.63	2871	9.19	20.91	206.59	2857	9.65	21.95	205.55	2843	10.10	22.99	204.51	2828
228	8.70	19.83	208.17	2879	9.15	20.87	207.13	2865	9.61	21.91	206.09	2850	10.06	22.95	205.05	2836
228.5	8.66	19.79	208.71	2886	9.12	20.83	207.67	2872	9.57	21.87	206.63	2858	10.02	22.91	205.59	2843
229	8.63	19.75	209.25	2894	9.08	20.79	208.21	2880	9.53	21.83	207.17	2865	9.98	22.86	206.14	2851
229.5	8.59	19.71	209.79	2901	9.04	20.75	208.75	2887	9.49	21.79	207.71	2873	9.94	22.82	206.68	2858
230	8.55	19.67	210.33	2909	9.00	20.71	209.29	2895	9.45	21.75	208.26	2880	9.91	22.78	207.22	2866
230.5	8.52	19.63	210.87	2916	8.97	20.67	209.83	2902	9.42	21.70	208.80	2888	9.87	22.74	207.76	2873
231	8.48	19.59	211.41	2924	8.93	20.63	210.37	2909	9.38	21.66	209.34	2895	9.83	22.70	208.30	2881
231.5	8.44	19.55	211.95	2931	8.89	20.58	210.92	2917	9.34	21.62	209.88	2903	9.79	22.66	208.84	2888
232	8.41	19.51	212.49	2939	8.85	20.54	211.46	2924	9.30	21.58	210.42	2910	9.75	22.62	209.38	2896
232.5	8.37	19.47	213.04	2946	8.82	20.50	212.00	2932	9.26	21.54	210.96	2918	9.71	22.58	209.92	2903
233	8.34	19.42	213.58	2954	8.78	20.46	212.54	2939	9.23	21.50	211.50	2925	9.67	22.54	210.46	2911
233.5	8.30	19.38	214.12	2961	8.75	20.42	213.08	2947	9.19	21.46	212.04	2933	9.63	22.50	211.00	2918
234	8.27	19.34	214.66	2969	8.71	20.38	213.62	2954	9.15	21.42	212.58	2940	9.60	22.45	211.55	2926
234.5	8.23	19.30	215.20	2976	8.67	20.34	214.16	2962	9.12	21.38	213.12	2948	9.56	22.41	212.09	2933
235	8.20	19.26	215.74	2984	8.64	20.30	214.70	2969	9.08	21.34	213.67	2955	9.52	22.37	212.63	2941
235.5	8.16	19.22	216.28	2991	8.60	20.26	215.24	2977	9.04	21.29	214.21	2962	9.48	22.33	213.17	2948
236	8.13	19.18	216.82	2999	8.57	20.22	215.78	2984	9.01	21.25	214.75	2970	9.45	22.29	213.71	2956
236.5	8.09	19.14	217.36	3006	8.53	20.17	216.33	2992	8.97	21.21	215.29	2977	9.41	22.25	214.25	2963
237	8.06	19.10	217.90	3014	8.50	20.13	216.87	2999	8.93	21.17	215.83	2985	9.37	22.21	214.79	2971
237.5	8.02	19.06	218.45	3021	8.46	20.09	217.41	3007	8.90	21.13	216.37	2992	9.33	22.17	215.33	2978
238	7.99	19.01	218.99	3029	8.42	20.05	217.95	3014	8.86	21.09	216.91	3000	9.30	22.13	215.87	2986
238.5	7.96	18.97	219.53	3036	8.39	20.01	218.49	3022	8.83	21.05	217.45	3007	9.26	22.09	216.41	2993
239	7.92	18.93	220.07	3044	8.36	19.97	219.03	3029	8.79	21.01	217.99	3015	9.22	22.04	216.96	3000
239.5	7.89	18.89	220.61	3051	8.32	19.93	219.57	3037	8.75	20.97	218.53	3022	9.19	22.00	217.50	3008
240	7.85	18.85	221.15	3059	8.29	19.89	220.11	3044	8.72	20.93	219.08	3030	9.15	21.96	218.04	3015
240.5	7.82	18.81	221.69	3066	8.25	19.85	220.65	3052	8.68	20.88	219.62	3037	9.11	21.92	218.58	3023
241	7.79	18.77	222.23	3073	8.22	19.81	221.19	3059	8.65	20.84	220.16	3045	9.08	21.88	219.12	3030
241.5	7.75	18.73	222.77	3081	8.18	19.76	221.74	3067	8.61	20.80	220.70	3052	9.04	21.84	219.66	3038
242	7.72	18.69	223.31	3088	8.15	19.72	222.28	3074	8.58	20.76	221.24	3060	9.01	21.80	220.20	3045
242.5	7.69	18.65	223.86	3096	8.12	19.68	222.82	3082	8.54	20.72	221.78	3067	8.97	21.76	220.74	3053
243	7.66	18.60	224.40	3103	8.08	19.64	223.36	3089	8.51	20.68	222.32	3075	8.94	21.72	221.28	3060
243.5	7.62	18.56	224.94	3111	8.05	19.60	223.90	3097	8.48	20.64	222.86	3082	8.90	21.68	221.82	3068
244	7.59	18.52	225.48	3118	8.02	19.56	224.44	3104	8.44	20.60	223.40	3090	8.87	21.63	222.37	3075
244.5	7.56	18.48	226.02	3126	7.98	19.52	224.98	3111	8.41	20.56	223.94	3097	8.83	21.59	222.91	3083
245	7.53	18.44	226.56	3133	7.95	19.48	225.52	3119	8.37	20.52	224.49	3105	8.80	21.55	223.45	3090
245.5	7.49	18.40	227.10	3141	7.92	19.44	226.06	3126	8.34	20.47	225.03	3112	8.76	21.51	223.99	3098
246	7.46	18.36	227.64	3148	7.88	19.40	226.60	3134	8.31	20.43	225.57	3120	8.73	21.47	224.53	3105
246.5	7.43	18.32	228.18	3156	7.85	19.35	227.15	3141	8.27	20.39	226.11	3127	8.69	21.43	225.07	3113
247	7.40	18.28	228.72	3163	7.82	19.31	227.69	3149	8.24	20.35	226.65	3135	8.66	21.39	225.61	3120
247.5	7.37	18.24	229.27	3171	7.79	19.27	228.23	3156	8.21	20.31	227.19	3142	8.63	21.35	226.15	3128

Body Composition   MALE   216-247.5 Lb.

Weight: Lb.	Waist: 34 inches Fat: %	Fat: Lb.	LBM: Lb.	RMR: Cal.	34.25 inches Fat: %	Fat: Lb.	LBM: Lb.	RMR: Cal.	34.5 inches Fat: %	Fat: Lb.	LBM: Lb.	RMR: Cal.	34.75 inches Fat: %	Fat: Lb.	LBM: Lb.	RMR: Cal.
216	11.56	24.97	191.03	2642	12.04	26.01	189.99	2628	12.52	27.04	188.96	2613	13.00	28.08	187.92	2599
216.5	11.51	24.93	191.57	2649	11.99	25.96	190.54	2635	12.47	27.00	189.50	2621	12.95	28.04	188.46	2606
217	11.47	24.89	192.11	2657	11.95	25.92	191.08	2643	12.42	26.96	190.04	2628	12.90	28.00	189.00	2614
217.5	11.42	24.85	192.66	2664	11.90	25.88	191.62	2650	12.38	26.92	190.58	2635	12.85	27.96	189.54	2621
218	11.38	24.80	193.20	2672	11.85	25.84	192.16	2658	12.33	26.88	191.12	2643	12.81	27.92	190.08	2629
218.5	11.33	24.76	193.74	2679	11.81	25.80	192.70	2665	12.28	26.84	191.66	2651	12.76	27.88	190.62	2636
219	11.29	24.72	194.28	2687	11.76	25.76	193.24	2673	12.24	26.80	192.20	2658	12.71	27.83	191.17	2644
219.5	11.24	24.68	194.82	2694	11.72	25.72	193.78	2680	12.19	26.76	192.74	2666	12.66	27.79	191.71	2651
220	11.20	24.64	195.36	2702	11.67	25.68	194.32	2687	12.14	26.72	193.29	2673	12.61	27.75	192.25	2659
220.5	11.16	24.60	195.90	2709	11.63	25.64	194.86	2695	12.10	26.67	193.83	2681	12.57	27.71	192.79	2666
221	11.11	24.56	196.44	2717	11.58	25.60	195.40	2702	12.05	26.63	194.37	2688	12.52	27.67	193.33	2674
221.5	11.07	24.52	196.98	2724	11.54	25.55	195.95	2710	12.01	26.59	194.91	2696	12.47	27.63	193.87	2681
222	11.03	24.48	197.52	2732	11.49	25.51	196.49	2717	11.96	26.55	195.45	2703	12.43	27.59	194.41	2689
222.5	10.98	24.44	198.07	2739	11.45	25.47	197.03	2725	11.91	26.51	195.99	2711	12.38	27.55	194.95	2696
223	10.94	24.39	198.61	2747	11.40	25.43	197.57	2732	11.87	26.47	196.53	2718	12.33	27.51	195.49	2704
223.5	10.90	24.35	199.15	2754	11.36	25.39	198.11	2740	11.82	26.43	197.07	2726	12.29	27.47	196.03	2711
224	10.85	24.31	199.69	2762	11.32	25.35	198.65	2747	11.78	26.39	197.61	2733	12.24	27.42	196.58	2719
224.5	10.81	24.27	200.23	2769	11.27	25.31	199.19	2755	11.74	26.35	198.15	2740	12.20	27.38	197.12	2726
225	10.77	24.23	200.77	2777	11.23	25.27	199.73	2762	11.69	26.31	198.70	2748	12.15	27.34	197.66	2734
225.5	10.73	24.19	201.31	2784	11.19	25.23	200.27	2770	11.65	26.26	199.24	2755	12.11	27.30	198.20	2741
226	10.68	24.15	201.85	2792	11.14	25.19	200.81	2777	11.60	26.22	199.78	2763	12.06	27.26	198.74	2749
226.5	10.64	24.11	202.39	2799	11.10	25.14	201.36	2785	11.56	26.18	200.32	2770	12.02	27.22	199.28	2756
227	10.60	24.07	202.93	2807	11.06	25.10	201.90	2792	11.52	26.14	200.86	2778	11.97	27.18	199.82	2764
227.5	10.56	24.03	203.48	2814	11.02	25.06	202.44	2800	11.47	26.10	201.40	2785	11.93	27.14	200.36	2771
228	10.52	23.98	204.02	2822	10.97	25.02	202.98	2807	11.43	26.06	201.94	2793	11.88	27.10	200.90	2778
228.5	10.48	23.94	204.56	2829	10.93	24.98	203.52	2815	11.39	26.02	202.48	2800	11.84	27.06	201.44	2786
229	10.44	23.90	205.10	2837	10.89	24.94	204.06	2822	11.34	25.98	203.02	2808	11.80	27.01	201.99	2793
229.5	10.40	23.86	205.64	2844	10.85	24.90	204.60	2830	11.30	25.94	203.56	2815	11.75	26.97	202.53	2801
230	10.36	23.82	206.18	2851	10.81	24.86	205.14	2837	11.26	25.90	204.11	2823	11.71	26.93	203.07	2808
230.5	10.32	23.78	206.72	2859	10.77	24.82	205.68	2845	11.22	25.85	204.65	2830	11.67	26.89	203.61	2816
231	10.28	23.74	207.26	2866	10.73	24.78	206.22	2852	11.17	25.81	205.19	2838	11.62	26.85	204.15	2823
231.5	10.24	23.70	207.80	2874	10.68	24.73	206.77	2860	11.13	25.77	205.73	2845	11.58	26.81	204.69	2831
232	10.20	23.66	208.34	2881	10.64	24.69	207.31	2867	11.09	25.73	206.27	2853	11.54	26.77	205.23	2838
232.5	10.16	23.62	208.89	2889	10.60	24.65	207.85	2875	11.05	25.69	206.81	2860	11.50	26.73	205.77	2846
233	10.12	23.57	209.43	2896	10.56	24.61	208.39	2882	11.01	25.65	207.35	2868	11.45	26.69	206.31	2853
233.5	10.08	23.53	209.97	2904	10.52	24.57	208.93	2889	10.97	25.61	207.89	2875	11.41	26.65	206.85	2861
234	10.04	23.49	210.51	2911	10.48	24.53	209.47	2897	10.93	25.57	208.43	2883	11.37	26.60	207.40	2868
234.5	10.00	23.45	211.05	2919	10.44	24.49	210.01	2904	10.89	25.53	208.97	2890	11.33	26.56	207.94	2876
235	9.96	23.41	211.59	2926	10.40	24.45	210.55	2912	10.84	25.49	209.52	2898	11.29	26.52	208.48	2883
235.5	9.92	23.37	212.13	2934	10.36	24.41	211.09	2919	10.80	25.44	210.06	2905	11.24	26.48	209.02	2891
236	9.88	23.33	212.67	2941	10.32	24.37	211.63	2927	10.76	25.40	210.60	2913	11.20	26.44	209.56	2898
236.5	9.85	23.29	213.21	2949	10.29	24.32	212.18	2934	10.72	25.36	211.14	2920	11.16	26.40	210.10	2906
237	9.81	23.25	213.75	2956	10.25	24.28	212.72	2942	10.68	25.32	211.68	2928	11.12	26.36	210.64	2913
237.5	9.77	23.21	214.30	2964	10.21	24.24	213.26	2949	10.64	25.28	212.22	2935	11.08	26.32	211.18	2921
238	9.73	23.16	214.84	2971	10.17	24.20	213.80	2957	10.60	25.24	212.76	2942	11.04	26.28	211.72	2928
238.5	9.70	23.12	215.38	2979	10.13	24.16	214.34	2964	10.57	25.20	213.30	2950	11.00	26.24	212.26	2936
239	9.66	23.08	215.92	2986	10.09	24.12	214.88	2972	10.53	25.16	213.84	2957	10.96	26.19	212.81	2943
239.5	9.62	23.04	216.46	2994	10.05	24.08	215.42	2979	10.49	25.12	214.38	2965	10.92	26.15	213.35	2951
240	9.58	23.00	217.00	3001	10.02	24.04	215.96	2987	10.45	25.08	214.93	2972	10.88	26.11	213.89	2958
240.5	9.55	22.96	217.54	3009	9.98	24.00	216.50	2994	10.41	25.03	215.47	2980	10.84	26.07	214.43	2966
241	9.51	22.92	218.08	3016	9.94	23.96	217.04	3002	10.37	24.99	216.01	2987	10.80	26.03	214.97	2973
241.5	9.47	22.88	218.62	3024	9.90	23.91	217.59	3009	10.33	24.95	216.55	2995	10.76	25.99	215.51	2981
242	9.44	22.84	219.16	3031	9.87	23.87	218.13	3017	10.29	24.91	217.09	3002	10.72	25.95	216.05	2988
242.5	9.40	22.80	219.71	3039	9.83	23.83	218.67	3024	10.26	24.87	217.63	3010	10.68	25.91	216.59	2995
243	9.36	22.75	220.25	3046	9.79	23.79	219.21	3032	10.22	24.83	218.17	3017	10.64	25.87	217.13	3003
243.5	9.33	22.71	220.79	3053	9.75	23.75	219.75	3039	10.18	24.79	218.71	3025	10.61	25.83	217.67	3010
244	9.29	22.67	221.33	3061	9.72	23.71	220.29	3047	10.14	24.75	219.25	3032	10.57	25.78	218.22	3018
244.5	9.26	22.63	221.87	3068	9.68	23.67	220.83	3054	10.10	24.71	219.79	3040	10.53	25.74	218.76	3025
245	9.22	22.59	222.41	3076	9.64	23.63	221.37	3062	10.07	24.67	220.34	3047	10.49	25.70	219.30	3033
245.5	9.18	22.55	222.95	3083	9.61	23.59	221.91	3069	10.03	24.62	220.88	3055	10.45	25.66	219.84	3040
246	9.15	22.51	223.49	3091	9.57	23.55	222.45	3077	9.99	24.58	221.42	3062	10.41	25.62	220.38	3048
246.5	9.11	22.47	224.03	3098	9.54	23.50	223.00	3084	9.96	24.54	221.96	3070	10.38	25.58	220.92	3055
247	9.08	22.43	224.57	3106	9.50	23.46	223.54	3092	9.92	24.50	222.50	3077	10.34	25.54	221.46	3063
247.5	9.04	22.39	225.12	3113	9.46	23.42	224.08	3099	9.88	24.46	223.04	3085	10.30	25.50	222.00	3070

Body Composition   MALE   216-247.5 Lb.

Weight: Lb.	Waist: 35 inches				35.25 inches				35.5 inches				35.75 inches			
	Fat: %	Fat: Lb.	LBM: Lb.	RMR: Cal.	Fat: %	Fat: Lb.	LBM: Lb.	RMR: Cal.	Fat: %	Fat: Lb.	LBM: Lb.	RMR: Cal.	Fat: %	Fat: Lb.	LBM: Lb.	RMR: Cal.
216	13.48	29.12	186.88	2585	13.96	30.16	185.84	2570	14.44	31.19	184.81	2556	14.92	32.23	183.77	2542
216.5	13.43	29.08	187.42	2592	13.91	30.11	186.39	2578	14.39	31.15	185.35	2563	14.87	32.19	184.31	2549
217	13.38	29.04	187.96	2600	13.86	30.07	186.93	2585	14.34	31.11	185.89	2571	14.81	32.15	184.85	2556
217.5	13.33	29.00	188.51	2607	13.81	30.03	187.47	2593	14.29	31.07	186.43	2578	14.76	32.11	185.39	2564
218	13.28	28.95	189.05	2615	13.76	29.99	188.01	2600	14.23	31.03	186.97	2586	14.71	32.07	185.93	2571
218.5	13.23	28.91	189.59	2622	13.71	29.95	188.55	2608	14.18	30.99	187.51	2593	14.66	32.03	186.47	2579
219	13.18	28.87	190.13	2629	13.66	29.91	189.09	2615	14.13	30.95	188.05	2601	14.60	31.98	187.02	2586
219.5	13.13	28.83	190.67	2637	13.61	29.87	189.63	2623	14.08	30.91	188.59	2608	14.55	31.94	187.56	2594
220	13.09	28.79	191.21	2644	13.56	29.83	190.17	2630	14.03	30.87	189.14	2616	14.50	31.90	188.10	2601
220.5	13.04	28.75	191.75	2652	13.51	29.79	190.71	2638	13.98	30.82	189.68	2623	14.45	31.86	188.64	2609
221	12.99	28.71	192.29	2659	13.46	29.75	191.25	2645	13.93	30.78	190.22	2631	14.40	31.82	189.18	2616
221.5	12.94	28.67	192.83	2667	13.41	29.70	191.80	2653	13.88	30.74	190.76	2638	14.35	31.78	189.72	2624
222	12.89	28.63	193.37	2674	13.36	29.66	192.34	2660	13.83	30.70	191.30	2646	14.30	31.74	190.26	2631
222.5	12.85	28.59	193.92	2682	13.31	29.62	192.88	2667	13.78	30.66	191.84	2653	14.25	31.70	190.80	2639
223	12.80	28.54	194.46	2689	13.27	29.58	193.42	2675	13.73	30.62	192.38	2661	14.20	31.66	191.34	2646
223.5	12.75	28.50	195.00	2697	13.22	29.54	193.96	2682	13.68	30.58	192.92	2668	14.15	31.62	191.88	2654
224	12.71	28.46	195.54	2704	13.17	29.50	194.50	2690	13.63	30.54	193.46	2676	14.10	31.57	192.43	2661
224.5	12.66	28.42	196.08	2712	13.12	29.46	195.04	2697	13.58	30.50	194.00	2683	14.05	31.53	192.97	2669
225	12.61	28.38	196.62	2719	13.07	29.42	195.58	2705	13.54	30.46	194.55	2691	14.00	31.49	193.51	2676
225.5	12.57	28.34	197.16	2727	13.03	29.38	196.12	2712	13.49	30.41	195.09	2698	13.95	31.45	194.05	2684
226	12.52	28.30	197.70	2734	12.98	29.34	196.66	2720	13.44	30.37	195.63	2706	13.90	31.41	194.59	2691
226.5	12.48	28.26	198.24	2742	12.93	29.29	197.21	2727	13.39	30.33	196.17	2713	13.85	31.37	195.13	2699
227	12.43	28.22	198.78	2749	12.89	29.25	197.75	2735	13.34	30.29	196.71	2720	13.80	31.33	195.67	2706
227.5	12.38	28.18	199.33	2757	12.84	29.21	198.29	2742	13.30	30.25	197.25	2728	13.75	31.29	196.21	2714
228	12.34	28.13	199.87	2764	12.79	29.17	198.83	2750	13.25	30.21	197.79	2735	13.70	31.25	196.75	2721
228.5	12.29	28.09	200.41	2772	12.75	29.13	199.37	2757	13.20	30.17	198.33	2743	13.66	31.21	197.29	2729
229	12.25	28.05	200.95	2779	12.70	29.09	199.91	2765	13.16	30.13	198.87	2750	13.61	31.16	197.84	2736
229.5	12.21	28.01	201.49	2787	12.66	29.05	200.45	2772	13.11	30.09	199.41	2758	13.56	31.12	198.38	2744
230	12.16	27.97	202.03	2794	12.61	29.01	200.99	2780	13.06	30.05	199.96	2765	13.51	31.08	198.92	2751
230.5	12.12	27.93	202.57	2802	12.57	28.97	201.53	2787	13.02	30.00	200.50	2773	13.47	31.04	199.46	2759
231	12.07	27.89	203.11	2809	12.52	28.93	202.07	2795	12.97	29.96	201.04	2780	13.42	31.00	200.00	2766
231.5	12.03	27.85	203.65	2817	12.48	28.88	202.62	2802	12.93	29.92	201.58	2788	13.37	30.96	200.54	2773
232	11.99	27.81	204.19	2824	12.43	28.84	203.16	2810	12.88	29.88	202.12	2795	13.33	30.92	201.08	2781
232.5	11.94	27.77	204.74	2831	12.39	28.80	203.70	2817	12.83	29.84	202.66	2803	13.28	30.88	201.62	2788
233	11.90	27.72	205.28	2839	12.34	28.76	204.24	2825	12.79	29.80	203.20	2810	13.23	30.84	202.16	2796
233.5	11.86	27.68	205.82	2846	12.30	28.72	204.78	2832	12.74	29.76	203.74	2818	13.19	30.80	202.70	2803
234	11.81	27.64	206.36	2854	12.26	28.68	205.32	2840	12.70	29.72	204.28	2825	13.14	30.75	203.25	2811
234.5	11.77	27.60	206.90	2861	12.21	28.64	205.86	2847	12.66	29.68	204.82	2833	13.10	30.71	203.79	2818
235	11.73	27.56	207.44	2869	12.17	28.60	206.40	2855	12.61	29.64	205.37	2840	13.05	30.67	204.33	2826
235.5	11.69	27.52	207.98	2876	12.13	28.56	206.94	2862	12.57	29.59	205.91	2848	13.01	30.63	204.87	2833
236	11.64	27.48	208.52	2884	12.08	28.52	207.48	2870	12.52	29.55	206.45	2855	12.96	30.59	205.41	2841
236.5	11.60	27.44	209.06	2891	12.04	28.47	208.03	2877	12.48	29.51	206.99	2863	12.92	30.55	205.95	2848
237	11.56	27.40	209.60	2899	12.00	28.43	208.57	2884	12.44	29.47	207.53	2870	12.87	30.51	206.49	2856
237.5	11.52	27.36	210.15	2906	11.95	28.39	209.11	2892	12.39	29.43	208.07	2878	12.83	30.47	207.03	2863
238	11.48	27.31	210.69	2914	11.91	28.35	209.65	2899	12.35	29.39	208.61	2885	12.78	30.43	207.57	2871
238.5	11.44	27.27	211.23	2921	11.87	28.31	210.19	2907	12.31	29.35	209.15	2893	12.74	30.39	208.11	2878
239	11.39	27.23	211.77	2929	11.83	28.27	210.73	2914	12.26	29.31	209.69	2900	12.70	30.34	208.66	2886
239.5	11.35	27.19	212.31	2936	11.79	28.23	211.27	2922	12.22	29.27	210.23	2908	12.65	30.30	209.20	2893
240	11.31	27.15	212.85	2944	11.74	28.19	211.81	2929	12.18	29.23	210.78	2915	12.61	30.26	209.74	2901
240.5	11.27	27.11	213.39	2951	11.70	28.15	212.35	2937	12.13	29.18	211.32	2923	12.57	30.22	210.28	2908
241	11.23	27.07	213.93	2959	11.66	28.11	212.89	2944	12.09	29.14	211.86	2930	12.52	30.18	210.82	2916
241.5	11.19	27.03	214.47	2966	11.62	28.06	213.44	2952	12.05	29.10	212.40	2937	12.48	30.14	211.36	2923
242	11.15	26.99	215.01	2974	11.58	28.02	213.98	2959	12.01	29.06	212.94	2945	12.44	30.10	211.90	2931
242.5	11.11	26.95	215.56	2981	11.54	27.98	214.52	2967	11.97	29.02	213.48	2952	12.39	30.06	212.44	2938
243	11.07	26.90	216.10	2989	11.50	27.94	215.06	2974	11.93	28.98	214.02	2960	12.35	30.02	212.98	2946
243.5	11.03	26.86	216.64	2996	11.46	27.90	215.60	2982	11.88	28.94	214.56	2967	12.31	29.98	213.52	2953
244	10.99	26.82	217.18	3004	11.42	27.86	216.14	2989	11.84	28.90	215.10	2975	12.27	29.93	214.07	2961
244.5	10.95	26.78	217.72	3011	11.38	27.82	216.68	2997	11.80	28.86	215.64	2982	12.23	29.89	214.61	2968
245	10.91	26.74	218.26	3019	11.34	27.78	217.22	3004	11.76	28.82	216.19	2990	12.18	29.85	215.15	2975
245.5	10.88	26.70	218.80	3026	11.30	27.74	217.76	3012	11.72	28.77	216.73	2997	12.14	29.81	215.69	2983
246	10.84	26.66	219.34	3033	11.26	27.70	218.30	3019	11.68	28.73	217.27	3005	12.10	29.77	216.23	2990
246.5	10.80	26.62	219.88	3041	11.22	27.65	218.85	3027	11.64	28.69	217.81	3012	12.06	29.73	216.77	2998
247	10.76	26.58	220.42	3048	11.18	27.61	219.39	3034	11.60	28.65	218.35	3020	12.02	29.69	217.31	3005
247.5	10.72	26.54	220.97	3056	11.14	27.57	219.93	3042	11.56	28.61	218.89	3027	11.98	29.65	217.85	3013

Body Composition MALE 216-247.5 Lb.

Weight: Lb.	Waist: 36 inches				36.25 inches				36.5 inches				36.75 inches			
	Fat: %	Fat: Lb.	LBM: Lb.	RMR: Cal.	Fat: %	Fat: Lb.	LBM: Lb.	RMR: Cal.	Fat: %	Fat: Lb.	LBM: Lb.	RMR: Cal.	Fat: %	Fat: Lb.	LBM: Lb.	RMR: Cal.
216	15.40	33.27	182.73	2527	15.88	34.31	181.69	2513	16.36	35.34	180.66	2498	16.84	36.38	179.62	2484
216.5	15.35	33.23	183.27	2535	15.83	34.26	182.24	2520	16.31	35.30	181.20	2506	16.78	36.34	180.16	2492
217	15.29	33.19	183.81	2542	15.77	34.22	182.78	2528	16.25	35.26	181.74	2513	16.73	36.30	180.70	2499
217.5	15.24	33.15	184.36	2550	15.72	34.18	183.32	2535	16.19	35.22	182.28	2521	16.67	36.26	181.24	2507
218	15.19	33.10	184.90	2557	15.66	34.14	183.86	2543	16.14	35.18	182.82	2528	16.61	36.22	181.78	2514
218.5	15.13	33.06	185.44	2565	15.61	34.10	184.40	2550	16.08	35.14	183.36	2536	16.56	36.18	182.32	2522
219	15.08	33.02	185.98	2572	15.55	34.06	184.94	2558	16.03	35.10	183.90	2543	16.50	36.13	182.87	2529
219.5	15.03	32.98	186.52	2580	15.50	34.02	185.48	2565	15.97	35.06	184.44	2551	16.44	36.09	183.41	2537
220	14.97	32.94	187.06	2587	15.44	33.98	186.02	2573	15.92	35.02	184.99	2558	16.39	36.05	183.95	2544
220.5	14.92	32.90	187.60	2595	15.39	33.94	186.56	2580	15.86	34.97	185.53	2566	16.33	36.01	184.49	2551
221	14.87	32.86	188.14	2602	15.34	33.90	187.10	2588	15.81	34.93	186.07	2573	16.28	35.97	185.03	2559
221.5	14.82	32.82	188.68	2609	15.28	33.85	187.65	2595	15.75	34.89	186.61	2581	16.22	35.93	185.57	2566
222	14.76	32.78	189.22	2617	15.23	33.81	188.19	2603	15.70	34.85	187.15	2588	16.17	35.89	186.11	2574
222.5	14.71	32.74	189.77	2624	15.18	33.77	188.73	2610	15.64	34.81	187.69	2596	16.11	35.85	186.65	2581
223	14.66	32.69	190.31	2632	15.13	33.73	189.27	2618	15.59	34.77	188.23	2603	16.06	35.81	187.19	2589
223.5	14.61	32.65	190.85	2639	15.07	33.69	189.81	2625	15.54	34.73	188.77	2611	16.00	35.77	187.73	2596
224	14.56	32.61	191.39	2647	15.02	33.65	190.35	2633	15.49	34.69	189.31	2618	15.95	35.72	188.28	2604
224.5	14.51	32.57	191.93	2654	14.97	33.61	190.89	2640	15.43	34.65	189.85	2626	15.89	35.68	188.82	2611
225	14.46	32.53	192.47	2662	14.92	33.57	191.43	2648	15.38	34.61	190.40	2633	15.84	35.64	189.36	2619
225.5	14.41	32.49	193.01	2669	14.87	33.53	191.97	2655	15.33	34.56	190.94	2641	15.79	35.60	189.90	2626
226	14.36	32.45	193.55	2677	14.82	33.49	192.51	2662	15.28	34.52	191.48	2648	15.73	35.56	190.44	2634
226.5	14.31	32.41	194.09	2684	14.77	33.44	193.06	2670	15.22	34.48	192.02	2656	15.68	35.52	190.98	2641
227	14.26	32.37	194.63	2692	14.72	33.40	193.60	2677	15.17	34.44	192.56	2663	15.63	35.48	191.52	2649
227.5	14.21	32.33	195.18	2699	14.66	33.36	194.14	2685	15.12	34.40	193.10	2671	15.58	35.44	192.06	2656
228	14.16	32.28	195.72	2707	14.61	33.32	194.68	2692	15.07	34.36	193.64	2678	15.52	35.40	192.60	2664
228.5	14.11	32.24	196.26	2714	14.56	33.28	195.22	2700	15.02	34.32	194.18	2686	15.47	35.36	193.14	2671
229	14.06	32.20	196.80	2722	14.52	33.24	195.76	2707	14.97	34.28	194.72	2693	15.42	35.31	193.69	2679
229.5	14.01	32.16	197.34	2729	14.47	33.20	196.30	2715	14.92	34.24	195.26	2701	15.37	35.27	194.23	2686
230	13.97	32.12	197.88	2737	14.42	33.16	196.84	2722	14.87	34.20	195.81	2708	15.32	35.23	194.77	2694
230.5	13.92	32.08	198.42	2744	14.37	33.12	197.38	2730	14.82	34.15	196.35	2715	15.27	35.19	195.31	2701
231	13.87	32.04	198.96	2752	14.32	33.08	197.92	2737	14.77	34.11	196.89	2723	15.22	35.15	195.85	2709
231.5	13.82	32.00	199.50	2759	14.27	33.03	198.47	2745	14.72	34.07	197.43	2730	15.17	35.11	196.39	2716
232	13.77	31.96	200.04	2767	14.22	32.99	199.01	2752	14.67	34.03	197.97	2738	15.12	35.07	196.93	2724
232.5	13.73	31.92	200.59	2774	14.17	32.95	199.55	2760	14.62	33.99	198.51	2745	15.07	35.03	197.47	2731
233	13.68	31.87	201.13	2782	14.13	32.91	200.09	2767	14.57	33.95	199.05	2753	15.02	34.99	198.01	2739
233.5	13.63	31.83	201.67	2789	14.08	32.87	200.63	2775	14.52	33.91	199.59	2760	14.97	34.95	198.55	2746
234	13.59	31.79	202.21	2797	14.03	32.83	201.17	2782	14.47	33.87	200.13	2768	14.92	34.90	199.10	2753
234.5	13.54	31.75	202.75	2804	13.98	32.79	201.71	2790	14.42	33.83	200.67	2775	14.87	34.86	199.64	2761
235	13.49	31.71	203.29	2812	13.94	32.75	202.25	2797	14.38	33.79	201.22	2783	14.82	34.82	200.18	2768
235.5	13.45	31.67	203.83	2819	13.89	32.71	202.79	2805	14.33	33.74	201.76	2790	14.77	34.78	200.72	2776
236	13.40	31.63	204.37	2826	13.84	32.67	203.33	2812	14.28	33.70	202.30	2798	14.72	34.74	201.26	2783
236.5	13.36	31.59	204.91	2834	13.79	32.62	203.88	2820	14.23	33.66	202.84	2805	14.67	34.70	201.80	2791
237	13.31	31.55	205.45	2841	13.75	32.58	204.42	2827	14.19	33.62	203.38	2813	14.62	34.66	202.34	2798
237.5	13.27	31.51	206.00	2849	13.70	32.54	204.96	2835	14.14	33.58	203.92	2820	14.58	34.62	202.88	2806
238	13.22	31.46	206.54	2856	13.66	32.50	205.50	2842	14.09	33.54	204.46	2828	14.53	34.58	203.42	2813
238.5	13.18	31.42	207.08	2864	13.61	32.46	206.04	2850	14.05	33.50	205.00	2835	14.48	34.54	203.96	2821
239	13.13	31.38	207.62	2871	13.56	32.42	206.58	2857	14.00	33.46	205.54	2843	14.43	34.49	204.51	2828
239.5	13.09	31.34	208.16	2879	13.52	32.38	207.12	2864	13.95	33.42	206.08	2850	14.39	34.45	205.05	2836
240	13.04	31.30	208.70	2886	13.47	32.34	207.66	2872	13.91	33.38	206.63	2858	14.34	34.41	205.59	2843
240.5	13.00	31.26	209.24	2894	13.43	32.30	208.20	2879	13.86	33.33	207.17	2865	14.29	34.37	206.13	2851
241	12.95	31.22	209.78	2901	13.38	32.26	208.74	2887	13.81	33.29	207.71	2873	14.25	34.33	206.67	2858
241.5	12.91	31.18	210.32	2909	13.34	32.21	209.29	2894	13.77	33.25	208.25	2880	14.20	34.29	207.21	2866
242	12.87	31.14	210.86	2916	13.29	32.17	209.83	2902	13.72	33.21	208.79	2888	14.15	34.25	207.75	2873
242.5	12.82	31.10	211.41	2924	13.25	32.13	210.37	2909	13.68	33.17	209.33	2895	14.11	34.21	208.29	2881
243	12.78	31.05	211.95	2931	13.21	32.09	210.91	2917	13.63	33.13	209.87	2903	14.06	34.17	208.83	2888
243.5	12.74	31.01	212.49	2939	13.16	32.05	211.45	2924	13.59	33.09	210.41	2910	14.01	34.13	209.37	2896
244	12.69	30.97	213.03	2946	13.12	32.01	211.99	2932	13.54	33.05	210.95	2917	13.97	34.08	209.92	2903
244.5	12.65	30.93	213.57	2954	13.08	31.97	212.53	2939	13.50	33.01	211.49	2925	13.92	34.04	210.46	2911
245	12.61	30.89	214.11	2961	13.03	31.93	213.07	2947	13.46	32.97	212.04	2932	13.88	34.00	211.00	2918
245.5	12.57	30.85	214.65	2969	12.99	31.89	213.61	2954	13.41	32.92	212.58	2940	13.83	33.96	211.54	2926
246	12.52	30.81	215.19	2976	12.95	31.85	214.15	2962	13.37	32.88	213.12	2947	13.79	33.92	212.08	2933
246.5	12.48	30.77	215.73	2984	12.90	31.80	214.70	2969	13.32	32.84	213.66	2955	13.74	33.88	212.62	2941
247	12.44	30.73	216.27	2991	12.86	31.76	215.24	2977	13.28	32.80	214.20	2962	13.70	33.84	213.16	2948
247.5	12.40	30.69	216.82	2999	12.82	31.72	215.78	2984	13.24	32.76	214.74	2970	13.66	33.80	213.70	2956

Body Composition MALE 216-247.5 Lb.

Weight: Lb.	Waist: 37 inches Fat: %	Fat: Lb.	LBM: Lb.	RMR: Cal.	37.25 inches Fat: %	Fat: Lb.	LBM: Lb.	RMR: Cal.	37.5 inches Fat: %	Fat: Lb.	LBM: Lb.	RMR: Cal.	37.75 inches Fat: %	Fat: Lb.	LBM: Lb.	RMR: Cal.
216	17.32	37.42	178.58	2470	17.80	38.46	177.54	2455	18.28	39.49	176.51	2441	18.76	40.53	175.47	2427
216.5	17.26	37.38	179.12	2477	17.74	38.41	178.09	2463	18.22	39.45	177.05	2449	18.70	40.49	176.01	2434
217	17.21	37.34	179.66	2485	17.68	38.37	178.63	2470	18.16	39.41	177.59	2456	18.64	40.45	176.55	2442
217.5	17.15	37.30	180.21	2492	17.62	38.33	179.17	2478	18.10	39.37	178.13	2464	18.58	40.41	177.09	2449
218	17.09	37.25	180.75	2500	17.56	38.29	179.71	2485	18.04	39.33	178.67	2471	18.52	40.37	177.63	2457
218.5	17.03	37.21	181.29	2507	17.51	38.25	180.25	2493	17.98	39.29	179.21	2479	18.46	40.33	178.17	2464
219	16.97	37.17	181.83	2515	17.45	38.21	180.79	2500	17.92	39.25	179.75	2486	18.39	40.28	178.72	2472
219.5	16.92	37.13	182.37	2522	17.39	38.17	181.33	2508	17.86	39.21	180.29	2493	18.33	40.24	179.26	2479
220	16.86	37.09	182.91	2530	17.33	38.13	181.87	2515	17.80	39.17	180.84	2501	18.27	40.20	179.80	2487
220.5	16.80	37.05	183.45	2537	17.27	38.09	182.41	2523	17.74	39.12	181.38	2508	18.21	40.16	180.34	2494
221	16.75	37.01	183.99	2545	17.22	38.05	182.95	2530	17.68	39.08	181.92	2516	18.15	40.12	180.88	2502
221.5	16.69	36.97	184.53	2552	17.16	38.00	183.50	2538	17.63	39.04	182.46	2523	18.09	40.08	181.42	2509
222	16.63	36.93	185.07	2560	17.10	37.96	184.04	2545	17.57	39.00	183.00	2531	18.04	40.04	181.96	2517
222.5	16.58	36.89	185.62	2567	17.04	37.92	184.58	2553	17.51	38.96	183.54	2538	17.98	40.00	182.50	2524
223	16.52	36.84	186.16	2575	16.99	37.88	185.12	2560	17.45	38.92	184.08	2546	17.92	39.96	183.04	2531
223.5	16.47	36.80	186.70	2582	16.93	37.84	185.66	2568	17.40	38.88	184.62	2553	17.86	39.92	183.58	2539
224	16.41	36.76	187.24	2590	16.87	37.80	186.20	2575	17.34	38.84	185.16	2561	17.80	39.87	184.13	2546
224.5	16.36	36.72	187.78	2597	16.82	37.76	186.74	2583	17.28	38.80	185.70	2568	17.74	39.83	184.67	2554
225	16.30	36.68	188.32	2604	16.76	37.72	187.28	2590	17.22	38.76	186.25	2576	17.69	39.79	185.21	2561
225.5	16.25	36.64	188.86	2612	16.71	37.68	187.82	2598	17.17	38.71	186.79	2583	17.63	39.75	185.75	2569
226	16.19	36.60	189.40	2619	16.65	37.64	188.36	2605	17.11	38.67	187.33	2591	17.57	39.71	186.29	2576
226.5	16.14	36.56	189.94	2627	16.60	37.59	188.91	2613	17.06	38.63	187.87	2598	17.51	39.67	186.83	2584
227	16.09	36.52	190.48	2634	16.54	37.55	189.45	2620	17.00	38.59	188.41	2606	17.46	39.63	187.37	2591
227.5	16.03	36.48	191.03	2642	16.49	37.51	189.99	2628	16.95	38.55	188.95	2613	17.40	39.59	187.91	2599
228	15.98	36.43	191.57	2649	16.43	37.47	190.53	2635	16.89	38.51	189.49	2621	17.34	39.55	188.45	2606
228.5	15.93	36.39	192.11	2657	16.38	37.43	191.07	2642	16.84	38.47	190.03	2628	17.29	39.51	188.99	2614
229	15.87	36.35	192.65	2664	16.33	37.39	191.61	2650	16.78	38.43	190.57	2636	17.23	39.46	189.54	2621
229.5	15.82	36.31	193.19	2672	16.27	37.35	192.15	2657	16.73	38.39	191.11	2643	17.18	39.42	190.08	2629
230	15.77	36.27	193.73	2679	16.22	37.31	192.69	2665	16.67	38.35	191.66	2651	17.12	39.38	190.62	2636
230.5	15.72	36.23	194.27	2687	16.17	37.27	193.23	2672	16.62	38.30	192.20	2658	17.07	39.34	191.16	2644
231	15.67	36.19	194.81	2694	16.11	37.23	193.77	2680	16.56	38.26	192.74	2666	17.01	39.30	191.70	2651
231.5	15.61	36.15	195.35	2702	16.06	37.18	194.32	2687	16.51	38.22	193.28	2673	16.96	39.26	192.24	2659
232	15.56	36.11	195.89	2709	16.01	37.14	194.86	2695	16.46	38.18	193.82	2681	16.90	39.22	192.78	2666
232.5	15.51	36.07	196.44	2717	15.96	37.10	195.40	2702	16.40	38.14	194.36	2688	16.85	39.18	193.32	2674
233	15.46	36.02	196.98	2724	15.91	37.06	195.94	2710	16.35	38.10	194.90	2695	16.80	39.14	193.86	2681
233.5	15.41	35.98	197.52	2732	15.85	37.02	196.48	2717	16.30	38.06	195.44	2703	16.74	39.10	194.40	2689
234	15.36	35.94	198.06	2739	15.80	36.98	197.02	2725	16.25	38.02	195.98	2710	16.69	39.05	194.95	2696
234.5	15.31	35.90	198.60	2747	15.75	36.94	197.56	2732	16.19	37.98	196.52	2718	16.64	39.01	195.49	2704
235	15.26	35.86	199.14	2754	15.70	36.90	198.10	2740	16.14	37.94	197.07	2725	16.58	38.97	196.03	2711
235.5	15.21	35.82	199.68	2762	15.65	36.86	198.64	2747	16.09	37.89	197.61	2733	16.53	38.93	196.57	2719
236	15.16	35.78	200.22	2769	15.60	36.82	199.18	2755	16.04	37.85	198.15	2740	16.48	38.89	197.11	2726
236.5	15.11	35.74	200.76	2777	15.55	36.77	199.73	2762	15.99	37.81	198.69	2748	16.43	38.85	197.65	2734
237	15.06	35.70	201.30	2784	15.50	36.73	200.27	2770	15.94	37.77	199.23	2755	16.37	38.81	198.19	2741
237.5	15.01	35.66	201.85	2792	15.45	36.69	200.81	2777	15.89	37.73	199.77	2763	16.32	38.77	198.73	2748
238	14.96	35.61	202.39	2799	15.40	36.65	201.35	2785	15.84	37.69	200.31	2770	16.27	38.73	199.27	2756
238.5	14.92	35.57	202.93	2806	15.35	36.61	201.89	2792	15.79	37.65	200.85	2778	16.22	38.69	199.81	2763
239	14.87	35.53	203.47	2814	15.30	36.57	202.43	2800	15.74	37.61	201.39	2785	16.17	38.64	200.36	2771
239.5	14.82	35.49	204.01	2821	15.25	36.53	202.97	2807	15.69	37.57	201.93	2793	16.12	38.60	200.90	2778
240	14.77	35.45	204.55	2829	15.20	36.49	203.51	2815	15.64	37.53	202.48	2800	16.07	38.56	201.44	2786
240.5	14.72	35.41	205.09	2836	15.15	36.45	204.05	2822	15.59	37.48	203.02	2808	16.02	38.52	201.98	2793
241	14.68	35.37	205.63	2844	15.11	36.41	204.59	2830	15.54	37.44	203.56	2815	15.97	38.48	202.52	2801
241.5	14.63	35.33	206.17	2851	15.06	36.36	205.14	2837	15.49	37.40	204.10	2823	15.92	38.44	203.06	2808
242	14.58	35.29	206.71	2859	15.01	36.32	205.68	2845	15.44	37.36	204.64	2830	15.87	38.40	203.60	2816
242.5	14.53	35.25	207.26	2866	14.96	36.28	206.22	2852	15.39	37.32	205.18	2838	15.82	38.36	204.14	2823
243	14.49	35.20	207.80	2874	14.91	36.24	206.76	2859	15.34	37.28	205.72	2845	15.77	38.32	204.68	2831
243.5	14.44	35.16	208.34	2881	14.87	36.20	207.30	2867	15.29	37.24	206.26	2853	15.72	38.28	205.22	2838
244	14.39	35.12	208.88	2889	14.82	36.16	207.84	2874	15.24	37.20	206.80	2860	15.67	38.23	205.77	2846
244.5	14.35	35.08	209.42	2896	14.77	36.12	208.38	2882	15.20	37.16	207.34	2868	15.62	38.19	206.31	2853
245	14.30	35.04	209.96	2904	14.73	36.08	208.92	2889	15.15	37.12	207.89	2875	15.57	38.15	206.85	2861
245.5	14.26	35.00	210.50	2911	14.68	36.04	209.46	2897	15.10	37.07	208.43	2883	15.52	38.11	207.39	2868
246	14.21	34.96	211.04	2919	14.63	36.00	210.00	2904	15.05	37.03	208.97	2890	15.48	38.07	207.93	2876
246.5	14.17	34.92	211.58	2926	14.59	35.95	210.55	2912	15.01	36.99	209.51	2897	15.43	38.03	208.47	2883
247	14.12	34.88	212.12	2934	14.54	35.91	211.09	2919	14.96	36.95	210.05	2905	15.38	37.99	209.01	2891
247.5	14.07	34.84	212.67	2941	14.49	35.87	211.63	2927	14.91	36.91	210.59	2912	15.33	37.95	209.55	2898

Body Composition   MALE   216-247.5 Lb.

Weight: Lb.	Waist: 38 inches				38.25 inches				38.5 inches				38.75 inches			
	Fat: %	Fat: Lb.	LBM: Lb.	RMR: Cal.	Fat: %	Fat: Lb.	LBM: Lb.	RMR: Cal.	Fat: %	Fat: Lb.	LBM: Lb.	RMR: Cal.	Fat: %	Fat: Lb.	LBM: Lb.	RMR: Cal.
216	19.24	41.57	174.43	2412	19.72	42.61	173.39	2398	20.21	43.64	172.36	2384	20.69	44.68	171.32	2369
216.5	19.18	41.53	174.97	2420	19.66	42.56	173.94	2406	20.14	43.60	172.90	2391	20.62	44.64	171.86	2377
217	19.12	41.49	175.51	2427	19.60	42.52	174.48	2413	20.07	43.56	173.44	2399	20.55	44.60	172.40	2384
217.5	19.06	41.45	176.06	2435	19.53	42.48	175.02	2420	20.01	43.52	173.98	2406	20.49	44.56	172.94	2392
218	18.99	41.40	176.60	2442	19.47	42.44	175.56	2428	19.94	43.48	174.52	2414	20.42	44.52	173.48	2399
218.5	18.93	41.36	177.14	2450	19.41	42.40	176.10	2435	19.88	43.44	175.06	2421	20.35	44.48	174.02	2407
219	18.87	41.32	177.68	2457	19.34	42.36	176.64	2443	19.82	43.40	175.60	2429	20.29	44.43	174.57	2414
219.5	18.81	41.28	178.22	2465	19.28	42.32	177.18	2450	19.75	43.36	176.14	2436	20.22	44.39	175.11	2422
220	18.75	41.24	178.76	2472	19.22	42.28	177.72	2458	19.69	43.32	176.69	2444	20.16	44.35	175.65	2429
220.5	18.68	41.20	179.30	2480	19.15	42.24	178.26	2465	19.63	43.27	177.23	2451	20.10	44.31	176.19	2437
221	18.62	41.16	179.84	2487	19.09	42.20	178.80	2473	19.56	43.23	177.77	2459	20.03	44.27	176.73	2444
221.5	18.56	41.12	180.38	2495	19.03	42.15	179.35	2480	19.50	43.19	178.31	2466	19.97	44.23	177.27	2452
222	18.50	41.08	180.92	2502	18.97	42.11	179.89	2488	19.44	43.15	178.85	2473	19.90	44.19	177.81	2459
222.5	18.44	41.04	181.47	2510	18.91	42.07	180.43	2495	19.38	43.11	179.39	2481	19.84	44.15	178.35	2467
223	18.38	40.99	182.01	2517	18.85	42.03	180.97	2503	19.31	43.07	179.93	2488	19.78	44.11	178.89	2474
223.5	18.32	40.95	182.55	2525	18.79	41.99	181.51	2510	19.25	43.03	180.47	2496	19.72	44.07	179.43	2482
224	18.26	40.91	183.09	2532	18.73	41.95	182.05	2518	19.19	42.99	181.01	2503	19.65	44.02	179.98	2489
224.5	18.21	40.87	183.63	2540	18.67	41.91	182.59	2525	19.13	42.95	181.55	2511	19.59	43.98	180.52	2497
225	18.15	40.83	184.17	2547	18.61	41.87	183.13	2533	19.07	42.91	182.10	2518	19.53	43.94	181.06	2504
225.5	18.09	40.79	184.71	2555	18.55	41.83	183.67	2540	19.01	42.86	182.64	2526	19.47	43.90	181.60	2512
226	18.03	40.75	185.25	2562	18.49	41.79	184.21	2548	18.95	42.82	183.18	2533	19.41	43.86	182.14	2519
226.5	17.97	40.71	185.79	2570	18.43	41.74	184.76	2555	18.89	42.78	183.72	2541	19.35	43.82	182.68	2526
227	17.91	40.67	186.33	2577	18.37	41.70	185.30	2563	18.83	42.74	184.26	2548	19.29	43.78	183.22	2534
227.5	17.86	40.63	186.88	2584	18.31	41.66	185.84	2570	18.77	42.70	184.80	2556	19.23	43.74	183.76	2541
228	17.80	40.58	187.42	2592	18.26	41.62	186.38	2578	18.71	42.66	185.34	2563	19.17	43.70	184.30	2549
228.5	17.74	40.54	187.96	2599	18.20	41.58	186.92	2585	18.65	42.62	185.88	2571	19.11	43.66	184.84	2556
229	17.69	40.50	188.50	2607	18.14	41.54	187.46	2593	18.59	42.58	186.42	2578	19.05	43.61	185.39	2564
229.5	17.63	40.46	189.04	2614	18.08	41.50	188.00	2600	18.53	42.54	186.96	2586	18.99	43.57	185.93	2571
230	17.57	40.42	189.58	2622	18.03	41.46	188.54	2608	18.48	42.50	187.51	2593	18.93	43.53	186.47	2579
230.5	17.52	40.38	190.12	2629	17.97	41.42	189.08	2615	18.42	42.45	188.05	2601	18.87	43.49	187.01	2586
231	17.46	40.34	190.66	2637	17.91	41.38	189.62	2623	18.36	42.41	188.59	2608	18.81	43.45	187.55	2594
231.5	17.41	40.30	191.20	2644	17.86	41.33	190.17	2630	18.30	42.37	189.13	2616	18.75	43.41	188.09	2601
232	17.35	40.26	191.74	2652	17.80	41.29	190.71	2637	18.25	42.33	189.67	2623	18.69	43.37	188.63	2609
232.5	17.30	40.22	192.29	2659	17.74	41.25	191.25	2645	18.19	42.29	190.21	2631	18.64	43.33	189.17	2616
233	17.24	40.17	192.83	2667	17.69	41.21	191.79	2652	18.13	42.25	190.75	2638	18.58	43.29	189.71	2624
233.5	17.19	40.13	193.37	2674	17.63	41.17	192.33	2660	18.08	42.21	191.29	2646	18.52	43.25	190.25	2631
234	17.13	40.09	193.91	2682	17.58	41.13	192.87	2667	18.02	42.17	191.83	2653	18.46	43.20	190.80	2639
234.5	17.08	40.05	194.45	2689	17.52	41.09	193.41	2675	17.96	42.13	192.37	2661	18.41	43.16	191.34	2646
235	17.03	40.01	194.99	2697	17.47	41.05	193.95	2682	17.91	42.09	192.92	2668	18.35	43.12	191.88	2654
235.5	16.97	39.97	195.53	2704	17.41	41.01	194.49	2690	17.85	42.04	193.46	2675	18.29	43.08	192.42	2661
236	16.92	39.93	196.07	2712	17.36	40.97	195.03	2697	17.80	42.00	194.00	2683	18.24	43.04	192.96	2669
236.5	16.87	39.89	196.61	2719	17.30	40.92	195.58	2705	17.74	41.96	194.54	2690	18.18	43.00	193.50	2676
237	16.81	39.85	197.15	2727	17.25	40.88	196.12	2712	17.69	41.92	195.08	2698	18.13	42.96	194.04	2684
237.5	16.76	39.81	197.70	2734	17.20	40.84	196.66	2720	17.63	41.88	195.62	2705	18.07	42.92	194.58	2691
238	16.71	39.76	198.24	2742	17.14	40.80	197.20	2727	17.58	41.84	196.16	2713	18.02	42.88	195.12	2699
238.5	16.66	39.72	198.78	2749	17.09	40.76	197.74	2735	17.53	41.80	196.70	2720	17.96	42.84	195.66	2706
239	16.60	39.68	199.32	2757	17.04	40.72	198.28	2742	17.47	41.76	197.24	2728	17.91	42.79	196.21	2714
239.5	16.55	39.64	199.86	2764	16.98	40.68	198.82	2750	17.42	41.72	197.78	2735	17.85	42.75	196.75	2721
240	16.50	39.60	200.40	2772	16.93	40.64	199.36	2757	17.36	41.68	198.33	2743	17.80	42.71	197.29	2728
240.5	16.45	39.56	200.94	2779	16.88	40.60	199.90	2765	17.31	41.63	198.87	2750	17.74	42.67	197.83	2736
241	16.40	39.52	201.48	2786	16.83	40.56	200.44	2772	17.26	41.59	199.41	2758	17.69	42.63	198.37	2743
241.5	16.35	39.48	202.02	2794	16.78	40.51	200.99	2780	17.21	41.55	199.95	2765	17.64	42.59	198.91	2751
242	16.30	39.44	202.56	2801	16.72	40.47	201.53	2787	17.15	41.51	200.49	2773	17.58	42.55	199.45	2758
242.5	16.25	39.40	203.11	2809	16.67	40.43	202.07	2795	17.10	41.47	201.03	2780	17.53	42.51	199.99	2766
243	16.20	39.35	203.65	2816	16.62	40.39	202.61	2802	17.05	41.43	201.57	2788	17.48	42.47	200.53	2773
243.5	16.14	39.31	204.19	2824	16.57	40.35	203.15	2810	17.00	41.39	202.11	2795	17.42	42.43	201.07	2781
244	16.10	39.27	204.73	2831	16.52	40.31	203.69	2817	16.95	41.35	202.65	2803	17.37	42.38	201.62	2788
244.5	16.05	39.23	205.27	2839	16.47	40.27	204.23	2825	16.89	41.31	203.19	2810	17.32	42.34	202.16	2796
245	16.00	39.19	205.81	2846	16.42	40.23	204.77	2832	16.84	41.27	203.74	2818	17.27	42.30	202.70	2803
245.5	15.95	39.15	206.35	2854	16.37	40.19	205.31	2839	16.79	41.22	204.28	2825	17.21	42.26	203.24	2811
246	15.90	39.11	206.89	2861	16.32	40.15	205.85	2847	16.74	41.18	204.82	2833	17.16	42.22	203.78	2818
246.5	15.85	39.07	207.43	2869	16.27	40.10	206.40	2854	16.69	41.14	205.36	2840	17.11	42.18	204.32	2826
247	15.80	39.03	207.97	2876	16.22	40.06	206.94	2862	16.64	41.10	205.90	2848	17.06	42.14	204.86	2833
247.5	15.75	38.99	208.52	2884	16.17	40.02	207.48	2869	16.59	41.06	206.44	2855	17.01	42.10	205.40	2841

Body Composition   MALE   216-247.5 Lb.

Weight: Lb.	Waist: 39 inches				39.25 inches				39.5 inches				39.75 inches			
	Fat: %	Fat: Lb.	LBM: Lb.	RMR: Cal.	Fat: %	Fat: Lb.	LBM: Lb.	RMR: Cal.	Fat: %	Fat: Lb.	LBM: Lb.	RMR: Cal.	Fat: %	Fat: Lb.	LBM: Lb.	RMR: Cal.
216	21.17	45.72	170.28	2355	21.65	46.76	169.24	2341	22.13	47.79	168.21	2326	22.61	48.83	167.17	2312
216.5	21.10	45.68	170.82	2362	21.58	46.71	169.79	2348	22.06	47.75	168.75	2334	22.54	48.79	167.71	2319
217	21.03	45.64	171.36	2370	21.51	46.67	170.33	2356	21.99	47.71	169.29	2341	22.46	48.75	168.25	2327
217.5	20.96	45.60	171.91	2377	21.44	46.63	170.87	2363	21.92	47.67	169.83	2349	22.39	48.71	168.79	2334
218	20.90	45.55	172.45	2385	21.37	46.59	171.41	2371	21.85	47.63	170.37	2356	22.32	48.67	169.33	2342
218.5	20.83	45.51	172.99	2392	21.30	46.55	171.95	2378	21.78	47.59	170.91	2364	22.25	48.63	169.87	2349
219	20.76	45.47	173.53	2400	21.24	46.51	172.49	2386	21.71	47.55	171.45	2371	22.18	48.58	170.42	2357
219.5	20.70	45.43	174.07	2407	21.17	46.47	173.03	2393	21.64	47.51	171.99	2379	22.12	48.54	170.96	2364
220	20.63	45.39	174.61	2415	21.10	46.43	173.57	2401	21.58	47.47	172.54	2386	22.05	48.50	171.50	2372
220.5	20.57	45.35	175.15	2422	21.04	46.39	174.11	2408	21.51	47.42	173.08	2394	21.98	48.46	172.04	2379
221	20.50	45.31	175.69	2430	20.97	46.35	174.65	2415	21.44	47.38	173.62	2401	21.91	48.42	172.58	2387
221.5	20.44	45.27	176.23	2437	20.90	46.30	175.20	2423	21.37	47.34	174.16	2409	21.84	48.38	173.12	2394
222	20.37	45.23	176.77	2445	20.84	46.26	175.74	2430	21.31	47.30	174.70	2416	21.77	48.34	173.66	2402
222.5	20.31	45.19	177.32	2452	20.77	46.22	176.28	2438	21.24	47.26	175.24	2424	21.71	48.30	174.20	2409
223	20.24	45.14	177.86	2460	20.71	46.18	176.82	2445	21.17	47.22	175.78	2431	21.64	48.26	174.74	2417
223.5	20.18	45.10	178.40	2467	20.64	46.14	177.36	2453	21.11	47.18	176.32	2439	21.57	48.22	175.28	2424
224	20.12	45.06	178.94	2475	20.58	46.10	177.90	2460	21.04	47.14	176.86	2446	21.51	48.17	175.83	2432
224.5	20.05	45.02	179.48	2482	20.52	46.06	178.44	2468	20.98	47.10	177.40	2453	21.44	48.13	176.37	2439
225	19.99	44.98	180.02	2490	20.45	46.02	178.98	2475	20.91	47.06	177.95	2461	21.37	48.09	176.91	2447
225.5	19.93	44.94	180.56	2497	20.39	45.98	179.52	2483	20.85	47.01	178.49	2468	21.31	48.05	177.45	2454
226	19.87	44.90	181.10	2505	20.33	45.94	180.06	2490	20.78	46.97	179.03	2476	21.24	48.01	177.99	2462
226.5	19.80	44.86	181.64	2512	20.26	45.89	180.61	2498	20.72	46.93	179.57	2483	21.18	47.97	178.53	2469
227	19.74	44.82	182.18	2520	20.20	45.85	181.15	2505	20.66	46.89	180.11	2491	21.11	47.93	179.07	2477
227.5	19.68	44.78	182.73	2527	20.14	45.81	181.69	2513	20.59	46.85	180.65	2498	21.05	47.89	179.61	2484
228	19.62	44.73	183.27	2535	20.08	45.77	182.23	2520	20.53	46.81	181.19	2506	20.99	47.85	180.15	2492
228.5	19.56	44.69	183.81	2542	20.01	45.73	182.77	2528	20.47	46.77	181.73	2513	20.92	47.81	180.69	2499
229	19.50	44.65	184.35	2550	19.95	45.69	183.31	2535	20.40	46.73	182.27	2521	20.86	47.76	181.24	2506
229.5	19.44	44.61	184.89	2557	19.89	45.65	183.85	2543	20.34	46.69	182.81	2528	20.79	47.72	181.78	2514
230	19.38	44.57	185.43	2564	19.83	45.61	184.39	2550	20.28	46.65	183.36	2536	20.73	47.68	182.32	2521
230.5	19.32	44.53	185.97	2572	19.77	45.57	184.93	2558	20.22	46.60	183.90	2543	20.67	47.64	182.86	2529
231	19.26	44.49	186.51	2579	19.71	45.53	185.47	2565	20.16	46.56	184.44	2551	20.61	47.60	183.40	2536
231.5	19.20	44.45	187.05	2587	19.65	45.48	186.02	2573	20.10	46.52	184.98	2558	20.54	47.56	183.94	2544
232	19.14	44.41	187.59	2594	19.59	45.44	186.56	2580	20.03	46.48	185.52	2566	20.48	47.52	184.48	2551
232.5	19.08	44.37	188.14	2602	19.53	45.40	187.10	2588	19.97	46.44	186.06	2573	20.42	47.48	185.02	2559
233	19.02	44.32	188.68	2609	19.47	45.36	187.64	2595	19.91	46.40	186.60	2581	20.36	47.44	185.56	2566
233.5	18.96	44.28	189.22	2617	19.41	45.32	188.18	2603	19.85	46.36	187.14	2588	20.30	47.40	186.10	2574
234	18.91	44.24	189.76	2624	19.35	45.28	188.72	2610	19.79	46.32	187.68	2596	20.24	47.35	186.65	2581
234.5	18.85	44.20	190.30	2632	19.29	45.24	189.26	2617	19.73	46.28	188.22	2603	20.18	47.31	187.19	2589
235	18.79	44.16	190.84	2639	19.23	45.20	189.80	2625	19.67	46.24	188.77	2611	20.12	47.27	187.73	2596
235.5	18.73	44.12	191.38	2647	19.17	45.16	190.34	2632	19.62	46.19	189.31	2618	20.06	47.23	188.27	2604
236	18.68	44.08	191.92	2654	19.12	45.12	190.88	2640	19.56	46.15	189.85	2626	20.00	47.19	188.81	2611
236.5	18.62	44.04	192.46	2662	19.06	45.07	191.43	2647	19.50	46.11	190.39	2633	19.94	47.15	189.35	2619
237	18.56	44.00	193.00	2669	19.00	45.03	191.97	2655	19.44	46.07	190.93	2641	19.88	47.11	189.89	2626
237.5	18.51	43.96	193.55	2677	18.94	44.99	192.51	2662	19.38	46.03	191.47	2648	19.82	47.07	190.43	2634
238	18.45	43.91	194.09	2684	18.89	44.95	193.05	2670	19.32	45.99	192.01	2656	19.76	47.03	190.97	2641
238.5	18.40	43.87	194.63	2692	18.83	44.91	193.59	2677	19.27	45.95	192.55	2663	19.70	46.99	191.51	2649
239	18.34	43.83	195.17	2699	18.77	44.87	194.13	2685	19.21	45.91	193.09	2670	19.64	46.94	192.06	2656
239.5	18.28	43.79	195.71	2707	18.72	44.83	194.67	2692	19.15	45.87	193.63	2678	19.58	46.90	192.60	2664
240	18.23	43.75	196.25	2714	18.66	44.79	195.21	2700	19.09	45.83	194.18	2685	19.53	46.86	193.14	2671
240.5	18.17	43.71	196.79	2722	18.61	44.75	195.75	2707	19.04	45.78	194.72	2693	19.47	46.82	193.68	2679
241	18.12	43.67	197.33	2729	18.55	44.71	196.29	2715	18.98	45.74	195.26	2700	19.41	46.78	194.22	2686
241.5	18.07	43.63	197.87	2737	18.49	44.66	196.84	2722	18.92	45.70	195.80	2708	19.35	46.74	194.76	2694
242	18.01	43.59	198.41	2744	18.44	44.62	197.38	2730	18.87	45.66	196.34	2715	19.30	46.70	195.30	2701
242.5	17.96	43.55	198.96	2752	18.38	44.58	197.92	2737	18.81	45.62	196.88	2723	19.24	46.66	195.84	2709
243	17.90	43.50	199.50	2759	18.33	44.54	198.46	2745	18.76	45.58	197.42	2730	19.18	46.62	196.38	2716
243.5	17.85	43.46	200.04	2767	18.28	44.50	199.00	2752	18.70	45.54	197.96	2738	19.13	46.58	196.92	2723
244	17.80	43.42	200.58	2774	18.22	44.46	199.54	2760	18.65	45.50	198.50	2745	19.07	46.53	197.47	2731
244.5	17.74	43.38	201.12	2781	18.17	44.42	200.08	2767	18.59	45.46	199.04	2753	19.02	46.49	198.01	2738
245	17.69	43.34	201.66	2789	18.11	44.38	200.62	2775	18.54	45.42	199.59	2760	18.96	46.45	198.55	2746
245.5	17.64	43.30	202.20	2796	18.06	44.34	201.16	2782	18.48	45.37	200.13	2768	18.90	46.41	199.09	2753
246	17.58	43.26	202.74	2804	18.01	44.30	201.70	2790	18.43	45.33	200.67	2775	18.85	46.37	199.63	2761
246.5	17.53	43.22	203.28	2811	17.95	44.25	202.25	2797	18.37	45.29	201.21	2783	18.79	46.33	200.17	2768
247	17.48	43.18	203.82	2819	17.90	44.21	202.79	2805	18.32	45.25	201.75	2790	18.74	46.29	200.71	2776
247.5	17.43	43.14	204.37	2826	17.85	44.17	203.33	2812	18.27	45.21	202.29	2798	18.69	46.25	201.25	2783

Body Composition   MALE   216-247.5 Lb.

Weight: Lb.	Waist: 40 inches Fat: %	Fat: Lb.	LBM: Lb.	RMR: Cal.	40.25 inches Fat: %	Fat: Lb.	LBM: Lb.	RMR: Cal.	40.5 inches Fat: %	Fat: Lb.	LBM: Lb.	RMR: Cal.	40.75 inches Fat: %	Fat: Lb.	LBM: Lb.	RMR: Cal.
216	23.09	49.87	166.13	2298	23.57	50.91	165.09	2283	24.05	51.94	164.06	2269	24.53	52.98	163.02	2255
216.5	23.01	49.83	166.67	2305	23.49	50.86	165.64	2291	23.97	51.90	164.60	2276	24.45	52.94	163.56	2262
217	22.94	49.79	167.21	2313	23.42	50.82	166.18	2298	23.90	51.86	165.14	2284	24.38	52.90	164.10	2270
217.5	22.87	49.75	167.76	2320	23.35	50.78	166.72	2306	23.83	51.82	165.68	2291	24.30	52.86	164.64	2277
218	22.80	49.70	168.30	2328	23.28	50.74	167.26	2313	23.75	51.78	166.22	2299	24.23	52.82	165.18	2284
218.5	22.73	49.66	168.84	2335	23.20	50.70	167.80	2321	23.68	51.74	166.76	2306	24.15	52.78	165.72	2292
219	22.66	49.62	169.38	2342	23.13	50.66	168.34	2328	23.61	51.70	167.30	2314	24.08	52.73	166.27	2299
219.5	22.59	49.58	169.92	2350	23.06	50.62	168.88	2336	23.53	51.66	167.84	2321	24.01	52.69	166.81	2307
220	22.52	49.54	170.46	2357	22.99	50.58	169.42	2343	23.46	51.62	168.39	2329	23.93	52.65	167.35	2314
220.5	22.45	49.50	171.00	2365	22.92	50.54	169.96	2351	23.39	51.57	168.93	2336	23.86	52.61	167.89	2322
221	22.38	49.46	171.54	2372	22.85	50.50	170.50	2358	23.32	51.53	169.47	2344	23.79	52.57	168.43	2329
221.5	22.31	49.42	172.08	2380	22.78	50.45	171.05	2366	23.25	51.49	170.01	2351	23.72	52.53	168.97	2337
222	22.24	49.38	172.62	2387	22.71	50.41	171.59	2373	23.18	51.45	170.55	2359	23.64	52.49	169.51	2344
222.5	22.17	49.34	173.17	2395	22.64	50.37	172.13	2381	23.11	51.41	171.09	2366	23.57	52.45	170.05	2352
223	22.10	49.29	173.71	2402	22.57	50.33	172.67	2388	23.04	51.37	171.63	2374	23.50	52.41	170.59	2359
223.5	22.04	49.25	174.25	2410	22.50	50.29	173.21	2395	22.97	51.33	172.17	2381	23.43	52.37	171.13	2367
224	21.97	49.21	174.79	2417	22.43	50.25	173.75	2403	22.90	51.29	172.71	2389	23.36	52.32	171.68	2374
224.5	21.90	49.17	175.33	2425	22.36	50.21	174.29	2410	22.83	51.25	173.25	2396	23.29	52.28	172.22	2382
225	21.84	49.13	175.87	2432	22.30	50.17	174.83	2418	22.76	51.21	173.80	2404	23.22	52.24	172.76	2389
225.5	21.77	49.09	176.41	2440	22.23	50.13	175.37	2425	22.69	51.16	174.34	2411	23.15	52.20	173.30	2397
226	21.70	49.05	176.95	2447	22.16	50.09	175.91	2433	22.62	51.12	174.88	2419	23.08	52.16	173.84	2404
226.5	21.64	49.01	177.49	2455	22.09	50.04	176.46	2440	22.55	51.08	175.42	2426	23.01	52.12	174.38	2412
227	21.57	48.97	178.03	2462	22.03	50.00	177.00	2448	22.49	51.04	175.96	2434	22.94	52.08	174.92	2419
227.5	21.51	48.93	178.58	2470	21.96	49.96	177.54	2455	22.42	51.00	176.50	2441	22.87	52.04	175.46	2427
228	21.44	48.88	179.12	2477	21.90	49.92	178.08	2463	22.35	50.96	177.04	2448	22.81	52.00	176.00	2434
228.5	21.38	48.84	179.66	2485	21.83	49.88	178.62	2470	22.28	50.92	177.58	2456	22.74	51.96	176.54	2442
229	21.31	48.80	180.20	2492	21.76	49.84	179.16	2478	22.22	50.88	178.12	2463	22.67	51.91	177.09	2449
229.5	21.25	48.76	180.74	2500	21.70	49.80	179.70	2485	22.15	50.84	178.66	2471	22.60	51.87	177.63	2457
230	21.18	48.72	181.28	2507	21.63	49.76	180.24	2493	22.08	50.80	179.21	2478	22.54	51.83	178.17	2464
230.5	21.12	48.68	181.82	2515	21.57	49.72	180.78	2500	22.02	50.75	179.75	2486	22.47	51.79	178.71	2472
231	21.06	48.64	182.36	2522	21.50	49.68	181.32	2508	21.95	50.71	180.29	2493	22.40	51.75	179.25	2479
231.5	20.99	48.60	182.90	2530	21.44	49.63	181.87	2515	21.89	50.67	180.83	2501	22.34	51.71	179.79	2487
232	20.93	48.56	183.44	2537	21.38	49.59	182.41	2523	21.82	50.63	181.37	2508	22.27	51.67	180.33	2494
232.5	20.87	48.52	183.99	2545	21.31	49.55	182.95	2530	21.76	50.59	181.91	2516	22.21	51.63	180.87	2501
233	20.80	48.47	184.53	2552	21.25	49.51	183.49	2538	21.69	50.55	182.45	2523	22.14	51.59	181.41	2509
233.5	20.74	48.43	185.07	2559	21.19	49.47	184.03	2545	21.63	50.51	182.99	2531	22.08	51.55	181.95	2516
234	20.68	48.39	185.61	2567	21.12	49.43	184.57	2553	21.57	50.47	183.53	2538	22.01	51.50	182.50	2524
234.5	20.62	48.35	186.15	2574	21.06	49.39	185.11	2560	21.50	50.43	184.07	2546	21.95	51.46	183.04	2531
235	20.56	48.31	186.69	2582	21.00	49.35	185.65	2568	21.44	50.39	184.62	2553	21.88	51.42	183.58	2539
235.5	20.50	48.27	187.23	2589	20.94	49.31	186.19	2575	21.38	50.34	185.16	2561	21.82	51.38	184.12	2546
236	20.44	48.23	187.77	2597	20.88	49.27	186.73	2583	21.31	50.30	185.70	2568	21.75	51.34	184.66	2554
236.5	20.38	48.19	188.31	2604	20.81	49.22	187.28	2590	21.25	50.26	186.24	2576	21.69	51.30	185.20	2561
237	20.31	48.15	188.85	2612	20.75	49.18	187.82	2598	21.19	50.22	186.78	2583	21.63	51.26	185.74	2569
237.5	20.25	48.11	189.40	2619	20.69	49.14	188.36	2605	21.13	50.18	187.32	2591	21.57	51.22	186.28	2576
238	20.19	48.06	189.94	2627	20.63	49.10	188.90	2612	21.07	50.14	187.86	2598	21.50	51.18	186.82	2584
238.5	20.14	48.02	190.48	2634	20.57	49.06	189.44	2620	21.01	50.10	188.40	2606	21.44	51.14	187.36	2591
239	20.08	47.98	191.02	2642	20.51	49.02	189.98	2627	20.94	50.06	188.94	2613	21.38	51.09	187.91	2599
239.5	20.02	47.94	191.56	2649	20.45	48.98	190.52	2635	20.88	50.02	189.48	2621	21.32	51.05	188.45	2606
240	19.96	47.90	192.10	2657	20.39	48.94	191.06	2642	20.82	49.98	190.03	2628	21.26	51.01	188.99	2614
240.5	19.90	47.86	192.64	2664	20.33	48.90	191.60	2650	20.76	49.93	190.57	2636	21.19	50.97	189.53	2621
241	19.84	47.82	193.18	2672	20.27	48.86	192.14	2657	20.70	49.89	191.11	2643	21.13	50.93	190.07	2629
241.5	19.78	47.78	193.72	2679	20.21	48.81	192.69	2665	20.64	49.85	191.65	2650	21.07	50.89	190.61	2636
242	19.73	47.74	194.26	2687	20.15	48.77	193.23	2672	20.58	49.81	192.19	2658	21.01	50.85	191.15	2644
242.5	19.67	47.70	194.81	2694	20.10	48.73	193.77	2680	20.52	49.77	192.73	2665	20.95	50.81	191.69	2651
243	19.61	47.65	195.35	2702	20.04	48.69	194.31	2687	20.46	49.73	193.27	2673	20.89	50.77	192.23	2659
243.5	19.55	47.61	195.89	2709	19.98	48.65	194.85	2695	20.41	49.69	193.81	2680	20.83	50.73	192.77	2666
244	19.50	47.57	196.43	2717	19.92	48.61	195.39	2702	20.35	49.65	194.35	2688	20.77	50.68	193.32	2674
244.5	19.44	47.53	196.97	2724	19.86	48.57	195.93	2710	20.29	49.61	194.89	2695	20.71	50.64	193.86	2681
245	19.38	47.49	197.51	2732	19.81	48.53	196.47	2717	20.23	49.57	195.44	2703	20.65	50.60	194.40	2689
245.5	19.33	47.45	198.05	2739	19.75	48.49	197.01	2725	20.17	49.52	195.98	2710	20.60	50.56	194.94	2696
246	19.27	47.41	198.59	2747	19.69	48.45	197.55	2732	20.12	49.48	196.52	2718	20.54	50.52	195.48	2703
246.5	19.22	47.37	199.13	2754	19.64	48.40	198.10	2740	20.06	49.44	197.06	2725	20.48	50.48	196.02	2711
247	19.16	47.33	199.67	2761	19.58	48.36	198.64	2747	20.00	49.40	197.60	2733	20.42	50.44	196.56	2718
247.5	19.11	47.29	200.22	2769	19.52	48.32	199.18	2755	19.94	49.36	198.14	2740	20.36	50.40	197.10	2726

Body Composition   MALE   216-247.5 Lb.

Weight: Lb.	Waist: 41 inches Fat: %	Fat: Lb.	LBM: Lb.	RMR: Cal.	41.25 inches Fat: %	Fat: Lb.	LBM: Lb.	RMR: Cal.	41.5 inches Fat: %	Fat: Lb.	LBM: Lb.	RMR: Cal.	41.75 inches Fat: %	Fat: Lb.	LBM: Lb.	RMR: Cal.
216	25.01	54.02	161.98	2240	25.49	55.06	160.94	2226	25.97	56.09	159.91	2212	26.45	57.13	158.87	2197
216.5	24.93	53.98	162.52	2248	25.41	55.01	161.49	2233	25.89	56.05	160.45	2219	26.37	57.09	159.41	2205
217	24.86	53.94	163.06	2255	25.33	54.97	162.03	2241	25.81	56.01	160.99	2226	26.29	57.05	159.95	2212
217.5	24.78	53.90	163.61	2263	25.26	54.93	162.57	2248	25.73	55.97	161.53	2234	26.21	57.01	160.49	2220
218	24.70	53.85	164.15	2270	25.18	54.89	163.11	2256	25.66	55.93	162.07	2241	26.13	56.97	161.03	2227
218.5	24.63	53.81	164.69	2278	25.10	54.85	163.65	2263	25.58	55.89	162.61	2249	26.05	56.93	161.57	2235
219	24.55	53.77	165.23	2285	25.03	54.81	164.19	2271	25.50	55.85	163.15	2256	25.97	56.88	162.12	2242
219.5	24.48	53.73	165.77	2293	24.95	54.77	164.73	2278	25.42	55.81	163.69	2264	25.90	56.84	162.66	2250
220	24.40	53.69	166.31	2300	24.88	54.73	165.27	2286	25.35	55.77	164.24	2271	25.82	56.80	163.20	2257
220.5	24.33	53.65	166.85	2308	24.80	54.69	165.81	2293	25.27	55.72	164.78	2279	25.74	56.76	163.74	2265
221	24.26	53.61	167.39	2315	24.73	54.65	166.35	2301	25.20	55.68	165.32	2286	25.67	56.72	164.28	2272
221.5	24.18	53.57	167.93	2323	24.65	54.60	166.90	2308	25.12	55.64	165.86	2294	25.59	56.68	164.82	2279
222	24.11	53.53	168.47	2330	24.58	54.56	167.44	2316	25.05	55.60	166.40	2301	25.51	56.64	165.36	2287
222.5	24.04	53.49	169.02	2337	24.50	54.52	167.98	2323	24.97	55.56	166.94	2309	25.44	56.60	165.90	2294
223	23.97	53.44	169.56	2345	24.43	54.48	168.52	2331	24.90	55.52	167.48	2316	25.36	56.56	166.44	2302
223.5	23.89	53.40	170.10	2352	24.36	54.44	169.06	2338	24.82	55.48	168.02	2324	25.29	56.52	166.98	2309
224	23.82	53.36	170.64	2360	24.29	54.40	169.60	2346	24.75	55.44	168.56	2331	25.21	56.47	167.53	2317
224.5	23.75	53.32	171.18	2367	24.21	54.36	170.14	2353	24.68	55.40	169.10	2339	25.14	56.43	168.07	2324
225	23.68	53.28	171.72	2375	24.14	54.32	170.68	2361	24.60	55.36	169.65	2346	25.06	56.39	168.61	2332
225.5	23.61	53.24	172.26	2382	24.07	54.28	171.22	2368	24.53	55.31	170.19	2354	24.99	56.35	169.15	2339
226	23.54	53.20	172.80	2390	24.00	54.24	171.76	2376	24.46	55.27	170.73	2361	24.92	56.31	169.69	2347
226.5	23.47	53.16	173.34	2397	23.93	54.19	172.31	2383	24.38	55.23	171.27	2369	24.84	56.27	170.23	2354
227	23.40	53.12	173.88	2405	23.86	54.15	172.85	2390	24.31	55.19	171.81	2376	24.77	56.23	170.77	2362
227.5	23.33	53.08	174.43	2412	23.79	54.11	173.39	2398	24.24	55.15	172.35	2384	24.70	56.19	171.31	2369
228	23.26	53.03	174.97	2420	23.72	54.07	173.93	2405	24.17	55.11	172.89	2391	24.63	56.15	171.85	2377
228.5	23.19	52.99	175.51	2427	23.65	54.03	174.47	2413	24.10	55.07	173.43	2399	24.55	56.11	172.39	2384
229	23.12	52.95	176.05	2435	23.58	53.99	175.01	2420	24.03	55.03	173.97	2406	24.48	56.06	172.94	2392
229.5	23.05	52.91	176.59	2442	23.51	53.95	175.55	2428	23.96	54.99	174.51	2414	24.41	56.02	173.48	2399
230	22.99	52.87	177.13	2450	23.44	53.91	176.09	2435	23.89	54.95	175.06	2421	24.34	55.98	174.02	2407
230.5	22.92	52.83	177.67	2457	23.37	53.87	176.63	2443	23.82	54.90	175.60	2428	24.27	55.94	174.56	2414
231	22.85	52.79	178.21	2465	23.30	53.83	177.17	2450	23.75	54.86	176.14	2436	24.20	55.90	175.10	2422
231.5	22.78	52.75	178.75	2472	23.23	53.78	177.72	2458	23.68	54.82	176.68	2443	24.13	55.86	175.64	2429
232	22.72	52.71	179.29	2480	23.17	53.74	178.26	2465	23.61	54.78	177.22	2451	24.06	55.82	176.18	2437
232.5	22.65	52.67	179.84	2487	23.10	53.70	178.80	2473	23.54	54.74	177.76	2458	23.99	55.78	176.72	2444
233	22.59	52.62	180.38	2495	23.03	53.66	179.34	2480	23.48	54.70	178.30	2466	23.92	55.74	177.26	2452
233.5	22.52	52.58	180.92	2502	22.96	53.62	179.88	2488	23.41	54.66	178.84	2473	23.85	55.70	177.80	2459
234	22.45	52.54	181.46	2510	22.90	53.58	180.42	2495	23.34	54.62	179.38	2481	23.78	55.65	178.35	2467
234.5	22.39	52.50	182.00	2517	22.83	53.54	180.96	2503	23.27	54.58	179.92	2488	23.72	55.61	178.89	2474
235	22.32	52.46	182.54	2525	22.76	53.50	181.50	2510	23.21	54.54	180.47	2496	23.65	55.57	179.43	2481
235.5	22.26	52.42	183.08	2532	22.70	53.46	182.04	2518	23.14	54.49	181.01	2503	23.58	55.53	179.97	2489
236	22.19	52.38	183.62	2539	22.63	53.42	182.58	2525	23.07	54.45	181.55	2511	23.51	55.49	180.51	2496
236.5	22.13	52.34	184.16	2547	22.57	53.37	183.13	2533	23.01	54.41	182.09	2518	23.45	55.45	181.05	2504
237	22.07	52.30	184.70	2554	22.50	53.33	183.67	2540	22.94	54.37	182.63	2526	23.38	55.41	181.59	2511
237.5	22.00	52.26	185.25	2562	22.44	53.29	184.21	2548	22.88	54.33	183.17	2533	23.31	55.37	182.13	2519
238	21.94	52.21	185.79	2569	22.37	53.25	184.75	2555	22.81	54.29	183.71	2541	23.25	55.33	182.67	2526
238.5	21.88	52.17	186.33	2577	22.31	53.21	185.29	2563	22.75	54.25	184.25	2548	23.18	55.29	183.21	2534
239	21.81	52.13	186.87	2584	22.25	53.17	185.83	2570	22.68	54.21	184.79	2556	23.11	55.24	183.76	2541
239.5	21.75	52.09	187.41	2592	22.18	53.13	186.37	2578	22.62	54.17	185.33	2563	23.05	55.20	184.30	2549
240	21.69	52.05	187.95	2599	22.12	53.09	186.91	2585	22.55	54.13	185.88	2571	22.98	55.16	184.84	2556
240.5	21.63	52.01	188.49	2607	22.06	53.05	187.45	2592	22.49	54.08	186.42	2578	22.92	55.12	185.38	2564
241	21.56	51.97	189.03	2614	21.99	53.01	187.99	2600	22.42	54.04	186.96	2586	22.85	55.08	185.92	2571
241.5	21.50	51.93	189.57	2622	21.93	52.96	188.54	2607	22.36	54.00	187.50	2593	22.79	55.04	186.46	2579
242	21.44	51.89	190.11	2629	21.87	52.92	189.08	2615	22.30	53.96	188.04	2601	22.73	55.00	187.00	2586
242.5	21.38	51.85	190.66	2637	21.81	52.88	189.62	2622	22.24	53.92	188.58	2608	22.66	54.96	187.54	2594
243	21.32	51.80	191.20	2644	21.75	52.84	190.16	2630	22.17	53.88	189.12	2616	22.60	54.92	188.08	2601
243.5	21.26	51.76	191.74	2652	21.68	52.80	190.70	2637	22.11	53.84	189.66	2623	22.54	54.88	188.62	2609
244	21.20	51.72	192.28	2659	21.62	52.76	191.24	2645	22.05	53.80	190.20	2631	22.47	54.83	189.17	2616
244.5	21.14	51.68	192.82	2667	21.56	52.72	191.78	2652	21.99	53.76	190.74	2638	22.41	54.79	189.71	2624
245	21.08	51.64	193.36	2674	21.50	52.68	192.32	2660	21.92	53.72	191.29	2645	22.35	54.75	190.25	2631
245.5	21.02	51.60	193.90	2682	21.44	52.64	192.86	2667	21.86	53.67	191.83	2653	22.29	54.71	190.79	2639
246	20.96	51.56	194.44	2689	21.38	52.60	193.40	2675	21.80	53.63	192.37	2660	22.22	54.67	191.33	2646
246.5	20.90	51.52	194.98	2697	21.32	52.55	193.95	2682	21.74	53.59	192.91	2668	22.16	54.63	191.87	2654
247	20.84	51.48	195.52	2704	21.26	52.51	194.49	2690	21.68	53.55	193.45	2675	22.10	54.59	192.41	2661
247.5	20.78	51.44	196.07	2712	21.20	52.47	195.03	2697	21.62	53.51	193.99	2683	22.04	54.55	192.95	2669

Body Composition MALE 216-247.5 Lb.

Weight: Lb.	Waist: 42 inches				42.25 inches				42.5 inches				42.75 inches			
	Fat: %	Fat: Lb.	LBM: Lb.	RMR: Cal.	Fat: %	Fat: Lb.	LBM: Lb.	RMR: Cal.	Fat: %	Fat: Lb.	LBM: Lb.	RMR: Cal.	Fat: %	Fat: Lb.	LBM: Lb.	RMR: Cal.
216	26.93	58.17	157.83	2183	27.41	59.21	156.79	2168	27.89	60.24	155.76	2154	28.37	61.28	154.72	2140
216.5	26.85	58.13	158.37	2190	27.33	59.16	157.34	2176	27.81	60.20	156.30	2162	28.29	61.24	155.26	2147
217	26.77	58.09	158.91	2198	27.25	59.12	157.88	2183	27.72	60.16	156.84	2169	28.20	61.20	155.80	2155
217.5	26.69	58.05	159.46	2205	27.16	59.08	158.42	2191	27.64	60.12	157.38	2177	28.12	61.16	156.34	2162
218	26.61	58.00	160.00	2213	27.08	59.04	158.96	2198	27.56	60.08	157.92	2184	28.04	61.12	156.88	2170
218.5	26.53	57.96	160.54	2220	27.00	59.00	159.50	2206	27.48	60.04	158.46	2192	27.95	61.08	157.42	2177
219	26.45	57.92	161.08	2228	26.92	58.96	160.04	2213	27.40	60.00	159.00	2199	27.87	61.03	157.97	2185
219.5	26.37	57.88	161.62	2235	26.84	58.92	160.58	2221	27.31	59.96	159.54	2206	27.79	60.99	158.51	2192
220	26.29	57.84	162.16	2243	26.76	58.88	161.12	2228	27.23	59.92	160.09	2214	27.71	60.95	159.05	2200
220.5	26.21	57.80	162.70	2250	26.68	58.84	161.66	2236	27.15	59.87	160.63	2221	27.62	60.91	159.59	2207
221	26.13	57.76	163.24	2258	26.60	58.80	162.20	2243	27.07	59.83	161.17	2229	27.54	60.87	160.13	2215
221.5	26.06	57.72	163.78	2265	26.53	58.75	162.75	2251	26.99	59.79	161.71	2236	27.46	60.83	160.67	2222
222	25.98	57.68	164.32	2273	26.45	58.71	163.29	2258	26.91	59.75	162.25	2244	27.38	60.79	161.21	2230
222.5	25.90	57.64	164.87	2280	26.37	58.67	163.83	2266	26.84	59.71	162.79	2251	27.30	60.75	161.75	2237
223	25.83	57.59	165.41	2288	26.29	58.63	164.37	2273	26.76	59.67	163.33	2259	27.22	60.71	162.29	2245
223.5	25.75	57.55	165.95	2295	26.21	58.59	164.91	2281	26.68	59.63	163.87	2266	27.14	60.67	162.83	2252
224	25.68	57.51	166.49	2303	26.14	58.55	165.45	2288	26.60	59.59	164.41	2274	27.06	60.62	163.38	2259
224.5	25.60	57.47	167.03	2310	26.06	58.51	165.99	2296	26.52	59.55	164.95	2281	26.99	60.58	163.92	2267
225	25.52	57.43	167.57	2317	25.99	58.47	166.53	2303	26.45	59.51	165.50	2289	26.91	60.54	164.46	2274
225.5	25.45	57.39	168.11	2325	25.91	58.43	167.07	2311	26.37	59.46	166.04	2296	26.83	60.50	165.00	2282
226	25.38	57.35	168.65	2332	25.83	58.39	167.61	2318	26.29	59.42	166.58	2304	26.75	60.46	165.54	2289
226.5	25.30	57.31	169.19	2340	25.76	58.34	168.16	2326	26.22	59.38	167.12	2311	26.68	60.42	166.08	2297
227	25.23	57.27	169.73	2347	25.68	58.30	168.70	2333	26.14	59.34	167.66	2319	26.60	60.38	166.62	2304
227.5	25.15	57.23	170.28	2355	25.61	58.26	169.24	2341	26.07	59.30	168.20	2326	26.52	60.34	167.16	2312
228	25.08	57.18	170.82	2362	25.54	58.22	169.78	2348	25.99	59.26	168.74	2334	26.45	60.30	167.70	2319
228.5	25.01	57.14	171.36	2370	25.46	58.18	170.32	2356	25.92	59.22	169.28	2341	26.37	60.26	168.24	2327
229	24.94	57.10	171.90	2377	25.39	58.14	170.86	2363	25.84	59.18	169.82	2349	26.29	60.21	168.79	2334
229.5	24.86	57.06	172.44	2385	25.32	58.10	171.40	2370	25.77	59.14	170.36	2356	26.22	60.17	169.33	2342
230	24.79	57.02	172.98	2392	25.24	58.06	171.94	2378	25.69	59.10	170.91	2364	26.14	60.13	169.87	2349
230.5	24.72	56.98	173.52	2400	25.17	58.02	172.48	2385	25.62	59.05	171.45	2371	26.07	60.09	170.41	2357
231	24.65	56.94	174.06	2407	25.10	57.98	173.02	2393	25.55	59.01	171.99	2379	26.00	60.05	170.95	2364
231.5	24.58	56.90	174.60	2415	25.03	57.93	173.57	2400	25.47	58.97	172.53	2386	25.92	60.01	171.49	2372
232	24.51	56.86	175.14	2422	24.95	57.89	174.11	2408	25.40	58.93	173.07	2394	25.85	59.97	172.03	2379
232.5	24.44	56.82	175.69	2430	24.88	57.85	174.65	2415	25.33	58.89	173.61	2401	25.78	59.93	172.57	2387
233	24.37	56.77	176.23	2437	24.81	57.81	175.19	2423	25.26	58.85	174.15	2409	25.70	59.89	173.11	2394
233.5	24.30	56.73	176.77	2445	24.74	57.77	175.73	2430	25.19	58.81	174.69	2416	25.63	59.85	173.65	2402
234	24.23	56.69	177.31	2452	24.67	57.73	176.27	2438	25.11	58.77	175.23	2423	25.56	59.80	174.20	2409
234.5	24.16	56.65	177.85	2460	24.60	57.69	176.81	2445	25.04	58.73	175.77	2431	25.49	59.76	174.74	2417
235	24.09	56.61	178.39	2467	24.53	57.65	177.35	2453	24.97	58.69	176.32	2438	25.41	59.72	175.28	2424
235.5	24.02	56.57	178.93	2475	24.46	57.61	177.89	2460	24.90	58.64	176.86	2446	25.34	59.68	175.82	2432
236	23.95	56.53	179.47	2482	24.39	57.57	178.43	2468	24.83	58.60	177.40	2453	25.27	59.64	176.36	2439
236.5	23.88	56.49	180.01	2490	24.32	57.52	178.98	2475	24.76	58.56	177.94	2461	25.20	59.60	176.90	2447
237	23.82	56.45	180.55	2497	24.25	57.48	179.52	2483	24.69	58.52	178.48	2468	25.13	59.56	177.44	2454
237.5	23.75	56.41	181.10	2505	24.19	57.44	180.06	2490	24.62	58.48	179.02	2476	25.06	59.52	177.98	2461
238	23.68	56.36	181.64	2512	24.12	57.40	180.60	2498	24.55	58.44	179.56	2483	24.99	59.48	178.52	2469
238.5	23.62	56.32	182.18	2520	24.05	57.36	181.14	2505	24.49	58.40	180.10	2491	24.92	59.44	179.06	2476
239	23.55	56.28	182.72	2527	23.98	57.32	181.68	2513	24.42	58.36	180.64	2498	24.85	59.39	179.61	2484
239.5	23.48	56.24	183.26	2534	23.92	57.28	182.22	2520	24.35	58.32	181.18	2506	24.78	59.35	180.15	2491
240	23.42	56.20	183.80	2542	23.85	57.24	182.76	2528	24.28	58.28	181.73	2513	24.71	59.31	180.69	2499
240.5	23.35	56.16	184.34	2549	23.78	57.20	183.30	2535	24.21	58.23	182.27	2521	24.65	59.27	181.23	2506
241	23.29	56.12	184.88	2557	23.72	57.16	183.84	2543	24.15	58.19	182.81	2528	24.58	59.23	181.77	2514
241.5	23.22	56.08	185.42	2564	23.65	57.11	184.39	2550	24.08	58.15	183.35	2536	24.51	59.19	182.31	2521
242	23.16	56.04	185.96	2572	23.58	57.07	184.93	2558	24.01	58.11	183.89	2543	24.44	59.15	182.85	2529
242.5	23.09	56.00	186.51	2579	23.52	57.03	185.47	2565	23.95	58.07	184.43	2551	24.37	59.11	183.39	2536
243	23.03	55.95	187.05	2587	23.45	56.99	186.01	2572	23.88	58.03	184.97	2558	24.31	59.07	183.93	2544
243.5	22.96	55.91	187.59	2594	23.39	56.95	186.55	2580	23.81	57.99	185.51	2566	24.24	59.03	184.47	2551
244	22.90	55.87	188.13	2602	23.32	56.91	187.09	2587	23.75	57.95	186.05	2573	24.17	58.98	185.02	2559
244.5	22.83	55.83	188.67	2609	23.26	56.87	187.63	2595	23.68	57.91	186.59	2581	24.11	58.94	185.56	2566
245	22.77	55.79	189.21	2617	23.19	56.83	188.17	2602	23.62	57.87	187.14	2588	24.04	58.90	186.10	2574
245.5	22.71	55.75	189.75	2624	23.13	56.79	188.71	2610	23.55	57.82	187.68	2596	23.98	58.86	186.64	2581
246	22.65	55.71	190.29	2632	23.07	56.75	189.25	2617	23.49	57.78	188.22	2603	23.91	58.82	187.18	2589
246.5	22.58	55.67	190.83	2639	23.00	56.70	189.80	2625	23.42	57.74	188.76	2611	23.85	58.78	187.72	2596
247	22.52	55.63	191.37	2647	22.94	56.66	190.34	2632	23.36	57.70	189.30	2618	23.78	58.74	188.26	2604
247.5	22.46	55.59	191.92	2654	22.88	56.62	190.88	2640	23.30	57.66	189.84	2625	23.72	58.70	188.80	2611

Body Composition MALE 216-247.5 Lb.

Weight: Lb.	Waist: 43 inches				43.25 inches				43.5 inches				43.75 inches			
	Fat: %	Fat: Lb.	LBM: Lb.	RMR: Cal.	Fat: %	Fat: Lb.	LBM: Lb.	RMR: Cal.	Fat: %	Fat: Lb.	LBM: Lb.	RMR: Cal.	Fat: %	Fat: Lb.	LBM: Lb.	RMR: Cal.
216	28.85	62.32	153.68	2125	29.33	63.36	152.64	2111	29.81	64.39	151.61	2097	30.29	65.43	150.57	2082
216.5	28.77	62.28	154.22	2133	29.24	63.31	153.19	2119	29.72	64.35	152.15	2104	30.20	65.39	151.11	2090
217	28.68	62.24	154.76	2140	29.16	63.27	153.73	2126	29.64	64.31	152.69	2112	30.11	65.35	151.65	2097
217.5	28.60	62.20	155.31	2148	29.07	63.23	154.27	2134	29.55	64.27	153.23	2119	30.03	65.31	152.19	2105
218	28.51	62.15	155.85	2155	28.99	63.19	154.81	2141	29.46	64.23	153.77	2127	29.94	65.27	152.73	2112
218.5	28.43	62.11	156.39	2163	28.90	63.15	155.35	2148	29.38	64.19	154.31	2134	29.85	65.23	153.27	2120
219	28.34	62.07	156.93	2170	28.82	63.11	155.89	2156	29.29	64.15	154.85	2142	29.76	65.18	153.82	2127
219.5	28.26	62.03	157.47	2178	28.73	63.07	156.43	2163	29.21	64.11	155.39	2149	29.68	65.14	154.36	2135
220	28.18	61.99	158.01	2185	28.65	63.03	156.97	2171	29.12	64.07	155.94	2157	29.59	65.10	154.90	2142
220.5	28.09	61.95	158.55	2193	28.57	62.99	157.51	2178	29.04	64.02	156.48	2164	29.51	65.06	155.44	2150
221	28.01	61.91	159.09	2200	28.48	62.95	158.05	2186	28.95	63.98	157.02	2172	29.42	65.02	155.98	2157
221.5	27.93	61.87	159.63	2208	28.40	62.90	158.60	2193	28.87	63.94	157.56	2179	29.34	64.98	156.52	2165
222	27.85	61.83	160.17	2215	28.32	62.86	159.14	2201	28.78	63.90	158.10	2187	29.25	64.94	157.06	2172
222.5	27.77	61.79	160.72	2223	28.23	62.82	159.68	2208	28.70	63.86	158.64	2194	29.17	64.90	157.60	2180
223	27.69	61.74	161.26	2230	28.15	62.78	160.22	2216	28.62	63.82	159.18	2201	29.08	64.86	158.14	2187
223.5	27.61	61.70	161.80	2238	28.07	62.74	160.76	2223	28.54	63.78	159.72	2209	29.00	64.82	158.68	2195
224	27.53	61.66	162.34	2245	27.99	62.70	161.30	2231	28.45	63.74	160.26	2216	28.92	64.77	159.23	2202
224.5	27.45	61.62	162.88	2253	27.91	62.66	161.84	2238	28.37	63.70	160.80	2224	28.83	64.73	159.77	2210
225	27.37	61.58	163.42	2260	27.83	62.62	162.38	2246	28.29	63.66	161.35	2231	28.75	64.69	160.31	2217
225.5	27.29	61.54	163.96	2268	27.75	62.58	162.92	2253	28.21	63.61	161.89	2239	28.67	64.65	160.85	2225
226	27.21	61.50	164.50	2275	27.67	62.54	163.46	2261	28.13	63.57	162.43	2246	28.59	64.61	161.39	2232
226.5	27.13	61.46	165.04	2283	27.59	62.49	164.01	2268	28.05	63.53	162.97	2254	28.51	64.57	161.93	2239
227	27.06	61.42	165.58	2290	27.51	62.45	164.55	2276	27.97	63.49	163.51	2261	28.43	64.53	162.47	2247
227.5	26.98	61.38	166.13	2298	27.43	62.41	165.09	2283	27.89	63.45	164.05	2269	28.35	64.49	163.01	2254
228	26.90	61.33	166.67	2305	27.36	62.37	165.63	2291	27.81	63.41	164.59	2276	28.27	64.45	163.55	2262
228.5	26.82	61.29	167.21	2312	27.28	62.33	166.17	2298	27.73	63.37	165.13	2284	28.19	64.41	164.09	2269
229	26.75	61.25	167.75	2320	27.20	62.29	166.71	2306	27.65	63.33	165.67	2291	28.11	64.36	164.64	2277
229.5	26.67	61.21	168.29	2327	27.12	62.25	167.25	2313	27.58	63.29	166.21	2299	28.03	64.32	165.18	2284
230	26.60	61.17	168.83	2335	27.05	62.21	167.79	2321	27.50	63.25	166.76	2306	27.95	64.28	165.72	2292
230.5	26.52	61.13	169.37	2342	26.97	62.17	168.33	2328	27.42	63.20	167.30	2314	27.87	64.24	166.26	2299
231	26.45	61.09	169.91	2350	26.89	62.13	168.87	2336	27.34	63.16	167.84	2321	27.79	64.20	166.80	2307
231.5	26.37	61.05	170.45	2357	26.82	62.08	169.42	2343	27.27	63.12	168.38	2329	27.71	64.16	167.34	2314
232	26.30	61.01	170.99	2365	26.74	62.04	169.96	2350	27.19	63.08	168.92	2336	27.64	64.12	167.88	2322
232.5	26.22	60.97	171.54	2372	26.67	62.00	170.50	2358	27.11	63.04	169.46	2344	27.56	64.08	168.42	2329
233	26.15	60.92	172.08	2380	26.59	61.96	171.04	2365	27.04	63.00	170.00	2351	27.48	64.04	168.96	2337
233.5	26.07	60.88	172.62	2387	26.52	61.92	171.58	2373	26.96	62.96	170.54	2359	27.41	64.00	169.50	2344
234	26.00	60.84	173.16	2395	26.44	61.88	172.12	2380	26.89	62.92	171.08	2366	27.33	63.95	170.05	2352
234.5	25.93	60.80	173.70	2402	26.37	61.84	172.66	2388	26.81	62.88	171.62	2374	27.26	63.91	170.59	2359
235	25.86	60.76	174.24	2410	26.30	61.80	173.20	2395	26.74	62.84	172.17	2381	27.18	63.87	171.13	2367
235.5	25.78	60.72	174.78	2417	26.22	61.76	173.74	2403	26.66	62.79	172.71	2389	27.10	63.83	171.67	2374
236	25.71	60.68	175.32	2425	26.15	61.72	174.28	2410	26.59	62.75	173.25	2396	27.03	63.79	172.21	2382
236.5	25.64	60.64	175.86	2432	26.08	61.67	174.83	2418	26.52	62.71	173.79	2403	26.96	63.75	172.75	2389
237	25.57	60.60	176.40	2440	26.01	61.63	175.37	2425	26.44	62.67	174.33	2411	26.88	63.71	173.29	2397
237.5	25.50	60.56	176.95	2447	25.93	61.59	175.91	2433	26.37	62.63	174.87	2418	26.81	63.67	173.83	2404
238	25.43	60.51	177.49	2455	25.86	61.55	176.45	2440	26.30	62.59	175.41	2426	26.73	63.63	174.37	2412
238.5	25.36	60.47	178.03	2462	25.79	61.51	176.99	2448	26.23	62.55	175.95	2433	26.66	63.59	174.91	2419
239	25.29	60.43	178.57	2470	25.72	61.47	177.53	2455	26.15	62.51	176.49	2441	26.59	63.54	175.46	2427
239.5	25.22	60.39	179.11	2477	25.65	61.43	178.07	2463	26.08	62.47	177.03	2448	26.52	63.50	176.00	2434
240	25.15	60.35	179.65	2485	25.58	61.39	178.61	2470	26.01	62.43	177.58	2456	26.44	63.46	176.54	2442
240.5	25.08	60.31	180.19	2492	25.51	61.35	179.15	2478	25.94	62.38	178.12	2463	26.37	63.42	177.08	2449
241	25.01	60.27	180.73	2500	25.44	61.31	179.69	2485	25.87	62.34	178.66	2471	26.30	63.38	177.62	2456
241.5	24.94	60.23	181.27	2507	25.37	61.26	180.24	2493	25.80	62.30	179.20	2478	26.23	63.34	178.16	2464
242	24.87	60.19	181.81	2514	25.30	61.22	180.78	2500	25.73	62.26	179.74	2486	26.16	63.30	178.70	2471
242.5	24.80	60.15	182.36	2522	25.23	61.18	181.32	2508	25.66	62.22	180.28	2493	26.09	63.26	179.24	2479
243	24.73	60.10	182.90	2529	25.16	61.14	181.86	2515	25.59	62.18	180.82	2501	26.02	63.22	179.78	2486
243.5	24.67	60.06	183.44	2537	25.09	61.10	182.40	2523	25.52	62.14	181.36	2508	25.94	63.18	180.32	2494
244	24.60	60.02	183.98	2544	25.02	61.06	182.94	2530	25.45	62.10	181.90	2516	25.87	63.13	180.87	2501
244.5	24.53	59.98	184.52	2552	24.96	61.02	183.48	2538	25.38	62.06	182.44	2523	25.81	63.09	181.41	2509
245	24.47	59.94	185.06	2559	24.89	60.98	184.02	2545	25.31	62.02	182.99	2531	25.74	63.05	181.95	2516
245.5	24.40	59.90	185.60	2567	24.82	60.94	184.56	2553	25.24	61.97	183.53	2538	25.67	63.01	182.49	2524
246	24.33	59.86	186.14	2574	24.75	60.90	185.10	2560	25.18	61.93	184.07	2546	25.60	62.97	183.03	2531
246.5	24.27	59.82	186.68	2582	24.69	60.85	185.65	2567	25.11	61.89	184.61	2553	25.53	62.93	183.57	2539
247	24.20	59.78	187.22	2589	24.62	60.81	186.19	2575	25.04	61.85	185.15	2561	25.46	62.89	184.11	2546
247.5	24.14	59.74	187.77	2597	24.55	60.77	186.73	2582	24.97	61.81	185.69	2568	25.39	62.85	184.65	2554

Body Composition MALE 216-247.5 Lb.

Weight: Lb.	Waist: 44 inches				44.25 inches				44.5 inches				44.75 inches			
	Fat: %	Fat: Lb.	LBM: Lb.	RMR: Cal.	Fat: %	Fat: Lb.	LBM: Lb.	RMR: Cal.	Fat: %	Fat: Lb.	LBM: Lb.	RMR: Cal.	Fat: %	Fat: Lb.	LBM: Lb.	RMR: Cal.
216	30.77	66.47	149.53	2068	31.25	67.51	148.49	2054	31.73	68.54	147.46	2039	32.21	69.58	146.42	2025
216.5	30.68	66.43	150.07	2076	31.16	67.46	149.04	2061	31.64	68.50	148.00	2047	32.12	69.54	146.96	2032
217	30.59	66.39	150.61	2083	31.07	67.42	149.58	2069	31.55	68.46	148.54	2054	32.03	69.50	147.50	2040
217.5	30.50	66.35	151.16	2090	30.98	67.38	150.12	2076	31.46	68.42	149.08	2062	31.93	69.46	148.04	2047
218	30.41	66.30	151.70	2098	30.89	67.34	150.66	2084	31.37	68.38	149.62	2069	31.84	69.42	148.58	2055
218.5	30.33	66.26	152.24	2105	30.80	67.30	151.20	2091	31.28	68.34	150.16	2077	31.75	69.38	149.12	2062
219	30.24	66.22	152.78	2113	30.71	67.26	151.74	2099	31.19	68.30	150.70	2084	31.66	69.33	149.67	2070
219.5	30.15	66.18	153.32	2120	30.62	67.22	152.28	2106	31.10	68.26	151.24	2092	31.57	69.29	150.21	2077
220	30.06	66.14	153.86	2128	30.54	67.18	152.82	2114	31.01	68.22	151.79	2099	31.48	69.25	150.75	2085
220.5	29.98	66.10	154.40	2135	30.45	67.14	153.36	2121	30.92	68.17	152.33	2107	31.39	69.21	151.29	2092
221	29.89	66.06	154.94	2143	30.36	67.10	153.90	2128	30.83	68.13	152.87	2114	31.30	69.17	151.83	2100
221.5	29.80	66.02	155.48	2150	30.27	67.05	154.45	2136	30.74	68.09	153.41	2122	31.21	69.13	152.37	2107
222	29.72	65.98	156.02	2158	30.19	67.01	154.99	2143	30.65	68.05	153.95	2129	31.12	69.09	152.91	2115
222.5	29.63	65.94	156.57	2165	30.10	66.97	155.53	2151	30.57	68.01	154.49	2137	31.03	69.05	153.45	2122
223	29.55	65.89	157.11	2173	30.01	66.93	156.07	2158	30.48	67.97	155.03	2144	30.94	69.01	153.99	2130
223.5	29.46	65.85	157.65	2180	29.93	66.89	156.61	2166	30.39	67.93	155.57	2152	30.86	68.97	154.53	2137
224	29.38	65.81	158.19	2188	29.84	66.85	157.15	2173	30.31	67.89	156.11	2159	30.77	68.92	155.08	2145
224.5	29.30	65.77	158.73	2195	29.76	66.81	157.69	2181	30.22	67.85	156.65	2167	30.68	68.88	155.62	2152
225	29.21	65.73	159.27	2203	29.67	66.77	158.23	2188	30.14	67.81	157.20	2174	30.60	68.84	156.16	2160
225.5	29.13	65.69	159.81	2210	29.59	66.73	158.77	2196	30.05	67.76	157.74	2181	30.51	68.80	156.70	2167
226	29.05	65.65	160.35	2218	29.51	66.69	159.31	2203	29.97	67.72	158.28	2189	30.43	68.76	157.24	2175
226.5	28.97	65.61	160.89	2225	29.42	66.64	159.86	2211	29.88	67.68	158.82	2196	30.34	68.72	157.78	2182
227	28.88	65.57	161.43	2233	29.34	66.60	160.40	2218	29.80	67.64	159.36	2204	30.25	68.68	158.32	2190
227.5	28.80	65.53	161.98	2240	29.26	66.56	160.94	2226	29.71	67.60	159.90	2211	30.17	68.64	158.86	2197
228	28.72	65.48	162.52	2248	29.18	66.52	161.48	2233	29.63	67.56	160.44	2219	30.09	68.60	159.40	2205
228.5	28.64	65.44	163.06	2255	29.09	66.48	162.02	2241	29.55	67.52	160.98	2226	30.00	68.56	159.94	2212
229	28.56	65.40	163.60	2263	29.01	66.44	162.56	2248	29.47	67.48	161.52	2234	29.92	68.51	160.49	2220
229.5	28.48	65.36	164.14	2270	28.93	66.40	163.10	2256	29.38	67.44	162.06	2241	29.84	68.47	161.03	2227
230	28.40	65.32	164.68	2278	28.85	66.36	163.64	2263	29.30	67.40	162.61	2249	29.75	68.43	161.57	2234
230.5	28.32	65.28	165.22	2285	28.77	66.32	164.18	2271	29.22	67.35	163.15	2256	29.67	68.39	162.11	2242
231	28.24	65.24	165.76	2292	28.69	66.28	164.72	2278	29.14	67.31	163.69	2264	29.59	68.35	162.65	2249
231.5	28.16	65.20	166.30	2300	28.61	66.23	165.27	2286	29.06	67.27	164.23	2271	29.51	68.31	163.19	2257
232	28.08	65.16	166.84	2307	28.53	66.19	165.81	2293	28.98	67.23	164.77	2279	29.43	68.27	163.73	2264
232.5	28.01	65.12	167.39	2315	28.45	66.15	166.35	2301	28.90	67.19	165.31	2286	29.35	68.23	164.27	2272
233	27.93	65.07	167.93	2322	28.37	66.11	166.89	2308	28.82	67.15	165.85	2294	29.26	68.19	164.81	2279
233.5	27.85	65.03	168.47	2330	28.30	66.07	167.43	2316	28.74	67.11	166.39	2301	29.18	68.15	165.35	2287
234	27.77	64.99	169.01	2337	28.22	66.03	167.97	2323	28.66	67.07	166.93	2309	29.10	68.10	165.90	2294
234.5	27.70	64.95	169.55	2345	28.14	65.99	168.51	2331	28.58	67.03	167.47	2316	29.02	68.06	166.44	2302
235	27.62	64.91	170.09	2352	28.06	65.95	169.05	2338	28.50	66.99	168.02	2324	28.95	68.02	166.98	2309
235.5	27.55	64.87	170.63	2360	27.99	65.91	169.59	2345	28.43	66.94	168.56	2331	28.87	67.98	167.52	2317
236	27.47	64.83	171.17	2367	27.91	65.87	170.13	2353	28.35	66.90	169.10	2339	28.79	67.94	168.06	2324
236.5	27.39	64.79	171.71	2375	27.83	65.82	170.68	2360	28.27	66.86	169.64	2346	28.71	67.90	168.60	2332
237	27.32	64.75	172.25	2382	27.76	65.78	171.22	2368	28.19	66.82	170.18	2354	28.63	67.86	169.14	2339
237.5	27.24	64.71	172.80	2390	27.68	65.74	171.76	2375	28.12	66.78	170.72	2361	28.55	67.82	169.68	2347
238	27.17	64.66	173.34	2397	27.61	65.70	172.30	2383	28.04	66.74	171.26	2369	28.48	67.78	170.22	2354
238.5	27.10	64.62	173.88	2405	27.53	65.66	172.84	2390	27.97	66.70	171.80	2376	28.40	67.74	170.76	2362
239	27.02	64.58	174.42	2412	27.46	65.62	173.38	2398	27.89	66.66	172.34	2384	28.32	67.69	171.31	2369
239.5	26.95	64.54	174.96	2420	27.38	65.58	173.92	2405	27.81	66.62	172.88	2391	28.25	67.65	171.85	2377
240	26.88	64.50	175.50	2427	27.31	65.54	174.46	2413	27.74	66.58	173.43	2398	28.17	67.61	172.39	2384
240.5	26.80	64.46	176.04	2435	27.23	65.50	175.00	2420	27.66	66.53	173.97	2406	28.10	67.57	172.93	2392
241	26.73	64.42	176.58	2442	27.16	65.46	175.54	2428	27.59	66.49	174.51	2413	28.02	67.53	173.47	2399
241.5	26.66	64.38	177.12	2450	27.09	65.41	176.09	2435	27.52	66.45	175.05	2421	27.95	67.49	174.01	2407
242	26.59	64.34	177.66	2457	27.01	65.37	176.63	2443	27.44	66.41	175.59	2428	27.87	67.45	174.55	2414
242.5	26.51	64.30	178.21	2465	26.94	65.33	177.17	2450	27.37	66.37	176.13	2436	27.80	67.41	175.09	2422
243	26.44	64.25	178.75	2472	26.87	65.29	177.71	2458	27.30	66.33	176.67	2443	27.72	67.37	175.63	2429
243.5	26.37	64.21	179.29	2480	26.80	65.25	178.25	2465	27.22	66.29	177.21	2451	27.65	67.33	176.17	2436
244	26.30	64.17	179.83	2487	26.73	65.21	178.79	2473	27.15	66.25	177.75	2458	27.58	67.28	176.72	2444
244.5	26.23	64.13	180.37	2495	26.65	65.17	179.33	2480	27.08	66.21	178.29	2466	27.50	67.24	177.26	2451
245	26.16	64.09	180.91	2502	26.58	65.13	179.87	2488	27.01	66.17	178.84	2473	27.43	67.20	177.80	2459
245.5	26.09	64.05	181.45	2509	26.51	65.09	180.41	2495	26.93	66.12	179.38	2481	27.36	67.16	178.34	2466
246	26.02	64.01	181.99	2517	26.44	65.05	180.95	2503	26.86	66.08	179.92	2488	27.28	67.12	178.88	2474
246.5	25.95	63.97	182.53	2524	26.37	65.00	181.50	2510	26.79	66.04	180.46	2496	27.21	67.08	179.42	2481
247	25.88	63.93	183.07	2532	26.30	64.96	182.04	2518	26.72	66.00	181.00	2503	27.14	67.04	179.96	2489
247.5	25.81	63.89	183.62	2539	26.23	64.92	182.58	2525	26.65	65.96	181.54	2511	27.07	67.00	180.50	2496

Body Composition MALE 216-247.5 Lb.

Weight: Lb.	Waist: 45 inches Fat: %	Fat: Lb.	LBM: Lb.	RMR: Cal.	45.25 inches Fat: %	Fat: Lb.	LBM: Lb.	RMR: Cal.	45.5 inches Fat: %	Fat: Lb.	LBM: Lb.	RMR: Cal.	45.75 inches Fat: %	Fat: Lb.	LBM: Lb.	RMR: Cal.
216	32.69	70.62	145.38	2011	33.17	71.66	144.34	1996	33.65	72.69	143.31	1982	34.13	73.73	142.27	1968
216.5	32.60	70.58	145.92	2018	33.08	71.61	144.89	2004	33.56	72.65	143.85	1989	34.04	73.69	142.81	1975
217	32.51	70.54	146.46	2026	32.98	71.57	145.43	2011	33.46	72.61	144.39	1997	33.94	73.65	143.35	1983
217.5	32.41	70.50	147.01	2033	32.89	71.53	145.97	2019	33.37	72.57	144.93	2004	33.84	73.61	143.89	1990
218	32.32	70.45	147.55	2041	32.79	71.49	146.51	2026	33.27	72.53	145.47	2012	33.75	73.57	144.43	1998
218.5	32.23	70.41	148.09	2048	32.70	71.45	147.05	2034	33.18	72.49	146.01	2019	33.65	73.53	144.97	2005
219	32.13	70.37	148.63	2056	32.61	71.41	147.59	2041	33.08	72.45	146.55	2027	33.55	73.48	145.52	2012
219.5	32.04	70.33	149.17	2063	32.51	71.37	148.13	2049	32.99	72.41	147.09	2034	33.46	73.44	146.06	2020
220	31.95	70.29	149.71	2070	32.42	71.33	148.67	2056	32.89	72.37	147.64	2042	33.36	73.40	146.60	2027
220.5	31.86	70.25	150.25	2078	32.33	71.29	149.21	2064	32.80	72.32	148.18	2049	33.27	73.36	147.14	2035
221	31.77	70.21	150.79	2085	32.24	71.25	149.75	2071	32.71	72.28	148.72	2057	33.18	73.32	147.68	2042
221.5	31.68	70.17	151.33	2093	32.15	71.20	150.30	2079	32.61	72.24	149.26	2064	33.08	73.28	148.22	2050
222	31.59	70.13	151.87	2100	32.06	71.16	150.84	2086	32.52	72.20	149.80	2072	32.99	73.24	148.76	2057
222.5	31.50	70.09	152.42	2108	31.97	71.12	151.38	2094	32.43	72.16	150.34	2079	32.90	73.20	149.30	2065
223	31.41	70.04	152.96	2115	31.88	71.08	151.92	2101	32.34	72.12	150.88	2087	32.81	73.16	149.84	2072
223.5	31.32	70.00	153.50	2123	31.79	71.04	152.46	2109	32.25	72.08	151.42	2094	32.71	73.12	150.38	2080
224	31.23	69.96	154.04	2130	31.70	71.00	153.00	2116	32.16	72.04	151.96	2102	32.62	73.07	150.93	2087
224.5	31.15	69.92	154.58	2138	31.61	70.96	153.54	2123	32.07	72.00	152.50	2109	32.53	73.03	151.47	2095
225	31.06	69.88	155.12	2145	31.52	70.92	154.08	2131	31.98	71.96	153.05	2117	32.44	72.99	152.01	2102
225.5	30.97	69.84	155.66	2153	31.43	70.88	154.62	2138	31.89	71.91	153.59	2124	32.35	72.95	152.55	2110
226	30.88	69.80	156.20	2160	31.34	70.84	155.16	2146	31.80	71.87	154.13	2132	32.26	72.91	153.09	2117
226.5	30.80	69.76	156.74	2168	31.26	70.79	155.71	2153	31.71	71.83	154.67	2139	32.17	72.87	153.63	2125
227	30.71	69.72	157.28	2175	31.17	70.75	156.25	2161	31.63	71.79	155.21	2147	32.08	72.83	154.17	2132
227.5	30.63	69.68	157.83	2183	31.08	70.71	156.79	2168	31.54	71.75	155.75	2154	31.99	72.79	154.71	2140
228	30.54	69.63	158.37	2190	31.00	70.67	157.33	2176	31.45	71.71	156.29	2162	31.91	72.75	155.25	2147
228.5	30.46	69.59	158.91	2198	30.91	70.63	157.87	2183	31.36	71.67	156.83	2169	31.82	72.71	155.79	2155
229	30.37	69.55	159.45	2205	30.83	70.59	158.41	2191	31.28	71.63	157.37	2176	31.73	72.66	156.34	2162
229.5	30.29	69.51	159.99	2213	30.74	70.55	158.95	2198	31.19	71.59	157.91	2184	31.64	72.62	156.88	2170
230	30.20	69.47	160.53	2220	30.66	70.51	159.49	2206	31.11	71.55	158.46	2191	31.56	72.58	157.42	2177
230.5	30.12	69.43	161.07	2228	30.57	70.47	160.03	2213	31.02	71.50	159.00	2199	31.47	72.54	157.96	2185
231	30.04	69.39	161.61	2235	30.49	70.43	160.57	2221	30.94	71.46	159.54	2206	31.39	72.50	158.50	2192
231.5	29.96	69.35	162.15	2243	30.40	70.38	161.12	2228	30.85	71.42	160.08	2214	31.30	72.46	159.04	2200
232	29.87	69.31	162.69	2250	30.32	70.34	161.66	2236	30.77	71.38	160.62	2221	31.21	72.42	159.58	2207
232.5	29.79	69.27	163.24	2258	30.24	70.30	162.20	2243	30.68	71.34	161.16	2229	31.13	72.38	160.12	2214
233	29.71	69.22	163.78	2265	30.16	70.26	162.74	2251	30.60	71.30	161.70	2236	31.05	72.34	160.66	2222
233.5	29.63	69.18	164.32	2273	30.07	70.22	163.28	2258	30.52	71.26	162.24	2244	30.96	72.30	161.20	2229
234	29.55	69.14	164.86	2280	29.99	70.18	163.82	2266	30.43	71.22	162.78	2251	30.88	72.25	161.75	2237
234.5	29.47	69.10	165.40	2287	29.91	70.14	164.36	2273	30.35	71.18	163.32	2259	30.79	72.21	162.29	2244
235	29.39	69.06	165.94	2295	29.83	70.10	164.90	2281	30.27	71.14	163.87	2266	30.71	72.17	162.83	2252
235.5	29.31	69.02	166.48	2302	29.75	70.06	165.44	2288	30.19	71.09	164.41	2274	30.63	72.13	163.37	2259
236	29.23	68.98	167.02	2310	29.67	70.02	165.98	2296	30.11	71.05	164.95	2281	30.55	72.09	163.91	2267
236.5	29.15	68.94	167.56	2317	29.59	69.97	166.53	2303	30.03	71.01	165.49	2289	30.46	72.05	164.45	2274
237	29.07	68.90	168.10	2325	29.51	69.93	167.07	2311	29.95	70.97	166.03	2296	30.38	72.01	164.99	2282
237.5	28.99	68.86	168.65	2332	29.43	69.89	167.61	2318	29.87	70.93	166.57	2304	30.30	71.97	165.53	2289
238	28.91	68.81	169.19	2340	29.35	69.85	168.15	2325	29.79	70.89	167.11	2311	30.22	71.93	166.07	2297
238.5	28.84	68.77	169.73	2347	29.27	69.81	168.69	2333	29.71	70.85	167.65	2319	30.14	71.89	166.61	2304
239	28.76	68.73	170.27	2355	29.19	69.77	169.23	2340	29.63	70.81	168.19	2326	30.06	71.84	167.16	2312
239.5	28.68	68.69	170.81	2362	29.11	69.73	169.77	2348	29.55	70.77	168.73	2334	29.98	71.80	167.70	2319
240	28.60	68.65	171.35	2370	29.04	69.69	170.31	2355	29.47	70.73	169.28	2341	29.90	71.76	168.24	2327
240.5	28.53	68.61	171.89	2377	28.96	69.65	170.85	2363	29.39	70.68	169.82	2349	29.82	71.72	168.78	2334
241	28.45	68.57	172.43	2385	28.88	69.61	171.39	2370	29.31	70.64	170.36	2356	29.74	71.68	169.32	2342
241.5	28.38	68.53	172.97	2392	28.81	69.56	171.94	2378	29.23	70.60	170.90	2364	29.66	71.64	169.86	2349
242	28.30	68.49	173.51	2400	28.73	69.52	172.48	2385	29.16	70.56	171.44	2371	29.59	71.60	170.40	2357
242.5	28.22	68.45	174.06	2407	28.65	69.48	173.02	2393	29.08	70.52	171.98	2378	29.51	71.56	170.94	2364
243	28.15	68.40	174.60	2415	28.50	69.44	173.56	2400	29.00	70.48	172.52	2386	29.43	71.52	171.48	2372
243.5	28.08	68.36	175.14	2422	28.50	69.40	174.10	2408	28.93	70.44	173.06	2393	29.35	71.48	172.02	2379
244	28.00	68.32	175.68	2430	28.43	69.36	174.64	2415	28.85	70.40	173.60	2401	29.28	71.43	172.57	2387
244.5	27.93	68.28	176.22	2437	28.35	69.32	175.18	2423	28.78	70.36	174.14	2408	29.20	71.39	173.11	2394
245	27.85	68.24	176.76	2445	28.28	69.28	175.72	2430	28.70	70.32	174.69	2416	29.12	71.35	173.65	2402
245.5	27.78	68.20	177.30	2452	28.20	69.24	176.26	2438	28.62	70.27	175.23	2423	29.05	71.31	174.19	2409
246	27.71	68.16	177.84	2460	28.13	69.20	176.80	2445	28.55	70.23	175.77	2431	28.97	71.27	174.73	2417
246.5	27.63	68.12	178.38	2467	28.05	69.15	177.35	2453	28.48	70.19	176.31	2438	28.90	71.23	175.27	2424
247	27.56	68.08	178.92	2475	27.98	69.11	177.89	2460	28.40	70.15	176.85	2446	28.82	71.19	175.81	2431
247.5	27.49	68.04	179.47	2482	27.91	69.07	178.43	2468	28.33	70.11	177.39	2453	28.75	71.15	176.35	2439

Body Composition MALE 216-247.5 Lb.

Weight: Lb.	Waist: 46 inches				46.25 inches				46.5 inches				46.75 inches			
	Fat: %	Fat: Lb.	LBM: Lb.	RMR: Cal.	Fat: %	Fat: Lb.	LBM: Lb.	RMR: Cal.	Fat: %	Fat: Lb.	LBM: Lb.	RMR: Cal.	Fat: %	Fat: Lb.	LBM: Lb.	RMR: Cal.
216	34.61	74.77	141.23	1953	35.10	75.81	140.19	1939	35.58	76.84	139.16	1925	36.06	77.88	138.12	1910
216.5	34.52	74.73	141.77	1961	35.00	75.76	140.74	1946	35.47	76.80	139.70	1932	35.95	77.84	138.66	1918
217	34.42	74.69	142.31	1968	34.90	75.72	141.28	1954	35.37	76.76	140.24	1940	35.85	77.80	139.20	1925
217.5	34.32	74.65	142.86	1976	34.80	75.68	141.82	1961	35.27	76.72	140.78	1947	35.75	77.76	139.74	1933
218	34.22	74.60	143.40	1983	34.70	75.64	142.36	1969	35.17	76.68	141.32	1954	35.65	77.72	140.28	1940
218.5	34.12	74.56	143.94	1991	34.60	75.60	142.90	1976	35.07	76.64	141.86	1962	35.55	77.68	140.82	1948
219	34.03	74.52	144.48	1998	34.50	75.56	143.44	1984	34.98	76.60	142.40	1969	35.45	77.63	141.37	1955
219.5	33.93	74.48	145.02	2006	34.40	75.52	143.98	1991	34.88	76.56	142.94	1977	35.35	77.59	141.91	1963
220	33.84	74.44	145.56	2013	34.31	75.48	144.52	1999	34.78	76.52	143.49	1984	35.25	77.55	142.45	1970
220.5	33.74	74.40	146.10	2021	34.21	75.44	145.06	2006	34.68	76.47	144.03	1992	35.15	77.51	142.99	1978
221	33.65	74.36	146.64	2028	34.12	75.40	145.60	2014	34.59	76.43	144.57	1999	35.05	77.47	143.53	1985
221.5	33.55	74.32	147.18	2036	34.02	75.35	146.15	2021	34.49	76.39	145.11	2007	34.96	77.43	144.07	1992
222	33.46	74.28	147.72	2043	33.93	75.31	146.69	2029	34.39	76.35	145.65	2014	34.86	77.39	144.61	2000
222.5	33.36	74.24	148.27	2051	33.83	75.27	147.23	2036	34.30	76.31	146.19	2022	34.76	77.35	145.15	2007
223	33.27	74.19	148.81	2058	33.74	75.23	147.77	2044	34.20	76.27	146.73	2029	34.67	77.31	145.69	2015
223.5	33.18	74.15	149.35	2065	33.64	75.19	148.31	2051	34.11	76.23	147.27	2037	34.57	77.27	146.23	2022
224	33.09	74.11	149.89	2073	33.55	75.15	148.85	2059	34.01	76.19	147.81	2044	34.48	77.22	146.78	2030
224.5	32.99	74.07	150.43	2080	33.46	75.11	149.39	2066	33.92	76.15	148.35	2052	34.38	77.18	147.32	2037
225	32.90	74.03	150.97	2088	33.36	75.07	149.93	2074	33.82	76.11	148.90	2059	34.29	77.14	147.86	2045
225.5	32.81	73.99	151.51	2095	33.27	75.03	150.47	2081	33.73	76.06	149.44	2067	34.19	77.10	148.40	2052
226	32.72	73.95	152.05	2103	33.18	74.99	151.01	2089	33.64	76.02	149.98	2074	34.10	77.06	148.94	2060
226.5	32.63	73.91	152.59	2110	33.09	74.94	151.56	2096	33.55	75.98	150.52	2082	34.00	77.02	149.48	2067
227	32.54	73.87	153.13	2118	33.00	74.90	152.10	2103	33.45	75.94	151.06	2089	33.91	76.98	150.02	2075
227.5	32.45	73.83	153.68	2125	32.91	74.86	152.64	2111	33.36	75.90	151.60	2097	33.82	76.94	150.56	2082
228	32.36	73.78	154.22	2133	32.82	74.82	153.18	2118	33.27	75.86	152.14	2104	33.73	76.90	151.10	2090
228.5	32.27	73.74	154.76	2140	32.73	74.78	153.72	2126	33.18	75.82	152.68	2112	33.63	76.86	151.64	2097
229	32.18	73.70	155.30	2148	32.64	74.74	154.26	2133	33.09	75.78	153.22	2119	33.54	76.81	152.19	2105
229.5	32.10	73.66	155.84	2155	32.55	74.70	154.80	2141	33.00	75.74	153.76	2127	33.45	76.77	152.73	2112
230	32.01	73.62	156.38	2163	32.46	74.66	155.34	2148	32.91	75.70	154.31	2134	33.36	76.73	153.27	2120
230.5	31.92	73.58	156.92	2170	32.37	74.62	155.88	2156	32.82	75.65	154.85	2142	33.27	76.69	153.81	2127
231	31.83	73.54	157.46	2178	32.28	74.58	156.42	2163	32.73	75.61	155.39	2149	33.18	76.65	154.35	2135
231.5	31.75	73.50	158.00	2185	32.20	74.53	156.97	2171	32.64	75.57	155.93	2156	33.09	76.61	154.89	2142
232	31.66	73.46	158.54	2193	32.11	74.49	157.51	2178	32.56	75.53	156.47	2164	33.00	76.57	155.43	2150
232.5	31.58	73.42	159.09	2200	32.02	74.45	158.05	2186	32.47	75.49	157.01	2171	32.92	76.53	155.97	2157
233	31.49	73.37	159.63	2208	31.94	74.41	158.59	2193	32.38	75.45	157.55	2179	32.83	76.49	156.51	2165
233.5	31.41	73.33	160.17	2215	31.85	74.37	159.13	2201	32.29	75.41	158.09	2186	32.74	76.45	157.05	2172
234	31.32	73.29	160.71	2223	31.76	74.33	159.67	2208	32.21	75.37	158.63	2194	32.65	76.40	157.60	2180
234.5	31.24	73.25	161.25	2230	31.68	74.29	160.21	2216	32.12	75.33	159.17	2201	32.56	76.36	158.14	2187
235	31.15	73.21	161.79	2238	31.59	74.25	160.75	2223	32.04	75.29	159.72	2209	32.48	76.32	158.68	2195
235.5	31.07	73.17	162.33	2245	31.51	74.21	161.29	2231	31.95	75.24	160.26	2216	32.39	76.28	159.22	2202
236	30.99	73.13	162.87	2253	31.43	74.17	161.83	2238	31.87	75.20	160.80	2224	32.31	76.24	159.76	2209
236.5	30.90	73.09	163.41	2260	31.34	74.12	162.38	2246	31.78	75.16	161.34	2231	32.22	76.20	160.30	2217
237	30.82	73.05	163.95	2267	31.26	74.08	162.92	2253	31.70	75.12	161.88	2239	32.13	76.16	160.84	2224
237.5	30.74	73.01	164.50	2275	31.18	74.04	163.46	2261	31.61	75.08	162.42	2246	32.05	76.12	161.38	2232
238	30.66	72.96	165.04	2282	31.09	74.00	164.00	2268	31.53	75.04	162.96	2254	31.96	76.08	161.92	2239
238.5	30.58	72.92	165.58	2290	31.01	73.96	164.54	2276	31.45	75.00	163.50	2261	31.88	76.04	162.46	2247
239	30.49	72.88	166.12	2297	30.93	73.92	165.08	2283	31.36	74.96	164.04	2269	31.80	75.99	163.01	2254
239.5	30.41	72.84	166.66	2305	30.85	73.88	165.62	2291	31.28	74.92	164.58	2276	31.71	75.95	163.55	2262
240	30.33	72.80	167.20	2312	30.77	73.84	166.16	2298	31.20	74.88	165.13	2284	31.63	75.91	164.09	2269
240.5	30.25	72.76	167.74	2320	30.68	73.80	166.70	2306	31.12	74.83	165.67	2291	31.55	75.87	164.63	2277
241	30.17	72.72	168.28	2327	30.60	73.76	167.24	2313	31.03	74.79	166.21	2299	31.46	75.83	165.17	2284
241.5	30.09	72.68	168.82	2335	30.52	73.71	167.79	2320	30.95	74.75	166.75	2306	31.38	75.79	165.71	2292
242	30.01	72.64	169.36	2342	30.44	73.67	168.33	2328	30.87	74.71	167.29	2314	31.30	75.75	166.25	2299
242.5	29.94	72.60	169.91	2350	30.36	73.63	168.87	2335	30.79	74.67	167.83	2321	31.22	75.71	166.79	2307
243	29.86	72.55	170.45	2357	30.28	73.59	169.41	2343	30.71	74.63	168.37	2329	31.14	75.67	167.33	2314
243.5	29.78	72.51	170.99	2365	30.21	73.55	169.95	2350	30.63	74.59	168.91	2336	31.06	75.63	167.87	2322
244	29.70	72.47	171.53	2372	30.13	73.51	170.49	2358	30.55	74.55	169.45	2344	30.98	75.58	168.42	2329
244.5	29.62	72.43	172.07	2380	30.05	73.47	171.03	2365	30.47	74.51	169.99	2351	30.90	75.54	168.96	2337
245	29.55	72.39	172.61	2387	29.97	73.43	171.57	2373	30.39	74.47	170.54	2358	30.82	75.50	169.50	2344
245.5	29.47	72.35	173.15	2395	29.89	73.39	172.11	2380	30.32	74.42	171.08	2366	30.74	75.46	170.04	2352
246	29.39	72.31	173.69	2402	29.82	73.35	172.65	2388	30.24	74.38	171.62	2373	30.66	75.42	170.58	2359
246.5	29.32	72.27	174.23	2410	29.74	73.30	173.20	2395	30.16	74.34	172.16	2381	30.58	75.38	171.12	2367
247	29.24	72.23	174.77	2417	29.66	73.26	173.74	2403	30.08	74.30	172.70	2388	30.50	75.34	171.66	2374
247.5	29.17	72.19	175.32	2425	29.58	73.22	174.28	2410	30.00	74.26	173.24	2396	30.42	75.30	172.20	2382

Body Composition MALE 216-247.5 Lb.

Weight: Lb.	Waist: 47 inches Fat: %	Fat: Lb.	LBM: Lb.	RMR: Cal.	47.25 inches Fat: %	Fat: Lb.	LBM: Lb.	RMR: Cal.	47.5 inches Fat: %	Fat: Lb.	LBM: Lb.	RMR: Cal.	47.75 inches Fat: %	Fat: Lb.	LBM: Lb.	RMR: Cal.
216	36.54	78.92	137.08	1896	37.02	79.96	136.04	1881	37.50	80.99	135.01	1867	37.98	82.03	133.97	1853
216.5	36.43	78.88	137.62	1903	36.91	79.91	136.59	1889	37.39	80.95	135.55	1875	37.87	81.99	134.51	1860
217	36.33	78.84	138.16	1911	36.81	79.87	137.13	1896	37.29	80.91	136.09	1882	37.76	81.95	135.05	1868
217.5	36.23	78.80	138.71	1918	36.70	79.83	137.67	1904	37.18	80.87	136.63	1890	37.66	81.91	135.59	1875
218	36.13	78.75	139.25	1926	36.60	79.79	138.21	1911	37.08	80.83	137.17	1897	37.55	81.87	136.13	1883
218.5	36.02	78.71	139.79	1933	36.50	79.75	138.75	1919	36.97	80.79	137.71	1905	37.45	81.83	136.67	1890
219	35.92	78.67	140.33	1941	36.40	79.71	139.29	1926	36.87	80.75	138.25	1912	37.34	81.78	137.22	1898
219.5	35.82	78.63	140.87	1948	36.30	79.67	139.83	1934	36.77	80.71	138.79	1920	37.24	81.74	137.76	1905
220	35.72	78.59	141.41	1956	36.19	79.63	140.37	1941	36.67	80.67	139.34	1927	37.14	81.70	138.30	1913
220.5	35.62	78.55	141.95	1963	36.09	79.59	140.91	1949	36.56	80.62	139.88	1934	37.03	81.66	138.84	1920
221	35.52	78.51	142.49	1971	35.99	79.55	141.45	1956	36.46	80.58	140.42	1942	36.93	81.62	139.38	1928
221.5	35.43	78.47	143.03	1978	35.89	79.50	142.00	1964	36.36	80.54	140.96	1949	36.83	81.58	139.92	1935
222	35.33	78.43	143.57	1986	35.79	79.46	142.54	1971	36.26	80.50	141.50	1957	36.73	81.54	140.46	1943
222.5	35.23	78.39	144.12	1993	35.70	79.42	143.08	1979	36.16	80.46	142.04	1964	36.63	81.50	141.00	1950
223	35.13	78.34	144.66	2001	35.60	79.38	143.62	1986	36.06	80.42	142.58	1972	36.53	81.46	141.54	1958
223.5	35.03	78.30	145.20	2008	35.50	79.34	144.16	1994	35.96	80.38	143.12	1979	36.43	81.42	142.08	1965
224	34.94	78.26	145.74	2016	35.40	79.30	144.70	2001	35.86	80.34	143.66	1987	36.33	81.37	142.63	1973
224.5	34.84	78.22	146.28	2023	35.30	79.26	145.24	2009	35.77	80.30	144.20	1994	36.23	81.33	143.17	1980
225	34.75	78.18	146.82	2031	35.21	79.22	145.78	2016	35.67	80.26	144.75	2002	36.13	81.29	143.71	1987
225.5	34.65	78.14	147.36	2038	35.11	79.18	146.32	2024	35.57	80.21	145.29	2009	36.03	81.25	144.25	1995
226	34.56	78.10	147.90	2045	35.02	79.14	146.86	2031	35.47	80.17	145.83	2017	35.93	81.21	144.79	2002
226.5	34.46	78.06	148.44	2053	34.92	79.09	147.41	2039	35.38	80.13	146.37	2024	35.84	81.17	145.33	2010
227	34.37	78.02	148.98	2060	34.83	79.05	147.95	2046	35.28	80.09	146.91	2032	35.74	81.13	145.87	2017
227.5	34.27	77.98	149.53	2068	34.73	79.01	148.49	2054	35.19	80.05	147.45	2039	35.64	81.09	146.41	2025
228	34.18	77.93	150.07	2075	34.64	78.97	149.03	2061	35.09	80.01	147.99	2047	35.55	81.05	146.95	2032
228.5	34.09	77.89	150.61	2083	34.54	78.93	149.57	2069	35.00	79.97	148.53	2054	35.45	81.01	147.49	2040
229	34.00	77.85	151.15	2090	34.45	78.89	150.11	2076	34.90	79.93	149.07	2062	35.36	80.96	148.04	2047
229.5	33.90	77.81	151.69	2098	34.36	78.85	150.65	2084	34.81	79.89	149.61	2069	35.26	80.92	148.58	2055
230	33.81	77.77	152.23	2105	34.26	78.81	151.19	2091	34.72	79.85	150.16	2077	35.17	80.88	149.12	2062
230.5	33.72	77.73	152.77	2113	34.17	78.77	151.73	2098	34.62	79.80	150.70	2084	35.07	80.84	149.66	2070
231	33.63	77.69	153.31	2120	34.08	78.73	152.27	2106	34.53	79.76	151.24	2092	34.98	80.80	150.20	2077
231.5	33.54	77.65	153.85	2128	33.99	78.68	152.82	2113	34.44	79.72	151.78	2099	34.89	80.76	150.74	2085
232	33.45	77.61	154.39	2135	33.90	78.64	153.36	2121	34.35	79.68	152.32	2107	34.79	80.72	151.28	2092
232.5	33.36	77.57	154.94	2143	33.81	78.60	153.90	2128	34.25	79.64	152.86	2114	34.70	80.68	151.82	2100
233	33.27	77.52	155.48	2150	33.72	78.56	154.44	2136	34.16	79.60	153.40	2122	34.61	80.64	152.36	2107
233.5	33.18	77.48	156.02	2158	33.63	78.52	154.98	2143	34.07	79.56	153.94	2129	34.52	80.60	152.90	2115
234	33.09	77.44	156.56	2165	33.54	78.48	155.52	2151	33.98	79.52	154.48	2136	34.43	80.55	153.45	2122
234.5	33.01	77.40	157.10	2173	33.45	78.44	156.06	2158	33.89	79.48	155.02	2144	34.33	80.51	153.99	2130
235	32.92	77.36	157.64	2180	33.36	78.40	156.60	2166	33.80	79.44	155.57	2151	34.24	80.47	154.53	2137
235.5	32.83	77.32	158.18	2188	33.27	78.36	157.14	2173	33.71	79.39	156.11	2159	34.15	80.43	155.07	2145
236	32.74	77.28	158.72	2195	33.18	78.32	157.68	2181	33.62	79.35	156.65	2166	34.06	80.39	155.61	2152
236.5	32.66	77.24	159.26	2203	33.10	78.27	158.23	2188	33.54	79.31	157.19	2174	33.97	80.35	156.15	2160
237	32.57	77.20	159.80	2210	33.01	78.23	158.77	2196	33.45	79.27	157.73	2181	33.89	80.31	156.69	2167
237.5	32.49	77.16	160.35	2218	32.92	78.19	159.31	2203	33.36	79.23	158.27	2189	33.80	80.27	157.23	2175
238	32.40	77.11	160.89	2225	32.84	78.15	159.85	2211	33.27	79.19	158.81	2196	33.71	80.23	157.77	2182
238.5	32.32	77.07	161.43	2233	32.75	78.11	160.39	2218	33.19	79.15	159.35	2204	33.62	80.19	158.31	2189
239	32.23	77.03	161.97	2240	32.67	78.07	160.93	2226	33.10	79.11	159.89	2211	33.53	80.14	158.86	2197
239.5	32.15	76.99	162.51	2247	32.58	78.03	161.47	2233	33.01	79.07	160.43	2219	33.45	80.10	159.40	2204
240	32.06	76.95	163.05	2255	32.49	77.99	162.01	2241	32.93	79.03	160.98	2226	33.36	80.06	159.94	2212
240.5	31.98	76.91	163.59	2262	32.41	77.95	162.55	2248	32.84	78.98	161.52	2234	33.27	80.02	160.48	2219
241	31.90	76.87	164.13	2270	32.33	77.91	163.09	2256	32.76	78.94	162.06	2241	33.19	79.98	161.02	2227
241.5	31.81	76.83	164.67	2277	32.24	77.86	163.64	2263	32.67	78.90	162.60	2249	33.10	79.94	161.56	2234
242	31.73	76.79	165.21	2285	32.16	77.82	164.18	2271	32.59	78.86	163.14	2256	33.02	79.90	162.10	2242
242.5	31.65	76.75	165.76	2292	32.08	77.78	164.72	2278	32.50	78.82	163.68	2264	32.93	79.86	162.64	2249
243	31.57	76.70	166.30	2300	31.99	77.74	165.26	2286	32.42	78.78	164.22	2271	32.85	79.82	163.18	2257
243.5	31.48	76.66	166.84	2307	31.91	77.70	165.80	2293	32.34	78.74	164.76	2279	32.76	79.78	163.72	2264
244	31.40	76.62	167.38	2315	31.83	77.66	166.34	2300	32.25	78.70	165.30	2286	32.68	79.73	164.27	2272
244.5	31.32	76.58	167.92	2322	31.75	77.62	166.88	2308	32.17	78.66	165.84	2294	32.59	79.69	164.81	2279
245	31.24	76.54	168.46	2330	31.66	77.58	167.42	2315	32.09	78.62	166.39	2301	32.51	79.65	165.35	2287
245.5	31.16	76.50	169.00	2337	31.58	77.54	167.96	2323	32.01	78.57	166.93	2309	32.43	79.61	165.89	2294
246	31.08	76.46	169.54	2345	31.50	77.50	168.50	2330	31.92	78.53	167.47	2316	32.35	79.57	166.43	2302
246.5	31.00	76.42	170.08	2352	31.42	77.45	169.05	2338	31.84	78.49	168.01	2324	32.26	79.53	166.97	2309
247	30.92	76.38	170.62	2360	31.34	77.41	169.59	2345	31.76	78.45	168.55	2331	32.18	79.49	167.51	2317
247.5	30.84	76.34	171.17	2367	31.26	77.37	170.13	2353	31.68	78.41	169.09	2339	32.10	79.45	168.05	2324

Body Composition MALE 216-247.5 Lb.

Weight: Lb.	Waist: 48 inches Fat: %	Fat: Lb.	LBM: Lb.	RMR: Cal.	48.25 inches Fat: %	Fat: Lb.	LBM: Lb.	RMR: Cal.	48.5 inches Fat: %	Fat: Lb.	LBM: Lb.	RMR: Cal.	48.75 inches Fat: %	Fat: Lb.	LBM: Lb.	RMR: Cal.
216	38.46	83.07	132.93	1838	38.94	84.11	131.89	1824	39.42	85.14	130.86	1810	39.90	86.18	129.82	1795
216.5	38.35	83.03	133.47	1846	38.83	84.06	132.44	1832	39.31	85.10	131.40	1817	39.79	86.14	130.36	1803
217	38.24	82.99	134.01	1853	38.72	84.02	132.98	1839	39.20	85.06	131.94	1825	39.68	86.10	130.90	1810
217.5	38.14	82.95	134.56	1861	38.61	83.98	133.52	1847	39.09	85.02	132.48	1832	39.57	86.06	131.44	1818
218	38.03	82.90	135.10	1868	38.51	83.94	134.06	1854	38.98	84.98	133.02	1840	39.46	86.02	131.98	1825
218.5	37.92	82.86	135.64	1876	38.40	83.90	134.60	1862	38.87	84.94	133.56	1847	39.35	85.98	132.52	1833
219	37.82	82.82	136.18	1883	38.29	83.86	135.14	1869	38.77	84.90	134.10	1855	39.24	85.93	133.07	1840
219.5	37.71	82.78	136.72	1891	38.19	83.82	135.68	1876	38.66	84.86	134.64	1862	39.13	85.89	133.61	1848
220	37.61	82.74	137.26	1898	38.08	83.78	136.22	1884	38.55	84.82	135.19	1870	39.02	85.85	134.15	1855
220.5	37.51	82.70	137.80	1906	37.98	83.74	136.76	1891	38.45	84.77	135.73	1877	38.92	85.81	134.69	1863
221	37.40	82.66	138.34	1913	37.87	83.70	137.30	1899	38.34	84.73	136.27	1885	38.81	85.77	135.23	1870
221.5	37.30	82.62	138.88	1921	37.77	83.65	137.85	1906	38.24	84.69	136.81	1892	38.70	85.73	135.77	1878
222	37.20	82.58	139.42	1928	37.66	83.61	138.39	1914	38.13	84.65	137.35	1900	38.60	85.69	136.31	1885
222.5	37.09	82.54	139.97	1936	37.56	83.57	138.93	1921	38.03	84.61	137.89	1907	38.49	85.65	136.85	1893
223	36.99	82.49	140.51	1943	37.46	83.53	139.47	1929	37.92	84.57	138.43	1915	38.39	85.61	137.39	1900
223.5	36.89	82.45	141.05	1951	37.36	83.49	140.01	1936	37.82	84.53	138.97	1922	38.28	85.57	137.93	1908
224	36.79	82.41	141.59	1958	37.25	83.45	140.55	1944	37.72	84.49	139.51	1929	38.18	85.52	138.48	1915
224.5	36.69	82.37	142.13	1966	37.15	83.41	141.09	1951	37.62	84.45	140.05	1937	38.08	85.48	139.02	1923
225	36.59	82.33	142.67	1973	37.05	83.37	141.63	1959	37.51	84.41	140.60	1944	37.97	85.44	139.56	1930
225.5	36.49	82.29	143.21	1981	36.95	83.33	142.17	1966	37.41	84.36	141.14	1952	37.87	85.40	140.10	1938
226	36.39	82.25	143.75	1988	36.85	83.29	142.71	1974	37.31	84.32	141.68	1959	37.77	85.36	140.64	1945
226.5	36.29	82.21	144.29	1996	36.75	83.24	143.26	1981	37.21	84.28	142.22	1967	37.67	85.32	141.18	1953
227	36.20	82.17	144.83	2003	36.65	83.20	143.80	1989	37.11	84.24	142.76	1974	37.57	85.28	141.72	1960
227.5	36.10	82.13	145.38	2011	36.55	83.16	144.34	1996	37.01	84.20	143.30	1982	37.47	85.24	142.26	1967
228	36.00	82.08	145.92	2018	36.46	83.12	144.88	2004	36.91	84.16	143.84	1989	37.37	85.20	142.80	1975
228.5	35.91	82.04	146.46	2026	36.36	83.08	145.42	2011	36.81	84.12	144.38	1997	37.27	85.16	143.34	1982
229	35.81	82.00	147.00	2033	36.26	83.04	145.96	2019	36.71	84.08	144.92	2004	37.17	85.11	143.89	1990
229.5	35.71	81.96	147.54	2040	36.16	83.00	146.50	2026	36.62	84.04	145.46	2012	37.07	85.07	144.43	1997
230	35.62	81.92	148.08	2048	36.07	82.96	147.04	2034	36.52	84.00	146.01	2019	36.97	85.03	144.97	2005
230.5	35.52	81.88	148.62	2055	35.97	82.92	147.58	2041	36.42	83.95	146.55	2027	36.87	84.99	145.51	2012
231	35.43	81.84	149.16	2063	35.88	82.88	148.12	2049	36.33	83.91	147.09	2034	36.78	84.95	146.05	2020
231.5	35.33	81.80	149.70	2070	35.78	82.83	148.67	2056	36.23	83.87	147.63	2042	36.68	84.91	146.59	2027
232	35.24	81.76	150.24	2078	35.69	82.79	149.21	2064	36.13	83.83	148.17	2049	36.58	84.87	147.13	2035
232.5	35.15	81.72	150.79	2085	35.59	82.75	149.75	2071	36.04	83.79	148.71	2057	36.48	84.83	147.67	2042
233	35.05	81.67	151.33	2093	35.50	82.71	150.29	2078	35.94	83.75	149.25	2064	36.39	84.79	148.21	2050
233.5	34.96	81.63	151.87	2100	35.40	82.67	150.83	2086	35.85	83.71	149.79	2072	36.29	84.75	148.75	2057
234	34.87	81.59	152.41	2108	35.31	82.63	151.37	2093	35.76	83.67	150.33	2079	36.20	84.70	149.30	2065
234.5	34.78	81.55	152.95	2115	35.22	82.59	151.91	2101	35.66	83.63	150.87	2087	36.10	84.66	149.84	2072
235	34.69	81.51	153.49	2123	35.13	82.55	152.45	2108	35.57	83.59	151.42	2094	36.01	84.62	150.38	2080
235.5	34.59	81.47	154.03	2130	35.03	82.51	152.99	2116	35.48	83.54	151.96	2102	35.92	84.58	150.92	2087
236	34.50	81.43	154.57	2138	34.94	82.47	153.53	2123	35.38	83.50	152.50	2109	35.82	84.54	151.46	2095
236.5	34.41	81.39	155.11	2145	34.85	82.42	154.08	2131	35.29	83.46	153.04	2117	35.73	84.50	152.00	2102
237	34.32	81.35	155.65	2153	34.76	82.38	154.62	2138	35.20	83.42	153.58	2124	35.64	84.46	152.54	2110
237.5	34.23	81.31	156.20	2160	34.67	82.34	155.16	2146	35.11	83.38	154.12	2131	35.54	84.42	153.08	2117
238	34.14	81.26	156.74	2168	34.58	82.30	155.70	2153	35.02	83.34	154.66	2139	35.45	84.38	153.62	2125
238.5	34.06	81.22	157.28	2175	34.49	82.26	156.24	2161	34.93	83.30	155.20	2146	35.36	84.34	154.16	2132
239	33.97	81.18	157.82	2183	34.40	82.22	156.78	2168	34.84	83.26	155.74	2154	35.27	84.29	154.71	2140
239.5	33.88	81.14	158.36	2190	34.31	82.18	157.32	2176	34.75	83.22	156.28	2161	35.18	84.25	155.25	2147
240	33.79	81.10	158.90	2198	34.22	82.14	157.86	2183	34.66	83.18	156.83	2169	35.09	84.21	155.79	2155
240.5	33.70	81.06	159.44	2205	34.14	82.10	158.40	2191	34.57	83.13	157.37	2176	35.00	84.17	156.33	2162
241	33.62	81.02	159.98	2213	34.05	82.06	158.94	2198	34.48	83.09	157.91	2184	34.91	84.13	156.87	2170
241.5	33.53	80.98	160.52	2220	33.96	82.01	159.49	2206	34.39	83.05	158.45	2191	34.82	84.09	157.41	2177
242	33.44	80.94	161.06	2228	33.87	81.97	160.03	2213	34.30	83.01	158.99	2199	34.73	84.05	157.95	2184
242.5	33.36	80.90	161.61	2235	33.79	81.93	160.57	2221	34.21	82.97	159.53	2206	34.64	84.01	158.49	2192
243	33.27	80.85	162.15	2242	33.70	81.89	161.11	2228	34.13	82.93	160.07	2214	34.55	83.97	159.03	2199
243.5	33.19	80.81	162.69	2250	33.61	81.85	161.65	2236	34.04	82.89	160.61	2221	34.47	83.93	159.57	2207
244	33.10	80.77	163.23	2257	33.53	81.81	162.19	2243	33.95	82.85	161.15	2229	34.38	83.88	160.12	2214
244.5	33.02	80.73	163.77	2265	33.44	81.77	162.73	2251	33.87	82.81	161.69	2236	34.29	83.84	160.66	2222
245	32.93	80.69	164.31	2272	33.36	81.73	163.27	2258	33.78	82.77	162.24	2244	34.21	83.80	161.20	2229
245.5	32.85	80.65	164.85	2280	33.27	81.69	163.81	2266	33.70	82.72	162.78	2251	34.12	83.76	161.74	2237
246	32.77	80.61	165.39	2287	33.19	81.65	164.35	2273	33.61	82.68	163.32	2259	34.03	83.72	162.28	2244
246.5	32.68	80.57	165.93	2295	33.11	81.60	164.90	2281	33.53	82.64	163.86	2266	33.95	83.68	162.82	2252
247	32.60	80.53	166.47	2302	33.02	81.56	165.44	2288	33.44	82.60	164.40	2274	33.86	83.64	163.36	2259
247.5	32.52	80.49	167.02	2310	32.94	81.52	165.98	2295	33.36	82.56	164.94	2281	33.78	83.60	163.90	2267

Body Composition   MALE   216-247.5 Lb.

Weight: Lb.	Waist: 49 inches				49.25 inches				49.5 inches				49.75 inches			
	Fat: %	Fat: Lb.	LBM: Lb.	RMR: Cal.	Fat: %	Fat: Lb.	LBM: Lb.	RMR: Cal.	Fat: %	Fat: Lb.	LBM: Lb.	RMR: Cal.	Fat: %	Fat: Lb.	LBM: Lb.	RMR: Cal.
216	40.38	87.22	128.78	1781	40.86	88.26	127.74	1767	41.34	89.29	126.71	1752	41.82	90.33	125.67	1738
216.5	40.27	87.18	129.32	1789	40.75	88.21	128.29	1774	41.22	89.25	127.25	1760	41.70	90.29	126.21	1745
217	40.15	87.14	129.86	1796	40.63	88.17	128.83	1782	41.11	89.21	127.79	1767	41.59	90.25	126.75	1753
217.5	40.04	87.10	130.41	1804	40.52	88.13	129.37	1789	41.00	89.17	128.33	1775	41.47	90.21	127.29	1760
218	39.93	87.05	130.95	1811	40.41	88.09	129.91	1797	40.88	89.13	128.87	1782	41.36	90.17	127.83	1768
218.5	39.82	87.01	131.49	1818	40.30	88.05	130.45	1804	40.77	89.09	129.41	1790	41.25	90.13	128.37	1775
219	39.71	86.97	132.03	1826	40.19	88.01	130.99	1812	40.66	89.05	129.95	1797	41.13	90.08	128.92	1783
219.5	39.60	86.93	132.57	1833	40.08	87.97	131.53	1819	40.55	89.01	130.49	1805	41.02	90.04	129.46	1790
220	39.50	86.89	133.11	1841	39.97	87.93	132.07	1827	40.44	88.97	131.04	1812	40.91	90.00	130.00	1798
220.5	39.39	86.85	133.65	1848	39.86	87.89	132.61	1834	40.33	88.92	131.58	1820	40.80	89.96	130.54	1805
221	39.28	86.81	134.19	1856	39.75	87.85	133.15	1842	40.22	88.88	132.12	1827	40.69	89.92	131.08	1813
221.5	39.17	86.77	134.73	1863	39.64	87.80	133.70	1849	40.11	88.84	132.66	1835	40.58	89.88	131.62	1820
222	39.07	86.73	135.27	1871	39.53	87.76	134.24	1856	40.00	88.80	133.20	1842	40.47	89.84	132.16	1828
222.5	38.96	86.69	135.82	1878	39.43	87.72	134.78	1864	39.89	88.76	133.74	1850	40.36	89.80	132.70	1835
223	38.85	86.64	136.36	1886	39.32	87.68	135.32	1871	39.78	88.72	134.28	1857	40.25	89.76	133.24	1843
223.5	38.75	86.60	136.90	1893	39.21	87.64	135.86	1879	39.68	88.68	134.82	1865	40.14	89.72	133.78	1850
224	38.64	86.56	137.44	1901	39.11	87.60	136.40	1886	39.57	88.64	135.36	1872	40.03	89.67	134.33	1858
224.5	38.54	86.52	137.98	1908	39.00	87.56	136.94	1894	39.46	88.60	135.90	1880	39.93	89.63	134.87	1865
225	38.44	86.48	138.52	1916	38.90	87.52	137.48	1901	39.36	88.56	136.45	1887	39.82	89.59	135.41	1873
225.5	38.33	86.44	139.06	1923	38.79	87.48	138.02	1909	39.25	88.51	136.99	1895	39.71	89.55	135.95	1880
226	38.23	86.40	139.60	1931	38.69	87.44	138.56	1916	39.15	88.47	137.53	1902	39.61	89.51	136.49	1888
226.5	38.13	86.36	140.14	1938	38.58	87.39	139.11	1924	39.04	88.43	138.07	1909	39.50	89.47	137.03	1895
227	38.02	86.32	140.68	1946	38.48	87.35	139.65	1931	38.94	88.39	138.61	1917	39.40	89.43	137.57	1903
227.5	37.92	86.28	141.23	1953	38.38	87.31	140.19	1939	38.84	88.35	139.15	1924	39.29	89.39	138.11	1910
228	37.82	86.23	141.77	1961	38.28	87.27	140.73	1946	38.73	88.31	139.69	1932	39.19	89.35	138.65	1918
228.5	37.72	86.19	142.31	1968	38.18	87.23	141.27	1954	38.63	88.27	140.23	1939	39.08	89.31	139.19	1925
229	37.62	86.15	142.85	1976	38.07	87.19	141.81	1961	38.53	88.23	140.77	1947	38.98	89.26	139.74	1933
229.5	37.52	86.11	143.39	1983	37.97	87.15	142.35	1969	38.43	88.19	141.31	1954	38.88	89.22	140.28	1940
230	37.42	86.07	143.93	1991	37.87	87.11	142.89	1976	38.32	88.15	141.86	1962	38.78	89.18	140.82	1948
230.5	37.32	86.03	144.47	1998	37.77	87.07	143.43	1984	38.22	88.10	142.40	1969	38.67	89.14	141.36	1955
231	37.22	85.99	145.01	2006	37.67	87.03	143.97	1991	38.12	88.06	142.94	1977	38.57	89.10	141.90	1962
231.5	37.13	85.95	145.55	2013	37.57	86.98	144.52	1999	38.02	88.02	143.48	1984	38.47	89.06	142.44	1970
232	37.03	85.91	146.09	2020	37.48	86.94	145.06	2006	37.92	87.98	144.02	1992	38.37	89.02	142.98	1977
232.5	36.93	85.87	146.64	2028	37.38	86.90	145.60	2014	37.82	87.94	144.56	1999	38.27	88.98	143.52	1985
233	36.83	85.82	147.18	2035	37.28	86.86	146.14	2021	37.72	87.90	145.10	2007	38.17	88.94	144.06	1992
233.5	36.74	85.78	147.72	2043	37.18	86.82	146.68	2029	37.63	87.86	145.64	2014	38.07	88.90	144.60	2000
234	36.64	85.74	148.26	2050	37.09	86.78	147.22	2036	37.53	87.82	146.18	2022	37.97	88.85	145.15	2007
234.5	36.55	85.70	148.80	2058	36.99	86.74	147.76	2044	37.43	87.78	146.72	2029	37.87	88.81	145.69	2015
235	36.45	85.66	149.34	2065	36.89	86.70	148.30	2051	37.33	87.74	147.27	2037	37.78	88.77	146.23	2022
235.5	36.36	85.62	149.88	2073	36.80	86.66	148.84	2059	37.24	87.69	147.81	2044	37.68	88.73	146.77	2030
236	36.26	85.58	150.42	2080	36.70	86.62	149.38	2066	37.14	87.65	148.35	2052	37.58	88.69	147.31	2037
236.5	36.17	85.54	150.96	2088	36.61	86.57	149.93	2073	37.05	87.61	148.89	2059	37.48	88.65	147.85	2045
237	36.07	85.50	151.50	2095	36.51	86.53	150.47	2081	36.95	87.57	149.43	2067	37.39	88.61	148.39	2052
237.5	35.98	85.46	152.05	2103	36.42	86.49	151.01	2088	36.85	87.53	149.97	2074	37.29	88.57	148.93	2060
238	35.89	85.41	152.59	2110	36.32	86.45	151.55	2096	36.76	87.49	150.51	2082	37.20	88.53	149.47	2067
238.5	35.80	85.37	153.13	2118	36.23	86.41	152.09	2103	36.67	87.45	151.05	2089	37.10	88.49	150.01	2075
239	35.70	85.33	153.67	2125	36.14	86.37	152.63	2111	36.57	87.41	151.59	2097	37.01	88.44	150.56	2082
239.5	35.61	85.29	154.21	2133	36.05	86.33	153.17	2118	36.48	87.37	152.13	2104	36.91	88.40	151.10	2090
240	35.52	85.25	154.75	2140	35.95	86.29	153.71	2126	36.39	87.33	152.68	2111	36.82	88.36	151.64	2097
240.5	35.43	85.21	155.29	2148	35.86	86.25	154.25	2133	36.29	87.28	153.22	2119	36.72	88.32	152.18	2105
241	35.34	85.17	155.83	2155	35.77	86.21	154.79	2141	36.20	87.24	153.76	2126	36.63	88.28	152.72	2112
241.5	35.25	85.13	156.37	2163	35.68	86.16	155.34	2148	36.11	87.20	154.30	2134	36.54	88.24	153.26	2120
242	35.16	85.09	156.91	2170	35.59	86.12	155.88	2156	36.02	87.16	154.84	2141	36.45	88.20	153.80	2127
242.5	35.07	85.05	157.46	2178	35.50	86.08	156.42	2163	35.93	87.12	155.38	2149	36.35	88.16	154.34	2135
243	34.98	85.00	158.00	2185	35.41	86.04	156.96	2171	35.83	87.08	155.92	2156	36.26	88.12	154.88	2142
243.5	34.89	84.96	158.54	2193	35.32	86.00	157.50	2178	35.74	87.04	156.46	2164	36.17	88.08	155.42	2150
244	34.80	84.92	159.08	2200	35.23	85.96	158.04	2186	35.65	87.00	157.00	2171	36.08	88.03	155.97	2157
244.5	34.72	84.88	159.62	2208	35.14	85.92	158.58	2193	35.56	86.96	157.54	2179	35.99	87.99	156.51	2164
245	34.63	84.84	160.16	2215	35.05	85.88	159.12	2201	35.48	86.92	158.09	2186	35.90	87.95	157.05	2172
245.5	34.54	84.80	160.70	2222	34.96	85.84	159.66	2208	35.39	86.87	158.63	2194	35.81	87.91	157.59	2179
246	34.45	84.76	161.24	2230	34.88	85.80	160.20	2216	35.30	86.83	159.17	2201	35.72	87.87	158.13	2187
246.5	34.37	84.72	161.78	2237	34.79	85.75	160.75	2223	35.21	86.79	159.71	2209	35.63	87.83	158.67	2194
247	34.28	84.68	162.32	2245	34.70	85.71	161.29	2231	35.12	86.75	160.25	2216	35.54	87.79	159.21	2202
247.5	34.20	84.64	162.87	2252	34.62	85.67	161.83	2238	35.03	86.71	160.79	2224	35.45	87.75	159.75	2209

Body Composition MALE 216-247.5 Lb.

Weight: Lb.	Waist: 50 inches				50.25 inches				50.5 inches				50.75 inches			
	Fat: %	Fat: Lb.	LBM: Lb.	RMR: Cal.	Fat: %	Fat: Lb.	LBM: Lb.	RMR: Cal.	Fat: %	Fat: Lb.	LBM: Lb.	RMR: Cal.	Fat: %	Fat: Lb.	LBM: Lb.	RMR: Cal.
216	42.30	91.37	124.63	1724	42.78	92.41	123.59	1709	43.26	93.44	122.56	1695	43.74	94.48	121.52	1681
216.5	42.18	91.33	125.17	1731	42.66	92.36	124.14	1717	43.14	93.40	123.10	1702	43.62	94.44	122.06	1688
217	42.07	91.29	125.71	1739	42.55	92.32	124.68	1724	43.02	93.36	123.64	1710	43.50	94.40	122.60	1696
217.5	41.95	91.25	126.26	1746	42.43	92.28	125.22	1732	42.91	93.32	124.18	1717	43.38	94.36	123.14	1703
218	41.84	91.20	126.80	1754	42.31	92.24	125.76	1739	42.79	93.28	124.72	1725	43.26	94.32	123.68	1711
218.5	41.72	91.16	127.34	1761	42.20	92.20	126.30	1747	42.67	93.24	125.26	1732	43.15	94.28	124.22	1718
219	41.61	91.12	127.88	1769	42.08	92.16	126.84	1754	42.56	93.20	125.80	1740	43.03	94.23	124.77	1726
219.5	41.49	91.08	128.42	1776	41.97	92.12	127.38	1762	42.44	93.16	126.34	1747	42.91	94.19	125.31	1733
220	41.38	91.04	128.96	1784	41.85	92.08	127.92	1769	42.33	93.12	126.89	1755	42.80	94.15	125.85	1740
220.5	41.27	91.00	129.50	1791	41.74	92.04	128.46	1777	42.21	93.07	127.43	1762	42.68	94.11	126.39	1748
221	41.16	90.96	130.04	1798	41.63	92.00	129.00	1784	42.10	93.03	127.97	1770	42.57	94.07	126.93	1755
221.5	41.05	90.92	130.58	1806	41.51	91.95	129.55	1792	41.98	92.99	128.51	1777	42.45	94.03	127.47	1763
222	40.94	90.88	131.12	1813	41.40	91.91	130.09	1799	41.87	92.95	129.05	1785	42.34	93.99	128.01	1770
222.5	40.82	90.84	131.67	1821	41.29	91.87	130.63	1807	41.76	92.91	129.59	1792	42.22	93.95	128.55	1778
223	40.71	90.79	132.21	1828	41.18	91.83	131.17	1814	41.65	92.87	130.13	1800	42.11	93.91	129.09	1785
223.5	40.61	90.75	132.75	1836	41.07	91.79	131.71	1822	41.53	92.83	130.67	1807	42.00	93.87	129.63	1793
224	40.50	90.71	133.29	1843	40.96	91.75	132.25	1829	41.42	92.79	131.21	1815	41.89	93.82	130.18	1800
224.5	40.39	90.67	133.83	1851	40.85	91.71	132.79	1837	41.31	92.75	131.75	1822	41.77	93.78	130.72	1808
225	40.28	90.63	134.37	1858	40.74	91.67	133.33	1844	41.20	92.71	132.30	1830	41.66	93.74	131.26	1815
225.5	40.17	90.59	134.91	1866	40.63	91.63	133.87	1851	41.09	92.66	132.84	1837	41.55	93.70	131.80	1823
226	40.07	90.55	135.45	1873	40.52	91.59	134.41	1859	40.98	92.62	133.38	1845	41.44	93.66	132.34	1830
226.5	39.96	90.51	135.99	1881	40.42	91.54	134.96	1866	40.88	92.58	133.92	1852	41.33	93.62	132.88	1838
227	39.85	90.47	136.53	1888	40.31	91.50	135.50	1874	40.77	92.54	134.46	1860	41.22	93.58	133.42	1845
227.5	39.75	90.43	137.08	1896	40.20	91.46	136.04	1881	40.66	92.50	135.00	1867	41.12	93.54	133.96	1853
228	39.64	90.38	137.62	1903	40.10	91.42	136.58	1889	40.55	92.46	135.54	1875	41.01	93.50	134.50	1860
228.5	39.54	90.34	138.16	1911	39.99	91.38	137.12	1896	40.45	92.42	136.08	1882	40.90	93.46	135.04	1868
229	39.43	90.30	138.70	1918	39.89	91.34	137.66	1904	40.34	92.38	136.62	1889	40.79	93.41	135.59	1875
229.5	39.33	90.26	139.24	1926	39.78	91.30	138.20	1911	40.23	92.34	137.16	1897	40.69	93.37	136.13	1883
230	39.23	90.22	139.78	1933	39.68	91.26	138.74	1919	40.13	92.30	137.71	1904	40.58	93.33	136.67	1890
230.5	39.12	90.18	140.32	1941	39.57	91.22	139.28	1926	40.02	92.25	138.25	1912	40.47	93.29	137.21	1898
231	39.02	90.14	140.86	1948	39.47	91.18	139.82	1934	39.92	92.21	138.79	1919	40.37	93.25	137.75	1905
231.5	38.92	90.10	141.40	1956	39.37	91.13	140.37	1941	39.82	92.17	139.33	1927	40.26	93.21	138.29	1913
232	38.82	90.06	141.94	1963	39.26	91.09	140.91	1949	39.71	92.13	139.87	1934	40.16	93.17	138.83	1920
232.5	38.72	90.02	142.49	1971	39.16	91.05	141.45	1956	39.61	92.09	140.41	1942	40.05	93.13	139.37	1928
233	38.62	89.97	143.03	1978	39.06	91.01	141.99	1964	39.51	92.05	140.95	1949	39.95	93.09	139.91	1935
233.5	38.52	89.93	143.57	1986	38.96	90.97	142.53	1971	39.40	92.01	141.49	1957	39.85	93.05	140.45	1942
234	38.42	89.89	144.11	1993	38.86	90.93	143.07	1979	39.30	91.97	142.03	1964	39.75	93.00	141.00	1950
234.5	38.32	89.85	144.65	2000	38.76	90.89	143.61	1986	39.20	91.93	142.57	1972	39.64	92.96	141.54	1957
235	38.22	89.81	145.19	2008	38.66	90.85	144.15	1994	39.10	91.89	143.12	1979	39.54	92.92	142.08	1965
235.5	38.12	89.77	145.73	2015	38.56	90.81	144.69	2001	39.00	91.84	143.66	1987	39.44	92.88	142.62	1972
236	38.02	89.73	146.27	2023	38.46	90.77	145.23	2009	38.90	91.80	144.20	1994	39.34	92.84	143.16	1980
236.5	37.92	89.69	146.81	2030	38.36	90.72	145.78	2016	38.80	91.76	144.74	2002	39.24	92.80	143.70	1987
237	37.83	89.65	147.35	2038	38.26	90.68	146.32	2024	38.70	91.72	145.28	2009	39.14	92.76	144.24	1995
237.5	37.73	89.61	147.90	2045	38.17	90.64	146.86	2031	38.60	91.68	145.82	2017	39.04	92.72	144.78	2002
238	37.63	89.56	148.44	2053	38.07	90.60	147.40	2039	38.50	91.64	146.36	2024	38.94	92.68	145.32	2010
238.5	37.54	89.52	148.98	2060	37.97	90.56	147.94	2046	38.41	91.60	146.90	2032	38.84	92.64	145.86	2017
239	37.44	89.48	149.52	2068	37.87	90.52	148.48	2053	38.31	91.56	147.44	2039	38.74	92.59	146.41	2025
239.5	37.34	89.44	150.06	2075	37.78	90.48	149.02	2061	38.21	91.52	147.98	2047	38.64	92.55	146.95	2032
240	37.25	89.40	150.60	2083	37.68	90.44	149.56	2068	38.11	91.48	148.53	2054	38.55	92.51	147.49	2040
240.5	37.16	89.36	151.14	2090	37.59	90.40	150.10	2076	38.02	91.43	149.07	2062	38.45	92.47	148.03	2047
241	37.06	89.32	151.68	2098	37.49	90.36	150.64	2083	37.92	91.39	149.61	2069	38.35	92.43	148.57	2055
241.5	36.97	89.28	152.22	2105	37.40	90.31	151.19	2091	37.83	91.35	150.15	2077	38.26	92.39	149.11	2062
242	36.87	89.24	152.76	2113	37.30	90.27	151.73	2098	37.73	91.31	150.69	2084	38.16	92.35	149.65	2070
242.5	36.78	89.20	153.31	2120	37.21	90.23	152.27	2106	37.64	91.27	151.23	2092	38.06	92.31	150.19	2077
243	36.69	89.15	153.85	2128	37.12	90.19	152.81	2113	37.54	91.23	151.77	2099	37.97	92.27	150.73	2085
243.5	36.60	89.11	154.39	2135	37.02	90.15	153.35	2121	37.45	91.19	152.31	2106	37.87	92.23	151.27	2092
244	36.50	89.07	154.93	2143	36.93	90.11	153.89	2128	37.36	91.15	152.85	2114	37.78	92.18	151.82	2100
244.5	36.41	89.03	155.47	2150	36.84	90.07	154.43	2136	37.26	91.11	153.39	2121	37.69	92.14	152.36	2107
245	36.32	88.99	156.01	2158	36.75	90.03	154.97	2143	37.17	91.07	153.94	2129	37.59	92.10	152.90	2115
245.5	36.23	88.95	156.55	2165	36.65	89.99	155.51	2151	37.08	91.02	154.48	2136	37.50	92.06	153.44	2122
246	36.14	88.91	157.09	2173	36.56	89.95	156.05	2158	36.98	90.98	155.02	2144	37.41	92.02	153.98	2130
246.5	36.05	88.87	157.63	2180	36.47	89.90	156.60	2166	36.89	90.94	155.56	2151	37.31	91.98	154.52	2137
247	35.96	88.83	158.17	2188	36.38	89.86	157.14	2173	36.80	90.90	156.10	2159	37.22	91.94	155.06	2145
247.5	35.87	88.79	158.72	2195	36.29	89.82	157.68	2181	36.71	90.86	156.64	2166	37.13	91.90	155.60	2152

Body Composition   MALE   216-247.5 Lb.

Weight: Lb.	Waist: 51 inches Fat: %	Fat: Lb.	LBM: Lb.	RMR: Cal.	51.25 inches Fat: %	Fat: Lb.	LBM: Lb.	RMR: Cal.	51.5 inches Fat: %	Fat: Lb.	LBM: Lb.	RMR: Cal.	51.75 inches Fat: %	Fat: Lb.	LBM: Lb.	RMR: Cal.
216	44.22	95.52	120.48	1666	44.70	96.56	119.44	1652	45.18	97.59	118.41	1638	45.66	98.63	117.37	1623
216.5	44.10	95.48	121.02	1674	44.58	96.51	119.99	1659	45.06	97.55	118.95	1645	45.54	98.59	117.91	1631
217	43.98	95.44	121.56	1681	44.46	96.47	120.53	1667	44.94	97.51	119.49	1653	45.41	98.55	118.45	1638
217.5	43.86	95.40	122.11	1689	44.34	96.43	121.07	1674	44.81	97.47	120.03	1660	45.29	98.51	118.99	1646
218	43.74	95.35	122.65	1696	44.22	96.39	121.61	1682	44.69	97.43	120.57	1667	45.17	98.47	119.53	1653
218.5	43.62	95.31	123.19	1704	44.10	96.35	122.15	1689	44.57	97.39	121.11	1675	45.05	98.43	120.07	1661
219	43.50	95.27	123.73	1711	43.98	96.31	122.69	1697	44.45	97.35	121.65	1682	44.92	98.38	120.62	1668
219.5	43.39	95.23	124.27	1719	43.86	96.27	123.23	1704	44.33	97.31	122.19	1690	44.80	98.34	121.16	1676
220	43.27	95.19	124.81	1726	43.74	96.23	123.77	1712	44.21	97.27	122.74	1697	44.68	98.30	121.70	1683
220.5	43.15	95.15	125.35	1734	43.62	96.19	124.31	1719	44.09	97.22	123.28	1705	44.56	98.26	122.24	1691
221	43.04	95.11	125.89	1741	43.50	96.15	124.85	1727	43.97	97.18	123.82	1712	44.44	98.22	122.78	1698
221.5	42.92	95.07	126.43	1749	43.39	96.10	125.40	1734	43.86	97.14	124.36	1720	44.32	98.18	123.32	1706
222	42.80	95.03	126.97	1756	43.27	96.06	125.94	1742	43.74	97.10	124.90	1727	44.21	98.14	123.86	1713
222.5	42.69	94.99	127.52	1764	43.16	96.02	126.48	1749	43.62	97.06	125.44	1735	44.09	98.10	124.40	1720
223	42.58	94.94	128.06	1771	43.04	95.98	127.02	1757	43.51	97.02	125.98	1742	43.97	98.06	124.94	1728
223.5	42.46	94.90	128.60	1778	42.93	95.94	127.56	1764	43.39	96.98	126.52	1750	43.85	98.02	125.48	1735
224	42.35	94.86	129.14	1786	42.81	95.90	128.10	1772	43.28	96.94	127.06	1757	43.74	97.97	126.03	1743
224.5	42.24	94.82	129.68	1793	42.70	95.86	128.64	1779	43.16	96.90	127.60	1765	43.62	97.93	126.57	1750
225	42.12	94.78	130.22	1801	42.59	95.82	129.18	1787	43.05	96.86	128.15	1772	43.51	97.89	127.11	1758
225.5	42.01	94.74	130.76	1808	42.47	95.78	129.72	1794	42.93	96.81	128.69	1780	43.39	97.85	127.65	1765
226	41.90	94.70	131.30	1816	42.36	95.74	130.26	1802	42.82	96.77	129.23	1787	43.28	97.81	128.19	1773
226.5	41.79	94.66	131.84	1823	42.25	95.69	130.81	1809	42.71	96.73	129.77	1795	43.17	97.77	128.73	1780
227	41.68	94.62	132.38	1831	42.14	95.65	131.35	1817	42.60	96.69	130.31	1802	43.05	97.73	129.27	1788
227.5	41.57	94.58	132.93	1838	42.03	95.61	131.89	1824	42.48	96.65	130.85	1810	42.94	97.69	129.81	1795
228	41.46	94.53	133.47	1846	41.92	95.57	132.43	1831	42.37	96.61	131.39	1817	42.83	97.65	130.35	1803
228.5	41.35	94.49	134.01	1853	41.81	95.53	132.97	1839	42.26	96.57	131.93	1825	42.72	97.61	130.89	1810
229	41.25	94.45	134.55	1861	41.70	95.49	133.51	1846	42.15	96.53	132.47	1832	42.60	97.56	131.44	1818
229.5	41.14	94.41	135.09	1868	41.59	95.45	134.05	1854	42.04	96.49	133.01	1840	42.49	97.52	131.98	1825
230	41.03	94.37	135.63	1876	41.48	95.41	134.59	1861	41.93	96.45	133.56	1847	42.38	97.48	132.52	1833
230.5	40.92	94.33	136.17	1883	41.37	95.37	135.13	1869	41.82	96.40	134.10	1855	42.27	97.44	133.06	1840
231	40.82	94.29	136.71	1891	41.27	95.33	135.67	1876	41.72	96.36	134.64	1862	42.16	97.40	133.60	1848
231.5	40.71	94.25	137.25	1898	41.16	95.28	136.22	1884	41.61	96.32	135.18	1870	42.06	97.36	134.14	1855
232	40.61	94.21	137.79	1906	41.05	95.24	136.76	1891	41.50	96.28	135.72	1877	41.95	97.32	134.68	1863
232.5	40.50	94.17	138.34	1913	40.95	95.20	137.30	1899	41.39	96.24	136.26	1884	41.84	97.28	135.22	1870
233	40.40	94.12	138.88	1921	40.84	95.16	137.84	1906	41.29	96.20	136.80	1892	41.73	97.24	135.76	1878
233.5	40.29	94.08	139.42	1928	40.74	95.12	138.38	1914	41.18	96.16	137.34	1899	41.63	97.20	136.30	1885
234	40.19	94.04	139.96	1936	40.63	95.08	138.92	1921	41.08	96.12	137.88	1907	41.52	97.15	136.85	1893
234.5	40.09	94.00	140.50	1943	40.53	95.04	139.46	1929	40.97	96.08	138.42	1914	41.41	97.11	137.39	1900
235	39.98	93.96	141.04	1951	40.42	95.00	140.00	1936	40.87	96.04	138.97	1922	41.31	97.07	137.93	1908
235.5	39.88	93.92	141.58	1958	40.32	94.96	140.54	1944	40.76	95.99	139.51	1929	41.20	97.03	138.47	1915
236	39.78	93.88	142.12	1966	40.22	94.92	141.08	1951	40.66	95.95	140.05	1937	41.10	96.99	139.01	1923
236.5	39.68	93.84	142.66	1973	40.12	94.87	141.63	1959	40.55	95.91	140.59	1944	40.99	96.95	139.55	1930
237	39.58	93.80	143.20	1981	40.01	94.83	142.17	1966	40.45	95.87	141.13	1952	40.89	96.91	140.09	1937
237.5	39.48	93.76	143.75	1988	39.91	94.79	142.71	1974	40.35	95.83	141.67	1959	40.79	96.87	140.63	1945
238	39.38	93.71	144.29	1995	39.81	94.75	143.25	1981	40.25	95.79	142.21	1967	40.68	96.83	141.17	1952
238.5	39.28	93.67	144.83	2003	39.71	94.71	143.79	1989	40.15	95.75	142.75	1974	40.58	96.79	141.71	1960
239	39.18	93.63	145.37	2010	39.61	94.67	144.33	1996	40.04	95.71	143.29	1982	40.48	96.74	142.26	1967
239.5	39.08	93.59	145.91	2018	39.51	94.63	144.87	2004	39.94	95.67	143.83	1989	40.38	96.70	142.80	1975
240	38.98	93.55	146.45	2025	39.41	94.59	145.41	2011	39.84	95.63	144.38	1997	40.28	96.66	143.34	1982
240.5	38.88	93.51	146.99	2033	39.31	94.55	145.95	2019	39.74	95.58	144.92	2004	40.18	96.62	143.88	1990
241	38.78	93.47	147.53	2040	39.21	94.51	146.49	2026	39.64	95.54	145.46	2012	40.07	96.58	144.42	1997
241.5	38.69	93.43	148.07	2048	39.12	94.46	147.04	2034	39.55	95.50	146.00	2019	39.97	96.54	144.96	2005
242	38.59	93.39	148.61	2055	39.02	94.42	147.58	2041	39.45	95.46	146.54	2027	39.88	96.50	145.50	2012
242.5	38.49	93.35	149.16	2063	38.92	94.38	148.12	2048	39.35	95.42	147.08	2034	39.78	96.46	146.04	2020
243	38.40	93.30	149.70	2070	38.82	94.34	148.66	2056	39.25	95.38	147.62	2042	39.68	96.42	146.58	2027
243.5	38.30	93.26	150.24	2078	38.73	94.30	149.20	2063	39.15	95.34	148.16	2049	39.58	96.38	147.12	2035
244	38.21	93.22	150.78	2085	38.63	94.26	149.74	2071	39.06	95.30	148.70	2057	39.48	96.33	147.67	2042
244.5	38.11	93.18	151.32	2093	38.54	94.22	150.28	2078	38.96	95.26	149.24	2064	39.38	96.29	148.21	2050
245	38.02	93.14	151.86	2100	38.44	94.18	150.82	2086	38.86	95.22	149.79	2072	39.29	96.25	148.75	2057
245.5	37.92	93.10	152.40	2108	38.34	94.14	151.36	2093	38.77	95.17	150.33	2079	39.19	96.21	149.29	2065
246	37.83	93.06	152.94	2115	38.25	94.10	151.90	2101	38.67	95.13	150.87	2086	39.09	96.17	149.83	2072
246.5	37.74	93.02	153.48	2123	38.16	94.05	152.45	2108	38.58	95.09	151.41	2094	39.00	96.13	150.37	2080
247	37.64	92.98	154.02	2130	38.06	94.01	152.99	2116	38.48	95.05	151.95	2101	38.90	96.09	150.91	2087
247.5	37.55	92.94	154.57	2138	37.97	93.97	153.53	2123	38.39	95.01	152.49	2109	38.81	96.05	151.45	2095

Body Composition MALE 216-247.5 Lb.

Weight: Lb.	Waist: 52 inches Fat: %	Fat: Lb.	LBM: Lb.	RMR: Cal.	52.25 inches Fat: %	Fat: Lb.	LBM: Lb.	RMR: Cal.	52.5 inches Fat: %	Fat: Lb.	LBM: Lb.	RMR: Cal.	52.75 inches Fat: %	Fat: Lb.	LBM: Lb.	RMR: Cal.
216	46.14	99.67	116.33	1609	46.62	100.71	115.29	1595	47.10	101.74	114.26	1580	47.58	102.78	113.22	1566
216.5	46.02	99.63	116.87	1616	46.50	100.66	115.84	1602	46.98	101.70	114.80	1588	47.45	102.74	113.76	1573
217	45.89	99.59	117.41	1624	46.37	100.62	116.38	1609	46.85	101.66	115.34	1595	47.33	102.70	114.30	1581
217.5	45.77	99.55	117.96	1631	46.24	100.58	116.92	1617	46.72	101.62	115.88	1603	47.20	102.66	114.84	1588
218	45.64	99.50	118.50	1639	46.12	100.54	117.46	1624	46.60	101.58	116.42	1610	47.07	102.62	115.38	1596
218.5	45.52	99.46	119.04	1646	46.00	100.50	118.00	1632	46.47	101.54	116.96	1618	46.95	102.58	115.92	1603
219	45.40	99.42	119.58	1654	45.87	100.46	118.54	1639	46.35	101.50	117.50	1625	46.82	102.53	116.47	1611
219.5	45.28	99.38	120.12	1661	45.75	100.42	119.08	1647	46.22	101.46	118.04	1633	46.69	102.49	117.01	1618
220	45.15	99.34	120.66	1669	45.63	100.38	119.62	1654	46.10	101.42	118.59	1640	46.57	102.45	117.55	1626
220.5	45.03	99.30	121.20	1676	45.50	100.34	120.16	1662	45.97	101.37	119.13	1648	46.45	102.41	118.09	1633
221	44.91	99.26	121.74	1684	45.38	100.30	120.70	1669	45.85	101.33	119.67	1655	46.32	102.37	118.63	1641
221.5	44.79	99.22	122.28	1691	45.26	100.25	121.25	1677	45.73	101.29	120.21	1662	46.20	102.33	119.17	1648
222	44.67	99.18	122.82	1699	45.14	100.21	121.79	1684	45.61	101.25	120.75	1670	46.08	102.29	119.71	1656
222.5	44.56	99.14	123.37	1706	45.02	100.17	122.33	1692	45.49	101.21	121.29	1677	45.95	102.25	120.25	1663
223	44.44	99.09	123.91	1714	44.90	100.13	122.87	1699	45.37	101.17	121.83	1685	45.83	102.21	120.79	1671
223.5	44.32	99.05	124.45	1721	44.78	100.09	123.41	1707	45.25	101.13	122.37	1692	45.71	102.17	121.33	1678
224	44.20	99.01	124.99	1729	44.66	100.05	123.95	1714	45.13	101.09	122.91	1700	45.59	102.12	121.88	1686
224.5	44.09	98.97	125.53	1736	44.55	100.01	124.49	1722	45.01	101.05	123.45	1707	45.47	102.08	122.42	1693
225	43.97	98.93	126.07	1744	44.43	99.97	125.03	1729	44.89	101.01	124.00	1715	45.35	102.04	122.96	1701
225.5	43.85	98.89	126.61	1751	44.31	99.93	125.57	1737	44.77	100.96	124.54	1722	45.23	102.00	123.50	1708
226	43.74	98.85	127.15	1759	44.20	99.89	126.11	1744	44.66	100.92	125.08	1730	45.12	101.96	124.04	1715
226.5	43.62	98.81	127.69	1766	44.08	99.84	126.66	1752	44.54	100.88	125.62	1737	45.00	101.92	124.58	1723
227	43.51	98.77	128.23	1773	43.97	99.80	127.20	1759	44.42	100.84	126.16	1745	44.88	101.88	125.12	1730
227.5	43.40	98.73	128.78	1781	43.85	99.76	127.74	1767	44.31	100.80	126.70	1752	44.76	101.84	125.66	1738
228	43.28	98.68	129.32	1788	43.74	99.72	128.28	1774	44.19	100.76	127.24	1760	44.65	101.80	126.20	1745
228.5	43.17	98.64	129.86	1796	43.62	99.68	128.82	1782	44.08	100.72	127.78	1767	44.53	101.76	126.74	1753
229	43.06	98.60	130.40	1803	43.51	99.64	129.36	1789	43.96	100.68	128.32	1775	44.42	101.71	127.29	1760
229.5	42.95	98.56	130.94	1811	43.40	99.60	129.90	1797	43.85	100.64	128.86	1782	44.30	101.67	127.83	1768
230	42.83	98.52	131.48	1818	43.29	99.56	130.44	1804	43.74	100.60	129.41	1790	44.19	101.63	128.37	1775
230.5	42.72	98.48	132.02	1826	43.17	99.52	130.98	1812	43.62	100.55	129.95	1797	44.07	101.59	128.91	1783
231	42.61	98.44	132.56	1833	43.06	99.48	131.52	1819	43.51	100.51	130.49	1805	43.96	101.55	129.45	1790
231.5	42.50	98.40	133.10	1841	42.95	99.43	132.07	1826	43.40	100.47	131.03	1812	43.85	101.51	129.99	1798
232	42.39	98.36	133.64	1848	42.84	99.39	132.61	1834	43.29	100.43	131.57	1820	43.74	101.47	130.53	1805
232.5	42.29	98.32	134.19	1856	42.73	99.35	133.15	1841	43.18	100.39	132.11	1827	43.62	101.43	131.07	1813
233	42.18	98.27	134.73	1863	42.62	99.31	133.69	1849	43.07	100.35	132.65	1835	43.51	101.39	131.61	1820
233.5	42.07	98.23	135.27	1871	42.51	99.27	134.23	1856	42.96	100.31	133.19	1842	43.40	101.35	132.15	1828
234	41.96	98.19	135.81	1878	42.41	99.23	134.77	1864	42.85	100.27	133.73	1850	43.29	101.30	132.70	1835
234.5	41.86	98.15	136.35	1886	42.30	99.19	135.31	1871	42.74	100.23	134.27	1857	43.18	101.26	133.24	1843
235	41.75	98.11	136.89	1893	42.19	99.15	135.85	1879	42.63	100.19	134.82	1864	43.07	101.22	133.78	1850
235.5	41.64	98.07	137.43	1901	42.08	99.11	136.39	1886	42.52	100.14	135.36	1872	42.96	101.18	134.32	1858
236	41.54	98.03	137.97	1908	41.98	99.07	136.93	1894	42.42	100.10	135.90	1879	42.86	101.14	134.86	1865
236.5	41.43	97.99	138.51	1916	41.87	99.02	137.48	1901	42.31	100.06	136.44	1887	42.75	101.10	135.40	1873
237	41.33	97.95	139.05	1923	41.77	98.98	138.02	1909	42.20	100.02	136.98	1894	42.64	101.06	135.94	1880
237.5	41.22	97.91	139.60	1931	41.66	98.94	138.56	1916	42.10	99.98	137.52	1902	42.53	101.02	136.48	1888
238	41.12	97.86	140.14	1938	41.56	98.90	139.10	1924	41.99	99.94	138.06	1909	42.43	100.98	137.02	1895
238.5	41.02	97.82	140.68	1946	41.45	98.86	139.64	1931	41.89	99.90	138.60	1917	42.32	100.94	137.56	1903
239	40.91	97.78	141.22	1953	41.35	98.82	140.18	1939	41.78	99.86	139.14	1924	42.22	100.89	138.11	1910
239.5	40.81	97.74	141.76	1961	41.24	98.78	140.72	1946	41.68	99.82	139.68	1932	42.11	100.85	138.65	1917
240	40.71	97.70	142.30	1968	41.14	98.74	141.26	1954	41.57	99.78	140.23	1939	42.01	100.81	139.19	1925
240.5	40.61	97.66	142.84	1975	41.04	98.70	141.80	1961	41.47	99.73	140.77	1947	41.90	100.77	139.73	1932
241	40.51	97.62	143.38	1983	40.94	98.66	142.34	1969	41.37	99.69	141.31	1954	41.80	100.73	140.27	1940
241.5	40.40	97.58	143.92	1990	40.83	98.61	142.89	1976	41.26	99.65	141.85	1962	41.69	100.69	140.81	1947
242	40.30	97.54	144.46	1998	40.73	98.57	143.43	1984	41.16	99.61	142.39	1969	41.59	100.65	141.35	1955
242.5	40.20	97.50	145.01	2005	40.63	98.53	143.97	1991	41.06	99.57	142.93	1977	41.49	100.61	141.89	1962
243	40.10	97.45	145.55	2013	40.53	98.49	144.51	1999	40.96	99.53	143.47	1984	41.39	100.57	142.43	1970
243.5	40.01	97.41	146.09	2020	40.43	98.45	145.05	2006	40.86	99.49	144.01	1992	41.28	100.53	142.97	1977
244	39.91	97.37	146.63	2028	40.33	98.41	145.59	2014	40.76	99.45	144.55	1999	41.18	100.48	143.52	1985
244.5	39.81	97.33	147.17	2035	40.23	98.37	146.13	2021	40.66	99.41	145.09	2007	41.08	100.44	144.06	1992
245	39.71	97.29	147.71	2043	40.13	98.33	146.67	2028	40.56	99.37	145.64	2014	40.98	100.40	144.60	2000
245.5	39.61	97.25	148.25	2050	40.04	98.29	147.21	2036	40.46	99.32	146.18	2022	40.88	100.36	145.14	2007
246	39.52	97.21	148.79	2058	39.94	98.25	147.75	2043	40.36	99.28	146.72	2029	40.78	100.32	145.68	2015
246.5	39.42	97.17	149.33	2065	39.84	98.20	148.30	2051	40.26	99.24	147.26	2037	40.68	100.28	146.22	2022
247	39.32	97.13	149.87	2073	39.74	98.16	148.84	2058	40.16	99.20	147.80	2044	40.58	100.24	146.76	2030
247.5	39.23	97.09	150.42	2080	39.65	98.12	149.38	2066	40.06	99.16	148.34	2052	40.48	100.20	147.30	2037

Body Composition   MALE   216-247.5 Lb.

Weight: Lb.	Waist: 53 inches Fat: %	Fat: Lb.	LBM: Lb.	RMR: Cal.	53.25 inches Fat: %	Fat: Lb.	LBM: Lb.	RMR: Cal.	53.5 inches Fat: %	Fat: Lb.	LBM: Lb.	RMR: Cal.	53.75 inches Fat: %	Fat: Lb.	LBM: Lb.	RMR: Cal.
216	48.06	103.82	112.18	1551	48.54	104.86	111.14	1537	49.02	105.89	110.11	1523	49.50	106.93	109.07	1508
216.5	47.93	103.78	112.72	1559	48.41	104.81	111.69	1545	48.89	105.85	110.65	1530	49.37	106.89	109.61	1516
217	47.80	103.74	113.26	1566	48.28	104.77	112.23	1552	48.76	105.81	111.19	1538	49.24	106.85	110.15	1523
217.5	47.68	103.70	113.81	1574	48.15	104.73	112.77	1560	48.63	105.77	111.73	1545	49.11	106.81	110.69	1531
218	47.55	103.65	114.35	1581	48.02	104.69	113.31	1567	48.50	105.73	112.27	1553	48.98	106.77	111.23	1538
218.5	47.42	103.61	114.89	1589	47.89	104.65	113.85	1575	48.37	105.69	112.81	1560	48.84	106.73	111.77	1546
219	47.29	103.57	115.43	1596	47.77	104.61	114.39	1582	48.24	105.65	113.35	1568	48.71	106.68	112.32	1553
219.5	47.17	103.53	115.97	1604	47.64	104.57	114.93	1590	48.11	105.61	113.89	1575	48.58	106.64	112.86	1561
220	47.04	103.49	116.51	1611	47.51	104.53	115.47	1597	47.98	105.57	114.44	1583	48.46	106.60	113.40	1568
220.5	46.92	103.45	117.05	1619	47.39	104.49	116.01	1604	47.86	105.52	114.98	1590	48.33	106.56	113.94	1576
221	46.79	103.41	117.59	1626	47.26	104.45	116.55	1612	47.73	105.48	115.52	1598	48.20	106.52	114.48	1583
221.5	46.67	103.37	118.13	1634	47.14	104.40	117.10	1619	47.60	105.44	116.06	1605	48.07	106.48	115.02	1591
222	46.54	103.33	118.67	1641	47.01	104.36	117.64	1627	47.48	105.40	116.60	1613	47.95	106.44	115.56	1598
222.5	46.42	103.29	119.22	1649	46.89	104.32	118.18	1634	47.35	105.36	117.14	1620	47.82	106.40	116.10	1606
223	46.30	103.24	119.76	1656	46.76	104.28	118.72	1642	47.23	105.32	117.68	1628	47.69	106.36	116.64	1613
223.5	46.18	103.20	120.30	1664	46.64	104.24	119.26	1649	47.10	105.28	118.22	1635	47.57	106.32	117.18	1621
224	46.05	103.16	120.84	1671	46.52	104.20	119.80	1657	46.98	105.24	118.76	1642	47.44	106.27	117.73	1628
224.5	45.93	103.12	121.38	1679	46.40	104.16	120.34	1664	46.86	105.20	119.30	1650	47.32	106.23	118.27	1636
225	45.81	103.08	121.92	1686	46.27	104.12	120.88	1672	46.74	105.16	119.85	1657	47.20	106.19	118.81	1643
225.5	45.69	103.04	122.46	1694	46.15	104.08	121.42	1679	46.61	105.11	120.39	1665	47.07	106.15	119.35	1651
226	45.57	103.00	123.00	1701	46.03	104.04	121.96	1687	46.49	105.07	120.93	1672	46.95	106.11	119.89	1658
226.5	45.46	102.96	123.54	1709	45.91	103.99	122.51	1694	46.37	105.03	121.47	1680	46.83	106.07	120.43	1666
227	45.34	102.92	124.08	1716	45.79	103.95	123.05	1702	46.25	104.99	122.01	1687	46.71	106.03	120.97	1673
227.5	45.22	102.88	124.63	1724	45.68	103.91	123.59	1709	46.13	104.95	122.55	1695	46.59	105.99	121.51	1681
228	45.10	102.83	125.17	1731	45.56	103.87	124.13	1717	46.01	104.91	123.09	1702	46.47	105.95	122.05	1688
228.5	44.99	102.79	125.71	1739	45.44	103.83	124.67	1724	45.89	104.87	123.63	1710	46.35	105.91	122.59	1695
229	44.87	102.75	126.25	1746	45.32	103.79	125.21	1732	45.78	104.83	124.17	1717	46.23	105.86	123.14	1703
229.5	44.75	102.71	126.79	1753	45.21	103.75	125.75	1739	45.66	104.79	124.71	1725	46.11	105.82	123.68	1710
230	44.64	102.67	127.33	1761	45.09	103.71	126.29	1747	45.54	104.75	125.26	1732	45.99	105.78	124.22	1718
230.5	44.52	102.63	127.87	1768	44.97	103.67	126.83	1754	45.42	104.70	125.80	1740	45.87	105.74	124.76	1725
231	44.41	102.59	128.41	1776	44.86	103.63	127.37	1762	45.31	104.66	126.34	1747	45.76	105.70	125.30	1733
231.5	44.30	102.55	128.95	1783	44.74	103.58	127.92	1769	45.19	104.62	126.88	1755	45.64	105.66	125.84	1740
232	44.18	102.51	129.49	1791	44.63	103.54	128.46	1777	45.08	104.58	127.42	1762	45.53	105.62	126.38	1748
232.5	44.07	102.47	130.04	1798	44.52	103.50	129.00	1784	44.96	104.54	127.96	1770	45.41	105.58	126.92	1755
233	43.96	102.42	130.58	1806	44.40	103.46	129.54	1792	44.85	104.50	128.50	1777	45.29	105.54	127.46	1763
233.5	43.85	102.38	131.12	1813	44.29	103.42	130.08	1799	44.74	104.46	129.04	1785	45.18	105.50	128.00	1770
234	43.74	102.34	131.66	1821	44.18	103.38	130.62	1806	44.62	104.42	129.58	1792	45.07	105.45	128.55	1778
234.5	43.63	102.30	132.20	1828	44.07	103.34	131.16	1814	44.51	104.38	130.12	1800	44.95	105.41	129.09	1785
235	43.51	102.26	132.74	1836	43.96	103.30	131.70	1821	44.40	104.34	130.67	1807	44.84	105.37	129.63	1793
235.5	43.41	102.22	133.28	1843	43.85	103.26	132.24	1829	44.29	104.29	131.21	1815	44.73	105.33	130.17	1800
236	43.30	102.18	133.82	1851	43.74	103.22	132.78	1836	44.18	104.25	131.75	1822	44.61	105.29	130.71	1808
236.5	43.19	102.14	134.36	1858	43.63	103.17	133.33	1844	44.06	104.21	132.29	1830	44.50	105.25	131.25	1815
237	43.08	102.10	134.90	1866	43.52	103.13	133.87	1851	43.95	104.17	132.83	1837	44.39	105.21	131.79	1823
237.5	42.97	102.06	135.45	1873	43.41	103.09	134.41	1859	43.84	104.13	133.37	1845	44.28	105.17	132.33	1830
238	42.86	102.01	135.99	1881	43.30	103.05	134.95	1866	43.73	104.09	133.91	1852	44.17	105.13	132.87	1838
238.5	42.76	101.97	136.53	1888	43.19	103.01	135.49	1874	43.63	104.05	134.45	1859	44.06	105.09	133.41	1845
239	42.65	101.93	137.07	1896	43.08	102.97	136.03	1881	43.52	104.01	134.99	1867	43.95	105.04	133.96	1853
239.5	42.54	101.89	137.61	1903	42.98	102.93	136.57	1889	43.41	103.97	135.53	1874	43.84	105.00	134.50	1860
240	42.44	101.85	138.15	1911	42.87	102.89	137.11	1896	43.30	103.93	136.08	1882	43.73	104.96	135.04	1868
240.5	42.33	101.81	138.69	1918	42.76	102.85	137.65	1904	43.20	103.88	136.62	1889	43.63	104.92	135.58	1875
241	42.23	101.77	139.23	1926	42.66	102.81	138.19	1911	43.09	103.84	137.16	1897	43.52	104.88	136.12	1883
241.5	42.12	101.73	139.77	1933	42.55	102.76	138.74	1919	42.98	103.80	137.70	1904	43.41	104.84	136.66	1890
242	42.02	101.69	140.31	1941	42.45	102.72	139.28	1926	42.88	103.76	138.24	1912	43.31	104.80	137.20	1897
242.5	41.92	101.65	140.86	1948	42.34	102.68	139.82	1934	42.77	103.72	138.78	1919	43.20	104.76	137.74	1905
243	41.81	101.60	141.40	1956	42.24	102.64	140.36	1941	42.67	103.68	139.32	1927	43.09	104.72	138.28	1912
243.5	41.71	101.56	141.94	1963	42.14	102.60	140.90	1949	42.56	103.64	139.86	1934	42.99	104.68	138.82	1920
244	41.61	101.52	142.48	1970	42.03	102.56	141.44	1956	42.46	103.60	140.40	1942	42.88	104.63	139.37	1927
244.5	41.51	101.48	143.02	1978	41.93	102.52	141.98	1964	42.35	103.56	140.94	1949	42.78	104.59	139.91	1935
245	41.40	101.44	143.56	1985	41.83	102.48	142.52	1971	42.25	103.52	141.49	1957	42.67	104.55	140.45	1942
245.5	41.30	101.40	144.10	1993	41.73	102.43	143.06	1979	42.15	103.47	142.03	1964	42.57	104.51	140.99	1950
246	41.20	101.36	144.64	2000	41.62	102.40	143.60	1986	42.05	103.43	142.57	1972	42.47	104.47	141.53	1957
246.5	41.10	101.32	145.18	2008	41.52	102.35	144.15	1994	41.94	103.39	143.11	1979	42.36	104.43	142.07	1965
247	41.00	101.28	145.72	2015	41.42	102.31	144.69	2001	41.84	103.35	143.65	1987	42.26	104.39	142.61	1972
247.5	40.90	101.24	146.27	2023	41.32	102.27	145.23	2008	41.74	103.31	144.19	1994	42.16	104.35	143.15	1980

Body Composition MALE 216-247.5 Lb.

Weight: Lb.	Waist: 54 inches Fat: %	Fat: Lb.	LBM: Lb.	RMR: Cal.	54.25 inches Fat: %	Fat: Lb.	LBM: Lb.	RMR: Cal.	54.5 inches Fat: %	Fat: Lb.	LBM: Lb.	RMR: Cal.	54.75 inches Fat: %	Fat: Lb.	LBM: Lb.	RMR: Cal.
216	49.99	107.97	108.03	1494	50.47	109.01	106.99	1480	50.95	110.04	105.96	1465	51.43	111.08	104.92	1451
216.5	49.85	107.93	108.57	1502	50.33	108.96	107.54	1487	50.81	110.00	106.50	1473	51.29	111.04	105.46	1459
217	49.72	107.89	109.11	1509	50.20	108.92	108.08	1495	50.67	109.96	107.04	1480	51.15	111.00	106.00	1466
217.5	49.58	107.85	109.66	1517	50.06	108.88	108.62	1502	50.54	109.92	107.58	1488	51.01	110.96	106.54	1473
218	49.45	107.80	110.20	1524	49.93	108.84	109.16	1510	50.40	109.88	108.12	1495	50.88	110.92	107.08	1481
218.5	49.32	107.76	110.74	1531	49.79	108.80	109.70	1517	50.27	109.84	108.66	1503	50.74	110.88	107.62	1488
219	49.19	107.72	111.28	1539	49.66	108.76	110.24	1525	50.14	109.80	109.20	1510	50.61	110.83	108.17	1496
219.5	49.06	107.68	111.82	1546	49.53	108.72	110.78	1532	50.00	109.76	109.74	1518	50.48	110.79	108.71	1503
220	48.93	107.64	112.36	1554	49.40	108.68	111.32	1540	49.87	109.72	110.29	1525	50.34	110.75	109.25	1511
220.5	48.80	107.60	112.90	1561	49.27	108.64	111.86	1547	49.74	109.67	110.83	1533	50.21	110.71	109.79	1518
221	48.67	107.56	113.44	1569	49.14	108.60	112.40	1555	49.61	109.63	111.37	1540	50.08	110.67	110.33	1526
221.5	48.54	107.52	113.98	1576	49.01	108.55	112.95	1562	49.48	109.59	111.91	1548	49.95	110.63	110.87	1533
222	48.41	107.48	114.52	1584	48.88	108.51	113.49	1570	49.35	109.55	112.45	1555	49.81	110.59	111.41	1541
222.5	48.29	107.44	115.07	1591	48.75	108.47	114.03	1577	49.22	109.51	112.99	1563	49.68	110.55	111.95	1548
223	48.16	107.39	115.61	1599	48.62	108.43	114.57	1584	49.09	109.47	113.53	1570	49.55	110.51	112.49	1556
223.5	48.03	107.35	116.15	1606	48.50	108.39	115.11	1592	48.96	109.43	114.07	1578	49.43	110.47	113.03	1563
224	47.91	107.31	116.69	1614	48.37	108.35	115.65	1599	48.83	109.39	114.61	1585	49.30	110.42	113.58	1571
224.5	47.78	107.27	117.23	1621	48.24	108.31	116.19	1607	48.71	109.35	115.15	1593	49.17	110.38	114.12	1578
225	47.66	107.23	117.77	1629	48.12	108.27	116.73	1614	48.58	109.31	115.70	1600	49.04	110.34	114.66	1586
225.5	47.53	107.19	118.31	1636	47.99	108.23	117.27	1622	48.45	109.26	116.24	1608	48.91	110.30	115.20	1593
226	47.41	107.15	118.85	1644	47.87	108.19	117.81	1629	48.33	109.22	116.78	1615	48.79	110.26	115.74	1601
226.5	47.29	107.11	119.39	1651	47.75	108.14	118.36	1637	48.20	109.18	117.32	1623	48.66	110.22	116.28	1608
227	47.17	107.07	119.93	1659	47.62	108.10	118.90	1644	48.08	109.14	117.86	1630	48.54	110.18	116.82	1616
227.5	47.04	107.03	120.48	1666	47.50	108.06	119.44	1652	47.96	109.10	118.40	1637	48.41	110.14	117.36	1623
228	46.92	106.98	121.02	1674	47.38	108.02	119.98	1659	47.83	109.06	118.94	1645	48.29	110.10	117.90	1631
228.5	46.80	106.94	121.56	1681	47.26	107.98	120.52	1667	47.71	109.02	119.48	1652	48.16	110.06	118.44	1638
229	46.68	106.90	122.10	1689	47.14	107.94	121.06	1674	47.59	108.98	120.02	1660	48.04	110.01	118.99	1646
229.5	46.56	106.86	122.64	1696	47.01	107.90	121.60	1682	47.47	108.94	120.56	1667	47.92	109.97	119.53	1653
230	46.44	106.82	123.18	1704	46.89	107.86	122.14	1689	47.35	108.90	121.11	1675	47.80	109.93	120.07	1661
230.5	46.32	106.78	123.72	1711	46.78	107.82	122.68	1697	47.23	108.85	121.65	1682	47.68	109.89	120.61	1668
231	46.21	106.74	124.26	1719	46.66	107.78	123.22	1704	47.11	108.81	122.19	1690	47.55	109.85	121.15	1675
231.5	46.09	106.70	124.80	1726	46.54	107.73	123.77	1712	46.99	108.77	122.73	1697	47.43	109.81	121.69	1683
232	45.97	106.66	125.34	1734	46.42	107.69	124.31	1719	46.87	108.73	123.27	1705	47.31	109.77	122.23	1690
232.5	45.86	106.62	125.89	1741	46.30	107.65	124.85	1727	46.75	108.69	123.81	1712	47.19	109.73	122.77	1698
233	45.74	106.57	126.43	1748	46.19	107.61	125.39	1734	46.63	108.65	124.35	1720	47.08	109.69	123.31	1705
233.5	45.62	106.53	126.97	1756	46.07	107.57	125.93	1742	46.51	108.61	124.89	1727	46.96	109.65	123.85	1713
234	45.51	106.49	127.51	1763	45.95	107.53	126.47	1749	46.40	108.57	125.43	1735	46.84	109.60	124.40	1720
234.5	45.39	106.45	128.05	1771	45.84	107.49	127.01	1757	46.28	108.53	125.97	1742	46.72	109.56	124.94	1728
235	45.28	106.41	128.59	1778	45.72	107.45	127.55	1764	46.16	108.49	126.52	1750	46.61	109.52	125.48	1735
235.5	45.17	106.37	129.13	1786	45.61	107.41	128.09	1772	46.05	108.44	127.06	1757	46.49	109.48	126.02	1743
236	45.05	106.33	129.67	1793	45.49	107.37	128.63	1779	45.93	108.40	127.60	1765	46.37	109.44	126.56	1750
236.5	44.94	106.29	130.21	1801	45.38	107.32	129.18	1786	45.82	108.36	128.14	1772	46.26	109.40	127.10	1758
237	44.83	106.25	130.75	1808	45.27	107.28	129.72	1794	45.71	108.32	128.68	1780	46.14	109.36	127.64	1765
237.5	44.72	106.21	131.30	1816	45.15	107.24	130.26	1801	45.59	108.28	129.22	1787	46.03	109.32	128.18	1773
238	44.61	106.16	131.84	1823	45.04	107.20	130.80	1809	45.48	108.24	129.76	1795	45.91	109.28	128.72	1780
238.5	44.50	106.12	132.38	1831	44.93	107.16	131.34	1816	45.37	108.20	130.30	1802	45.80	109.24	129.26	1788
239	44.39	106.08	132.92	1838	44.82	107.12	131.88	1824	45.25	108.16	130.84	1810	45.69	109.19	129.81	1795
239.5	44.28	106.04	133.46	1846	44.71	107.08	132.42	1831	45.14	108.12	131.38	1817	45.58	109.15	130.35	1803
240	44.17	106.00	134.00	1853	44.60	107.04	132.96	1839	45.03	108.08	131.93	1825	45.46	109.11	130.89	1810
240.5	44.06	105.96	134.54	1861	44.49	107.00	133.50	1846	44.92	108.03	132.47	1832	45.35	109.07	131.43	1818
241	43.95	105.92	135.08	1868	44.38	106.96	134.04	1854	44.81	107.99	133.01	1839	45.24	109.03	131.97	1825
241.5	43.84	105.88	135.62	1876	44.27	106.91	134.59	1861	44.70	107.95	133.55	1847	45.13	108.99	132.51	1833
242	43.73	105.84	136.16	1883	44.16	106.87	135.13	1869	44.59	107.91	134.09	1854	45.02	108.95	133.05	1840
242.5	43.63	105.80	136.71	1891	44.05	106.83	135.67	1876	44.48	107.87	134.63	1862	44.91	108.91	133.59	1848
243	43.52	105.75	137.25	1898	43.95	106.79	136.21	1884	44.37	107.83	135.17	1869	44.80	108.87	134.13	1855
243.5	43.41	105.71	137.79	1906	43.84	106.75	136.75	1891	44.27	107.79	135.71	1877	44.69	108.83	134.67	1863
244	43.31	105.67	138.33	1913	43.73	106.71	137.29	1899	44.16	107.75	136.25	1884	44.58	108.78	135.22	1870
244.5	43.20	105.63	138.87	1921	43.63	106.67	137.83	1906	44.05	107.71	136.79	1892	44.48	108.74	135.76	1878
245	43.10	105.59	139.41	1928	43.52	106.63	138.37	1914	43.94	107.67	137.34	1899	44.37	108.70	136.30	1885
245.5	42.99	105.55	139.95	1936	43.42	106.59	138.91	1921	43.84	107.62	137.88	1907	44.26	108.66	136.84	1892
246	42.89	105.51	140.49	1943	43.31	106.55	139.45	1929	43.73	107.58	138.42	1914	44.15	108.62	137.38	1900
246.5	42.79	105.47	141.03	1950	43.21	106.50	140.00	1936	43.63	107.54	138.96	1922	44.05	108.58	137.92	1907
247	42.68	105.43	141.57	1958	43.10	106.46	140.54	1944	43.52	107.50	139.50	1929	43.94	108.54	138.46	1915
247.5	42.58	105.39	142.12	1965	43.00	106.42	141.08	1951	43.42	107.46	140.04	1937	43.84	108.50	139.00	1922

Body Composition MALE 248-279.5 Lb.

Weight: Lb.	Waist: 31 inches Fat: %	Fat: Lb.	LBM: Lb.	RMR: Cal.	31.25 inches Fat: %	Fat: Lb.	LBM: Lb.	RMR: Cal.	31.5 inches Fat: %	Fat: Lb.	LBM: Lb.	RMR: Cal.	31.75 inches Fat: %	Fat: Lb.	LBM: Lb.	RMR: Cal.
248	3.99	9.89	238.11	3293	4.41	10.93	237.07	3279	4.83	11.97	236.03	3264	5.24	13.01	234.99	3250
248.5	3.96	9.85	238.65	3300	4.38	10.89	237.61	3286	4.80	11.93	236.57	3272	5.22	12.97	235.53	3257
249	3.94	9.81	239.19	3308	4.36	10.85	238.15	3294	4.77	11.89	237.11	3279	5.19	12.92	236.08	3265
249.5	3.92	9.77	239.73	3315	4.33	10.81	238.69	3301	4.75	11.85	237.65	3287	5.16	12.88	236.62	3272
250	3.89	9.73	240.27	3323	4.31	10.77	239.23	3309	4.72	11.81	238.20	3294	5.14	12.84	237.16	3280
250.5	3.87	9.69	240.81	3330	4.28	10.73	239.77	3316	4.70	11.76	238.74	3302	5.11	12.80	237.70	3287
251	3.84	9.65	241.35	3338	4.26	10.69	240.31	3324	4.67	11.72	239.28	3309	5.08	12.76	238.24	3295
251.5	3.82	9.61	241.89	3345	4.23	10.64	240.86	3331	4.64	11.68	239.82	3317	5.06	12.72	238.78	3302
252	3.80	9.57	242.43	3353	4.21	10.60	241.40	3339	4.62	11.64	240.36	3324	5.03	12.68	239.32	3310
252.5	3.77	9.52	242.98	3360	4.18	10.56	241.94	3346	4.59	11.60	240.90	3332	5.00	12.64	239.86	3317
253	3.75	9.48	243.52	3368	4.16	10.52	242.48	3353	4.57	11.56	241.44	3339	4.98	12.60	240.40	3325
253.5	3.73	9.44	244.06	3375	4.13	10.48	243.02	3361	4.54	11.52	241.98	3347	4.95	12.56	240.94	3332
254	3.70	9.40	244.60	3383	4.11	10.44	243.56	3368	4.52	11.48	242.52	3354	4.93	12.51	241.49	3340
254.5	3.68	9.36	245.14	3390	4.09	10.40	244.10	3376	4.49	11.44	243.06	3362	4.90	12.47	242.03	3347
255	3.65	9.32	245.68	3398	4.06	10.36	244.64	3383	4.47	11.40	243.61	3369	4.88	12.43	242.57	3355
255.5	3.63	9.28	246.22	3405	4.04	10.32	245.18	3391	4.44	11.35	244.15	3377	4.85	12.39	243.11	3362
256	3.61	9.24	246.76	3413	4.01	10.28	245.72	3398	4.42	11.31	244.69	3384	4.82	12.35	243.65	3370
256.5	3.59	9.20	247.30	3420	3.99	10.23	246.27	3406	4.39	11.27	245.23	3392	4.80	12.31	244.19	3377
257	3.56	9.16	247.84	3428	3.97	10.19	246.81	3413	4.37	11.23	245.77	3399	4.77	12.27	244.73	3385
257.5	3.54	9.12	248.39	3435	3.94	10.15	247.35	3421	4.35	11.19	246.31	3406	4.75	12.23	245.27	3392
258	3.52	9.07	248.93	3443	3.92	10.11	247.89	3428	4.32	11.15	246.85	3414	4.72	12.19	245.81	3400
258.5	3.49	9.03	249.47	3450	3.90	10.07	248.43	3436	4.30	11.11	247.39	3421	4.70	12.15	246.35	3407
259	3.47	8.99	250.01	3458	3.87	10.03	248.97	3443	4.27	11.07	247.93	3429	4.67	12.10	246.90	3415
259.5	3.45	8.95	250.55	3465	3.85	9.99	249.51	3451	4.25	11.03	248.47	3436	4.65	12.06	247.44	3422
260	3.43	8.91	251.09	3473	3.83	9.95	250.05	3458	4.23	10.99	249.02	3444	4.62	12.02	247.98	3430
260.5	3.40	8.87	251.63	3480	3.80	9.91	250.59	3466	4.20	10.94	249.56	3451	4.60	11.98	248.52	3437
261	3.38	8.83	252.17	3488	3.78	9.87	251.13	3473	4.18	10.90	250.10	3459	4.57	11.94	249.06	3444
261.5	3.36	8.79	252.71	3495	3.76	9.82	251.68	3481	4.15	10.86	250.64	3466	4.55	11.90	249.60	3452
262	3.34	8.75	253.25	3503	3.73	9.78	252.22	3488	4.13	10.82	251.18	3474	4.53	11.86	250.14	3459
262.5	3.32	8.70	253.80	3510	3.71	9.74	252.76	3496	4.11	10.78	251.72	3481	4.50	11.82	250.68	3467
263	3.29	8.66	254.34	3517	3.69	9.70	253.30	3503	4.08	10.74	252.26	3489	4.48	11.78	251.22	3474
263.5	3.27	8.62	254.88	3525	3.67	9.66	253.84	3511	4.06	10.70	252.80	3496	4.45	11.74	251.76	3482
264	3.25	8.58	255.42	3532	3.64	9.62	254.38	3518	4.04	10.66	253.34	3504	4.43	11.69	252.31	3489
264.5	3.23	8.54	255.96	3540	3.62	9.58	254.92	3526	4.01	10.62	253.88	3511	4.41	11.65	252.85	3497
265	3.21	8.50	256.50	3547	3.60	9.54	255.46	3533	3.99	10.58	254.43	3519	4.38	11.61	253.39	3504
265.5	3.19	8.46	257.04	3555	3.58	9.50	256.00	3541	3.97	10.53	254.97	3526	4.36	11.57	253.93	3512
266	3.16	8.42	257.58	3562	3.55	9.46	256.54	3548	3.94	10.49	255.51	3534	4.33	11.53	254.47	3519
266.5	3.14	8.38	258.12	3570	3.53	9.41	257.09	3555	3.92	10.45	256.05	3541	4.31	11.49	255.01	3527
267	3.12	8.34	258.66	3577	3.51	9.37	257.63	3563	3.90	10.41	256.59	3549	4.29	11.45	255.55	3534
267.5	3.10	8.30	259.21	3585	3.49	9.33	258.17	3570	3.88	10.37	257.13	3556	4.26	11.41	256.09	3542
268	3.08	8.25	259.75	3592	3.47	9.29	258.71	3578	3.85	10.33	257.67	3564	4.24	11.37	256.63	3549
268.5	3.06	8.21	260.29	3600	3.45	9.25	259.25	3585	3.83	10.29	258.21	3571	4.22	11.33	257.17	3557
269	3.04	8.17	260.83	3607	3.42	9.21	259.79	3593	3.81	10.25	258.75	3579	4.19	11.28	257.72	3564
269.5	3.02	8.13	261.37	3615	3.40	9.17	260.33	3600	3.79	10.21	259.29	3586	4.17	11.24	258.26	3572
270	3.00	8.09	261.91	3622	3.38	9.13	260.87	3608	3.76	10.17	259.84	3594	4.15	11.20	258.80	3579
270.5	2.98	8.05	262.45	3630	3.36	9.09	261.41	3615	3.74	10.12	260.38	3601	4.13	11.16	259.34	3587
271	2.95	8.01	262.99	3637	3.34	9.05	261.95	3623	3.72	10.08	260.92	3608	4.10	11.12	259.88	3594
271.5	2.93	7.97	263.53	3645	3.32	9.00	262.50	3630	3.70	10.04	261.46	3616	4.08	11.08	260.42	3602
272	2.91	7.93	264.07	3652	3.30	8.96	263.04	3638	3.68	10.00	262.00	3623	4.06	11.04	260.96	3609
272.5	2.89	7.88	264.62	3660	3.27	8.92	263.58	3645	3.66	9.96	262.54	3631	4.04	11.00	261.50	3617
273	2.87	7.84	265.16	3667	3.25	8.88	264.12	3653	3.63	9.92	263.08	3638	4.01	10.96	262.04	3624
273.5	2.85	7.80	265.70	3675	3.23	8.84	264.66	3660	3.61	9.88	263.62	3646	3.99	10.92	262.58	3632
274	2.83	7.76	266.24	3682	3.21	8.80	265.20	3668	3.59	9.84	264.16	3653	3.97	10.87	263.13	3639
274.5	2.81	7.72	266.78	3690	3.19	8.76	265.74	3675	3.57	9.80	264.70	3661	3.95	10.83	263.67	3647
275	2.79	7.68	267.32	3697	3.17	8.72	266.28	3683	3.55	9.76	265.25	3668	3.92	10.79	264.21	3654
275.5	2.77	7.64	267.86	3705	3.15	8.68	266.82	3690	3.53	9.71	265.79	3676	3.90	10.75	264.75	3661
276	2.75	7.60	268.40	3712	3.13	8.64	267.36	3698	3.50	9.67	266.33	3683	3.88	10.71	265.29	3669
276.5	2.73	7.56	268.94	3719	3.11	8.59	267.91	3705	3.48	9.63	266.87	3691	3.86	10.67	265.83	3676
277	2.71	7.52	269.48	3727	3.09	8.55	268.45	3713	3.46	9.59	267.41	3698	3.84	10.63	266.37	3684
277.5	2.69	7.48	270.03	3734	3.07	8.51	268.99	3720	3.44	9.55	267.95	3706	3.82	10.59	266.91	3691
278	2.67	7.43	270.57	3742	3.05	8.47	269.53	3728	3.42	9.51	268.49	3713	3.79	10.55	267.45	3699
278.5	2.65	7.39	271.11	3749	3.03	8.43	270.07	3735	3.40	9.47	269.03	3721	3.77	10.51	267.99	3706
279	2.64	7.35	271.65	3757	3.01	8.39	270.61	3743	3.38	9.43	269.57	3728	3.75	10.46	268.54	3714
279.5	2.62	7.31	272.19	3764	2.99	8.35	271.15	3750	3.36	9.39	270.11	3736	3.73	10.42	269.08	3721

Body Composition   MALE   248-279.5 Lb.

Waist:	32 inches			32.25 inches			32.5 inches			32.75 inches		
Weight: Lb.	Fat: %	Fat: Lb.	LBM: Lb.	RMR: Cal.	Fat: %	Fat: Lb.	LBM: Lb.	RMR: Cal.	Fat: %	Fat: Lb.	LBM: Lb.	RMR: Cal.	Fat: %	Fat: Lb.	LBM: Lb.	RMR: Cal.
248	5.66	14.04	233.96	3236	6.08	15.08	232.92	3221	6.50	16.12	231.88	3207	6.92	17.16	230.84	3193
248.5	5.64	14.00	234.50	3243	6.05	15.04	233.46	3229	6.47	16.08	232.42	3214	6.89	17.12	231.38	3200
249	5.61	13.96	235.04	3251	6.02	15.00	234.00	3236	6.44	16.04	232.96	3222	6.86	17.07	231.93	3208
249.5	5.58	13.92	235.58	3258	6.00	14.96	234.54	3244	6.41	16.00	233.50	3229	6.83	17.03	232.47	3215
250	5.55	13.88	236.12	3266	5.97	14.92	235.08	3251	6.38	15.96	234.05	3237	6.80	16.99	233.01	3222
250.5	5.52	13.84	236.66	3273	5.94	14.88	235.62	3259	6.35	15.91	234.59	3244	6.77	16.95	233.55	3230
251	5.50	13.80	237.20	3281	5.91	14.84	236.16	3266	6.32	15.87	235.13	3252	6.74	16.91	234.09	3237
251.5	5.47	13.76	237.74	3288	5.88	14.79	236.71	3274	6.30	15.83	235.67	3259	6.71	16.87	234.63	3245
252	5.44	13.72	238.28	3295	5.85	14.75	237.25	3281	6.27	15.79	236.21	3267	6.68	16.83	235.17	3252
252.5	5.42	13.68	238.83	3303	5.83	14.71	237.79	3289	6.24	15.75	236.75	3274	6.65	16.79	235.71	3260
253	5.39	13.63	239.37	3310	5.80	14.67	238.33	3296	6.21	15.71	237.29	3282	6.62	16.75	236.25	3267
253.5	5.36	13.59	239.91	3318	5.77	14.63	238.87	3304	6.18	15.67	237.83	3289	6.59	16.71	236.79	3275
254	5.34	13.55	240.45	3325	5.74	14.59	239.41	3311	6.15	15.63	238.37	3297	6.56	16.66	237.34	3282
254.5	5.31	13.51	240.99	3333	5.72	14.55	239.95	3319	6.12	15.59	238.91	3304	6.53	16.62	237.88	3290
255	5.28	13.47	241.53	3340	5.69	14.51	240.49	3326	6.10	15.55	239.46	3312	6.50	16.58	238.42	3297
255.5	5.26	13.43	242.07	3348	5.66	14.47	241.03	3333	6.07	15.50	240.00	3319	6.47	16.54	238.96	3305
256	5.23	13.39	242.61	3355	5.63	14.43	241.57	3341	6.04	15.46	240.54	3327	6.45	16.50	239.50	3312
256.5	5.20	13.35	243.15	3363	5.61	14.38	242.12	3348	6.01	15.42	241.08	3334	6.42	16.46	240.04	3320
257	5.18	13.31	243.69	3370	5.58	14.34	242.66	3356	5.98	15.38	241.62	3342	6.39	16.42	240.58	3327
257.5	5.15	13.27	244.24	3378	5.55	14.30	243.20	3363	5.96	15.34	242.16	3349	6.36	16.38	241.12	3335
258	5.13	13.22	244.78	3385	5.53	14.26	243.74	3371	5.93	15.30	242.70	3357	6.33	16.34	241.66	3342
258.5	5.10	13.18	245.32	3393	5.50	14.22	244.28	3378	5.90	15.26	243.24	3364	6.30	16.30	242.20	3350
259	5.07	13.14	245.86	3400	5.47	14.18	244.82	3386	5.88	15.22	243.78	3372	6.28	16.25	242.75	3357
259.5	5.05	13.10	246.40	3408	5.45	14.14	245.36	3393	5.85	15.18	244.32	3379	6.25	16.21	243.29	3365
260	5.02	13.06	246.94	3415	5.42	14.10	245.90	3401	5.82	15.14	244.87	3386	6.22	16.17	243.83	3372
260.5	5.00	13.02	247.48	3423	5.40	14.06	246.44	3408	5.79	15.09	245.41	3394	6.19	16.13	244.37	3380
261	4.97	12.98	248.02	3430	5.37	14.02	246.98	3416	5.77	15.05	245.95	3401	6.16	16.09	244.91	3387
261.5	4.95	12.94	248.56	3438	5.34	13.97	247.53	3423	5.74	15.01	246.49	3409	6.14	16.05	245.45	3395
262	4.92	12.90	249.10	3445	5.32	13.93	248.07	3431	5.71	14.97	247.03	3416	6.11	16.01	245.99	3402
262.5	4.90	12.86	249.65	3453	5.29	13.89	248.61	3438	5.69	14.93	247.57	3424	6.08	15.97	246.53	3410
263	4.87	12.81	250.19	3460	5.27	13.85	249.15	3446	5.66	14.89	248.11	3431	6.06	15.93	247.07	3417
263.5	4.85	12.77	250.73	3468	5.24	13.81	249.69	3453	5.63	14.85	248.65	3439	6.03	15.89	247.61	3425
264	4.82	12.73	251.27	3475	5.22	13.77	250.23	3461	5.61	14.81	249.19	3446	6.00	15.84	248.16	3432
264.5	4.80	12.69	251.81	3483	5.19	13.73	250.77	3468	5.58	14.77	249.73	3454	5.97	15.80	248.70	3439
265	4.77	12.65	252.35	3490	5.17	13.69	251.31	3476	5.56	14.73	250.28	3461	5.95	15.76	249.24	3447
265.5	4.75	12.61	252.89	3497	5.14	13.65	251.85	3483	5.53	14.68	250.82	3469	5.92	15.72	249.78	3454
266	4.72	12.57	253.43	3505	5.11	13.61	252.39	3491	5.50	14.64	251.36	3476	5.89	15.68	250.32	3462
266.5	4.70	12.53	253.97	3512	5.09	13.56	252.94	3498	5.48	14.60	251.90	3484	5.87	15.64	250.86	3469
267	4.68	12.49	254.51	3520	5.06	13.52	253.48	3506	5.45	14.56	252.44	3491	5.84	15.60	251.40	3477
267.5	4.65	12.45	255.06	3527	5.04	13.48	254.02	3513	5.43	14.52	252.98	3499	5.82	15.56	251.94	3484
268	4.63	12.40	255.60	3535	5.02	13.44	254.56	3521	5.40	14.48	253.52	3506	5.79	15.52	252.48	3492
268.5	4.60	12.36	256.14	3542	4.99	13.40	255.10	3528	5.38	14.44	254.06	3514	5.76	15.48	253.02	3499
269	4.58	12.32	256.68	3550	4.97	13.36	255.64	3536	5.35	14.40	254.60	3521	5.74	15.43	253.57	3507
269.5	4.56	12.28	257.22	3557	4.94	13.32	256.18	3543	5.33	14.36	255.14	3529	5.71	15.39	254.11	3514
270	4.53	12.24	257.76	3565	4.92	13.28	256.72	3550	5.30	14.31	255.69	3536	5.69	15.35	254.65	3522
270.5	4.51	12.20	258.30	3572	4.89	13.24	257.26	3558	5.28	14.27	256.23	3544	5.66	15.31	255.19	3529
271	4.49	12.16	258.84	3580	4.87	13.20	257.80	3565	5.25	14.23	256.77	3551	5.63	15.27	255.73	3537
271.5	4.46	12.12	259.38	3587	4.85	13.15	258.35	3573	5.23	14.19	257.31	3559	5.61	15.23	256.27	3544
272	4.44	12.08	259.92	3595	4.82	13.11	258.89	3580	5.20	14.15	257.85	3566	5.58	15.19	256.81	3552
272.5	4.42	12.04	260.47	3602	4.80	13.07	259.43	3588	5.18	14.11	258.39	3574	5.56	15.15	257.35	3559
273	4.39	11.99	261.01	3610	4.77	13.03	259.97	3595	5.15	14.07	258.93	3581	5.53	15.11	257.89	3567
273.5	4.37	11.95	261.55	3617	4.75	12.99	260.51	3603	5.13	14.03	259.47	3588	5.51	15.07	258.43	3574
274	4.35	11.91	262.09	3625	4.73	12.95	261.05	3610	5.10	13.99	260.01	3596	5.48	15.02	258.98	3582
274.5	4.32	11.87	262.63	3632	4.70	12.91	261.59	3618	5.08	13.95	260.55	3603	5.46	14.98	259.52	3589
275	4.30	11.83	263.17	3640	4.68	12.87	262.13	3625	5.06	13.91	261.10	3611	5.43	14.94	260.06	3597
275.5	4.28	11.79	263.71	3647	4.66	12.83	262.67	3633	5.03	13.86	261.64	3618	5.41	14.90	260.60	3604
276	4.26	11.75	264.25	3655	4.63	12.79	263.21	3640	5.01	13.82	262.18	3626	5.38	14.86	261.14	3612
276.5	4.23	11.71	264.79	3662	4.61	12.74	263.76	3648	4.98	13.78	262.72	3633	5.36	14.82	261.68	3619
277	4.21	11.67	265.33	3670	4.59	12.70	264.30	3655	4.96	13.74	263.26	3641	5.34	14.78	262.22	3627
277.5	4.19	11.63	265.88	3677	4.56	12.66	264.84	3663	4.94	13.70	263.80	3648	5.31	14.74	262.76	3634
278	4.17	11.58	266.42	3685	4.54	12.62	265.38	3670	4.91	13.66	264.34	3656	5.29	14.70	263.30	3641
278.5	4.14	11.54	266.96	3692	4.52	12.58	265.92	3678	4.89	13.62	264.88	3663	5.26	14.66	263.84	3649
279	4.12	11.50	267.50	3699	4.49	12.54	266.46	3685	4.87	13.58	265.42	3671	5.24	14.61	264.39	3656
279.5	4.10	11.46	268.04	3707	4.47	12.50	267.00	3693	4.84	13.54	265.96	3678	5.21	14.57	264.93	3664

Body Composition   MALE   248-279.5 Lb.

Weight: Lb.	Waist: 33 inches				33.25 inches				33.5 inches				33.75 inches			
	Fat: %	Fat: Lb.	LBM: Lb.	RMR: Cal.	Fat: %	Fat: Lb.	LBM: Lb.	RMR: Cal.	Fat: %	Fat: Lb.	LBM: Lb.	RMR: Cal.	Fat: %	Fat: Lb.	LBM: Lb.	RMR: Cal.
248	7.34	18.19	229.81	3178	7.75	19.23	228.77	3164	8.17	20.27	227.73	3150	8.59	21.31	226.69	3135
248.5	7.31	18.15	230.35	3186	7.72	19.19	229.31	3171	8.14	20.23	228.27	3157	8.56	21.27	227.23	3143
249	7.27	18.11	230.89	3193	7.69	19.15	229.85	3179	8.11	20.19	228.81	3164	8.52	21.22	227.78	3150
249.5	7.24	18.07	231.43	3201	7.66	19.11	230.39	3186	8.07	20.15	229.35	3172	8.49	21.18	228.32	3158
250	7.21	18.03	231.97	3208	7.63	19.07	230.93	3194	8.04	20.11	229.90	3179	8.46	21.14	228.86	3165
250.5	7.18	17.99	232.51	3216	7.60	19.03	231.47	3201	8.01	20.06	230.44	3187	8.42	21.10	229.40	3173
251	7.15	17.95	233.05	3223	7.56	18.99	232.01	3209	7.98	20.02	230.98	3194	8.39	21.06	229.94	3180
251.5	7.12	17.91	233.59	3231	7.53	18.94	232.56	3216	7.95	19.98	231.52	3202	8.36	21.02	230.48	3188
252	7.09	17.87	234.13	3238	7.50	18.90	233.10	3224	7.91	19.94	232.06	3209	8.32	20.98	231.02	3195
252.5	7.06	17.83	234.68	3246	7.47	18.86	233.64	3231	7.88	19.90	232.60	3217	8.29	20.94	231.56	3203
253	7.03	17.78	235.22	3253	7.44	18.82	234.18	3239	7.85	19.86	233.14	3224	8.26	20.90	232.10	3210
253.5	7.00	17.74	235.76	3261	7.41	18.78	234.72	3246	7.82	19.82	233.68	3232	8.23	20.86	232.64	3217
254	6.97	17.70	236.30	3268	7.38	18.74	235.26	3254	7.79	19.78	234.22	3239	8.19	20.81	233.19	3225
254.5	6.94	17.66	236.84	3275	7.35	18.70	235.80	3261	7.75	19.74	234.76	3247	8.16	20.77	233.73	3232
255	6.91	17.62	237.38	3283	7.32	18.66	236.34	3269	7.72	19.70	235.31	3254	8.13	20.73	234.27	3240
255.5	6.88	17.58	237.92	3290	7.29	18.62	236.88	3276	7.69	19.65	235.85	3262	8.10	20.69	234.81	3247
256	6.85	17.54	238.46	3298	7.26	18.58	237.42	3284	7.66	19.61	236.39	3269	8.07	20.65	235.35	3255
256.5	6.82	17.50	239.00	3305	7.23	18.53	237.97	3291	7.63	19.57	236.93	3277	8.03	20.61	235.89	3262
257	6.79	17.46	239.54	3313	7.20	18.49	238.51	3299	7.60	19.53	237.47	3284	8.00	20.57	236.43	3270
257.5	6.76	17.42	240.09	3320	7.17	18.45	239.05	3306	7.57	19.49	238.01	3292	7.97	20.53	236.97	3277
258	6.73	17.37	240.63	3328	7.14	18.41	239.59	3314	7.54	19.45	238.55	3299	7.94	20.49	237.51	3285
258.5	6.71	17.33	241.17	3335	7.11	18.37	240.13	3321	7.51	19.41	239.09	3307	7.91	20.45	238.05	3292
259	6.68	17.29	241.71	3343	7.08	18.33	240.67	3328	7.48	19.37	239.63	3314	7.88	20.40	238.60	3300
259.5	6.65	17.25	242.25	3350	7.05	18.29	241.21	3336	7.45	19.33	240.17	3322	7.85	20.36	239.14	3307
260	6.62	17.21	242.79	3358	7.02	18.25	241.75	3343	7.42	19.29	240.72	3329	7.82	20.32	239.68	3315
260.5	6.59	17.17	243.33	3365	6.99	18.21	242.29	3351	7.39	19.24	241.26	3337	7.79	20.28	240.22	3322
261	6.56	17.13	243.87	3373	6.96	18.17	242.83	3358	7.36	19.20	241.80	3344	7.75	20.24	240.76	3330
261.5	6.53	17.09	244.41	3380	6.93	18.12	243.38	3366	7.33	19.16	242.34	3352	7.72	20.20	241.30	3337
262	6.51	17.05	244.95	3388	6.90	18.08	243.92	3373	7.30	19.12	242.88	3359	7.69	20.16	241.84	3345
262.5	6.48	17.01	245.50	3395	6.87	18.04	244.46	3381	7.27	19.08	243.42	3366	7.66	20.12	242.38	3352
263	6.45	16.96	246.04	3403	6.84	18.00	245.00	3388	7.24	19.04	243.96	3374	7.63	20.08	242.92	3360
263.5	6.42	16.92	246.58	3410	6.82	17.96	245.54	3396	7.21	19.00	244.50	3381	7.60	20.04	243.46	3367
264	6.39	16.88	247.12	3418	6.79	17.92	246.08	3403	7.18	18.96	245.04	3389	7.57	19.99	244.01	3375
264.5	6.37	16.84	247.66	3425	6.76	17.88	246.62	3411	7.15	18.92	245.58	3396	7.54	19.95	244.55	3382
265	6.34	16.80	248.20	3433	6.73	17.84	247.16	3418	7.12	18.88	246.13	3404	7.51	19.91	245.09	3390
265.5	6.31	16.76	248.74	3440	6.70	17.80	247.70	3426	7.09	18.83	246.67	3411	7.48	19.87	245.63	3397
266	6.28	16.72	249.28	3448	6.67	17.76	248.24	3433	7.07	18.79	247.21	3419	7.46	19.83	246.17	3405
266.5	6.26	16.68	249.82	3455	6.65	17.71	248.79	3441	7.04	18.75	247.75	3426	7.43	19.79	246.71	3412
267	6.23	16.64	250.36	3463	6.62	17.67	249.33	3448	7.01	18.71	248.29	3434	7.40	19.75	247.25	3419
267.5	6.20	16.60	250.91	3470	6.59	17.63	249.87	3456	6.98	18.67	248.83	3441	7.37	19.71	247.79	3427
268	6.18	16.55	251.45	3477	6.56	17.59	250.41	3463	6.95	18.63	249.37	3449	7.34	19.67	248.33	3434
268.5	6.15	16.51	251.99	3485	6.54	17.55	250.95	3471	6.92	18.59	249.91	3456	7.31	19.63	248.87	3442
269	6.12	16.47	252.53	3492	6.51	17.51	251.49	3478	6.89	18.55	250.45	3464	7.28	19.58	249.42	3449
269.5	6.10	16.43	253.07	3500	6.48	17.47	252.03	3486	6.87	18.51	250.99	3471	7.25	19.54	249.96	3457
270	6.07	16.39	253.61	3507	6.45	17.43	252.57	3493	6.84	18.47	251.54	3479	7.22	19.50	250.50	3464
270.5	6.04	16.35	254.15	3515	6.43	17.39	253.11	3501	6.81	18.42	252.08	3486	7.19	19.46	251.04	3472
271	6.02	16.31	254.69	3522	6.40	17.35	253.65	3508	6.78	18.38	252.62	3494	7.17	19.42	251.58	3479
271.5	5.99	16.27	255.23	3530	6.37	17.30	254.20	3516	6.76	18.34	253.16	3501	7.14	19.38	252.12	3487
272	5.97	16.23	255.77	3537	6.35	17.26	254.74	3523	6.73	18.30	253.70	3509	7.11	19.34	252.66	3494
272.5	5.94	16.19	256.32	3545	6.32	17.22	255.28	3530	6.70	18.26	254.24	3516	7.08	19.30	253.20	3502
273	5.91	16.14	256.86	3552	6.29	17.18	255.82	3538	6.67	18.22	254.78	3524	7.05	19.26	253.74	3509
273.5	5.89	16.10	257.40	3560	6.27	17.14	256.36	3545	6.65	18.18	255.32	3531	7.03	19.22	254.28	3517
274	5.86	16.06	257.94	3567	6.24	17.10	256.90	3553	6.62	18.14	255.86	3539	7.00	19.17	254.83	3524
274.5	5.84	16.02	258.48	3575	6.21	17.06	257.44	3560	6.59	18.10	256.40	3546	6.97	19.13	255.37	3532
275	5.81	15.98	259.02	3582	6.19	17.02	257.98	3568	6.57	18.06	256.95	3554	6.94	19.09	255.91	3539
275.5	5.79	15.94	259.56	3590	6.16	16.98	258.52	3575	6.54	18.01	257.49	3561	6.92	19.05	256.45	3547
276	5.76	15.90	260.10	3597	6.14	16.94	259.06	3583	6.51	17.97	258.03	3569	6.89	19.01	256.99	3554
276.5	5.73	15.86	260.64	3605	6.11	16.89	259.61	3590	6.49	17.93	258.57	3576	6.86	18.97	257.53	3562
277	5.71	15.82	261.18	3612	6.08	16.85	260.15	3598	6.46	17.89	259.11	3583	6.83	18.93	258.07	3569
277.5	5.68	15.78	261.73	3620	6.06	16.81	260.69	3605	6.43	17.85	259.65	3591	6.81	18.89	258.61	3577
278	5.66	15.73	262.27	3627	6.03	16.77	261.23	3613	6.41	17.81	260.19	3598	6.78	18.85	259.15	3584
278.5	5.63	15.69	262.81	3635	6.01	16.73	261.77	3620	6.38	17.77	260.73	3606	6.75	18.81	259.69	3592
279	5.61	15.65	263.35	3642	5.98	16.69	262.31	3628	6.35	17.73	261.27	3613	6.73	18.76	260.24	3599
279.5	5.59	15.61	263.89	3650	5.96	16.65	262.85	3635	6.33	17.69	261.81	3621	6.70	18.72	260.78	3607

Body Composition   MALE   248-279.5 Lb.

Weight: Lb.	Waist: 34 inches Fat: %	Fat: Lb.	LBM: Lb.	RMR: Cal.	34.25 inches Fat: %	Fat: Lb.	LBM: Lb.	RMR: Cal.	34.5 inches Fat: %	Fat: Lb.	LBM: Lb.	RMR: Cal.	34.75 inches Fat: %	Fat: Lb.	LBM: Lb.	RMR: Cal.
248	9.01	22.34	225.66	3121	9.43	23.38	224.62	3106	9.85	24.42	223.58	3092	10.26	25.46	222.54	3078
248.5	8.98	22.30	226.20	3128	9.39	23.34	225.16	3114	9.81	24.38	224.12	3100	10.23	25.42	223.08	3085
249	8.94	22.26	226.74	3136	9.36	23.30	225.70	3121	9.77	24.34	224.66	3107	10.19	25.37	223.63	3093
249.5	8.91	22.22	227.28	3143	9.32	23.26	226.24	3129	9.74	24.30	225.20	3115	10.15	25.33	224.17	3100
250	8.87	22.18	227.82	3151	9.29	23.22	226.78	3136	9.70	24.26	225.75	3122	10.12	25.29	224.71	3108
250.5	8.84	22.14	228.36	3158	9.25	23.18	227.32	3144	9.67	24.21	226.29	3130	10.08	25.25	225.25	3115
251	8.80	22.10	228.90	3166	9.22	23.14	227.86	3151	9.63	24.17	226.83	3137	10.04	25.21	225.79	3123
251.5	8.77	22.06	229.44	3173	9.18	23.09	228.41	3159	9.60	24.13	227.37	3144	10.01	25.17	226.33	3130
252	8.74	22.02	229.98	3181	9.15	23.05	228.95	3166	9.56	24.09	227.91	3152	9.97	25.13	226.87	3138
252.5	8.70	21.98	230.53	3188	9.11	23.01	229.49	3174	9.52	24.05	228.45	3159	9.94	25.09	227.41	3145
253	8.67	21.93	231.07	3196	9.08	22.97	230.03	3181	9.49	24.01	228.99	3167	9.90	25.05	227.95	3153
253.5	8.64	21.89	231.61	3203	9.05	22.93	230.57	3189	9.45	23.97	229.53	3174	9.86	25.01	228.49	3160
254	8.60	21.85	232.15	3211	9.01	22.89	231.11	3196	9.42	23.93	230.07	3182	9.83	24.96	229.04	3168
254.5	8.57	21.81	232.69	3218	8.98	22.85	231.65	3204	9.39	23.89	230.61	3189	9.79	24.92	229.58	3175
255	8.54	21.77	233.23	3226	8.94	22.81	232.19	3211	9.35	23.85	231.16	3197	9.76	24.88	230.12	3183
255.5	8.50	21.73	233.77	3233	8.91	22.77	232.73	3219	9.32	23.80	231.70	3204	9.72	24.84	230.66	3190
256	8.47	21.69	234.31	3241	8.88	22.73	233.27	3226	9.28	23.76	232.24	3212	9.69	24.80	231.20	3197
256.5	8.44	21.65	234.85	3248	8.84	22.68	233.82	3234	9.25	23.72	232.78	3219	9.65	24.76	231.74	3205
257	8.41	21.61	235.39	3255	8.81	22.64	234.36	3241	9.21	23.68	233.32	3227	9.62	24.72	232.28	3212
257.5	8.37	21.57	235.94	3263	8.78	22.60	234.90	3249	9.18	23.64	233.86	3234	9.58	24.68	232.82	3220
258	8.34	21.52	236.48	3270	8.74	22.56	235.44	3256	9.15	23.60	234.40	3242	9.55	24.64	233.36	3227
258.5	8.31	21.48	237.02	3278	8.71	22.52	235.98	3264	9.11	23.56	234.94	3249	9.51	24.60	233.90	3235
259	8.28	21.44	237.56	3285	8.68	22.48	236.52	3271	9.08	23.52	235.48	3257	9.48	24.55	234.45	3242
259.5	8.25	21.40	238.10	3293	8.65	22.44	237.06	3279	9.05	23.48	236.02	3264	9.45	24.51	234.99	3250
260	8.22	21.36	238.64	3300	8.61	22.40	237.60	3286	9.01	23.44	236.57	3272	9.41	24.47	235.53	3257
260.5	8.18	21.32	239.18	3308	8.58	22.36	238.14	3294	8.98	23.39	237.11	3279	9.38	24.43	236.07	3265
261	8.15	21.28	239.72	3315	8.55	22.32	238.68	3301	8.95	23.35	237.65	3287	9.35	24.39	236.61	3272
261.5	8.12	21.24	240.26	3323	8.52	22.27	239.23	3308	8.91	23.31	238.19	3294	9.31	24.35	237.15	3280
262	8.09	21.20	240.80	3330	8.49	22.23	239.77	3316	8.88	23.27	238.73	3302	9.28	24.31	237.69	3287
262.5	8.06	21.16	241.35	3338	8.45	22.19	240.31	3323	8.85	23.23	239.27	3309	9.24	24.27	238.23	3295
263	8.03	21.11	241.89	3345	8.42	22.15	240.85	3331	8.82	23.19	239.81	3317	9.21	24.23	238.77	3302
263.5	8.00	21.07	242.43	3353	8.39	22.11	241.39	3338	8.78	23.15	240.35	3324	9.18	24.19	239.31	3310
264	7.97	21.03	242.97	3360	8.36	22.07	241.93	3346	8.75	23.11	240.89	3332	9.15	24.14	239.86	3317
264.5	7.94	20.99	243.51	3368	8.33	22.03	242.47	3353	8.72	23.07	241.43	3339	9.11	24.10	240.40	3325
265	7.91	20.95	244.05	3375	8.30	21.99	243.01	3361	8.69	23.03	241.98	3347	9.08	24.06	240.94	3332
265.5	7.88	20.91	244.59	3383	8.27	21.95	243.55	3368	8.66	22.98	242.52	3354	9.05	24.02	241.48	3340
266	7.85	20.87	245.13	3390	8.24	21.91	244.09	3376	8.63	22.94	243.06	3361	9.02	23.98	242.02	3347
266.5	7.82	20.83	245.67	3398	8.20	21.86	244.64	3383	8.59	22.90	243.60	3369	8.98	23.94	242.56	3355
267	7.79	20.79	246.21	3405	8.17	21.82	245.18	3391	8.56	22.86	244.14	3376	8.95	23.90	243.10	3362
267.5	7.76	20.75	246.76	3413	8.14	21.78	245.72	3398	8.53	22.82	244.68	3384	8.92	23.86	243.64	3370
268	7.73	20.70	247.30	3420	8.11	21.74	246.26	3406	8.50	22.78	245.22	3391	8.89	23.82	244.18	3377
268.5	7.70	20.66	247.84	3428	8.08	21.70	246.80	3413	8.47	22.74	245.76	3399	8.85	23.78	244.72	3385
269	7.67	20.62	248.38	3435	8.05	21.66	247.34	3421	8.44	22.70	246.30	3406	8.82	23.73	245.27	3392
269.5	7.64	20.58	248.92	3443	8.02	21.62	247.88	3428	8.41	22.66	246.84	3414	8.79	23.69	245.81	3400
270	7.61	20.54	249.46	3450	7.99	21.58	248.42	3436	8.38	22.62	247.39	3421	8.76	23.65	246.35	3407
270.5	7.58	20.50	250.00	3458	7.96	21.54	248.96	3443	8.35	22.57	247.93	3429	8.73	23.61	246.89	3414
271	7.55	20.46	250.54	3465	7.93	21.50	249.50	3451	8.31	22.53	248.47	3436	8.70	23.57	247.43	3422
271.5	7.52	20.42	251.08	3472	7.90	21.45	250.05	3458	8.28	22.49	249.01	3444	8.67	23.53	247.97	3429
272	7.49	20.38	251.62	3480	7.87	21.41	250.59	3466	8.25	22.45	249.55	3451	8.64	23.49	248.51	3437
272.5	7.46	20.34	252.17	3487	7.84	21.37	251.13	3473	8.22	22.41	250.09	3459	8.60	23.45	249.05	3444
273	7.43	20.29	252.71	3495	7.81	21.33	251.67	3481	8.19	22.37	250.63	3466	8.57	23.41	249.59	3452
273.5	7.41	20.25	253.25	3502	7.78	21.29	252.21	3488	8.16	22.33	251.17	3474	8.54	23.37	250.13	3459
274	7.38	20.21	253.79	3510	7.76	21.25	252.75	3496	8.13	22.29	251.71	3481	8.51	23.32	250.68	3467
274.5	7.35	20.17	254.33	3517	7.73	21.21	253.29	3503	8.10	22.25	252.25	3489	8.48	23.28	251.22	3474
275	7.32	20.13	254.87	3525	7.70	21.17	253.83	3511	8.07	22.21	252.80	3496	8.45	23.24	251.76	3482
275.5	7.29	20.09	255.41	3532	7.67	21.13	254.37	3518	8.05	22.16	253.34	3504	8.42	23.20	252.30	3489
276	7.26	20.05	255.95	3540	7.64	21.09	254.91	3525	8.02	22.12	253.88	3511	8.39	23.16	252.84	3497
276.5	7.24	20.01	256.49	3547	7.61	21.04	255.46	3533	7.99	22.08	254.42	3519	8.36	23.12	253.38	3504
277	7.21	19.97	257.03	3555	7.58	21.00	256.00	3540	7.96	22.04	254.96	3526	8.33	23.08	253.92	3512
277.5	7.18	19.93	257.58	3562	7.55	20.96	256.54	3548	7.93	22.00	255.50	3534	8.30	23.04	254.46	3519
278	7.15	19.88	258.12	3570	7.53	20.92	257.08	3555	7.90	21.96	256.04	3541	8.27	23.00	255.00	3527
278.5	7.12	19.84	258.66	3577	7.50	20.88	257.62	3563	7.87	21.92	256.58	3549	8.24	22.96	255.54	3534
279	7.10	19.80	259.20	3585	7.47	20.84	258.16	3570	7.84	21.88	257.12	3556	8.21	22.91	256.09	3542
279.5	7.07	19.76	259.74	3592	7.44	20.80	258.70	3578	7.81	21.84	257.66	3563	8.18	22.87	256.63	3549

Body Composition   MALE   248-279.5 Lb.

Weight: Lb.	Waist: 35 inches Fat: %	Fat: Lb.	LBM: Lb.	RMR: Cal.	35.25 inches Fat: %	Fat: Lb.	LBM: Lb.	RMR: Cal.	35.5 inches Fat: %	Fat: Lb.	LBM: Lb.	RMR: Cal.	35.75 inches Fat: %	Fat: Lb.	LBM: Lb.	RMR: Cal.
248	10.68	26.49	221.51	3063	11.10	27.53	220.47	3049	11.52	28.57	219.43	3035	11.94	29.61	218.39	3020
248.5	10.65	26.45	222.05	3071	11.06	27.49	221.01	3057	11.48	28.53	219.97	3042	11.90	29.57	218.93	3028
249	10.61	26.41	222.59	3078	11.02	27.45	221.55	3064	11.44	28.49	220.51	3050	11.86	29.52	219.48	3035
249.5	10.57	26.37	223.13	3086	10.99	27.41	222.09	3072	11.40	28.45	221.05	3057	11.82	29.48	220.02	3043
250	10.53	26.33	223.67	3093	10.95	27.37	222.63	3079	11.36	28.41	221.60	3065	11.78	29.44	220.56	3050
250.5	10.49	26.29	224.21	3101	10.91	27.33	223.17	3086	11.32	28.36	222.14	3072	11.74	29.40	221.10	3058
251	10.46	26.25	224.75	3108	10.87	27.29	223.71	3094	11.28	28.32	222.68	3080	11.70	29.36	221.64	3065
251.5	10.42	26.21	225.29	3116	10.83	27.24	224.26	3101	11.25	28.28	223.22	3087	11.66	29.32	222.18	3073
252	10.38	26.17	225.83	3123	10.80	27.20	224.80	3109	11.21	28.24	223.76	3095	11.62	29.28	222.72	3080
252.5	10.35	26.12	226.38	3131	10.76	27.16	225.34	3116	11.17	28.20	224.30	3102	11.58	29.24	223.26	3088
253	10.31	26.08	226.92	3138	10.72	27.12	225.88	3124	11.13	28.16	224.84	3110	11.54	29.20	223.80	3095
253.5	10.27	26.04	227.46	3146	10.68	27.08	226.42	3131	11.09	28.12	225.38	3117	11.50	29.16	224.34	3103
254	10.24	26.00	228.00	3153	10.65	27.04	226.96	3139	11.05	28.08	225.92	3125	11.46	29.11	224.89	3110
254.5	10.20	25.96	228.54	3161	10.61	27.00	227.50	3146	11.02	28.04	226.46	3132	11.42	29.07	225.43	3118
255	10.16	25.92	229.08	3168	10.57	26.96	228.04	3154	10.98	28.00	227.01	3139	11.39	29.03	225.97	3125
255.5	10.13	25.88	229.62	3176	10.53	26.92	228.58	3161	10.94	27.95	227.55	3147	11.35	28.99	226.51	3133
256	10.09	25.84	230.16	3183	10.50	26.88	229.12	3169	10.90	27.91	228.09	3154	11.31	28.95	227.05	3140
256.5	10.06	25.80	230.70	3191	10.46	26.83	229.67	3176	10.87	27.87	228.63	3162	11.27	28.91	227.59	3148
257	10.02	25.76	231.24	3198	10.43	26.79	230.21	3184	10.83	27.83	229.17	3169	11.23	28.87	228.13	3155
257.5	9.99	25.72	231.79	3206	10.39	26.75	230.75	3191	10.79	27.79	229.71	3177	11.20	28.83	228.67	3163
258	9.95	25.67	232.33	3213	10.35	26.71	231.29	3199	10.76	27.75	230.25	3184	11.16	28.79	229.21	3170
258.5	9.92	25.63	232.87	3221	10.32	26.67	231.83	3206	10.72	27.71	230.79	3192	11.12	28.75	229.75	3178
259	9.88	25.59	233.41	3228	10.28	26.63	232.37	3214	10.68	27.67	231.33	3199	11.08	28.70	230.30	3185
259.5	9.85	25.55	233.95	3236	10.25	26.59	232.91	3221	10.65	27.63	231.87	3207	11.05	28.66	230.84	3192
260	9.81	25.51	234.49	3243	10.21	26.55	233.45	3229	10.61	27.59	232.42	3214	11.01	28.62	231.38	3200
260.5	9.78	25.47	235.03	3250	10.18	26.51	233.99	3236	10.57	27.54	232.96	3222	10.97	28.58	231.92	3207
261	9.74	25.43	235.57	3258	10.14	26.47	234.53	3244	10.54	27.50	233.50	3229	10.94	28.54	232.46	3215
261.5	9.71	25.39	236.11	3265	10.10	26.42	235.08	3251	10.50	27.46	234.04	3237	10.90	28.50	233.00	3222
262	9.67	25.35	236.65	3273	10.07	26.38	235.62	3259	10.47	27.42	234.58	3244	10.86	28.46	233.54	3230
262.5	9.64	25.30	237.20	3280	10.04	26.34	236.16	3266	10.43	27.38	235.12	3252	10.83	28.42	234.08	3237
263	9.61	25.26	237.74	3288	10.00	26.30	236.70	3274	10.40	27.34	235.66	3259	10.79	28.38	234.62	3245
263.5	9.57	25.22	238.28	3295	9.97	26.26	237.24	3281	10.36	27.30	236.20	3267	10.75	28.34	235.16	3252
264	9.54	25.18	238.82	3303	9.93	26.22	237.78	3289	10.32	27.26	236.74	3274	10.72	28.29	235.71	3260
264.5	9.51	25.14	239.36	3310	9.90	26.18	238.32	3296	10.29	27.22	237.28	3282	10.68	28.25	236.25	3267
265	9.47	25.10	239.90	3318	9.86	26.14	238.86	3303	10.25	27.18	237.83	3289	10.65	28.21	236.79	3275
265.5	9.44	25.06	240.44	3325	9.83	26.10	239.40	3311	10.22	27.13	238.37	3297	10.61	28.17	237.33	3282
266	9.41	25.02	240.98	3333	9.80	26.06	239.94	3318	10.19	27.09	238.91	3304	10.58	28.13	237.87	3290
266.5	9.37	24.98	241.52	3340	9.76	26.01	240.49	3326	10.15	27.05	239.45	3312	10.54	28.09	238.41	3297
267	9.34	24.94	242.06	3348	9.73	25.97	241.03	3333	10.12	27.01	239.99	3319	10.51	28.05	238.95	3305
267.5	9.31	24.90	242.61	3355	9.69	25.93	241.57	3341	10.08	26.97	240.53	3327	10.47	28.01	239.49	3312
268	9.27	24.85	243.15	3363	9.66	25.89	242.11	3348	10.05	26.93	241.07	3334	10.44	27.97	240.03	3320
268.5	9.24	24.81	243.69	3370	9.63	25.85	242.65	3356	10.01	26.89	241.61	3341	10.40	27.93	240.57	3327
269	9.21	24.77	244.23	3378	9.59	25.81	243.19	3363	9.98	26.85	242.15	3349	10.37	27.88	241.12	3335
269.5	9.18	24.73	244.77	3385	9.56	25.77	243.73	3371	9.95	26.81	242.69	3356	10.33	27.84	241.66	3342
270	9.14	24.69	245.31	3393	9.53	25.73	244.27	3378	9.91	26.77	243.24	3364	10.30	27.80	242.20	3350
270.5	9.11	24.65	245.85	3400	9.50	25.69	244.81	3386	9.88	26.72	243.78	3371	10.26	27.76	242.74	3357
271	9.08	24.61	246.39	3408	9.46	25.65	245.35	3393	9.85	26.68	244.32	3379	10.23	27.72	243.28	3365
271.5	9.05	24.57	246.93	3415	9.43	25.60	245.90	3401	9.81	26.64	244.86	3386	10.20	27.68	243.82	3372
272	9.02	24.53	247.47	3423	9.40	25.56	246.44	3408	9.78	26.60	245.40	3394	10.16	27.64	244.36	3380
272.5	8.99	24.49	248.02	3430	9.37	25.52	246.98	3416	9.75	26.56	245.94	3401	10.13	27.60	244.90	3387
273	8.95	24.44	248.56	3438	9.33	25.48	247.52	3423	9.71	26.52	246.48	3409	10.09	27.56	245.44	3394
273.5	8.92	24.40	249.10	3445	9.30	25.44	248.06	3431	9.68	26.48	247.02	3416	10.06	27.52	245.98	3402
274	8.89	24.36	249.64	3452	9.27	25.40	248.60	3438	9.65	26.44	247.56	3424	10.03	27.47	246.53	3409
274.5	8.86	24.32	250.18	3460	9.24	25.36	249.14	3446	9.62	26.40	248.10	3431	9.99	27.43	247.07	3417
275	8.83	24.28	250.72	3467	9.21	25.32	249.68	3453	9.58	26.36	248.65	3439	9.96	27.39	247.61	3424
275.5	8.80	24.24	251.26	3475	9.17	25.28	250.22	3461	9.55	26.31	249.19	3446	9.93	27.35	248.15	3432
276	8.77	24.20	251.80	3482	9.14	25.24	250.76	3468	9.52	26.27	249.73	3454	9.90	27.31	248.69	3439
276.5	8.74	24.16	252.34	3490	9.11	25.19	251.31	3476	9.49	26.23	250.27	3461	9.86	27.27	249.23	3447
277	8.71	24.12	252.88	3497	9.08	25.15	251.85	3483	9.46	26.19	250.81	3469	9.83	27.23	249.77	3454
277.5	8.68	24.08	253.43	3505	9.05	25.11	252.39	3491	9.42	26.15	251.35	3476	9.80	27.19	250.31	3462
278	8.65	24.03	253.97	3512	9.02	25.07	252.93	3498	9.39	26.11	251.89	3484	9.76	27.15	250.85	3469
278.5	8.62	23.99	254.51	3520	8.99	25.03	253.47	3505	9.36	26.07	252.43	3491	9.73	27.11	251.39	3477
279	8.58	23.95	255.05	3527	8.96	24.99	254.01	3513	9.33	26.03	252.97	3499	9.70	27.06	251.94	3484
279.5	8.55	23.91	255.59	3535	8.93	24.95	254.55	3520	9.30	25.99	253.51	3506	9.67	27.02	252.48	3492

Body Composition   MALE   248-279.5 Lb.

Weight: Lb.	Waist: 36 inches Fat: %	Fat: Lb.	LBM: Lb.	RMR: Cal.	36.25 inches Fat: %	Fat: Lb.	LBM: Lb.	RMR: Cal.	36.5 inches Fat: %	Fat: Lb.	LBM: Lb.	RMR: Cal.	36.75 inches Fat: %	Fat: Lb.	LBM: Lb.	RMR: Cal.
248	12.36	30.64	217.36	3006	12.77	31.68	216.32	2992	13.19	32.72	215.28	2977	13.61	33.76	214.24	2963
248.5	12.32	30.60	217.90	3014	12.73	31.64	216.86	2999	13.15	32.68	215.82	2985	13.57	33.72	214.78	2970
249	12.27	30.56	218.44	3021	12.69	31.60	217.40	3007	13.11	32.64	216.36	2992	13.52	33.67	215.33	2978
249.5	12.23	30.52	218.98	3028	12.65	31.56	217.94	3014	13.06	32.60	216.90	3000	13.48	33.63	215.87	2985
250	12.19	30.48	219.52	3036	12.61	31.52	218.48	3022	13.02	32.56	217.45	3007	13.44	33.59	216.41	2993
250.5	12.15	30.44	220.06	3043	12.57	31.48	219.02	3029	12.98	32.51	217.99	3015	13.39	33.55	216.95	3000
251	12.11	30.40	220.60	3051	12.52	31.44	219.56	3037	12.94	32.47	218.53	3022	13.35	33.51	217.49	3008
251.5	12.07	30.36	221.14	3058	12.48	31.39	220.11	3044	12.90	32.43	219.07	3030	13.31	33.47	218.03	3015
252	12.03	30.32	221.68	3066	12.44	31.35	220.65	3052	12.85	32.39	219.61	3037	13.27	33.43	218.57	3023
252.5	11.99	30.28	222.23	3073	12.40	31.31	221.19	3059	12.81	32.35	220.15	3045	13.22	33.39	219.11	3030
253	11.95	30.23	222.77	3081	12.36	31.27	221.73	3067	12.77	32.31	220.69	3052	13.18	33.35	219.65	3038
253.5	11.91	30.19	223.31	3088	12.32	31.23	222.27	3074	12.73	32.27	221.23	3060	13.14	33.31	220.19	3045
254	11.87	30.15	223.85	3096	12.28	31.19	222.81	3081	12.69	32.23	221.77	3067	13.10	33.26	220.74	3053
254.5	11.83	30.11	224.39	3103	12.24	31.15	223.35	3089	12.65	32.19	222.31	3075	13.05	33.22	221.28	3060
255	11.79	30.07	224.93	3111	12.20	31.11	223.89	3096	12.61	32.15	222.86	3082	13.01	33.18	221.82	3068
255.5	11.75	30.03	225.47	3118	12.16	31.07	224.43	3104	12.57	32.10	223.40	3090	12.97	33.14	222.36	3075
256	11.71	29.99	226.01	3126	12.12	31.03	224.97	3111	12.52	32.06	223.94	3097	12.93	33.10	222.90	3083
256.5	11.68	29.95	226.55	3133	12.08	30.98	225.52	3119	12.48	32.02	224.48	3105	12.89	33.06	223.44	3090
257	11.64	29.91	227.09	3141	12.04	30.94	226.06	3126	12.44	31.98	225.02	3112	12.85	33.02	223.98	3098
257.5	11.60	29.87	227.64	3148	12.00	30.90	226.60	3134	12.40	31.94	225.56	3119	12.81	32.98	224.52	3105
258	11.56	29.82	228.18	3156	11.96	30.86	227.14	3141	12.36	31.90	226.10	3127	12.77	32.94	225.06	3113
258.5	11.52	29.78	228.72	3163	11.92	30.82	227.68	3149	12.32	31.86	226.64	3134	12.73	32.90	225.60	3120
259	11.48	29.74	229.26	3171	11.88	30.78	228.22	3156	12.28	31.82	227.18	3142	12.69	32.85	226.15	3128
259.5	11.45	29.70	229.80	3178	11.85	30.74	228.76	3164	12.25	31.78	227.72	3149	12.64	32.81	226.69	3135
260	11.41	29.66	230.34	3186	11.81	30.70	229.30	3171	12.21	31.74	228.27	3157	12.60	32.77	227.23	3143
260.5	11.37	29.62	230.88	3193	11.77	30.66	229.84	3179	12.17	31.69	228.81	3164	12.56	32.73	227.77	3150
261	11.33	29.58	231.42	3201	11.73	30.62	230.38	3186	12.13	31.65	229.35	3172	12.53	32.69	228.31	3158
261.5	11.30	29.54	231.96	3208	11.69	30.57	230.93	3194	12.09	31.61	229.89	3179	12.49	32.65	228.85	3165
262	11.26	29.50	232.50	3216	11.65	30.53	231.47	3201	12.05	31.57	230.43	3187	12.45	32.61	229.39	3172
262.5	11.22	29.46	233.05	3223	11.62	30.49	232.01	3209	12.01	31.53	230.97	3194	12.41	32.57	229.93	3180
263	11.18	29.41	233.59	3230	11.58	30.45	232.55	3216	11.97	31.49	231.51	3202	12.37	32.53	230.47	3187
263.5	11.15	29.37	234.13	3238	11.54	30.41	233.09	3224	11.93	31.45	232.05	3209	12.33	32.49	231.01	3195
264	11.11	29.33	234.67	3245	11.50	30.37	233.63	3231	11.90	31.41	232.59	3217	12.29	32.44	231.56	3202
264.5	11.07	29.29	235.21	3253	11.47	30.33	234.17	3239	11.86	31.37	233.13	3224	12.25	32.40	232.10	3210
265	11.04	29.25	235.75	3260	11.43	30.29	234.71	3246	11.82	31.33	233.68	3232	12.21	32.36	232.64	3217
265.5	11.00	29.21	236.29	3268	11.39	30.25	235.25	3254	11.78	31.28	234.22	3239	12.17	32.32	233.18	3225
266	10.97	29.17	236.83	3275	11.36	30.21	235.79	3261	11.75	31.24	234.76	3247	12.14	32.28	233.72	3232
266.5	10.93	29.13	237.37	3283	11.32	30.16	236.34	3269	11.71	31.20	235.30	3254	12.10	32.24	234.26	3240
267	10.89	29.09	237.91	3290	11.28	30.12	236.88	3276	11.67	31.16	235.84	3262	12.06	32.20	234.80	3247
267.5	10.86	29.05	238.46	3298	11.25	30.08	237.42	3283	11.63	31.12	236.38	3269	12.02	32.16	235.34	3255
268	10.82	29.00	239.00	3305	11.21	30.04	237.96	3291	11.60	31.08	236.92	3277	11.98	32.12	235.88	3262
268.5	10.79	28.96	239.54	3313	11.17	30.00	238.50	3298	11.56	31.04	237.46	3284	11.95	32.08	236.42	3270
269	10.75	28.92	240.08	3320	11.14	29.96	239.04	3306	11.52	31.00	238.00	3292	11.91	32.03	236.97	3277
269.5	10.72	28.88	240.62	3328	11.10	29.92	239.58	3313	11.49	30.96	238.54	3299	11.87	31.99	237.51	3285
270	10.68	28.84	241.16	3335	11.07	29.88	240.12	3321	11.45	30.92	239.09	3307	11.83	31.95	238.05	3292
270.5	10.65	28.80	241.70	3343	11.03	29.84	240.66	3328	11.41	30.87	239.63	3314	11.80	31.91	238.59	3300
271	10.61	28.76	242.24	3350	10.99	29.80	241.20	3336	11.38	30.83	240.17	3322	11.76	31.87	239.13	3307
271.5	10.58	28.72	242.78	3358	10.96	29.75	241.75	3343	11.34	30.79	240.71	3329	11.72	31.83	239.67	3315
272	10.54	28.68	243.32	3365	10.92	29.71	242.29	3351	11.31	30.75	241.25	3336	11.69	31.79	240.21	3322
272.5	10.51	28.64	243.87	3373	10.89	29.67	242.83	3358	11.27	30.71	241.79	3344	11.65	31.75	240.75	3330
273	10.47	28.59	244.41	3380	10.85	29.63	243.37	3366	11.23	30.67	242.33	3351	11.61	31.71	241.29	3337
273.5	10.44	28.55	244.95	3388	10.82	29.59	243.91	3373	11.20	30.63	242.87	3359	11.58	31.67	241.83	3345
274	10.41	28.51	245.49	3395	10.78	29.55	244.45	3381	11.16	30.59	243.41	3366	11.54	31.62	242.38	3352
274.5	10.37	28.47	246.03	3403	10.75	29.51	244.99	3388	11.13	30.55	243.95	3374	11.51	31.58	242.92	3360
275	10.34	28.43	246.57	3410	10.72	29.47	245.53	3396	11.09	30.51	244.50	3381	11.47	31.54	243.46	3367
275.5	10.30	28.39	247.11	3418	10.68	29.43	246.07	3403	11.06	30.46	245.04	3389	11.43	31.50	244.00	3374
276	10.27	28.35	247.65	3425	10.65	29.39	246.61	3411	11.02	30.42	245.58	3396	11.40	31.46	244.54	3382
276.5	10.24	28.31	248.19	3433	10.61	29.34	247.16	3418	10.99	30.38	246.12	3404	11.36	31.42	245.08	3389
277	10.20	28.27	248.73	3440	10.58	29.30	247.70	3426	10.95	30.34	246.66	3411	11.33	31.38	245.62	3397
277.5	10.17	28.23	249.28	3447	10.55	29.26	248.24	3433	10.92	30.30	247.20	3419	11.29	31.34	246.16	3404
278	10.14	28.18	249.82	3455	10.51	29.22	248.78	3441	10.88	30.26	247.74	3426	11.26	31.30	246.70	3412
278.5	10.11	28.14	250.36	3462	10.48	29.18	249.32	3448	10.85	30.22	248.28	3434	11.22	31.26	247.24	3419
279	10.07	28.10	250.90	3470	10.44	29.14	249.86	3456	10.82	30.18	248.82	3441	11.19	31.21	247.79	3427
279.5	10.04	28.06	251.44	3477	10.41	29.10	250.40	3463	10.78	30.14	249.36	3449	11.15	31.17	248.33	3434

Body Composition MALE 248-279.5 Lb.

Weight: Lb.	Waist: 37 inches Fat: %	Fat: Lb.	LBM: Lb.	RMR: Cal.	37.25 inches Fat: %	Fat: Lb.	LBM: Lb.	RMR: Cal.	37.5 inches Fat: %	Fat: Lb.	LBM: Lb.	RMR: Cal.	37.75 inches Fat: %	Fat: Lb.	LBM: Lb.	RMR: Cal.
248	14.03	34.79	213.21	2949	14.45	35.83	212.17	2934	14.87	36.87	211.13	2920	15.28	37.91	210.09	2906
248.5	13.99	34.75	213.75	2956	14.40	35.79	212.71	2942	14.82	36.83	211.67	2927	15.24	37.87	210.63	2913
249	13.94	34.71	214.29	2964	14.36	35.75	213.25	2949	14.77	36.79	212.21	2935	15.19	37.82	211.18	2921
249.5	13.90	34.67	214.83	2971	14.31	35.71	213.79	2957	14.73	36.75	212.75	2942	15.14	37.78	211.72	2928
250	13.85	34.63	215.37	2979	14.27	35.67	214.33	2964	14.68	36.71	213.30	2950	15.10	37.74	212.26	2936
250.5	13.81	34.59	215.91	2986	14.22	35.63	214.87	2972	14.64	36.66	213.84	2957	15.05	37.70	212.80	2943
251	13.76	34.55	216.45	2994	14.18	35.59	215.41	2979	14.59	36.62	214.38	2965	15.00	37.66	213.34	2950
251.5	13.72	34.51	216.99	3001	14.13	35.54	215.96	2987	14.55	36.58	214.92	2972	14.96	37.62	213.88	2958
252	13.68	34.47	217.53	3008	14.09	35.50	216.50	2994	14.50	36.54	215.46	2980	14.91	37.58	214.42	2965
252.5	13.63	34.43	218.08	3016	14.04	35.46	217.04	3002	14.46	36.50	216.00	2987	14.87	37.54	214.96	2973
253	13.59	34.38	218.62	3023	14.00	35.42	217.58	3009	14.41	36.46	216.54	2995	14.82	37.50	215.50	2980
253.5	13.55	34.34	219.16	3031	13.96	35.38	218.12	3017	14.37	36.42	217.08	3002	14.78	37.46	216.04	2988
254	13.50	34.30	219.70	3038	13.91	35.34	218.66	3024	14.32	36.38	217.62	3010	14.73	37.41	216.59	2995
254.5	13.46	34.26	220.24	3046	13.87	35.30	219.20	3032	14.28	36.34	218.16	3017	14.69	37.37	217.13	3003
255	13.42	34.22	220.78	3053	13.83	35.26	219.74	3039	14.23	36.30	218.71	3025	14.64	37.33	217.67	3010
255.5	13.38	34.18	221.32	3061	13.78	35.22	220.28	3047	14.19	36.25	219.25	3032	14.60	37.29	218.21	3018
256	13.34	34.14	221.86	3068	13.74	35.18	220.82	3054	14.15	36.21	219.79	3040	14.55	37.25	218.75	3025
256.5	13.29	34.10	222.40	3076	13.70	35.13	221.37	3061	14.10	36.17	220.33	3047	14.51	37.21	219.29	3033
257	13.25	34.06	222.94	3083	13.66	35.09	221.91	3069	14.06	36.13	220.87	3055	14.46	37.17	219.83	3040
257.5	13.21	34.02	223.49	3091	13.61	35.05	222.45	3076	14.02	36.09	221.41	3062	14.42	37.13	220.37	3048
258	13.17	33.97	224.03	3098	13.57	35.01	222.99	3084	13.97	36.05	221.95	3070	14.37	37.09	220.91	3055
258.5	13.13	33.93	224.57	3106	13.53	34.97	223.53	3091	13.93	36.01	222.49	3077	14.33	37.05	221.45	3063
259	13.09	33.89	225.11	3113	13.49	34.93	224.07	3099	13.89	35.97	223.03	3085	14.29	37.00	222.00	3070
259.5	13.04	33.85	225.65	3121	13.44	34.89	224.61	3106	13.84	35.93	223.57	3092	14.24	36.96	222.54	3078
260	13.00	33.81	226.19	3128	13.40	34.85	225.15	3114	13.80	35.89	224.12	3100	14.20	36.92	223.08	3085
260.5	12.96	33.77	226.73	3136	13.36	34.81	225.69	3121	13.76	35.84	224.66	3107	14.16	36.88	223.62	3093
261	12.92	33.73	227.27	3143	13.32	34.77	226.23	3129	13.72	35.80	225.20	3114	14.12	36.84	224.16	3100
261.5	12.88	33.69	227.81	3151	13.28	34.72	226.78	3136	13.68	35.76	225.74	3122	14.07	36.80	224.70	3108
262	12.84	33.65	228.35	3158	13.24	34.68	227.32	3144	13.63	35.72	226.28	3129	14.03	36.76	225.24	3115
262.5	12.80	33.61	228.90	3166	13.20	34.64	227.86	3151	13.59	35.68	226.82	3137	13.99	36.72	225.78	3123
263	12.76	33.56	229.44	3173	13.16	34.60	228.40	3159	13.55	35.64	227.36	3144	13.95	36.68	226.32	3130
263.5	12.72	33.52	229.98	3181	13.12	34.56	228.94	3166	13.51	35.60	227.90	3152	13.90	36.64	226.86	3138
264	12.68	33.48	230.52	3188	13.08	34.52	229.48	3174	13.47	35.56	228.44	3159	13.86	36.59	227.41	3145
264.5	12.64	33.44	231.06	3196	13.04	34.48	230.02	3181	13.43	35.52	228.98	3167	13.82	36.55	227.95	3153
265	12.60	33.40	231.60	3203	13.00	34.44	230.56	3189	13.39	35.48	229.53	3174	13.78	36.51	228.49	3160
265.5	12.56	33.36	232.14	3211	12.96	34.40	231.10	3196	13.35	35.43	230.07	3182	13.74	36.47	229.03	3167
266	12.53	33.32	232.68	3218	12.92	34.36	231.64	3204	13.31	35.39	230.61	3189	13.70	36.43	229.57	3175
266.5	12.49	33.28	233.22	3225	12.88	34.31	232.19	3211	13.27	35.35	231.15	3197	13.65	36.39	230.11	3182
267	12.45	33.24	233.76	3233	12.84	34.27	232.73	3219	13.23	35.31	231.69	3204	13.61	36.35	230.65	3190
267.5	12.41	33.20	234.31	3240	12.80	34.23	233.27	3226	13.19	35.27	232.23	3212	13.57	36.31	231.19	3197
268	12.37	33.15	234.85	3248	12.76	34.19	233.81	3234	13.15	35.23	232.77	3219	13.53	36.27	231.73	3205
268.5	12.33	33.11	235.39	3255	12.72	34.15	234.35	3241	13.11	35.19	233.31	3227	13.49	36.23	232.27	3212
269	12.29	33.07	235.93	3263	12.68	34.11	234.89	3249	13.07	35.15	233.85	3234	13.45	36.18	232.82	3220
269.5	12.26	33.03	236.47	3270	12.64	34.07	235.43	3256	13.03	35.11	234.39	3242	13.41	36.14	233.36	3227
270	12.22	32.99	237.01	3278	12.60	34.03	235.97	3263	12.99	35.06	234.94	3249	13.37	36.10	233.90	3235
270.5	12.18	32.95	237.55	3285	12.56	33.99	236.51	3271	12.95	35.02	235.48	3257	13.33	36.06	234.44	3242
271	12.14	32.91	238.09	3293	12.53	33.95	237.05	3278	12.91	34.98	236.02	3264	13.29	36.02	234.98	3250
271.5	12.11	32.87	238.63	3300	12.49	33.90	237.60	3286	12.87	34.94	236.56	3272	13.25	35.98	235.52	3257
272	12.07	32.83	239.17	3308	12.45	33.86	238.14	3293	12.83	34.90	237.10	3279	13.21	35.94	236.06	3265
272.5	12.03	32.79	239.72	3315	12.41	33.82	238.68	3301	12.79	34.86	237.64	3287	13.17	35.90	236.60	3272
273	11.99	32.74	240.26	3323	12.37	33.78	239.22	3308	12.75	34.82	238.18	3294	13.13	35.86	237.14	3280
273.5	11.96	32.70	240.80	3330	12.34	33.74	239.76	3316	12.72	34.78	238.72	3302	13.10	35.82	237.68	3287
274	11.92	32.66	241.34	3338	12.30	33.70	240.30	3323	12.68	34.74	239.26	3309	13.06	35.77	238.23	3295
274.5	11.88	32.62	241.88	3345	12.26	33.66	240.84	3331	12.64	34.70	239.80	3316	13.02	35.73	238.77	3302
275	11.85	32.58	242.42	3353	12.22	33.62	241.38	3338	12.60	34.66	240.35	3324	12.98	35.69	239.31	3310
275.5	11.81	32.54	242.96	3360	12.19	33.58	241.92	3346	12.56	34.61	240.89	3331	12.94	35.65	239.85	3317
276	11.77	32.50	243.50	3368	12.15	33.54	242.46	3353	12.53	34.57	241.43	3339	12.90	35.61	240.39	3325
276.5	11.74	32.46	244.04	3375	12.11	33.49	243.01	3361	12.49	34.53	241.97	3346	12.86	35.57	240.93	3332
277	11.70	32.42	244.58	3383	12.08	33.45	243.55	3368	12.45	34.49	242.51	3354	12.83	35.53	241.47	3340
277.5	11.67	32.38	245.13	3390	12.04	33.41	244.09	3376	12.41	34.45	243.05	3361	12.79	35.49	242.01	3347
278	11.63	32.33	245.67	3398	12.00	33.37	244.63	3383	12.38	34.41	243.59	3369	12.75	35.45	242.55	3355
278.5	11.60	32.29	246.21	3405	11.97	33.33	245.17	3391	12.34	34.37	244.13	3376	12.71	35.41	243.09	3362
279	11.56	32.25	246.75	3413	11.93	33.29	245.71	3398	12.30	34.33	244.67	3384	12.68	35.36	243.64	3369
279.5	11.52	32.21	247.29	3420	11.90	33.25	246.25	3406	12.27	34.29	245.21	3391	12.64	35.32	244.18	3377

Body Composition MALE 248-279.5 Lb.

Weight: Lb.	Waist: 38 inches Fat: %	Fat: Lb.	LBM: Lb.	RMR: Cal.	38.25 inches Fat: %	Fat: Lb.	LBM: Lb.	RMR: Cal.	38.5 inches Fat: %	Fat: Lb.	LBM: Lb.	RMR: Cal.	38.75 inches Fat: %	Fat: Lb.	LBM: Lb.	RMR: Cal.
248	15.70	38.94	209.06	2891	16.12	39.98	208.02	2877	16.54	41.02	206.98	2863	16.96	42.06	205.94	2848
248.5	15.66	38.90	209.60	2899	16.07	39.94	208.56	2884	16.49	40.98	207.52	2870	16.91	42.02	206.48	2856
249	15.61	38.86	210.14	2906	16.02	39.90	209.10	2892	16.44	40.94	208.06	2878	16.86	41.97	207.03	2863
249.5	15.56	38.82	210.68	2914	15.98	39.86	209.64	2899	16.39	40.90	208.60	2885	16.81	41.93	207.57	2871
250	15.51	38.78	211.22	2921	15.93	39.82	210.18	2907	16.34	40.86	209.15	2892	16.76	41.89	208.11	2878
250.5	15.46	38.74	211.76	2929	15.88	39.78	210.72	2914	16.29	40.81	209.69	2900	16.71	41.85	208.65	2886
251	15.42	38.70	212.30	2936	15.83	39.74	211.26	2922	16.24	40.77	210.23	2907	16.66	41.81	209.19	2893
251.5	15.37	38.66	212.84	2944	15.78	39.69	211.81	2929	16.20	40.73	210.77	2915	16.61	41.77	209.73	2901
252	15.32	38.62	213.38	2951	15.74	39.65	212.35	2937	16.15	40.69	211.31	2922	16.56	41.73	210.27	2908
252.5	15.28	38.58	213.93	2959	15.69	39.61	212.89	2944	16.10	40.65	211.85	2930	16.51	41.69	210.81	2916
253	15.23	38.53	214.47	2966	15.64	39.57	213.43	2952	16.05	40.61	212.39	2937	16.46	41.65	211.35	2923
253.5	15.18	38.49	215.01	2974	15.59	39.53	213.97	2959	16.00	40.57	212.93	2945	16.41	41.61	211.89	2931
254	15.14	38.45	215.55	2981	15.55	39.49	214.51	2967	15.96	40.53	213.47	2952	16.36	41.56	212.44	2938
254.5	15.09	38.41	216.09	2989	15.50	39.45	215.05	2974	15.91	40.49	214.01	2960	16.32	41.52	212.98	2945
255	15.05	38.37	216.63	2996	15.45	39.41	215.59	2982	15.86	40.45	214.56	2967	16.27	41.48	213.52	2953
255.5	15.00	38.33	217.17	3003	15.41	39.37	216.13	2989	15.81	40.40	215.10	2975	16.22	41.44	214.06	2960
256	14.96	38.29	217.71	3011	15.36	39.33	216.67	2997	15.77	40.36	215.64	2982	16.17	41.40	214.60	2968
256.5	14.91	38.25	218.25	3018	15.32	39.28	217.22	3004	15.72	40.32	216.18	2990	16.12	41.36	215.14	2975
257	14.87	38.21	218.79	3026	15.27	39.24	217.76	3012	15.67	40.28	216.72	2997	16.08	41.32	215.68	2983
257.5	14.82	38.17	219.34	3033	15.22	39.20	218.30	3019	15.63	40.24	217.26	3005	16.03	41.28	216.22	2990
258	14.78	38.12	219.88	3041	15.18	39.16	218.84	3027	15.58	40.20	217.80	3012	15.98	41.24	216.76	2998
258.5	14.73	38.08	220.42	3048	15.13	39.12	219.38	3034	15.54	40.16	218.34	3020	15.94	41.20	217.30	3005
259	14.69	38.04	220.96	3056	15.09	39.08	219.92	3042	15.49	40.12	218.88	3027	15.89	41.15	217.85	3013
259.5	14.64	38.00	221.50	3063	15.04	39.04	220.46	3049	15.44	40.08	219.42	3035	15.84	41.11	218.39	3020
260	14.60	37.96	222.04	3071	15.00	39.00	221.00	3056	15.40	40.04	219.97	3042	15.80	41.07	218.93	3028
260.5	14.56	37.92	222.58	3078	14.95	38.96	221.54	3064	15.35	39.99	220.51	3050	15.75	41.03	219.47	3035
261	14.51	37.88	223.12	3086	14.91	38.92	222.08	3071	15.31	39.95	221.05	3057	15.71	40.99	220.01	3043
261.5	14.47	37.84	223.66	3093	14.87	38.87	222.63	3079	15.26	39.91	221.59	3065	15.66	40.95	220.55	3050
262	14.43	37.80	224.20	3101	14.82	38.83	223.17	3086	15.22	39.87	222.13	3072	15.61	40.91	221.09	3058
262.5	14.38	37.76	224.75	3108	14.78	38.79	223.71	3094	15.17	39.83	222.67	3080	15.57	40.87	221.63	3065
263	14.34	37.71	225.29	3116	14.73	38.75	224.25	3101	15.13	39.79	223.21	3087	15.52	40.83	222.17	3073
263.5	14.30	37.67	225.83	3123	14.69	38.71	224.79	3109	15.08	39.75	223.75	3094	15.48	40.79	222.71	3080
264	14.25	37.63	226.37	3131	14.65	38.67	225.33	3116	15.04	39.71	224.29	3102	15.43	40.74	223.26	3088
264.5	14.21	37.59	226.91	3138	14.60	38.63	225.87	3124	15.00	39.67	224.83	3109	15.39	40.70	223.80	3095
265	14.17	37.55	227.45	3146	14.56	38.59	226.41	3131	14.95	39.63	225.38	3117	15.34	40.66	224.34	3103
265.5	14.13	37.51	227.99	3153	14.52	38.55	226.95	3139	14.91	39.58	225.92	3124	15.30	40.62	224.88	3110
266	14.09	37.47	228.53	3161	14.48	38.51	227.49	3146	14.87	39.54	226.46	3132	15.26	40.58	225.42	3118
266.5	14.04	37.43	229.07	3168	14.43	38.46	228.04	3154	14.82	39.50	227.00	3139	15.21	40.54	225.96	3125
267	14.00	37.39	229.61	3176	14.39	38.42	228.58	3161	14.78	39.46	227.54	3147	15.17	40.50	226.50	3133
267.5	13.96	37.35	230.16	3183	14.35	38.38	229.12	3169	14.74	39.42	228.08	3154	15.12	40.46	227.04	3140
268	13.92	37.30	230.70	3191	14.31	38.34	229.66	3176	14.69	39.38	228.62	3162	15.08	40.42	227.58	3147
268.5	13.88	37.26	231.24	3198	14.26	38.30	230.20	3184	14.65	39.34	229.16	3169	15.04	40.38	228.12	3155
269	13.84	37.22	231.78	3205	14.22	38.26	230.74	3191	14.61	39.30	229.70	3177	14.99	40.33	228.67	3162
269.5	13.80	37.18	232.32	3213	14.18	38.22	231.28	3199	14.57	39.26	230.24	3184	14.95	40.29	229.21	3170
270	13.76	37.14	232.86	3220	14.14	38.18	231.82	3206	14.52	39.22	230.79	3192	14.91	40.25	229.75	3177
270.5	13.71	37.10	233.40	3228	14.10	38.14	232.36	3214	14.48	39.17	231.33	3199	14.87	40.21	230.29	3185
271	13.67	37.06	233.94	3235	14.06	38.10	232.90	3221	14.44	39.13	231.87	3207	14.82	40.17	230.83	3192
271.5	13.63	37.02	234.48	3243	14.02	38.05	233.45	3229	14.40	39.09	232.41	3214	14.78	40.13	231.37	3200
272	13.59	36.98	235.02	3250	13.98	38.01	233.99	3236	14.36	39.05	232.95	3222	14.74	40.09	231.91	3207
272.5	13.55	36.94	235.57	3258	13.93	37.97	234.53	3244	14.32	39.01	233.49	3229	14.70	40.05	232.45	3215
273	13.51	36.89	236.11	3265	13.89	37.93	235.07	3251	14.27	38.97	234.03	3237	14.65	40.01	232.99	3222
273.5	13.47	36.85	236.65	3273	13.85	37.89	235.61	3258	14.23	38.93	234.57	3244	14.61	39.97	233.53	3230
274	13.44	36.81	237.19	3280	13.81	37.85	236.15	3266	14.19	38.89	235.11	3252	14.57	39.92	234.08	3237
274.5	13.40	36.77	237.73	3288	13.77	37.81	236.69	3273	14.15	38.85	235.65	3259	14.53	39.88	234.62	3245
275	13.36	36.73	238.27	3295	13.73	37.77	237.23	3281	14.11	38.81	236.20	3267	14.49	39.84	235.16	3252
275.5	13.32	36.69	238.81	3303	13.69	37.73	237.77	3288	14.07	38.77	236.74	3274	14.45	39.80	235.70	3260
276	13.28	36.65	239.35	3310	13.65	37.69	238.31	3296	14.03	38.72	237.28	3282	14.41	39.76	236.24	3267
276.5	13.24	36.61	239.89	3318	13.61	37.64	238.86	3303	13.99	38.68	237.82	3289	14.37	39.72	236.78	3275
277	13.20	36.57	240.43	3325	13.58	37.60	239.40	3311	13.95	38.64	238.36	3297	14.32	39.68	237.32	3282
277.5	13.16	36.53	240.98	3333	13.54	37.56	239.94	3318	13.91	38.60	238.90	3304	14.28	39.64	237.86	3290
278	13.12	36.48	241.52	3340	13.50	37.52	240.48	3326	13.87	38.56	239.44	3311	14.24	39.60	238.40	3297
278.5	13.09	36.44	242.06	3348	13.46	37.48	241.02	3333	13.83	38.52	239.98	3319	14.20	39.56	238.94	3305
279	13.05	36.40	242.60	3355	13.42	37.44	241.56	3341	13.79	38.48	240.52	3326	14.16	39.51	239.49	3312
279.5	13.01	36.36	243.14	3363	13.38	37.40	242.10	3348	13.75	38.44	241.06	3334	14.12	39.47	240.03	3320

Body Composition MALE 248-279.5 Lb.

Weight: Lb.	Waist: 39 inches Fat: %	Fat: Lb.	LBM: Lb.	RMR: Cal.	39.25 inches Fat: %	Fat: Lb.	LBM: Lb.	RMR: Cal.	39.5 inches Fat: %	Fat: Lb.	LBM: Lb.	RMR: Cal.	39.75 inches Fat: %	Fat: Lb.	LBM: Lb.	RMR: Cal.
248	17.38	43.09	204.91	2834	17.79	44.13	203.87	2820	18.21	45.17	202.83	2805	18.63	46.21	201.79	2791
248.5	17.33	43.05	205.45	2841	17.74	44.09	204.41	2827	18.16	45.13	203.37	2813	18.58	46.17	202.33	2798
249	17.27	43.01	205.99	2849	17.69	44.05	204.95	2834	18.11	45.09	203.91	2820	18.52	46.12	202.88	2806
249.5	17.22	42.97	206.53	2856	17.64	44.01	205.49	2842	18.05	45.05	204.45	2828	18.47	46.08	203.42	2813
250	17.17	42.93	207.07	2864	17.59	43.97	206.03	2849	18.00	45.01	205.00	2835	18.42	46.04	203.96	2821
250.5	17.12	42.89	207.61	2871	17.54	43.93	206.57	2857	17.95	44.96	205.54	2843	18.36	46.00	204.50	2828
251	17.07	42.85	208.15	2879	17.48	43.89	207.11	2864	17.90	44.92	206.08	2850	18.31	45.96	205.04	2836
251.5	17.02	42.81	208.69	2886	17.43	43.84	207.66	2872	17.85	44.88	206.62	2858	18.26	45.92	205.58	2843
252	16.97	42.77	209.23	2894	17.38	43.80	208.20	2879	17.79	44.84	207.16	2865	18.21	45.88	206.12	2851
252.5	16.92	42.73	209.78	2901	17.33	43.76	208.74	2887	17.74	44.80	207.70	2872	18.15	45.84	206.66	2858
253	16.87	42.68	210.32	2909	17.28	43.72	209.28	2894	17.69	44.76	208.24	2880	18.10	45.80	207.20	2866
253.5	16.82	42.64	210.86	2916	17.23	43.68	209.82	2902	17.64	44.72	208.78	2887	18.05	45.76	207.74	2873
254	16.77	42.60	211.40	2924	17.18	43.64	210.36	2909	17.59	44.68	209.32	2895	18.00	45.71	208.29	2881
254.5	16.72	42.56	211.94	2931	17.13	43.60	210.90	2917	17.54	44.64	209.86	2902	17.95	45.67	208.83	2888
255	16.67	42.52	212.48	2939	17.08	43.56	211.44	2924	17.49	44.60	210.41	2910	17.90	45.63	209.37	2896
255.5	16.63	42.48	213.02	2946	17.03	43.52	211.98	2932	17.44	44.55	210.95	2917	17.84	45.59	209.91	2903
256	16.58	42.44	213.56	2954	16.98	43.48	212.52	2939	17.39	44.51	211.49	2925	17.79	45.55	210.45	2911
256.5	16.53	42.40	214.10	2961	16.93	43.43	213.07	2947	17.34	44.47	212.03	2932	17.74	45.51	210.99	2918
257	16.48	42.36	214.64	2969	16.88	43.39	213.61	2954	17.29	44.43	212.57	2940	17.69	45.47	211.53	2925
257.5	16.43	42.32	215.19	2976	16.84	43.35	214.15	2962	17.24	44.39	213.11	2947	17.64	45.43	212.07	2933
258	16.39	42.27	215.73	2983	16.79	43.31	214.69	2969	17.19	44.35	213.65	2955	17.59	45.39	212.61	2940
258.5	16.34	42.23	216.27	2991	16.74	43.27	215.23	2977	17.14	44.31	214.19	2962	17.54	45.35	213.15	2948
259	16.29	42.19	216.81	2998	16.69	43.23	215.77	2984	17.09	44.27	214.73	2970	17.49	45.30	213.70	2955
259.5	16.24	42.15	217.35	3006	16.64	43.19	216.31	2992	17.04	44.23	215.27	2977	17.44	45.26	214.24	2963
260	16.20	42.11	217.89	3013	16.60	43.15	216.85	2999	16.99	44.19	215.82	2985	17.39	45.22	214.78	2970
260.5	16.15	42.07	218.43	3021	16.55	43.11	217.39	3007	16.95	44.14	216.36	2992	17.34	45.18	215.32	2978
261	16.10	42.03	218.97	3028	16.50	43.07	217.93	3014	16.90	44.10	216.90	3000	17.30	45.14	215.86	2985
261.5	16.06	41.99	219.51	3036	16.45	43.02	218.48	3022	16.85	44.06	217.44	3007	17.25	45.10	216.40	2993
262	16.01	41.95	220.05	3043	16.41	42.98	219.02	3029	16.80	44.02	217.98	3015	17.20	45.06	216.94	3000
262.5	15.96	41.91	220.60	3051	16.36	42.94	219.56	3036	16.75	43.98	218.52	3022	17.15	45.02	217.48	3008
263	15.92	41.86	221.14	3058	16.31	42.90	220.10	3044	16.71	43.94	219.06	3030	17.10	44.98	218.02	3015
263.5	15.87	41.82	221.68	3066	16.27	42.86	220.64	3051	16.66	43.90	219.60	3037	17.05	44.94	218.56	3023
264	15.83	41.78	222.22	3073	16.22	42.82	221.18	3059	16.61	43.86	220.14	3045	17.01	44.89	219.11	3030
264.5	15.78	41.74	222.76	3081	16.17	42.78	221.72	3066	16.57	43.82	220.68	3052	16.96	44.85	219.65	3038
265	15.74	41.70	223.30	3088	16.13	42.74	222.26	3074	16.52	43.78	221.23	3060	16.91	44.81	220.19	3045
265.5	15.69	41.66	223.84	3096	16.08	42.70	222.80	3081	16.47	43.73	221.77	3067	16.86	44.77	220.73	3053
266	15.65	41.62	224.38	3103	16.04	42.66	223.34	3089	16.43	43.69	222.31	3075	16.82	44.73	221.27	3060
266.5	15.60	41.58	224.92	3111	15.99	42.61	223.89	3096	16.38	43.65	222.85	3082	16.77	44.69	221.81	3068
267	15.56	41.54	225.46	3118	15.95	42.57	224.43	3104	16.33	43.61	223.39	3089	16.72	44.65	222.35	3075
267.5	15.51	41.50	226.01	3126	15.90	42.53	224.97	3111	16.29	43.57	223.93	3097	16.68	44.61	222.89	3083
268	15.47	41.45	226.55	3133	15.86	42.49	225.51	3119	16.24	43.53	224.47	3104	16.63	44.57	223.43	3090
268.5	15.42	41.41	227.09	3141	15.81	42.45	226.05	3126	16.20	43.49	225.01	3112	16.58	44.53	223.97	3098
269	15.38	41.37	227.63	3148	15.77	42.41	226.59	3134	16.15	43.45	225.55	3119	16.54	44.48	224.52	3105
269.5	15.34	41.33	228.17	3156	15.72	42.37	227.13	3141	16.11	43.41	226.09	3127	16.49	44.44	225.06	3113
270	15.29	41.29	228.71	3163	15.68	42.33	227.67	3149	16.06	43.37	226.64	3134	16.45	44.40	225.60	3120
270.5	15.25	41.25	229.25	3171	15.63	42.29	228.21	3156	16.02	43.32	227.18	3142	16.40	44.36	226.14	3127
271	15.21	41.21	229.79	3178	15.59	42.25	228.75	3164	15.97	43.28	227.72	3149	16.35	44.32	226.68	3135
271.5	15.16	41.17	230.33	3186	15.54	42.20	229.30	3171	15.93	43.24	228.26	3157	16.31	44.28	227.22	3142
272	15.12	41.13	230.87	3193	15.50	42.16	229.84	3179	15.88	43.20	228.80	3164	16.26	44.24	227.76	3150
272.5	15.08	41.09	231.42	3200	15.46	42.12	230.38	3186	15.84	43.16	229.34	3172	16.22	44.20	228.30	3157
273	15.03	41.04	231.96	3208	15.41	42.08	230.92	3194	15.79	43.12	229.88	3179	16.17	44.16	228.84	3165
273.5	14.99	41.00	232.50	3215	15.37	42.04	231.46	3201	15.75	43.08	230.42	3187	16.13	44.12	229.38	3172
274	14.95	40.96	233.04	3223	15.33	42.00	232.00	3209	15.71	43.04	230.96	3194	16.09	44.07	229.93	3180
274.5	14.91	40.92	233.58	3230	15.29	41.96	232.54	3216	15.66	43.00	231.50	3202	16.04	44.03	230.47	3187
275	14.87	40.88	234.12	3238	15.24	41.92	233.08	3224	15.62	42.96	232.05	3209	16.00	43.99	231.01	3195
275.5	14.82	40.84	234.66	3245	15.20	41.88	233.62	3231	15.58	42.91	232.59	3217	15.95	43.95	231.55	3202
276	14.78	40.80	235.20	3253	15.16	41.84	234.16	3238	15.53	42.87	233.13	3224	15.91	43.91	232.09	3210
276.5	14.74	40.76	235.74	3260	15.12	41.79	234.71	3246	15.49	42.83	233.67	3232	15.87	43.87	232.63	3217
277	14.70	40.72	236.28	3268	15.07	41.75	235.25	3253	15.45	42.79	234.21	3239	15.82	43.83	233.17	3225
277.5	14.66	40.68	236.83	3275	15.03	41.71	235.79	3261	15.41	42.75	234.75	3247	15.78	43.79	233.71	3232
278	14.62	40.63	237.37	3283	14.99	41.67	236.33	3268	15.36	42.71	235.29	3254	15.74	43.75	234.25	3240
278.5	14.58	40.59	237.91	3290	14.95	41.63	236.87	3276	15.32	42.67	235.83	3262	15.69	43.71	234.79	3247
279	14.53	40.55	238.45	3298	14.91	41.59	237.41	3283	15.28	42.63	236.37	3269	15.65	43.66	235.34	3255
279.5	14.49	40.51	238.99	3305	14.87	41.55	237.95	3291	15.24	42.59	236.91	3277	15.61	43.62	235.88	3262

Body Composition   MALE   248-279.5 Lb.

Weight: Lb.	Waist: 40 inches				40.25 inches				40.5 inches				40.75 inches			
	Fat: %	Fat: Lb.	LBM: Lb.	RMR: Cal.	Fat: %	Fat: Lb.	LBM: Lb.	RMR: Cal.	Fat: %	Fat: Lb.	LBM: Lb.	RMR: Cal.	Fat: %	Fat: Lb.	LBM: Lb.	RMR: Cal.
248	19.05	47.24	200.76	2776	19.47	48.28	199.72	2762	19.89	49.32	198.68	2748	20.31	50.36	197.64	2733
248.5	19.00	47.20	201.30	2784	19.41	48.24	200.26	2770	19.83	49.28	199.22	2755	20.25	50.32	198.18	2741
249	18.94	47.16	201.84	2791	19.36	48.20	200.80	2777	19.77	49.24	199.76	2763	20.19	50.27	198.73	2748
249.5	18.89	47.12	202.38	2799	19.30	48.16	201.34	2785	19.72	49.20	200.30	2770	20.13	50.23	199.27	2756
250	18.83	47.08	202.92	2806	19.25	48.12	201.88	2792	19.66	49.16	200.85	2778	20.08	50.19	199.81	2763
250.5	18.78	47.04	203.46	2814	19.19	48.08	202.42	2800	19.61	49.11	201.39	2785	20.02	50.15	200.35	2771
251	18.72	47.00	204.00	2821	19.14	48.04	202.96	2807	19.55	49.07	201.93	2793	19.96	50.11	200.89	2778
251.5	18.67	46.96	204.54	2829	19.08	47.99	203.51	2814	19.50	49.03	202.47	2800	19.91	50.07	201.43	2786
252	18.62	46.92	205.08	2836	19.03	47.95	204.05	2822	19.44	48.99	203.01	2808	19.85	50.03	201.97	2793
252.5	18.56	46.87	205.63	2844	18.98	47.91	204.59	2829	19.39	48.95	203.55	2815	19.80	49.99	202.51	2801
253	18.51	46.83	206.17	2851	18.92	47.87	205.13	2837	19.33	48.91	204.09	2823	19.74	49.95	203.05	2808
253.5	18.46	46.79	206.71	2859	18.87	47.83	205.67	2844	19.28	48.87	204.63	2830	19.69	49.91	203.59	2816
254	18.41	46.75	207.25	2866	18.81	47.79	206.21	2852	19.22	48.83	205.17	2838	19.63	49.86	204.14	2823
254.5	18.35	46.71	207.79	2874	18.76	47.75	206.75	2859	19.17	48.79	205.71	2845	19.58	49.82	204.68	2831
255	18.30	46.67	208.33	2881	18.71	47.71	207.29	2867	19.12	48.75	206.26	2853	19.52	49.78	205.22	2838
255.5	18.25	46.63	208.87	2889	18.66	47.67	207.83	2874	19.06	48.70	206.80	2860	19.47	49.74	205.76	2846
256	18.20	46.59	209.41	2896	18.60	47.63	208.37	2882	19.01	48.66	207.34	2867	19.41	49.70	206.30	2853
256.5	18.15	46.55	209.95	2904	18.55	47.58	208.92	2889	18.96	48.62	207.88	2875	19.36	49.66	206.84	2861
257	18.10	46.51	210.49	2911	18.50	47.54	209.46	2897	18.90	48.58	208.42	2882	19.31	49.62	207.38	2868
257.5	18.04	46.47	211.04	2919	18.45	47.50	210.00	2904	18.85	48.54	208.96	2890	19.25	49.58	207.92	2876
258	17.99	46.42	211.58	2926	18.40	47.46	210.54	2912	18.80	48.50	209.50	2897	19.20	49.54	208.46	2883
258.5	17.94	46.38	212.12	2934	18.34	47.42	211.08	2919	18.75	48.46	210.04	2905	19.15	49.50	209.00	2891
259	17.89	46.34	212.66	2941	18.29	47.38	211.62	2927	18.69	48.42	210.58	2912	19.09	49.45	209.55	2898
259.5	17.84	46.30	213.20	2949	18.24	47.34	212.16	2934	18.64	48.38	211.12	2920	19.04	49.41	210.09	2905
260	17.79	46.26	213.74	2956	18.19	47.30	212.70	2942	18.59	48.34	211.67	2927	18.99	49.37	210.63	2913
260.5	17.74	46.22	214.28	2964	18.14	47.26	213.24	2949	18.54	48.29	212.21	2935	18.94	49.33	211.17	2920
261	17.69	46.18	214.82	2971	18.09	47.22	213.78	2957	18.49	48.25	212.75	2942	18.89	49.29	211.71	2928
261.5	17.64	46.14	215.36	2978	18.04	47.17	214.33	2964	18.44	48.21	213.29	2950	18.83	49.25	212.25	2935
262	17.59	46.10	215.90	2986	17.99	47.13	214.87	2972	18.39	48.17	213.83	2957	18.78	49.21	212.79	2943
262.5	17.54	46.05	216.45	2993	17.94	47.09	215.41	2979	18.34	48.13	214.37	2965	18.73	49.17	213.33	2950
263	17.50	46.01	216.99	3001	17.89	47.05	215.95	2987	18.28	48.09	214.91	2972	18.68	49.13	213.87	2958
263.5	17.45	45.97	217.53	3008	17.84	47.01	216.49	2994	18.23	48.05	215.45	2980	18.63	49.09	214.41	2965
264	17.40	45.93	218.07	3016	17.79	46.97	217.03	3002	18.18	48.01	215.99	2987	18.58	49.04	214.96	2973
264.5	17.35	45.89	218.61	3023	17.74	46.93	217.57	3009	18.13	47.97	216.53	2995	18.53	49.00	215.50	2980
265	17.30	45.85	219.15	3031	17.69	46.89	218.11	3016	18.08	47.93	217.08	3002	18.48	48.96	216.04	2988
265.5	17.25	45.81	219.69	3038	17.64	46.85	218.65	3024	18.04	47.88	217.62	3010	18.43	48.92	216.58	2995
266	17.21	45.77	220.23	3046	17.60	46.81	219.19	3031	17.99	47.84	218.16	3017	18.38	48.88	217.12	3003
266.5	17.16	45.73	220.77	3053	17.55	46.76	219.74	3039	17.94	47.80	218.70	3025	18.33	48.84	217.66	3010
267	17.11	45.69	221.31	3061	17.50	46.72	220.28	3046	17.89	47.76	219.24	3032	18.28	48.80	218.20	3018
267.5	17.06	45.65	221.86	3068	17.45	46.68	220.82	3054	17.84	47.72	219.78	3040	18.23	48.76	218.74	3025
268	17.02	45.60	222.40	3076	17.40	46.64	221.36	3061	17.79	47.68	220.32	3047	18.18	48.72	219.28	3033
268.5	16.97	45.56	222.94	3083	17.36	46.60	221.90	3069	17.74	47.64	220.86	3055	18.13	48.68	219.82	3040
269	16.92	45.52	223.48	3091	17.31	46.56	222.44	3076	17.69	47.60	221.40	3062	18.08	48.63	220.37	3048
269.5	16.88	45.48	224.02	3098	17.26	46.52	222.98	3084	17.65	47.56	221.94	3069	18.03	48.59	220.91	3055
270	16.83	45.44	224.56	3106	17.21	46.48	223.52	3091	17.60	47.52	222.49	3077	17.98	48.55	221.45	3063
270.5	16.78	45.40	225.10	3113	17.17	46.44	224.06	3099	17.55	47.47	223.03	3084	17.93	48.51	221.99	3070
271	16.74	45.36	225.64	3121	17.12	46.40	224.60	3106	17.50	47.43	223.57	3092	17.89	48.47	222.53	3078
271.5	16.69	45.32	226.18	3128	17.07	46.35	225.15	3114	17.46	47.39	224.11	3099	17.84	48.43	223.07	3085
272	16.65	45.28	226.72	3136	17.03	46.31	225.69	3121	17.41	47.35	224.65	3107	17.79	48.39	223.61	3093
272.5	16.60	45.24	227.27	3143	16.98	46.27	226.23	3129	17.36	47.31	225.19	3114	17.74	48.35	224.15	3100
273	16.55	45.19	227.81	3151	16.93	46.23	226.77	3136	17.31	47.27	225.73	3122	17.69	48.31	224.69	3108
273.5	16.51	45.15	228.35	3158	16.89	46.19	227.31	3144	17.27	47.23	226.27	3129	17.65	48.27	225.23	3115
274	16.46	45.11	228.89	3166	16.84	46.15	227.85	3151	17.22	47.19	226.81	3137	17.60	48.22	225.78	3122
274.5	16.42	45.07	229.43	3173	16.80	46.11	228.39	3159	17.18	47.15	227.35	3144	17.55	48.18	226.32	3130
275	16.37	45.03	229.97	3180	16.75	46.07	228.93	3166	17.13	47.11	227.90	3152	17.51	48.14	226.86	3137
275.5	16.33	44.99	230.51	3188	16.71	46.03	229.47	3174	17.08	47.06	228.44	3159	17.46	48.10	227.40	3145
276	16.29	44.95	231.05	3195	16.66	45.99	230.01	3181	17.04	47.02	228.98	3167	17.41	48.06	227.94	3152
276.5	16.24	44.91	231.59	3203	16.62	45.94	230.56	3189	16.99	46.98	229.52	3174	17.37	48.02	228.48	3160
277	16.20	44.87	232.13	3210	16.57	45.90	231.10	3196	16.95	46.94	230.06	3182	17.32	47.98	229.02	3167
277.5	16.15	44.83	232.68	3218	16.53	45.86	231.64	3204	16.90	46.90	230.60	3189	17.27	47.94	229.56	3175
278	16.11	44.78	233.22	3225	16.48	45.82	232.18	3211	16.86	46.86	231.14	3197	17.23	47.90	230.10	3182
278.5	16.07	44.74	233.76	3233	16.44	45.78	232.72	3219	16.81	46.82	231.68	3204	17.18	47.86	230.64	3190
279	16.02	44.70	234.30	3240	16.39	45.74	233.26	3226	16.77	46.78	232.22	3212	17.14	47.81	231.19	3197
279.5	15.98	44.66	234.84	3248	16.35	45.70	233.80	3233	16.72	46.74	232.76	3219	17.09	47.77	231.73	3205

Body Composition MALE 248-279.5 Lb.

Weight: Lb.	Waist: 41 inches Fat: %	Fat: Lb.	LBM: Lb.	RMR: Cal.	41.25 inches Fat: %	Fat: Lb.	LBM: Lb.	RMR: Cal.	41.5 inches Fat: %	Fat: Lb.	LBM: Lb.	RMR: Cal.	41.75 inches Fat: %	Fat: Lb.	LBM: Lb.	RMR: Cal.
248	20.72	51.39	196.61	2719	21.14	52.43	195.57	2705	21.56	53.47	194.53	2690	21.98	54.51	193.49	2676
248.5	20.67	51.35	197.15	2727	21.08	52.39	196.11	2712	21.50	53.43	195.07	2698	21.92	54.47	194.03	2683
249	20.61	51.31	197.69	2734	21.02	52.35	196.65	2720	21.44	53.39	195.61	2705	21.86	54.42	194.58	2691
249.5	20.55	51.27	198.23	2742	20.97	52.31	197.19	2727	21.38	53.35	196.15	2713	21.80	54.38	195.12	2698
250	20.49	51.23	198.77	2749	20.91	52.27	197.73	2735	21.32	53.31	196.70	2720	21.74	54.34	195.66	2706
250.5	20.43	51.19	199.31	2756	20.85	52.23	198.27	2742	21.26	53.26	197.24	2728	21.68	54.30	196.20	2713
251	20.38	51.15	199.85	2764	20.79	52.19	198.81	2750	21.20	53.22	197.78	2735	21.62	54.26	196.74	2721
251.5	20.32	51.11	200.39	2771	20.73	52.14	199.36	2757	21.15	53.18	198.32	2743	21.56	54.22	197.28	2728
252	20.26	51.07	200.93	2779	20.68	52.10	199.90	2765	21.09	53.14	198.86	2750	21.50	54.18	197.82	2736
252.5	20.21	51.03	201.48	2786	20.62	52.06	200.44	2772	21.03	53.10	199.40	2758	21.44	54.14	198.36	2743
253	20.15	50.98	202.02	2794	20.56	52.02	200.98	2780	20.97	53.06	199.94	2765	21.38	54.10	198.90	2751
253.5	20.10	50.94	202.56	2801	20.51	51.98	201.52	2787	20.91	53.02	200.48	2773	21.32	54.06	199.44	2758
254	20.04	50.90	203.10	2809	20.45	51.94	202.06	2794	20.86	52.98	201.02	2780	21.27	54.01	199.99	2766
254.5	19.98	50.86	203.64	2816	20.39	51.90	202.60	2802	20.80	52.94	201.56	2788	21.21	53.97	200.53	2773
255	19.93	50.82	204.18	2824	20.34	51.86	203.14	2809	20.74	52.90	202.11	2795	21.15	53.93	201.07	2781
255.5	19.87	50.78	204.72	2831	20.28	51.82	203.68	2817	20.69	52.85	202.65	2803	21.09	53.89	201.61	2788
256	19.82	50.74	205.26	2839	20.22	51.78	204.22	2824	20.63	52.81	203.19	2810	21.04	53.85	202.15	2796
256.5	19.76	50.70	205.80	2846	20.17	51.73	204.77	2832	20.57	52.77	203.73	2818	20.98	53.81	202.69	2803
257	19.71	50.66	206.34	2854	20.11	51.69	205.31	2839	20.52	52.73	204.27	2825	20.92	53.77	203.23	2811
257.5	19.66	50.62	206.89	2861	20.06	51.65	205.85	2847	20.46	52.69	204.81	2833	20.87	53.73	203.77	2818
258	19.60	50.57	207.43	2869	20.00	51.61	206.39	2854	20.41	52.65	205.35	2840	20.81	53.69	204.31	2826
258.5	19.55	50.53	207.97	2876	19.95	51.57	206.93	2862	20.35	52.61	205.89	2847	20.75	53.65	204.85	2833
259	19.49	50.49	208.51	2884	19.90	51.53	207.47	2869	20.30	52.57	206.43	2855	20.70	53.60	205.40	2841
259.5	19.44	50.45	209.05	2891	19.84	51.49	208.01	2877	20.24	52.53	206.97	2862	20.64	53.56	205.94	2848
260	19.39	50.41	209.59	2899	19.79	51.45	208.55	2884	20.19	52.49	207.52	2870	20.59	53.52	206.48	2856
260.5	19.34	50.37	210.13	2906	19.73	51.41	209.09	2892	20.13	52.44	208.06	2877	20.53	53.48	207.02	2863
261	19.28	50.33	210.67	2914	19.68	51.37	209.63	2899	20.08	52.40	208.60	2885	20.48	53.44	207.56	2871
261.5	19.23	50.29	211.21	2921	19.63	51.32	210.18	2907	20.02	52.36	209.14	2892	20.42	53.40	208.10	2878
262	19.18	50.25	211.75	2929	19.57	51.28	210.72	2914	19.97	52.32	209.68	2900	20.37	53.36	208.64	2886
262.5	19.13	50.21	212.30	2936	19.52	51.24	211.26	2922	19.92	52.28	210.22	2907	20.31	53.32	209.18	2893
263	19.07	50.16	212.84	2944	19.47	51.20	211.80	2929	19.86	52.24	210.76	2915	20.26	53.28	209.72	2900
263.5	19.02	50.12	213.38	2951	19.42	51.16	212.34	2937	19.81	52.20	211.30	2922	20.20	53.24	210.26	2908
264	18.97	50.08	213.92	2958	19.36	51.12	212.88	2944	19.76	52.16	211.84	2930	20.15	53.19	210.81	2915
264.5	18.92	50.04	214.46	2966	19.31	51.08	213.42	2952	19.70	52.12	212.38	2937	20.10	53.15	211.35	2923
265	18.87	50.00	215.00	2973	19.26	51.04	213.96	2959	19.65	52.08	212.93	2945	20.04	53.11	211.89	2930
265.5	18.82	49.96	215.54	2981	19.21	51.00	214.50	2967	19.60	52.03	213.47	2952	19.99	53.07	212.43	2938
266	18.77	49.92	216.08	2988	19.16	50.96	215.04	2974	19.55	51.99	214.01	2960	19.94	53.03	212.97	2945
266.5	18.72	49.88	216.62	2996	19.10	50.91	215.59	2982	19.49	51.95	214.55	2967	19.88	52.99	213.51	2953
267	18.67	49.84	217.16	3003	19.05	50.87	216.13	2989	19.44	51.91	215.09	2975	19.83	52.95	214.05	2960
267.5	18.61	49.80	217.71	3011	19.00	50.83	216.67	2997	19.39	51.87	215.63	2982	19.78	52.91	214.59	2968
268	18.56	49.75	218.25	3018	18.95	50.79	217.21	3004	19.34	51.83	216.17	2990	19.73	52.87	215.13	2975
268.5	18.52	49.71	218.79	3026	18.90	50.75	217.75	3011	19.29	51.79	216.71	2997	19.67	52.83	215.67	2983
269	18.47	49.67	219.33	3033	18.85	50.71	218.29	3019	19.24	51.75	217.25	3005	19.62	52.78	216.22	2990
269.5	18.42	49.63	219.87	3041	18.80	50.67	218.83	3026	19.19	51.71	217.79	3012	19.57	52.74	216.76	2998
270	18.37	49.59	220.41	3048	18.75	50.63	219.37	3034	19.14	51.67	218.34	3020	19.52	52.70	217.30	3005
270.5	18.32	49.55	220.95	3056	18.70	50.59	219.91	3041	19.08	51.62	218.88	3027	19.47	52.66	217.84	3013
271	18.27	49.51	221.49	3063	18.65	50.55	220.45	3049	19.03	51.58	219.42	3035	19.42	52.62	218.38	3020
271.5	18.22	49.47	222.03	3071	18.60	50.50	221.00	3056	18.98	51.54	219.96	3042	19.37	52.58	218.92	3028
272	18.17	49.43	222.57	3078	18.55	50.46	221.54	3064	18.93	51.50	220.50	3050	19.32	52.54	219.46	3035
272.5	18.12	49.39	223.12	3086	18.50	50.42	222.08	3071	18.88	51.46	221.04	3057	19.27	52.50	220.00	3043
273	18.07	49.34	223.66	3093	18.45	50.38	222.62	3079	18.83	51.42	221.58	3064	19.21	52.46	220.54	3050
273.5	18.03	49.30	224.20	3101	18.41	50.34	223.16	3086	18.79	51.38	222.12	3072	19.16	52.42	221.08	3058
274	17.98	49.26	224.74	3108	18.36	50.30	223.70	3094	18.74	51.34	222.66	3079	19.11	52.37	221.63	3065
274.5	17.93	49.22	225.28	3116	18.31	50.26	224.24	3101	18.69	51.30	223.20	3087	19.07	52.33	222.17	3073
275	17.88	49.18	225.82	3123	18.26	50.22	224.78	3109	18.64	51.26	223.75	3094	19.02	52.29	222.71	3080
275.5	17.84	49.14	226.36	3131	18.21	50.18	225.32	3116	18.59	51.21	224.29	3102	18.97	52.25	223.25	3088
276	17.79	49.10	226.90	3138	18.17	50.14	225.86	3124	18.54	51.17	224.83	3109	18.92	52.21	223.79	3095
276.5	17.74	49.06	227.44	3146	18.12	50.09	226.41	3131	18.49	51.13	225.37	3117	18.87	52.17	224.33	3102
277	17.70	49.02	227.98	3153	18.07	50.05	226.95	3139	18.44	51.09	225.91	3124	18.82	52.13	224.87	3110
277.5	17.65	48.98	228.53	3161	18.02	50.01	227.49	3146	18.40	51.05	226.45	3132	18.77	52.09	225.41	3117
278	17.60	48.93	229.07	3168	17.98	49.97	228.03	3154	18.35	51.01	226.99	3139	18.72	52.05	225.95	3125
278.5	17.56	48.89	229.61	3175	17.93	49.93	228.57	3161	18.30	50.97	227.53	3147	18.67	52.01	226.49	3132
279	17.51	48.85	230.15	3183	17.88	49.89	229.11	3169	18.25	50.93	228.07	3154	18.63	51.96	227.04	3140
279.5	17.46	48.81	230.69	3190	17.83	49.85	229.65	3176	18.21	50.89	228.61	3162	18.58	51.92	227.58	3147

THE BODY FAT GUIDE

Body Composition   MALE   248-279.5 Lb.

Weight: Lb.	Waist: 42 inches				42.25 inches				42.5 inches				42.75 inches			
	Fat: %	Fat: Lb.	LBM: Lb.	RMR: Cal.	Fat: %	Fat: Lb.	LBM: Lb.	RMR: Cal.	Fat: %	Fat: Lb.	LBM: Lb.	RMR: Cal.	Fat: %	Fat: Lb.	LBM: Lb.	RMR: Cal.
248	22.40	55.54	192.46	2662	22.82	56.58	191.42	2647	23.23	57.62	190.38	2633	23.65	58.66	189.34	2619
248.5	22.34	55.50	193.00	2669	22.75	56.54	191.96	2655	23.17	57.58	190.92	2640	23.59	58.62	189.88	2626
249	22.27	55.46	193.54	2677	22.69	56.50	192.50	2662	23.11	57.54	191.46	2648	23.52	58.57	190.43	2634
249.5	22.21	55.42	194.08	2684	22.63	56.46	193.04	2670	23.04	57.50	192.00	2655	23.46	58.53	190.97	2641
250	22.15	55.38	194.62	2692	22.57	56.42	193.58	2677	22.98	57.46	192.55	2663	23.40	58.49	191.51	2649
250.5	22.09	55.34	195.16	2699	22.51	56.38	194.12	2685	22.92	57.41	193.09	2670	23.33	58.45	192.05	2656
251	22.03	55.30	195.70	2707	22.44	56.34	194.66	2692	22.86	57.37	193.63	2678	23.27	58.41	192.59	2664
251.5	21.97	55.26	196.24	2714	22.38	56.29	195.21	2700	22.80	57.33	194.17	2685	23.21	58.37	193.13	2671
252	21.91	55.22	196.78	2722	22.32	56.25	195.75	2707	22.73	57.29	194.71	2693	23.15	58.33	193.67	2678
252.5	21.85	55.18	197.33	2729	22.26	56.21	196.29	2715	22.67	57.25	195.25	2700	23.08	58.29	194.21	2686
253	21.79	55.13	197.87	2736	22.20	56.17	196.83	2722	22.61	57.21	195.79	2708	23.02	58.25	194.75	2693
253.5	21.73	55.09	198.41	2744	22.14	56.13	197.37	2730	22.55	57.17	196.33	2715	22.96	58.21	195.29	2701
254	21.67	55.05	198.95	2751	22.08	56.09	197.91	2737	22.49	57.13	196.87	2723	22.90	58.16	195.84	2708
254.5	21.62	55.01	199.49	2759	22.02	56.05	198.45	2745	22.43	57.09	197.41	2730	22.84	58.12	196.38	2716
255	21.56	54.97	200.03	2766	21.96	56.01	198.99	2752	22.37	57.05	197.96	2738	22.78	58.08	196.92	2723
255.5	21.50	54.93	200.57	2774	21.90	55.97	199.53	2760	22.31	57.00	198.50	2745	22.72	58.04	197.46	2731
256	21.44	54.89	201.11	2781	21.85	55.93	200.07	2767	22.25	56.96	199.04	2753	22.66	58.00	198.00	2738
256.5	21.38	54.85	201.65	2789	21.79	55.88	200.62	2775	22.19	56.92	199.58	2760	22.60	57.96	198.54	2746
257	21.33	54.81	202.19	2796	21.73	55.84	201.16	2782	22.13	56.88	200.12	2768	22.54	57.92	199.08	2753
257.5	21.27	54.77	202.74	2804	21.67	55.80	201.70	2789	22.07	56.84	200.66	2775	22.48	57.88	199.62	2761
258	21.21	54.72	203.28	2811	21.61	55.76	202.24	2797	22.02	56.80	201.20	2783	22.42	57.84	200.16	2768
258.5	21.15	54.68	203.82	2819	21.56	55.72	202.78	2804	21.96	56.76	201.74	2790	22.36	57.80	200.70	2776
259	21.10	54.64	204.36	2826	21.50	55.68	203.32	2812	21.90	56.72	202.28	2798	22.30	57.75	201.25	2783
259.5	21.04	54.60	204.90	2834	21.44	55.64	203.86	2819	21.84	56.68	202.82	2805	22.24	57.71	201.79	2791
260	20.98	54.56	205.44	2841	21.38	55.60	204.40	2827	21.78	56.64	203.37	2813	22.18	57.67	202.33	2798
260.5	20.93	54.52	205.98	2849	21.33	55.56	204.94	2834	21.73	56.59	203.91	2820	22.12	57.63	202.87	2806
261	20.87	54.48	206.52	2856	21.27	55.52	205.48	2842	21.67	56.55	204.45	2828	22.07	57.59	203.41	2813
261.5	20.82	54.44	207.06	2864	21.21	55.47	206.03	2849	21.61	56.51	204.99	2835	22.01	57.55	203.95	2821
262	20.76	54.40	207.60	2871	21.16	55.43	206.57	2857	21.55	56.47	205.53	2842	21.95	57.51	204.49	2828
262.5	20.71	54.36	208.15	2879	21.10	55.39	207.11	2864	21.50	56.43	206.07	2850	21.89	57.47	205.03	2836
263	20.65	54.31	208.69	2886	21.05	55.35	207.65	2872	21.44	56.39	206.61	2857	21.84	57.43	205.57	2843
263.5	20.60	54.27	209.23	2894	20.99	55.31	208.19	2879	21.38	56.35	207.15	2865	21.78	57.39	206.11	2851
264	20.54	54.23	209.77	2901	20.94	55.27	208.73	2887	21.33	56.31	207.69	2872	21.72	57.34	206.66	2858
264.5	20.49	54.19	210.31	2909	20.88	55.23	209.27	2894	21.27	56.27	208.23	2880	21.66	57.30	207.20	2866
265	20.43	54.15	210.85	2916	20.83	55.19	209.81	2902	21.22	56.23	208.78	2887	21.61	57.26	207.74	2873
265.5	20.38	54.11	211.39	2924	20.77	55.15	210.35	2909	21.16	56.18	209.32	2895	21.55	57.22	208.28	2880
266	20.33	54.07	211.93	2931	20.72	55.11	210.89	2917	21.11	56.14	209.86	2902	21.50	57.18	208.82	2888
266.5	20.27	54.03	212.47	2939	20.66	55.06	211.44	2924	21.05	56.10	210.40	2910	21.44	57.14	209.36	2895
267	20.22	53.99	213.01	2946	20.61	55.02	211.98	2932	21.00	56.06	210.94	2917	21.39	57.10	209.90	2903
267.5	20.17	53.95	213.56	2953	20.55	54.98	212.52	2939	20.94	56.02	211.48	2925	21.33	57.06	210.44	2910
268	20.11	53.90	214.10	2961	20.50	54.94	213.06	2947	20.89	55.98	212.02	2932	21.27	57.02	210.98	2918
268.5	20.06	53.86	214.64	2968	20.45	54.90	213.60	2954	20.83	55.94	212.56	2940	21.22	56.98	211.52	2925
269	20.01	53.82	215.18	2976	20.39	54.86	214.14	2962	20.78	55.90	213.10	2947	21.17	56.93	212.07	2933
269.5	19.96	53.78	215.72	2983	20.34	54.82	214.68	2969	20.73	55.86	213.64	2955	21.11	56.89	212.61	2940
270	19.90	53.74	216.26	2991	20.29	54.78	215.22	2977	20.67	55.82	214.19	2962	21.06	56.85	213.15	2948
270.5	19.85	53.70	216.80	2998	20.24	54.74	215.76	2984	20.62	55.77	214.73	2970	21.00	56.81	213.69	2955
271	19.80	53.66	217.34	3006	20.18	54.70	216.30	2991	20.57	55.73	215.27	2977	20.95	56.77	214.23	2963
271.5	19.75	53.62	217.88	3013	20.13	54.65	216.85	2999	20.51	55.69	215.81	2985	20.89	56.73	214.77	2970
272	19.70	53.58	218.42	3021	20.08	54.61	217.39	3006	20.46	55.65	216.35	2992	20.84	56.69	215.31	2978
272.5	19.65	53.54	218.97	3028	20.03	54.57	217.93	3014	20.41	55.61	216.89	3000	20.79	56.65	215.85	2985
273	19.59	53.49	219.51	3036	19.97	54.53	218.47	3021	20.35	55.57	217.43	3007	20.73	56.61	216.39	2993
273.5	19.54	53.45	220.05	3043	19.92	54.49	219.01	3029	20.30	55.53	217.97	3015	20.68	56.57	216.93	3000
274	19.49	53.41	220.59	3051	19.87	54.45	219.55	3036	20.25	55.49	218.51	3022	20.63	56.52	217.48	3008
274.5	19.44	53.37	221.13	3058	19.82	54.41	220.09	3044	20.20	55.45	219.05	3030	20.58	56.48	218.02	3015
275	19.39	53.33	221.67	3066	19.77	54.37	220.63	3051	20.15	55.41	219.60	3037	20.52	56.44	218.56	3023
275.5	19.34	53.29	222.21	3073	19.72	54.33	221.17	3059	20.10	55.36	220.14	3044	20.47	56.40	219.10	3030
276	19.29	53.25	222.75	3081	19.67	54.29	221.71	3066	20.04	55.32	220.68	3052	20.42	56.36	219.64	3038
276.5	19.24	53.21	223.29	3088	19.62	54.24	222.26	3074	19.99	55.28	221.22	3059	20.37	56.32	220.18	3045
277	19.19	53.17	223.83	3096	19.57	54.20	222.80	3081	19.94	55.24	221.76	3067	20.32	56.28	220.72	3053
277.5	19.14	53.13	224.38	3103	19.52	54.16	223.34	3089	19.89	55.20	222.30	3074	20.27	56.24	221.26	3060
278	19.09	53.08	224.92	3111	19.47	54.12	223.88	3096	19.84	55.16	222.84	3082	20.21	56.20	221.80	3068
278.5	19.05	53.04	225.46	3118	19.42	54.08	224.42	3104	19.79	55.12	223.38	3089	20.16	56.16	222.34	3075
279	19.00	53.00	226.00	3126	19.37	54.04	224.96	3111	19.74	55.08	223.92	3097	20.11	56.11	222.89	3083
279.5	18.95	52.96	226.54	3133	19.32	54.00	225.50	3119	19.69	55.04	224.46	3104	20.06	56.07	223.43	3090

Body Composition MALE 248-279.5 Lb.

Weight: Lb.	Waist: 43 inches				43.25 inches				43.5 inches				43.75 inches			
	Fat: %	Fat: Lb.	LBM: Lb.	RMR: Cal.	Fat: %	Fat: Lb.	LBM: Lb.	RMR: Cal.	Fat: %	Fat: Lb.	LBM: Lb.	RMR: Cal.	Fat: %	Fat: Lb.	LBM: Lb.	RMR: Cal.
248	24.07	59.69	188.31	2604	24.49	60.73	187.27	2590	24.91	61.77	186.23	2576	25.33	62.81	185.19	2561
248.5	24.01	59.65	188.85	2612	24.42	60.69	187.81	2597	24.84	61.73	186.77	2583	25.26	62.77	185.73	2569
249	23.94	59.61	189.39	2619	24.36	60.65	188.35	2605	24.77	61.69	187.31	2591	25.19	62.72	186.28	2576
249.5	23.88	59.57	189.93	2627	24.29	60.61	188.89	2612	24.71	61.65	187.85	2598	25.12	62.68	186.82	2584
250	23.81	59.53	190.47	2634	24.23	60.57	189.43	2620	24.64	61.61	188.40	2606	25.06	62.64	187.36	2591
250.5	23.75	59.49	191.01	2642	24.16	60.53	189.97	2627	24.58	61.56	188.94	2613	24.99	62.60	187.90	2599
251	23.68	59.45	191.55	2649	24.10	60.49	190.51	2635	24.51	61.52	189.48	2620	24.92	62.56	188.44	2606
251.5	23.62	59.41	192.09	2657	24.03	60.44	191.06	2642	24.45	61.48	190.02	2628	24.86	62.52	188.98	2614
252	23.56	59.37	192.63	2664	23.97	60.40	191.60	2650	24.38	61.44	190.56	2635	24.79	62.48	189.52	2621
252.5	23.50	59.33	193.18	2672	23.91	60.36	192.14	2657	24.32	61.40	191.10	2643	24.73	62.44	190.06	2629
253	23.43	59.28	193.72	2679	23.84	60.32	192.68	2665	24.25	61.36	191.64	2650	24.66	62.40	190.60	2636
253.5	23.37	59.24	194.26	2687	23.78	60.28	193.22	2672	24.19	61.32	192.18	2658	24.60	62.36	191.14	2644
254	23.31	59.20	194.80	2694	23.72	60.24	193.76	2680	24.12	61.28	192.72	2665	24.53	62.31	191.69	2651
254.5	23.25	59.16	195.34	2702	23.65	60.20	194.30	2687	24.06	61.24	193.26	2673	24.47	62.27	192.23	2658
255	23.18	59.12	195.88	2709	23.59	60.16	194.84	2695	24.00	61.20	193.81	2680	24.40	62.23	192.77	2666
255.5	23.12	59.08	196.42	2717	23.53	60.12	195.38	2702	23.94	61.15	194.35	2688	24.34	62.19	193.31	2673
256	23.06	59.04	196.96	2724	23.47	60.08	195.92	2710	23.87	61.11	194.89	2695	24.28	62.15	193.85	2681
256.5	23.00	59.00	197.50	2731	23.41	60.03	196.47	2717	23.81	61.07	195.43	2703	24.21	62.11	194.39	2688
257	22.94	58.96	198.04	2739	23.34	59.99	197.01	2725	23.75	61.03	195.97	2710	24.15	62.07	194.93	2696
257.5	22.88	58.92	198.59	2746	23.28	59.95	197.55	2732	23.69	60.99	196.51	2718	24.09	62.03	195.47	2703
258	22.82	58.87	199.13	2754	23.22	59.91	198.09	2740	23.62	60.95	197.05	2725	24.03	61.99	196.01	2711
258.5	22.76	58.83	199.67	2761	23.16	59.87	198.63	2747	23.56	60.91	197.59	2733	23.96	61.95	196.55	2718
259	22.70	58.79	200.21	2769	23.10	59.83	199.17	2755	23.50	60.87	198.13	2740	23.90	61.90	197.10	2726
259.5	22.64	58.75	200.75	2776	23.04	59.79	199.71	2762	23.44	60.83	198.67	2748	23.84	61.86	197.64	2733
260	22.58	58.71	201.29	2784	22.98	59.75	200.25	2769	23.38	60.79	199.22	2755	23.78	61.82	198.18	2741
260.5	22.52	58.67	201.83	2791	22.92	59.71	200.79	2777	23.32	60.74	199.76	2763	23.72	61.78	198.72	2748
261	22.46	58.63	202.37	2799	22.86	59.67	201.33	2784	23.26	60.70	200.30	2770	23.66	61.74	199.26	2756
261.5	22.40	58.59	202.91	2806	22.80	59.62	201.88	2792	23.20	60.66	200.84	2778	23.59	61.70	199.80	2763
262	22.35	58.55	203.45	2814	22.74	59.58	202.42	2799	23.14	60.62	201.38	2785	23.53	61.66	200.34	2771
262.5	22.29	58.51	204.00	2821	22.68	59.54	202.96	2807	23.08	60.58	201.92	2793	23.47	61.62	200.88	2778
263	22.23	58.46	204.54	2829	22.62	59.50	203.50	2814	23.02	60.54	202.46	2800	23.41	61.58	201.42	2786
263.5	22.17	58.42	205.08	2836	22.57	59.46	204.04	2822	22.96	60.50	203.00	2808	23.35	61.54	201.96	2793
264	22.11	58.38	205.62	2844	22.51	59.42	204.58	2829	22.90	60.46	203.54	2815	23.29	61.49	202.51	2801
264.5	22.06	58.34	206.16	2851	22.45	59.38	205.12	2837	22.84	60.42	204.08	2822	23.23	61.45	203.05	2808
265	22.00	58.30	206.70	2859	22.39	59.34	205.66	2844	22.78	60.38	204.63	2830	23.17	61.41	203.59	2816
265.5	21.94	58.26	207.24	2866	22.33	59.30	206.20	2852	22.72	60.33	205.17	2837	23.12	61.37	204.13	2823
266	21.89	58.22	207.78	2874	22.28	59.26	206.74	2859	22.67	60.29	205.71	2845	23.06	61.33	204.67	2831
266.5	21.83	58.18	208.32	2881	22.22	59.21	207.29	2867	22.61	60.25	206.25	2852	23.00	61.29	205.21	2838
267	21.77	58.14	208.86	2889	22.16	59.17	207.83	2874	22.55	60.21	206.79	2860	22.94	61.25	205.75	2846
267.5	21.72	58.10	209.41	2896	22.11	59.13	208.37	2882	22.49	60.17	207.33	2867	22.88	61.21	206.29	2853
268	21.66	58.05	209.95	2904	22.05	59.09	208.91	2889	22.44	60.13	207.87	2875	22.82	61.17	206.83	2861
268.5	21.61	58.01	210.49	2911	21.99	59.05	209.45	2897	22.38	60.09	208.41	2882	22.77	61.13	207.37	2868
269	21.55	57.97	211.03	2919	21.94	59.01	209.99	2904	22.32	60.05	208.95	2890	22.71	61.08	207.92	2875
269.5	21.50	57.93	211.57	2926	21.88	58.97	210.53	2912	22.27	60.01	209.49	2897	22.65	61.04	208.46	2883
270	21.44	57.89	212.11	2933	21.83	58.93	211.07	2919	22.21	59.97	210.04	2905	22.59	61.00	209.00	2890
270.5	21.39	57.85	212.65	2941	21.77	58.89	211.61	2927	22.15	59.92	210.58	2912	22.54	60.96	209.54	2898
271	21.33	57.81	213.19	2948	21.71	58.85	212.15	2934	22.10	59.88	211.12	2920	22.48	60.92	210.08	2905
271.5	21.28	57.77	213.73	2956	21.66	58.80	212.70	2942	22.04	59.84	211.66	2927	22.42	60.88	210.62	2913
272	21.22	57.73	214.27	2963	21.60	58.76	213.24	2949	21.99	59.80	212.20	2935	22.37	60.84	211.16	2920
272.5	21.17	57.69	214.82	2971	21.55	58.72	213.78	2957	21.93	59.76	212.74	2942	22.31	60.80	211.70	2928
273	21.12	57.64	215.36	2978	21.50	58.68	214.32	2964	21.88	59.72	213.28	2950	22.26	60.76	212.24	2935
273.5	21.06	57.60	215.90	2986	21.44	58.64	214.86	2972	21.82	59.68	213.82	2957	22.20	60.72	212.78	2943
274	21.01	57.56	216.44	2993	21.39	58.60	215.40	2979	21.77	59.64	214.36	2965	22.14	60.67	213.33	2950
274.5	20.95	57.52	216.98	3001	21.33	58.56	215.94	2986	21.71	59.60	214.90	2972	22.09	60.63	213.87	2958
275	20.90	57.48	217.52	3008	21.28	58.52	216.48	2994	21.66	59.56	215.45	2980	22.03	60.59	214.41	2965
275.5	20.85	57.44	218.06	3016	21.23	58.48	217.02	3001	21.60	59.51	215.99	2987	21.98	60.55	214.95	2973
276	20.80	57.40	218.60	3023	21.17	58.44	217.56	3009	21.55	59.47	216.53	2995	21.92	60.51	215.49	2980
276.5	20.74	57.36	219.14	3031	21.12	58.39	218.11	3016	21.49	59.43	217.07	3002	21.87	60.47	216.03	2988
277	20.69	57.32	219.68	3038	21.07	58.35	218.65	3024	21.44	59.39	217.61	3010	21.82	60.43	216.57	2995
277.5	20.64	57.28	220.23	3046	21.01	58.31	219.19	3031	21.39	59.35	218.15	3017	21.76	60.39	217.11	3003
278	20.59	57.23	220.77	3053	20.96	58.27	219.73	3039	21.33	59.31	218.69	3024	21.71	60.35	217.65	3010
278.5	20.54	57.19	221.31	3061	20.91	58.23	220.27	3046	21.28	59.27	219.23	3032	21.65	60.31	218.19	3018
279	20.48	57.15	221.85	3068	20.86	58.19	220.81	3054	21.23	59.23	219.77	3039	21.60	60.26	218.74	3025
279.5	20.43	57.11	222.39	3076	20.80	58.15	221.35	3061	21.18	59.19	220.31	3047	21.55	60.22	219.28	3033

Body Composition MALE 248-279.5 Lb.

Weight: Lb.	Waist: 44 inches				44.25 inches				44.5 inches				44.75 inches			
	Fat: %	Fat: Lb.	LBM: Lb.	RMR: Cal.	Fat: %	Fat: Lb.	LBM: Lb.	RMR: Cal.	Fat: %	Fat: Lb.	LBM: Lb.	RMR: Cal.	Fat: %	Fat: Lb.	LBM: Lb.	RMR: Cal.
248	25.74	63.84	184.16	2547	26.16	64.88	183.12	2533	26.58	65.92	182.08	2518	27.00	66.96	181.04	2504
248.5	25.68	63.80	184.70	2554	26.09	64.84	183.66	2540	26.51	65.88	182.62	2526	26.93	66.92	181.58	2511
249	25.61	63.76	185.24	2562	26.02	64.80	184.20	2547	26.44	65.84	183.16	2533	26.86	66.87	182.13	2519
249.5	25.54	63.72	185.78	2569	25.96	64.76	184.74	2555	26.37	65.80	183.70	2541	26.79	66.83	182.67	2526
250	25.47	63.68	186.32	2577	25.89	64.72	185.28	2562	26.30	65.76	184.25	2548	26.72	66.79	183.21	2534
250.5	25.40	63.64	186.86	2584	25.82	64.68	185.82	2570	26.23	65.71	184.79	2556	26.65	66.75	183.75	2541
251	25.34	63.60	187.40	2592	25.75	64.64	186.36	2577	26.16	65.67	185.33	2563	26.58	66.71	184.29	2549
251.5	25.27	63.56	187.94	2599	25.68	64.59	186.91	2585	26.10	65.63	185.87	2571	26.51	66.67	184.83	2556
252	25.20	63.52	188.48	2607	25.62	64.55	187.45	2592	26.03	65.59	186.41	2578	26.44	66.63	185.37	2564
252.5	25.14	63.48	189.03	2614	25.55	64.51	187.99	2600	25.96	65.55	186.95	2586	26.37	66.59	185.91	2571
253	25.07	63.43	189.57	2622	25.48	64.47	188.53	2607	25.89	65.51	187.49	2593	26.30	66.55	186.45	2579
253.5	25.01	63.39	190.11	2629	25.42	64.43	189.07	2615	25.83	65.47	188.03	2600	26.23	66.51	186.99	2586
254	24.94	63.35	190.65	2637	25.35	64.39	189.61	2622	25.76	65.43	188.57	2608	26.17	66.46	187.54	2594
254.5	24.88	63.31	191.19	2644	25.28	64.35	190.15	2630	25.69	65.39	189.11	2615	26.10	66.42	188.08	2601
255	24.81	63.27	191.73	2652	25.22	64.31	190.69	2637	25.63	65.35	189.66	2623	26.03	66.38	188.62	2609
255.5	24.75	63.23	192.27	2659	25.15	64.27	191.23	2645	25.56	65.30	190.20	2630	25.97	66.34	189.16	2616
256	24.68	63.19	192.81	2667	25.09	64.23	191.77	2652	25.49	65.26	190.74	2638	25.90	66.30	189.70	2624
256.5	24.62	63.15	193.35	2674	25.02	64.18	192.32	2660	25.43	65.22	191.28	2645	25.83	66.26	190.24	2631
257	24.55	63.11	193.89	2682	24.96	64.14	192.86	2667	25.36	65.18	191.82	2653	25.77	66.22	190.78	2639
257.5	24.49	63.07	194.44	2689	24.89	64.10	193.40	2675	25.30	65.14	192.36	2660	25.70	66.18	191.32	2646
258	24.43	63.02	194.98	2697	24.83	64.06	193.94	2682	25.23	65.10	192.90	2668	25.63	66.14	191.86	2653
258.5	24.36	62.98	195.52	2704	24.77	64.02	194.48	2690	25.17	65.06	193.44	2675	25.57	66.10	192.40	2661
259	24.30	62.94	196.06	2711	24.70	63.98	195.02	2697	25.10	65.02	193.98	2683	25.50	66.05	192.95	2668
259.5	24.24	62.90	196.60	2719	24.64	63.94	195.56	2705	25.04	64.98	194.52	2690	25.44	66.01	193.49	2676
260	24.18	62.86	197.14	2726	24.58	63.90	196.10	2712	24.98	64.94	195.07	2698	25.37	65.97	194.03	2683
260.5	24.11	62.82	197.68	2734	24.51	63.86	196.64	2720	24.91	64.89	195.61	2705	25.31	65.93	194.57	2691
261	24.05	62.78	198.22	2741	24.45	63.82	197.18	2727	24.85	64.85	196.15	2713	25.25	65.89	195.11	2698
261.5	23.99	62.74	198.76	2749	24.39	63.77	197.73	2735	24.78	64.81	196.69	2720	25.18	65.85	195.65	2706
262	23.93	62.70	199.30	2756	24.33	63.73	198.27	2742	24.72	64.77	197.23	2728	25.12	65.81	196.19	2713
262.5	23.87	62.66	199.85	2764	24.26	63.69	198.81	2750	24.66	64.73	197.77	2735	25.05	65.77	196.73	2721
263	23.81	62.61	200.39	2771	24.20	63.65	199.35	2757	24.60	64.69	198.31	2743	24.99	65.73	197.27	2728
263.5	23.75	62.57	200.93	2779	24.14	63.61	199.89	2764	24.53	64.65	198.85	2750	24.93	65.69	197.81	2736
264	23.69	62.53	201.47	2786	24.08	63.57	200.43	2772	24.47	64.61	199.39	2758	24.87	65.64	198.36	2743
264.5	23.63	62.49	202.01	2794	24.02	63.53	200.97	2779	24.41	64.57	199.93	2765	24.80	65.60	198.90	2751
265	23.57	62.45	202.55	2801	23.96	63.49	201.51	2787	24.35	64.53	200.48	2773	24.74	65.56	199.44	2758
265.5	23.51	62.41	203.09	2809	23.90	63.45	202.05	2794	24.29	64.48	201.02	2780	24.68	65.52	199.98	2766
266	23.45	62.37	203.63	2816	23.84	63.41	202.59	2802	24.23	64.44	201.56	2788	24.62	65.48	200.52	2773
266.5	23.39	62.33	204.17	2824	23.78	63.36	203.14	2809	24.17	64.40	202.10	2795	24.56	65.44	201.06	2781
267	23.33	62.29	204.71	2831	23.72	63.32	203.68	2817	24.11	64.36	202.64	2802	24.49	65.40	201.60	2788
267.5	23.27	62.25	205.26	2839	23.66	63.28	204.22	2824	24.04	64.32	203.18	2810	24.43	65.36	202.14	2796
268	23.21	62.20	205.80	2846	23.60	63.24	204.76	2832	23.98	64.28	203.72	2817	24.37	65.32	202.68	2803
268.5	23.15	62.16	206.34	2854	23.54	63.20	205.30	2839	23.92	64.24	204.26	2825	24.31	65.28	203.22	2811
269	23.09	62.12	206.88	2861	23.48	63.16	205.84	2847	23.87	64.20	204.80	2832	24.25	65.23	203.77	2818
269.5	23.04	62.08	207.42	2869	23.42	63.12	206.38	2854	23.81	64.16	205.34	2840	24.19	65.19	204.31	2826
270	22.98	62.04	207.96	2876	23.36	63.08	206.92	2862	23.75	64.12	205.89	2847	24.13	65.15	204.85	2833
270.5	22.92	62.00	208.50	2884	23.30	63.04	207.46	2869	23.69	64.07	206.43	2855	24.07	65.11	205.39	2841
271	22.86	61.96	209.04	2891	23.25	63.00	208.00	2877	23.63	64.03	206.97	2862	24.01	65.07	205.93	2848
271.5	22.81	61.92	209.58	2899	23.19	62.95	208.55	2884	23.57	63.99	207.51	2870	23.95	65.03	206.47	2855
272	22.75	61.88	210.12	2906	23.13	62.91	209.09	2892	23.51	63.95	208.05	2877	23.89	64.99	207.01	2863
272.5	22.69	61.84	210.67	2913	23.07	62.87	209.63	2899	23.45	63.91	208.59	2885	23.83	64.95	207.55	2870
273	22.64	61.79	211.21	2921	23.02	62.83	210.17	2907	23.40	63.87	209.13	2892	23.78	64.91	208.09	2878
273.5	22.58	61.75	211.75	2928	22.96	62.79	210.71	2914	23.34	63.83	209.67	2900	23.72	64.87	208.63	2885
274	22.52	61.71	212.29	2936	22.90	62.75	211.25	2922	23.28	63.79	210.21	2907	23.66	64.82	209.18	2893
274.5	22.47	61.67	212.83	2943	22.84	62.71	211.79	2929	23.22	63.75	210.75	2915	23.60	64.78	209.72	2900
275	22.41	61.63	213.37	2951	22.79	62.67	212.33	2937	23.17	63.71	211.30	2922	23.54	64.74	210.26	2908
275.5	22.36	61.59	213.91	2958	22.73	62.63	212.87	2944	23.11	63.66	211.84	2930	23.49	64.70	210.80	2915
276	22.30	61.55	214.45	2966	22.68	62.59	213.41	2952	23.05	63.62	212.38	2937	23.43	64.66	211.34	2923
276.5	22.24	61.51	214.99	2973	22.62	62.54	213.96	2959	23.00	63.58	212.92	2945	23.37	64.62	211.88	2930
277	22.19	61.47	215.53	2981	22.56	62.50	214.50	2966	22.94	63.54	213.46	2952	23.31	64.58	212.42	2938
277.5	22.14	61.43	216.08	2988	22.51	62.46	215.04	2974	22.88	63.50	214.00	2960	23.26	64.54	212.96	2945
278	22.08	61.38	216.62	2996	22.45	62.42	215.58	2981	22.83	63.46	214.54	2967	23.20	64.50	213.50	2953
278.5	22.03	61.34	217.16	3003	22.40	62.38	216.12	2989	22.77	63.42	215.08	2975	23.14	64.46	214.04	2960
279	21.97	61.30	217.70	3011	22.34	62.34	216.66	2996	22.72	63.38	215.62	2982	23.09	64.41	214.59	2968
279.5	21.92	61.26	218.24	3018	22.29	62.30	217.20	3004	22.66	63.34	216.16	2990	23.03	64.37	215.13	2975

Body Composition MALE 248-279.5 Lb.

Weight: Lb.	Waist: 45 inches Fat: %	Fat: Lb.	LBM: Lb.	RMR: Cal.	45.25 inches Fat: %	Fat: Lb.	LBM: Lb.	RMR: Cal.	45.5 inches Fat: %	Fat: Lb.	LBM: Lb.	RMR: Cal.	45.75 inches Fat: %	Fat: Lb.	LBM: Lb.	RMR: Cal.
248	27.42	67.99	180.01	2489	27.84	69.03	178.97	2475	28.25	70.07	177.93	2461	28.67	71.11	176.89	2446
248.5	27.35	67.95	180.55	2497	27.76	68.99	179.51	2483	28.18	70.03	178.47	2468	28.60	71.07	177.43	2454
249	27.27	67.91	181.09	2504	27.69	68.95	180.05	2490	28.11	69.99	179.01	2476	28.52	71.02	177.98	2461
249.5	27.20	67.87	181.63	2512	27.62	68.91	180.59	2498	28.03	69.95	179.55	2483	28.45	70.98	178.52	2469
250	27.13	67.83	182.17	2519	27.55	68.87	181.13	2505	27.96	69.91	180.10	2491	28.38	70.94	179.06	2476
250.5	27.06	67.79	182.71	2527	27.48	68.83	181.67	2513	27.89	69.86	180.64	2498	28.30	70.90	179.60	2484
251	26.99	67.75	183.25	2534	27.40	68.79	182.21	2520	27.82	69.82	181.18	2506	28.23	70.86	180.14	2491
251.5	26.92	67.71	183.79	2542	27.33	68.74	182.76	2528	27.75	69.78	181.72	2513	28.16	70.82	180.68	2499
252	26.85	67.67	184.33	2549	27.26	68.70	183.30	2535	27.68	69.74	182.26	2521	28.09	70.78	181.22	2506
252.5	26.78	67.63	184.88	2557	27.19	68.66	183.84	2542	27.60	69.70	182.80	2528	28.01	70.74	181.76	2514
253	26.71	67.58	185.42	2564	27.12	68.62	184.38	2550	27.53	69.66	183.34	2536	27.94	70.70	182.30	2521
253.5	26.64	67.54	185.96	2572	27.05	68.58	184.92	2557	27.46	69.62	183.88	2543	27.87	70.66	182.84	2529
254	26.58	67.50	186.50	2579	26.98	68.54	185.46	2565	27.39	69.58	184.42	2551	27.80	70.61	183.39	2536
254.5	26.51	67.46	187.04	2587	26.91	68.50	186.00	2572	27.32	69.54	184.96	2558	27.73	70.57	183.93	2544
255	26.44	67.42	187.58	2594	26.85	68.46	186.54	2580	27.25	69.50	185.51	2566	27.66	70.53	184.47	2551
255.5	26.37	67.38	188.12	2602	26.78	68.42	187.08	2587	27.18	69.45	186.05	2573	27.59	70.49	185.01	2559
256	26.30	67.34	188.66	2609	26.71	68.38	187.62	2595	27.11	69.41	186.59	2580	27.52	70.45	185.55	2566
256.5	26.24	67.30	189.20	2617	26.64	68.33	188.17	2602	27.05	69.37	187.13	2588	27.45	70.41	186.09	2574
257	26.17	67.26	189.74	2624	26.57	68.29	188.71	2610	26.98	69.33	187.67	2595	27.38	70.37	186.63	2581
257.5	26.10	67.22	190.29	2632	26.51	68.25	189.25	2617	26.91	69.29	188.21	2603	27.31	70.33	187.17	2589
258	26.04	67.17	190.83	2639	26.44	68.21	189.79	2625	26.84	69.25	188.75	2610	27.24	70.29	187.71	2596
258.5	25.97	67.13	191.37	2647	26.37	68.17	190.33	2632	26.77	69.21	189.29	2618	27.17	70.25	188.25	2604
259	25.90	67.09	191.91	2654	26.30	68.13	190.87	2640	26.71	69.17	189.83	2625	27.11	70.20	188.80	2611
259.5	25.84	67.05	192.45	2662	26.24	68.09	191.41	2647	26.64	69.13	190.37	2633	27.04	70.16	189.34	2619
260	25.77	67.01	192.99	2669	26.17	68.05	191.95	2655	26.57	69.09	190.92	2640	26.97	70.12	189.88	2626
260.5	25.71	66.97	193.53	2677	26.11	68.01	192.49	2662	26.50	69.04	191.46	2648	26.90	70.08	190.42	2633
261	25.64	66.93	194.07	2684	26.04	67.97	193.03	2670	26.44	69.00	192.00	2655	26.84	70.04	190.96	2641
261.5	25.58	66.89	194.61	2691	25.97	67.92	193.58	2677	26.37	68.96	192.54	2663	26.77	70.00	191.50	2648
262	25.51	66.85	195.15	2699	25.91	67.88	194.12	2685	26.31	68.92	193.08	2670	26.70	69.96	192.04	2656
262.5	25.45	66.81	195.70	2706	25.84	67.84	194.66	2692	26.24	68.88	193.62	2678	26.64	69.92	192.58	2663
263	25.39	66.76	196.24	2714	25.78	67.80	195.20	2700	26.17	68.84	194.16	2685	26.57	69.88	193.12	2671
263.5	25.32	66.72	196.78	2721	25.72	67.76	195.74	2707	26.11	68.80	194.70	2693	26.50	69.84	193.66	2678
264	25.26	66.68	197.32	2729	25.65	67.72	196.28	2715	26.04	68.76	195.24	2700	26.44	69.79	194.21	2686
264.5	25.20	66.64	197.86	2736	25.59	67.68	196.82	2722	25.98	68.72	195.78	2708	26.37	69.75	194.75	2693
265	25.13	66.60	198.40	2744	25.52	67.64	197.36	2730	25.92	68.68	196.33	2715	26.31	69.71	195.29	2701
265.5	25.07	66.56	198.94	2751	25.46	67.60	197.90	2737	25.85	68.63	196.87	2723	26.24	69.67	195.83	2708
266	25.01	66.52	199.48	2759	25.40	67.56	198.44	2744	25.79	68.59	197.41	2730	26.18	69.63	196.37	2716
266.5	24.94	66.48	200.02	2766	25.33	67.51	198.99	2752	25.72	68.55	197.95	2738	26.11	69.59	196.91	2723
267	24.88	66.44	200.56	2774	25.27	67.47	199.53	2759	25.66	68.51	198.49	2745	26.05	69.55	197.45	2731
267.5	24.82	66.40	201.11	2781	25.21	67.43	200.07	2767	25.60	68.47	199.03	2753	25.98	69.51	197.99	2738
268	24.76	66.35	201.65	2789	25.15	67.39	200.61	2774	25.53	68.43	199.57	2760	25.92	69.47	198.53	2746
268.5	24.70	66.31	202.19	2796	25.08	67.35	201.15	2782	25.47	68.39	200.11	2768	25.86	69.43	199.07	2753
269	24.64	66.27	202.73	2804	25.02	67.31	201.69	2789	25.41	68.35	200.65	2775	25.79	69.38	199.62	2761
269.5	24.58	66.23	203.27	2811	24.96	67.27	202.23	2797	25.35	68.31	201.19	2783	25.73	69.34	200.16	2768
270	24.51	66.19	203.81	2819	24.90	67.23	202.77	2804	25.28	68.27	201.74	2790	25.67	69.30	200.70	2776
270.5	24.45	66.15	204.35	2826	24.84	67.19	203.31	2812	25.22	68.22	202.28	2797	25.60	69.26	201.24	2783
271	24.39	66.11	204.89	2834	24.78	67.15	203.85	2819	25.16	68.18	202.82	2805	25.54	69.22	201.78	2791
271.5	24.33	66.07	205.43	2841	24.72	67.10	204.40	2827	25.10	68.14	203.36	2812	25.48	69.18	202.32	2798
272	24.27	66.03	205.97	2849	24.66	67.06	204.94	2834	25.04	68.10	203.90	2820	25.42	69.14	202.86	2806
272.5	24.21	65.99	206.52	2856	24.60	67.02	205.48	2842	24.98	68.06	204.44	2827	25.36	69.10	203.40	2813
273	24.16	65.94	207.06	2864	24.54	66.98	206.02	2849	24.92	68.02	204.98	2835	25.30	69.06	203.94	2821
273.5	24.10	65.90	207.60	2871	24.48	66.94	206.56	2857	24.85	67.98	205.52	2842	25.23	69.02	204.48	2828
274	24.04	65.86	208.14	2879	24.42	66.90	207.10	2864	24.79	67.94	206.06	2850	25.17	68.97	205.03	2836
274.5	23.98	65.82	208.68	2886	24.36	66.86	207.64	2872	24.73	67.90	206.60	2857	25.11	68.93	205.57	2843
275	23.92	65.78	209.22	2894	24.30	66.82	208.18	2879	24.67	67.86	207.15	2865	25.05	68.89	206.11	2850
275.5	23.86	65.74	209.76	2901	24.24	66.78	208.72	2887	24.61	67.81	207.69	2872	24.99	68.85	206.65	2858
276	23.80	65.70	210.30	2908	24.18	66.74	209.26	2894	24.56	67.77	208.23	2880	24.93	68.81	207.19	2865
276.5	23.75	65.66	210.84	2916	24.12	66.69	209.81	2902	24.50	67.73	208.77	2887	24.87	68.77	207.73	2873
277	23.69	65.62	211.38	2923	24.06	66.65	210.35	2909	24.44	67.69	209.31	2895	24.81	68.73	208.27	2880
277.5	23.63	65.58	211.93	2931	24.00	66.61	210.89	2917	24.38	67.65	209.85	2902	24.75	68.69	208.81	2888
278	23.57	65.53	212.47	2938	23.95	66.57	211.43	2924	24.32	67.61	210.39	2910	24.69	68.65	209.35	2895
278.5	23.52	65.49	213.01	2946	23.89	66.53	211.97	2932	24.26	67.57	210.93	2917	24.63	68.61	209.89	2903
279	23.46	65.45	213.55	2953	23.83	66.49	212.51	2939	24.20	67.53	211.47	2925	24.58	68.56	210.44	2910
279.5	23.40	65.41	214.09	2961	23.77	66.45	213.05	2947	24.15	67.49	212.01	2932	24.52	68.52	210.98	2918

Body Composition   MALE   248-279.5 Lb.

Weight: Lb.	Waist: 46 inches Fat: %	Fat: Lb.	LBM: Lb.	RMR: Cal.	46.25 inches Fat: %	Fat: Lb.	LBM: Lb.	RMR: Cal.	46.5 inches Fat: %	Fat: Lb.	LBM: Lb.	RMR: Cal.	46.75 inches Fat: %	Fat: Lb.	LBM: Lb.	RMR: Cal.
248	29.09	72.14	175.86	2432	29.51	73.18	174.82	2418	29.93	74.22	173.78	2403	30.35	75.26	172.74	2389
248.5	29.02	72.10	176.40	2440	29.43	73.14	175.36	2425	29.85	74.18	174.32	2411	30.27	75.22	173.28	2397
249	28.94	72.06	176.94	2447	29.36	73.10	175.90	2433	29.77	74.14	174.86	2418	30.19	75.17	173.83	2404
249.5	28.87	72.02	177.48	2455	29.28	73.06	176.44	2440	29.70	74.10	175.40	2426	30.11	75.13	174.37	2411
250	28.79	71.98	178.02	2462	29.21	73.02	176.98	2448	29.62	74.06	175.95	2433	30.04	75.09	174.91	2419
250.5	28.72	71.94	178.56	2469	29.13	72.98	177.52	2455	29.55	74.01	176.49	2441	29.96	75.05	175.45	2426
251	28.64	71.90	179.10	2477	29.06	72.94	178.06	2463	29.47	73.97	177.03	2448	29.88	75.01	175.99	2434
251.5	28.57	71.86	179.64	2484	28.98	72.89	178.61	2470	29.40	73.93	177.57	2456	29.81	74.97	176.53	2441
252	28.50	71.82	180.18	2492	28.91	72.85	179.15	2478	29.32	73.89	178.11	2463	29.73	74.93	177.07	2449
252.5	28.43	71.78	180.73	2499	28.84	72.81	179.69	2485	29.25	73.85	178.65	2471	29.66	74.89	177.61	2456
253	28.35	71.73	181.27	2507	28.76	72.77	180.23	2493	29.17	73.81	179.19	2478	29.58	74.85	178.15	2464
253.5	28.28	71.69	181.81	2514	28.69	72.73	180.77	2500	29.10	73.77	179.73	2486	29.51	74.81	178.69	2471
254	28.21	71.65	182.35	2522	28.62	72.69	181.31	2508	29.03	73.73	180.27	2493	29.43	74.76	179.24	2479
254.5	28.14	71.61	182.89	2529	28.55	72.65	181.85	2515	28.95	73.69	180.81	2501	29.36	74.72	179.78	2486
255	28.07	71.57	183.43	2537	28.47	72.61	182.39	2522	28.88	73.65	181.36	2508	29.29	74.68	180.32	2494
255.5	28.00	71.53	183.97	2544	28.40	72.57	182.93	2530	28.81	73.61	181.90	2516	29.21	74.64	180.86	2501
256	27.93	71.49	184.51	2552	28.33	72.53	183.47	2537	28.74	73.56	182.44	2523	29.14	74.60	181.40	2509
256.5	27.85	71.45	185.05	2559	28.26	72.48	184.02	2545	28.66	73.52	182.98	2531	29.07	74.56	181.94	2516
257	27.78	71.41	185.59	2567	28.19	72.44	184.56	2552	28.59	73.48	183.52	2538	29.00	74.52	182.48	2524
257.5	27.71	71.37	186.14	2574	28.12	72.40	185.10	2560	28.52	73.44	184.06	2546	28.92	74.48	183.02	2531
258	27.64	71.32	186.68	2582	28.05	72.36	185.64	2567	28.45	73.40	184.60	2553	28.85	74.44	183.56	2539
258.5	27.58	71.28	187.22	2589	27.98	72.32	186.18	2575	28.38	73.36	185.14	2561	28.78	74.40	184.10	2546
259	27.51	71.24	187.76	2597	27.91	72.28	186.72	2582	28.31	73.32	185.68	2568	28.71	74.35	184.65	2554
259.5	27.44	71.20	188.30	2604	27.84	72.24	187.26	2590	28.24	73.28	186.22	2575	28.64	74.31	185.19	2561
260	27.37	71.16	188.84	2612	27.77	72.20	187.80	2597	28.17	73.24	186.77	2583	28.57	74.27	185.73	2569
260.5	27.30	71.12	189.38	2619	27.70	72.16	188.34	2605	28.10	73.19	187.31	2590	28.50	74.23	186.27	2576
261	27.23	71.08	189.92	2627	27.63	72.12	188.88	2612	28.03	73.15	187.85	2598	28.43	74.19	186.81	2584
261.5	27.17	71.04	190.46	2634	27.56	72.07	189.43	2620	27.96	73.11	188.39	2605	28.36	74.15	187.35	2591
262	27.10	71.00	191.00	2642	27.49	72.03	189.97	2627	27.89	73.07	188.93	2613	28.29	74.11	187.89	2599
262.5	27.03	70.96	191.55	2649	27.43	71.99	190.51	2635	27.82	73.03	189.47	2620	28.22	74.07	188.43	2606
263	26.96	70.91	192.09	2657	27.36	71.95	191.05	2642	27.75	72.99	190.01	2628	28.15	74.03	188.97	2614
263.5	26.90	70.87	192.63	2664	27.29	71.91	191.59	2650	27.68	72.95	190.55	2635	28.08	73.99	189.51	2621
264	26.83	70.83	193.17	2672	27.22	71.87	192.13	2657	27.62	72.91	191.09	2643	28.01	73.94	190.06	2628
264.5	26.76	70.79	193.71	2679	27.16	71.83	192.67	2665	27.55	72.87	191.63	2650	27.94	73.90	190.60	2636
265	26.70	70.75	194.25	2686	27.09	71.79	193.21	2672	27.48	72.83	192.18	2658	27.87	73.86	191.14	2643
265.5	26.63	70.71	194.79	2694	27.02	71.75	193.75	2680	27.41	72.78	192.72	2665	27.80	73.82	191.68	2651
266	26.57	70.67	195.33	2701	26.96	71.71	194.29	2687	27.35	72.74	193.26	2673	27.74	73.78	192.22	2658
266.5	26.50	70.63	195.87	2709	26.89	71.66	194.84	2695	27.28	72.70	193.80	2680	27.67	73.74	192.76	2666
267	26.44	70.59	196.41	2716	26.83	71.62	195.38	2702	27.21	72.66	194.34	2688	27.60	73.70	193.30	2673
267.5	26.37	70.55	196.96	2724	26.76	71.58	195.92	2710	27.15	72.62	194.88	2695	27.54	73.66	193.84	2681
268	26.31	70.50	197.50	2731	26.69	71.54	196.46	2717	27.08	72.58	195.42	2703	27.47	73.62	194.38	2688
268.5	26.24	70.46	198.04	2739	26.63	71.50	197.00	2725	27.02	72.54	195.96	2710	27.40	73.58	194.92	2696
269	26.18	70.42	198.58	2746	26.56	71.46	197.54	2732	26.95	72.50	196.50	2718	27.34	73.53	195.47	2703
269.5	26.12	70.38	199.12	2754	26.50	71.42	198.08	2739	26.89	72.46	197.04	2725	27.27	73.49	196.01	2711
270	26.05	70.34	199.66	2761	26.44	71.38	198.62	2747	26.82	72.42	197.59	2733	27.20	73.45	196.55	2718
270.5	25.99	70.30	200.20	2769	26.37	71.34	199.16	2754	26.76	72.37	198.13	2740	27.14	73.41	197.09	2726
271	25.93	70.26	200.74	2776	26.31	71.30	199.70	2762	26.69	72.33	198.67	2748	27.07	73.37	197.63	2733
271.5	25.86	70.22	201.28	2784	26.24	71.25	200.25	2769	26.63	72.29	199.21	2755	27.01	73.33	198.17	2741
272	25.80	70.18	201.82	2791	26.18	71.21	200.79	2777	26.56	72.25	199.75	2763	26.94	73.29	198.71	2748
272.5	25.74	70.14	202.37	2799	26.12	71.17	201.33	2784	26.50	72.21	200.29	2770	26.88	73.25	199.25	2756
273	25.68	70.09	202.91	2806	26.06	71.13	201.87	2792	26.44	72.17	200.83	2777	26.82	73.21	199.79	2763
273.5	25.61	70.05	203.45	2814	25.99	71.09	202.41	2799	26.37	72.13	201.37	2785	26.75	73.17	200.33	2771
274	25.55	70.01	203.99	2821	25.93	71.05	202.95	2807	26.31	72.09	201.91	2792	26.69	73.12	200.88	2778
274.5	25.49	69.97	204.53	2829	25.87	71.01	203.49	2814	26.25	72.05	202.45	2800	26.62	73.08	201.42	2786
275	25.43	69.93	205.07	2836	25.81	70.97	204.03	2822	26.18	72.01	203.00	2807	26.56	73.04	201.96	2793
275.5	25.37	69.89	205.61	2844	25.74	70.93	204.57	2829	26.12	71.96	203.54	2815	26.50	73.00	202.50	2801
276	25.31	69.85	206.15	2851	25.68	70.89	205.11	2837	26.06	71.92	204.08	2822	26.43	72.96	203.04	2808
276.5	25.25	69.81	206.69	2859	25.62	70.84	205.66	2844	26.00	71.88	204.62	2830	26.37	72.92	203.58	2816
277	25.19	69.77	207.23	2866	25.56	70.80	206.20	2852	25.94	71.84	205.16	2837	26.31	72.88	204.12	2823
277.5	25.13	69.73	207.78	2874	25.50	70.76	206.74	2859	25.87	71.80	205.70	2845	26.25	72.84	204.66	2830
278	25.07	69.68	208.32	2881	25.44	70.72	207.28	2867	25.81	71.76	206.24	2852	26.19	72.80	205.20	2838
278.5	25.01	69.64	208.86	2888	25.38	70.68	207.82	2874	25.75	71.72	206.78	2860	26.12	72.76	205.74	2845
279	24.95	69.60	209.40	2896	25.32	70.64	208.36	2882	25.69	71.68	207.32	2867	26.06	72.71	206.29	2853
279.5	24.89	69.56	209.94	2903	25.26	70.60	208.90	2889	25.63	71.64	207.86	2875	26.00	72.67	206.83	2860

Body Composition MALE 248-279.5 Lb.

Weight: Lb.	Waist: 47 inches Fat: %	Fat: Lb.	LBM: Lb.	RMR: Cal.	47.25 inches Fat: %	Fat: Lb.	LBM: Lb.	RMR: Cal.	47.5 inches Fat: %	Fat: Lb.	LBM: Lb.	RMR: Cal.	47.75 inches Fat: %	Fat: Lb.	LBM: Lb.	RMR: Cal.
248	30.76	76.29	171.71	2375	31.18	77.33	170.67	2360	31.60	78.37	169.63	2346	32.02	79.41	168.59	2332
248.5	30.69	76.25	172.25	2382	31.10	77.29	171.21	2368	31.52	78.33	170.17	2353	31.94	79.37	169.13	2339
249	30.61	76.21	172.79	2390	31.02	77.25	171.75	2375	31.44	78.29	170.71	2361	31.86	79.32	169.68	2347
249.5	30.53	76.17	173.33	2397	30.95	77.21	172.29	2383	31.36	78.25	171.25	2368	31.78	79.28	170.22	2354
250	30.45	76.13	173.87	2405	30.87	77.17	172.83	2390	31.28	78.21	171.80	2376	31.70	79.24	170.76	2362
250.5	30.37	76.09	174.41	2412	30.79	77.13	173.37	2398	31.20	78.16	172.34	2383	31.62	79.20	171.30	2369
251	30.30	76.05	174.95	2420	30.71	77.09	173.91	2405	31.12	78.12	172.88	2391	31.54	79.16	171.84	2377
251.5	30.22	76.01	175.49	2427	30.63	77.04	174.46	2413	31.05	78.08	173.42	2398	31.46	79.12	172.38	2384
252	30.15	75.97	176.03	2435	30.56	77.00	175.00	2420	30.97	78.04	173.96	2406	31.38	79.08	172.92	2392
252.5	30.07	75.93	176.58	2442	30.48	76.96	175.54	2428	30.89	78.00	174.50	2413	31.30	79.04	173.46	2399
253	29.99	75.88	177.12	2450	30.40	76.92	176.08	2435	30.81	77.96	175.04	2421	31.22	79.00	174.00	2406
253.5	29.92	75.84	177.66	2457	30.33	76.88	176.62	2443	30.74	77.92	175.58	2428	31.15	78.96	174.54	2414
254	29.84	75.80	178.20	2464	30.25	76.84	177.16	2450	30.66	77.88	176.12	2436	31.07	78.91	175.09	2421
254.5	29.77	75.76	178.74	2472	30.18	76.80	177.70	2458	30.58	77.84	176.66	2443	30.99	78.87	175.63	2429
255	29.69	75.72	179.28	2479	30.10	76.76	178.24	2465	30.51	77.80	177.21	2451	30.91	78.83	176.17	2436
255.5	29.62	75.68	179.82	2487	30.03	76.72	178.78	2473	30.43	77.75	177.75	2458	30.84	78.79	176.71	2444
256	29.55	75.64	180.36	2494	29.95	76.68	179.32	2480	30.36	77.71	178.29	2466	30.76	78.75	177.25	2451
256.5	29.47	75.60	180.90	2502	29.88	76.63	179.87	2488	30.28	77.67	178.83	2473	30.69	78.71	177.70	2460
257	29.40	75.56	181.44	2509	29.80	76.59	180.41	2495	30.21	77.63	179.37	2481	30.61	78.67	178.33	2466
257.5	29.33	75.52	181.99	2517	29.73	76.55	180.95	2503	30.13	77.59	179.91	2488	30.53	78.63	178.87	2474
258	29.25	75.47	182.53	2524	29.66	76.51	181.49	2510	30.06	77.55	180.45	2496	30.46	78.59	179.41	2481
258.5	29.18	75.43	183.07	2532	29.58	76.47	182.03	2517	29.98	77.51	180.99	2503	30.39	78.55	179.95	2489
259	29.11	75.39	183.61	2539	29.51	76.43	182.57	2525	29.91	77.47	181.53	2511	30.31	78.50	180.50	2496
259.5	29.04	75.35	184.15	2547	29.44	76.39	183.11	2532	29.84	77.43	182.07	2518	30.24	78.46	181.04	2504
260	28.97	75.31	184.69	2554	29.36	76.35	183.65	2540	29.76	77.39	182.62	2526	30.16	78.42	181.58	2511
260.5	28.89	75.27	185.23	2562	29.29	76.31	184.19	2547	29.69	77.34	183.16	2533	30.09	78.38	182.12	2519
261	28.82	75.23	185.77	2569	29.22	76.27	184.73	2555	29.62	77.30	183.70	2541	30.02	78.34	182.66	2526
261.5	28.75	75.19	186.31	2577	29.15	76.22	185.28	2562	29.55	77.26	184.24	2548	29.94	78.30	183.20	2534
262	28.68	75.15	186.85	2584	29.08	76.18	185.82	2570	29.47	77.22	184.78	2555	29.87	78.26	183.74	2541
262.5	28.61	75.11	187.40	2592	29.01	76.14	186.36	2577	29.40	77.18	185.32	2563	29.80	78.22	184.28	2549
263	28.54	75.06	187.94	2599	28.94	76.10	186.90	2585	29.33	77.14	185.86	2570	29.72	78.18	184.82	2556
263.5	28.47	75.02	188.48	2607	28.87	76.06	187.44	2592	29.26	77.10	186.40	2578	29.65	78.14	185.36	2564
264	28.40	74.98	189.02	2614	28.80	76.02	187.98	2600	29.19	77.06	186.94	2585	29.58	78.09	185.91	2571
264.5	28.33	74.94	189.56	2622	28.73	75.98	188.52	2607	29.12	77.02	187.48	2593	29.51	78.05	186.45	2579
265	28.26	74.90	190.10	2629	28.66	75.94	189.06	2615	29.05	76.98	188.03	2600	29.44	78.01	186.99	2586
265.5	28.20	74.86	190.64	2637	28.59	75.90	189.60	2622	28.98	76.93	188.57	2608	29.37	77.97	187.53	2594
266	28.13	74.82	191.18	2644	28.52	75.86	190.14	2630	28.91	76.89	189.11	2615	29.30	77.93	188.07	2601
266.5	28.06	74.78	191.72	2652	28.45	75.81	190.69	2637	28.84	76.85	189.65	2623	29.23	77.89	188.61	2608
267	27.99	74.74	192.26	2659	28.38	75.77	191.23	2645	28.77	76.81	190.19	2630	29.16	77.85	189.15	2616
267.5	27.92	74.70	192.81	2666	28.31	75.73	191.77	2652	28.70	76.77	190.73	2638	29.09	77.81	189.69	2623
268	27.86	74.65	193.35	2674	28.24	75.69	192.31	2660	28.63	76.73	191.27	2645	29.02	77.77	190.23	2631
268.5	27.79	74.61	193.89	2681	28.18	75.65	192.85	2667	28.56	76.69	191.81	2653	28.95	77.73	190.77	2638
269	27.72	74.57	194.43	2689	28.11	75.61	193.39	2675	28.49	76.65	192.35	2660	28.88	77.68	191.32	2646
269.5	27.66	74.53	194.97	2696	28.04	75.57	193.93	2682	28.43	76.61	192.89	2668	28.81	77.64	191.86	2653
270	27.59	74.49	195.51	2704	27.97	75.53	194.47	2690	28.36	76.57	193.44	2675	28.74	77.60	192.40	2661
270.5	27.52	74.45	196.05	2711	27.91	75.49	195.01	2697	28.29	76.52	193.98	2683	28.67	77.56	192.94	2668
271	27.46	74.41	196.59	2719	27.84	75.45	195.55	2705	28.22	76.48	194.52	2690	28.61	77.52	193.48	2676
271.5	27.39	74.37	197.13	2726	27.77	75.40	196.10	2712	28.16	76.44	195.06	2698	28.54	77.48	194.02	2683
272	27.33	74.33	197.67	2734	27.71	75.36	196.64	2719	28.09	76.40	195.60	2705	28.47	77.44	194.56	2691
272.5	27.26	74.29	198.22	2741	27.64	75.32	197.18	2727	28.02	76.36	196.14	2713	28.40	77.40	195.10	2698
273	27.20	74.24	198.76	2749	27.58	75.28	197.72	2734	27.96	76.32	196.68	2720	28.34	77.36	195.64	2706
273.5	27.13	74.20	199.30	2756	27.51	75.24	198.26	2742	27.89	76.28	197.22	2728	28.27	77.32	196.18	2713
274	27.07	74.16	199.84	2764	27.45	75.20	198.80	2749	27.82	76.24	197.76	2735	28.20	77.27	196.73	2721
274.5	27.00	74.12	200.38	2771	27.38	75.16	199.34	2757	27.76	76.20	198.30	2743	28.14	77.23	197.27	2728
275	26.94	74.08	200.92	2779	27.32	75.12	199.88	2764	27.69	76.16	198.85	2750	28.07	77.19	197.81	2736
275.5	26.87	74.04	201.46	2786	27.25	75.08	200.42	2772	27.63	76.11	199.39	2758	28.00	77.15	198.35	2743
276	26.81	74.00	202.00	2794	27.19	75.04	200.96	2779	27.56	76.07	199.93	2765	27.94	77.11	198.89	2751
276.5	26.75	73.96	202.54	2801	27.12	74.99	201.51	2787	27.50	76.03	200.47	2772	27.87	77.07	199.43	2758
277	26.68	73.92	203.08	2809	27.06	74.95	202.05	2794	27.43	75.99	201.01	2780	27.81	77.03	199.97	2766
277.5	26.62	73.88	203.63	2816	27.00	74.91	202.59	2802	27.37	75.95	201.55	2787	27.74	76.99	200.51	2773
278	26.56	73.83	204.17	2824	26.93	74.87	203.13	2809	27.31	75.91	202.09	2795	27.68	76.95	201.05	2781
278.5	26.50	73.79	204.71	2831	26.87	74.83	203.67	2817	27.24	75.87	202.63	2802	27.61	76.91	201.59	2788
279	26.43	73.75	205.25	2839	26.81	74.79	204.21	2824	27.18	75.83	203.17	2810	27.55	76.86	202.14	2796
279.5	26.37	73.71	205.79	2846	26.74	74.75	204.75	2832	27.11	75.79	203.71	2817	27.49	76.82	202.68	2803

Body Composition　MALE　248-279.5 Lb.

Weight: Lb.	Waist: 48 inches				48.25 inches				48.5 inches				48.75 inches			
	Fat: %	Fat: Lb.	LBM: Lb.	RMR: Cal.	Fat: %	Fat: Lb.	LBM: Lb.	RMR: Cal.	Fat: %	Fat: Lb.	LBM: Lb.	RMR: Cal.	Fat: %	Fat: Lb.	LBM: Lb.	RMR: Cal.
248	32.44	80.44	167.56	2317	32.86	81.48	166.52	2303	33.27	82.52	165.48	2289	33.69	83.56	164.44	2274
248.5	32.36	80.40	168.10	2325	32.77	81.44	167.06	2310	33.19	82.48	166.02	2296	33.61	83.52	164.98	2282
249	32.27	80.36	168.64	2332	32.69	81.40	167.60	2318	33.11	82.44	166.56	2304	33.52	83.47	165.53	2289
249.5	32.19	80.32	169.18	2340	32.61	81.36	168.14	2325	33.02	82.40	167.10	2311	33.44	83.43	166.07	2297
250	32.11	80.28	169.72	2347	32.53	81.32	168.68	2333	32.94	82.36	167.65	2319	33.36	83.39	166.61	2304
250.5	32.03	80.24	170.26	2355	32.45	81.28	169.22	2340	32.86	82.31	168.19	2326	33.27	83.35	167.15	2312
251	31.95	80.20	170.80	2362	32.36	81.24	169.76	2348	32.78	82.27	168.73	2333	33.19	83.31	167.69	2319
251.5	31.87	80.16	171.34	2370	32.28	81.19	170.31	2355	32.70	82.23	169.27	2341	33.11	83.27	168.23	2327
252	31.79	80.12	171.88	2377	32.20	81.15	170.85	2363	32.62	82.19	169.81	2348	33.03	83.23	168.77	2334
252.5	31.71	80.08	172.43	2385	32.12	81.11	171.39	2370	32.53	82.15	170.35	2356	32.95	83.19	169.31	2342
253	31.63	80.03	172.97	2392	32.04	81.07	171.93	2378	32.45	82.11	170.89	2363	32.86	83.15	169.85	2349
253.5	31.56	79.99	173.51	2400	31.96	81.03	172.47	2385	32.37	82.07	171.43	2371	32.78	83.11	170.39	2357
254	31.48	79.95	174.05	2407	31.89	80.99	173.01	2393	32.29	82.03	171.97	2378	32.70	83.06	170.94	2364
254.5	31.40	79.91	174.59	2415	31.81	80.95	173.55	2400	32.21	81.99	172.51	2386	32.62	83.02	171.48	2372
255	31.32	79.87	175.13	2422	31.73	80.91	174.09	2408	32.14	81.95	173.06	2393	32.54	82.98	172.02	2379
255.5	31.24	79.83	175.67	2430	31.65	80.87	174.63	2415	32.06	81.90	173.60	2401	32.46	82.94	172.56	2386
256	31.17	79.79	176.21	2437	31.57	80.83	175.17	2423	31.98	81.86	174.14	2408	32.38	82.90	173.10	2394
256.5	31.09	79.75	176.75	2444	31.49	80.78	175.72	2430	31.90	81.82	174.68	2416	32.30	82.86	173.64	2401
257	31.01	79.71	177.29	2452	31.42	80.74	176.26	2438	31.82	81.78	175.22	2423	32.23	82.82	174.18	2409
257.5	30.94	79.67	177.84	2459	31.34	80.70	176.80	2445	31.74	81.74	175.76	2431	32.15	82.78	174.72	2416
258	30.86	79.62	178.38	2467	31.26	80.66	177.34	2453	31.67	81.70	176.30	2438	32.07	82.74	175.26	2424
258.5	30.79	79.58	178.92	2474	31.19	80.62	177.88	2460	31.59	81.66	176.84	2446	31.99	82.70	175.80	2431
259	30.71	79.54	179.46	2482	31.11	80.58	178.42	2468	31.51	81.62	177.38	2453	31.91	82.65	176.35	2439
259.5	30.64	79.50	180.00	2489	31.04	80.54	178.96	2475	31.44	81.58	177.92	2461	31.84	82.61	176.89	2446
260	30.56	79.46	180.54	2497	30.96	80.50	179.50	2483	31.36	81.54	178.47	2468	31.76	82.57	177.43	2454
260.5	30.49	79.42	181.08	2504	30.89	80.46	180.04	2490	31.28	81.49	179.01	2476	31.68	82.53	177.97	2461
261	30.41	79.38	181.62	2512	30.81	80.42	180.58	2497	31.21	81.45	179.55	2483	31.61	82.49	178.51	2469
261.5	30.34	79.34	182.16	2519	30.74	80.37	181.13	2505	31.13	81.41	180.09	2491	31.53	82.45	179.05	2476
262	30.27	79.30	182.70	2527	30.66	80.33	181.67	2512	31.06	81.37	180.63	2498	31.45	82.41	179.59	2484
262.5	30.19	79.26	183.25	2534	30.59	80.29	182.21	2520	30.98	81.33	181.17	2506	31.38	82.37	180.13	2491
263	30.12	79.21	183.79	2542	30.51	80.25	182.75	2527	30.91	81.29	181.71	2513	31.30	82.33	180.67	2499
263.5	30.05	79.17	184.33	2549	30.44	80.21	183.29	2535	30.83	81.25	182.25	2521	31.23	82.29	181.21	2506
264	29.97	79.13	184.87	2557	30.37	80.17	183.83	2542	30.76	81.21	182.79	2528	31.15	82.24	181.76	2514
264.5	29.90	79.09	185.41	2564	30.29	80.13	184.37	2550	30.69	81.17	183.33	2536	31.08	82.20	182.30	2521
265	29.83	79.05	185.95	2572	30.22	80.09	184.91	2557	30.61	81.13	183.88	2543	31.00	82.16	182.84	2529
265.5	29.76	79.01	186.49	2579	30.15	80.05	185.45	2565	30.54	81.08	184.42	2550	30.93	82.12	183.38	2536
266	29.69	78.97	187.03	2587	30.08	80.01	185.99	2572	30.47	81.04	184.96	2558	30.86	82.08	183.92	2544
266.5	29.62	78.93	187.57	2594	30.01	79.96	186.54	2580	30.39	81.00	185.50	2565	30.78	82.04	184.46	2551
267	29.55	78.89	188.11	2602	29.93	79.92	187.08	2587	30.32	80.96	186.04	2573	30.71	82.00	185.00	2559
267.5	29.47	78.85	188.66	2609	29.86	79.88	187.62	2595	30.25	80.92	186.58	2580	30.64	81.96	185.54	2566
268	29.40	78.80	189.20	2617	29.79	79.84	188.16	2602	30.18	80.88	187.12	2588	30.57	81.92	186.08	2574
268.5	29.33	78.76	189.74	2624	29.72	79.80	188.70	2610	30.11	80.84	187.66	2595	30.49	81.88	186.62	2581
269	29.26	78.72	190.28	2632	29.65	79.76	189.24	2617	30.04	80.80	188.20	2603	30.42	81.83	187.17	2588
269.5	29.20	78.68	190.82	2639	29.58	79.72	189.78	2625	29.97	80.76	188.74	2610	30.35	81.79	187.71	2596
270	29.13	78.64	191.36	2647	29.51	79.68	190.32	2632	29.89	80.72	189.29	2618	30.28	81.75	188.25	2603
270.5	29.06	78.60	191.90	2654	29.44	79.64	190.86	2640	29.82	80.67	189.83	2625	30.21	81.71	188.79	2611
271	28.99	78.56	192.44	2661	29.37	79.60	191.40	2647	29.75	80.63	190.37	2633	30.14	81.67	189.33	2618
271.5	28.92	78.52	192.98	2669	29.30	79.55	191.95	2655	29.68	80.59	190.91	2640	30.07	81.63	189.87	2626
272	28.85	78.48	193.52	2676	29.23	79.51	192.49	2662	29.61	80.55	191.45	2648	30.00	81.59	190.41	2633
272.5	28.78	78.44	194.07	2684	29.16	79.47	193.03	2670	29.54	80.51	191.99	2655	29.93	81.55	190.95	2641
273	28.72	78.39	194.61	2691	29.10	79.43	193.57	2677	29.48	80.47	192.53	2663	29.86	81.51	191.49	2648
273.5	28.65	78.35	195.15	2699	29.03	79.39	194.11	2685	29.41	80.43	193.07	2670	29.79	81.47	192.03	2656
274	28.58	78.31	195.69	2706	28.96	79.35	194.65	2692	29.34	80.39	193.61	2678	29.72	81.42	192.58	2663
274.5	28.51	78.27	196.23	2714	28.89	79.31	195.19	2699	29.27	80.35	194.15	2685	29.65	81.38	193.12	2671
275	28.45	78.23	196.77	2721	28.82	79.27	195.73	2707	29.20	80.31	194.70	2693	29.58	81.34	193.66	2678
275.5	28.38	78.19	197.31	2729	28.76	79.23	196.27	2714	29.13	80.26	195.24	2700	29.51	81.30	194.20	2686
276	28.31	78.15	197.85	2736	28.69	79.19	196.81	2722	29.07	80.22	195.78	2708	29.44	81.26	194.74	2693
276.5	28.25	78.11	198.39	2744	28.62	79.14	197.36	2729	29.00	80.18	196.32	2715	29.37	81.22	195.28	2701
277	28.18	78.07	198.93	2751	28.56	79.10	197.90	2737	28.93	80.14	196.86	2723	29.31	81.18	195.82	2708
277.5	28.12	78.03	199.48	2759	28.49	79.06	198.44	2744	28.86	80.10	197.40	2730	29.24	81.14	196.36	2716
278	28.05	77.98	200.02	2766	28.43	79.02	198.98	2752	28.80	80.06	197.94	2738	29.17	81.10	196.90	2723
278.5	27.99	77.94	200.56	2774	28.36	78.98	199.52	2759	28.73	80.02	198.48	2745	29.10	81.06	197.44	2731
279	27.92	77.90	201.10	2781	28.29	78.94	200.06	2767	28.67	79.98	199.02	2752	29.04	81.01	197.99	2738
279.5	27.86	77.86	201.64	2789	28.23	78.90	200.60	2774	28.60	79.94	199.56	2760	28.97	80.97	198.53	2746

Body Composition MALE 248-279.5 Lb.

Weight: Lb.	Waist: 49 inches Fat: %	Fat: Lb.	LBM: Lb.	RMR: Cal.	49.25 inches Fat: %	Fat: Lb.	LBM: Lb.	RMR: Cal.	49.5 inches Fat: %	Fat: Lb.	LBM: Lb.	RMR: Cal.	49.75 inches Fat: %	Fat: Lb.	LBM: Lb.	RMR: Cal.
248	34.11	84.59	163.41	2260	34.53	85.63	162.37	2246	34.95	86.67	161.33	2231	35.37	87.71	160.29	2217
248.5	34.03	84.55	163.95	2267	34.44	85.59	162.91	2253	34.86	86.63	161.87	2239	35.28	87.67	160.83	2224
249	33.94	84.51	164.49	2275	34.36	85.55	163.45	2261	34.77	86.59	162.41	2246	35.19	87.62	161.38	2232
249.5	33.86	84.47	165.03	2282	34.27	85.51	163.99	2268	34.69	86.55	162.95	2254	35.10	87.58	161.92	2239
250	33.77	84.43	165.57	2290	34.19	85.47	164.53	2275	34.60	86.51	163.50	2261	35.02	87.54	162.46	2247
250.5	33.69	84.39	166.11	2297	34.10	85.43	165.07	2283	34.52	86.46	164.04	2269	34.93	87.50	163.00	2254
251	33.60	84.35	166.65	2305	34.02	85.39	165.61	2290	34.43	86.42	164.58	2276	34.84	87.46	163.54	2262
251.5	33.52	84.31	167.19	2312	33.93	85.34	166.16	2298	34.35	86.38	165.12	2284	34.76	87.42	164.08	2269
252	33.44	84.27	167.73	2320	33.85	85.30	166.70	2305	34.26	86.34	165.66	2291	34.67	87.38	164.62	2277
252.5	33.36	84.23	168.28	2327	33.77	85.26	167.24	2313	34.18	86.30	166.20	2299	34.59	87.34	165.16	2284
253	33.27	84.18	168.82	2335	33.68	85.22	167.78	2320	34.09	86.26	166.74	2306	34.50	87.30	165.70	2292
253.5	33.19	84.14	169.36	2342	33.60	85.18	168.32	2328	34.01	86.22	167.28	2314	34.42	87.26	166.24	2299
254	33.11	84.10	169.90	2350	33.52	85.14	168.86	2335	33.93	86.18	167.82	2321	34.34	87.21	166.79	2307
254.5	33.03	84.06	170.44	2357	33.44	85.10	169.40	2343	33.85	86.14	168.36	2328	34.25	87.17	167.33	2314
255	32.95	84.02	170.98	2365	33.36	85.06	169.94	2350	33.76	86.10	168.91	2336	34.17	87.13	167.87	2322
255.5	32.87	83.98	171.52	2372	33.27	85.02	170.48	2358	33.68	86.05	169.45	2343	34.09	87.09	168.41	2329
256	32.79	83.94	172.06	2380	33.19	84.98	171.02	2365	33.60	86.01	169.99	2351	34.00	87.05	168.95	2337
256.5	32.71	83.90	172.60	2387	33.11	84.93	171.57	2373	33.52	85.97	170.53	2358	33.92	87.01	169.49	2344
257	32.63	83.86	173.14	2395	33.03	84.89	172.11	2380	33.44	85.93	171.07	2366	33.84	86.97	170.03	2352
257.5	32.55	83.82	173.69	2402	32.95	84.85	172.65	2388	33.36	85.89	171.61	2373	33.76	86.93	170.57	2359
258	32.47	83.77	174.23	2410	32.87	84.81	173.19	2395	33.27	85.85	172.15	2381	33.68	86.89	171.11	2366
258.5	32.39	83.73	174.77	2417	32.79	84.77	173.73	2403	33.19	85.81	172.69	2388	33.60	86.85	171.65	2374
259	32.31	83.69	175.31	2425	32.71	84.73	174.27	2410	33.11	85.77	173.23	2396	33.52	86.80	172.20	2381
259.5	32.24	83.65	175.85	2432	32.64	84.69	174.81	2418	33.04	85.73	173.77	2403	33.43	86.76	172.74	2389
260	32.16	83.61	176.39	2439	32.56	84.65	175.35	2425	32.96	85.69	174.32	2411	33.35	86.72	173.28	2396
260.5	32.08	83.57	176.93	2447	32.48	84.61	175.89	2433	32.88	85.64	174.86	2418	33.28	86.68	173.82	2404
261	32.00	83.53	177.47	2454	32.40	84.57	176.43	2440	32.80	85.60	175.40	2426	33.20	86.64	174.36	2411
261.5	31.93	83.49	178.01	2462	32.32	84.52	176.98	2448	32.72	85.56	175.94	2433	33.12	86.60	174.90	2419
262	31.85	83.45	178.55	2469	32.25	84.48	177.52	2455	32.64	85.52	176.48	2441	33.04	86.56	175.44	2426
262.5	31.77	83.41	179.10	2477	32.17	84.44	178.06	2463	32.56	85.48	177.02	2448	32.96	86.52	175.98	2434
263	31.70	83.36	179.64	2484	32.09	84.40	178.60	2470	32.49	85.44	177.56	2456	32.88	86.48	176.52	2441
263.5	31.62	83.32	180.18	2492	32.02	84.36	179.14	2477	32.41	85.40	178.10	2463	32.80	86.44	177.06	2449
264	31.55	83.28	180.72	2499	31.94	84.32	179.68	2485	32.33	85.36	178.64	2471	32.73	86.39	177.61	2456
264.5	31.47	83.24	181.26	2507	31.86	84.28	180.22	2492	32.26	85.32	179.18	2478	32.65	86.35	178.15	2464
265	31.40	83.20	181.80	2514	31.79	84.24	180.76	2500	32.18	85.28	179.73	2486	32.57	86.31	178.69	2471
265.5	31.32	83.16	182.34	2522	31.71	84.20	181.30	2507	32.10	85.23	180.27	2493	32.49	86.27	179.23	2479
266	31.25	83.12	182.88	2529	31.64	84.16	181.84	2515	32.03	85.19	180.81	2501	32.42	86.23	179.77	2486
266.5	31.17	83.08	183.42	2537	31.56	84.11	182.39	2522	31.95	85.15	181.35	2508	32.34	86.19	180.31	2494
267	31.10	83.04	183.96	2544	31.49	84.07	182.93	2530	31.88	85.11	181.89	2516	32.27	86.15	180.85	2501
267.5	31.03	83.00	184.51	2552	31.41	84.03	183.47	2537	31.80	85.07	182.43	2523	32.19	86.11	181.39	2509
268	30.95	82.95	185.05	2559	31.34	83.99	184.01	2545	31.73	85.03	182.97	2530	32.11	86.07	181.93	2516
268.5	30.88	82.91	185.59	2567	31.27	83.95	184.55	2552	31.65	84.99	183.51	2538	32.04	86.03	182.47	2524
269	30.81	82.87	186.13	2574	31.19	83.91	185.09	2560	31.58	84.95	184.05	2545	31.96	85.98	183.02	2531
269.5	30.74	82.83	186.67	2582	31.12	83.87	185.63	2567	31.51	84.91	184.59	2553	31.89	85.94	183.56	2539
270	30.66	82.79	187.21	2589	31.05	83.83	186.17	2575	31.43	84.87	185.14	2560	31.82	85.90	184.10	2546
270.5	30.59	82.75	187.75	2597	30.97	83.79	186.71	2582	31.36	84.82	185.68	2568	31.74	85.86	184.64	2554
271	30.52	82.71	188.29	2604	30.90	83.75	187.25	2590	31.29	84.78	186.22	2575	31.67	85.82	185.18	2561
271.5	30.45	82.67	188.83	2612	30.83	83.70	187.80	2597	31.21	84.74	186.76	2583	31.59	85.78	185.72	2569
272	30.38	82.63	189.37	2619	30.76	83.66	188.34	2605	31.14	84.70	187.30	2590	31.52	85.74	186.26	2576
272.5	30.31	82.59	189.92	2627	30.69	83.62	188.88	2612	31.07	84.66	187.84	2598	31.45	85.70	186.80	2583
273	30.24	82.54	190.46	2634	30.62	83.58	189.42	2620	31.00	84.62	188.38	2605	31.38	85.66	187.34	2591
273.5	30.17	82.50	191.00	2641	30.54	83.54	189.96	2627	30.92	84.58	188.92	2613	31.30	85.62	187.88	2598
274	30.10	82.46	191.54	2649	30.47	83.50	190.50	2635	30.85	84.54	189.46	2620	31.23	85.57	188.43	2606
274.5	30.03	82.42	192.08	2656	30.40	83.46	191.04	2642	30.78	84.50	190.00	2628	31.16	85.53	188.97	2613
275	29.96	82.38	192.62	2664	30.33	83.42	191.58	2650	30.71	84.46	190.55	2635	31.09	85.49	189.51	2621
275.5	29.89	82.34	193.16	2671	30.26	83.38	192.12	2657	30.64	84.41	191.09	2643	31.02	85.45	190.05	2628
276	29.82	82.30	193.70	2679	30.19	83.34	192.66	2665	30.57	84.37	191.63	2650	30.95	85.41	190.59	2636
276.5	29.75	82.26	194.24	2686	30.12	83.29	193.21	2672	30.50	84.33	192.17	2658	30.88	85.37	191.13	2643
277	29.68	82.22	194.78	2694	30.06	83.25	193.75	2680	30.43	84.29	192.71	2665	30.80	85.33	191.67	2651
277.5	29.61	82.18	195.33	2701	29.99	83.21	194.29	2687	30.36	84.25	193.25	2673	30.73	85.29	192.21	2658
278	29.54	82.13	195.87	2709	29.92	83.17	194.83	2694	30.29	84.21	193.79	2680	30.66	85.25	192.75	2666
278.5	29.48	82.09	196.41	2716	29.85	83.13	195.37	2702	30.22	84.17	194.33	2688	30.59	85.21	193.29	2673
279	29.41	82.05	196.95	2724	29.78	83.09	195.91	2709	30.15	84.13	194.87	2695	30.52	85.16	193.84	2681
279.5	29.34	82.01	197.49	2731	29.71	83.05	196.45	2717	30.08	84.09	195.41	2703	30.46	85.12	194.38	2688

Body Composition MALE 248-279.5 Lb.

Weight: Lb.	Waist: 50 inches Fat: %	Fat: Lb.	LBM: Lb.	RMR: Cal.	50.25 inches Fat: %	Fat: Lb.	LBM: Lb.	RMR: Cal.	50.5 inches Fat: %	Fat: Lb.	LBM: Lb.	RMR: Cal.	50.75 inches Fat: %	Fat: Lb.	LBM: Lb.	RMR: Cal.
248	35.78	88.74	159.26	2203	36.20	89.78	158.22	2188	36.62	90.82	157.18	2174	37.04	91.86	156.14	2159
248.5	35.70	88.70	159.80	2210	36.11	89.74	158.76	2196	36.53	90.78	157.72	2181	36.95	91.82	156.68	2167
249	35.61	88.66	160.34	2217	36.02	89.70	159.30	2203	36.44	90.74	158.26	2189	36.86	91.77	157.23	2174
249.5	35.52	88.62	160.88	2225	35.94	89.66	159.84	2211	36.35	90.70	158.80	2196	36.77	91.73	157.77	2182
250	35.43	88.58	161.42	2232	35.85	89.62	160.38	2218	36.26	90.66	159.35	2204	36.68	91.69	158.31	2189
250.5	35.34	88.54	161.96	2240	35.76	89.58	160.92	2226	36.17	90.61	159.89	2211	36.59	91.65	158.85	2197
251	35.26	88.50	162.50	2247	35.67	89.54	161.46	2233	36.08	90.57	160.43	2219	36.50	91.61	159.39	2204
251.5	35.17	88.46	163.04	2255	35.58	89.49	162.01	2241	36.00	90.53	160.97	2226	36.41	91.57	159.93	2212
252	35.09	88.42	163.58	2262	35.50	89.45	162.55	2248	35.91	90.49	161.51	2234	36.32	91.53	160.47	2219
252.5	35.00	88.38	164.13	2270	35.41	89.41	163.09	2256	35.82	90.45	162.05	2241	36.23	91.49	161.01	2227
253	34.91	88.33	164.67	2277	35.32	89.37	163.63	2263	35.73	90.41	162.59	2249	36.14	91.45	161.55	2234
253.5	34.83	88.29	165.21	2285	35.24	89.33	164.17	2270	35.65	90.37	163.13	2256	36.06	91.41	162.09	2242
254	34.74	88.25	165.75	2292	35.15	89.29	164.71	2278	35.56	90.33	163.67	2264	35.97	91.36	162.64	2249
254.5	34.66	88.21	166.29	2300	35.07	89.25	165.25	2285	35.48	90.29	164.21	2271	35.88	91.32	163.18	2257
255	34.58	88.17	166.83	2307	34.98	89.21	165.79	2293	35.39	90.25	164.76	2279	35.80	91.28	163.72	2264
255.5	34.49	88.13	167.37	2315	34.90	89.17	166.33	2300	35.30	90.20	165.30	2286	35.71	91.24	164.26	2272
256	34.41	88.09	167.91	2322	34.81	89.13	166.87	2308	35.22	90.16	165.84	2294	35.63	91.20	164.80	2279
256.5	34.33	88.05	168.45	2330	34.73	89.08	167.42	2315	35.14	90.12	166.38	2301	35.54	91.16	165.34	2287
257	34.24	88.01	168.99	2337	34.65	89.04	167.96	2323	35.05	90.08	166.92	2308	35.45	91.12	165.88	2294
257.5	34.16	87.97	169.54	2345	34.56	89.00	168.50	2330	34.97	90.04	167.46	2316	35.37	91.08	166.42	2302
258	34.08	87.92	170.08	2352	34.48	88.96	169.04	2338	34.88	90.00	168.00	2323	35.29	91.04	166.96	2309
258.5	34.00	87.88	170.62	2360	34.40	88.92	169.58	2345	34.80	89.96	168.54	2331	35.20	91.00	167.50	2317
259	33.92	87.84	171.16	2367	34.32	88.88	170.12	2353	34.72	89.92	169.08	2338	35.12	90.95	168.05	2324
259.5	33.83	87.80	171.70	2375	34.23	88.84	170.66	2360	34.63	89.88	169.62	2346	35.03	90.91	168.59	2332
260	33.75	87.76	172.24	2382	34.15	88.80	171.20	2368	34.55	89.84	170.17	2353	34.95	90.87	169.13	2339
260.5	33.67	87.72	172.78	2390	34.07	88.76	171.74	2375	34.47	89.79	170.71	2361	34.87	90.83	169.67	2347
261	33.59	87.68	173.32	2397	33.99	88.72	172.28	2383	34.39	89.75	171.25	2368	34.79	90.79	170.21	2354
261.5	33.51	87.64	173.86	2405	33.91	88.67	172.83	2390	34.31	89.71	171.79	2376	34.70	90.75	170.75	2361
262	33.43	87.60	174.40	2412	33.83	88.63	173.37	2398	34.23	89.67	172.33	2383	34.62	90.71	171.29	2369
262.5	33.35	87.56	174.95	2419	33.75	88.59	173.91	2405	34.14	89.63	172.87	2391	34.54	90.67	171.83	2376
263	33.28	87.51	175.49	2427	33.67	88.55	174.45	2413	34.06	89.59	173.41	2398	34.46	90.63	172.37	2384
263.5	33.20	87.47	176.03	2434	33.59	88.51	174.99	2420	33.98	89.55	173.95	2406	34.38	90.59	172.91	2391
264	33.12	87.43	176.57	2442	33.51	88.47	175.53	2428	33.90	89.51	174.49	2413	34.30	90.54	173.46	2399
264.5	33.04	87.39	177.11	2449	33.43	88.43	176.07	2435	33.82	89.47	175.03	2421	34.22	90.50	174.00	2406
265	32.96	87.35	177.65	2457	33.35	88.39	176.61	2443	33.75	89.43	175.58	2428	34.14	90.46	174.54	2414
265.5	32.88	87.31	178.19	2464	33.28	88.35	177.15	2450	33.67	89.38	176.12	2436	34.06	90.42	175.08	2421
266	32.81	87.27	178.73	2472	33.20	88.31	177.69	2458	33.59	89.34	176.66	2443	33.98	90.38	175.62	2429
266.5	32.73	87.23	179.27	2479	33.12	88.26	178.24	2465	33.51	89.30	177.20	2451	33.90	90.34	176.16	2436
267	32.65	87.19	179.81	2487	33.04	88.22	178.78	2472	33.43	89.26	177.74	2458	33.82	90.30	176.70	2444
267.5	32.58	87.15	180.36	2494	32.97	88.18	179.32	2480	33.35	89.22	178.28	2466	33.74	90.26	177.24	2451
268	32.50	87.10	180.90	2502	32.89	88.14	179.86	2487	33.28	89.18	178.82	2473	33.66	90.22	177.78	2459
268.5	32.43	87.06	181.44	2509	32.81	88.10	180.40	2495	33.20	89.14	179.36	2481	33.58	90.18	178.32	2466
269	32.35	87.02	181.98	2517	32.74	88.06	180.94	2502	33.12	89.10	179.90	2488	33.51	90.13	178.87	2474
269.5	32.27	86.98	182.52	2524	32.66	88.02	181.48	2510	33.04	89.06	180.44	2496	33.43	90.09	179.41	2481
270	32.20	86.94	183.06	2532	32.58	87.98	182.02	2517	32.97	89.02	180.99	2503	33.35	90.05	179.95	2489
270.5	32.13	86.90	183.60	2539	32.51	87.94	182.56	2525	32.89	88.97	181.53	2511	33.28	90.01	180.49	2496
271	32.05	86.86	184.14	2547	32.43	87.90	183.10	2532	32.82	88.93	182.07	2518	33.20	89.97	181.03	2504
271.5	31.98	86.82	184.68	2554	32.36	87.85	183.65	2540	32.74	88.89	182.61	2525	33.12	89.93	181.57	2511
272	31.90	86.78	185.22	2562	32.28	87.81	184.19	2547	32.67	88.85	183.15	2533	33.05	89.89	182.11	2519
272.5	31.83	86.74	185.77	2569	32.21	87.77	184.73	2555	32.59	88.81	183.69	2540	32.97	89.85	182.65	2526
273	31.76	86.69	186.31	2577	32.14	87.73	185.27	2562	32.52	88.77	184.23	2548	32.90	89.81	183.19	2534
273.5	31.68	86.65	186.85	2584	32.06	87.69	185.81	2570	32.44	88.73	184.77	2555	32.82	89.77	183.73	2541
274	31.61	86.61	187.39	2592	31.99	87.65	186.35	2577	32.37	88.69	185.31	2563	32.75	89.72	184.28	2549
274.5	31.54	86.57	187.93	2599	31.92	87.61	186.89	2585	32.29	88.65	185.85	2570	32.67	89.68	184.82	2556
275	31.47	86.53	188.47	2607	31.84	87.57	187.43	2592	32.22	88.61	186.40	2578	32.60	89.64	185.36	2563
275.5	31.39	86.49	189.01	2614	31.77	87.53	187.97	2600	32.15	88.56	186.94	2585	32.52	89.60	185.90	2571
276	31.32	86.45	189.55	2622	31.70	87.49	188.51	2607	32.07	88.52	187.48	2593	32.45	89.56	186.44	2578
276.5	31.25	86.41	190.09	2629	31.63	87.44	189.06	2615	32.00	88.48	188.02	2600	32.38	89.52	186.98	2586
277	31.18	86.37	190.63	2636	31.55	87.40	189.60	2622	31.93	88.44	188.56	2608	32.30	89.48	187.52	2593
277.5	31.11	86.33	191.18	2644	31.48	87.36	190.14	2630	31.86	88.40	189.10	2615	32.23	89.44	188.06	2601
278	31.04	86.28	191.72	2651	31.41	87.32	190.68	2637	31.78	88.36	189.64	2623	32.16	89.40	188.60	2608
278.5	30.97	86.24	192.26	2659	31.34	87.28	191.22	2645	31.71	88.32	190.18	2630	32.08	89.36	189.14	2616
279	30.90	86.20	192.80	2666	31.27	87.24	191.76	2652	31.64	88.28	190.72	2638	32.01	89.31	189.69	2623
279.5	30.83	86.16	193.34	2674	31.20	87.20	192.30	2660	31.57	88.24	191.26	2645	31.94	89.27	190.23	2631

Body Composition MALE 248-279.5 Lb.

Weight: Lb.	Waist: 51 inches				51.25 inches				51.5 inches				51.75 inches			
	Fat: %	Fat: Lb.	LBM: Lb.	RMR: Cal.	Fat: %	Fat: Lb.	LBM: Lb.	RMR: Cal.	Fat: %	Fat: Lb.	LBM: Lb.	RMR: Cal.	Fat: %	Fat: Lb.	LBM: Lb.	RMR: Cal.
248	37.46	92.89	155.11	2145	37.88	93.93	154.07	2131	38.29	94.97	153.03	2116	38.71	96.01	151.99	2102
248.5	37.37	92.85	155.65	2153	37.78	93.89	154.61	2138	38.20	94.93	153.57	2124	38.62	95.97	152.53	2110
249	37.27	92.81	156.19	2160	37.69	93.85	155.15	2146	38.11	94.89	154.11	2131	38.52	95.92	153.08	2117
249.5	37.18	92.77	156.73	2168	37.60	93.81	155.69	2153	38.01	94.85	154.65	2139	38.43	95.88	153.62	2125
250	37.09	92.73	157.27	2175	37.51	93.77	156.23	2161	37.92	94.81	155.20	2146	38.34	95.84	154.16	2132
250.5	37.00	92.69	157.81	2183	37.42	93.73	156.77	2168	37.83	94.76	155.74	2154	38.24	95.80	154.70	2139
251	36.91	92.65	158.35	2190	37.32	93.69	157.31	2176	37.74	94.72	156.28	2161	38.15	95.76	155.24	2147
251.5	36.82	92.61	158.89	2197	37.23	93.64	157.86	2183	37.65	94.68	156.82	2169	38.06	95.72	155.78	2154
252	36.73	92.57	159.43	2205	37.14	93.60	158.40	2191	37.56	94.64	157.36	2176	37.97	95.68	156.32	2162
252.5	36.64	92.53	159.98	2212	37.05	93.56	158.94	2198	37.47	94.60	157.90	2184	37.88	95.64	156.86	2169
253	36.55	92.48	160.52	2220	36.97	93.52	159.48	2206	37.38	94.56	158.44	2191	37.79	95.60	157.40	2177
253.5	36.47	92.44	161.06	2227	36.88	93.48	160.02	2213	37.29	94.52	158.98	2199	37.69	95.56	157.94	2184
254	36.38	92.40	161.60	2235	36.79	93.44	160.56	2221	37.20	94.48	159.52	2206	37.60	95.51	158.49	2192
254.5	36.29	92.36	162.14	2242	36.70	93.40	161.10	2228	37.11	94.44	160.06	2214	37.51	95.47	159.03	2199
255	36.20	92.32	162.68	2250	36.61	93.36	161.64	2236	37.02	94.40	160.61	2221	37.42	95.43	159.57	2207
255.5	36.12	92.28	163.22	2257	36.52	93.32	162.18	2243	36.93	94.35	161.15	2229	37.34	95.39	160.11	2214
256	36.03	92.24	163.76	2265	36.44	93.28	162.72	2250	36.84	94.31	161.69	2236	37.25	95.35	160.65	2222
256.5	35.94	92.20	164.30	2272	36.35	93.23	163.27	2258	36.75	94.27	162.23	2244	37.16	95.31	161.19	2229
257	35.86	92.16	164.84	2280	36.26	93.19	163.81	2265	36.67	94.23	162.77	2251	37.07	95.27	161.73	2237
257.5	35.77	92.12	165.39	2287	36.18	93.15	164.35	2273	36.58	94.19	163.31	2259	36.98	95.23	162.27	2244
258	35.69	92.07	165.93	2295	36.09	93.11	164.89	2280	36.49	94.15	163.85	2266	36.89	95.19	162.81	2252
258.5	35.60	92.03	166.47	2302	36.00	93.07	165.43	2288	36.41	94.11	164.39	2274	36.81	95.15	163.35	2259
259	35.52	91.99	167.01	2310	35.92	93.03	165.97	2295	36.32	94.07	164.93	2281	36.72	95.10	163.90	2267
259.5	35.43	91.95	167.55	2317	35.83	92.99	166.51	2303	36.23	94.03	165.47	2289	36.63	95.06	164.44	2274
260	35.35	91.91	168.09	2325	35.75	92.95	167.05	2310	36.15	93.99	166.02	2296	36.55	95.02	164.98	2282
260.5	35.27	91.87	168.63	2332	35.66	92.91	167.59	2318	36.06	93.94	166.56	2303	36.46	94.98	165.52	2289
261	35.18	91.83	169.17	2340	35.58	92.87	168.13	2325	35.98	93.90	167.10	2311	36.38	94.94	166.06	2297
261.5	35.10	91.79	169.71	2347	35.50	92.82	168.68	2333	35.89	93.86	167.64	2318	36.29	94.90	166.60	2304
262	35.02	91.75	170.25	2355	35.41	92.78	169.22	2340	35.81	93.82	168.18	2326	36.21	94.86	167.14	2312
262.5	34.94	91.71	170.80	2362	35.33	92.74	169.76	2348	35.73	93.78	168.72	2333	36.12	94.82	167.68	2319
263	34.85	91.66	171.34	2370	35.25	92.70	170.30	2355	35.64	93.74	169.26	2341	36.04	94.78	168.22	2327
263.5	34.77	91.62	171.88	2377	35.17	92.66	170.84	2363	35.56	93.70	169.80	2348	35.95	94.74	168.76	2334
264	34.69	91.58	172.42	2385	35.08	92.62	171.38	2370	35.48	93.66	170.34	2356	35.87	94.69	169.31	2341
264.5	34.61	91.54	172.96	2392	35.00	92.58	171.92	2378	35.39	93.62	170.88	2363	35.79	94.65	169.85	2349
265	34.53	91.50	173.50	2400	34.92	92.54	172.46	2385	35.31	93.58	171.43	2371	35.70	94.61	170.39	2356
265.5	34.45	91.46	174.04	2407	34.84	92.50	173.00	2393	35.23	93.53	171.97	2378	35.62	94.57	170.93	2364
266	34.37	91.42	174.58	2414	34.76	92.46	173.54	2400	35.15	93.49	172.51	2386	35.54	94.53	171.47	2371
266.5	34.29	91.38	175.12	2422	34.68	92.41	174.09	2408	35.07	93.45	173.05	2393	35.46	94.49	172.01	2379
267	34.21	91.34	175.66	2429	34.60	92.37	174.63	2415	34.99	93.41	173.59	2401	35.37	94.45	172.55	2386
267.5	34.13	91.30	176.21	2437	34.52	92.33	175.17	2423	34.90	93.37	174.13	2408	35.29	94.41	173.09	2394
268	34.05	91.25	176.75	2444	34.44	92.29	175.71	2430	34.82	93.33	174.67	2416	35.21	94.37	173.63	2401
268.5	33.97	91.21	177.29	2452	34.36	92.25	176.25	2438	34.74	93.29	175.21	2423	35.13	94.33	174.17	2409
269	33.89	91.17	177.83	2459	34.28	92.21	176.79	2445	34.66	93.25	175.75	2431	35.05	94.28	174.72	2416
269.5	33.81	91.13	178.37	2467	34.20	92.17	177.33	2452	34.58	93.21	176.29	2438	34.97	94.24	175.26	2424
270	33.74	91.09	178.91	2474	34.12	92.13	177.87	2460	34.51	93.17	176.84	2446	34.89	94.20	175.80	2431
270.5	33.66	91.05	179.45	2482	34.04	92.09	178.41	2467	34.43	93.12	177.38	2453	34.81	94.16	176.34	2439
271	33.58	91.01	179.99	2489	33.97	92.05	178.95	2475	34.35	93.08	177.92	2461	34.73	94.12	176.88	2446
271.5	33.51	90.97	180.53	2497	33.89	92.00	179.50	2482	34.27	93.04	178.46	2468	34.65	94.08	177.42	2454
272	33.43	90.93	181.07	2504	33.81	91.96	180.04	2490	34.19	93.00	179.00	2476	34.57	94.04	177.96	2461
272.5	33.35	90.89	181.62	2512	33.73	91.92	180.58	2497	34.11	92.96	179.54	2483	34.49	94.00	178.50	2469
273	33.28	90.84	182.16	2519	33.66	91.88	181.12	2505	34.04	92.92	180.08	2491	34.42	93.96	179.04	2476
273.5	33.20	90.80	182.70	2527	33.58	91.84	181.66	2512	33.96	92.88	180.62	2498	34.34	93.92	179.58	2484
274	33.12	90.76	183.24	2534	33.50	91.80	182.20	2520	33.88	92.84	181.16	2505	34.26	93.87	180.13	2491
274.5	33.05	90.72	183.78	2542	33.43	91.76	182.74	2527	33.81	92.80	181.70	2513	34.18	93.83	180.67	2499
275	32.97	90.68	184.32	2549	33.35	91.72	183.28	2535	33.73	92.76	182.25	2520	34.11	93.79	181.21	2506
275.5	32.90	90.64	184.86	2557	33.28	91.68	183.82	2542	33.65	92.71	182.79	2528	34.03	93.75	181.75	2514
276	32.83	90.60	185.40	2564	33.20	91.64	184.36	2550	33.58	92.67	183.33	2535	33.95	93.71	182.29	2521
276.5	32.75	90.56	185.94	2572	33.13	91.59	184.91	2557	33.50	92.63	183.87	2543	33.88	93.67	182.83	2529
277	32.68	90.52	186.48	2579	33.05	91.55	185.45	2565	33.43	92.59	184.41	2550	33.80	93.63	183.37	2536
277.5	32.60	90.48	187.03	2587	32.98	91.51	185.99	2572	33.35	92.55	184.95	2558	33.73	93.59	183.91	2544
278	32.53	90.43	187.57	2594	32.90	91.47	186.53	2580	33.28	92.51	185.49	2565	33.65	93.55	184.45	2551
278.5	32.46	90.39	188.11	2602	32.83	91.43	187.07	2587	33.20	92.47	186.03	2573	33.57	93.51	184.99	2558
279	32.38	90.35	188.65	2609	32.76	91.39	187.61	2595	33.13	92.43	186.57	2580	33.50	93.46	185.54	2566
279.5	32.31	90.31	189.19	2616	32.68	91.35	188.15	2602	33.05	92.39	187.11	2588	33.43	93.42	186.08	2573

Body Composition MALE 248-279.5 Lb.

Weight: Lb.	Waist: 52 inches Fat: %	Fat: Lb.	LBM: Lb.	RMR: Cal.	52.25 inches Fat: %	Fat: Lb.	LBM: Lb.	RMR: Cal.	52.5 inches Fat: %	Fat: Lb.	LBM: Lb.	RMR: Cal.	52.75 inches Fat: %	Fat: Lb.	LBM: Lb.	RMR: Cal.
248	39.13	97.04	150.96	2088	39.55	98.08	149.92	2073	39.97	99.12	148.88	2059	40.39	100.16	147.84	2045
248.5	39.04	97.00	151.50	2095	39.45	98.04	150.46	2081	39.87	99.08	149.42	2067	40.29	100.12	148.38	2052
249	38.94	96.96	152.04	2103	39.36	98.00	151.00	2088	39.77	99.04	149.96	2074	40.19	100.07	148.93	2060
249.5	38.85	96.92	152.58	2110	39.26	97.96	151.54	2096	39.68	99.00	150.50	2081	40.09	100.03	149.47	2067
250	38.75	96.88	153.12	2118	39.17	97.92	152.08	2103	39.58	98.96	151.05	2089	40.00	99.99	150.01	2075
250.5	38.66	96.84	153.66	2125	39.07	97.88	152.62	2111	39.49	98.91	151.59	2096	39.90	99.95	150.55	2082
251	38.56	96.80	154.20	2133	38.98	97.84	153.16	2118	39.39	98.87	152.13	2104	39.80	99.91	151.09	2090
251.5	38.47	96.76	154.74	2140	38.88	97.79	153.71	2126	39.30	98.83	152.67	2111	39.71	99.87	151.63	2097
252	38.38	96.72	155.28	2148	38.79	97.75	154.25	2133	39.20	98.79	153.21	2119	39.61	99.83	152.17	2105
252.5	38.29	96.68	155.83	2155	38.70	97.71	154.79	2141	39.11	98.75	153.75	2126	39.52	99.79	152.71	2112
253	38.20	96.63	156.37	2163	38.61	97.67	155.33	2148	39.02	98.71	154.29	2134	39.43	99.75	153.25	2119
253.5	38.10	96.59	156.91	2170	38.51	97.63	155.87	2156	38.92	98.67	154.83	2141	39.33	99.71	153.79	2127
254	38.01	96.55	157.45	2178	38.42	97.59	156.41	2163	38.83	98.63	155.37	2149	39.24	99.66	154.34	2134
254.5	37.92	96.51	157.99	2185	38.33	97.55	156.95	2171	38.74	98.59	155.91	2156	39.14	99.62	154.88	2142
255	37.83	96.47	158.53	2192	38.24	97.51	157.49	2178	38.65	98.55	156.46	2164	39.05	99.58	155.42	2149
255.5	37.74	96.43	159.07	2200	38.15	97.47	158.03	2186	38.55	98.50	157.00	2171	38.96	99.54	155.96	2157
256	37.65	96.39	159.61	2207	38.06	97.43	158.57	2193	38.46	98.46	157.54	2179	38.87	99.50	156.50	2164
256.5	37.56	96.35	160.15	2215	37.97	97.38	159.12	2201	38.37	98.42	158.08	2186	38.78	99.46	157.04	2172
257	37.47	96.31	160.69	2222	37.88	97.34	159.66	2208	38.28	98.38	158.62	2194	38.68	99.42	157.58	2179
257.5	37.38	96.27	161.24	2230	37.79	97.30	160.20	2216	38.19	98.34	159.16	2201	38.59	99.38	158.12	2187
258	37.30	96.22	161.78	2237	37.70	97.26	160.74	2223	38.10	98.30	159.70	2209	38.50	99.34	158.66	2194
258.5	37.21	96.18	162.32	2245	37.61	97.22	161.28	2230	38.01	98.26	160.24	2216	38.41	99.30	159.20	2202
259	37.12	96.14	162.86	2252	37.52	97.18	161.82	2238	37.92	98.22	160.78	2224	38.32	99.25	159.75	2209
259.5	37.03	96.10	163.40	2260	37.43	97.14	162.36	2245	37.83	98.18	161.32	2231	38.23	99.21	160.29	2217
260	36.95	96.06	163.94	2267	37.35	97.10	162.90	2253	37.74	98.14	161.87	2239	38.14	99.17	160.83	2224
260.5	36.86	96.02	164.48	2275	37.26	97.06	163.44	2260	37.66	98.09	162.41	2246	38.05	99.13	161.37	2232
261	36.77	95.98	165.02	2282	37.17	97.02	163.98	2268	37.57	98.05	162.95	2254	37.97	99.09	161.91	2239
261.5	36.69	95.94	165.56	2290	37.08	96.97	164.53	2275	37.48	98.01	163.49	2261	37.88	99.05	162.45	2247
262	36.60	95.90	166.10	2297	37.00	96.93	165.07	2283	37.39	97.97	164.03	2269	37.79	99.01	162.99	2254
262.5	36.52	95.86	166.65	2305	36.91	96.89	165.61	2290	37.31	97.93	164.57	2276	37.70	98.97	163.53	2262
263	36.43	95.81	167.19	2312	36.83	96.85	166.15	2298	37.22	97.89	165.11	2283	37.61	98.93	164.07	2269
263.5	36.35	95.77	167.73	2320	36.74	96.81	166.69	2305	37.13	97.85	165.65	2291	37.53	98.89	164.61	2277
264	36.26	95.73	168.27	2327	36.66	96.77	167.23	2313	37.05	97.81	166.19	2298	37.44	98.84	165.16	2284
264.5	36.18	95.69	168.81	2335	36.57	96.73	167.77	2320	36.96	97.77	166.73	2306	37.35	98.80	165.70	2292
265	36.09	95.65	169.35	2342	36.49	96.69	168.31	2328	36.88	97.73	167.28	2313	37.27	98.76	166.24	2299
265.5	36.01	95.61	169.89	2350	36.40	96.65	168.85	2335	36.79	97.68	167.82	2321	37.18	98.72	166.78	2307
266	35.93	95.57	170.43	2357	36.32	96.61	169.39	2343	36.71	97.64	168.36	2328	37.10	98.68	167.32	2314
266.5	35.85	95.53	170.97	2365	36.23	96.56	169.94	2350	36.62	97.60	168.90	2336	37.01	98.64	167.86	2322
267	35.76	95.49	171.51	2372	36.15	96.52	170.48	2358	36.54	97.56	169.44	2343	36.93	98.60	168.40	2329
267.5	35.68	95.45	172.06	2380	36.07	96.48	171.02	2365	36.46	97.52	169.98	2351	36.84	98.56	168.94	2336
268	35.60	95.40	172.60	2387	35.99	96.44	171.56	2373	36.37	97.48	170.52	2358	36.76	98.52	169.48	2344
268.5	35.52	95.36	173.14	2394	35.90	96.40	172.10	2380	36.29	97.44	171.06	2366	36.68	98.48	170.02	2351
269	35.44	95.32	173.68	2402	35.82	96.36	172.64	2388	36.21	97.40	171.60	2373	36.59	98.43	170.57	2359
269.5	35.35	95.28	174.22	2409	35.74	96.32	173.18	2395	36.12	97.36	172.14	2381	36.51	98.39	171.11	2366
270	35.27	95.24	174.76	2417	35.66	96.28	173.72	2403	36.04	97.32	172.69	2388	36.43	98.35	171.65	2374
270.5	35.19	95.20	175.30	2424	35.58	96.24	174.26	2410	35.96	97.27	173.23	2396	36.34	98.31	172.19	2381
271	35.11	95.16	175.84	2432	35.50	96.20	174.80	2418	35.88	97.23	173.77	2403	36.26	98.27	172.73	2389
271.5	35.03	95.12	176.38	2439	35.42	96.15	175.35	2425	35.80	97.19	174.31	2411	36.18	98.23	173.27	2396
272	34.95	95.08	176.92	2447	35.34	96.11	175.89	2433	35.72	97.15	174.85	2418	36.10	98.19	173.81	2404
272.5	34.88	95.04	177.47	2454	35.26	96.07	176.43	2440	35.64	97.11	175.39	2426	36.02	98.15	174.35	2411
273	34.80	94.99	178.01	2462	35.18	96.03	176.97	2447	35.56	97.07	175.93	2433	35.94	98.11	174.89	2419
273.5	34.72	94.95	178.55	2469	35.10	95.99	177.51	2455	35.48	97.03	176.47	2441	35.86	98.07	175.43	2426
274	34.64	94.91	179.09	2477	35.02	95.95	178.05	2462	35.40	96.99	177.01	2448	35.78	98.02	175.98	2434
274.5	34.56	94.87	179.63	2484	34.94	95.91	178.59	2470	35.32	96.95	177.55	2456	35.70	97.98	176.52	2441
275	34.48	94.83	180.17	2492	34.86	95.87	179.13	2477	35.24	96.91	178.10	2463	35.62	97.94	177.06	2449
275.5	34.41	94.79	180.71	2499	34.78	95.83	179.67	2485	35.16	96.86	178.64	2471	35.54	97.90	177.60	2456
276	34.33	94.75	181.25	2507	34.70	95.79	180.21	2492	35.08	96.82	179.18	2478	35.46	97.86	178.14	2464
276.5	34.25	94.71	181.79	2514	34.63	95.74	180.76	2500	35.00	96.78	179.72	2485	35.38	97.82	178.68	2471
277	34.18	94.67	182.33	2522	34.55	95.70	181.30	2507	34.92	96.74	180.26	2493	35.30	97.78	179.22	2479
277.5	34.10	94.63	182.88	2529	34.47	95.66	181.84	2515	34.85	96.70	180.80	2500	35.22	97.74	179.76	2486
278	34.02	94.58	183.42	2537	34.40	95.62	182.38	2522	34.77	96.66	181.34	2508	35.14	97.70	180.30	2494
278.5	33.95	94.54	183.96	2544	34.32	95.58	182.92	2530	34.69	96.62	181.88	2515	35.06	97.66	180.84	2501
279	33.87	94.50	184.50	2552	34.24	95.54	183.46	2537	34.62	96.58	182.42	2523	34.99	97.61	181.39	2509
279.5	33.80	94.46	185.04	2559	34.17	95.50	184.00	2545	34.54	96.54	182.96	2530	34.91	97.57	181.93	2516

Body Composition   MALE   248-279.5 Lb.

Weight: Lb.	Waist: 53 inches Fat: %	Fat: Lb.	LBM: Lb.	RMR: Cal.	53.25 inches Fat: %	Fat: Lb.	LBM: Lb.	RMR: Cal.	53.5 inches Fat: %	Fat: Lb.	LBM: Lb.	RMR: Cal.	53.75 inches Fat: %	Fat: Lb.	LBM: Lb.	RMR: Cal.
248	40.80	101.19	146.81	2030	41.22	102.23	145.77	2016	41.64	103.27	144.73	2002	42.06	104.31	143.69	1987
248.5	40.71	101.15	147.35	2038	41.12	102.19	146.31	2023	41.54	103.23	145.27	2009	41.96	104.27	144.23	1995
249	40.61	101.11	147.89	2045	41.02	102.15	146.85	2031	41.44	103.19	145.81	2017	41.86	104.22	144.78	2002
249.5	40.51	101.07	148.43	2053	40.93	102.11	147.39	2038	41.34	103.15	146.35	2024	41.76	104.18	145.32	2010
250	40.41	101.03	148.97	2060	40.83	102.07	147.93	2046	41.24	103.11	146.90	2032	41.66	104.14	145.86	2017
250.5	40.31	100.99	149.51	2068	40.73	102.03	148.47	2053	41.14	103.06	147.44	2039	41.56	104.10	146.40	2025
251	40.22	100.95	150.05	2075	40.63	101.99	149.01	2061	41.05	103.02	147.98	2047	41.46	104.06	146.94	2032
251.5	40.12	100.91	150.59	2083	40.53	101.94	149.56	2068	40.95	102.98	148.52	2054	41.36	104.02	147.48	2040
252	40.03	100.87	151.13	2090	40.44	101.90	150.10	2076	40.85	102.94	149.06	2061	41.26	103.98	148.02	2047
252.5	39.93	100.83	151.68	2098	40.34	101.86	150.64	2083	40.75	102.90	149.60	2069	41.16	103.94	148.56	2055
253	39.84	100.78	152.22	2105	40.25	101.82	151.18	2091	40.66	102.86	150.14	2076	41.07	103.90	149.10	2062
253.5	39.74	100.74	152.76	2113	40.15	101.78	151.72	2098	40.56	102.82	150.68	2084	40.97	103.86	149.64	2070
254	39.65	100.70	153.30	2120	40.05	101.74	152.26	2106	40.46	102.78	151.22	2091	40.87	103.81	150.19	2077
254.5	39.55	100.66	153.84	2128	39.96	101.70	152.80	2113	40.37	102.74	151.76	2099	40.78	103.77	150.73	2085
255	39.46	100.62	154.38	2135	39.87	101.66	153.34	2121	40.27	102.70	152.31	2106	40.68	103.73	151.27	2092
255.5	39.37	100.58	154.92	2143	39.77	101.62	153.88	2128	40.18	102.65	152.85	2114	40.58	103.69	151.81	2100
256	39.27	100.54	155.46	2150	39.68	101.58	154.42	2136	40.08	102.61	153.39	2121	40.49	103.65	152.35	2107
256.5	39.18	100.50	156.00	2158	39.58	101.53	154.97	2143	39.99	102.57	153.93	2129	40.39	103.61	152.89	2114
257	39.09	100.46	156.54	2165	39.49	101.49	155.51	2151	39.90	102.53	154.47	2136	40.30	103.57	153.43	2122
257.5	39.00	100.42	157.09	2172	39.40	101.45	156.05	2158	39.80	102.49	155.01	2144	40.20	103.53	153.97	2129
258	38.90	100.37	157.63	2180	39.31	101.41	156.59	2166	39.71	102.45	155.55	2151	40.11	103.49	154.51	2137
258.5	38.81	100.33	158.17	2187	39.21	101.37	157.13	2173	39.62	102.41	156.09	2159	40.02	103.45	155.05	2144
259	38.72	100.29	158.71	2195	39.12	101.33	157.67	2181	39.52	102.37	156.63	2166	39.92	103.40	155.60	2152
259.5	38.63	100.25	159.25	2202	39.03	101.29	158.21	2188	39.43	102.33	157.17	2174	39.83	103.36	156.14	2159
260	38.54	100.21	159.79	2210	38.94	101.25	158.75	2196	39.34	102.29	157.72	2181	39.74	103.32	156.68	2167
260.5	38.45	100.17	160.33	2217	38.85	101.21	159.29	2203	39.25	102.24	158.26	2189	39.65	103.28	157.22	2174
261	38.36	100.13	160.87	2225	38.76	101.17	159.83	2211	39.16	102.20	158.80	2196	39.56	103.24	157.76	2182
261.5	38.27	100.09	161.41	2232	38.67	101.12	160.38	2218	39.07	102.16	159.34	2204	39.46	103.20	158.30	2189
262	38.19	100.05	161.95	2240	38.58	101.08	160.92	2225	38.98	102.12	159.88	2211	39.37	103.16	158.84	2197
262.5	38.10	100.01	162.50	2247	38.49	101.04	161.46	2233	38.89	102.08	160.42	2219	39.28	103.12	159.38	2204
263	38.01	99.96	163.04	2255	38.40	101.00	162.00	2240	38.80	102.04	160.96	2226	39.19	103.08	159.92	2212
263.5	37.92	99.92	163.58	2262	38.32	100.96	162.54	2248	38.71	102.00	161.50	2234	39.10	103.04	160.46	2219
264	37.83	99.88	164.12	2270	38.23	100.92	163.08	2255	38.62	101.96	162.04	2241	39.01	102.99	161.01	2227
264.5	37.75	99.84	164.66	2277	38.14	100.88	163.62	2263	38.53	101.92	162.58	2249	38.92	102.95	161.55	2234
265	37.66	99.80	165.20	2285	38.05	100.84	164.16	2270	38.44	101.88	163.13	2256	38.83	102.91	162.09	2242
265.5	37.57	99.76	165.74	2292	37.96	100.80	164.70	2278	38.36	101.83	163.67	2264	38.75	102.87	162.63	2249
266	37.49	99.72	166.28	2300	37.88	100.76	165.24	2285	38.27	101.79	164.21	2271	38.66	102.83	163.17	2257
266.5	37.40	99.68	166.82	2307	37.79	100.72	165.79	2293	38.18	101.75	164.75	2278	38.57	102.79	163.71	2264
267	37.32	99.64	167.36	2315	37.71	100.67	166.33	2300	38.09	101.71	165.29	2286	38.48	102.75	164.25	2272
267.5	37.23	99.60	167.91	2322	37.62	100.63	166.87	2308	38.01	101.67	165.83	2293	38.40	102.71	164.79	2279
268	37.15	99.55	168.45	2330	37.53	100.59	167.41	2315	37.92	101.63	166.37	2301	38.31	102.67	165.33	2287
268.5	37.06	99.51	168.99	2337	37.45	100.55	167.95	2323	37.84	101.59	166.91	2308	38.22	102.63	165.87	2294
269	36.98	99.47	169.53	2345	37.36	100.51	168.49	2330	37.75	101.55	167.45	2316	38.14	102.58	166.42	2302
269.5	36.89	99.43	170.07	2352	37.28	100.47	169.03	2338	37.66	101.51	167.99	2323	38.05	102.54	166.96	2309
270	36.81	99.39	170.61	2360	37.20	100.43	169.57	2345	37.58	101.47	168.54	2331	37.96	102.50	167.50	2316
270.5	36.73	99.35	171.15	2367	37.11	100.39	170.11	2353	37.50	101.42	169.08	2338	37.88	102.46	168.04	2324
271	36.65	99.31	171.69	2375	37.03	100.35	170.65	2360	37.41	101.38	169.62	2346	37.79	102.42	168.58	2331
271.5	36.56	99.27	172.23	2382	36.94	100.31	171.20	2368	37.33	101.34	170.16	2353	37.71	102.38	169.12	2339
272	36.48	99.23	172.77	2389	36.86	100.26	171.74	2375	37.24	101.30	170.70	2361	37.62	102.34	169.66	2346
272.5	36.40	99.19	173.32	2397	36.78	100.22	172.28	2383	37.16	101.26	171.24	2368	37.54	102.30	170.20	2354
273	36.32	99.14	173.86	2404	36.70	100.18	172.82	2390	37.08	101.22	171.78	2376	37.46	102.26	170.74	2361
273.5	36.24	99.10	174.40	2412	36.61	100.14	173.36	2398	36.99	101.18	172.32	2383	37.37	102.22	171.28	2369
274	36.15	99.06	174.94	2419	36.53	100.10	173.90	2405	36.91	101.14	172.86	2391	37.29	102.17	171.83	2376
274.5	36.07	99.02	175.48	2427	36.45	100.06	174.44	2413	36.83	101.10	173.40	2398	37.21	102.13	172.37	2384
275	35.99	98.98	176.02	2434	36.37	100.02	174.98	2420	36.75	101.06	173.95	2406	37.12	102.09	172.91	2391
275.5	35.91	98.94	176.56	2442	36.29	99.98	175.52	2427	36.67	101.01	174.49	2413	37.04	102.05	173.45	2399
276	35.83	98.90	177.10	2449	36.21	99.94	176.06	2435	36.58	100.97	175.03	2421	36.96	102.01	173.99	2406
276.5	35.75	98.86	177.64	2457	36.13	99.89	176.61	2442	36.50	100.93	175.57	2428	36.88	101.97	174.53	2414
277	35.67	98.82	178.18	2464	36.05	99.85	177.15	2450	36.42	100.89	176.11	2436	36.80	101.93	175.07	2421
277.5	35.59	98.78	178.73	2472	35.97	99.81	177.69	2457	36.34	100.85	176.65	2443	36.72	101.89	175.61	2429
278	35.52	98.73	179.27	2479	35.89	99.77	178.23	2465	36.26	100.81	177.19	2451	36.64	101.85	176.15	2436
278.5	35.44	98.69	179.81	2487	35.81	99.73	178.77	2472	36.18	100.77	177.73	2458	36.55	101.81	176.69	2444
279	35.36	98.65	180.35	2494	35.73	99.69	179.31	2480	36.10	100.73	178.27	2466	36.47	101.76	177.24	2451
279.5	35.28	98.61	180.89	2502	35.65	99.65	179.85	2487	36.02	100.69	178.81	2473	36.39	101.72	177.78	2459

Body Composition   MALE   248-279.5 Lb.

Weight: Lb.	Waist: 54 inches Fat: %	Fat: Lb.	LBM: Lb.	RMR: Cal.	54.25 inches Fat: %	Fat: Lb.	LBM: Lb.	RMR: Cal.	54.5 inches Fat: %	Fat: Lb.	LBM: Lb.	RMR: Cal.	54.75 inches Fat: %	Fat: Lb.	LBM: Lb.	RMR: Cal.
248	42.48	105.34	142.66	1973	42.90	106.38	141.62	1959	43.31	107.42	140.58	1944	43.73	108.46	139.54	1930
248.5	42.38	105.30	143.20	1980	42.79	106.34	142.16	1966	43.21	107.38	141.12	1952	43.63	108.42	140.08	1937
249	42.27	105.26	143.74	1988	42.69	106.30	142.70	1974	43.11	107.34	141.66	1959	43.52	108.37	140.63	1945
249.5	42.17	105.22	144.28	1995	42.59	106.26	143.24	1981	43.00	107.30	142.20	1967	43.42	108.33	141.17	1952
250	42.07	105.18	144.82	2003	42.49	106.22	143.78	1989	42.90	107.26	142.75	1974	43.32	108.29	141.71	1960
250.5	41.97	105.14	145.36	2010	42.39	106.18	144.32	1996	42.80	107.21	143.29	1982	43.21	108.25	142.25	1967
251	41.87	105.10	145.90	2018	42.29	106.14	144.86	2003	42.70	107.17	143.83	1989	43.11	108.21	142.79	1975
251.5	41.77	105.06	146.44	2025	42.18	106.09	145.41	2011	42.60	107.13	144.37	1997	43.01	108.17	143.33	1982
252	41.67	105.02	146.98	2033	42.08	106.05	145.95	2018	42.50	107.09	144.91	2004	42.91	108.13	143.87	1990
252.5	41.57	104.98	147.53	2040	41.99	106.01	146.49	2026	42.40	107.05	145.45	2012	42.81	108.09	144.41	1997
253	41.48	104.93	148.07	2048	41.89	105.97	147.03	2033	42.30	107.01	145.99	2019	42.71	108.05	144.95	2005
253.5	41.38	104.89	148.61	2055	41.79	105.93	147.57	2041	42.20	106.97	146.53	2027	42.61	108.01	145.49	2012
254	41.28	104.85	149.15	2063	41.69	105.89	148.11	2048	42.10	106.93	147.07	2034	42.51	107.96	146.04	2020
254.5	41.18	104.81	149.69	2070	41.59	105.85	148.65	2056	42.00	106.89	147.61	2042	42.41	107.92	146.58	2027
255	41.09	104.77	150.23	2078	41.49	105.81	149.19	2063	41.90	106.85	148.16	2049	42.31	107.88	147.12	2035
255.5	40.99	104.73	150.77	2085	41.40	105.77	149.73	2071	41.80	106.80	148.70	2056	42.21	107.84	147.66	2042
256	40.89	104.69	151.31	2093	41.30	105.73	150.27	2078	41.70	106.76	149.24	2064	42.11	107.80	148.20	2050
256.5	40.80	104.65	151.85	2100	41.20	105.68	150.82	2086	41.61	106.72	149.78	2071	42.01	107.76	148.74	2057
257	40.70	104.61	152.39	2108	41.11	105.64	151.36	2093	41.51	106.68	150.32	2079	41.91	107.72	149.28	2065
257.5	40.61	104.57	152.94	2115	41.01	105.60	151.90	2101	41.41	106.64	150.86	2086	41.82	107.68	149.82	2072
258	40.51	104.52	153.48	2123	40.92	105.56	152.44	2108	41.32	106.60	151.40	2094	41.72	107.64	150.36	2080
258.5	40.42	104.48	154.02	2130	40.82	105.52	152.98	2116	41.22	106.56	151.94	2101	41.62	107.60	150.90	2087
259	40.33	104.44	154.56	2138	40.73	105.48	153.52	2123	41.13	106.52	152.48	2109	41.53	107.55	151.45	2094
259.5	40.23	104.40	155.10	2145	40.63	105.44	154.06	2131	41.03	106.48	153.02	2116	41.43	107.51	151.99	2102
260	40.14	104.36	155.64	2153	40.54	105.40	154.60	2138	40.94	106.44	153.57	2124	41.34	107.47	152.53	2109
260.5	40.05	104.32	156.18	2160	40.44	105.36	155.14	2146	40.84	106.39	154.11	2131	41.24	107.43	153.07	2117
261	39.95	104.28	156.72	2167	40.35	105.32	155.68	2153	40.75	106.35	154.65	2139	41.15	107.39	153.61	2124
261.5	39.86	104.24	157.26	2175	40.26	105.27	156.23	2161	40.65	106.31	155.19	2146	41.05	107.35	154.15	2132
262	39.77	104.20	157.80	2182	40.17	105.23	156.77	2168	40.56	106.27	155.73	2154	40.96	107.31	154.69	2139
262.5	39.68	104.16	158.35	2190	40.07	105.19	157.31	2176	40.47	106.23	156.27	2161	40.86	107.27	155.23	2147
263	39.59	104.11	158.89	2197	39.98	105.15	157.85	2183	40.38	106.19	156.81	2169	40.77	107.23	155.77	2154
263.5	39.50	104.07	159.43	2205	39.89	105.11	158.39	2191	40.28	106.15	157.35	2176	40.68	107.19	156.31	2162
264	39.41	104.03	159.97	2212	39.80	105.07	158.93	2198	40.19	106.11	157.89	2184	40.59	107.14	156.86	2169
264.5	39.32	103.99	160.51	2220	39.71	105.03	159.47	2205	40.10	106.07	158.43	2191	40.49	107.10	157.40	2177
265	39.23	103.95	161.05	2227	39.62	104.99	160.01	2213	40.01	106.03	158.98	2199	40.40	107.06	157.94	2184
265.5	39.14	103.91	161.59	2235	39.53	104.95	160.55	2220	39.92	105.98	159.52	2206	40.31	107.02	158.48	2192
266	39.05	103.87	162.13	2242	39.44	104.91	161.09	2228	39.83	105.94	160.06	2214	40.22	106.98	159.02	2199
266.5	38.96	103.83	162.67	2250	39.35	104.86	161.64	2235	39.74	105.90	160.60	2221	40.13	106.94	159.56	2207
267	38.87	103.79	163.21	2257	39.26	104.82	162.18	2243	39.65	105.86	161.14	2229	40.04	106.90	160.10	2214
267.5	38.78	103.75	163.76	2265	39.17	104.78	162.72	2250	39.56	105.82	161.68	2236	39.95	106.86	160.64	2222
268	38.70	103.70	164.30	2272	39.08	104.74	163.26	2258	39.47	105.78	162.22	2244	39.86	106.82	161.18	2229
268.5	38.61	103.66	164.84	2280	38.99	104.70	163.80	2265	39.38	105.74	162.76	2251	39.77	106.78	161.72	2237
269	38.52	103.62	165.38	2287	38.91	104.66	164.34	2273	39.29	105.70	163.30	2258	39.68	106.73	162.27	2244
269.5	38.43	103.58	165.92	2295	38.82	104.62	164.88	2280	39.20	105.66	163.84	2266	39.59	106.69	162.81	2252
270	38.35	103.54	166.46	2302	38.73	104.58	165.42	2288	39.12	105.62	164.39	2273	39.50	106.65	163.35	2259
270.5	38.26	103.50	167.00	2310	38.65	104.54	165.96	2295	39.03	105.57	164.93	2281	39.41	106.61	163.89	2267
271	38.18	103.46	167.54	2317	38.56	104.50	166.50	2303	38.94	105.53	165.47	2288	39.32	106.57	164.43	2274
271.5	38.09	103.42	168.08	2325	38.47	104.45	167.05	2310	38.86	105.49	166.01	2296	39.24	106.53	164.97	2282
272	38.01	103.38	168.62	2332	38.39	104.41	167.59	2318	38.77	105.45	166.55	2303	39.15	106.49	165.51	2289
272.5	37.92	103.34	169.17	2340	38.30	104.37	168.13	2325	38.68	105.41	167.09	2311	39.06	106.45	166.05	2297
273	37.84	103.29	169.71	2347	38.22	104.33	168.67	2333	38.60	105.37	167.63	2318	38.98	106.41	166.59	2304
273.5	37.75	103.25	170.25	2355	38.13	104.29	169.21	2340	38.51	105.33	168.17	2326	38.89	106.37	167.13	2311
274	37.67	103.21	170.79	2362	38.05	104.25	169.75	2348	38.43	105.29	168.71	2333	38.80	106.32	167.68	2319
274.5	37.59	103.17	171.33	2369	37.96	104.21	170.29	2355	38.34	105.25	169.25	2341	38.72	106.28	168.22	2326
275	37.50	103.13	171.87	2377	37.88	104.17	170.83	2363	38.26	105.21	169.80	2348	38.63	106.24	168.76	2334
275.5	37.42	103.09	172.41	2384	37.80	104.13	171.37	2370	38.17	105.16	170.34	2356	38.55	106.20	169.30	2341
276	37.34	103.05	172.95	2392	37.71	104.09	171.91	2378	38.09	105.12	170.88	2363	38.46	106.16	169.84	2349
276.5	37.25	103.01	173.49	2399	37.63	104.04	172.46	2385	38.00	105.08	171.42	2371	38.38	106.12	170.38	2356
277	37.17	102.97	174.03	2407	37.55	104.00	173.00	2393	37.92	105.04	171.96	2378	38.30	106.08	170.92	2364
277.5	37.09	102.93	174.58	2414	37.46	103.96	173.54	2400	37.84	105.00	172.50	2386	38.21	106.04	171.46	2371
278	37.01	102.88	175.12	2422	37.38	103.92	174.08	2408	37.76	104.96	173.04	2393	38.13	106.00	172.00	2379
278.5	36.93	102.84	175.66	2429	37.30	103.88	174.62	2415	37.67	104.92	173.58	2401	38.05	105.96	172.54	2386
279	36.85	102.80	176.20	2437	37.22	103.84	175.16	2422	37.59	104.88	174.12	2408	37.96	105.91	173.09	2394
279.5	36.77	102.76	176.74	2444	37.14	103.80	175.70	2430	37.51	104.84	174.66	2416	37.88	105.87	173.63	2401

Body Composition MALE 248-279.5 Lb.

Weight: Lb.	Waist: 55 inches				55.25 inches				55.5 inches				55.75 inches			
	Fat: %	Fat: Lb.	LBM: Lb.	RMR: Cal.	Fat: %	Fat: Lb.	LBM: Lb.	RMR: Cal.	Fat: %	Fat: Lb.	LBM: Lb.	RMR: Cal.	Fat: %	Fat: Lb.	LBM: Lb.	RMR: Cal.
248	44.15	109.49	138.51	1916	44.57	110.53	137.47	1901	44.99	111.57	136.43	1887	45.41	112.61	135.39	1872
248.5	44.05	109.45	139.05	1923	44.46	110.49	138.01	1909	44.88	111.53	136.97	1894	45.30	112.57	135.93	1880
249	43.94	109.41	139.59	1931	44.36	110.45	138.55	1916	44.77	111.49	137.51	1902	45.19	112.52	136.48	1887
249.5	43.84	109.37	140.13	1938	44.25	110.41	139.09	1924	44.67	111.45	138.05	1909	45.08	112.48	137.02	1895
250	43.73	109.33	140.67	1945	44.15	110.37	139.63	1931	44.56	111.41	138.60	1917	44.98	112.44	137.56	1902
250.5	43.63	109.29	141.21	1953	44.04	110.33	140.17	1939	44.46	111.36	139.14	1924	44.87	112.40	138.10	1910
251	43.53	109.25	141.75	1960	43.94	110.29	140.71	1946	44.35	111.32	139.68	1932	44.77	112.36	138.64	1917
251.5	43.42	109.21	142.29	1968	43.83	110.24	141.26	1954	44.25	111.28	140.22	1939	44.66	112.32	139.18	1925
252	43.32	109.17	142.83	1975	43.73	110.20	141.80	1961	44.14	111.24	140.76	1947	44.55	112.28	139.72	1932
252.5	43.22	109.13	143.38	1983	43.63	110.16	142.34	1969	44.04	111.20	141.30	1954	44.45	112.24	140.26	1940
253	43.12	109.08	143.92	1990	43.53	110.12	142.88	1976	43.94	111.16	141.84	1962	44.35	112.20	140.80	1947
253.5	43.01	109.04	144.46	1998	43.42	110.08	143.42	1983	43.83	111.12	142.38	1969	44.24	112.16	141.34	1955
254	42.91	109.00	145.00	2005	43.32	110.04	143.96	1991	43.73	111.08	142.92	1977	44.14	112.11	141.89	1962
254.5	42.81	108.96	145.54	2013	43.22	110.00	144.50	1998	43.63	111.04	143.46	1984	44.04	112.07	142.43	1970
255	42.71	108.92	146.08	2020	43.12	109.96	145.04	2006	43.53	111.00	144.01	1992	43.93	112.03	142.97	1977
255.5	42.61	108.88	146.62	2028	43.02	109.92	145.58	2013	43.43	110.95	144.55	1999	43.83	111.99	143.51	1985
256	42.51	108.84	147.16	2035	42.92	109.88	146.12	2021	43.33	110.91	145.09	2007	43.73	111.95	144.05	1992
256.5	42.42	108.80	147.70	2043	42.82	109.83	146.67	2028	43.23	110.87	145.63	2014	43.63	111.91	144.59	2000
257	42.32	108.76	148.24	2050	42.72	109.79	147.21	2036	43.12	110.83	146.17	2022	43.53	111.87	145.13	2007
257.5	42.22	108.72	148.79	2058	42.62	109.75	147.75	2043	43.03	110.79	146.71	2029	43.43	111.83	145.67	2015
258	42.12	108.67	149.33	2065	42.52	109.71	148.29	2051	42.93	110.75	147.25	2036	43.33	111.79	146.21	2022
258.5	42.02	108.63	149.87	2073	42.43	109.67	148.83	2058	42.83	110.71	147.79	2044	43.23	111.75	146.75	2030
259	41.93	108.59	150.41	2080	42.33	109.63	149.37	2066	42.73	110.67	148.33	2051	43.13	111.70	147.30	2037
259.5	41.83	108.55	150.95	2088	42.23	109.59	149.91	2073	42.63	110.63	148.87	2059	43.03	111.66	147.84	2045
260	41.73	108.51	151.49	2095	42.13	109.55	150.45	2081	42.53	110.59	149.42	2066	42.93	111.62	148.38	2052
260.5	41.64	108.47	152.03	2103	42.04	109.51	150.99	2088	42.44	110.54	149.96	2074	42.83	111.58	148.92	2060
261	41.54	108.43	152.57	2110	41.94	109.47	151.53	2096	42.34	110.50	150.50	2081	42.74	111.54	149.46	2067
261.5	41.45	108.39	153.11	2118	41.84	109.42	152.08	2103	42.24	110.46	151.04	2089	42.64	111.50	150.00	2075
262	41.35	108.35	153.65	2125	41.75	109.38	152.62	2111	42.15	110.42	151.58	2096	42.54	111.46	150.54	2082
262.5	41.26	108.31	154.20	2133	41.65	109.34	153.16	2118	42.05	110.38	152.12	2104	42.44	111.42	151.08	2089
263	41.17	108.26	154.74	2140	41.56	109.30	153.70	2126	41.95	110.34	152.66	2111	42.35	111.38	151.62	2097
263.5	41.07	108.22	155.28	2147	41.47	109.26	154.24	2133	41.86	110.30	153.20	2119	42.25	111.34	152.16	2104
264	40.98	108.18	155.82	2155	41.37	109.22	154.78	2141	41.76	110.26	153.74	2126	42.16	111.29	152.71	2112
264.5	40.89	108.14	156.36	2162	41.28	109.18	155.32	2148	41.67	110.22	154.28	2134	42.06	111.25	153.25	2119
265	40.79	108.10	156.90	2170	41.18	109.14	155.86	2156	41.58	110.18	154.83	2141	41.97	111.21	153.79	2127
265.5	40.70	108.06	157.44	2177	41.09	109.10	156.40	2163	41.48	110.13	155.37	2149	41.87	111.17	154.33	2134
266	40.61	108.02	157.98	2185	41.00	109.06	156.94	2171	41.39	110.09	155.91	2156	41.78	111.13	154.87	2142
266.5	40.52	107.98	158.52	2192	40.91	109.01	157.49	2178	41.30	110.05	156.45	2164	41.68	111.09	155.41	2149
267	40.43	107.94	159.06	2200	40.81	108.97	158.03	2186	41.20	110.01	156.99	2171	41.59	111.05	155.95	2157
267.5	40.33	107.90	159.61	2207	40.72	108.93	158.57	2193	41.11	109.97	157.53	2179	41.50	111.01	156.49	2164
268	40.24	107.85	160.15	2215	40.63	108.89	159.11	2200	41.02	109.93	158.07	2186	41.41	110.97	157.03	2172
268.5	40.15	107.81	160.69	2222	40.54	108.85	159.65	2208	40.93	109.89	158.61	2194	41.31	110.93	157.57	2179
269	40.06	107.77	161.23	2230	40.45	108.81	160.19	2215	40.84	109.85	159.15	2201	41.22	110.88	158.12	2187
269.5	39.97	107.73	161.77	2237	40.36	108.77	160.73	2223	40.74	109.81	159.69	2209	41.13	110.84	158.66	2194
270	39.89	107.69	162.31	2245	40.27	108.73	161.27	2230	40.65	109.77	160.24	2216	41.04	110.80	159.20	2202
270.5	39.80	107.65	162.85	2252	40.18	108.69	161.81	2238	40.56	109.72	160.78	2224	40.95	110.76	159.74	2209
271	39.71	107.61	163.39	2260	40.09	108.65	162.35	2245	40.47	109.68	161.32	2231	40.86	110.72	160.28	2217
271.5	39.62	107.57	163.93	2267	40.00	108.60	162.90	2253	40.38	109.64	161.86	2238	40.77	110.68	160.82	2224
272	39.53	107.53	164.47	2275	39.91	108.56	163.44	2260	40.29	109.60	162.40	2246	40.68	110.64	161.36	2232
272.5	39.44	107.49	165.02	2282	39.82	108.52	163.98	2268	40.21	109.56	162.94	2253	40.59	110.60	161.90	2239
273	39.36	107.44	165.56	2290	39.74	108.48	164.52	2275	40.12	109.52	163.48	2261	40.50	110.56	162.44	2247
273.5	39.27	107.40	166.10	2297	39.65	108.44	165.06	2283	40.03	109.48	164.02	2268	40.41	110.52	162.98	2254
274	39.18	107.36	166.64	2305	39.56	108.40	165.60	2290	39.94	109.44	164.56	2276	40.32	110.47	163.53	2262
274.5	39.10	107.32	167.18	2312	39.47	108.36	166.14	2298	39.85	109.40	165.10	2283	40.23	110.43	164.07	2269
275	39.01	107.28	167.72	2320	39.39	108.32	166.68	2305	39.77	109.36	165.65	2291	40.14	110.39	164.61	2277
275.5	38.93	107.24	168.26	2327	39.30	108.28	167.22	2313	39.68	109.31	166.19	2298	40.05	110.35	165.15	2284
276	38.84	107.20	168.80	2335	39.22	108.24	167.76	2320	39.59	109.27	166.73	2306	39.97	110.31	165.69	2291
276.5	38.75	107.16	169.34	2342	39.13	108.19	168.31	2328	39.51	109.23	167.27	2313	39.88	110.27	166.23	2299
277	38.67	107.12	169.88	2349	39.04	108.15	168.85	2335	39.42	109.19	167.81	2321	39.79	110.23	166.77	2306
277.5	38.59	107.08	170.43	2357	38.96	108.11	169.39	2343	39.33	109.15	168.35	2328	39.71	110.19	167.31	2314
278	38.50	107.03	170.97	2364	38.87	108.07	169.93	2350	39.25	109.11	168.89	2336	39.62	110.15	167.85	2321
278.5	38.42	106.99	171.51	2372	38.79	108.03	170.47	2358	39.16	109.07	169.43	2343	39.54	110.11	168.39	2329
279	38.33	106.95	172.05	2379	38.71	107.99	171.01	2365	39.08	109.03	169.97	2351	39.45	110.06	168.94	2336
279.5	38.25	106.91	172.59	2387	38.62	107.95	171.55	2373	38.99	108.99	170.51	2358	39.36	110.02	169.48	2344

Body Composition　MALE　248-279.5 Lb.

Weight: Lb.	Waist: 56 inches Fat: %	Fat: Lb.	LBM: Lb.	RMR: Cal.	56.25 inches Fat: %	Fat: Lb.	LBM: Lb.	RMR: Cal.	56.5 inches Fat: %	Fat: Lb.	LBM: Lb.	RMR: Cal.	56.75 inches Fat: %	Fat: Lb.	LBM: Lb.	RMR: Cal.
248	45.82	113.64	134.36	1858	46.24	114.68	133.32	1844	46.66	115.72	132.28	1829	47.08	116.76	131.24	1815
248.5	45.72	113.60	134.90	1866	46.13	114.64	133.86	1851	46.55	115.68	132.82	1837	46.97	116.72	131.78	1823
249	45.61	113.56	135.44	1873	46.02	114.60	134.40	1859	46.44	115.64	133.36	1844	46.86	116.67	132.33	1830
249.5	45.50	113.52	135.98	1881	45.92	114.56	134.94	1866	46.33	115.60	133.90	1852	46.75	116.63	132.87	1838
250	45.39	113.48	136.52	1888	45.81	114.52	135.48	1874	46.22	115.56	134.45	1859	46.64	116.59	133.41	1845
250.5	45.29	113.44	137.06	1896	45.70	114.48	136.02	1881	46.11	115.51	134.99	1867	46.53	116.55	133.95	1853
251	45.18	113.40	137.60	1903	45.59	114.44	136.56	1889	46.01	115.47	135.53	1874	46.42	116.51	134.49	1860
251.5	45.07	113.36	138.14	1911	45.48	114.39	137.11	1896	45.90	115.43	136.07	1882	46.31	116.47	135.03	1867
252	44.97	113.32	138.68	1918	45.38	114.35	137.65	1904	45.79	115.39	136.61	1889	46.20	116.43	135.57	1875
252.5	44.86	113.28	139.23	1925	45.27	114.31	138.19	1911	45.68	115.35	137.15	1897	46.09	116.39	136.11	1882
253	44.76	113.23	139.77	1933	45.17	114.27	138.73	1919	45.58	115.31	137.69	1904	45.99	116.35	136.65	1890
253.5	44.65	113.19	140.31	1940	45.06	114.23	139.27	1926	45.47	115.27	138.23	1912	45.88	116.31	137.19	1897
254	44.55	113.15	140.85	1948	44.96	114.19	139.81	1934	45.36	115.23	138.77	1919	45.77	116.26	137.74	1905
254.5	44.44	113.11	141.39	1955	44.85	114.15	140.35	1941	45.26	115.19	139.31	1927	45.67	116.22	138.28	1912
255	44.34	113.07	141.93	1963	44.75	114.11	140.89	1949	45.15	115.15	139.86	1934	45.56	116.18	138.82	1920
255.5	44.24	113.03	142.47	1970	44.64	114.07	141.43	1956	45.05	115.10	140.40	1942	45.46	116.14	139.36	1927
256	44.14	112.99	143.01	1978	44.54	114.03	141.97	1964	44.95	115.06	140.94	1949	45.35	116.10	139.90	1935
256.5	44.03	112.95	143.55	1985	44.44	113.98	142.52	1971	44.84	115.02	141.48	1957	45.25	116.06	140.44	1942
257	43.93	112.91	144.09	1993	44.34	113.94	143.06	1978	44.74	114.98	142.02	1964	45.14	116.02	140.98	1950
257.5	43.83	112.87	144.64	2000	44.23	113.90	143.60	1986	44.64	114.94	142.56	1972	45.04	115.98	141.52	1957
258	43.73	112.82	145.18	2008	44.13	113.86	144.14	1993	44.53	114.90	143.10	1979	44.94	115.94	142.06	1965
258.5	43.63	112.78	145.72	2015	44.03	113.82	144.68	2001	44.43	114.86	143.64	1987	44.83	115.90	142.60	1972
259	43.53	112.74	146.26	2023	43.93	113.78	145.22	2008	44.33	114.82	144.18	1994	44.73	115.85	143.15	1980
259.5	43.43	112.70	146.80	2030	43.83	113.74	145.76	2016	44.23	114.78	144.72	2002	44.63	115.81	143.69	1987
260	43.33	112.66	147.34	2038	43.73	113.70	146.30	2023	44.13	114.74	145.27	2009	44.53	115.77	144.23	1995
260.5	43.23	112.62	147.88	2045	43.63	113.66	146.84	2031	44.03	114.69	145.81	2016	44.43	115.73	144.77	2002
261	43.13	112.58	148.42	2053	43.53	113.62	147.38	2038	43.93	114.65	146.35	2024	44.33	115.69	145.31	2010
261.5	43.04	112.54	148.96	2060	43.43	113.57	147.93	2046	43.83	114.61	146.89	2031	44.23	115.65	145.85	2017
262	42.94	112.50	149.50	2068	43.33	113.53	148.47	2053	43.73	114.57	147.43	2039	44.13	115.61	146.39	2025
262.5	42.84	112.46	150.05	2075	43.24	113.49	149.01	2061	43.63	114.53	147.97	2046	44.03	115.57	146.93	2032
263	42.74	112.41	150.59	2083	43.14	113.45	149.55	2068	43.53	114.49	148.51	2054	43.93	115.53	147.47	2040
263.5	42.65	112.37	151.13	2090	43.04	113.41	150.09	2076	43.43	114.45	149.05	2061	43.83	115.49	148.01	2047
264	42.55	112.33	151.67	2098	42.94	113.37	150.63	2083	43.34	114.41	149.59	2069	43.73	115.44	148.56	2055
264.5	42.45	112.29	152.21	2105	42.85	113.33	151.17	2091	43.24	114.37	150.13	2076	43.63	115.40	149.10	2062
265	42.36	112.25	152.75	2113	42.75	113.29	151.71	2098	43.14	114.33	150.68	2084	43.53	115.36	149.64	2069
265.5	42.26	112.21	153.29	2120	42.65	113.25	152.25	2106	43.04	114.28	151.22	2091	43.44	115.32	150.18	2077
266	42.17	112.17	153.83	2127	42.56	113.21	152.79	2113	42.95	114.24	151.76	2099	43.34	115.28	150.72	2084
266.5	42.07	112.13	154.37	2135	42.46	113.16	153.34	2121	42.85	114.20	152.30	2106	43.24	115.24	151.26	2092
267	41.98	112.09	154.91	2142	42.37	113.12	153.88	2128	42.76	114.16	152.84	2114	43.15	115.20	151.80	2099
267.5	41.89	112.05	155.46	2150	42.27	113.08	154.42	2136	42.66	114.12	153.38	2121	43.05	115.16	152.34	2107
268	41.79	112.00	156.00	2157	42.18	113.04	154.96	2143	42.57	114.08	153.92	2129	42.95	115.12	152.88	2114
268.5	41.70	111.96	156.54	2165	42.09	113.00	155.50	2151	42.47	114.04	154.46	2136	42.86	115.08	153.42	2122
269	41.61	111.92	157.08	2172	41.99	112.96	156.04	2158	42.38	114.00	155.00	2144	42.76	115.03	153.97	2129
269.5	41.51	111.88	157.62	2180	41.90	112.92	156.58	2166	42.28	113.96	155.54	2151	42.67	114.99	154.51	2137
270	41.42	111.84	158.16	2187	41.81	112.88	157.12	2173	42.19	113.92	156.09	2159	42.58	114.95	155.05	2144
270.5	41.33	111.80	158.70	2195	41.71	112.84	157.66	2180	42.10	113.87	156.63	2166	42.48	114.91	155.59	2152
271	41.24	111.76	159.24	2202	41.62	112.80	158.20	2188	42.00	113.83	157.17	2174	42.39	114.87	156.13	2159
271.5	41.15	111.72	159.78	2210	41.53	112.75	158.75	2195	41.91	113.79	157.71	2181	42.29	114.83	156.67	2167
272	41.06	111.68	160.32	2217	41.44	112.71	159.29	2203	41.82	113.75	158.25	2189	42.20	114.79	157.21	2174
272.5	40.97	111.64	160.87	2225	41.35	112.67	159.83	2210	41.73	113.71	158.79	2196	42.11	114.75	157.75	2182
273	40.88	111.59	161.41	2232	41.26	112.63	160.37	2218	41.64	113.67	159.33	2204	42.02	114.71	158.29	2189
273.5	40.79	111.55	161.95	2240	41.17	112.59	160.91	2225	41.55	113.63	159.87	2211	41.93	114.67	158.83	2197
274	40.70	111.51	162.49	2247	41.08	112.55	161.45	2233	41.46	113.59	160.41	2219	41.83	114.62	159.38	2204
274.5	40.61	111.47	163.03	2255	40.99	112.51	161.99	2240	41.36	113.55	160.95	2226	41.74	114.58	159.92	2212
275	40.52	111.43	163.57	2262	40.90	112.47	162.53	2248	41.27	113.51	161.50	2233	41.65	114.54	160.46	2219
275.5	40.43	111.39	164.11	2270	40.81	112.43	163.07	2255	41.18	113.46	162.04	2241	41.56	114.50	161.00	2227
276	40.34	111.35	164.65	2277	40.72	112.39	163.61	2263	41.10	113.42	162.58	2248	41.47	114.46	161.54	2234
276.5	40.26	111.31	165.19	2285	40.63	112.34	164.16	2270	41.01	113.38	163.12	2256	41.38	114.42	162.08	2242
277	40.17	111.27	165.73	2292	40.54	112.30	164.70	2278	40.92	113.34	163.66	2263	41.29	114.38	162.62	2249
277.5	40.08	111.23	166.28	2300	40.45	112.26	165.24	2285	40.83	113.30	164.20	2271	41.20	114.34	163.16	2257
278	39.99	111.18	166.82	2307	40.37	112.22	165.78	2293	40.74	113.26	164.74	2278	41.11	114.30	163.70	2264
278.5	39.91	111.14	167.36	2315	40.28	112.18	166.32	2300	40.65	113.22	165.28	2286	41.03	114.26	164.24	2272
279	39.82	111.10	167.90	2322	40.19	112.14	166.86	2308	40.57	113.18	165.82	2293	40.94	114.21	164.79	2279
279.5	39.74	111.06	168.44	2330	40.11	112.10	167.40	2315	40.48	113.14	166.36	2301	40.85	114.17	165.33	2286

Body Composition   MALE   248-279.5 Lb.

Weight: Lb.	Waist: 57 inches				57.25 inches				57.5 inches				57.75 inches			
	Fat: %	Fat: Lb.	LBM: Lb.	RMR: Cal.	Fat: %	Fat: Lb.	LBM: Lb.	RMR: Cal.	Fat: %	Fat: Lb.	LBM: Lb.	RMR: Cal.	Fat: %	Fat: Lb.	LBM: Lb.	RMR: Cal.
248	47.50	117.79	130.21	1801	47.92	118.83	129.17	1786	48.33	119.87	128.13	1772	48.75	120.91	127.09	1758
248.5	47.39	117.75	130.75	1808	47.80	118.79	129.71	1794	48.22	119.83	128.67	1780	48.64	120.87	127.63	1765
249	47.27	117.71	131.29	1816	47.69	118.75	130.25	1801	48.11	119.79	129.21	1787	48.52	120.82	128.18	1773
249.5	47.16	117.67	131.83	1823	47.58	118.71	130.79	1809	47.99	119.75	129.75	1794	48.41	120.78	128.72	1780
250	47.05	117.63	132.37	1831	47.47	118.67	131.33	1816	47.88	119.71	130.30	1802	48.30	120.74	129.26	1788
250.5	46.94	117.59	132.91	1838	47.36	118.63	131.87	1824	47.77	119.66	130.84	1809	48.18	120.70	129.80	1795
251	46.83	117.55	133.45	1846	47.25	118.59	132.41	1831	47.66	119.62	131.38	1817	48.07	120.66	130.34	1803
251.5	46.72	117.51	133.99	1853	47.13	118.54	132.96	1839	47.55	119.58	131.92	1824	47.96	120.62	130.88	1810
252	46.61	117.47	134.53	1861	47.03	118.50	133.50	1846	47.44	119.54	132.46	1832	47.85	120.58	131.42	1818
252.5	46.50	117.43	135.08	1868	46.92	118.46	134.04	1854	47.33	119.50	133.00	1839	47.74	120.54	131.96	1825
253	46.40	117.38	135.62	1876	46.81	118.42	134.58	1861	47.22	119.46	133.54	1847	47.63	120.50	132.50	1833
253.5	46.29	117.34	136.16	1883	46.70	118.38	135.12	1869	47.11	119.42	134.08	1854	47.52	120.46	133.04	1840
254	46.18	117.30	136.70	1891	46.59	118.34	135.66	1876	47.00	119.38	134.62	1862	47.41	120.41	133.59	1847
254.5	46.08	117.26	137.24	1898	46.48	118.30	136.20	1884	46.89	119.34	135.16	1869	47.30	120.37	134.13	1855
255	45.97	117.22	137.78	1905	46.38	118.26	136.74	1891	46.78	119.30	135.71	1877	47.19	120.33	134.67	1862
255.5	45.86	117.18	138.32	1913	46.27	118.22	137.28	1899	46.67	119.25	136.25	1884	47.08	120.29	135.21	1870
256	45.76	117.14	138.86	1920	46.16	118.18	137.82	1906	46.57	119.21	136.79	1892	46.97	120.25	135.75	1877
256.5	45.65	117.10	139.40	1928	46.06	118.13	138.37	1914	46.46	119.17	137.33	1899	46.87	120.21	136.29	1885
257	45.55	117.06	139.94	1935	45.95	118.09	138.91	1921	46.35	119.13	137.87	1907	46.76	120.17	136.83	1892
257.5	45.44	117.02	140.49	1943	45.85	118.05	139.45	1929	46.25	119.09	138.41	1914	46.65	120.13	137.37	1900
258	45.34	116.97	141.03	1950	45.74	118.01	139.99	1936	46.14	119.05	138.95	1922	46.55	120.09	137.91	1907
258.5	45.24	116.93	141.57	1958	45.64	117.97	140.53	1944	46.04	119.01	139.49	1929	46.44	120.05	138.45	1915
259	45.13	116.89	142.11	1965	45.53	117.93	141.07	1951	45.93	118.97	140.03	1937	46.33	120.00	139.00	1922
259.5	45.03	116.85	142.65	1973	45.43	117.89	141.61	1958	45.83	118.93	140.57	1944	46.23	119.96	139.54	1930
260	44.93	116.81	143.19	1980	45.33	117.85	142.15	1966	45.73	118.89	141.12	1952	46.12	119.92	140.08	1937
260.5	44.82	116.77	143.73	1988	45.22	117.81	142.69	1973	45.62	118.84	141.66	1959	46.02	119.88	140.62	1945
261	44.72	116.73	144.27	1995	45.12	117.77	143.23	1981	45.52	118.80	142.20	1967	45.92	119.84	141.16	1952
261.5	44.62	116.69	144.81	2003	45.02	117.72	143.78	1988	45.42	118.76	142.74	1974	45.81	119.80	141.70	1960
262	44.52	116.65	145.35	2010	44.92	117.68	144.32	1996	45.31	118.72	143.28	1982	45.71	119.76	142.24	1967
262.5	44.42	116.61	145.90	2018	44.82	117.64	144.86	2003	45.21	118.68	143.82	1989	45.61	119.72	142.78	1975
263	44.32	116.56	146.44	2025	44.72	117.60	145.40	2011	45.11	118.64	144.36	1997	45.50	119.68	143.32	1982
263.5	44.22	116.52	146.98	2033	44.61	117.56	145.94	2018	45.01	118.60	144.90	2004	45.40	119.64	143.86	1990
264	44.12	116.48	147.52	2040	44.51	117.52	146.48	2026	44.91	118.56	145.44	2011	45.30	119.59	144.41	1997
264.5	44.02	116.44	148.06	2048	44.42	117.48	147.02	2033	44.81	118.52	145.98	2019	45.20	119.55	144.95	2005
265	43.92	116.40	148.60	2055	44.32	117.44	147.56	2041	44.71	118.48	146.53	2026	45.10	119.51	145.49	2012
265.5	43.83	116.36	149.14	2063	44.22	117.40	148.10	2048	44.61	118.43	147.07	2034	45.00	119.47	146.03	2020
266	43.73	116.32	149.68	2070	44.12	117.36	148.64	2056	44.51	118.39	147.61	2041	44.90	119.43	146.57	2027
266.5	43.63	116.28	150.22	2078	44.02	117.31	149.19	2063	44.41	118.35	148.15	2049	44.80	119.39	147.11	2035
267	43.53	116.24	150.76	2085	43.92	117.27	149.73	2071	44.31	118.31	148.69	2056	44.70	119.35	147.65	2042
267.5	43.44	116.20	151.31	2093	43.83	117.23	150.27	2078	44.21	118.27	149.23	2064	44.60	119.31	148.19	2050
268	43.34	116.15	151.85	2100	43.73	117.19	150.81	2086	44.12	118.23	149.77	2071	44.50	119.27	148.73	2057
268.5	43.25	116.11	152.39	2108	43.63	117.15	151.35	2093	44.02	118.19	150.31	2079	44.40	119.23	149.27	2064
269	43.15	116.07	152.93	2115	43.54	117.11	151.89	2101	43.92	118.15	150.85	2086	44.31	119.18	149.82	2072
269.5	43.05	116.03	153.47	2122	43.44	117.07	152.43	2108	43.82	118.11	151.39	2094	44.21	119.14	150.36	2079
270	42.96	115.99	154.01	2130	43.34	117.03	152.97	2116	43.73	118.07	151.94	2101	44.11	119.10	150.90	2087
270.5	42.86	115.95	154.55	2137	43.25	116.99	153.51	2123	43.63	118.02	152.48	2109	44.02	119.06	151.44	2094
271	42.77	115.91	155.09	2145	43.15	116.95	154.05	2131	43.54	117.98	153.02	2116	43.92	119.02	151.98	2102
271.5	42.68	115.87	155.63	2152	43.06	116.90	154.60	2138	43.44	117.94	153.56	2124	43.82	118.98	152.52	2109
272	42.58	115.83	156.17	2160	42.96	116.86	155.14	2146	43.35	117.90	154.10	2131	43.73	118.94	153.06	2117
272.5	42.49	115.79	156.72	2167	42.87	116.82	155.68	2153	43.25	117.86	154.64	2139	43.63	118.90	153.60	2124
273	42.40	115.74	157.26	2175	42.78	116.78	156.22	2161	43.16	117.82	155.18	2146	43.54	118.86	154.14	2132
273.5	42.30	115.70	157.80	2182	42.68	116.74	156.76	2168	43.06	117.78	155.72	2154	43.44	118.82	154.68	2139
274	42.21	115.66	158.34	2190	42.59	116.70	157.30	2175	42.97	117.74	156.26	2161	43.35	118.77	155.23	2147
274.5	42.12	115.62	158.88	2197	42.50	116.66	157.84	2183	42.88	117.70	156.80	2169	43.25	118.73	155.77	2154
275	42.03	115.58	159.42	2205	42.41	116.62	158.38	2190	42.78	117.66	157.35	2176	43.16	118.69	156.31	2162
275.5	41.94	115.54	159.96	2212	42.31	116.58	158.92	2198	42.69	117.61	157.89	2184	43.07	118.65	156.85	2169
276	41.85	115.50	160.50	2220	42.22	116.54	159.46	2205	42.60	117.57	158.43	2191	42.97	118.61	157.39	2177
276.5	41.76	115.46	161.04	2227	42.13	116.49	160.01	2213	42.51	117.53	158.97	2199	42.88	118.57	157.93	2184
277	41.67	115.42	161.58	2235	42.04	116.45	160.55	2220	42.42	117.49	159.51	2206	42.79	118.53	158.47	2192
277.5	41.58	115.38	162.13	2242	41.95	116.41	161.09	2228	42.32	117.45	160.05	2213	42.70	118.49	159.01	2199
278	41.49	115.33	162.67	2250	41.86	116.37	161.63	2235	42.23	117.41	160.59	2221	42.61	118.45	159.55	2207
278.5	41.40	115.29	163.21	2257	41.77	116.33	162.17	2243	42.14	117.37	161.13	2228	42.52	118.41	160.09	2214
279	41.31	115.25	163.75	2265	41.68	116.29	162.71	2250	42.05	117.33	161.67	2236	42.42	118.36	160.64	2222
279.5	41.22	115.21	164.29	2272	41.59	116.25	163.25	2258	41.96	117.29	162.21	2243	42.33	118.32	161.18	2229

Body Composition   MALE   248-279.5 Lb.

Weight: Lb.	Waist: 58 inches Fat: %	Fat: Lb.	LBM: Lb.	RMR: Cal.	58.25 inches Fat: %	Fat: Lb.	LBM: Lb.	RMR: Cal.	58.5 inches Fat: %	Fat: Lb.	LBM: Lb.	RMR: Cal.	58.75 inches Fat: %	Fat: Lb.	LBM: Lb.	RMR: Cal.
248	49.17	121.94	126.06	1743	49.59	122.98	125.02	1729	50.01	124.02	123.98	1715	50.43	125.06	122.94	1700
248.5	49.06	121.90	126.60	1751	49.47	122.94	125.56	1736	49.89	123.98	124.52	1722	50.31	125.02	123.48	1708
249	48.94	121.86	127.14	1758	49.36	122.90	126.10	1744	49.77	123.94	125.06	1730	50.19	124.97	124.03	1715
249.5	48.83	121.82	127.68	1766	49.24	122.86	126.64	1751	49.66	123.90	125.60	1737	50.07	124.93	124.57	1723
250	48.71	121.78	128.22	1773	49.13	122.82	127.18	1759	49.54	123.86	126.15	1745	49.96	124.89	125.11	1730
250.5	48.60	121.74	128.76	1781	49.01	122.78	127.72	1766	49.43	123.81	126.69	1752	49.84	124.85	125.65	1738
251	48.49	121.70	129.30	1788	48.90	122.74	128.26	1774	49.31	123.77	127.23	1760	49.73	124.81	126.19	1745
251.5	48.37	121.66	129.84	1796	48.79	122.69	128.81	1781	49.20	123.73	127.77	1767	49.61	124.77	126.73	1753
252	48.26	121.62	130.38	1803	48.67	122.65	129.35	1789	49.08	123.69	128.31	1775	49.50	124.73	127.27	1760
252.5	48.15	121.58	130.93	1811	48.56	122.61	129.89	1796	48.97	123.65	128.85	1782	49.38	124.69	127.81	1768
253	48.04	121.53	131.47	1818	48.45	122.57	130.43	1804	48.86	123.61	129.39	1789	49.27	124.65	128.35	1775
253.5	47.93	121.49	132.01	1826	48.34	122.53	130.97	1811	48.74	123.57	129.93	1797	49.15	124.61	128.89	1783
254	47.82	121.45	132.55	1833	48.22	122.49	131.51	1819	48.63	123.53	130.47	1804	49.04	124.56	129.44	1790
254.5	47.71	121.41	133.09	1841	48.11	122.45	132.05	1826	48.52	123.49	131.01	1812	48.93	124.52	129.98	1798
255	47.60	121.37	133.63	1848	48.00	122.41	132.59	1834	48.41	123.45	131.56	1819	48.82	124.48	130.52	1805
255.5	47.49	121.33	134.17	1856	47.89	122.37	133.13	1841	48.30	123.40	132.10	1827	48.71	124.44	131.06	1813
256	47.38	121.29	134.71	1863	47.78	122.33	133.67	1849	48.19	123.36	132.64	1834	48.59	124.40	131.60	1820
256.5	47.27	121.25	135.25	1871	47.67	122.28	134.22	1856	48.08	123.32	133.18	1842	48.48	124.36	132.14	1828
257	47.16	121.21	135.79	1878	47.57	122.24	134.76	1864	47.97	123.28	133.72	1849	48.37	124.32	132.68	1835
257.5	47.05	121.17	136.34	1886	47.46	122.20	135.30	1871	47.86	123.24	134.26	1857	48.26	124.28	133.22	1842
258	46.95	121.12	136.88	1893	47.35	122.16	135.84	1879	47.75	123.20	134.80	1864	48.15	124.24	133.76	1850
258.5	46.84	121.08	137.42	1900	47.24	122.12	136.38	1886	47.64	123.16	135.34	1872	48.04	124.20	134.30	1857
259	46.73	121.04	137.96	1908	47.13	122.08	136.92	1894	47.54	123.12	135.88	1879	47.94	124.15	134.85	1865
259.5	46.63	121.00	138.50	1915	47.03	122.04	137.46	1901	47.43	123.08	136.42	1887	47.83	124.11	135.39	1872
260	46.52	120.96	139.04	1923	46.92	122.00	138.00	1909	47.32	123.04	136.97	1894	47.72	124.07	135.93	1880
260.5	46.42	120.92	139.58	1930	46.82	121.96	138.54	1916	47.21	122.99	137.51	1902	47.61	124.03	136.47	1887
261	46.31	120.88	140.12	1938	46.71	121.92	139.08	1924	47.11	122.95	138.05	1909	47.51	123.99	137.01	1895
261.5	46.21	120.84	140.66	1945	46.61	121.87	139.63	1931	47.00	122.91	138.59	1917	47.40	123.95	137.55	1902
262	46.11	120.80	141.20	1953	46.50	121.83	140.17	1939	46.90	122.87	139.13	1924	47.29	123.91	138.09	1910
262.5	46.00	120.76	141.75	1960	46.40	121.79	140.71	1946	46.79	122.83	139.67	1932	47.19	123.87	138.63	1917
263	45.90	120.71	142.29	1968	46.29	121.75	141.25	1953	46.69	122.79	140.21	1939	47.08	123.83	139.17	1925
263.5	45.80	120.67	142.83	1975	46.19	121.71	141.79	1961	46.58	122.75	140.75	1947	46.98	123.79	139.71	1932
264	45.69	120.63	143.37	1983	46.09	121.67	142.33	1968	46.48	122.71	141.29	1954	46.87	123.74	140.26	1940
264.5	45.59	120.59	143.91	1990	45.98	121.63	142.87	1976	46.38	122.67	141.83	1962	46.77	123.70	140.80	1947
265	45.49	120.55	144.45	1998	45.88	121.59	143.41	1983	46.27	122.63	142.38	1969	46.67	123.66	141.34	1955
265.5	45.39	120.51	144.99	2005	45.78	121.55	143.95	1991	46.17	122.58	142.92	1977	46.56	123.62	141.88	1962
266	45.29	120.47	145.53	2013	45.68	121.51	144.49	1998	46.07	122.54	143.46	1984	46.46	123.58	142.42	1970
266.5	45.19	120.43	146.07	2020	45.58	121.46	145.04	2006	45.97	122.50	144.00	1991	46.36	123.54	142.96	1977
267	45.09	120.39	146.61	2028	45.48	121.42	145.58	2013	45.87	122.46	144.54	1999	46.25	123.50	143.50	1985
267.5	44.99	120.35	147.16	2035	45.38	121.38	146.12	2021	45.76	122.42	145.08	2006	46.15	123.46	144.04	1992
268	44.89	120.30	147.70	2043	45.28	121.34	146.66	2028	45.66	122.38	145.62	2014	46.05	123.42	144.58	2000
268.5	44.79	120.26	148.24	2050	45.18	121.30	147.20	2036	45.56	122.34	146.16	2021	45.95	123.38	145.12	2007
269	44.69	120.22	148.78	2058	45.08	121.26	147.74	2043	45.46	122.30	146.70	2029	45.85	123.33	145.67	2015
269.5	44.59	120.18	149.32	2065	44.98	121.22	148.28	2051	45.36	122.26	147.24	2036	45.75	123.29	146.21	2022
270	44.50	120.14	149.86	2073	44.88	121.18	148.82	2058	45.26	122.22	147.79	2044	45.65	123.25	146.75	2030
270.5	44.40	120.10	150.40	2080	44.78	121.14	149.36	2066	45.17	122.17	148.33	2051	45.55	123.21	147.29	2037
271	44.30	120.06	150.94	2088	44.68	121.10	149.90	2073	45.07	122.13	148.87	2059	45.45	123.17	147.83	2044
271.5	44.21	120.02	151.48	2095	44.59	121.05	150.45	2081	44.97	122.09	149.41	2066	45.35	123.13	148.37	2052
272	44.11	119.98	152.02	2102	44.49	121.01	150.99	2088	44.87	122.05	149.95	2074	45.25	123.09	148.91	2059
272.5	44.01	119.94	152.57	2110	44.39	120.97	151.53	2096	44.77	122.01	150.49	2081	45.16	123.05	149.45	2067
273	43.92	119.89	153.11	2117	44.30	120.93	152.07	2103	44.68	121.97	151.03	2089	45.06	123.01	149.99	2074
273.5	43.82	119.85	153.65	2125	44.20	120.89	152.61	2111	44.58	121.93	151.57	2096	44.96	122.97	150.53	2082
274	43.73	119.81	154.19	2132	44.11	120.85	153.15	2118	44.48	121.89	152.11	2104	44.86	122.92	151.08	2089
274.5	43.63	119.77	154.73	2140	44.01	120.81	153.69	2126	44.39	121.85	152.65	2111	44.77	122.88	151.62	2097
275	43.54	119.73	155.27	2147	43.92	120.77	154.23	2133	44.29	121.81	153.20	2119	44.67	122.84	152.16	2104
275.5	43.44	119.69	155.81	2155	43.82	120.73	154.77	2141	44.20	121.76	153.74	2126	44.57	122.80	152.70	2112
276	43.35	119.65	156.35	2162	43.73	120.69	155.31	2148	44.10	121.72	154.28	2134	44.48	122.76	153.24	2119
276.5	43.26	119.61	156.89	2170	43.63	120.64	155.86	2155	44.01	121.68	154.82	2141	44.38	122.72	153.78	2127
277	43.16	119.57	157.43	2177	43.54	120.60	156.40	2163	43.91	121.64	155.36	2149	44.29	122.68	154.32	2134
277.5	43.07	119.53	157.98	2185	43.45	120.56	156.94	2170	43.82	121.60	155.90	2156	44.19	122.64	154.86	2142
278	42.98	119.48	158.52	2192	43.35	120.52	157.48	2178	43.73	121.56	156.44	2164	44.10	122.60	155.40	2149
278.5	42.89	119.44	159.06	2200	43.26	120.48	158.02	2185	43.63	121.52	156.98	2171	44.01	122.56	155.94	2157
279	42.80	119.40	159.60	2207	43.17	120.44	158.56	2193	43.54	121.48	157.52	2179	43.91	122.51	156.49	2164
279.5	42.71	119.36	160.14	2215	43.08	120.40	159.10	2200	43.45	121.44	158.06	2186	43.82	122.47	157.03	2172

Body Composition   MALE   248-279.5 Lb.

Weight: Lb.	Waist: 59 inches Fat: %	Fat: Lb.	LBM: Lb.	RMR: Cal.	59.25 inches Fat: %	Fat: Lb.	LBM: Lb.	RMR: Cal.	59.5 inches Fat: %	Fat: Lb.	LBM: Lb.	RMR: Cal.	59.75 inches Fat: %	Fat: Lb.	LBM: Lb.	RMR: Cal.
248	50.84	126.09	121.91	1686	51.26	127.13	120.87	1672	51.68	128.17	119.83	1657	52.10	129.21	118.79	1643
248.5	50.73	126.05	122.45	1693	51.14	127.09	121.41	1679	51.56	128.13	120.37	1665	51.98	129.17	119.33	1650
249	50.61	126.01	122.99	1701	51.02	127.05	121.95	1687	51.44	128.09	120.91	1672	51.86	129.12	119.88	1658
249.5	50.49	125.97	123.53	1708	50.91	127.01	122.49	1694	51.32	128.05	121.45	1680	51.74	129.08	120.42	1665
250	50.37	125.93	124.07	1716	50.79	126.97	123.03	1702	51.20	128.01	122.00	1687	51.62	129.04	120.96	1673
250.5	50.26	125.89	124.61	1723	50.67	126.93	123.57	1709	51.08	127.96	122.54	1695	51.50	129.00	121.50	1680
251	50.14	125.85	125.15	1731	50.55	126.89	124.11	1717	50.97	127.92	123.08	1702	51.38	128.96	122.04	1688
251.5	50.02	125.81	125.69	1738	50.44	126.84	124.66	1724	50.85	127.88	123.62	1710	51.26	128.92	122.58	1695
252	49.91	125.77	126.23	1746	50.32	126.80	125.20	1731	50.73	127.84	124.16	1717	51.14	128.88	123.12	1703
252.5	49.79	125.73	126.78	1753	50.20	126.76	125.74	1739	50.61	127.80	124.70	1725	51.02	128.84	123.66	1710
253	49.68	125.68	127.32	1761	50.09	126.72	126.28	1746	50.50	127.76	125.24	1732	50.91	128.80	124.20	1718
253.5	49.56	125.64	127.86	1768	49.97	126.68	126.82	1754	50.38	127.72	125.78	1740	50.79	128.76	124.74	1725
254	49.45	125.60	128.40	1776	49.86	126.64	127.36	1761	50.27	127.68	126.32	1747	50.68	128.71	125.29	1733
254.5	49.34	125.56	128.94	1783	49.74	126.60	127.90	1769	50.15	127.64	126.86	1755	50.56	128.67	125.83	1740
255	49.22	125.52	129.48	1791	49.63	126.56	128.44	1776	50.04	127.60	127.41	1762	50.44	128.63	126.37	1748
255.5	49.11	125.48	130.02	1798	49.52	126.52	128.98	1784	49.92	127.55	127.95	1769	50.33	128.59	126.91	1755
256	49.00	125.44	130.56	1806	49.40	126.48	129.52	1791	49.81	127.51	128.49	1777	50.22	128.55	127.45	1763
256.5	48.89	125.40	131.10	1813	49.29	126.43	130.07	1799	49.70	127.47	129.03	1784	50.10	128.51	127.99	1770
257	48.78	125.36	131.64	1821	49.18	126.39	130.61	1806	49.58	127.43	129.57	1792	49.99	128.47	128.53	1778
257.5	48.67	125.32	132.19	1828	49.07	126.35	131.15	1814	49.47	127.39	130.11	1799	49.87	128.43	129.07	1785
258	48.56	125.27	132.73	1836	48.96	126.31	131.69	1821	49.36	127.35	130.65	1807	49.76	128.39	129.61	1793
258.5	48.45	125.23	133.27	1843	48.85	126.27	132.23	1829	49.25	127.31	131.19	1814	49.65	128.35	130.15	1800
259	48.34	125.19	133.81	1851	48.74	126.23	132.77	1836	49.14	127.27	131.73	1822	49.54	128.30	130.70	1808
259.5	48.23	125.15	134.35	1858	48.63	126.19	133.31	1844	49.03	127.23	132.27	1829	49.43	128.26	131.24	1815
260	48.12	125.11	134.89	1866	48.52	126.15	133.85	1851	48.92	127.19	132.82	1837	49.32	128.22	131.78	1822
260.5	48.01	125.07	135.43	1873	48.41	126.11	134.39	1859	48.81	127.14	133.36	1844	49.21	128.18	132.32	1830
261	47.90	125.03	135.97	1880	48.30	126.07	134.93	1866	48.70	127.10	133.90	1852	49.10	128.14	132.86	1837
261.5	47.80	124.99	136.51	1888	48.19	126.02	135.48	1874	48.59	127.06	134.44	1859	48.99	128.10	133.40	1845
262	47.69	124.95	137.05	1895	48.09	125.98	136.02	1881	48.48	127.02	134.98	1867	48.88	128.06	133.94	1852
262.5	47.58	124.91	137.60	1903	47.98	125.94	136.56	1889	48.37	126.98	135.52	1874	48.77	128.02	134.48	1860
263	47.48	124.86	138.14	1910	47.87	125.90	137.10	1896	48.27	126.94	136.06	1882	48.66	127.98	135.02	1867
263.5	47.37	124.82	138.68	1918	47.76	125.86	137.64	1904	48.16	126.90	136.60	1889	48.55	127.94	135.56	1875
264	47.27	124.78	139.22	1925	47.66	125.82	138.18	1911	48.05	126.86	137.14	1897	48.44	127.89	136.11	1882
264.5	47.16	124.74	139.76	1933	47.55	125.78	138.72	1919	47.95	126.82	137.68	1904	48.34	127.85	136.65	1890
265	47.06	124.70	140.30	1940	47.45	125.74	139.26	1926	47.84	126.78	138.23	1912	48.23	127.81	137.19	1897
265.5	46.95	124.66	140.84	1948	47.34	125.70	139.80	1933	47.73	126.73	138.77	1919	48.12	127.77	137.73	1905
266	46.85	124.62	141.38	1955	47.24	125.66	140.34	1941	47.63	126.69	139.31	1927	48.02	127.73	138.27	1912
266.5	46.75	124.58	141.92	1963	47.13	125.61	140.89	1948	47.52	126.65	139.85	1934	47.91	127.69	138.81	1920
267	46.64	124.54	142.46	1970	47.03	125.57	141.43	1956	47.42	126.61	140.39	1942	47.81	127.65	139.35	1927
267.5	46.54	124.50	143.01	1978	46.93	125.53	141.97	1963	47.32	126.57	140.93	1949	47.70	127.61	139.89	1935
268	46.44	124.45	143.55	1985	46.83	125.49	142.51	1971	47.21	126.53	141.47	1957	47.60	127.57	140.43	1942
268.5	46.34	124.41	144.09	1993	46.72	125.45	143.05	1978	47.11	126.49	142.01	1964	47.50	127.53	140.97	1950
269	46.23	124.37	144.63	2000	46.62	125.41	143.59	1986	47.01	126.45	142.55	1972	47.39	127.48	141.52	1957
269.5	46.13	124.33	145.17	2008	46.52	125.37	144.13	1993	46.90	126.41	143.09	1979	47.29	127.44	142.06	1965
270	46.03	124.29	145.71	2015	46.42	125.33	144.67	2001	46.80	126.37	143.64	1986	47.19	127.40	142.60	1972
270.5	45.93	124.25	146.25	2023	46.32	125.29	145.21	2008	46.70	126.32	144.18	1994	47.08	127.36	143.14	1980
271	45.83	124.21	146.79	2030	46.22	125.25	145.75	2016	46.60	126.28	144.72	2001	46.98	127.32	143.68	1987
271.5	45.73	124.17	147.33	2038	46.12	125.20	146.30	2023	46.50	126.24	145.26	2009	46.88	127.28	144.22	1995
272	45.63	124.13	147.87	2045	46.02	125.16	146.84	2031	46.40	126.20	145.80	2016	46.78	127.24	144.76	2002
272.5	45.54	124.09	148.42	2053	45.92	125.12	147.38	2038	46.30	126.16	146.34	2024	46.68	127.20	145.30	2010
273	45.44	124.04	148.96	2060	45.82	125.08	147.92	2046	46.20	126.12	146.88	2031	46.58	127.16	145.84	2017
273.5	45.34	124.00	149.50	2068	45.72	125.04	148.46	2053	46.10	126.08	147.42	2039	46.48	127.12	146.38	2024
274	45.24	123.96	150.04	2075	45.62	125.00	149.00	2061	46.00	126.04	147.96	2046	46.38	127.07	146.93	2032
274.5	45.14	123.92	150.58	2083	45.52	124.96	149.54	2068	45.90	126.00	148.50	2054	46.28	127.03	147.47	2039
275	45.05	123.88	151.12	2090	45.42	124.92	150.08	2076	45.80	125.96	149.05	2061	46.18	126.99	148.01	2047
275.5	44.95	123.84	151.66	2097	45.33	124.88	150.62	2083	45.70	125.91	149.59	2069	46.08	126.95	148.55	2054
276	44.85	123.80	152.20	2105	45.23	124.84	151.16	2091	45.61	125.87	150.13	2076	45.98	126.91	149.09	2062
276.5	44.76	123.76	152.74	2112	45.13	124.79	151.71	2098	45.51	125.83	150.67	2084	45.88	126.87	149.63	2069
277	44.66	123.72	153.28	2120	45.04	124.75	152.25	2106	45.41	125.79	151.21	2091	45.79	126.83	150.17	2077
277.5	44.57	123.68	153.83	2127	44.94	124.71	152.79	2113	45.32	125.75	151.75	2099	45.69	126.79	150.71	2084
278	44.47	123.63	154.37	2135	44.85	124.67	153.33	2121	45.22	125.71	152.29	2106	45.59	126.75	151.25	2092
278.5	44.38	123.59	154.91	2142	44.75	124.63	153.87	2128	45.12	125.67	152.83	2114	45.50	126.71	151.79	2099
279	44.28	123.55	155.45	2150	44.66	124.59	154.41	2135	45.03	125.63	153.37	2121	45.40	126.66	152.34	2107
279.5	44.19	123.51	155.99	2157	44.56	124.55	154.95	2143	44.93	125.59	153.91	2129	45.30	126.62	152.88	2114

THE BODY FAT GUIDE

Body Composition   MALE   248-279.5 Lb.

Weight: Lb.	Waist: 60 inches				60.25 inches				60.5 inches				60.75 inches			
	Fat: %	Fat: Lb.	LBM: Lb.	RMR: Cal.	Fat: %	Fat: Lb.	LBM: Lb.	RMR: Cal.	Fat: %	Fat: Lb.	LBM: Lb.	RMR: Cal.	Fat: %	Fat: Lb.	LBM: Lb.	RMR: Cal.
248	52.52	130.24	117.76	1629	52.94	131.28	116.72	1614	53.35	132.32	115.68	1600	53.77	133.36	114.64	1586
248.5	52.40	130.20	118.30	1636	52.81	131.24	117.26	1622	53.23	132.28	116.22	1607	53.65	133.32	115.18	1593
249	52.27	130.16	118.84	1644	52.69	131.20	117.80	1629	53.11	132.24	116.76	1615	53.52	133.27	115.73	1600
249.5	52.15	130.12	119.38	1651	52.57	131.16	118.34	1637	52.98	132.20	117.30	1622	53.40	133.23	116.27	1608
250	52.03	130.08	119.92	1658	52.45	131.12	118.88	1644	52.86	132.16	117.85	1630	53.28	133.19	116.81	1615
250.5	51.91	130.04	120.46	1666	52.33	131.08	119.42	1652	52.74	132.11	118.39	1637	53.15	133.15	117.35	1623
251	51.79	130.00	121.00	1673	52.21	131.04	119.96	1659	52.62	132.07	118.93	1645	53.03	133.11	117.89	1630
251.5	51.67	129.96	121.54	1681	52.09	130.99	120.51	1667	52.50	132.03	119.47	1652	52.91	133.07	118.43	1638
252	51.55	129.92	122.08	1688	51.97	130.95	121.05	1674	52.38	131.99	120.01	1660	52.79	133.03	118.97	1645
252.5	51.44	129.88	122.63	1696	51.85	130.91	121.59	1682	52.26	131.95	120.55	1667	52.67	132.99	119.51	1653
253	51.32	129.83	123.17	1703	51.73	130.87	122.13	1689	52.14	131.91	121.09	1675	52.55	132.95	120.05	1660
253.5	51.20	129.79	123.71	1711	51.61	130.83	122.67	1697	52.02	131.87	121.63	1682	52.43	132.91	120.59	1668
254	51.08	129.75	124.25	1718	51.49	130.79	123.21	1704	51.90	131.83	122.17	1690	52.31	132.86	121.14	1675
254.5	50.97	129.71	124.79	1726	51.37	130.75	123.75	1711	51.78	131.79	122.71	1697	52.19	132.82	121.68	1683
255	50.85	129.67	125.33	1733	51.26	130.71	124.29	1719	51.66	131.75	123.26	1705	52.07	132.78	122.22	1690
255.5	50.74	129.63	125.87	1741	51.14	130.67	124.83	1726	51.55	131.70	123.80	1712	51.95	132.74	122.76	1698
256	50.62	129.59	126.41	1748	51.03	130.63	125.37	1734	51.43	131.66	124.34	1720	51.84	132.70	123.30	1705
256.5	50.51	129.55	126.95	1756	50.91	130.58	125.92	1741	51.31	131.62	124.88	1727	51.72	132.66	123.84	1713
257	50.39	129.51	127.49	1763	50.80	130.54	126.46	1749	51.20	131.58	125.42	1735	51.60	132.62	124.38	1720
257.5	50.28	129.47	128.04	1771	50.68	130.50	127.00	1756	51.08	131.54	125.96	1742	51.49	132.58	124.92	1728
258	50.16	129.42	128.58	1778	50.57	130.46	127.54	1764	50.97	131.50	126.50	1750	51.37	132.54	125.46	1735
258.5	50.05	129.38	129.12	1786	50.45	130.42	128.08	1771	50.85	131.46	127.04	1757	51.26	132.50	126.00	1743
259	49.94	129.34	129.66	1793	50.34	130.38	128.62	1779	50.74	131.42	127.58	1764	51.14	132.45	126.55	1750
259.5	49.83	129.30	130.20	1801	50.23	130.34	129.16	1786	50.63	131.38	128.12	1772	51.03	132.41	127.09	1758
260	49.72	129.26	130.74	1808	50.11	130.30	129.70	1794	50.51	131.34	128.67	1779	50.91	132.37	127.63	1765
260.5	49.60	129.22	131.28	1816	50.00	130.26	130.24	1801	50.40	131.29	129.21	1787	50.80	132.33	128.17	1773
261	49.49	129.18	131.82	1823	49.89	130.22	130.78	1809	50.29	131.25	129.75	1794	50.69	132.29	128.71	1780
261.5	49.38	129.14	132.36	1831	49.78	130.17	131.33	1816	50.18	131.21	130.29	1802	50.57	132.25	129.25	1788
262	49.27	129.10	132.90	1838	49.67	130.13	131.87	1824	50.07	131.17	130.83	1809	50.46	132.21	129.79	1795
262.5	49.16	129.06	133.45	1846	49.56	130.09	132.41	1831	49.95	131.13	131.37	1817	50.35	132.17	130.33	1802
263	49.05	129.01	133.99	1853	49.45	130.05	132.95	1839	49.84	131.09	131.91	1824	50.24	132.13	130.87	1810
263.5	48.95	128.97	134.53	1861	49.34	130.01	133.49	1846	49.73	131.05	132.45	1832	50.13	132.09	131.41	1817
264	48.84	128.93	135.07	1868	49.23	129.97	134.03	1854	49.62	131.01	132.99	1839	50.02	132.04	131.96	1825
264.5	48.73	128.89	135.61	1875	49.12	129.93	134.57	1861	49.51	130.97	133.53	1847	49.91	132.00	132.50	1832
265	48.62	128.85	136.15	1883	49.01	129.89	135.11	1869	49.41	130.93	134.08	1854	49.80	131.96	133.04	1840
265.5	48.52	128.81	136.69	1890	48.91	129.85	135.65	1876	49.30	130.88	134.62	1862	49.69	131.92	133.58	1847
266	48.41	128.77	137.23	1898	48.80	129.81	136.19	1884	49.19	130.84	135.16	1869	49.58	131.88	134.12	1855
266.5	48.30	128.73	137.77	1905	48.69	129.76	136.74	1891	49.08	130.80	135.70	1877	49.47	131.84	134.66	1862
267	48.20	128.69	138.31	1913	48.59	129.72	137.28	1899	48.97	130.76	136.24	1884	49.36	131.80	135.20	1870
267.5	48.09	128.65	138.86	1920	48.48	129.68	137.82	1906	48.87	130.72	136.78	1892	49.26	131.76	135.74	1877
268	47.99	128.60	139.40	1928	48.37	129.64	138.36	1913	48.76	130.68	137.32	1899	49.15	131.72	136.28	1885
268.5	47.88	128.56	139.94	1935	48.27	129.60	138.90	1921	48.65	130.64	137.86	1907	49.04	131.68	136.82	1892
269	47.78	128.52	140.48	1943	48.16	129.56	139.44	1928	48.55	130.60	138.40	1914	48.93	131.63	137.37	1900
269.5	47.67	128.48	141.02	1950	48.06	129.52	139.98	1936	48.44	130.56	138.94	1922	48.83	131.59	137.91	1907
270	47.57	128.44	141.56	1958	47.95	129.48	140.52	1943	48.34	130.52	139.49	1929	48.72	131.55	138.45	1915
270.5	47.47	128.40	142.10	1965	47.85	129.44	141.06	1951	48.23	130.47	140.03	1937	48.62	131.51	138.99	1922
271	47.36	128.36	142.64	1973	47.75	129.40	141.60	1958	48.13	130.43	140.57	1944	48.51	131.47	139.53	1930
271.5	47.26	128.32	143.18	1980	47.64	129.35	142.15	1966	48.03	130.39	141.11	1952	48.41	131.43	140.07	1937
272	47.16	128.28	143.72	1988	47.54	129.31	142.69	1973	47.92	130.35	141.65	1959	48.30	131.39	140.61	1945
272.5	47.06	128.24	144.27	1995	47.44	129.27	143.23	1981	47.82	130.31	142.19	1966	48.20	131.35	141.15	1952
273	46.96	128.19	144.81	2003	47.34	129.23	143.77	1988	47.72	130.27	142.73	1974	48.10	131.31	141.69	1960
273.5	46.86	128.15	145.35	2010	47.24	129.19	144.31	1996	47.62	130.23	143.27	1981	47.99	131.27	142.23	1967
274	46.76	128.11	145.89	2018	47.13	129.15	144.85	2003	47.51	130.19	143.81	1989	47.89	131.22	142.78	1975
274.5	46.66	128.07	146.43	2025	47.03	129.11	145.39	2011	47.41	130.15	144.35	1996	47.79	131.18	143.32	1982
275	46.56	128.03	146.97	2033	46.93	129.07	145.93	2018	47.31	130.11	144.90	2004	47.69	131.14	143.86	1990
275.5	46.46	127.99	147.51	2040	46.83	129.03	146.47	2026	47.21	130.06	145.44	2011	47.59	131.10	144.40	1997
276	46.36	127.95	148.05	2048	46.73	128.99	147.01	2033	47.11	130.02	145.98	2019	47.49	131.06	144.94	2005
276.5	46.26	127.91	148.59	2055	46.63	128.94	147.56	2041	47.01	129.98	146.52	2026	47.38	131.02	145.48	2012
277	46.16	127.87	149.13	2063	46.54	128.90	148.10	2048	46.91	129.94	147.06	2034	47.28	130.98	146.02	2019
277.5	46.06	127.83	149.68	2070	46.44	128.86	148.64	2056	46.81	129.90	147.60	2041	47.18	130.94	146.56	2027
278	45.97	127.78	150.22	2077	46.34	128.82	149.18	2063	46.71	129.86	148.14	2049	47.09	130.90	147.10	2034
278.5	45.87	127.74	150.76	2085	46.24	128.78	149.72	2071	46.61	129.82	148.68	2056	46.99	130.86	147.64	2042
279	45.77	127.70	151.30	2092	46.14	128.74	150.26	2078	46.52	129.78	149.22	2064	46.89	130.81	148.19	2049
279.5	45.67	127.66	151.84	2100	46.05	128.70	150.80	2086	46.42	129.74	149.76	2071	46.79	130.77	148.73	2057

Body Composition MALE 280-311.5 Lb.

Weight: Lb.	Waist: 32 inches Fat: %	Fat: Lb.	LBM: Lb.	RMR: Cal.	32.25 inches Fat: %	Fat: Lb.	LBM: Lb.	RMR: Cal.	32.5 inches Fat: %	Fat: Lb.	LBM: Lb.	RMR: Cal.	32.75 inches Fat: %	Fat: Lb.	LBM: Lb.	RMR: Cal.
280	4.08	11.42	268.58	3714	4.45	12.46	267.54	3700	4.82	13.49	266.51	3686	5.19	14.53	265.47	3671
280.5	4.06	11.38	269.12	3722	4.43	12.42	268.08	3708	4.80	13.45	267.05	3693	5.17	14.49	266.01	3679
281	4.03	11.34	269.66	3729	4.40	12.38	268.62	3715	4.77	13.41	267.59	3701	5.14	14.45	266.55	3686
281.5	4.01	11.30	270.20	3737	4.38	12.33	269.17	3723	4.75	13.37	268.13	3708	5.12	14.41	267.09	3694
282	3.99	11.26	270.74	3744	4.36	12.29	269.71	3730	4.73	13.33	268.67	3716	5.10	14.37	267.63	3701
282.5	3.97	11.22	271.29	3752	4.34	12.25	270.25	3738	4.70	13.29	269.21	3723	5.07	14.33	268.17	3709
283	3.95	11.17	271.83	3759	4.32	12.21	270.79	3745	4.68	13.25	269.75	3731	5.05	14.29	268.71	3716
283.5	3.93	11.13	272.37	3767	4.29	12.17	271.33	3752	4.66	13.21	270.29	3738	5.02	14.25	269.25	3724
284	3.91	11.09	272.91	3774	4.27	12.13	271.87	3760	4.64	13.17	270.83	3746	5.00	14.20	269.80	3731
284.5	3.88	11.05	273.45	3782	4.25	12.09	272.41	3767	4.61	13.13	271.37	3753	4.98	14.16	270.34	3739
285	3.86	11.01	273.99	3789	4.23	12.05	272.95	3775	4.59	13.09	271.92	3761	4.96	14.12	270.88	3746
285.5	3.84	10.97	274.53	3797	4.21	12.01	273.49	3782	4.57	13.04	272.46	3768	4.93	14.08	271.42	3754
286	3.82	10.93	275.07	3804	4.18	11.97	274.03	3790	4.55	13.00	273.00	3776	4.91	14.04	271.96	3761
286.5	3.80	10.89	275.61	3812	4.16	11.92	274.58	3797	4.52	12.96	273.54	3783	4.89	14.00	272.50	3769
287	3.78	10.85	276.15	3819	4.14	11.88	275.12	3805	4.50	12.92	274.08	3791	4.86	13.96	273.04	3776
287.5	3.76	10.80	276.70	3827	4.12	11.84	275.66	3812	4.48	12.88	274.62	3798	4.84	13.92	273.58	3784
288	3.74	10.76	277.24	3834	4.10	11.80	276.20	3820	4.46	12.84	275.16	3805	4.82	13.88	274.12	3791
288.5	3.72	10.72	277.78	3842	4.08	11.76	276.74	3827	4.44	12.80	276.70	3813	4.80	13.84	274.66	3799
289	3.70	10.68	278.32	3849	4.06	11.72	277.28	3835	4.41	12.76	276.24	3820	4.77	13.79	275.21	3806
289.5	3.68	10.64	278.86	3857	4.03	11.68	277.82	3842	4.39	12.72	276.78	3828	4.75	13.75	275.75	3814
290	3.66	10.60	279.40	3864	4.01	11.64	278.36	3850	4.37	12.68	277.33	3835	4.73	13.71	276.29	3821
290.5	3.63	10.56	279.94	3872	3.99	11.60	278.90	3857	4.35	12.63	277.87	3843	4.71	13.67	276.83	3829
291	3.61	10.52	280.48	3879	3.97	11.56	279.44	3865	4.33	12.59	278.41	3850	4.68	13.63	277.37	3836
291.5	3.59	10.48	281.02	3887	3.95	11.51	279.99	3872	4.31	12.55	278.95	3858	4.66	13.59	277.91	3844
292	3.57	10.44	281.56	3894	3.93	11.47	280.53	3880	4.28	12.51	279.49	3865	4.64	13.55	278.45	3851
292.5	3.55	10.40	282.11	3902	3.91	11.43	281.07	3887	4.26	12.47	280.03	3873	4.62	13.51	278.99	3858
293	3.53	10.35	282.65	3909	3.89	11.39	281.61	3895	4.24	12.43	280.57	3880	4.60	13.47	279.53	3866
293.5	3.51	10.31	283.19	3916	3.87	11.35	282.15	3902	4.22	12.39	281.11	3888	4.57	13.43	280.07	3873
294	3.49	10.27	283.73	3924	3.85	11.31	282.69	3909	4.20	12.35	281.65	3895	4.55	13.38	280.62	3881
294.5	3.47	10.23	284.27	3931	3.83	11.27	283.23	3917	4.18	12.31	282.19	3903	4.53	13.34	281.16	3888
295	3.45	10.19	284.81	3939	3.81	11.23	283.77	3925	4.16	12.27	282.74	3910	4.51	13.30	281.70	3896
295.5	3.43	10.15	285.35	3946	3.79	11.19	284.31	3932	4.14	12.22	283.28	3918	4.49	13.26	282.24	3903
296	3.41	10.11	285.89	3954	3.77	11.15	284.85	3940	4.12	12.18	283.82	3925	4.47	13.22	282.78	3911
296.5	3.40	10.07	286.43	3961	3.75	11.10	285.40	3947	4.10	12.14	284.36	3933	4.45	13.18	283.32	3918
297	3.38	10.03	286.97	3969	3.73	11.06	285.94	3955	4.07	12.10	284.90	3940	4.42	13.14	283.86	3926
297.5	3.36	9.98	287.52	3976	3.71	11.02	286.48	3962	4.05	12.06	285.44	3948	4.40	13.10	284.40	3933
298	3.34	9.94	288.06	3984	3.69	10.98	287.02	3969	4.03	12.02	285.98	3955	4.38	13.06	284.94	3941
298.5	3.32	9.90	288.60	3991	3.67	10.94	287.56	3977	4.01	11.98	286.52	3963	4.36	13.02	285.48	3948
299	3.30	9.86	289.14	3999	3.65	10.90	288.10	3984	3.99	11.94	287.06	3970	4.34	12.97	286.03	3956
299.5	3.28	9.82	289.68	4006	3.63	10.86	288.64	3992	3.97	11.90	287.60	3978	4.32	12.93	286.57	3963
300	3.26	9.78	290.22	4014	3.61	10.82	289.18	3999	3.95	11.86	288.15	3985	4.30	12.89	287.11	3971
300.5	3.24	9.74	290.76	4021	3.59	10.78	289.72	4007	3.93	11.81	288.69	3993	4.28	12.85	287.65	3978
301	3.22	9.70	291.30	4029	3.57	10.74	290.26	4014	3.91	11.77	289.23	4000	4.26	12.81	288.19	3986
301.5	3.20	9.66	291.84	4036	3.55	10.69	290.81	4022	3.89	11.73	289.77	4007	4.24	12.77	288.73	3993
302	3.18	9.62	292.38	4044	3.53	10.65	291.35	4029	3.87	11.69	290.31	4015	4.21	12.73	289.27	4001
302.5	3.17	9.57	292.93	4051	3.51	10.61	291.89	4037	3.85	11.65	290.85	4022	4.19	12.69	289.81	4008
303	3.15	9.53	293.47	4059	3.49	10.57	292.43	4044	3.83	11.61	291.39	4030	4.17	12.65	290.35	4016
303.5	3.13	9.49	294.01	4066	3.47	10.53	292.97	4052	3.81	11.57	291.93	4037	4.15	12.61	290.89	4023
304	3.11	9.45	294.55	4074	3.45	10.49	293.51	4059	3.79	11.53	292.47	4045	4.13	12.56	291.44	4031
304.5	3.09	9.41	295.09	4081	3.43	10.45	294.05	4067	3.77	11.49	293.01	4052	4.11	12.52	291.98	4038
305	3.07	9.37	295.63	4089	3.41	10.41	294.59	4074	3.75	11.44	293.56	4060	4.09	12.48	292.52	4046
305.5	3.05	9.33	296.17	4096	3.39	10.37	295.13	4082	3.73	11.40	294.10	4067	4.07	12.44	293.06	4053
306	3.04	9.29	296.71	4104	3.37	10.33	295.67	4089	3.71	11.36	294.64	4075	4.05	12.40	293.60	4060
306.5	3.02	9.25	297.25	4111	3.36	10.28	296.22	4097	3.69	11.32	295.18	4082	4.03	12.36	294.14	4068
307	3.00	9.21	297.79	4118	3.34	10.24	296.76	4104	3.67	11.28	295.72	4090	4.01	12.32	294.68	4075
307.5	2.98	9.16	298.34	4126	3.32	10.20	297.30	4112	3.66	11.24	296.26	4097	3.99	12.28	295.22	4083
308	2.96	9.12	298.88	4133	3.30	10.16	297.84	4119	3.64	11.20	296.80	4105	3.97	12.24	295.76	4090
308.5	2.94	9.08	299.42	4141	3.28	10.12	298.38	4127	3.62	11.16	297.34	4112	3.95	12.20	296.30	4098
309	2.93	9.04	299.96	4148	3.26	10.08	298.92	4134	3.60	11.12	297.88	4120	3.93	12.15	296.85	4105
309.5	2.91	9.00	300.50	4156	3.24	10.04	299.46	4142	3.58	11.08	298.42	4127	3.91	12.11	297.39	4113
310	2.89	8.96	301.04	4163	3.23	10.00	300.00	4149	3.56	11.04	298.97	4135	3.89	12.07	297.93	4120
310.5	2.87	8.92	301.58	4171	3.21	9.96	300.54	4157	3.54	10.99	299.51	4142	3.87	12.03	298.47	4128
311	2.85	8.88	302.12	4178	3.19	9.92	301.08	4164	3.52	10.95	300.05	4150	3.86	11.99	299.01	4135
311.5	2.84	8.84	302.66	4186	3.17	9.87	301.63	4171	3.50	10.91	300.59	4157	3.84	11.95	299.55	4143

Body Composition   MALE   280-311.5 Lb.

Weight: Lb.	Waist: Fat: %	33 inches Fat: Lb.	LBM: Lb.	RMR: Cal.	Fat: %	33.25 inches Fat: Lb.	LBM: Lb.	RMR: Cal.	Fat: %	33.5 inches Fat: Lb.	LBM: Lb.	RMR: Cal.	Fat: %	33.75 inches Fat: Lb.	LBM: Lb.	RMR: Cal.
280	5.56	15.57	264.43	3657	5.93	16.61	263.39	3643	6.30	17.65	262.36	3628	6.67	18.68	261.32	3614
280.5	5.54	15.53	264.97	3665	5.91	16.57	263.93	3650	6.28	17.60	262.90	3636	6.65	18.64	261.86	3622
281	5.51	15.49	265.51	3672	5.88	16.53	264.47	3658	6.25	17.56	263.44	3643	6.62	18.60	262.40	3629
281.5	5.49	15.45	266.05	3680	5.86	16.48	265.02	3665	6.22	17.52	263.98	3651	6.59	18.56	262.94	3636
282	5.46	15.41	266.59	3687	5.83	16.44	265.56	3673	6.20	17.48	264.52	3658	6.57	18.52	263.48	3644
282.5	5.44	15.37	267.14	3694	5.81	16.40	266.10	3680	6.17	17.44	265.06	3666	6.54	18.48	264.02	3651
283	5.41	15.32	267.68	3702	5.78	16.36	266.64	3688	6.15	17.40	265.60	3673	6.51	18.44	264.56	3659
283.5	5.39	15.28	268.22	3709	5.76	16.32	267.18	3695	6.12	17.36	266.14	3681	6.49	18.40	265.10	3666
284	5.37	15.24	268.76	3717	5.73	16.28	267.72	3703	6.10	17.32	266.68	3688	6.46	18.35	265.65	3674
284.5	5.34	15.20	269.30	3724	5.71	16.24	268.26	3710	6.07	17.28	267.22	3696	6.44	18.31	266.19	3681
285	5.32	15.16	269.84	3732	5.68	16.20	268.80	3718	6.05	17.24	267.77	3703	6.41	18.27	266.73	3689
285.5	5.30	15.12	270.38	3739	5.66	16.16	269.34	3725	6.02	17.19	268.31	3711	6.39	18.23	267.27	3696
286	5.27	15.08	270.92	3747	5.63	16.12	269.88	3733	6.00	17.15	268.85	3718	6.36	18.19	267.81	3704
286.5	5.25	15.04	271.46	3754	5.61	16.07	270.43	3740	5.97	17.11	269.39	3726	6.33	18.15	268.35	3711
287	5.23	15.00	272.00	3762	5.59	16.03	270.97	3747	5.95	17.07	269.93	3733	6.31	18.11	268.89	3719
287.5	5.20	14.96	272.55	3769	5.56	15.99	271.51	3755	5.92	17.03	270.47	3741	6.28	18.07	269.43	3726
288	5.18	14.91	273.09	3777	5.54	15.95	272.05	3762	5.90	16.99	271.01	3748	6.26	18.03	269.97	3734
288.5	5.16	14.87	273.63	3784	5.51	15.91	272.59	3770	5.87	16.95	271.55	3756	6.23	17.99	270.51	3741
289	5.13	14.83	274.17	3792	5.49	15.87	273.13	3777	5.85	16.91	272.09	3763	6.21	17.94	271.06	3749
289.5	5.11	14.79	274.71	3799	5.47	15.83	273.67	3785	5.83	16.87	272.63	3771	6.18	17.90	271.60	3756
290	5.09	14.75	275.25	3807	5.44	15.79	274.21	3792	5.80	16.83	273.18	3778	6.16	17.86	272.14	3764
290.5	5.06	14.71	275.79	3814	5.42	15.75	274.75	3800	5.78	16.78	273.72	3785	6.13	17.82	272.68	3771
291	5.04	14.67	276.33	3822	5.40	15.71	275.29	3807	5.75	16.74	274.26	3793	6.11	17.78	273.22	3779
291.5	5.02	14.63	276.87	3829	5.37	15.66	275.84	3815	5.73	16.70	274.80	3800	6.09	17.74	273.76	3786
292	5.00	14.59	277.41	3837	5.35	15.62	276.38	3822	5.71	16.66	275.34	3808	6.06	17.70	274.30	3794
292.5	4.97	14.55	277.96	3844	5.33	15.58	276.92	3830	5.68	16.62	275.88	3815	6.04	17.66	274.84	3801
293	4.95	14.50	278.50	3852	5.30	15.54	277.46	3837	5.66	16.58	276.42	3823	6.01	17.62	275.38	3809
293.5	4.93	14.46	279.04	3859	5.28	15.50	278.00	3845	5.63	16.54	276.96	3830	5.99	17.58	275.92	3816
294	4.91	14.42	279.58	3867	5.26	15.46	278.54	3852	5.61	16.50	277.50	3838	5.96	17.53	276.47	3824
294.5	4.88	14.38	280.12	3874	5.24	15.42	279.08	3860	5.59	16.46	278.04	3845	5.94	17.49	277.01	3831
295	4.86	14.34	280.66	3882	5.21	15.38	279.62	3867	5.56	16.42	278.59	3853	5.92	17.45	277.55	3838
295.5	4.84	14.30	281.20	3889	5.19	15.34	280.16	3875	5.54	16.37	279.13	3860	5.89	17.41	278.09	3846
296	4.82	14.26	281.74	3896	5.17	15.30	280.70	3882	5.52	16.33	279.67	3868	5.87	17.37	278.63	3853
296.5	4.79	14.22	282.28	3904	5.14	15.25	281.25	3890	5.49	16.29	280.21	3875	5.84	17.33	279.17	3861
297	4.77	14.18	282.82	3911	5.12	15.21	281.79	3897	5.47	16.25	280.75	3883	5.82	17.29	279.71	3868
297.5	4.75	14.14	283.37	3919	5.10	15.17	282.33	3905	5.45	16.21	281.29	3890	5.80	17.25	280.25	3876
298	4.73	14.09	283.91	3926	5.08	15.13	282.87	3912	5.43	16.17	281.83	3898	5.77	17.21	280.79	3883
298.5	4.71	14.05	284.45	3934	5.06	15.09	283.41	3920	5.40	16.13	282.37	3905	5.75	17.17	281.33	3891
299	4.69	14.01	284.99	3941	5.03	15.05	283.95	3927	5.38	16.09	282.91	3913	5.73	17.12	281.88	3898
299.5	4.66	13.97	285.53	3949	5.01	15.01	284.49	3935	5.36	16.05	283.45	3920	5.70	17.08	282.42	3906
300	4.64	13.93	286.07	3956	4.99	14.97	285.03	3942	5.34	16.01	284.00	3928	5.68	17.04	282.96	3913
300.5	4.62	13.89	286.61	3964	4.97	14.93	285.57	3949	5.31	15.96	284.54	3935	5.66	17.00	283.50	3921
301	4.60	13.85	287.15	3971	4.95	14.89	286.11	3957	5.29	15.92	285.08	3943	5.63	16.96	284.04	3928
301.5	4.58	13.81	287.69	3979	4.92	14.84	286.66	3964	5.27	15.88	285.62	3950	5.61	16.92	284.58	3936
302	4.56	13.77	288.23	3986	4.90	14.80	287.20	3972	5.25	15.84	286.16	3958	5.59	16.88	285.12	3943
302.5	4.54	13.73	288.78	3994	4.88	14.76	287.74	3979	5.22	15.80	286.70	3965	5.57	16.84	285.66	3951
303	4.52	13.68	289.32	4001	4.86	14.72	288.28	3987	5.20	15.76	287.24	3973	5.54	16.80	286.20	3958
303.5	4.50	13.64	289.86	4009	4.84	14.68	288.82	3994	5.18	15.72	287.78	3980	5.52	16.76	286.74	3966
304	4.47	13.60	290.40	4016	4.82	14.64	289.36	4002	5.16	15.68	288.32	3988	5.50	16.71	287.29	3973
304.5	4.45	13.56	290.94	4024	4.79	14.60	289.90	4009	5.13	15.64	288.86	3995	5.48	16.67	287.83	3981
305	4.43	13.52	291.48	4031	4.77	14.56	290.44	4017	5.11	15.60	289.41	4002	5.45	16.63	288.37	3988
305.5	4.41	13.48	292.02	4039	4.75	14.52	290.98	4024	5.09	15.55	289.95	4010	5.43	16.59	288.91	3996
306	4.39	13.44	292.56	4046	4.73	14.48	291.52	4032	5.07	15.51	290.49	4017	5.41	16.55	289.45	4003
306.5	4.37	13.40	293.10	4054	4.71	14.43	292.07	4039	5.05	15.47	291.03	4025	5.39	16.51	289.99	4011
307	4.35	13.36	293.64	4061	4.69	14.39	292.61	4047	5.03	15.43	291.57	4032	5.36	16.47	290.53	4018
307.5	4.33	13.32	294.19	4069	4.67	14.35	293.15	4054	5.00	15.39	292.11	4040	5.34	16.43	291.07	4026
308	4.31	13.27	294.73	4076	4.65	14.31	293.69	4062	4.98	15.35	292.65	4047	5.32	16.39	291.61	4033
308.5	4.29	13.23	295.27	4084	4.63	14.27	294.23	4069	4.96	15.31	293.19	4055	5.30	16.35	292.15	4040
309	4.27	13.19	295.81	4091	4.61	14.23	294.77	4077	4.94	15.27	293.73	4062	5.28	16.30	292.70	4048
309.5	4.25	13.15	296.35	4099	4.58	14.19	295.31	4084	4.92	15.23	294.27	4070	5.25	16.26	293.24	4055
310	4.23	13.11	296.89	4106	4.56	14.15	295.85	4092	4.90	15.19	294.82	4077	5.23	16.22	293.78	4063
310.5	4.21	13.07	297.43	4113	4.54	14.11	296.39	4099	4.88	15.14	295.36	4085	5.21	16.18	294.32	4070
311	4.19	13.03	297.97	4121	4.52	14.07	296.93	4107	4.86	15.10	295.90	4092	5.19	16.14	294.86	4078
311.5	4.17	12.99	298.51	4128	4.50	14.02	297.48	4114	4.84	15.06	296.44	4100	5.17	16.10	295.40	4085

Body Composition MALE 280-311.5 Lb.

Weight: Lb.	Waist: 34 inches Fat: %	Fat: Lb.	LBM: Lb.	RMR: Cal.	34.25 inches Fat: %	Fat: Lb.	LBM: Lb.	RMR: Cal.	34.5 inches Fat: %	Fat: Lb.	LBM: Lb.	RMR: Cal.	34.75 inches Fat: %	Fat: Lb.	LBM: Lb.	RMR: Cal.
280	7.04	19.72	260.28	3600	7.41	20.76	259.24	3585	7.78	21.80	258.21	3571	8.15	22.83	257.17	3557
280.5	7.02	19.68	260.82	3607	7.39	20.72	259.78	3593	7.76	21.75	258.75	3578	8.13	22.79	257.71	3564
281	6.99	19.64	261.36	3615	7.36	20.68	260.32	3600	7.73	21.71	259.29	3586	8.10	22.75	258.25	3572
281.5	6.96	19.60	261.90	3622	7.33	20.63	260.87	3608	7.70	21.67	259.83	3593	8.07	22.71	258.79	3579
282	6.93	19.56	262.44	3630	7.30	20.59	261.41	3615	7.67	21.63	260.37	3601	8.04	22.67	259.33	3587
282.5	6.91	19.52	262.99	3637	7.28	20.55	261.95	3623	7.64	21.59	260.91	3608	8.01	22.63	259.87	3594
283	6.88	19.47	263.53	3645	7.25	20.51	262.49	3630	7.61	21.55	261.45	3616	7.98	22.59	260.41	3602
283.5	6.85	19.43	264.07	3652	7.22	20.47	263.03	3638	7.59	21.51	261.99	3623	7.95	22.55	260.95	3609
284	6.83	19.39	264.61	3660	7.19	20.43	263.57	3645	7.56	21.47	262.53	3631	7.92	22.50	261.50	3616
284.5	6.80	19.35	265.15	3667	7.17	20.39	264.11	3653	7.53	21.43	263.07	3638	7.90	22.46	262.04	3624
285	6.78	19.31	265.69	3674	7.14	20.35	264.65	3660	7.50	21.39	263.62	3646	7.87	22.42	262.58	3631
285.5	6.75	19.27	266.23	3682	7.11	20.31	265.19	3668	7.48	21.34	264.16	3653	7.84	22.38	263.12	3639
286	6.72	19.23	266.77	3689	7.09	20.27	265.73	3675	7.45	21.30	264.70	3661	7.81	22.34	263.66	3646
286.5	6.70	19.19	267.31	3697	7.06	20.22	266.28	3683	7.42	21.26	265.24	3668	7.78	22.30	264.20	3654
287	6.67	19.15	267.85	3704	7.03	20.18	266.82	3690	7.39	21.22	265.78	3676	7.76	22.26	264.74	3661
287.5	6.65	19.11	268.40	3712	7.01	20.14	267.36	3698	7.37	21.18	266.32	3683	7.73	22.22	265.28	3669
288	6.62	19.06	268.94	3719	6.98	20.10	267.90	3705	7.34	21.14	266.86	3691	7.70	22.18	265.82	3676
288.5	6.59	19.02	269.48	3727	6.95	20.06	268.44	3713	7.31	21.10	267.40	3698	7.67	22.14	266.36	3684
289	6.57	18.98	270.02	3734	6.93	20.02	268.98	3720	7.29	21.06	267.94	3706	7.65	22.09	266.91	3691
289.5	6.54	18.94	270.56	3742	6.90	19.98	269.52	3727	7.26	21.02	268.48	3713	7.62	22.05	267.45	3699
290	6.52	18.90	271.10	3749	6.88	19.94	270.06	3735	7.23	20.98	269.03	3721	7.59	22.01	267.99	3706
290.5	6.49	18.86	271.64	3757	6.85	19.90	270.60	3742	7.21	20.93	269.57	3728	7.56	21.97	268.53	3714
291	6.47	18.82	272.18	3764	6.82	19.86	271.14	3750	7.18	20.89	270.11	3736	7.54	21.93	269.07	3721
291.5	6.44	18.78	272.72	3772	6.80	19.81	271.69	3757	7.15	20.85	270.65	3743	7.51	21.89	269.61	3729
292	6.42	18.74	273.26	3779	6.77	19.77	272.23	3765	7.13	20.81	271.19	3751	7.48	21.85	270.15	3736
292.5	6.39	18.70	273.81	3787	6.75	19.73	272.77	3772	7.10	20.77	271.73	3758	7.46	21.81	270.69	3744
293	6.37	18.65	274.35	3794	6.72	19.69	273.31	3780	7.07	20.73	272.27	3766	7.43	21.77	271.23	3751
293.5	6.34	18.61	274.89	3802	6.70	19.65	273.85	3787	7.05	20.69	272.81	3773	7.40	21.73	271.77	3759
294	6.32	18.57	275.43	3809	6.67	19.61	274.39	3795	7.02	20.65	273.35	3780	7.38	21.68	272.32	3766
294.5	6.29	18.53	275.97	3817	6.64	19.57	274.93	3802	7.00	20.61	273.89	3788	7.35	21.64	272.86	3774
295	6.27	18.49	276.51	3824	6.62	19.53	275.47	3810	6.97	20.57	274.44	3795	7.32	21.60	273.40	3781
295.5	6.24	18.45	277.05	3832	6.59	19.49	276.01	3817	6.95	20.52	274.98	3803	7.30	21.56	273.94	3789
296	6.22	18.41	277.59	3839	6.57	19.45	276.55	3825	6.92	20.48	275.52	3810	7.27	21.52	274.48	3796
296.5	6.19	18.37	278.13	3847	6.54	19.40	277.10	3832	6.89	20.44	276.06	3818	7.24	21.48	275.02	3804
297	6.17	18.33	278.67	3854	6.52	19.36	277.64	3840	6.87	20.40	276.60	3825	7.22	21.44	275.56	3811
297.5	6.15	18.29	279.22	3862	6.49	19.32	278.18	3847	6.84	20.36	277.14	3833	7.19	21.40	276.10	3818
298	6.12	18.24	279.76	3869	6.47	19.28	278.72	3855	6.82	20.32	277.68	3840	7.17	21.36	276.64	3826
298.5	6.10	18.20	280.30	3877	6.45	19.24	279.26	3862	6.79	20.28	278.22	3848	7.14	21.32	277.18	3833
299	6.07	18.16	280.84	3884	6.42	19.20	279.80	3870	6.77	20.24	278.76	3855	7.12	21.27	277.73	3841
299.5	6.05	18.12	281.38	3891	6.40	19.16	280.34	3877	6.74	20.20	279.30	3863	7.09	21.23	278.27	3848
300	6.03	18.08	281.92	3899	6.37	19.12	280.88	3885	6.72	20.16	279.85	3870	7.06	21.19	278.81	3856
300.5	6.00	18.04	282.46	3906	6.35	19.08	281.42	3892	6.69	20.11	280.39	3878	7.04	21.15	279.35	3863
301	5.98	18.00	283.00	3914	6.32	19.04	281.96	3900	6.67	20.07	280.93	3885	7.01	21.11	279.89	3871
301.5	5.96	17.96	283.54	3921	6.30	18.99	282.51	3907	6.64	20.03	281.47	3893	6.99	21.07	280.43	3878
302	5.93	17.92	284.08	3929	6.28	18.95	283.05	3915	6.62	19.99	282.01	3900	6.96	21.03	280.97	3886
302.5	5.91	17.88	284.63	3936	6.25	18.91	283.59	3922	6.60	19.95	282.55	3908	6.94	20.99	281.51	3893
303	5.89	17.83	285.17	3944	6.23	18.87	284.13	3929	6.57	19.91	283.09	3915	6.91	20.95	282.05	3901
303.5	5.86	17.79	285.71	3951	6.20	18.83	284.67	3937	6.55	19.87	283.63	3923	6.89	20.91	282.59	3908
304	5.84	17.75	286.25	3959	6.18	18.79	285.21	3944	6.52	19.83	284.17	3930	6.86	20.86	283.14	3916
304.5	5.82	17.71	286.79	3966	6.16	18.75	285.75	3952	6.50	19.79	284.71	3938	6.84	20.82	283.68	3923
305	5.79	17.67	287.33	3974	6.13	18.71	286.29	3959	6.47	19.74	285.26	3945	6.81	20.78	284.22	3931
305.5	5.77	17.63	287.87	3981	6.11	18.67	286.83	3967	6.45	19.70	285.80	3953	6.79	20.74	284.76	3938
306	5.75	17.59	288.41	3989	6.09	18.63	287.37	3974	6.43	19.66	286.34	3960	6.76	20.70	285.30	3946
306.5	5.72	17.55	288.95	3996	6.06	18.58	287.92	3982	6.40	19.62	286.88	3968	6.74	20.66	285.84	3953
307	5.70	17.51	289.49	4004	6.04	18.54	288.46	3989	6.38	19.58	287.42	3975	6.72	20.62	286.38	3961
307.5	5.68	17.47	290.04	4011	6.02	18.50	289.00	3997	6.35	19.54	287.96	3982	6.69	20.58	286.92	3968
308	5.66	17.42	290.58	4019	5.99	18.46	289.54	4004	6.33	19.50	288.50	3990	6.67	20.54	287.46	3976
308.5	5.63	17.38	291.12	4026	5.97	18.42	290.08	4012	6.31	19.46	289.04	3997	6.64	20.50	288.00	3983
309	5.61	17.34	291.66	4034	5.95	18.38	290.62	4019	6.28	19.42	289.58	4005	6.62	20.45	288.55	3991
309.5	5.59	17.30	292.20	4041	5.93	18.34	291.16	4027	6.26	19.38	290.12	4012	6.60	20.41	289.09	3998
310	5.57	17.26	292.74	4049	5.90	18.30	291.70	4034	6.24	19.34	290.67	4020	6.57	20.37	289.63	4006
310.5	5.55	17.22	293.28	4056	5.88	18.26	292.24	4042	6.21	19.29	291.21	4027	6.55	20.33	290.17	4013
311	5.52	17.18	293.82	4064	5.86	18.22	292.78	4049	6.19	19.25	291.75	4035	6.52	20.29	290.71	4021
311.5	5.50	17.14	294.36	4071	5.83	18.17	293.33	4057	6.17	19.21	292.29	4042	6.50	20.25	291.25	4028

Body Composition MALE 280-311.5 Lb.

Weight: Lb.	Waist: 35 inches Fat: %	Fat: Lb.	LBM: Lb.	RMR: Cal.	35.25 inches Fat: %	Fat: Lb.	LBM: Lb.	RMR: Cal.	35.5 inches Fat: %	Fat: Lb.	LBM: Lb.	RMR: Cal.	35.75 inches Fat: %	Fat: Lb.	LBM: Lb.	RMR: Cal.
280	8.52	23.87	256.13	3542	8.90	24.91	255.09	3528	9.27	25.95	254.06	3514	9.64	26.98	253.02	3499
280.5	8.50	23.83	256.67	3550	8.87	24.87	255.63	3535	9.23	25.90	254.60	3521	9.60	26.94	253.56	3507
281	8.47	23.79	257.21	3557	8.83	24.83	256.17	3543	9.20	25.86	255.14	3529	9.57	26.90	254.10	3514
281.5	8.44	23.75	257.75	3565	8.80	24.78	256.72	3550	9.17	25.82	255.68	3536	9.54	26.86	254.64	3522
282	8.41	23.71	258.29	3572	8.77	24.74	257.26	3558	9.14	25.78	256.22	3544	9.51	26.82	255.18	3529
282.5	8.38	23.67	258.84	3580	8.74	24.70	257.80	3565	9.11	25.74	256.76	3551	9.48	26.78	255.72	3537
283	8.35	23.62	259.38	3587	8.71	24.66	258.34	3573	9.08	25.70	257.30	3558	9.45	26.74	256.26	3544
283.5	8.32	23.58	259.92	3595	8.68	24.62	258.88	3580	9.05	25.66	257.84	3566	9.42	26.70	256.80	3552
284	8.29	23.54	260.46	3602	8.65	24.58	259.42	3588	9.02	25.62	258.38	3573	9.39	26.65	257.35	3559
284.5	8.26	23.50	261.00	3610	8.63	24.54	259.96	3595	8.99	25.58	258.92	3581	9.35	26.61	257.89	3567
285	8.23	23.46	261.54	3617	8.60	24.50	260.50	3603	8.96	25.54	259.47	3588	9.32	26.57	258.43	3574
285.5	8.20	23.42	262.08	3625	8.57	24.46	261.04	3610	8.93	25.49	260.01	3596	9.29	26.53	258.97	3582
286	8.17	23.38	262.62	3632	8.54	24.42	261.58	3618	8.90	25.45	260.55	3603	9.26	26.49	259.51	3589
286.5	8.15	23.34	263.16	3640	8.51	24.37	262.13	3625	8.87	25.41	261.09	3611	9.23	26.45	260.05	3596
287	8.12	23.30	263.70	3647	8.48	24.33	262.67	3633	8.84	25.37	261.63	3618	9.20	26.41	260.59	3604
287.5	8.09	23.25	264.25	3655	8.45	24.29	263.21	3640	8.81	25.33	262.17	3626	9.17	26.37	261.13	3611
288	8.06	23.21	264.79	3662	8.42	24.25	263.75	3648	8.78	25.29	262.71	3633	9.14	26.33	261.67	3619
288.5	8.03	23.17	265.33	3669	8.39	24.21	264.29	3655	8.75	25.25	263.25	3641	9.11	26.29	262.21	3626
289	8.00	23.13	265.87	3677	8.36	24.17	264.83	3663	8.72	25.21	263.79	3648	9.08	26.24	262.76	3634
289.5	7.98	23.09	266.41	3684	8.33	24.13	265.37	3670	8.69	25.17	264.33	3656	9.05	26.20	263.30	3641
290	7.95	23.05	266.95	3692	8.31	24.09	265.91	3678	8.66	25.13	264.88	3663	9.02	26.16	263.84	3649
290.5	7.92	23.01	267.49	3699	8.28	24.05	266.45	3685	8.63	25.08	265.42	3671	8.99	26.12	264.38	3656
291	7.89	22.97	268.03	3707	8.25	24.01	266.99	3693	8.61	25.04	265.96	3678	8.96	26.08	264.92	3664
291.5	7.87	22.93	268.57	3714	8.22	23.96	267.54	3700	8.58	25.00	266.50	3686	8.93	26.04	265.46	3671
292	7.84	22.89	269.11	3722	8.19	23.92	268.08	3707	8.55	24.96	267.04	3693	8.90	26.00	266.00	3679
292.5	7.81	22.85	269.66	3729	8.16	23.88	268.62	3715	8.52	24.92	267.58	3701	8.87	25.96	266.54	3686
293	7.78	22.80	270.20	3737	8.14	23.84	269.16	3722	8.49	24.88	268.12	3708	8.85	25.92	267.08	3694
293.5	7.76	22.76	270.74	3744	8.11	23.80	269.70	3730	8.46	24.84	268.66	3716	8.82	25.88	267.62	3701
294	7.73	22.72	271.28	3752	8.08	23.76	270.24	3737	8.43	24.80	269.20	3723	8.79	25.83	268.17	3709
294.5	7.70	22.68	271.82	3759	8.05	23.72	270.78	3745	8.41	24.76	269.74	3731	8.76	25.79	268.71	3716
295	7.67	22.64	272.36	3767	8.03	23.68	271.32	3752	8.38	24.72	270.29	3738	8.73	25.75	269.25	3724
295.5	7.65	22.60	272.90	3774	8.00	23.64	271.86	3760	8.35	24.67	270.83	3746	8.70	25.71	269.79	3731
296	7.62	22.56	273.44	3782	7.97	23.60	272.40	3767	8.32	24.63	271.37	3753	8.67	25.67	270.33	3739
296.5	7.59	22.52	273.98	3789	7.94	23.55	272.95	3775	8.29	24.59	271.91	3760	8.64	25.63	270.87	3746
297	7.57	22.48	274.52	3797	7.92	23.51	273.49	3782	8.27	24.55	272.45	3768	8.62	25.59	271.41	3754
297.5	7.54	22.43	275.07	3804	7.89	23.47	274.03	3790	8.24	24.51	272.99	3775	8.59	25.55	271.95	3761
298	7.51	22.39	275.61	3812	7.86	23.43	274.57	3797	8.21	24.47	273.53	3783	8.56	25.51	272.49	3769
298.5	7.49	22.35	276.15	3819	7.84	23.39	275.11	3805	8.18	24.43	274.07	3790	8.53	25.47	273.03	3776
299	7.46	22.31	276.69	3827	7.81	23.35	275.65	3812	8.16	24.39	274.61	3798	8.50	25.42	273.58	3784
299.5	7.44	22.27	277.23	3834	7.78	23.31	276.19	3820	8.13	24.35	275.15	3805	8.48	25.38	274.12	3791
300	7.41	22.23	277.77	3842	7.76	23.27	276.73	3827	8.10	24.31	275.70	3813	8.45	25.34	274.66	3799
300.5	7.38	22.19	278.31	3849	7.73	23.23	277.27	3835	8.07	24.26	276.24	3820	8.42	25.30	275.20	3806
301	7.36	22.15	278.85	3857	7.70	23.19	277.81	3842	8.05	24.22	276.78	3828	8.39	25.26	275.74	3813
301.5	7.33	22.11	279.39	3864	7.68	23.14	278.36	3850	8.02	24.18	277.32	3835	8.36	25.22	276.28	3821
302	7.31	22.07	279.93	3871	7.65	23.10	278.90	3857	7.99	24.14	277.86	3843	8.34	25.18	276.82	3828
302.5	7.28	22.03	280.48	3879	7.62	23.06	279.44	3865	7.97	24.10	278.40	3850	8.31	25.14	277.36	3836
303	7.26	21.98	281.02	3886	7.60	23.02	279.98	3872	7.94	24.06	278.94	3858	8.28	25.10	277.90	3843
303.5	7.23	21.94	281.56	3894	7.57	22.98	280.52	3880	7.91	24.02	279.48	3865	8.26	25.06	278.44	3851
304	7.20	21.90	282.10	3901	7.55	22.94	281.06	3887	7.89	23.98	280.02	3873	8.23	25.01	278.99	3858
304.5	7.18	21.86	282.64	3909	7.52	22.90	281.60	3895	7.86	23.94	280.56	3880	8.20	24.97	279.53	3866
305	7.15	21.82	283.18	3916	7.49	22.86	282.14	3902	7.83	23.90	281.11	3888	8.17	24.93	280.07	3873
305.5	7.13	21.78	283.72	3924	7.47	22.82	282.68	3910	7.81	23.85	281.65	3895	8.15	24.89	280.61	3881
306	7.10	21.74	284.26	3931	7.44	22.78	283.22	3917	7.78	23.81	282.19	3903	8.12	24.85	281.15	3888
306.5	7.08	21.70	284.80	3939	7.42	22.73	283.77	3924	7.76	23.77	282.73	3910	8.09	24.81	281.69	3896
307	7.05	21.66	285.34	3946	7.39	22.69	284.31	3932	7.73	23.73	283.27	3918	8.07	24.77	282.23	3903
307.5	7.03	21.62	285.89	3954	7.37	22.65	284.85	3939	7.70	23.69	283.81	3925	8.04	24.73	282.77	3911
308	7.00	21.57	286.43	3961	7.34	22.61	285.39	3947	7.68	23.65	284.35	3933	8.02	24.69	283.31	3918
308.5	6.98	21.53	286.97	3969	7.32	22.57	285.93	3954	7.65	23.61	284.89	3940	7.99	24.65	283.85	3926
309	6.96	21.49	287.51	3976	7.29	22.53	286.47	3962	7.63	23.57	285.43	3948	7.96	24.60	284.40	3933
309.5	6.93	21.45	288.05	3984	7.27	22.49	287.01	3969	7.60	23.53	285.97	3955	7.94	24.56	284.94	3941
310	6.91	21.41	288.59	3991	7.24	22.45	287.55	3977	7.58	23.49	286.52	3963	7.91	24.52	285.48	3948
310.5	6.88	21.37	289.13	3999	7.22	22.41	288.09	3984	7.55	23.44	287.06	3970	7.88	24.48	286.02	3956
311	6.86	21.33	289.67	4006	7.19	22.37	288.63	3992	7.53	23.40	287.60	3977	7.86	24.44	286.56	3963
311.5	6.83	21.29	290.21	4014	7.17	22.32	289.18	3999	7.50	23.36	288.14	3985	7.83	24.40	287.10	3971

Body Composition   MALE   280-311.5 Lb.

Weight: Lb.	Waist: 36 inches Fat: %	Fat: Lb.	LBM: Lb.	RMR: Cal.	36.25 inches Fat: %	Fat: Lb.	LBM: Lb.	RMR: Cal.	36.5 inches Fat: %	Fat: Lb.	LBM: Lb.	RMR: Cal.	36.75 inches Fat: %	Fat: Lb.	LBM: Lb.	RMR: Cal.
280	10.01	28.02	251.98	3485	10.38	29.06	250.94	3471	10.75	30.10	249.91	3456	11.12	31.13	248.87	3442
280.5	9.97	27.98	252.52	3492	10.34	29.02	251.48	3478	10.71	30.05	250.45	3464	11.08	31.09	249.41	3449
281	9.94	27.94	253.06	3500	10.31	28.98	252.02	3485	10.68	30.01	250.99	3471	11.05	31.05	249.95	3457
281.5	9.91	27.90	253.60	3507	10.28	28.93	252.57	3493	10.65	29.97	251.53	3479	11.02	31.01	250.49	3464
282	9.88	27.86	254.14	3515	10.25	28.89	253.11	3500	10.61	29.93	252.07	3486	10.98	30.97	251.03	3472
282.5	9.85	27.82	254.69	3522	10.21	28.85	253.65	3508	10.58	29.89	252.61	3494	10.95	30.93	251.57	3479
283	9.81	27.77	255.23	3530	10.18	28.81	254.19	3515	10.55	29.85	253.15	3501	10.91	30.89	252.11	3487
283.5	9.78	27.73	255.77	3537	10.15	28.77	254.73	3523	10.51	29.81	253.69	3509	10.88	30.85	252.65	3494
284	9.75	27.69	256.31	3545	10.12	28.73	255.27	3530	10.48	29.77	254.23	3516	10.85	30.80	253.20	3502
284.5	9.72	27.65	256.85	3552	10.08	28.69	255.81	3538	10.45	29.73	254.77	3524	10.81	30.76	253.74	3509
285	9.69	27.61	257.39	3560	10.05	28.65	256.35	3545	10.42	29.69	255.32	3531	10.78	30.72	254.28	3517
285.5	9.66	27.57	257.93	3567	10.02	28.61	256.89	3553	10.38	29.64	255.86	3538	10.75	30.68	254.82	3524
286	9.63	27.53	258.47	3575	9.99	28.57	257.43	3560	10.35	29.60	256.40	3546	10.71	30.64	255.36	3532
286.5	9.59	27.49	259.01	3582	9.96	28.52	257.98	3568	10.32	29.56	256.94	3553	10.68	30.60	255.90	3539
287	9.56	27.45	259.55	3590	9.92	28.48	258.52	3575	10.29	29.52	257.48	3561	10.65	30.56	256.44	3547
287.5	9.53	27.41	260.10	3597	9.89	28.44	259.06	3583	10.25	29.48	258.02	3568	10.61	30.52	256.98	3554
288	9.50	27.36	260.64	3605	9.86	28.40	259.60	3590	10.22	29.44	258.56	3576	10.58	30.48	257.52	3562
288.5	9.47	27.32	261.18	3612	9.83	28.36	260.14	3598	10.19	29.40	259.10	3583	10.55	30.44	258.06	3569
289	9.44	27.28	261.72	3620	9.80	28.32	260.68	3605	10.16	29.36	259.64	3591	10.52	30.39	258.61	3577
289.5	9.41	27.24	262.26	3627	9.77	28.28	261.22	3613	10.13	29.32	260.18	3598	10.48	30.35	259.15	3584
290	9.38	27.20	262.80	3635	9.74	28.24	261.76	3620	10.09	29.28	260.73	3606	10.45	30.31	259.69	3591
290.5	9.35	27.16	263.34	3642	9.71	28.20	262.30	3628	10.06	29.23	261.27	3613	10.42	30.27	260.23	3599
291	9.32	27.12	263.88	3649	9.68	28.16	262.84	3635	10.03	29.19	261.81	3621	10.39	30.23	260.77	3606
291.5	9.29	27.08	264.42	3657	9.64	28.11	263.39	3643	10.00	29.15	262.35	3628	10.36	30.19	261.31	3614
292	9.26	27.04	264.96	3664	9.61	28.07	263.93	3650	9.97	29.11	262.89	3636	10.32	30.15	261.85	3621
292.5	9.23	27.00	265.51	3672	9.58	28.03	264.47	3658	9.94	29.07	263.43	3643	10.29	30.11	262.39	3629
293	9.20	26.95	266.05	3679	9.55	27.99	265.01	3665	9.91	29.03	263.97	3651	10.26	30.07	262.93	3636
293.5	9.17	26.91	266.59	3687	9.52	27.95	265.55	3673	9.88	28.99	264.51	3658	10.23	30.03	263.47	3644
294	9.14	26.87	267.13	3694	9.49	27.91	266.09	3680	9.85	28.95	265.05	3666	10.20	29.98	264.02	3651
294.5	9.11	26.83	267.67	3702	9.46	27.87	266.63	3688	9.82	28.91	265.59	3673	10.17	29.94	264.56	3659
295	9.08	26.79	268.21	3709	9.43	27.83	267.17	3695	9.78	28.87	266.14	3681	10.14	29.90	265.10	3666
295.5	9.05	26.75	268.75	3717	9.40	27.79	267.71	3702	9.75	28.82	266.68	3688	10.11	29.86	265.64	3674
296	9.02	26.71	269.29	3724	9.37	27.75	268.25	3710	9.72	28.78	267.22	3696	10.07	29.82	266.18	3681
296.5	8.99	26.67	269.83	3732	9.34	27.70	268.80	3717	9.69	28.74	267.76	3703	10.04	29.78	266.72	3689
297	8.96	26.63	270.37	3739	9.31	27.66	269.34	3725	9.66	28.70	268.30	3711	10.01	29.74	267.26	3696
297.5	8.94	26.59	270.92	3747	9.28	27.62	269.88	3732	9.63	28.66	268.84	3718	9.98	29.70	267.80	3704
298	8.91	26.54	271.46	3754	9.26	27.58	270.42	3740	9.60	28.62	269.38	3726	9.95	29.66	268.34	3711
298.5	8.88	26.50	272.00	3762	9.23	27.54	270.96	3747	9.57	28.58	269.92	3733	9.92	29.62	268.88	3719
299	8.85	26.46	272.54	3769	9.20	27.50	271.50	3755	9.54	28.54	270.46	3741	9.89	29.57	269.43	3726
299.5	8.82	26.42	273.08	3777	9.17	27.46	272.04	3762	9.51	28.50	271.00	3748	9.86	29.53	269.97	3734
300	8.79	26.38	273.62	3784	9.14	27.42	272.58	3770	9.48	28.46	271.55	3755	9.83	29.49	270.51	3741
300.5	8.77	26.34	274.16	3792	9.11	27.38	273.12	3777	9.46	28.41	272.09	3763	9.80	29.45	271.05	3749
301	8.74	26.30	274.70	3799	9.08	27.34	273.66	3785	9.43	28.37	272.63	3770	9.77	29.41	271.59	3756
301.5	8.71	26.26	275.24	3807	9.05	27.29	274.21	3792	9.40	28.33	273.17	3778	9.74	29.37	272.13	3764
302	8.68	26.22	275.78	3814	9.02	27.25	274.75	3800	9.37	28.29	273.71	3785	9.71	29.33	272.67	3771
302.5	8.65	26.18	276.33	3822	9.00	27.21	275.29	3807	9.34	28.25	274.25	3793	9.68	29.29	273.21	3779
303	8.63	26.13	276.87	3829	8.97	27.17	275.83	3815	9.31	28.21	274.79	3800	9.65	29.25	273.75	3786
303.5	8.60	26.09	277.41	3837	8.94	27.13	276.37	3822	9.28	28.17	275.33	3808	9.62	29.21	274.29	3793
304	8.57	26.05	277.95	3844	8.91	27.09	276.91	3830	9.25	28.13	275.87	3815	9.59	29.16	274.84	3801
304.5	8.54	26.01	278.49	3852	8.88	27.05	277.45	3837	9.22	28.09	276.41	3823	9.56	29.12	275.38	3808
305	8.51	25.97	279.03	3859	8.85	27.01	277.99	3845	9.20	28.05	276.96	3830	9.54	29.08	275.92	3816
305.5	8.49	25.93	279.57	3866	8.83	26.97	278.53	3852	9.17	28.00	277.50	3838	9.51	29.04	276.46	3823
306	8.46	25.89	280.11	3874	8.80	26.93	279.07	3860	9.14	27.96	278.04	3845	9.48	29.00	277.00	3831
306.5	8.43	25.85	280.65	3881	8.77	26.88	279.62	3867	9.11	27.92	278.58	3853	9.45	28.96	277.54	3838
307	8.41	25.81	281.19	3889	8.74	26.84	280.16	3875	9.08	27.88	279.12	3860	9.42	28.92	278.08	3846
307.5	8.38	25.77	281.74	3896	8.72	26.80	280.70	3882	9.05	27.84	279.66	3868	9.39	28.88	278.62	3853
308	8.35	25.72	282.28	3904	8.69	26.76	281.24	3890	9.03	27.80	280.20	3875	9.36	28.84	279.16	3861
308.5	8.33	25.68	282.82	3911	8.66	26.72	281.78	3897	9.00	27.76	280.74	3883	9.33	28.80	279.70	3868
309	8.30	25.64	283.36	3919	8.63	26.68	282.32	3904	8.97	27.72	281.28	3890	9.31	28.75	280.25	3876
309.5	8.27	25.60	283.90	3926	8.61	26.64	282.86	3912	8.94	27.68	281.82	3898	9.28	28.71	280.79	3883
310	8.25	25.56	284.44	3934	8.58	26.60	283.40	3919	8.91	27.64	282.37	3905	9.25	28.67	281.33	3891
310.5	8.22	25.52	284.98	3941	8.55	26.56	283.94	3927	8.89	27.59	282.91	3913	9.22	28.63	281.87	3898
311	8.19	25.48	285.52	3949	8.53	26.52	284.48	3934	8.86	27.55	283.45	3920	9.19	28.59	282.41	3906
311.5	8.17	25.44	286.06	3956	8.50	26.47	285.03	3942	8.83	27.51	283.99	3928	9.17	28.55	282.95	3913

Body Composition MALE 280-311.5 Lb.

Weight: Lb.	Waist: 37 inches				37.25 inches				37.5 inches				37.75 inches			
	Fat: %	Fat: Lb.	LBM: Lb.	RMR: Cal.	Fat: %	Fat: Lb.	LBM: Lb.	RMR: Cal.	Fat: %	Fat: Lb.	LBM: Lb.	RMR: Cal.	Fat: %	Fat: Lb.	LBM: Lb.	RMR: Cal.
280	11.49	32.17	247.83	3427	11.86	33.21	246.79	3413	12.23	34.24	245.76	3399	12.60	35.28	244.72	3384
280.5	11.45	32.13	248.37	3435	11.82	33.17	247.33	3421	12.19	34.20	246.30	3406	12.56	35.24	245.26	3392
281	11.42	32.09	248.91	3442	11.79	33.13	247.87	3428	12.16	34.16	246.84	3414	12.53	35.20	245.80	3399
281.5	11.38	32.05	249.45	3450	11.75	33.08	248.42	3436	12.12	34.12	247.38	3421	12.49	35.16	246.34	3407
282	11.35	32.01	249.99	3457	11.72	33.04	248.96	3443	12.09	34.08	247.92	3429	12.45	35.12	246.88	3414
282.5	11.32	31.97	250.54	3465	11.68	33.00	249.50	3451	12.05	34.04	248.46	3436	12.42	35.08	247.42	3422
283	11.28	31.92	251.08	3472	11.65	32.96	250.04	3458	12.01	34.00	249.00	3444	12.38	35.04	247.96	3429
283.5	11.25	31.88	251.62	3480	11.61	32.92	250.58	3466	11.98	33.96	249.54	3451	12.34	35.00	248.50	3437
284	11.21	31.84	252.16	3487	11.58	32.88	251.12	3473	11.94	33.92	250.08	3459	12.31	34.95	249.05	3444
284.5	11.18	31.80	252.70	3495	11.54	32.84	251.66	3480	11.91	33.88	250.62	3466	12.27	34.91	249.59	3452
285	11.14	31.76	253.24	3502	11.51	32.80	252.20	3488	11.87	33.84	251.17	3474	12.24	34.87	250.13	3459
285.5	11.11	31.72	253.78	3510	11.47	32.76	252.74	3495	11.84	33.79	251.71	3481	12.20	34.83	250.67	3467
286	11.08	31.68	254.32	3517	11.44	32.72	253.28	3503	11.80	33.75	252.25	3489	12.16	34.79	251.21	3474
286.5	11.04	31.64	254.86	3525	11.40	32.67	253.83	3510	11.77	33.71	252.79	3496	12.13	34.75	251.75	3482
287	11.01	31.60	255.40	3532	11.37	32.63	254.37	3518	11.73	33.67	253.33	3504	12.09	34.71	252.29	3489
287.5	10.98	31.55	255.95	3540	11.34	32.59	254.91	3525	11.70	33.63	253.87	3511	12.06	34.67	252.83	3497
288	10.94	31.51	256.49	3547	11.30	32.55	255.45	3533	11.66	33.59	254.41	3519	12.02	34.63	253.37	3504
288.5	10.91	31.47	257.03	3555	11.27	32.51	255.99	3540	11.63	33.55	254.95	3526	11.99	34.59	253.91	3512
289	10.88	31.43	257.57	3562	11.24	32.47	256.53	3548	11.59	33.51	255.49	3533	11.95	34.54	254.46	3519
289.5	10.84	31.39	258.11	3570	11.20	32.43	257.07	3555	11.56	33.47	256.03	3541	11.92	34.50	255.00	3527
290	10.81	31.35	258.65	3577	11.17	32.39	257.61	3563	11.53	33.43	256.58	3548	11.88	34.46	255.54	3534
290.5	10.78	31.31	259.19	3585	11.13	32.35	258.15	3570	11.49	33.38	257.12	3556	11.85	34.42	256.08	3542
291	10.75	31.27	259.73	3592	11.10	32.31	258.69	3578	11.46	33.34	257.66	3563	11.81	34.38	256.62	3549
291.5	10.71	31.23	260.27	3600	11.07	32.26	259.24	3585	11.42	33.30	258.20	3571	11.78	34.34	257.16	3557
292	10.68	31.19	260.81	3607	11.04	32.22	259.78	3593	11.39	33.26	258.74	3578	11.75	34.30	257.70	3564
292.5	10.65	31.15	261.36	3615	11.00	32.18	260.32	3600	11.36	33.22	259.28	3586	11.71	34.26	258.24	3571
293	10.62	31.10	261.90	3622	10.97	32.14	260.86	3608	11.32	33.18	259.82	3593	11.68	34.22	258.78	3579
293.5	10.58	31.06	262.44	3630	10.94	32.10	261.40	3615	11.29	33.14	260.36	3601	11.64	34.18	259.32	3586
294	10.55	31.02	262.98	3637	10.90	32.06	261.94	3623	11.26	33.10	260.90	3608	11.61	34.13	259.87	3594
294.5	10.52	30.98	263.52	3644	10.87	32.02	262.48	3630	11.22	33.06	261.44	3616	11.58	34.09	260.41	3601
295	10.49	30.94	264.06	3652	10.84	31.98	263.02	3638	11.19	33.02	261.99	3623	11.54	34.05	260.95	3609
295.5	10.46	30.90	264.60	3659	10.81	31.94	263.56	3645	11.16	32.97	262.53	3631	11.51	34.01	261.49	3616
296	10.43	30.86	265.14	3667	10.78	31.90	264.10	3653	11.13	32.93	263.07	3638	11.48	33.97	262.03	3624
296.5	10.39	30.82	265.68	3674	10.74	31.85	264.65	3660	11.09	32.89	263.61	3646	11.44	33.93	262.57	3631
297	10.36	30.78	266.22	3682	10.71	31.81	265.19	3668	11.06	32.85	264.15	3653	11.41	33.89	263.11	3639
297.5	10.33	30.74	266.77	3689	10.68	31.77	265.73	3675	11.03	32.81	264.69	3661	11.38	33.85	263.65	3646
298	10.30	30.69	267.31	3697	10.65	31.73	266.27	3682	11.00	32.77	265.23	3668	11.34	33.81	264.19	3654
298.5	10.27	30.65	267.85	3704	10.62	31.69	266.81	3690	10.96	32.73	265.77	3676	11.31	33.77	264.73	3661
299	10.24	30.61	268.39	3712	10.59	31.65	267.35	3697	10.93	32.69	266.31	3683	11.28	33.72	265.28	3669
299.5	10.21	30.57	268.93	3719	10.55	31.61	267.89	3705	10.90	32.65	266.85	3691	11.25	33.68	265.82	3676
300	10.18	30.53	269.47	3727	10.52	31.57	268.43	3712	10.87	32.61	267.40	3698	11.21	33.64	266.36	3684
300.5	10.15	30.49	270.01	3734	10.49	31.53	268.97	3720	10.84	32.56	267.94	3706	11.18	33.60	266.90	3691
301	10.12	30.45	270.55	3742	10.46	31.49	269.51	3727	10.80	32.52	268.48	3713	11.15	33.56	267.44	3699
301.5	10.09	30.41	271.09	3749	10.43	31.44	270.06	3735	10.77	32.48	269.02	3721	11.12	33.52	267.98	3706
302	10.05	30.37	271.63	3757	10.40	31.40	270.60	3742	10.74	32.44	269.56	3728	11.09	33.48	268.52	3714
302.5	10.02	30.33	272.18	3764	10.37	31.36	271.14	3750	10.71	32.40	270.10	3735	11.05	33.44	269.06	3721
303	9.99	30.28	272.72	3772	10.34	31.32	271.68	3757	10.68	32.36	270.64	3743	11.02	33.40	269.60	3729
303.5	9.96	30.24	273.26	3779	10.31	31.28	272.22	3765	10.65	32.32	271.18	3750	10.99	33.36	270.14	3736
304	9.93	30.20	273.80	3787	10.28	31.24	272.76	3772	10.62	32.28	271.72	3758	10.96	33.31	270.69	3744
304.5	9.91	30.16	274.34	3794	10.25	31.20	273.30	3780	10.59	32.24	272.26	3765	10.93	33.27	271.23	3751
305	9.88	30.12	274.88	3802	10.22	31.16	273.84	3787	10.56	32.19	272.81	3773	10.90	33.23	271.77	3759
305.5	9.85	30.08	275.42	3809	10.19	31.12	274.38	3795	10.53	32.15	273.35	3780	10.86	33.19	272.31	3766
306	9.82	30.04	275.96	3817	10.16	31.08	274.92	3802	10.49	32.11	273.89	3788	10.83	33.15	272.85	3774
306.5	9.79	30.00	276.50	3824	10.13	31.03	275.47	3810	10.46	32.07	274.43	3795	10.80	33.11	273.39	3781
307	9.76	29.96	277.04	3832	10.10	30.99	276.01	3817	10.43	32.03	274.97	3803	10.77	33.07	273.93	3788
307.5	9.73	29.92	277.59	3839	10.07	30.95	276.55	3825	10.40	31.99	275.51	3810	10.74	33.03	274.47	3796
308	9.70	29.87	278.13	3846	10.04	30.91	277.09	3832	10.37	31.95	276.05	3818	10.71	32.99	275.01	3803
308.5	9.67	29.83	278.67	3854	10.01	30.87	277.63	3840	10.34	31.91	276.59	3825	10.68	32.95	275.55	3811
309	9.64	29.79	279.21	3861	9.98	30.83	278.17	3847	10.31	31.87	277.13	3833	10.65	32.90	276.10	3818
309.5	9.61	29.75	279.75	3869	9.95	30.79	278.71	3855	10.28	31.83	277.67	3840	10.62	32.86	276.64	3826
310	9.58	29.71	280.29	3876	9.92	30.75	279.25	3862	10.25	31.79	278.22	3848	10.59	32.82	277.18	3833
310.5	9.56	29.67	280.83	3884	9.89	30.71	279.79	3870	10.22	31.74	278.76	3855	10.56	32.78	277.72	3841
311	9.53	29.63	281.37	3891	9.86	30.67	280.33	3877	10.19	31.70	279.30	3863	10.53	32.74	278.26	3848
311.5	9.50	29.59	281.91	3899	9.83	30.62	280.88	3885	10.16	31.66	279.84	3870	10.50	32.70	278.80	3856

Body Composition MALE 280-311.5 Lb.

Weight: Lb.	Waist: 38 inches				38.25 inches				38.5 inches				38.75 inches			
	Fat: %	Fat: Lb.	LBM: Lb.	RMR: Cal.	Fat: %	Fat: Lb.	LBM: Lb.	RMR: Cal.	Fat: %	Fat: Lb.	LBM: Lb.	RMR: Cal.	Fat: %	Fat: Lb.	LBM: Lb.	RMR: Cal.
280	12.97	36.32	243.68	3370	13.34	37.36	242.64	3356	13.71	38.40	241.61	3341	14.08	39.43	240.57	3327
280.5	12.93	36.28	244.22	3378	13.30	37.32	243.18	3363	13.67	38.35	242.15	3349	14.04	39.39	241.11	3335
281	12.90	36.24	244.76	3385	13.27	37.28	243.72	3371	13.63	38.31	242.69	3356	14.00	39.35	241.65	3342
281.5	12.86	36.20	245.30	3393	13.23	37.23	244.27	3378	13.60	38.27	243.23	3364	13.96	39.31	242.19	3349
282	12.82	36.16	245.84	3400	13.19	37.19	244.81	3386	13.56	38.23	243.77	3371	13.93	39.27	242.73	3357
282.5	12.78	36.12	246.39	3408	13.15	37.15	245.35	3393	13.52	38.19	244.31	3379	13.89	39.23	243.27	3364
283	12.75	36.07	246.93	3415	13.11	37.11	245.89	3401	13.48	38.15	244.85	3386	13.85	39.19	243.81	3372
283.5	12.71	36.03	247.47	3422	13.08	37.07	246.43	3408	13.44	38.11	245.39	3394	13.81	39.15	244.35	3379
284	12.67	35.99	248.01	3430	13.04	37.03	246.97	3416	13.40	38.07	245.93	3401	13.77	39.10	244.90	3387
284.5	12.64	35.95	248.55	3437	13.00	36.99	247.51	3423	13.37	38.03	246.47	3409	13.73	39.06	245.44	3394
285	12.60	35.91	249.09	3445	12.96	36.95	248.05	3431	13.33	37.99	247.02	3416	13.69	39.02	245.98	3402
285.5	12.56	35.87	249.63	3452	12.93	36.91	248.59	3438	13.29	37.94	247.56	3424	13.65	38.98	246.52	3409
286	12.53	35.83	250.17	3460	12.89	36.87	249.13	3446	13.25	37.90	248.10	3431	13.62	38.94	247.06	3417
286.5	12.49	35.79	250.71	3467	12.85	36.82	249.68	3453	13.22	37.86	248.64	3439	13.58	38.90	247.60	3424
287	12.46	35.75	251.25	3475	12.82	36.78	250.22	3460	13.18	37.82	249.18	3446	13.54	38.86	248.14	3432
287.5	12.42	35.71	251.80	3482	12.78	36.74	250.76	3468	13.14	37.78	249.72	3454	13.50	38.82	248.68	3439
288	12.38	35.66	252.34	3490	12.74	36.70	251.30	3475	13.10	37.74	250.26	3461	13.46	38.78	249.22	3447
288.5	12.35	35.62	252.88	3497	12.71	36.66	251.84	3483	13.07	37.70	250.80	3469	13.43	38.74	249.76	3454
289	12.31	35.58	253.42	3505	12.67	36.62	252.38	3490	13.03	37.66	251.34	3476	13.39	38.69	250.31	3462
289.5	12.28	35.54	253.96	3512	12.64	36.58	252.92	3498	12.99	37.62	251.88	3484	13.35	38.65	250.85	3469
290	12.24	35.50	254.50	3520	12.60	36.54	253.46	3505	12.96	37.58	252.43	3491	13.31	38.61	251.39	3477
290.5	12.21	35.46	255.04	3527	12.56	36.50	254.00	3513	12.92	37.53	252.97	3499	13.28	38.57	251.93	3484
291	12.17	35.42	255.58	3535	12.53	36.46	254.54	3520	12.88	37.49	253.51	3506	13.24	38.53	252.47	3492
291.5	12.14	35.38	256.12	3542	12.49	36.41	255.09	3528	12.85	37.45	254.05	3513	13.20	38.49	253.01	3499
292	12.10	35.34	256.66	3550	12.46	36.37	255.63	3535	12.81	37.41	254.59	3521	13.17	38.45	253.55	3507
292.5	12.07	35.30	257.21	3557	12.42	36.33	256.17	3543	12.78	37.37	255.13	3528	13.13	38.41	254.09	3514
293	12.03	35.25	257.75	3565	12.39	36.29	256.71	3550	12.74	37.33	255.67	3536	13.09	38.37	254.63	3522
293.5	12.00	35.21	258.29	3572	12.35	36.25	257.25	3558	12.70	37.29	256.21	3543	13.06	38.33	255.17	3529
294	11.96	35.17	258.83	3580	12.32	36.21	257.79	3565	12.67	37.25	256.75	3551	13.02	38.28	255.72	3537
294.5	11.93	35.13	259.37	3587	12.28	36.17	258.33	3573	12.63	37.21	257.29	3558	12.99	38.24	256.26	3544
295	11.89	35.09	259.91	3595	12.25	36.13	258.87	3580	12.60	37.17	257.84	3566	12.95	38.20	256.80	3552
295.5	11.86	35.05	260.45	3602	12.21	36.09	259.41	3588	12.56	37.12	258.38	3573	12.91	38.16	257.34	3559
296	11.83	35.01	260.99	3610	12.18	36.05	259.95	3595	12.53	37.08	258.92	3581	12.88	38.12	257.88	3566
296.5	11.79	34.97	261.53	3617	12.14	36.00	260.50	3603	12.49	37.04	259.46	3588	12.84	38.08	258.42	3574
297	11.76	34.93	262.07	3624	12.11	35.96	261.04	3610	12.46	37.00	260.00	3596	12.81	38.04	258.96	3581
297.5	11.73	34.89	262.62	3632	12.07	35.92	261.58	3618	12.42	36.96	260.54	3603	12.77	38.00	259.50	3589
298	11.69	34.84	263.16	3639	12.04	35.88	262.12	3625	12.39	36.92	261.08	3611	12.74	37.96	260.04	3596
298.5	11.66	34.80	263.70	3647	12.01	35.84	262.66	3633	12.35	36.88	261.62	3618	12.70	37.92	260.58	3604
299	11.63	34.76	264.24	3654	11.97	35.80	263.20	3640	12.32	36.84	262.16	3626	12.67	37.87	261.13	3611
299.5	11.59	34.72	264.78	3662	11.94	35.76	263.74	3648	12.29	36.80	262.70	3633	12.63	37.83	261.67	3619
300	11.56	34.68	265.32	3669	11.91	35.72	264.28	3655	12.25	36.76	263.25	3641	12.60	37.79	262.21	3626
300.5	11.53	34.64	265.86	3677	11.87	35.68	264.82	3663	12.22	36.71	263.79	3648	12.56	37.75	262.75	3634
301	11.49	34.60	266.40	3684	11.84	35.64	265.36	3670	12.18	36.67	264.33	3656	12.53	37.71	263.29	3641
301.5	11.46	34.56	266.94	3692	11.81	35.59	265.91	3677	12.15	36.63	264.87	3663	12.49	37.67	263.83	3649
302	11.43	34.52	267.48	3699	11.77	35.55	266.45	3685	12.12	36.59	265.41	3671	12.46	37.63	264.37	3656
302.5	11.40	34.48	268.03	3707	11.74	35.51	266.99	3692	12.08	36.55	265.95	3678	12.43	37.59	264.91	3664
303	11.36	34.43	268.57	3714	11.71	35.47	267.53	3700	12.05	36.51	266.49	3686	12.39	37.55	265.45	3671
303.5	11.33	34.39	269.11	3722	11.67	35.43	268.07	3707	12.02	36.47	267.03	3693	12.36	37.51	265.99	3679
304	11.30	34.35	269.65	3729	11.64	35.39	268.61	3715	11.98	36.43	267.57	3701	12.32	37.46	266.54	3686
304.5	11.27	34.31	270.19	3737	11.61	35.35	269.15	3722	11.95	36.39	268.11	3708	12.29	37.42	267.08	3694
305	11.24	34.27	270.73	3744	11.58	35.31	269.69	3730	11.92	36.35	268.66	3715	12.26	37.38	267.62	3701
305.5	11.20	34.23	271.27	3752	11.54	35.27	270.23	3737	11.88	36.30	269.20	3723	12.22	37.34	268.16	3709
306	11.17	34.19	271.81	3759	11.51	35.23	270.77	3745	11.85	36.26	269.74	3730	12.19	37.30	268.70	3716
306.5	11.14	34.15	272.35	3767	11.48	35.18	271.32	3752	11.82	36.22	270.28	3738	12.16	37.26	269.24	3724
307	11.11	34.11	272.89	3774	11.45	35.14	271.86	3760	11.79	36.18	270.82	3745	12.12	37.22	269.78	3731
307.5	11.08	34.07	273.44	3782	11.42	35.10	272.40	3767	11.75	36.14	271.36	3753	12.09	37.18	270.32	3739
308	11.05	34.02	273.98	3789	11.38	35.06	272.94	3775	11.72	36.10	271.90	3760	12.06	37.14	270.86	3746
308.5	11.02	33.98	274.52	3797	11.35	35.02	273.48	3782	11.69	36.06	272.44	3768	12.02	37.10	271.40	3754
309	10.98	33.94	275.06	3804	11.32	34.98	274.02	3790	11.66	36.02	272.98	3775	11.99	37.05	271.95	3761
309.5	10.95	33.90	275.60	3812	11.29	34.94	274.56	3797	11.62	35.98	273.52	3783	11.96	37.01	272.49	3768
310	10.92	33.86	276.14	3819	11.26	34.90	275.10	3805	11.59	35.94	274.07	3790	11.93	36.97	273.03	3776
310.5	10.89	33.82	276.68	3826	11.23	34.86	275.64	3812	11.56	35.89	274.61	3798	11.89	36.93	273.57	3783
311	10.86	33.78	277.22	3834	11.19	34.82	276.18	3820	11.53	35.85	275.15	3805	11.86	36.89	274.11	3791
311.5	10.83	33.74	277.76	3841	11.16	34.77	276.73	3827	11.50	35.81	275.69	3813	11.83	36.85	274.65	3798

Body Composition   MALE   280-311.5 Lb.

Weight: Lb.	Waist: 39 inches Fat: %	Fat: Lb.	LBM: Lb.	RMR: Cal.	39.25 inches Fat: %	Fat: Lb.	LBM: Lb.	RMR: Cal.	39.5 inches Fat: %	Fat: Lb.	LBM: Lb.	RMR: Cal.	39.75 inches Fat: %	Fat: Lb.	LBM: Lb.	RMR: Cal.
280	14.45	40.47	239.53	3313	14.82	41.51	238.49	3298	15.19	42.55	237.46	3284	15.57	43.58	236.42	3270
280.5	14.41	40.43	240.07	3320	14.78	41.47	239.03	3306	15.15	42.50	238.00	3291	15.52	43.54	236.96	3277
281	14.37	40.39	240.61	3328	14.74	41.43	239.57	3313	15.11	42.46	238.54	3299	15.48	43.50	237.50	3285
281.5	14.33	40.35	241.15	3335	14.70	41.38	240.12	3321	15.07	42.42	239.08	3306	15.44	43.46	238.04	3292
282	14.29	40.31	241.69	3343	14.66	41.34	240.66	3328	15.03	42.38	239.62	3314	15.40	43.42	238.58	3300
282.5	14.25	40.27	242.24	3350	14.62	41.30	241.20	3336	14.99	42.34	240.16	3321	15.35	43.38	239.12	3307
283	14.21	40.22	242.78	3358	14.58	41.26	241.74	3343	14.95	42.30	240.70	3329	15.31	43.34	239.66	3315
283.5	14.17	40.18	243.32	3365	14.54	41.22	242.28	3351	14.91	42.26	241.24	3336	15.27	43.30	240.20	3322
284	14.13	40.14	243.86	3373	14.50	41.18	242.82	3358	14.87	42.22	241.78	3344	15.23	43.25	240.75	3330
284.5	14.10	40.10	244.40	3380	14.46	41.14	243.36	3366	14.82	42.18	242.32	3351	15.19	43.21	241.29	3337
285	14.06	40.06	244.94	3388	14.42	41.10	243.90	3373	14.78	42.14	242.87	3359	15.15	43.17	241.83	3344
285.5	14.02	40.02	245.48	3395	14.38	41.06	244.44	3381	14.74	42.09	243.41	3366	15.11	43.13	242.37	3352
286	13.98	39.98	246.02	3402	14.34	41.02	244.98	3388	14.70	42.05	243.95	3374	15.07	43.09	242.91	3359
286.5	13.94	39.94	246.56	3410	14.30	40.97	245.53	3396	14.66	42.01	244.49	3381	15.03	43.05	243.45	3367
287	13.90	39.90	247.10	3417	14.26	40.93	246.07	3403	14.62	41.97	245.03	3389	14.99	43.01	243.99	3374
287.5	13.86	39.86	247.65	3425	14.22	40.89	246.61	3411	14.58	41.93	245.57	3396	14.95	42.97	244.53	3382
288	13.82	39.81	248.19	3432	14.18	40.85	247.15	3418	14.54	41.89	246.11	3404	14.91	42.93	245.07	3389
288.5	13.79	39.77	248.73	3440	14.15	40.81	247.69	3426	14.51	41.85	246.65	3411	14.86	42.89	245.61	3397
289	13.75	39.73	249.27	3447	14.11	40.77	248.23	3433	14.47	41.81	247.19	3419	14.83	42.84	246.16	3404
289.5	13.71	39.69	249.81	3455	14.07	40.73	248.77	3441	14.43	41.77	247.73	3426	14.79	42.80	246.70	3412
290	13.67	39.65	250.35	3462	14.03	40.69	249.31	3448	14.39	41.73	248.28	3434	14.75	42.76	247.24	3419
290.5	13.63	39.61	250.89	3470	13.99	40.65	249.85	3455	14.35	41.68	248.82	3441	14.71	42.72	247.78	3427
291	13.60	39.57	251.43	3477	13.95	40.61	250.39	3463	14.31	41.64	249.36	3449	14.67	42.68	248.32	3434
291.5	13.56	39.53	251.97	3485	13.92	40.56	250.94	3470	14.27	41.60	249.90	3456	14.63	42.64	248.86	3442
292	13.52	39.49	252.51	3492	13.88	40.52	251.48	3478	14.23	41.56	250.44	3464	14.59	42.60	249.40	3449
292.5	13.49	39.45	253.06	3500	13.84	40.48	252.02	3485	14.19	41.52	250.98	3471	14.55	42.56	249.94	3457
293	13.45	39.40	253.60	3507	13.80	40.44	252.56	3493	14.16	41.48	251.52	3479	14.51	42.52	250.48	3464
293.5	13.41	39.36	254.14	3515	13.77	40.40	253.10	3500	14.12	41.44	252.06	3486	14.47	42.48	251.02	3472
294	13.37	39.32	254.68	3522	13.73	40.36	253.64	3508	14.08	41.40	252.60	3493	14.43	42.43	251.57	3479
294.5	13.34	39.28	255.22	3530	13.69	40.32	254.18	3515	14.04	41.36	253.14	3501	14.40	42.39	252.11	3487
295	13.30	39.24	255.76	3537	13.65	40.28	254.72	3523	14.01	41.32	253.69	3508	14.36	42.35	252.65	3494
295.5	13.27	39.20	256.30	3545	13.62	40.24	255.26	3530	13.97	41.27	254.23	3516	14.32	42.31	253.19	3502
296	13.23	39.16	256.84	3552	13.58	40.20	255.80	3538	13.93	41.23	254.77	3523	14.28	42.27	253.73	3509
296.5	13.19	39.12	257.38	3560	13.54	40.15	256.35	3545	13.89	41.19	255.31	3531	14.24	42.23	254.27	3517
297	13.16	39.08	257.92	3567	13.51	40.11	256.89	3553	13.86	41.15	255.85	3538	14.20	42.19	254.81	3524
297.5	13.12	39.04	258.47	3575	13.47	40.07	257.43	3560	13.82	41.11	256.39	3546	14.17	42.15	255.35	3532
298	13.09	38.99	259.01	3582	13.43	40.03	257.97	3568	13.78	41.07	256.93	3553	14.13	42.11	255.89	3539
298.5	13.05	38.95	259.55	3590	13.40	39.99	258.51	3575	13.74	41.03	257.47	3561	14.09	42.07	256.43	3546
299	13.01	38.91	260.09	3597	13.36	39.95	259.05	3583	13.71	40.99	258.01	3568	14.06	42.02	256.98	3554
299.5	12.98	38.87	260.63	3604	13.33	39.91	259.59	3590	13.67	40.95	258.55	3576	14.02	41.98	257.52	3561
300	12.94	38.83	261.17	3612	13.29	39.87	260.13	3598	13.64	40.91	259.10	3583	13.98	41.94	258.06	3569
300.5	12.91	38.79	261.71	3619	13.25	39.83	260.67	3605	13.60	40.86	259.64	3591	13.94	41.90	258.60	3576
301	12.87	38.75	262.25	3627	13.22	39.79	261.21	3613	13.56	40.82	260.18	3598	13.91	41.86	259.14	3584
301.5	12.84	38.71	262.79	3634	13.18	39.74	261.76	3620	13.53	40.78	260.72	3606	13.87	41.82	259.68	3591
302	12.80	38.67	263.33	3642	13.15	39.70	262.30	3628	13.49	40.74	261.26	3613	13.83	41.78	260.22	3599
302.5	12.77	38.63	263.88	3649	13.11	39.66	262.84	3635	13.45	40.70	261.80	3621	13.80	41.74	260.76	3606
303	12.73	38.58	264.42	3657	13.08	39.62	263.38	3643	13.42	40.66	262.34	3628	13.76	41.70	261.30	3614
303.5	12.70	38.54	264.96	3664	13.04	39.58	263.92	3650	13.38	40.62	262.88	3636	13.73	41.66	261.84	3621
304	12.67	38.50	265.50	3672	13.01	39.54	264.46	3657	13.35	40.58	263.42	3643	13.69	41.61	262.39	3629
304.5	12.63	38.46	266.04	3679	12.97	39.50	265.00	3665	13.31	40.54	263.96	3651	13.65	41.57	262.93	3636
305	12.60	38.42	266.58	3687	12.94	39.46	265.54	3672	13.28	40.49	264.51	3658	13.62	41.53	263.47	3644
305.5	12.56	38.38	267.12	3694	12.90	39.42	266.08	3680	13.24	40.45	265.05	3666	13.58	41.49	264.01	3651
306	12.53	38.34	267.66	3702	12.87	39.38	266.62	3687	13.21	40.41	265.59	3673	13.55	41.45	264.55	3659
306.5	12.49	38.30	268.20	3709	12.83	39.33	267.17	3695	13.17	40.37	266.13	3681	13.51	41.41	265.09	3666
307	12.46	38.26	268.74	3717	12.80	39.29	267.71	3702	13.14	40.33	266.67	3688	13.48	41.37	265.63	3674
307.5	12.43	38.22	269.29	3724	12.77	39.25	268.25	3710	13.10	40.29	267.21	3696	13.44	41.33	266.17	3681
308	12.39	38.17	269.83	3732	12.73	39.21	268.79	3717	13.07	40.25	267.75	3703	13.40	41.29	266.71	3689
308.5	12.36	38.13	270.37	3739	12.70	39.17	269.33	3725	13.03	40.21	268.29	3710	13.37	41.25	267.25	3696
309	12.33	38.09	270.91	3747	12.66	39.13	269.87	3732	13.00	40.17	268.83	3718	13.33	41.20	267.80	3704
309.5	12.29	38.05	271.45	3754	12.63	39.09	270.41	3740	12.96	40.13	269.37	3725	13.30	41.16	268.34	3711
310	12.26	38.01	271.99	3762	12.60	39.05	270.95	3747	12.93	40.09	269.92	3733	13.27	41.12	268.88	3719
310.5	12.23	37.97	272.53	3769	12.56	39.01	271.49	3755	12.90	40.04	270.46	3740	13.23	41.08	269.42	3726
311	12.20	37.93	273.07	3777	12.53	38.97	272.03	3762	12.86	40.00	271.00	3748	13.20	41.04	269.96	3734
311.5	12.16	37.89	273.61	3784	12.50	38.92	272.58	3770	12.83	39.96	271.54	3755	13.16	41.00	270.50	3741

Body Composition MALE 280-311.5 Lb.

Weight: Lb.	Waist: 40 inches Fat: %	Fat: Lb.	LBM: Lb.	RMR: Cal.	40.25 inches Fat: %	Fat: Lb.	LBM: Lb.	RMR: Cal.	40.5 inches Fat: %	Fat: Lb.	LBM: Lb.	RMR: Cal.	40.75 inches Fat: %	Fat: Lb.	LBM: Lb.	RMR: Cal.
280	15.94	44.62	235.38	3255	16.31	45.66	234.34	3241	16.68	46.70	233.31	3227	17.05	47.73	232.27	3212
280.5	15.89	44.58	235.92	3263	16.26	45.62	234.88	3248	16.63	46.65	233.85	3234	17.00	47.69	232.81	3220
281	15.85	44.54	236.46	3270	16.22	45.58	235.42	3256	16.59	46.61	234.39	3242	16.96	47.65	233.35	3227
281.5	15.81	44.50	237.00	3278	16.18	45.53	235.97	3263	16.54	46.57	234.93	3249	16.91	47.61	233.89	3235
282	15.76	44.46	237.54	3285	16.13	45.49	236.51	3271	16.50	46.53	235.47	3257	16.87	47.57	234.43	3242
282.5	15.72	44.42	238.09	3293	16.09	45.45	237.05	3278	16.46	46.49	236.01	3264	16.82	47.53	234.97	3250
283	15.68	44.37	238.63	3300	16.05	45.41	237.59	3286	16.41	46.45	236.55	3272	16.78	47.49	235.51	3257
283.5	15.64	44.33	239.17	3308	16.00	45.37	238.13	3293	16.37	46.41	237.09	3279	16.74	47.45	236.05	3265
284	15.60	44.29	239.71	3315	15.96	45.33	238.67	3301	16.33	46.37	237.63	3286	16.69	47.40	236.60	3272
284.5	15.55	44.25	240.25	3323	15.92	45.29	239.21	3308	16.28	46.33	238.17	3294	16.65	47.36	237.14	3280
285	15.51	44.21	240.79	3330	15.88	45.25	239.75	3316	16.24	46.29	238.72	3301	16.60	47.32	237.68	3287
285.5	15.47	44.17	241.33	3338	15.83	45.21	240.29	3323	16.20	46.24	239.26	3309	16.56	47.28	238.22	3295
286	15.43	44.13	241.87	3345	15.79	45.17	240.83	3331	16.15	46.20	239.80	3316	16.52	47.24	238.76	3302
286.5	15.39	44.09	242.41	3353	15.75	45.12	241.38	3338	16.11	46.16	240.34	3324	16.47	47.20	239.30	3310
287	15.35	44.05	242.95	3360	15.71	45.08	241.92	3346	16.07	46.12	240.88	3331	16.43	47.16	239.84	3317
287.5	15.31	44.01	243.50	3368	15.67	45.04	242.46	3353	16.03	46.08	241.42	3339	16.39	47.12	240.38	3324
288	15.27	43.96	244.04	3375	15.63	45.00	243.00	3361	15.99	46.04	241.96	3346	16.35	47.08	240.92	3332
288.5	15.22	43.92	244.58	3382	15.58	44.96	243.54	3368	15.94	46.00	242.50	3354	16.30	47.04	241.46	3339
289	15.18	43.88	245.12	3390	15.54	44.92	244.08	3376	15.90	45.96	243.04	3361	16.26	46.99	242.01	3347
289.5	15.14	43.84	245.66	3397	15.50	44.88	244.62	3383	15.86	45.92	243.58	3369	16.22	46.95	242.55	3354
290	15.10	43.80	246.20	3405	15.46	44.84	245.16	3391	15.82	45.88	244.13	3376	16.18	46.91	243.09	3362
290.5	15.06	43.76	246.74	3412	15.42	44.80	245.70	3398	15.78	45.83	244.67	3384	16.13	46.87	243.63	3369
291	15.02	43.72	247.28	3420	15.38	44.76	246.24	3406	15.74	45.79	245.21	3391	16.09	46.83	244.17	3377
291.5	14.98	43.68	247.82	3427	15.34	44.71	246.79	3413	15.70	45.75	245.75	3399	16.05	46.79	244.71	3384
292	14.94	43.64	248.36	3435	15.30	44.67	247.33	3421	15.65	45.71	246.29	3406	16.01	46.75	245.25	3392
292.5	14.90	43.60	248.91	3442	15.26	44.63	247.87	3428	15.61	45.67	246.83	3414	15.97	46.71	245.79	3399
293	14.86	43.55	249.45	3450	15.22	44.59	248.41	3435	15.57	45.63	247.37	3421	15.93	46.67	246.33	3407
293.5	14.83	43.51	249.99	3457	15.18	44.55	248.95	3443	15.53	45.59	247.91	3429	15.89	46.63	246.87	3414
294	14.79	43.47	250.53	3465	15.14	44.51	249.49	3450	15.49	45.55	248.45	3436	15.85	46.58	247.42	3422
294.5	14.75	43.43	251.07	3472	15.10	44.47	250.03	3458	15.45	45.51	248.99	3444	15.80	46.54	247.96	3429
295	14.71	43.39	251.61	3480	15.06	44.43	250.57	3465	15.41	45.47	249.54	3451	15.76	46.50	248.50	3437
295.5	14.67	43.35	252.15	3487	15.02	44.39	251.11	3473	15.37	45.42	250.08	3459	15.72	46.46	249.04	3444
296	14.63	43.31	252.69	3495	14.98	44.35	251.65	3480	15.33	45.38	250.62	3466	15.68	46.42	249.58	3452
296.5	14.59	43.27	253.23	3502	14.94	44.30	252.20	3488	15.29	45.34	251.16	3474	15.64	46.38	250.12	3459
297	14.55	43.23	253.77	3510	14.90	44.26	252.74	3495	15.25	45.30	251.70	3481	15.60	46.34	250.66	3467
297.5	14.52	43.18	254.32	3517	14.86	44.22	253.28	3503	15.21	45.26	252.24	3488	15.56	46.30	251.20	3474
298	14.48	43.14	254.86	3525	14.83	44.18	253.82	3510	15.17	45.22	252.78	3496	15.52	46.26	251.74	3482
298.5	14.44	43.10	255.40	3532	14.79	44.14	254.36	3518	15.14	45.18	253.32	3503	15.48	46.22	252.28	3489
299	14.40	43.06	255.94	3540	14.75	44.10	254.90	3525	15.10	45.14	253.86	3511	15.44	46.17	252.83	3497
299.5	14.36	43.02	256.48	3547	14.71	44.06	255.44	3533	15.06	45.10	254.40	3518	15.40	46.13	253.37	3504
300	14.33	42.98	257.02	3555	14.67	44.02	255.98	3540	15.02	45.06	254.95	3526	15.36	46.09	253.91	3512
300.5	14.29	42.94	257.56	3562	14.63	43.98	256.52	3548	14.98	45.01	255.49	3533	15.32	46.05	254.45	3519
301	14.25	42.90	258.10	3570	14.60	43.94	257.06	3555	14.94	44.97	256.03	3541	15.29	46.01	254.99	3527
301.5	14.21	42.86	258.64	3577	14.56	43.89	257.61	3563	14.90	44.93	256.57	3548	15.25	45.97	255.53	3534
302	14.18	42.82	259.18	3585	14.52	43.85	258.15	3570	14.86	44.89	257.11	3556	15.21	45.93	256.07	3541
302.5	14.14	42.78	259.73	3592	14.48	43.81	258.69	3578	14.83	44.85	257.65	3563	15.17	45.89	256.61	3549
303	14.10	42.73	260.27	3599	14.45	43.77	259.23	3585	14.79	44.81	258.19	3571	15.13	45.85	257.15	3556
303.5	14.07	42.69	260.81	3607	14.41	43.73	259.77	3593	14.75	44.77	258.73	3578	15.09	45.81	257.69	3564
304	14.03	42.65	261.35	3614	14.37	43.69	260.31	3600	14.71	44.73	259.27	3586	15.05	45.76	258.24	3571
304.5	13.99	42.61	261.89	3622	14.33	43.65	260.85	3608	14.68	44.69	259.81	3593	15.02	45.72	258.78	3579
305	13.96	42.57	262.43	3629	14.30	43.61	261.39	3615	14.64	44.65	260.36	3601	14.98	45.68	259.32	3586
305.5	13.92	42.53	262.97	3637	14.26	43.57	261.93	3623	14.60	44.60	260.90	3608	14.94	45.64	259.86	3594
306	13.88	42.49	263.51	3644	14.22	43.53	262.47	3630	14.56	44.56	261.44	3616	14.90	45.60	260.40	3601
306.5	13.85	42.45	264.05	3652	14.19	43.48	263.02	3638	14.53	44.52	261.98	3623	14.86	45.56	260.94	3609
307	13.81	42.41	264.59	3659	14.15	43.44	263.56	3645	14.49	44.48	262.52	3631	14.83	45.52	261.48	3616
307.5	13.78	42.37	265.14	3667	14.11	43.40	264.10	3652	14.45	44.44	263.06	3638	14.79	45.48	262.02	3624
308	13.74	42.32	265.68	3674	14.08	43.36	264.64	3660	14.42	44.40	263.60	3646	14.75	45.44	262.56	3631
308.5	13.71	42.28	266.22	3682	14.04	43.32	265.18	3667	14.38	44.36	264.14	3653	14.71	45.40	263.10	3639
309	13.67	42.24	266.76	3689	14.01	43.28	265.72	3675	14.34	44.32	264.68	3661	14.68	45.35	263.65	3646
309.5	13.64	42.20	267.30	3697	13.97	43.24	266.26	3682	14.31	44.28	265.22	3668	14.64	45.31	264.19	3654
310	13.60	42.16	267.84	3704	13.93	43.20	266.80	3690	14.27	44.24	265.77	3676	14.60	45.27	264.73	3661
310.5	13.56	42.12	268.38	3712	13.90	43.16	267.34	3697	14.23	44.19	266.31	3683	14.57	45.23	265.27	3669
311	13.53	42.08	268.92	3719	13.86	43.12	267.88	3705	14.20	44.15	266.85	3690	14.53	45.19	265.81	3676
311.5	13.50	42.04	269.46	3727	13.83	43.07	268.43	3712	14.16	44.11	267.39	3698	14.49	45.15	266.35	3684

Body Composition   MALE   280-311.5 Lb.

Weight: Lb.	Waist: 41 inches				41.25 inches				41.5 inches				41.75 inches			
	Fat: %	Fat: Lb.	LBM: Lb.	RMR: Cal.	Fat: %	Fat: Lb.	LBM: Lb.	RMR: Cal.	Fat: %	Fat: Lb.	LBM: Lb.	RMR: Cal.	Fat: %	Fat: Lb.	LBM: Lb.	RMR: Cal.
280	17.42	48.77	231.23	3198	17.79	49.81	230.19	3184	18.16	50.85	229.16	3169	18.53	51.88	228.12	3155
280.5	17.37	48.73	231.77	3205	17.74	49.77	230.73	3191	18.11	50.80	229.70	3177	18.48	51.84	228.66	3162
281	17.33	48.69	232.31	3213	17.70	49.73	231.27	3199	18.07	50.76	230.24	3184	18.43	51.80	229.20	3170
281.5	17.28	48.65	232.85	3220	17.65	49.68	231.82	3206	18.02	50.72	230.78	3192	18.39	51.76	229.74	3177
282	17.24	48.61	233.39	3228	17.60	49.64	232.36	3213	17.97	50.68	231.32	3199	18.34	51.72	230.28	3185
282.5	17.19	48.57	233.94	3235	17.56	49.60	232.90	3221	17.93	50.64	231.86	3207	18.29	51.68	230.82	3192
283	17.15	48.52	234.48	3243	17.51	49.56	233.44	3228	17.88	50.60	232.40	3214	18.25	51.64	231.36	3200
283.5	17.10	48.48	235.02	3250	17.47	49.52	233.98	3236	17.83	50.56	232.94	3222	18.20	51.60	231.90	3207
284	17.06	48.44	235.56	3258	17.42	49.48	234.52	3243	17.79	50.52	233.48	3229	18.15	51.55	232.45	3215
284.5	17.01	48.40	236.10	3265	17.38	49.44	235.06	3251	17.74	50.48	234.02	3237	18.11	51.51	232.99	3222
285	16.97	48.36	236.64	3273	17.33	49.40	235.60	3258	17.70	50.44	234.57	3244	18.06	51.47	233.53	3230
285.5	16.92	48.32	237.18	3280	17.29	49.36	236.14	3266	17.65	50.39	235.11	3252	18.01	51.43	234.07	3237
286	16.88	48.28	237.72	3288	17.24	49.32	236.68	3273	17.61	50.35	235.65	3259	17.97	51.39	234.61	3245
286.5	16.84	48.24	238.26	3295	17.20	49.27	237.23	3281	17.56	50.31	236.19	3266	17.92	51.35	235.15	3252
287	16.79	48.20	238.80	3303	17.15	49.23	237.77	3288	17.52	50.27	236.73	3274	17.88	51.31	235.69	3260
287.5	16.75	48.16	239.35	3310	17.11	49.19	238.31	3296	17.47	50.23	237.27	3281	17.83	51.27	236.23	3267
288	16.71	48.11	239.89	3318	17.07	49.15	238.85	3303	17.43	50.19	237.81	3289	17.79	51.23	236.77	3275
288.5	16.66	48.07	240.43	3325	17.02	49.11	239.39	3311	17.38	50.15	238.35	3296	17.74	51.19	237.31	3282
289	16.62	48.03	240.97	3333	16.98	49.07	239.93	3318	17.34	50.11	238.89	3304	17.70	51.14	237.86	3290
289.5	16.58	47.99	241.51	3340	16.94	49.03	240.47	3326	17.29	50.07	239.43	3311	17.65	51.10	238.40	3297
290	16.53	47.95	242.05	3348	16.89	48.99	241.01	3333	17.25	50.03	239.98	3319	17.61	51.06	238.94	3305
290.5	16.49	47.91	242.59	3355	16.85	48.95	241.55	3341	17.21	49.98	240.52	3326	17.56	51.02	239.48	3312
291	16.45	47.87	243.13	3363	16.81	48.91	242.09	3348	17.16	49.94	241.06	3334	17.52	50.98	240.02	3319
291.5	16.41	47.83	243.67	3370	16.76	48.86	242.64	3356	17.12	49.90	241.60	3341	17.47	50.94	240.56	3327
292	16.37	47.79	244.21	3377	16.72	48.82	243.18	3363	17.08	49.86	242.14	3349	17.43	50.90	241.10	3334
292.5	16.32	47.75	244.76	3385	16.68	48.78	243.72	3371	17.03	49.82	242.68	3356	17.39	50.86	241.64	3342
293	16.28	47.70	245.30	3392	16.64	48.74	244.26	3378	16.99	49.78	243.22	3364	17.34	50.82	242.18	3349
293.5	16.24	47.66	245.84	3400	16.59	48.70	244.80	3386	16.95	49.74	243.76	3371	17.30	50.78	242.72	3357
294	16.20	47.62	246.38	3407	16.55	48.66	245.34	3393	16.90	49.70	244.30	3379	17.26	50.73	243.27	3364
294.5	16.16	47.58	246.92	3415	16.51	48.62	245.88	3401	16.86	49.66	244.84	3386	17.21	50.69	243.81	3372
295	16.12	47.54	247.46	3422	16.47	48.58	246.42	3408	16.82	49.62	245.39	3394	17.17	50.65	244.35	3379
295.5	16.07	47.50	248.00	3430	16.43	48.54	246.96	3416	16.78	49.57	245.93	3401	17.13	50.61	244.89	3387
296	16.03	47.46	248.54	3437	16.38	48.50	247.50	3423	16.73	49.53	246.47	3409	17.08	50.57	245.43	3394
296.5	15.99	47.42	249.08	3445	16.34	48.45	248.05	3430	16.69	49.49	247.01	3416	17.04	50.53	245.97	3402
297	15.95	47.38	249.62	3452	16.30	48.41	248.59	3438	16.65	49.45	247.55	3424	17.00	50.49	246.51	3409
297.5	15.91	47.34	250.17	3460	16.26	48.37	249.13	3445	16.61	49.41	248.09	3431	16.96	50.45	247.05	3417
298	15.87	47.29	250.71	3467	16.22	48.33	249.67	3453	16.57	49.37	248.63	3439	16.91	50.41	247.59	3424
298.5	15.83	47.25	251.25	3475	16.18	48.29	250.21	3460	16.53	49.33	249.17	3446	16.87	50.37	248.13	3432
299	15.79	47.21	251.79	3482	16.14	48.25	250.75	3468	16.48	49.29	249.71	3454	16.83	50.32	248.68	3439
299.5	15.75	47.17	252.33	3490	16.10	48.21	251.29	3475	16.44	49.25	250.25	3461	16.79	50.28	249.22	3447
300	15.71	47.13	252.87	3497	16.06	48.17	251.83	3483	16.40	49.21	250.80	3468	16.75	50.24	249.76	3454
300.5	15.67	47.09	253.41	3505	16.02	48.13	252.37	3490	16.36	49.16	251.34	3476	16.71	50.20	250.30	3462
301	15.63	47.05	253.95	3512	15.98	48.09	252.91	3498	16.32	49.12	251.88	3483	16.66	50.16	250.84	3469
301.5	15.59	47.01	254.49	3520	15.94	48.04	253.46	3505	16.28	49.08	252.42	3491	16.62	50.12	251.38	3477
302	15.55	46.97	255.03	3527	15.90	48.00	254.00	3513	16.24	49.04	252.96	3498	16.58	50.08	251.92	3484
302.5	15.51	46.93	255.58	3535	15.86	47.96	254.54	3520	16.20	49.00	253.50	3506	16.54	50.04	252.46	3492
303	15.47	46.88	256.12	3542	15.82	47.92	255.08	3528	16.16	48.96	254.04	3513	16.50	50.00	253.00	3499
303.5	15.43	46.84	256.66	3550	15.78	47.88	255.62	3535	16.12	48.92	254.58	3521	16.46	49.96	253.54	3507
304	15.40	46.80	257.20	3557	15.74	47.84	256.16	3543	16.08	48.88	255.12	3528	16.42	49.91	254.09	3514
304.5	15.36	46.76	257.74	3565	15.70	47.80	256.70	3550	16.04	48.84	255.66	3536	16.38	49.87	254.63	3521
305	15.32	46.72	258.28	3572	15.66	47.76	257.24	3558	16.00	48.80	256.21	3543	16.34	49.83	255.17	3529
305.5	15.28	46.68	258.82	3579	15.62	47.72	257.78	3565	15.96	48.75	256.75	3551	16.30	49.79	255.71	3536
306	15.24	46.64	259.36	3587	15.58	47.68	258.32	3573	15.92	48.71	257.29	3558	16.26	49.75	256.25	3544
306.5	15.20	46.60	259.90	3594	15.54	47.63	258.87	3580	15.88	48.67	257.83	3566	16.22	49.71	256.79	3551
307	15.16	46.56	260.44	3602	15.50	47.59	259.41	3588	15.84	48.63	258.37	3573	16.18	49.67	257.33	3559
307.5	15.13	46.52	260.99	3609	15.46	47.55	259.95	3595	15.80	48.59	258.91	3581	16.14	49.63	257.87	3566
308	15.09	46.47	261.53	3617	15.43	47.51	260.49	3603	15.76	48.55	259.45	3588	16.10	49.59	258.41	3574
308.5	15.05	46.43	262.07	3624	15.39	47.47	261.03	3610	15.72	48.51	259.99	3596	16.06	49.55	258.95	3581
309	15.01	46.39	262.61	3632	15.35	47.43	261.57	3618	15.69	48.47	260.53	3603	16.02	49.50	259.50	3589
309.5	14.98	46.35	263.15	3639	15.31	47.39	262.11	3625	15.65	48.43	261.07	3611	15.98	49.46	260.04	3596
310	14.94	46.31	263.69	3647	15.27	47.35	262.65	3632	15.61	48.39	261.62	3618	15.94	49.42	260.58	3604
310.5	14.90	46.27	264.23	3654	15.24	47.31	263.19	3640	15.57	48.34	262.16	3626	15.90	49.38	261.12	3611
311	14.86	46.23	264.77	3662	15.20	47.27	263.73	3647	15.53	48.30	262.70	3633	15.87	49.34	261.66	3619
311.5	14.83	46.19	265.31	3669	15.16	47.22	264.28	3655	15.49	48.26	263.24	3641	15.83	49.30	262.20	3626

Body Composition MALE 280-311.5 Lb.

Weight: Lb.	42 inches Fat: %	Fat: Lb.	LBM: Lb.	RMR: Cal.	42.25 inches Fat: %	Fat: Lb.	LBM: Lb.	RMR: Cal.	42.5 inches Fat: %	Fat: Lb.	LBM: Lb.	RMR: Cal.	42.75 inches Fat: %	Fat: Lb.	LBM: Lb.	RMR: Cal.
280	18.90	52.92	227.08	3141	19.27	53.96	226.04	3126	19.64	55.00	225.01	3112	20.01	56.03	223.97	3097
280.5	18.85	52.88	227.62	3148	19.22	53.92	226.58	3134	19.59	54.95	225.55	3119	19.96	55.99	224.51	3105
281	18.80	52.84	228.16	3155	19.17	53.88	227.12	3141	19.54	54.91	226.09	3127	19.91	55.95	225.05	3112
281.5	18.76	52.80	228.70	3163	19.12	53.83	227.67	3149	19.49	54.87	226.63	3134	19.86	55.91	225.59	3120
282	18.71	52.76	229.24	3170	19.08	53.79	228.21	3156	19.44	54.83	227.17	3142	19.81	55.87	226.13	3127
282.5	18.66	52.72	229.79	3178	19.03	53.75	228.75	3164	19.39	54.79	227.71	3149	19.76	55.83	226.67	3135
283	18.61	52.67	230.33	3185	18.98	53.71	229.29	3171	19.35	54.75	228.25	3157	19.71	55.79	227.21	3142
283.5	18.57	52.63	230.87	3193	18.93	53.67	229.83	3179	19.30	54.71	228.79	3164	19.66	55.75	227.75	3150
284	18.52	52.59	231.41	3200	18.88	53.63	230.37	3186	19.25	54.67	229.33	3172	19.61	55.70	228.30	3157
284.5	18.47	52.55	231.95	3208	18.84	53.59	230.91	3194	19.20	54.63	229.87	3179	19.57	55.66	228.84	3165
285	18.42	52.51	232.49	3215	18.79	53.55	231.45	3201	19.15	54.59	230.42	3187	19.52	55.62	229.38	3172
285.5	18.38	52.47	233.03	3223	18.74	53.51	231.99	3208	19.10	54.54	230.96	3194	19.47	55.58	229.92	3180
286	18.33	52.43	233.57	3230	18.69	53.47	232.53	3216	19.06	54.50	231.50	3202	19.42	55.54	230.46	3187
286.5	18.29	52.39	234.11	3238	18.65	53.42	233.08	3223	19.01	54.46	232.04	3209	19.37	55.50	231.00	3195
287	18.24	52.35	234.65	3245	18.60	53.38	233.62	3231	18.96	54.42	232.58	3217	19.32	55.46	231.54	3202
287.5	18.19	52.30	235.20	3253	18.55	53.34	234.16	3238	18.91	54.38	233.12	3224	19.28	55.42	232.08	3210
288	18.15	52.26	235.74	3260	18.51	53.30	234.70	3246	18.87	54.34	233.66	3232	19.23	55.38	232.62	3217
288.5	18.10	52.22	236.28	3268	18.46	53.26	235.24	3253	18.82	54.30	234.20	3239	19.18	55.34	233.16	3225
289	18.06	52.18	236.82	3275	18.42	53.22	235.78	3261	18.77	54.26	234.74	3246	19.13	55.29	233.71	3232
289.5	18.01	52.14	237.36	3283	18.37	53.18	236.32	3268	18.73	54.22	235.28	3254	19.09	55.25	234.25	3240
290	17.97	52.10	237.90	3290	18.32	53.14	236.86	3276	18.68	54.18	235.83	3261	19.04	55.21	234.79	3247
290.5	17.92	52.06	238.44	3298	18.28	53.10	237.40	3283	18.63	54.13	236.37	3269	18.99	55.17	235.33	3255
291	17.88	52.02	238.98	3305	18.23	53.06	237.94	3291	18.59	54.09	236.91	3276	18.95	55.13	235.87	3262
291.5	17.83	51.98	239.52	3313	18.19	53.01	238.49	3298	18.54	54.05	237.45	3284	18.90	55.09	236.41	3270
292	17.79	51.94	240.06	3320	18.14	52.97	239.03	3306	18.50	54.01	237.99	3291	18.85	55.05	236.95	3277
292.5	17.74	51.90	240.61	3328	18.10	52.93	239.57	3313	18.45	53.97	238.53	3299	18.81	55.01	237.49	3285
293	17.70	51.85	241.15	3335	18.05	52.89	240.11	3321	18.41	53.93	239.07	3306	18.76	54.97	238.03	3292
293.5	17.65	51.81	241.69	3343	18.01	52.85	240.65	3328	18.36	53.89	239.61	3314	18.71	54.93	238.57	3299
294	17.61	51.77	242.23	3350	17.96	52.81	241.19	3336	18.32	53.85	240.15	3321	18.67	54.88	239.12	3307
294.5	17.57	51.73	242.77	3357	17.92	52.77	241.73	3343	18.27	53.81	240.69	3329	18.62	54.84	239.66	3314
295	17.52	51.69	243.31	3365	17.87	52.73	242.27	3351	18.23	53.77	241.24	3336	18.58	54.80	240.20	3322
295.5	17.48	51.65	243.85	3372	17.83	52.69	242.81	3358	18.18	53.72	241.78	3344	18.53	54.76	240.74	3329
296	17.44	51.61	244.39	3380	17.79	52.65	243.35	3366	18.14	53.68	242.32	3351	18.49	54.72	241.28	3337
296.5	17.39	51.57	244.93	3387	17.74	52.60	243.90	3373	18.09	53.64	242.86	3359	18.44	54.68	241.82	3344
297	17.35	51.53	245.47	3395	17.70	52.56	244.44	3381	18.05	53.60	243.40	3366	18.40	54.64	242.36	3352
297.5	17.31	51.49	246.02	3402	17.65	52.52	244.98	3388	18.00	53.56	243.94	3374	18.35	54.60	242.90	3359
298	17.26	51.44	246.56	3410	17.61	52.48	245.52	3396	17.96	53.52	244.48	3381	18.31	54.56	243.44	3367
298.5	17.22	51.40	247.10	3417	17.57	52.44	246.06	3403	17.92	53.48	245.02	3389	18.26	54.52	243.98	3374
299	17.18	51.36	247.64	3425	17.52	52.40	246.60	3410	17.87	53.44	245.56	3396	18.22	54.47	244.53	3382
299.5	17.14	51.32	248.18	3432	17.48	52.36	247.14	3418	17.83	53.40	246.10	3404	18.17	54.43	245.07	3389
300	17.09	51.28	248.72	3440	17.44	52.32	247.68	3425	17.79	53.36	246.65	3411	18.13	54.39	245.61	3397
300.5	17.05	51.24	249.26	3447	17.40	52.28	248.22	3433	17.74	53.31	247.19	3419	18.09	54.35	246.15	3404
301	17.01	51.20	249.80	3455	17.35	52.24	248.76	3440	17.70	53.27	247.73	3426	18.04	54.31	246.69	3412
301.5	16.97	51.16	250.34	3462	17.31	52.19	249.31	3448	17.66	53.23	248.27	3434	18.00	54.27	247.23	3419
302	16.93	51.12	250.88	3470	17.27	52.15	249.85	3455	17.61	53.19	248.81	3441	17.96	54.23	247.77	3427
302.5	16.88	51.08	251.43	3477	17.23	52.11	250.39	3463	17.57	53.15	249.35	3449	17.91	54.19	248.31	3434
303	16.84	51.03	251.97	3485	17.19	52.07	250.93	3470	17.53	53.11	249.89	3456	17.87	54.15	248.85	3442
303.5	16.80	50.99	252.51	3492	17.14	52.03	251.47	3478	17.49	53.07	250.43	3463	17.83	54.11	249.39	3449
304	16.76	50.95	253.05	3500	17.10	51.99	252.01	3485	17.44	53.03	250.97	3471	17.78	54.06	249.94	3457
304.5	16.72	50.91	253.59	3507	17.06	51.95	252.55	3493	17.40	52.99	251.51	3478	17.74	54.02	250.48	3464
305	16.68	50.87	254.13	3515	17.02	51.91	253.09	3500	17.36	52.95	252.06	3486	17.70	53.98	251.02	3472
305.5	16.64	50.83	254.67	3522	16.98	51.87	253.63	3508	17.32	52.90	252.60	3493	17.66	53.94	251.56	3479
306	16.60	50.79	255.21	3530	16.94	51.83	254.17	3515	17.28	52.86	253.14	3501	17.61	53.90	252.10	3487
306.5	16.56	50.75	255.75	3537	16.90	51.78	254.72	3523	17.23	52.82	253.68	3508	17.57	53.86	252.64	3494
307	16.52	50.71	256.29	3545	16.85	51.74	255.26	3530	17.19	52.78	254.22	3516	17.53	53.82	253.18	3502
307.5	16.48	50.67	256.84	3552	16.81	51.70	255.80	3538	17.15	52.74	254.76	3523	17.49	53.78	253.72	3509
308	16.44	50.62	257.38	3560	16.77	51.66	256.34	3545	17.11	52.70	255.30	3531	17.45	53.74	254.26	3516
308.5	16.40	50.58	257.92	3567	16.73	51.62	256.88	3553	17.07	52.66	255.84	3538	17.41	53.70	254.80	3524
309	16.36	50.54	258.46	3574	16.69	51.58	257.42	3560	17.03	52.62	256.38	3546	17.36	53.65	255.35	3531
309.5	16.32	50.50	259.00	3582	16.65	51.54	257.96	3568	16.99	52.58	256.92	3553	17.32	53.61	255.89	3539
310	16.28	50.46	259.54	3589	16.61	51.50	258.50	3575	16.95	52.54	257.47	3561	17.28	53.57	256.43	3546
310.5	16.24	50.42	260.08	3597	16.57	51.46	259.04	3583	16.91	52.49	258.01	3568	17.24	53.53	256.97	3554
311	16.20	50.38	260.62	3604	16.53	51.42	259.58	3590	16.87	52.45	258.55	3576	17.20	53.49	257.51	3561
311.5	16.16	50.34	261.16	3612	16.49	51.37	260.13	3598	16.83	52.41	259.09	3583	17.16	53.45	258.05	3569

Body Composition MALE 280-311.5 Lb.

Weight: Lb.	Waist: 43 inches				43.25 inches				43.5 inches				43.75 inches			
	Fat: %	Fat: Lb.	LBM: Lb.	RMR: Cal.	Fat: %	Fat: Lb.	LBM: Lb.	RMR: Cal.	Fat: %	Fat: Lb.	LBM: Lb.	RMR: Cal.	Fat: %	Fat: Lb.	LBM: Lb.	RMR: Cal.
280	20.38	57.07	222.93	3083	20.75	58.11	221.89	3069	21.12	59.15	220.86	3054	21.49	60.18	219.82	3040
280.5	20.33	57.03	223.47	3091	20.70	58.07	222.43	3076	21.07	59.10	221.40	3062	21.44	60.14	220.36	3048
281	20.28	56.99	224.01	3098	20.65	58.03	222.97	3084	21.02	59.06	221.94	3069	21.39	60.10	220.90	3055
281.5	20.23	56.95	224.55	3106	20.60	57.98	223.52	3091	20.97	59.02	222.48	3077	21.34	60.06	221.44	3063
282	20.18	56.91	225.09	3113	20.55	57.94	224.06	3099	20.92	58.98	223.02	3084	21.28	60.02	221.98	3070
282.5	20.13	56.87	225.64	3121	20.50	57.90	224.60	3106	20.86	58.94	223.56	3092	21.23	59.98	222.52	3077
283	20.08	56.82	226.18	3128	20.45	57.86	225.14	3114	20.81	58.90	224.10	3099	21.18	59.94	223.06	3085
283.5	20.03	56.78	226.72	3135	20.40	57.82	225.68	3121	20.76	58.86	224.64	3107	21.13	59.90	223.60	3092
284	19.98	56.74	227.26	3143	20.34	57.78	226.22	3129	20.71	58.82	225.18	3114	21.08	59.85	224.15	3100
284.5	19.93	56.70	227.80	3150	20.29	57.74	226.76	3136	20.66	58.78	225.72	3122	21.02	59.81	224.69	3107
285	19.88	56.66	228.34	3158	20.24	57.70	227.30	3144	20.61	58.74	226.27	3129	20.97	59.77	225.23	3115
285.5	19.83	56.62	228.88	3165	20.19	57.66	227.84	3151	20.56	58.69	226.81	3137	20.92	59.73	225.77	3122
286	19.78	56.58	229.42	3173	20.15	57.62	228.38	3159	20.51	58.65	227.35	3144	20.87	59.69	226.31	3130
286.5	19.73	56.54	229.96	3180	20.10	57.57	228.93	3166	20.46	58.61	227.89	3152	20.82	59.65	226.85	3137
287	19.69	56.50	230.50	3188	20.05	57.53	229.47	3174	20.41	58.57	228.43	3159	20.77	59.61	227.39	3145
287.5	19.64	56.46	231.05	3195	20.00	57.49	230.01	3181	20.36	58.53	228.97	3167	20.72	59.57	227.93	3152
288	19.59	56.41	231.59	3203	19.95	57.45	230.55	3188	20.31	58.49	229.51	3174	20.67	59.53	228.47	3160
288.5	19.54	56.37	232.13	3210	19.90	57.41	231.09	3196	20.26	58.45	230.05	3182	20.62	59.49	229.01	3167
289	19.49	56.33	232.67	3218	19.85	57.37	231.63	3203	20.21	58.41	230.59	3189	20.57	59.44	229.56	3175
289.5	19.44	56.29	233.21	3225	19.80	57.33	232.17	3211	20.16	58.37	231.13	3197	20.52	59.40	230.10	3182
290	19.40	56.25	233.75	3233	19.75	57.29	232.71	3218	20.11	58.33	231.68	3204	20.47	59.36	230.64	3190
290.5	19.35	56.21	234.29	3240	19.71	57.25	233.25	3226	20.06	58.28	232.22	3212	20.42	59.32	231.18	3197
291	19.30	56.17	234.83	3248	19.66	57.21	233.79	3233	20.01	58.24	232.76	3219	20.37	59.28	231.72	3205
291.5	19.25	56.13	235.37	3255	19.61	57.16	234.34	3241	19.97	58.20	233.30	3227	20.32	59.24	232.26	3212
292	19.21	56.09	235.91	3263	19.56	57.12	234.88	3248	19.92	58.16	233.84	3234	20.27	59.20	232.80	3220
292.5	19.16	56.05	236.46	3270	19.52	57.08	235.42	3256	19.87	58.12	234.38	3241	20.22	59.16	233.34	3227
293	19.11	56.00	237.00	3278	19.47	57.04	235.96	3263	19.82	58.08	234.92	3249	20.18	59.12	233.88	3235
293.5	19.07	55.96	237.54	3285	19.42	57.00	236.50	3271	19.77	58.04	235.46	3256	20.13	59.08	234.42	3242
294	19.02	55.92	238.08	3293	19.37	56.96	237.04	3278	19.73	58.00	236.00	3264	20.08	59.03	234.97	3250
294.5	18.97	55.88	238.62	3300	19.33	56.92	237.58	3286	19.68	57.96	236.54	3271	20.03	58.99	235.51	3257
295	18.93	55.84	239.16	3308	19.28	56.88	238.12	3293	19.63	57.92	237.09	3279	19.98	58.95	236.05	3265
295.5	18.88	55.80	239.70	3315	19.23	56.84	238.66	3301	19.59	57.87	237.63	3286	19.94	58.91	236.59	3272
296	18.84	55.76	240.24	3323	19.19	56.80	239.20	3308	19.54	57.83	238.17	3294	19.89	58.87	237.13	3280
296.5	18.79	55.72	240.78	3330	19.14	56.75	239.75	3316	19.49	57.79	238.71	3301	19.84	58.83	237.67	3287
297	18.75	55.68	241.32	3338	19.10	56.71	240.29	3323	19.44	57.75	239.25	3309	19.79	58.79	238.21	3294
297.5	18.70	55.64	241.87	3345	19.05	56.67	240.83	3331	19.40	57.71	239.79	3316	19.75	58.75	238.75	3302
298	18.66	55.59	242.41	3352	19.00	56.63	241.37	3338	19.35	57.67	240.33	3324	19.70	58.71	239.29	3309
298.5	18.61	55.55	242.95	3360	18.96	56.59	241.91	3346	19.31	57.63	240.87	3331	19.65	58.67	239.83	3317
299	18.57	55.51	243.49	3367	18.91	56.55	242.45	3353	19.26	57.59	241.41	3339	19.61	58.62	240.38	3324
299.5	18.52	55.47	244.03	3375	18.87	56.51	242.99	3361	19.21	57.55	241.95	3346	19.56	58.58	240.92	3332
300	18.48	55.43	244.57	3382	18.82	56.47	243.53	3368	19.17	57.51	242.50	3354	19.51	58.54	241.46	3339
300.5	18.43	55.39	245.11	3390	18.78	56.43	244.07	3376	19.12	57.46	243.04	3361	19.47	58.50	242.00	3347
301	18.39	55.35	245.65	3397	18.73	56.39	244.61	3383	19.08	57.42	243.58	3369	19.42	58.46	242.54	3354
301.5	18.34	55.31	246.19	3405	18.69	56.34	245.16	3391	19.03	57.38	244.12	3376	19.38	58.42	243.08	3362
302	18.30	55.27	246.73	3412	18.64	56.30	245.70	3398	18.99	57.34	244.66	3384	19.33	58.38	243.62	3369
302.5	18.26	55.23	247.28	3420	18.60	56.26	246.24	3405	18.94	57.30	245.20	3391	19.29	58.34	244.16	3377
303	18.21	55.18	247.82	3427	18.55	56.22	246.78	3413	18.90	57.26	245.74	3399	19.24	58.30	244.70	3384
303.5	18.17	55.14	248.36	3435	18.51	56.18	247.32	3420	18.85	57.22	246.28	3406	19.19	58.26	245.24	3392
304	18.13	55.10	248.90	3442	18.47	56.14	247.86	3428	18.81	57.18	246.82	3414	19.15	58.21	245.79	3399
304.5	18.08	55.06	249.44	3450	18.42	56.10	248.40	3435	18.76	57.14	247.36	3421	19.10	58.17	246.33	3407
305	18.04	55.02	249.98	3457	18.38	56.06	248.94	3443	18.72	57.10	247.91	3429	19.06	58.13	246.87	3414
305.5	18.00	54.98	250.52	3465	18.34	56.02	249.48	3450	18.68	57.05	248.45	3436	19.02	58.09	247.41	3422
306	17.95	54.94	251.06	3472	18.29	55.98	250.02	3458	18.63	57.01	248.99	3443	18.97	58.05	247.95	3429
306.5	17.91	54.90	251.60	3480	18.25	55.93	250.57	3465	18.59	56.97	249.53	3451	18.93	58.01	248.49	3437
307	17.87	54.86	252.14	3487	18.21	55.89	251.11	3473	18.54	56.93	250.07	3458	18.88	57.97	249.03	3444
307.5	17.83	54.82	252.69	3495	18.16	55.85	251.65	3480	18.50	56.89	250.61	3466	18.84	57.93	249.57	3452
308	17.78	54.77	253.23	3502	18.12	55.81	252.19	3488	18.46	56.85	251.15	3473	18.79	57.89	250.11	3459
308.5	17.74	54.73	253.77	3510	18.08	55.77	252.73	3495	18.41	56.81	251.69	3481	18.75	57.85	250.65	3467
309	17.70	54.69	254.31	3517	18.04	55.73	253.27	3503	18.37	56.77	252.23	3488	18.71	57.80	251.20	3474
309.5	17.66	54.65	254.85	3525	17.99	55.69	253.81	3510	18.33	56.73	252.77	3496	18.66	57.76	251.74	3482
310	17.62	54.61	255.39	3532	17.95	55.65	254.35	3518	18.29	56.69	253.32	3503	18.62	57.72	252.28	3489
310.5	17.57	54.57	255.93	3540	17.91	55.61	254.89	3525	18.24	56.64	253.86	3511	18.58	57.68	252.82	3496
311	17.53	54.53	256.47	3547	17.87	55.57	255.43	3533	18.20	56.60	254.40	3518	18.53	57.64	253.36	3504
311.5	17.49	54.49	257.01	3554	17.82	55.52	255.98	3540	18.16	56.56	254.94	3526	18.49	57.60	253.90	3511

Body Composition MALE 280-311.5 Lb.

Weight: Lb.	Waist: 44 inches				44.25 inches				44.5 inches				44.75 inches			
	Fat: %	Fat: Lb.	LBM: Lb.	RMR: Cal.	Fat: %	Fat: Lb.	LBM: Lb.	RMR: Cal.	Fat: %	Fat: Lb.	LBM: Lb.	RMR: Cal.	Fat: %	Fat: Lb.	LBM: Lb.	RMR: Cal.
280	21.86	61.22	218.78	3026	22.23	62.26	217.74	3011	22.61	63.30	216.71	2997	22.98	64.33	215.67	2983
280.5	21.81	61.18	219.32	3033	22.18	62.22	218.28	3019	22.55	63.25	217.25	3005	22.92	64.29	216.21	2990
281	21.76	61.14	219.86	3041	22.13	62.18	218.82	3026	22.50	63.21	217.79	3012	22.86	64.25	216.75	2998
281.5	21.70	61.10	220.40	3048	22.07	62.13	219.37	3034	22.44	63.17	218.33	3019	22.81	64.21	217.29	3005
282	21.65	61.06	220.94	3056	22.02	62.09	219.91	3041	22.39	63.13	218.87	3027	22.75	64.17	217.83	3013
282.5	21.60	61.02	221.49	3063	21.97	62.05	220.45	3049	22.33	63.09	219.41	3034	22.70	64.13	218.37	3020
283	21.55	60.97	222.03	3071	21.91	62.01	220.99	3056	22.28	63.05	219.95	3042	22.65	64.09	218.91	3028
283.5	21.49	60.93	222.57	3078	21.86	61.97	221.53	3064	22.23	63.01	220.49	3049	22.59	64.05	219.45	3035
284	21.44	60.89	223.11	3086	21.81	61.93	222.07	3071	22.17	62.97	221.03	3057	22.54	64.00	220.00	3043
284.5	21.39	60.85	223.65	3093	21.75	61.89	222.61	3079	22.12	62.93	221.57	3064	22.48	63.96	220.54	3050
285	21.34	60.81	224.19	3101	21.70	61.85	223.15	3086	22.06	62.89	222.12	3072	22.43	63.92	221.08	3058
285.5	21.29	60.77	224.73	3108	21.65	61.81	223.69	3094	22.01	62.84	222.66	3079	22.38	63.88	221.62	3065
286	21.23	60.73	225.27	3116	21.60	61.77	224.23	3101	21.96	62.80	223.20	3087	22.32	63.84	222.16	3072
286.5	21.18	60.69	225.81	3123	21.54	61.72	224.78	3109	21.91	62.76	223.74	3094	22.27	63.80	222.70	3080
287	21.13	60.65	226.35	3130	21.49	61.68	225.32	3116	21.85	62.72	224.28	3102	22.22	63.76	223.24	3087
287.5	21.08	60.61	226.90	3138	21.44	61.64	225.86	3124	21.80	62.68	224.82	3109	22.16	63.72	223.78	3095
288	21.03	60.56	227.44	3145	21.39	61.60	226.40	3131	21.75	62.64	225.36	3117	22.11	63.68	224.32	3102
288.5	20.98	60.52	227.98	3153	21.34	61.56	226.94	3139	21.70	62.60	225.90	3124	22.06	63.64	224.86	3110
289	20.93	60.48	228.52	3160	21.29	61.52	227.48	3146	21.65	62.56	226.44	3132	22.01	63.59	225.41	3117
289.5	20.88	60.44	229.06	3168	21.24	61.48	228.02	3154	21.59	62.52	226.98	3139	21.95	63.55	225.95	3125
290	20.83	60.40	229.60	3175	21.19	61.44	228.56	3161	21.54	62.48	227.53	3147	21.90	63.51	226.49	3132
290.5	20.78	60.36	230.14	3183	21.13	61.40	229.10	3169	21.49	62.43	228.07	3154	21.85	63.47	227.03	3140
291	20.73	60.32	230.68	3190	21.08	61.36	229.64	3176	21.44	62.39	228.61	3162	21.80	63.43	227.57	3147
291.5	20.68	60.28	231.22	3198	21.03	61.31	230.19	3183	21.39	62.35	229.15	3169	21.75	63.39	228.11	3155
292	20.63	60.24	231.76	3205	20.98	61.27	230.73	3191	21.34	62.31	229.69	3177	21.69	63.35	228.65	3162
292.5	20.58	60.20	232.31	3213	20.93	61.23	231.27	3198	21.29	62.27	230.23	3184	21.64	63.31	229.19	3170
293	20.53	60.15	232.85	3220	20.88	61.19	231.81	3206	21.24	62.23	230.77	3192	21.59	63.27	229.73	3177
293.5	20.48	60.11	233.39	3228	20.83	61.15	232.35	3213	21.19	62.19	231.31	3199	21.54	63.23	230.27	3185
294	20.43	60.07	233.93	3235	20.79	61.11	232.89	3221	21.14	62.15	231.85	3207	21.49	63.18	230.82	3192
294.5	20.38	60.03	234.47	3243	20.74	61.07	233.43	3228	21.09	62.11	232.39	3214	21.44	63.14	231.36	3200
295	20.34	59.99	235.01	3250	20.69	61.03	233.97	3236	21.04	62.07	232.94	3221	21.39	63.10	231.90	3207
295.5	20.29	59.95	235.55	3258	20.64	60.99	234.51	3243	20.99	62.02	233.48	3229	21.34	63.06	232.44	3215
296	20.24	59.91	236.09	3265	20.59	60.95	235.05	3251	20.94	61.98	234.02	3236	21.29	63.02	232.98	3222
296.5	20.19	59.87	236.63	3273	20.54	60.90	235.60	3258	20.89	61.94	234.56	3244	21.24	62.98	233.52	3230
297	20.14	59.83	237.17	3280	20.49	60.86	236.14	3266	20.84	61.90	235.10	3251	21.19	62.94	234.06	3237
297.5	20.10	59.79	237.72	3288	20.44	60.82	236.68	3273	20.79	61.86	235.64	3259	21.14	62.90	234.60	3245
298	20.05	59.74	238.26	3295	20.40	60.78	237.22	3281	20.74	61.82	236.18	3266	21.09	62.86	235.14	3252
298.5	20.00	59.70	238.80	3303	20.35	60.74	237.76	3288	20.70	61.78	236.72	3274	21.04	62.82	235.68	3260
299	19.95	59.66	239.34	3310	20.30	60.70	238.30	3296	20.65	61.74	237.26	3281	20.99	62.77	236.23	3267
299.5	19.91	59.62	239.88	3318	20.25	60.66	238.84	3303	20.60	61.70	237.80	3289	20.95	62.73	236.77	3274
300	19.86	59.58	240.42	3325	20.21	60.62	239.38	3311	20.55	61.66	238.35	3296	20.90	62.69	237.31	3282
300.5	19.81	59.54	240.96	3332	20.16	60.58	239.92	3318	20.50	61.61	238.89	3304	20.85	62.65	237.85	3289
301	19.77	59.50	241.50	3340	20.11	60.54	240.46	3326	20.46	61.57	239.43	3311	20.80	62.61	238.39	3297
301.5	19.72	59.46	242.04	3347	20.06	60.49	241.01	3333	20.41	61.53	239.97	3319	20.75	62.57	238.93	3304
302	19.67	59.42	242.58	3355	20.02	60.45	241.55	3341	20.36	61.49	240.51	3326	20.70	62.53	239.47	3312
302.5	19.63	59.38	243.13	3362	19.97	60.41	242.09	3348	20.31	61.45	241.05	3334	20.66	62.49	240.01	3319
303	19.58	59.33	243.67	3370	19.92	60.37	242.63	3356	20.27	61.41	241.59	3341	20.61	62.45	240.55	3327
303.5	19.54	59.29	244.21	3377	19.88	60.33	243.17	3363	20.22	61.37	242.13	3349	20.56	62.41	241.09	3334
304	19.49	59.25	244.75	3385	19.83	60.29	243.71	3371	20.17	61.33	242.67	3356	20.51	62.36	241.64	3342
304.5	19.45	59.21	245.29	3392	19.79	60.25	244.25	3378	20.13	61.29	243.21	3364	20.47	62.32	242.18	3349
305	19.40	59.17	245.83	3400	19.74	60.21	244.79	3385	20.08	61.24	243.76	3371	20.42	62.28	242.72	3357
305.5	19.35	59.13	246.37	3407	19.69	60.17	245.33	3393	20.03	61.20	244.30	3379	20.37	62.24	243.26	3364
306	19.31	59.09	246.91	3415	19.65	60.13	245.87	3400	19.99	61.16	244.84	3386	20.33	62.20	243.80	3372
306.5	19.26	59.05	247.45	3422	19.60	60.08	246.42	3408	19.94	61.12	245.38	3394	20.28	62.16	244.34	3379
307	19.22	59.01	247.99	3430	19.56	60.04	246.96	3415	19.90	61.08	245.92	3401	20.23	62.12	244.88	3387
307.5	19.18	58.97	248.54	3437	19.51	60.00	247.50	3423	19.85	61.04	246.46	3409	20.19	62.08	245.42	3394
308	19.13	58.92	249.08	3445	19.47	59.96	248.04	3430	19.80	61.00	247.00	3416	20.14	62.04	245.96	3402
308.5	19.09	58.88	249.62	3452	19.42	59.92	248.58	3438	19.76	60.96	247.54	3424	20.10	62.00	246.50	3409
309	19.04	58.84	250.16	3460	19.38	59.88	249.12	3445	19.71	60.92	248.08	3431	20.05	61.95	247.05	3417
309.5	19.00	58.80	250.70	3467	19.33	59.84	249.66	3453	19.67	60.88	248.62	3438	20.00	61.91	247.59	3424
310	18.95	58.76	251.24	3475	19.29	59.80	250.20	3460	19.62	60.84	249.17	3446	19.96	61.87	248.13	3432
310.5	18.91	58.72	251.78	3482	19.25	59.76	250.74	3468	19.58	60.79	249.71	3453	19.91	61.83	248.67	3439
311	18.87	58.68	252.32	3490	19.20	59.72	251.28	3475	19.53	60.75	250.25	3461	19.87	61.79	249.21	3447
311.5	18.82	58.64	252.86	3497	19.16	59.67	251.83	3483	19.49	60.71	250.79	3468	19.82	61.75	249.75	3454

Body Composition   MALE   280-311.5 Lb.

Weight: Lb.	Waist: 45 inches Fat: %	Fat: Lb.	LBM: Lb.	RMR: Cal.	45.25 inches Fat: %	Fat: Lb.	LBM: Lb.	RMR: Cal.	45.5 inches Fat: %	Fat: Lb.	LBM: Lb.	RMR: Cal.	45.75 inches Fat: %	Fat: Lb.	LBM: Lb.	RMR: Cal.
280	23.35	65.37	214.63	2968	23.72	66.41	213.59	2954	24.09	67.45	212.56	2940	24.46	68.48	211.52	2925
280.5	23.29	65.33	215.17	2976	23.66	66.37	214.13	2961	24.03	67.40	213.10	2947	24.40	68.44	212.06	2933
281	23.23	65.29	215.71	2983	23.60	66.33	214.67	2969	23.97	67.36	213.64	2955	24.34	68.40	212.60	2940
281.5	23.18	65.25	216.25	2991	23.55	66.28	215.22	2976	23.92	67.32	214.18	2962	24.28	68.36	213.14	2948
282	23.12	65.21	216.79	2998	23.49	66.24	215.76	2984	23.86	67.28	214.72	2970	24.23	68.32	213.68	2955
282.5	23.07	65.17	217.34	3006	23.43	66.20	216.30	2991	23.80	67.24	215.26	2977	24.17	68.28	214.22	2963
283	23.01	65.12	217.88	3013	23.38	66.16	216.84	2999	23.75	67.20	215.80	2985	24.11	68.24	214.76	2970
283.5	22.96	65.08	218.42	3021	23.32	66.12	217.38	3006	23.69	67.16	216.34	2992	24.05	68.20	215.30	2978
284	22.90	65.04	218.96	3028	23.27	66.08	217.92	3014	23.63	67.12	216.88	2999	24.00	68.15	215.85	2985
284.5	22.85	65.00	219.50	3036	23.21	66.04	218.46	3021	23.58	67.08	217.42	3007	23.94	68.11	216.39	2993
285	22.79	64.96	220.04	3043	23.16	66.00	219.00	3029	23.52	67.04	217.97	3014	23.89	68.07	216.93	3000
285.5	22.74	64.92	220.58	3051	23.10	65.96	219.54	3036	23.47	66.99	218.51	3022	23.83	68.03	217.47	3008
286	22.68	64.88	221.12	3058	23.05	65.92	220.08	3044	23.41	66.95	219.05	3029	23.77	67.99	218.01	3015
286.5	22.63	64.84	221.66	3066	22.99	65.87	220.63	3051	23.35	66.91	219.59	3037	23.72	67.95	218.55	3023
287	22.58	64.80	222.20	3073	22.94	65.83	221.17	3059	23.30	66.87	220.13	3044	23.66	67.91	219.09	3030
287.5	22.52	64.76	222.75	3081	22.88	65.79	221.71	3066	23.25	66.83	220.67	3052	23.61	67.87	219.63	3038
288	22.47	64.71	223.29	3088	22.83	65.75	222.25	3074	23.19	66.79	221.21	3059	23.55	67.83	220.17	3045
288.5	22.42	64.67	223.83	3096	22.78	65.71	222.79	3081	23.14	66.75	221.75	3067	23.50	67.79	220.71	3052
289	22.36	64.63	224.37	3103	22.72	65.67	223.33	3089	23.08	66.71	222.29	3074	23.44	67.74	221.26	3060
289.5	22.31	64.59	224.91	3110	22.67	65.63	223.87	3096	23.03	66.67	222.83	3082	23.39	67.70	221.80	3067
290	22.26	64.55	225.45	3118	22.62	65.59	224.41	3104	22.97	66.63	223.38	3089	23.33	67.66	222.34	3075
290.5	22.21	64.51	225.99	3125	22.56	65.55	224.95	3111	22.92	66.58	223.92	3097	23.28	67.62	222.88	3082
291	22.15	64.47	226.53	3133	22.51	65.51	225.49	3119	22.87	66.54	224.46	3104	23.22	67.58	223.42	3090
291.5	22.10	64.43	227.07	3140	22.46	65.46	226.04	3126	22.81	66.50	225.00	3112	23.17	67.54	223.96	3097
292	22.05	64.39	227.61	3148	22.41	65.42	226.58	3134	22.76	66.46	225.54	3119	23.12	67.50	224.50	3105
292.5	22.00	64.35	228.16	3155	22.35	65.38	227.12	3141	22.71	66.42	226.08	3127	23.06	67.46	225.04	3112
293	21.95	64.30	228.70	3163	22.30	65.34	227.66	3149	22.65	66.38	226.62	3134	23.01	67.42	225.58	3120
293.5	21.90	64.26	229.24	3170	22.25	65.30	228.20	3156	22.60	66.34	227.16	3142	22.96	67.38	226.12	3127
294	21.84	64.22	229.78	3178	22.20	65.26	228.74	3163	22.55	66.30	227.70	3149	22.90	67.33	226.67	3135
294.5	21.79	64.18	230.32	3185	22.15	65.22	229.28	3171	22.50	66.26	228.24	3157	22.85	67.29	227.21	3142
295	21.74	64.14	230.86	3193	22.09	65.18	229.82	3178	22.45	66.22	228.79	3164	22.80	67.25	227.75	3150
295.5	21.69	64.10	231.40	3200	22.04	65.14	230.36	3186	22.39	66.17	229.33	3172	22.75	67.21	228.29	3157
296	21.64	64.06	231.94	3208	21.99	65.10	230.90	3193	22.34	66.13	229.87	3179	22.69	67.17	228.83	3165
296.5	21.59	64.02	232.48	3215	21.94	65.05	231.45	3201	22.29	66.09	230.41	3187	22.64	67.13	229.37	3172
297	21.54	63.98	233.02	3223	21.89	65.01	231.99	3208	22.24	66.05	230.95	3194	22.59	67.09	229.91	3180
297.5	21.49	63.94	233.57	3230	21.84	64.97	232.53	3216	22.19	66.01	231.49	3202	22.54	67.05	230.45	3187
298	21.44	63.89	234.11	3238	21.79	64.93	233.07	3223	22.14	65.97	232.03	3209	22.49	67.01	230.99	3195
298.5	21.39	63.85	234.65	3245	21.74	64.89	233.61	3231	22.09	65.93	232.57	3216	22.43	66.97	231.53	3202
299	21.34	63.81	235.19	3253	21.69	64.85	234.15	3238	22.04	65.89	233.11	3224	22.38	66.92	232.08	3210
299.5	21.29	63.77	235.73	3260	21.64	64.81	234.69	3246	21.99	65.85	233.65	3231	22.33	66.88	232.62	3217
300	21.24	63.73	236.27	3268	21.59	64.77	235.23	3253	21.94	65.81	234.20	3239	22.28	66.84	233.16	3225
300.5	21.19	63.69	236.81	3275	21.54	64.73	235.77	3261	21.88	65.76	234.74	3246	22.23	66.80	233.70	3232
301	21.15	63.65	237.35	3283	21.49	64.69	236.31	3268	21.83	65.72	235.28	3254	22.18	66.76	234.24	3240
301.5	21.10	63.61	237.89	3290	21.44	64.64	236.86	3276	21.79	65.68	235.82	3261	22.13	66.72	234.78	3247
302	21.05	63.57	238.43	3298	21.39	64.60	237.40	3283	21.74	65.64	236.36	3269	22.08	66.68	235.32	3254
302.5	21.00	63.53	238.98	3305	21.34	64.56	237.94	3291	21.69	65.60	236.90	3276	22.03	66.64	235.86	3262
303	20.95	63.48	239.52	3313	21.29	64.52	238.48	3298	21.64	65.56	237.44	3284	21.98	66.60	236.40	3269
303.5	20.90	63.44	240.06	3320	21.25	64.48	239.02	3306	21.59	65.52	237.98	3291	21.93	66.56	236.94	3277
304	20.86	63.40	240.60	3327	21.20	64.44	239.56	3313	21.54	65.48	238.52	3299	21.88	66.51	237.49	3284
304.5	20.81	63.36	241.14	3335	21.15	64.40	240.10	3321	21.49	65.44	239.06	3306	21.83	66.47	238.03	3292
305	20.76	63.32	241.68	3342	21.10	64.36	240.64	3328	21.44	65.40	239.61	3314	21.78	66.43	238.57	3299
305.5	20.71	63.28	242.22	3350	21.05	64.32	241.18	3336	21.39	65.35	240.15	3321	21.73	66.39	239.11	3307
306	20.67	63.24	242.76	3357	21.01	64.28	241.72	3343	21.34	65.31	240.69	3329	21.68	66.35	239.65	3314
306.5	20.62	63.20	243.30	3365	20.96	64.23	242.27	3351	21.30	65.27	241.23	3336	21.63	66.31	240.19	3322
307	20.57	63.16	243.84	3372	20.91	64.19	242.81	3358	21.25	65.23	241.77	3344	21.59	66.27	240.73	3329
307.5	20.53	63.12	244.39	3380	20.86	64.15	243.35	3365	21.20	65.19	242.31	3351	21.54	66.23	241.27	3337
308	20.48	63.07	244.93	3387	20.82	64.11	243.89	3373	21.15	65.15	242.85	3359	21.49	66.19	241.81	3344
308.5	20.43	63.03	245.47	3395	20.77	64.07	244.43	3380	21.10	65.11	243.39	3366	21.44	66.15	242.35	3352
309	20.39	62.99	246.01	3402	20.72	64.03	244.97	3388	21.06	65.07	243.93	3374	21.39	66.10	242.90	3359
309.5	20.34	62.95	246.55	3410	20.67	63.99	245.51	3395	21.01	65.03	244.47	3381	21.35	66.06	243.44	3367
310	20.29	62.91	247.09	3417	20.63	63.95	246.05	3403	20.96	64.99	245.02	3389	21.30	66.02	243.98	3374
310.5	20.25	62.87	247.63	3425	20.58	63.91	246.59	3410	20.92	64.94	245.56	3396	21.25	65.98	244.52	3382
311	20.20	62.83	248.17	3432	20.54	63.87	247.13	3418	20.87	64.90	246.10	3404	21.20	65.94	245.06	3389
311.5	20.16	62.79	248.71	3440	20.49	63.82	247.68	3425	20.82	64.86	246.64	3411	21.16	65.90	245.60	3397

Body Composition MALE 280-311.5 Lb.

Weight: Lb.	Waist: 46 inches Fat: %	Fat: Lb.	LBM: Lb.	RMR: Cal.	46.25 inches Fat: %	Fat: Lb.	LBM: Lb.	RMR: Cal.	46.5 inches Fat: %	Fat: Lb.	LBM: Lb.	RMR: Cal.	46.75 inches Fat: %	Fat: Lb.	LBM: Lb.	RMR: Cal.
280	24.83	69.52	210.48	2911	25.20	70.56	209.44	2897	25.57	71.60	208.41	2882	25.94	72.63	207.37	2868
280.5	24.77	69.48	211.02	2918	25.14	70.52	209.98	2904	25.51	71.55	208.95	2890	25.88	72.59	207.91	2875
281	24.71	69.44	211.56	2926	25.08	70.48	210.52	2912	25.45	71.51	209.49	2897	25.82	72.55	208.45	2883
281.5	24.65	69.40	212.10	2933	25.02	70.43	211.07	2919	25.39	71.47	210.03	2905	25.76	72.51	208.99	2890
282	24.59	69.36	212.64	2941	24.96	70.39	211.61	2927	25.33	71.43	210.57	2912	25.70	72.47	209.53	2898
282.5	24.54	69.32	213.19	2948	24.90	70.35	212.15	2934	25.27	71.39	211.11	2920	25.64	72.43	210.07	2905
283	24.48	69.27	213.73	2956	24.85	70.31	212.69	2941	25.21	71.35	211.65	2927	25.58	72.39	210.61	2913
283.5	24.42	69.23	214.27	2963	24.79	70.27	213.23	2949	25.15	71.31	212.19	2935	25.52	72.35	211.15	2920
284	24.36	69.19	214.81	2971	24.73	70.23	213.77	2956	25.09	71.27	212.73	2942	25.46	72.30	211.70	2928
284.5	24.31	69.15	215.35	2978	24.67	70.19	214.31	2964	25.04	71.23	213.27	2950	25.40	72.26	212.24	2935
285	24.25	69.11	215.89	2986	24.61	70.15	214.85	2971	24.98	71.19	213.82	2957	25.34	72.22	212.78	2943
285.5	24.19	69.07	216.43	2993	24.56	70.11	215.39	2979	24.92	71.14	214.36	2965	25.28	72.18	213.32	2950
286	24.14	69.03	216.97	3001	24.50	70.07	215.93	2986	24.86	71.10	214.90	2972	25.22	72.14	213.86	2958
286.5	24.08	68.99	217.51	3008	24.44	70.02	216.48	2994	24.80	71.06	215.44	2980	25.17	72.10	214.40	2965
287	24.02	68.95	218.05	3016	24.38	69.98	217.02	3001	24.75	71.02	215.98	2987	25.11	72.06	214.94	2973
287.5	23.97	68.91	218.60	3023	24.33	69.94	217.56	3009	24.69	70.98	216.52	2994	25.05	72.02	215.48	2980
288	23.91	68.86	219.14	3031	24.27	69.90	218.10	3016	24.63	70.94	217.06	3002	24.99	71.98	216.02	2988
288.5	23.86	68.82	219.68	3038	24.22	69.86	218.64	3024	24.57	70.90	217.60	3009	24.93	71.94	216.56	2995
289	23.80	68.78	220.22	3046	24.16	69.82	219.18	3031	24.52	70.86	218.14	3017	24.88	71.89	217.11	3003
289.5	23.74	68.74	220.76	3053	24.10	69.78	219.72	3039	24.46	70.82	218.68	3024	24.82	71.85	217.65	3010
290	23.69	68.70	221.30	3061	24.05	69.74	220.26	3046	24.41	70.78	219.23	3032	24.76	71.81	218.19	3018
290.5	23.63	68.66	221.84	3068	23.99	69.70	220.80	3054	24.35	70.73	219.77	3039	24.71	71.77	218.73	3025
291	23.58	68.62	222.38	3076	23.94	69.66	221.34	3061	24.29	70.69	220.31	3047	24.65	71.73	219.27	3032
291.5	23.53	68.58	222.92	3083	23.88	69.61	221.89	3069	24.24	70.65	220.85	3054	24.59	71.69	219.81	3040
292	23.47	68.54	223.46	3091	23.83	69.57	222.43	3076	24.18	70.61	221.39	3062	24.54	71.65	220.35	3047
292.5	23.42	68.50	224.01	3098	23.77	69.53	222.97	3084	24.13	70.57	221.93	3069	24.48	71.61	220.89	3055
293	23.36	68.45	224.55	3105	23.72	69.49	223.51	3091	24.07	70.53	222.47	3077	24.43	71.57	221.43	3062
293.5	23.31	68.41	225.09	3113	23.66	69.45	224.05	3099	24.02	70.49	223.01	3084	24.37	71.53	221.97	3070
294	23.26	68.37	225.63	3120	23.61	69.41	224.59	3106	23.96	70.45	223.55	3092	24.31	71.48	222.52	3077
294.5	23.20	68.33	226.17	3128	23.55	69.37	225.13	3114	23.91	70.41	224.09	3099	24.26	71.44	223.06	3085
295	23.15	68.29	226.71	3135	23.50	69.33	225.67	3121	23.85	70.37	224.64	3107	24.20	71.40	223.60	3092
295.5	23.10	68.25	227.25	3143	23.45	69.29	226.21	3129	23.80	70.32	225.18	3114	24.15	71.36	224.14	3100
296	23.04	68.21	227.79	3150	23.39	69.25	226.75	3136	23.74	70.28	225.72	3122	24.09	71.32	224.68	3107
296.5	22.99	68.17	228.33	3158	23.34	69.20	227.30	3143	23.69	70.24	226.26	3129	24.04	71.28	225.22	3115
297	22.94	68.13	228.87	3165	23.29	69.16	227.84	3151	23.64	70.20	226.80	3137	23.99	71.24	225.76	3122
297.5	22.89	68.09	229.42	3173	23.23	69.12	228.38	3158	23.58	70.16	227.34	3144	23.93	71.20	226.30	3130
298	22.83	68.04	229.96	3180	23.18	69.08	228.92	3166	23.53	70.12	227.88	3152	23.88	71.16	226.84	3137
298.5	22.78	68.00	230.50	3188	23.13	69.04	229.46	3173	23.48	70.08	228.42	3159	23.82	71.12	227.38	3145
299	22.73	67.96	231.04	3195	23.08	69.00	230.00	3181	23.42	70.04	228.96	3167	23.77	71.07	227.93	3152
299.5	22.68	67.92	231.58	3203	23.02	68.96	230.54	3188	23.37	70.00	229.50	3174	23.72	71.03	228.47	3160
300	22.63	67.88	232.12	3210	22.97	68.92	231.08	3196	23.32	69.96	230.05	3182	23.66	70.99	229.01	3167
300.5	22.58	67.84	232.66	3218	22.92	68.88	231.62	3203	23.27	69.91	230.59	3189	23.61	70.95	229.55	3175
301	22.52	67.80	233.20	3225	22.87	68.84	232.16	3211	23.21	69.87	231.13	3196	23.56	70.91	230.09	3182
301.5	22.47	67.76	233.74	3233	22.82	68.79	232.71	3218	23.16	69.83	231.67	3204	23.51	70.87	230.63	3190
302	22.42	67.72	234.28	3240	22.77	68.75	233.25	3226	23.11	69.79	232.21	3211	23.45	70.83	231.17	3197
302.5	22.37	67.68	234.83	3248	22.71	68.71	233.79	3233	23.06	69.75	232.75	3219	23.40	70.79	231.71	3205
303	22.32	67.63	235.37	3255	22.66	68.67	234.33	3241	23.01	69.71	233.29	3226	23.35	70.75	232.25	3212
303.5	22.27	67.59	235.91	3263	22.61	68.63	234.87	3248	22.95	69.67	233.83	3234	23.30	70.71	232.79	3220
304	22.22	67.55	236.45	3270	22.56	68.59	235.41	3256	22.90	69.63	234.37	3241	23.24	70.66	233.34	3227
304.5	22.17	67.51	236.99	3278	22.51	68.55	235.95	3263	22.85	69.59	234.91	3249	23.19	70.62	233.88	3235
305	22.12	67.47	237.53	3285	22.46	68.51	236.49	3271	22.80	69.55	235.46	3256	23.14	70.58	234.42	3242
305.5	22.07	67.43	238.07	3293	22.41	68.47	237.03	3278	22.75	69.50	236.00	3264	23.09	70.54	234.96	3249
306	22.02	67.39	238.61	3300	22.36	68.43	237.57	3286	22.70	69.46	236.54	3271	23.04	70.50	235.50	3257
306.5	21.97	67.35	239.15	3307	22.31	68.38	238.12	3293	22.65	69.42	237.08	3279	22.99	70.46	236.04	3264
307	21.92	67.31	239.69	3315	22.26	68.34	238.66	3301	22.60	69.38	237.62	3286	22.94	70.42	236.58	3272
307.5	21.87	67.27	240.24	3322	22.21	68.30	239.20	3308	22.55	69.34	238.16	3294	22.89	70.38	237.12	3279
308	21.83	67.22	240.78	3330	22.16	68.26	239.74	3316	22.50	69.30	238.70	3301	22.84	70.34	237.66	3287
308.5	21.78	67.18	241.32	3337	22.11	68.22	240.28	3323	22.45	69.26	239.24	3309	22.79	70.30	238.20	3294
309	21.73	67.14	241.86	3345	22.06	68.18	240.82	3331	22.40	69.22	239.78	3316	22.74	70.25	238.75	3302
309.5	21.68	67.10	242.40	3352	22.02	68.14	241.36	3338	22.35	69.18	240.32	3324	22.69	70.21	239.29	3309
310	21.63	67.06	242.94	3360	21.97	68.10	241.90	3346	22.30	69.14	240.87	3331	22.64	70.17	239.83	3317
310.5	21.58	67.02	243.48	3367	21.92	68.06	242.44	3353	22.25	69.09	241.41	3339	22.59	70.13	240.37	3324
311	21.54	66.98	244.02	3375	21.87	68.02	242.98	3360	22.20	69.05	241.95	3346	22.54	70.09	240.91	3332
311.5	21.49	66.94	244.56	3382	21.82	67.97	243.53	3368	22.15	69.01	242.49	3354	22.49	70.05	241.45	3339

Body Composition MALE 280-311.5 Lb.

Weight: Lb.	Waist: 47 inches				47.25 inches				47.5 inches				47.75 inches			
	Fat: %	Fat: Lb.	LBM: Lb.	RMR: Cal.	Fat: %	Fat: Lb.	LBM: Lb.	RMR: Cal.	Fat: %	Fat: Lb.	LBM: Lb.	RMR: Cal.	Fat: %	Fat: Lb.	LBM: Lb.	RMR: Cal.
280	26.31	73.67	206.33	2854	26.68	74.71	205.29	2839	27.05	75.75	204.26	2825	27.42	76.78	203.22	2810
280.5	26.25	73.63	206.87	2861	26.62	74.67	205.83	2847	26.99	75.70	204.80	2832	27.36	76.74	203.76	2818
281	26.19	73.59	207.41	2869	26.56	74.63	206.37	2854	26.93	75.66	205.34	2840	27.30	76.70	204.30	2825
281.5	26.13	73.55	207.95	2876	26.50	74.58	206.92	2862	26.86	75.62	205.88	2847	27.23	76.66	204.84	2833
282	26.07	73.51	208.49	2883	26.43	74.54	207.46	2869	26.80	75.58	206.42	2855	27.17	76.62	205.38	2840
282.5	26.01	73.47	209.04	2891	26.37	74.50	208.00	2877	26.74	75.54	206.96	2862	27.11	76.58	205.92	2848
283	25.94	73.42	209.58	2898	26.31	74.46	208.54	2884	26.68	75.50	207.50	2870	27.04	76.54	206.46	2855
283.5	25.88	73.38	210.12	2906	26.25	74.42	209.08	2892	26.62	75.46	208.04	2877	26.98	76.50	207.00	2863
284	25.82	73.34	210.66	2913	26.19	74.38	209.62	2899	26.56	75.42	208.58	2885	26.92	76.45	207.55	2870
284.5	25.76	73.30	211.20	2921	26.13	74.34	210.16	2907	26.49	75.38	209.12	2892	26.86	76.41	208.09	2878
285	25.71	73.26	211.74	2928	26.07	74.30	210.70	2914	26.43	75.34	209.67	2900	26.80	76.37	208.63	2885
285.5	25.65	73.22	212.28	2936	26.01	74.26	211.24	2921	26.37	75.29	210.21	2907	26.74	76.33	209.17	2893
286	25.59	73.18	212.82	2943	25.95	74.22	211.78	2929	26.31	75.25	210.75	2915	26.68	76.29	209.71	2900
286.5	25.53	73.14	213.36	2951	25.89	74.17	212.33	2936	26.25	75.21	211.29	2922	26.61	76.25	210.25	2908
287	25.47	73.10	213.90	2958	25.83	74.13	212.87	2944	26.19	75.17	211.83	2930	26.55	76.21	210.79	2915
287.5	25.41	73.05	214.45	2966	25.77	74.09	213.41	2951	26.13	75.13	212.37	2937	26.49	76.17	211.33	2923
288	25.35	73.01	214.99	2973	25.71	74.05	213.95	2959	26.07	75.09	212.91	2945	26.43	76.13	211.87	2930
288.5	25.29	72.97	215.53	2981	25.65	74.01	214.49	2966	26.01	75.05	213.45	2952	26.37	76.09	212.41	2938
289	25.24	72.93	216.07	2988	25.59	73.97	215.03	2974	25.95	75.01	213.99	2960	26.31	76.04	212.96	2945
289.5	25.18	72.89	216.61	2996	25.54	73.93	215.57	2981	25.89	74.97	214.53	2967	26.25	76.00	213.50	2953
290	25.12	72.85	217.15	3003	25.48	73.89	216.11	2989	25.84	74.93	215.08	2974	26.19	75.96	214.04	2960
290.5	25.06	72.81	217.69	3011	25.42	73.85	216.65	2996	25.78	74.88	215.62	2982	26.13	75.92	214.58	2968
291	25.01	72.77	218.23	3018	25.36	73.81	217.19	3004	25.72	74.84	216.16	2989	26.08	75.88	215.12	2975
291.5	24.95	72.73	218.77	3026	25.31	73.76	217.74	3011	25.66	74.80	216.70	2997	26.02	75.84	215.66	2983
292	24.89	72.69	219.31	3033	25.25	73.72	218.28	3019	25.60	74.76	217.24	3004	25.96	75.80	216.20	2990
292.5	24.84	72.65	219.86	3041	25.19	73.68	218.82	3026	25.55	74.72	217.78	3012	25.90	75.76	216.74	2998
293	24.78	72.60	220.40	3048	25.13	73.64	219.36	3034	25.49	74.68	218.32	3019	25.84	75.72	217.28	3005
293.5	24.72	72.56	220.94	3056	25.08	73.60	219.90	3041	25.43	74.64	218.86	3027	25.78	75.68	217.82	3013
294	24.67	72.52	221.48	3063	25.02	73.56	220.44	3049	25.37	74.60	219.40	3034	25.73	75.63	218.37	3020
294.5	24.61	72.48	222.02	3071	24.96	73.52	220.98	3056	25.32	74.56	219.94	3042	25.67	75.59	218.91	3027
295	24.56	72.44	222.56	3078	24.91	73.48	221.52	3064	25.26	74.52	220.49	3049	25.61	75.55	219.45	3035
295.5	24.50	72.40	223.10	3085	24.85	73.44	222.06	3071	25.20	74.47	221.03	3057	25.55	75.51	219.99	3042
296	24.45	72.36	223.64	3093	24.80	73.40	222.60	3079	25.15	74.43	221.57	3064	25.50	75.47	220.53	3050
296.5	24.39	72.32	224.18	3100	24.74	73.35	223.15	3086	25.09	74.39	222.11	3072	25.44	75.43	221.07	3057
297	24.34	72.28	224.72	3108	24.68	73.31	223.69	3094	25.03	74.35	222.65	3079	25.38	75.39	221.61	3065
297.5	24.28	72.24	225.27	3115	24.63	73.27	224.23	3101	24.98	74.31	223.19	3087	25.33	75.35	222.15	3072
298	24.23	72.19	225.81	3123	24.57	73.23	224.77	3109	24.92	74.27	223.73	3094	25.27	75.31	222.69	3080
298.5	24.17	72.15	226.35	3130	24.52	73.19	225.31	3116	24.87	74.23	224.27	3102	25.21	75.27	223.23	3087
299	24.12	72.11	226.89	3138	24.46	73.15	225.85	3124	24.81	74.19	224.81	3109	25.16	75.22	223.78	3095
299.5	24.06	72.07	227.43	3145	24.41	73.11	226.39	3131	24.76	74.15	225.35	3117	25.10	75.18	224.32	3102
300	24.01	72.03	227.97	3153	24.36	73.07	226.93	3138	24.70	74.11	225.90	3124	25.05	75.14	224.86	3110
300.5	23.96	71.99	228.51	3160	24.30	73.03	227.47	3146	24.65	74.06	226.44	3132	24.99	75.10	225.40	3117
301	23.90	71.95	229.05	3168	24.25	72.99	228.01	3153	24.59	74.02	226.98	3139	24.94	75.06	225.94	3125
301.5	23.85	71.91	229.59	3175	24.19	72.94	228.56	3161	24.54	73.98	227.52	3147	24.88	75.02	226.48	3132
302	23.80	71.87	230.13	3183	24.14	72.90	229.10	3168	24.48	73.94	228.06	3154	24.83	74.98	227.02	3140
302.5	23.74	71.83	230.68	3190	24.09	72.86	229.64	3176	24.43	73.90	228.60	3162	24.77	74.94	227.56	3147
303	23.69	71.78	231.22	3198	24.03	72.82	230.18	3183	24.38	73.86	229.14	3169	24.72	74.90	228.10	3155
303.5	23.64	71.74	231.76	3205	23.98	72.78	230.72	3191	24.32	73.82	229.68	3177	24.66	74.86	228.64	3162
304	23.59	71.70	232.30	3213	23.93	72.74	231.26	3198	24.27	73.78	230.22	3184	24.61	74.81	229.19	3170
304.5	23.53	71.66	232.84	3220	23.87	72.70	231.80	3206	24.22	73.74	230.76	3191	24.56	74.77	229.73	3177
305	23.48	71.62	233.38	3228	23.82	72.66	232.34	3213	24.16	73.70	231.31	3199	24.50	74.73	230.27	3185
305.5	23.43	71.58	233.92	3235	23.77	72.62	232.88	3221	24.11	73.65	231.85	3206	24.45	74.69	230.81	3192
306	23.38	71.54	234.46	3243	23.72	72.58	233.42	3228	24.06	73.61	232.39	3214	24.40	74.65	231.35	3200
306.5	23.33	71.50	235.00	3250	23.67	72.53	233.97	3236	24.00	73.57	232.93	3221	24.34	74.61	231.89	3207
307	23.28	71.46	235.54	3258	23.61	72.49	234.51	3243	23.95	73.53	233.47	3229	24.29	74.57	232.43	3215
307.5	23.22	71.42	236.09	3265	23.56	72.45	235.05	3251	23.90	73.49	234.01	3236	24.24	74.53	232.97	3222
308	23.17	71.37	236.63	3273	23.51	72.41	235.59	3258	23.85	73.45	234.55	3244	24.18	74.49	233.51	3229
308.5	23.12	71.33	237.17	3280	23.46	72.37	236.13	3266	23.80	73.41	235.09	3251	24.13	74.45	234.05	3237
309	23.07	71.29	237.71	3288	23.41	72.33	236.67	3273	23.74	73.37	235.63	3259	24.08	74.40	234.60	3244
309.5	23.02	71.25	238.25	3295	23.36	72.29	237.21	3281	23.69	73.33	236.17	3266	24.03	74.36	235.14	3252
310	22.97	71.21	238.79	3302	23.31	72.25	237.75	3288	23.64	73.29	236.72	3274	23.98	74.32	235.68	3259
310.5	22.92	71.17	239.33	3310	23.25	72.21	238.29	3296	23.59	73.24	237.26	3281	23.92	74.28	236.22	3267
311	22.87	71.13	239.87	3317	23.20	72.17	238.83	3303	23.54	73.20	237.80	3289	23.87	74.24	236.76	3274
311.5	22.82	71.09	240.41	3325	23.15	72.12	239.38	3311	23.49	73.16	238.34	3296	23.82	74.20	237.30	3282

Body Composition MALE 280-311.5 Lb.

Weight: Lb.	Waist: 48 inches				48.25 inches				48.5 inches				48.75 inches			
	Fat: %	Fat: Lb.	LBM: Lb.	RMR: Cal.	Fat: %	Fat: Lb.	LBM: Lb.	RMR: Cal.	Fat: %	Fat: Lb.	LBM: Lb.	RMR: Cal.	Fat: %	Fat: Lb.	LBM: Lb.	RMR: Cal.
280	27.79	77.82	202.18	2796	28.16	78.86	201.14	2782	28.53	79.90	200.11	2767	28.90	80.93	199.07	2753
280.5	27.73	77.78	202.72	2804	28.10	78.82	201.68	2789	28.47	79.85	200.65	2775	28.84	80.89	199.61	2761
281	27.66	77.74	203.26	2811	28.03	78.78	202.22	2797	28.40	79.81	201.19	2782	28.77	80.85	200.15	2768
281.5	27.60	77.70	203.80	2819	27.97	78.73	202.77	2804	28.34	79.77	201.73	2790	28.71	80.81	200.69	2776
282	27.54	77.66	204.34	2826	27.91	78.69	203.31	2812	28.27	79.73	202.27	2797	28.64	80.77	201.23	2783
282.5	27.47	77.62	204.89	2834	27.84	78.65	203.85	2819	28.21	79.69	202.81	2805	28.58	80.73	201.77	2791
283	27.41	77.57	205.43	2841	27.78	78.61	204.39	2827	28.14	79.65	203.35	2812	28.51	80.69	202.31	2798
283.5	27.35	77.53	205.97	2849	27.71	78.57	204.93	2834	28.08	79.61	203.89	2820	28.45	80.65	202.85	2805
284	27.29	77.49	206.51	2856	27.65	78.53	205.47	2842	28.02	79.57	204.43	2827	28.38	80.60	203.40	2813
284.5	27.22	77.45	207.05	2863	27.59	78.49	206.01	2849	27.95	79.53	204.97	2835	28.32	80.56	203.94	2820
285	27.16	77.41	207.59	2871	27.53	78.45	206.55	2857	27.89	79.49	205.52	2842	28.25	80.52	204.48	2828
285.5	27.10	77.37	208.13	2878	27.46	78.41	207.09	2864	27.83	79.44	206.06	2850	28.19	80.48	205.02	2835
286	27.04	77.33	208.67	2886	27.40	78.37	207.63	2872	27.76	79.40	206.60	2857	28.13	80.44	205.56	2843
286.5	26.98	77.29	209.21	2893	27.34	78.32	208.18	2879	27.70	79.36	207.14	2865	28.06	80.40	206.10	2850
287	26.91	77.25	209.75	2901	27.28	78.28	208.72	2887	27.64	79.32	207.68	2872	28.00	80.36	206.64	2858
287.5	26.85	77.21	210.30	2908	27.21	78.24	209.26	2894	27.58	79.28	208.22	2880	27.94	80.32	207.18	2865
288	26.79	77.16	210.84	2916	27.15	78.20	209.80	2902	27.51	79.24	208.76	2887	27.87	80.28	207.72	2873
288.5	26.73	77.12	211.00	2923	27.09	78.10	210.34	2909	27.45	79.20	209.30	2895	27.81	80.24	208.26	2880
289	26.67	77.08	211.92	2931	27.03	78.12	210.88	2916	27.39	79.16	209.84	2902	27.75	80.19	208.81	2888
289.5	26.61	77.04	212.46	2938	26.97	78.08	211.42	2924	27.33	79.12	210.38	2910	27.69	80.15	209.35	2895
290	26.55	77.00	213.00	2946	26.91	78.04	211.96	2931	27.27	79.08	210.93	2917	27.63	80.11	209.89	2903
290.5	26.49	76.96	213.54	2953	26.85	78.00	212.50	2939	27.21	79.03	211.47	2925	27.56	80.07	210.43	2910
291	26.43	76.92	214.08	2961	26.79	77.96	213.04	2946	27.15	78.99	212.01	2932	27.50	80.03	210.97	2918
291.5	26.37	76.88	214.62	2968	26.73	77.91	213.59	2954	27.08	78.95	212.55	2940	27.44	79.99	211.51	2925
292	26.31	76.84	215.16	2976	26.67	77.87	214.13	2961	27.02	78.91	213.09	2947	27.38	79.95	212.05	2933
292.5	26.25	76.80	215.71	2983	26.61	77.83	214.67	2969	26.96	78.87	213.63	2955	27.32	79.91	212.59	2940
293	26.20	76.75	216.25	2991	26.55	77.79	215.21	2976	26.90	78.83	214.17	2962	27.26	79.87	213.13	2948
293.5	26.14	76.71	216.79	2998	26.49	77.75	215.75	2984	26.84	78.79	214.71	2969	27.20	79.83	213.67	2955
294	26.08	76.67	217.33	3006	26.43	77.71	216.29	2991	26.78	78.75	215.25	2977	27.14	79.78	214.22	2963
294.5	26.02	76.63	217.87	3013	26.37	77.67	216.83	2999	26.73	78.71	215.79	2984	27.08	79.74	214.76	2970
295	25.96	76.59	218.41	3021	26.31	77.63	217.37	3006	26.67	78.67	216.34	2992	27.02	79.70	215.30	2978
295.5	25.90	76.55	218.95	3028	26.26	77.59	217.91	3014	26.61	78.62	216.88	2999	26.96	79.66	215.84	2985
296	25.85	76.51	219.49	3036	26.20	77.55	218.45	3021	26.55	78.58	217.42	3007	26.90	79.62	216.38	2993
296.5	25.79	76.47	220.03	3043	26.14	77.50	219.00	3029	26.49	78.54	217.96	3014	26.84	79.58	216.92	3000
297	25.73	76.43	220.57	3051	26.08	77.46	219.54	3036	26.43	78.50	218.50	3022	26.78	79.54	217.46	3007
297.5	25.68	76.39	221.12	3058	26.02	77.42	220.08	3044	26.37	78.46	219.04	3029	26.72	79.50	218.00	3015
298	25.62	76.34	221.66	3066	25.97	77.38	220.62	3051	26.32	78.42	219.58	3037	26.66	79.46	218.54	3022
298.5	25.56	76.30	222.20	3073	25.91	77.34	221.16	3059	26.26	78.38	220.12	3044	26.60	79.42	219.08	3030
299	25.51	76.26	222.74	3080	25.85	77.30	221.70	3066	26.20	78.34	220.66	3052	26.55	79.37	219.63	3037
299.5	25.45	76.22	223.28	3088	25.80	77.26	222.24	3074	26.14	78.30	221.20	3059	26.49	79.33	220.17	3045
300	25.39	76.18	223.82	3095	25.74	77.22	222.78	3081	26.09	78.26	221.75	3067	26.43	79.29	220.71	3052
300.5	25.34	76.14	224.36	3103	25.68	77.18	223.32	3089	26.03	78.21	222.29	3074	26.37	79.25	221.25	3060
301	25.28	76.10	224.90	3110	25.63	77.14	223.86	3096	25.97	78.17	222.83	3082	26.32	79.21	221.79	3067
301.5	25.23	76.06	225.44	3118	25.57	77.09	224.41	3104	25.91	78.13	223.37	3089	26.26	79.17	222.33	3075
302	25.17	76.02	225.98	3125	25.51	77.05	224.95	3111	25.86	78.09	223.91	3097	26.20	79.13	222.87	3082
302.5	25.12	75.98	226.53	3133	25.46	77.01	225.49	3118	25.80	78.05	224.45	3104	26.14	79.09	223.41	3090
303	25.06	75.93	227.07	3140	25.40	76.97	226.03	3126	25.75	78.01	224.99	3112	26.09	79.05	223.95	3097
303.5	25.01	75.89	227.61	3148	25.35	76.93	226.57	3133	25.69	77.97	225.53	3119	26.03	79.01	224.49	3105
304	24.95	75.85	228.15	3155	25.29	76.89	227.11	3141	25.63	77.93	226.07	3127	25.98	78.96	225.04	3112
304.5	24.90	75.81	228.69	3163	25.24	76.85	227.65	3148	25.58	77.89	226.61	3134	25.92	78.92	225.58	3120
305	24.84	75.77	229.23	3170	25.18	76.81	228.19	3156	25.52	77.85	227.16	3142	25.86	78.88	226.12	3127
305.5	24.79	75.73	229.77	3178	25.13	76.77	228.73	3163	25.47	77.80	227.70	3149	25.81	78.84	226.66	3135
306	24.73	75.69	230.31	3185	25.07	76.73	229.27	3171	25.41	77.76	228.24	3157	25.75	78.80	227.20	3142
306.5	24.68	75.65	230.85	3193	25.02	76.68	229.82	3178	25.36	77.72	228.78	3164	25.70	78.76	227.74	3150
307	24.63	75.61	231.39	3200	24.97	76.64	230.36	3186	25.30	77.68	229.32	3171	25.64	78.72	228.28	3157
307.5	24.57	75.57	231.94	3208	24.91	76.60	230.90	3193	25.25	77.64	229.86	3179	25.59	78.68	228.82	3165
308	24.52	75.52	232.48	3215	24.86	76.56	231.44	3201	25.19	77.60	230.40	3186	25.53	78.64	229.36	3172
308.5	24.47	75.48	233.02	3223	24.80	76.52	231.98	3208	25.14	77.56	230.94	3194	25.48	78.60	229.90	3180
309	24.41	75.44	233.56	3230	24.75	76.48	232.52	3216	25.09	77.52	231.48	3201	25.42	78.55	230.45	3187
309.5	24.36	75.40	234.10	3238	24.70	76.44	233.06	3223	25.03	77.48	232.02	3209	25.37	78.51	230.99	3195
310	24.31	75.36	234.64	3245	24.64	76.40	233.60	3231	24.98	77.44	232.57	3216	25.31	78.47	231.53	3202
310.5	24.26	75.32	235.18	3253	24.59	76.36	234.14	3238	24.93	77.39	233.11	3224	25.26	78.43	232.07	3210
311	24.21	75.28	235.72	3260	24.54	76.32	234.68	3246	24.87	77.35	233.65	3231	25.21	78.39	232.61	3217
311.5	24.15	75.24	236.26	3268	24.49	76.27	235.23	3253	24.82	77.31	234.19	3239	25.15	78.35	233.15	3224

Body Composition   MALE   280-311.5 Lb.

Waist:	49 inches				49.25 inches				49.5 inches				49.75 inches			
Weight: Lb.	Fat: %	Fat: Lb.	LBM: Lb.	RMR: Cal.	Fat: %	Fat: Lb.	LBM: Lb.	RMR: Cal.	Fat: %	Fat: Lb.	LBM: Lb.	RMR: Cal.	Fat: %	Fat: Lb.	LBM: Lb.	RMR: Cal.
280	29.28	81.97	198.03	2739	29.65	83.01	196.99	2724	30.02	84.05	195.96	2710	30.39	85.08	194.92	2696
280.5	29.21	81.93	198.57	2746	29.58	82.97	197.53	2732	29.95	84.00	196.50	2718	30.32	85.04	195.46	2703
281	29.14	81.89	199.11	2754	29.51	82.93	198.07	2739	29.88	83.96	197.04	2725	30.25	85.00	196.00	2711
281.5	29.08	81.85	199.65	2761	29.44	82.88	198.62	2747	29.81	83.92	197.58	2733	30.18	84.96	196.54	2718
282	29.01	81.81	200.19	2769	29.38	82.84	199.16	2754	29.75	83.88	198.12	2740	30.11	84.92	197.08	2726
282.5	28.94	81.77	200.74	2776	29.31	82.80	199.70	2762	29.68	83.84	198.66	2747	30.05	84.88	197.62	2733
283	28.88	81.72	201.28	2784	29.24	82.76	200.24	2769	29.61	83.80	199.20	2755	29.98	84.84	198.16	2741
283.5	28.81	81.68	201.82	2791	29.18	82.72	200.78	2777	29.54	83.76	199.74	2762	29.91	84.80	198.70	2748
284	28.75	81.64	202.36	2799	29.11	82.68	201.32	2784	29.48	83.72	200.28	2770	29.84	84.75	199.25	2756
284.5	28.68	81.60	202.90	2806	29.05	82.64	201.86	2792	29.41	83.68	200.82	2777	29.78	84.71	199.79	2763
285	28.62	81.56	203.44	2814	28.98	82.60	202.40	2799	29.35	83.64	201.37	2785	29.71	84.67	200.33	2771
285.5	28.55	81.52	203.98	2821	28.92	82.56	202.94	2807	29.28	83.59	201.91	2792	29.64	84.63	200.87	2778
286	28.49	81.48	204.52	2829	28.85	82.52	203.48	2814	29.21	83.55	202.45	2800	29.58	84.59	201.41	2785
286.5	28.42	81.44	205.06	2836	28.79	82.47	204.03	2822	29.15	83.51	202.99	2807	29.51	84.55	201.95	2793
287	28.36	81.40	205.60	2844	28.72	82.43	204.57	2829	29.08	83.47	203.53	2815	29.45	84.51	202.49	2800
287.5	28.30	81.36	206.15	2851	28.66	82.39	205.11	2837	29.02	83.43	204.07	2822	29.38	84.47	203.03	2808
288	28.23	81.31	206.69	2858	28.59	82.35	205.65	2844	28.95	83.39	204.61	2830	29.31	84.43	203.57	2815
288.5	28.17	81.27	207.23	2866	28.53	82.31	206.19	2852	28.89	83.35	205.15	2837	29.25	84.39	204.11	2823
289	28.11	81.23	207.77	2873	28.47	82.27	206.73	2859	28.83	83.31	205.69	2845	29.18	84.34	204.66	2830
289.5	28.05	81.19	208.31	2881	28.40	82.23	207.27	2867	28.76	83.27	206.23	2852	29.12	84.30	205.20	2838
290	27.98	81.15	208.85	2888	28.34	82.19	207.81	2874	28.70	83.23	206.78	2860	29.06	84.26	205.74	2845
290.5	27.92	81.11	209.39	2896	28.28	82.15	208.35	2882	28.63	83.18	207.32	2867	28.99	84.22	206.28	2853
291	27.86	81.07	209.93	2903	28.21	82.11	208.89	2889	28.57	83.14	207.86	2875	28.93	84.18	206.82	2860
291.5	27.80	81.03	210.47	2911	28.15	82.06	209.44	2896	28.51	83.10	208.40	2882	28.86	84.14	207.36	2868
292	27.73	80.99	211.01	2918	28.09	82.02	209.98	2904	28.45	83.06	208.94	2890	28.80	84.10	207.90	2875
292.5	27.67	80.95	211.56	2926	28.03	81.98	210.52	2911	28.38	83.02	209.48	2897	28.74	84.06	208.44	2883
293	27.61	80.90	212.10	2933	27.97	81.94	211.06	2919	28.32	82.98	210.02	2905	28.67	84.02	208.98	2890
293.5	27.55	80.86	212.64	2941	27.90	81.90	211.60	2926	28.26	82.94	210.56	2912	28.61	83.98	209.52	2898
294	27.49	80.82	213.18	2948	27.84	81.86	212.14	2934	28.20	82.90	211.10	2920	28.55	83.93	210.07	2905
294.5	27.43	80.78	213.72	2956	27.78	81.82	212.68	2941	28.13	82.86	211.64	2927	28.49	83.89	210.61	2913
295	27.37	80.74	214.26	2963	27.72	81.78	213.22	2949	28.07	82.82	212.19	2935	28.42	83.85	211.15	2920
295.5	27.31	80.70	214.80	2971	27.66	81.74	213.76	2956	28.01	82.77	212.73	2942	28.36	83.81	211.69	2928
296	27.25	80.66	215.34	2978	27.60	81.70	214.30	2964	27.95	82.73	213.27	2949	28.30	83.77	212.23	2935
296.5	27.19	80.62	215.88	2986	27.54	81.65	214.85	2971	27.89	82.69	213.81	2957	28.24	83.73	212.77	2943
297	27.13	80.58	216.42	2993	27.48	81.61	215.39	2979	27.83	82.65	214.35	2964	28.18	83.69	213.31	2950
297.5	27.07	80.54	216.97	3001	27.42	81.57	215.93	2986	27.77	82.61	214.89	2972	28.12	83.65	213.85	2958
298	27.01	80.49	217.51	3008	27.36	81.53	216.47	2994	27.71	82.57	215.43	2979	28.06	83.61	214.39	2965
298.5	26.95	80.45	218.05	3016	27.30	81.49	217.01	3001	27.65	82.53	215.97	2987	28.00	83.57	214.93	2973
299	26.89	80.41	218.59	3023	27.24	81.45	217.55	3009	27.59	82.49	216.51	2994	27.93	83.52	215.48	2980
299.5	26.84	80.37	219.13	3031	27.18	81.41	218.09	3016	27.53	82.45	217.05	3002	27.87	83.48	216.02	2988
300	26.78	80.33	219.67	3038	27.12	81.37	218.63	3024	27.47	82.41	217.60	3009	27.81	83.44	216.56	2995
300.5	26.72	80.29	220.21	3046	27.06	81.33	219.17	3031	27.41	82.36	218.14	3017	27.75	83.40	217.10	3002
301	26.66	80.25	220.75	3053	27.01	81.29	219.71	3039	27.35	82.32	218.68	3024	27.69	83.36	217.64	3010
301.5	26.60	80.21	221.29	3060	26.95	81.24	220.26	3046	27.29	82.28	219.22	3032	27.63	83.32	218.18	3017
302	26.55	80.17	221.83	3068	26.89	81.20	220.80	3054	27.23	82.24	219.76	3039	27.58	83.28	218.72	3025
302.5	26.49	80.13	222.38	3075	26.83	81.16	221.34	3061	27.17	82.20	220.30	3047	27.52	83.24	219.26	3032
303	26.43	80.08	222.92	3083	26.77	81.12	221.88	3069	27.12	82.16	220.84	3054	27.46	83.20	219.80	3040
303.5	26.37	80.04	223.46	3090	26.72	81.08	222.42	3076	27.06	82.12	221.38	3062	27.40	83.16	220.34	3047
304	26.32	80.00	224.00	3098	26.66	81.04	222.96	3084	27.00	82.08	221.92	3069	27.34	83.11	220.89	3055
304.5	26.26	79.96	224.54	3105	26.60	81.00	223.50	3091	26.94	82.04	222.46	3077	27.28	83.07	221.43	3062
305	26.20	79.92	225.08	3113	26.54	80.96	224.04	3099	26.88	81.99	223.01	3084	27.22	83.03	221.97	3070
305.5	26.15	79.88	225.62	3120	26.49	80.92	224.58	3106	26.83	81.95	223.55	3092	27.17	82.99	222.51	3077
306	26.09	79.84	226.16	3128	26.43	80.88	225.12	3113	26.77	81.91	224.09	3099	27.11	82.95	223.05	3085
306.5	26.03	79.80	226.70	3135	26.37	80.83	225.67	3121	26.71	81.87	224.63	3107	27.05	82.91	223.59	3092
307	25.98	79.76	227.24	3143	26.32	80.79	226.21	3128	26.66	81.83	225.17	3114	26.99	82.87	224.13	3100
307.5	25.92	79.72	227.79	3150	26.26	80.75	226.75	3136	26.60	81.79	225.71	3122	26.94	82.83	224.67	3107
308	25.87	79.67	228.33	3158	26.21	80.71	227.29	3143	26.54	81.75	226.25	3129	26.88	82.79	225.21	3115
308.5	25.81	79.63	228.87	3165	26.15	80.67	227.83	3151	26.49	81.71	226.79	3137	26.82	82.75	225.75	3122
309	25.76	79.59	229.41	3173	26.09	80.63	228.37	3158	26.43	81.67	227.33	3144	26.77	82.70	226.30	3130
309.5	25.70	79.55	229.95	3180	26.04	80.59	228.91	3166	26.37	81.63	227.87	3151	26.71	82.66	226.84	3137
310	25.65	79.51	230.49	3188	25.98	80.55	229.45	3173	26.32	81.59	228.42	3159	26.65	82.62	227.38	3145
310.5	25.59	79.47	231.03	3195	25.93	80.51	229.99	3181	26.26	81.54	228.96	3166	26.60	82.58	227.92	3152
311	25.54	79.43	231.57	3203	25.87	80.47	230.53	3188	26.21	81.50	229.50	3174	26.54	82.54	228.46	3160
311.5	25.49	79.39	232.11	3210	25.82	80.42	231.08	3196	26.15	81.46	230.04	3181	26.48	82.50	229.00	3167

Body Composition   MALE   280-311.5 Lb.

Weight: Lb.	Waist: 50 inches				50.25 inches				50.5 inches				50.75 inches			
	Fat: %	Fat: Lb.	LBM: Lb.	RMR: Cal.	Fat: %	Fat: Lb.	LBM: Lb.	RMR: Cal.	Fat: %	Fat: Lb.	LBM: Lb.	RMR: Cal.	Fat: %	Fat: Lb.	LBM: Lb.	RMR: Cal.
280	30.76	86.12	193.88	2681	31.13	87.16	192.84	2667	31.50	88.20	191.81	2653	31.87	89.23	190.77	2638
280.5	30.69	86.08	194.42	2689	31.06	87.12	193.38	2674	31.43	88.15	192.35	2660	31.80	89.19	191.31	2646
281	30.62	86.04	194.96	2696	30.99	87.08	193.92	2682	31.36	88.11	192.89	2668	31.73	89.15	191.85	2653
281.5	30.55	86.00	195.50	2704	30.92	87.03	194.47	2689	31.29	88.07	193.43	2675	31.66	89.11	192.39	2661
282	30.48	85.96	196.04	2711	30.85	86.99	195.01	2697	31.22	88.03	193.97	2683	31.58	89.07	192.93	2668
282.5	30.41	85.92	196.59	2719	30.78	86.95	195.55	2704	31.15	87.99	194.51	2690	31.51	89.03	193.47	2676
283	30.34	85.87	197.13	2726	30.71	86.91	196.09	2712	31.08	87.95	195.05	2698	31.44	88.99	194.01	2683
283.5	30.28	85.83	197.67	2734	30.64	86.87	196.63	2719	31.01	87.91	195.59	2705	31.37	88.95	194.55	2691
284	30.21	85.79	198.21	2741	30.57	86.83	197.17	2727	30.94	87.87	196.13	2713	31.30	88.90	195.10	2698
284.5	30.14	85.75	198.75	2749	30.51	86.79	197.71	2734	30.87	87.83	196.67	2720	31.23	88.86	195.64	2706
285	30.07	85.71	199.29	2756	30.44	86.75	198.25	2742	30.80	87.79	197.22	2727	31.17	88.82	196.18	2713
285.5	30.01	85.67	199.83	2764	30.37	86.71	198.79	2749	30.73	87.74	197.76	2735	31.10	88.78	196.72	2721
286	29.94	85.63	200.37	2771	30.30	86.67	199.33	2757	30.67	87.70	198.30	2742	31.03	88.74	197.26	2728
286.5	29.87	85.59	200.91	2779	30.24	86.62	199.88	2764	30.60	87.66	198.84	2750	30.96	88.70	197.80	2736
287	29.81	85.55	201.45	2786	30.17	86.58	200.42	2772	30.53	87.62	199.38	2757	30.89	88.66	198.34	2743
287.5	29.74	85.51	202.00	2794	30.10	86.54	200.96	2779	30.46	87.58	199.92	2765	30.82	88.62	198.88	2751
288	29.68	85.46	202.54	2801	30.04	86.50	201.50	2787	30.40	87.54	200.46	2772	30.76	88.58	199.42	2758
288.5	29.61	85.42	203.08	2809	29.97	86.46	202.04	2794	30.33	87.50	201.00	2780	30.69	88.54	199.96	2766
289	29.54	85.38	203.62	2816	29.90	86.42	202.58	2802	30.26	87.46	201.54	2787	30.62	88.49	200.51	2773
289.5	29.48	85.34	204.16	2824	29.84	86.38	203.12	2809	30.20	87.42	202.08	2795	30.55	88.45	201.05	2780
290	29.41	85.30	204.70	2831	29.77	86.34	203.66	2817	30.13	87.38	202.63	2802	30.49	88.41	201.59	2788
290.5	29.35	85.26	205.24	2838	29.71	86.30	204.20	2824	30.06	87.33	203.17	2810	30.42	88.37	202.13	2795
291	29.28	85.22	205.78	2846	29.64	86.26	204.74	2832	30.00	87.29	203.71	2817	30.35	88.33	202.67	2803
291.5	29.22	85.18	206.32	2853	29.58	86.21	205.29	2839	29.93	87.25	204.25	2825	30.29	88.29	203.21	2810
292	29.16	85.14	206.86	2861	29.51	86.17	205.83	2847	29.87	87.21	204.79	2832	30.22	88.25	203.75	2818
292.5	29.09	85.10	207.41	2868	29.45	86.13	206.37	2854	29.80	87.17	205.33	2840	30.16	88.21	204.29	2825
293	29.03	85.05	207.95	2876	29.38	86.09	206.91	2862	29.74	87.13	205.87	2847	30.09	88.17	204.83	2833
293.5	28.97	85.01	208.49	2883	29.32	86.05	207.45	2869	29.67	87.09	206.41	2855	30.03	88.13	205.37	2840
294	28.90	84.97	209.03	2891	29.25	86.01	207.99	2877	29.61	87.05	206.95	2862	29.96	88.08	205.92	2848
294.5	28.84	84.93	209.57	2898	29.19	85.97	208.53	2884	29.54	87.01	207.49	2870	29.90	88.04	206.46	2855
295	28.78	84.89	210.11	2906	29.13	85.93	209.07	2891	29.48	86.97	208.04	2877	29.83	88.00	207.00	2863
295.5	28.71	84.85	210.65	2913	29.06	85.89	209.61	2899	29.42	86.92	208.58	2885	29.77	87.96	207.54	2870
296	28.65	84.81	211.19	2921	29.00	85.85	210.15	2906	29.35	86.88	209.12	2892	29.70	87.92	208.08	2878
296.5	28.59	84.77	211.73	2928	28.94	85.80	210.70	2914	29.29	86.84	209.66	2900	29.64	87.88	208.62	2885
297	28.53	84.73	212.27	2936	28.88	85.76	211.24	2921	29.23	86.80	210.20	2907	29.58	87.84	209.16	2893
297.5	28.47	84.69	212.82	2943	28.81	85.72	211.78	2929	29.16	86.76	210.74	2915	29.51	87.80	209.70	2900
298	28.40	84.64	213.36	2951	28.75	85.68	212.32	2936	29.10	86.72	211.28	2922	29.45	87.76	210.24	2908
298.5	28.34	84.60	213.90	2958	28.69	85.64	212.86	2944	29.04	86.68	211.82	2929	29.39	87.72	210.78	2915
299	28.28	84.56	214.44	2966	28.63	85.60	213.40	2951	28.98	86.64	212.36	2937	29.32	87.67	211.33	2923
299.5	28.22	84.52	214.98	2973	28.57	85.56	213.94	2959	28.91	86.60	212.90	2944	29.26	87.63	211.87	2930
300	28.16	84.48	215.52	2981	28.51	85.52	214.48	2966	28.85	86.56	213.45	2952	29.20	87.59	212.41	2938
300.5	28.10	84.44	216.06	2988	28.44	85.48	215.02	2974	28.79	86.51	213.99	2959	29.14	87.55	212.95	2945
301	28.04	84.40	216.60	2996	28.38	85.44	215.56	2981	28.73	86.47	214.53	2967	29.07	87.51	213.49	2953
301.5	27.98	84.36	217.14	3003	28.32	85.39	216.11	2989	28.67	86.43	215.07	2974	29.01	87.47	214.03	2960
302	27.92	84.32	217.68	3011	28.26	85.35	216.65	2996	28.61	86.39	215.61	2982	28.95	87.43	214.57	2968
302.5	27.86	84.28	218.23	3018	28.20	85.31	217.19	3004	28.55	86.35	216.15	2989	28.89	87.39	215.11	2975
303	27.80	84.23	218.77	3026	28.14	85.27	217.73	3011	28.48	86.31	216.69	2997	28.83	87.35	215.65	2982
303.5	27.74	84.19	219.31	3033	28.08	85.23	218.27	3019	28.42	86.27	217.23	3004	28.77	87.31	216.19	2990
304	27.68	84.15	219.85	3040	28.02	85.19	218.81	3026	28.36	86.23	217.77	3012	28.71	87.26	216.74	2997
304.5	27.62	84.11	220.39	3048	27.96	85.15	219.35	3034	28.30	86.19	218.31	3019	28.64	87.22	217.28	3005
305	27.56	84.07	220.93	3055	27.90	85.11	219.89	3041	28.24	86.15	218.86	3027	28.58	87.18	217.82	3012
305.5	27.51	84.03	221.47	3063	27.85	85.07	220.43	3049	28.18	86.10	219.40	3034	28.52	87.14	218.36	3020
306	27.45	83.99	222.01	3070	27.79	85.03	220.97	3056	28.13	86.06	219.94	3042	28.46	87.10	218.90	3027
306.5	27.39	83.95	222.55	3078	27.73	84.98	221.52	3064	28.07	86.02	220.48	3049	28.40	87.06	219.44	3035
307	27.33	83.91	223.09	3085	27.67	84.94	222.06	3071	28.01	85.98	221.02	3057	28.34	87.02	219.98	3042
307.5	27.27	83.87	223.64	3093	27.61	84.90	222.60	3079	27.95	85.94	221.56	3064	28.29	86.98	220.52	3050
308	27.22	83.82	224.18	3100	27.55	84.86	223.14	3086	27.89	85.90	222.10	3072	28.23	86.94	221.06	3057
308.5	27.16	83.78	224.72	3108	27.49	84.82	223.68	3093	27.83	85.86	222.64	3079	28.17	86.90	221.60	3065
309	27.10	83.74	225.26	3115	27.44	84.78	224.22	3101	27.77	85.82	223.18	3087	28.11	86.85	222.15	3072
309.5	27.04	83.70	225.80	3123	27.38	84.74	224.76	3108	27.71	85.78	223.72	3094	28.05	86.81	222.69	3080
310	26.99	83.66	226.34	3130	27.32	84.70	225.30	3116	27.66	85.74	224.27	3102	27.99	86.77	223.23	3087
310.5	26.93	83.62	226.88	3138	27.26	84.66	225.84	3123	27.60	85.69	224.81	3109	27.93	86.73	223.77	3095
311	26.87	83.58	227.42	3145	27.21	84.62	226.38	3131	27.54	85.65	225.35	3117	27.87	86.69	224.31	3102
311.5	26.82	83.54	227.96	3153	27.15	84.57	226.93	3138	27.48	85.61	225.89	3124	27.82	86.65	224.85	3110

Body Composition   MALE   280-311.5 Lb.

Waist:	51 inches				51.25 inches				51.5 inches				51.75 inches			
Weight: Lb.	Fat: %	Fat: Lb.	LBM: Lb.	RMR: Cal.	Fat: %	Fat: Lb.	LBM: Lb.	RMR: Cal.	Fat: %	Fat: Lb.	LBM: Lb.	RMR: Cal.	Fat: %	Fat: Lb.	LBM: Lb.	RMR: Cal.
280	32.24	90.27	189.73	2624	32.61	91.31	188.69	2610	32.98	92.35	187.66	2595	33.35	93.38	186.62	2581
280.5	32.17	90.23	190.27	2631	32.54	91.27	189.23	2617	32.91	92.30	188.20	2603	33.28	93.34	187.16	2588
281	32.10	90.19	190.81	2639	32.46	91.23	189.77	2625	32.83	92.26	188.74	2610	33.20	93.30	187.70	2596
281.5	32.02	90.15	191.35	2646	32.39	91.18	190.32	2632	32.76	92.22	189.28	2618	33.13	93.26	188.24	2603
282	31.95	90.11	191.89	2654	32.32	91.14	190.86	2640	32.69	92.18	189.82	2625	33.06	93.22	188.78	2611
282.5	31.88	90.07	192.44	2661	32.25	91.10	191.40	2647	32.62	92.14	190.36	2633	32.98	93.18	189.32	2618
283	31.81	90.02	192.98	2669	32.18	91.06	191.94	2655	32.54	92.10	190.90	2640	32.91	93.14	189.86	2626
283.5	31.74	89.98	193.52	2676	32.11	91.02	192.48	2662	32.47	92.06	191.44	2648	32.84	93.10	190.40	2633
284	31.67	89.94	194.06	2684	32.04	90.98	193.02	2669	32.40	92.02	191.98	2655	32.77	93.05	190.95	2641
284.5	31.60	89.90	194.60	2691	31.96	90.94	193.56	2677	32.33	91.98	192.52	2663	32.69	93.01	191.49	2648
285	31.53	89.86	195.14	2699	31.89	90.90	194.10	2684	32.26	91.94	193.07	2670	32.62	92.97	192.03	2656
285.5	31.46	89.82	195.68	2706	31.82	90.86	194.64	2692	32.19	91.89	193.61	2678	32.55	92.93	192.57	2663
286	31.39	89.78	196.22	2714	31.75	90.82	195.18	2699	32.12	91.85	194.15	2685	32.48	92.89	193.11	2671
286.5	31.32	89.74	196.76	2721	31.68	90.77	195.73	2707	32.05	91.81	194.69	2693	32.41	92.85	193.65	2678
287	31.25	89.70	197.30	2729	31.61	90.73	196.27	2714	31.98	91.77	195.23	2700	32.34	92.81	194.19	2686
287.5	31.18	89.66	197.85	2736	31.55	90.69	196.81	2722	31.91	91.73	195.77	2707	32.27	92.77	194.73	2693
288	31.12	89.61	198.39	2744	31.48	90.65	197.35	2729	31.84	91.69	196.31	2715	32.20	92.73	195.27	2701
288.5	31.05	89.57	198.93	2751	31.41	90.61	197.89	2737	31.77	91.65	196.85	2722	32.13	92.69	195.81	2708
289	30.98	89.53	199.47	2759	31.34	90.57	198.43	2744	31.70	91.61	197.39	2730	32.06	92.64	196.36	2716
289.5	30.91	89.49	200.01	2766	31.27	90.53	198.97	2752	31.63	91.57	197.93	2737	31.99	92.60	196.90	2723
290	30.84	89.45	200.55	2774	31.20	90.49	199.51	2759	31.56	91.53	198.48	2745	31.92	92.56	197.44	2731
290.5	30.78	89.41	201.09	2781	31.13	90.45	200.05	2767	31.49	91.48	199.02	2752	31.85	92.52	197.98	2738
291	30.71	89.37	201.63	2789	31.07	90.41	200.59	2774	31.42	91.44	199.56	2760	31.78	92.48	198.52	2746
291.5	30.64	89.33	202.17	2796	31.00	90.36	201.14	2782	31.36	91.40	200.10	2767	31.71	92.44	199.06	2753
292	30.58	89.29	202.71	2804	30.93	90.32	201.68	2789	31.29	91.36	200.64	2775	31.64	92.40	199.60	2760
292.5	30.51	89.25	203.26	2811	30.87	90.28	202.22	2797	31.22	91.32	201.18	2782	31.58	92.36	200.14	2768
293	30.45	89.20	203.80	2818	30.80	90.24	202.76	2804	31.15	91.28	201.72	2790	31.51	92.32	200.68	2775
293.5	30.38	89.16	204.34	2826	30.73	90.20	203.30	2812	31.09	91.24	202.26	2797	31.44	92.28	201.22	2783
294	30.31	89.12	204.88	2833	30.67	90.16	203.84	2819	31.02	91.20	202.80	2805	31.37	92.23	201.77	2790
294.5	30.25	89.08	205.42	2841	30.60	90.12	204.38	2827	30.95	91.16	203.34	2812	31.31	92.19	202.31	2798
295	30.18	89.04	205.96	2848	30.53	90.08	204.92	2834	30.89	91.12	203.89	2820	31.24	92.15	202.85	2805
295.5	30.12	89.00	206.50	2856	30.47	90.04	205.46	2842	30.82	91.07	204.43	2827	31.17	92.11	203.39	2813
296	30.05	88.96	207.04	2863	30.40	90.00	206.00	2849	30.75	91.03	204.97	2835	31.10	92.07	203.93	2820
296.5	29.99	88.92	207.58	2871	30.34	89.95	206.55	2857	30.69	90.99	205.51	2842	31.04	92.03	204.47	2828
297	29.92	88.88	208.12	2878	30.27	89.91	207.09	2864	30.62	90.95	206.05	2850	30.97	91.99	205.01	2835
297.5	29.86	88.84	208.67	2886	30.21	89.87	207.63	2871	30.56	90.91	206.59	2857	30.91	91.95	205.55	2843
298	29.80	88.79	209.21	2893	30.14	89.83	208.17	2879	30.49	90.87	207.13	2865	30.84	91.91	206.09	2850
298.5	29.73	88.75	209.75	2901	30.08	89.79	208.71	2886	30.43	90.83	207.67	2872	30.78	91.87	206.63	2858
299	29.67	88.71	210.29	2908	30.02	89.75	209.25	2894	30.36	90.79	208.21	2880	30.71	91.82	207.18	2865
299.5	29.61	88.67	210.83	2916	29.95	89.71	209.79	2901	30.30	90.75	208.75	2887	30.65	91.78	207.72	2873
300	29.54	88.63	211.37	2923	29.89	89.67	210.33	2909	30.24	90.71	209.30	2895	30.58	91.74	208.26	2880
300.5	29.48	88.59	211.91	2931	29.83	89.63	210.87	2916	30.17	90.66	209.84	2902	30.52	91.70	208.80	2888
301	29.42	88.55	212.45	2938	29.76	89.59	211.41	2924	30.11	90.62	210.38	2910	30.45	91.66	209.34	2895
301.5	29.36	88.51	212.99	2946	29.70	89.54	211.96	2931	30.04	90.58	210.92	2917	30.39	91.62	209.88	2903
302	29.29	88.47	213.53	2953	29.64	89.50	212.50	2939	29.98	90.54	211.46	2924	30.32	91.58	210.42	2910
302.5	29.23	88.43	214.08	2961	29.57	89.46	213.04	2946	29.92	90.50	212.00	2932	30.26	91.54	210.96	2918
303	29.17	88.38	214.62	2968	29.51	89.42	213.58	2954	29.85	90.46	212.54	2939	30.20	91.50	211.50	2925
303.5	29.11	88.34	215.16	2976	29.45	89.38	214.12	2961	29.79	90.42	213.08	2947	30.13	91.46	212.04	2933
304	29.05	88.30	215.70	2983	29.39	89.34	214.66	2969	29.73	90.38	213.62	2954	30.07	91.41	212.59	2940
304.5	28.99	88.26	216.24	2991	29.33	89.30	215.20	2976	29.67	90.34	214.16	2962	30.01	91.37	213.13	2948
305	28.92	88.22	216.78	2998	29.26	89.26	215.74	2984	29.60	90.30	214.71	2969	29.95	91.33	213.67	2955
305.5	28.86	88.18	217.32	3006	29.20	89.22	216.28	2991	29.54	90.25	215.25	2977	29.88	91.29	214.21	2963
306	28.80	88.14	217.86	3013	29.14	89.18	216.82	2999	29.48	90.21	215.79	2984	29.82	91.25	214.75	2970
306.5	28.74	88.10	218.40	3021	29.08	89.13	217.37	3006	29.42	90.17	216.33	2992	29.76	91.21	215.29	2977
307	28.68	88.06	218.94	3028	29.02	89.09	217.91	3014	29.36	90.13	216.87	2999	29.70	91.17	215.83	2985
307.5	28.62	88.02	219.49	3035	28.96	89.05	218.45	3021	29.30	90.09	217.41	3007	29.63	91.13	216.37	2992
308	28.56	87.97	220.03	3043	28.90	89.01	218.99	3029	29.24	90.05	217.95	3014	29.57	91.09	216.91	3000
308.5	28.50	87.93	220.57	3050	28.84	88.97	219.53	3036	29.18	90.01	218.49	3022	29.51	91.05	217.45	3007
309	28.44	87.89	221.11	3058	28.78	88.93	220.07	3044	29.12	89.97	219.03	3029	29.45	91.01	218.00	3015
309.5	28.38	87.85	221.65	3065	28.72	88.89	220.61	3051	29.06	89.93	219.57	3037	29.39	90.96	218.54	3022
310	28.33	87.81	222.19	3073	28.66	88.85	221.15	3059	29.00	89.89	220.12	3044	29.33	90.92	219.08	3030
310.5	28.27	87.77	222.73	3080	28.60	88.81	221.69	3066	28.94	89.84	220.66	3052	29.27	90.88	219.62	3037
311	28.21	87.73	223.27	3088	28.54	88.77	222.23	3074	28.88	89.80	221.20	3059	29.21	90.84	220.16	3045
311.5	28.15	87.69	223.81	3095	28.48	88.72	222.78	3081	28.82	89.76	221.74	3067	29.15	90.80	220.70	3052

Body Composition MALE 280-311.5 Lb.

Weight: Lb.	Waist: 52 inches Fat: %	Fat: Lb.	LBM: Lb.	RMR: Cal.	52.25 inches Fat: %	Fat: Lb.	LBM: Lb.	RMR: Cal.	52.5 inches Fat: %	Fat: Lb.	LBM: Lb.	RMR: Cal.	52.75 inches Fat: %	Fat: Lb.	LBM: Lb.	RMR: Cal.
280	33.72	94.42	185.58	2567	34.09	95.46	184.54	2552	34.46	96.50	183.51	2538	34.83	97.53	182.47	2524
280.5	33.65	94.38	186.12	2574	34.02	95.42	185.08	2560	34.39	96.45	184.05	2545	34.76	97.49	183.01	2531
281	33.57	94.34	186.66	2582	33.94	95.38	185.62	2567	34.31	96.41	184.59	2553	34.68	97.45	183.55	2538
281.5	33.50	94.30	187.20	2589	33.87	95.33	186.17	2575	34.24	96.37	185.13	2560	34.60	97.41	184.09	2546
282	33.42	94.26	187.74	2596	33.79	95.29	186.71	2582	34.16	96.33	185.67	2568	34.53	97.37	184.63	2553
282.5	33.35	94.22	188.29	2604	33.72	95.25	187.25	2590	34.08	96.29	186.21	2575	34.45	97.33	185.17	2561
283	33.28	94.17	188.83	2611	33.64	95.21	187.79	2597	34.01	96.25	186.75	2583	34.38	97.29	185.71	2568
283.5	33.20	94.13	189.37	2619	33.57	95.17	188.33	2605	33.94	96.21	187.29	2590	34.30	97.25	186.25	2576
284	33.13	94.09	189.91	2626	33.50	95.13	188.87	2612	33.86	96.17	187.83	2598	34.23	97.20	186.80	2583
284.5	33.06	94.05	190.45	2634	33.42	95.09	189.41	2620	33.79	96.13	188.37	2605	34.15	97.16	187.34	2591
285	32.99	94.01	190.99	2641	33.35	95.05	189.95	2627	33.71	96.09	188.92	2613	34.08	97.12	187.88	2598
285.5	32.91	93.97	191.53	2649	33.28	95.01	190.49	2635	33.64	96.04	189.46	2620	34.00	97.08	188.42	2606
286	32.84	93.93	192.07	2656	33.20	94.97	191.03	2642	33.57	96.00	190.00	2628	33.93	97.04	188.96	2613
286.5	32.77	93.89	192.61	2664	33.13	94.92	191.58	2649	33.49	95.96	190.54	2635	33.86	97.00	189.50	2621
287	32.70	93.85	193.15	2671	33.06	94.88	192.12	2657	33.42	95.92	191.08	2643	33.78	96.96	190.04	2628
287.5	32.63	93.80	193.70	2679	32.99	94.84	192.66	2664	33.35	95.88	191.62	2650	33.71	96.92	190.58	2636
288	32.56	93.76	194.24	2686	32.92	94.80	193.20	2672	33.28	95.84	192.16	2658	33.64	96.88	191.12	2643
288.5	32.49	93.72	194.78	2694	32.85	94.76	193.74	2679	33.21	95.80	192.70	2665	33.57	96.84	191.66	2651
289	32.42	93.68	195.32	2701	32.77	94.72	194.28	2687	33.13	95.76	193.24	2673	33.49	96.79	192.21	2658
289.5	32.35	93.64	195.86	2709	32.70	94.68	194.82	2694	33.06	95.72	193.78	2680	33.42	96.75	192.75	2666
290	32.28	93.60	196.40	2716	32.63	94.64	195.36	2702	32.99	95.68	194.33	2688	33.35	96.71	193.29	2673
290.5	32.21	93.56	196.94	2724	32.56	94.60	195.90	2709	32.92	95.63	194.87	2695	33.28	96.67	193.83	2681
291	32.14	93.52	197.48	2731	32.49	94.56	196.44	2717	32.85	95.59	195.41	2702	33.21	96.63	194.37	2688
291.5	32.07	93.48	198.02	2739	32.42	94.51	196.99	2724	32.78	95.55	195.95	2710	33.14	96.59	194.91	2696
292	32.00	93.44	198.56	2746	32.35	94.47	197.53	2732	32.71	95.51	196.49	2717	33.06	96.55	195.45	2703
292.5	31.93	93.40	199.11	2754	32.28	94.43	198.07	2739	32.64	95.47	197.03	2725	32.99	96.51	195.99	2711
293	31.86	93.35	199.65	2761	32.22	94.39	198.61	2747	32.57	95.43	197.57	2732	32.92	96.47	196.53	2718
293.5	31.79	93.31	200.19	2769	32.15	94.35	199.15	2754	32.50	95.39	198.11	2740	32.85	96.43	197.07	2726
294	31.73	93.27	200.73	2776	32.08	94.31	199.69	2762	32.43	95.35	198.65	2747	32.78	96.38	197.62	2733
294.5	31.66	93.23	201.27	2784	32.01	94.27	200.23	2769	32.36	95.31	199.19	2755	32.71	96.34	198.16	2741
295	31.59	93.19	201.81	2791	31.94	94.23	200.77	2777	32.29	95.27	199.74	2762	32.64	96.30	198.70	2748
295.5	31.52	93.15	202.35	2799	31.87	94.19	201.31	2784	32.22	95.22	200.28	2770	32.58	96.26	199.24	2755
296	31.46	93.11	202.89	2806	31.81	94.15	201.85	2792	32.16	95.18	200.82	2777	32.51	96.22	199.78	2763
296.5	31.39	93.07	203.43	2813	31.74	94.10	202.40	2799	32.09	95.14	201.36	2785	32.44	96.18	200.32	2770
297	31.32	93.03	203.97	2821	31.67	94.06	202.94	2807	32.02	95.10	201.90	2792	32.37	96.14	200.86	2778
297.5	31.26	92.99	204.52	2828	31.60	94.02	203.48	2814	31.95	95.06	202.44	2800	32.30	96.10	201.40	2785
298	31.19	92.94	205.06	2836	31.54	93.98	204.02	2822	31.89	95.02	202.98	2807	32.23	96.06	201.94	2793
298.5	31.12	92.90	205.60	2843	31.47	93.94	204.56	2829	31.82	94.98	203.52	2815	32.17	96.02	202.48	2800
299	31.06	92.86	206.14	2851	31.40	93.90	205.10	2837	31.75	94.94	204.06	2822	32.10	95.97	203.03	2808
299.5	30.99	92.82	206.68	2858	31.34	93.86	205.64	2844	31.68	94.90	204.60	2830	32.03	95.93	203.57	2815
300	30.93	92.78	207.22	2866	31.27	93.82	206.18	2852	31.62	94.86	205.15	2837	31.96	95.89	204.11	2823
300.5	30.86	92.74	207.76	2873	31.21	93.78	206.72	2859	31.55	94.81	205.69	2845	31.90	95.85	204.65	2830
301	30.80	92.70	208.30	2881	31.14	93.74	207.26	2866	31.49	94.77	206.23	2852	31.83	95.81	205.19	2838
301.5	30.73	92.66	208.84	2888	31.08	93.69	207.81	2874	31.42	94.73	206.77	2860	31.76	95.77	205.73	2845
302	30.67	92.62	209.38	2896	31.01	93.65	208.35	2881	31.35	94.69	207.31	2867	31.70	95.73	206.27	2853
302.5	30.60	92.58	209.93	2903	30.95	93.61	208.89	2889	31.29	94.65	207.85	2875	31.63	95.69	206.81	2860
303	30.54	92.53	210.47	2911	30.88	93.57	209.43	2896	31.22	94.61	208.39	2882	31.57	95.65	207.35	2868
303.5	30.48	92.49	211.01	2918	30.82	93.53	209.97	2904	31.16	94.57	208.93	2890	31.50	95.61	207.89	2875
304	30.41	92.45	211.55	2926	30.75	93.49	210.51	2911	31.09	94.53	209.47	2897	31.44	95.56	208.44	2883
304.5	30.35	92.41	212.09	2933	30.69	93.45	211.05	2919	31.03	94.49	210.01	2904	31.37	95.52	208.98	2890
305	30.29	92.37	212.63	2941	30.63	93.41	211.59	2926	30.97	94.45	210.56	2912	31.31	95.48	209.52	2898
305.5	30.22	92.33	213.17	2948	30.56	93.37	212.13	2934	30.90	94.40	211.10	2919	31.24	95.44	210.06	2905
306	30.16	92.29	213.71	2956	30.50	93.33	212.67	2941	30.84	94.36	211.64	2927	31.18	95.40	210.60	2913
306.5	30.10	92.25	214.25	2963	30.44	93.28	213.22	2949	30.77	94.32	212.18	2934	31.11	95.36	211.14	2920
307	30.03	92.21	214.79	2971	30.37	93.24	213.76	2956	30.71	94.28	212.72	2942	31.05	95.32	211.68	2928
307.5	29.97	92.17	215.34	2978	30.31	93.20	214.30	2964	30.65	94.24	213.26	2949	30.98	95.28	212.22	2935
308	29.91	92.12	215.88	2986	30.25	93.16	214.84	2971	30.58	94.20	213.80	2957	30.92	95.24	212.76	2943
308.5	29.85	92.08	216.42	2993	30.18	93.12	215.38	2979	30.52	94.16	214.34	2964	30.86	95.20	213.30	2950
309	29.79	92.04	216.96	3001	30.12	93.08	215.92	2986	30.46	94.12	214.88	2972	30.79	95.15	213.85	2957
309.5	29.73	92.00	217.50	3008	30.06	93.04	216.46	2994	30.40	94.08	215.42	2979	30.73	95.11	214.39	2965
310	29.66	91.96	218.04	3015	30.00	93.00	217.00	3001	30.33	94.04	215.97	2987	30.67	95.07	214.93	2972
310.5	29.60	91.92	218.58	3023	29.94	92.96	217.54	3009	30.27	93.99	216.51	2994	30.61	95.03	215.47	2980
311	29.54	91.88	219.12	3030	29.88	92.92	218.08	3016	30.21	93.95	217.05	3002	30.54	94.99	216.01	2987
311.5	29.48	91.84	219.66	3038	29.82	92.87	218.63	3024	30.15	93.91	217.59	3009	30.48	94.95	216.55	2995

Body Composition MALE 280-311.5 Lb.

Weight: Lb.	Waist: 53 inches				53.25 inches				53.5 inches				53.75 inches			
	Fat: %	Fat: Lb.	LBM: Lb.	RMR: Cal.	Fat: %	Fat: Lb.	LBM: Lb.	RMR: Cal.	Fat: %	Fat: Lb.	LBM: Lb.	RMR: Cal.	Fat: %	Fat: Lb.	LBM: Lb.	RMR: Cal.
280	35.20	98.57	181.43	2509	35.57	99.61	180.39	2495	35.94	100.65	179.36	2480	36.32	101.68	178.32	2466
280.5	35.13	98.53	181.97	2517	35.50	99.57	180.93	2502	35.87	100.60	179.90	2488	36.24	101.64	178.86	2474
281	35.05	98.49	182.51	2524	35.42	99.53	181.47	2510	35.79	100.56	180.44	2495	36.16	101.60	179.40	2481
281.5	34.97	98.45	183.05	2532	35.34	99.48	182.02	2517	35.71	100.52	180.98	2503	36.08	101.56	179.94	2489
282	34.90	98.41	183.59	2539	35.26	99.44	182.56	2525	35.63	100.48	181.52	2510	36.00	101.52	180.48	2496
282.5	34.82	98.37	184.14	2547	35.19	99.40	183.10	2532	35.55	100.44	182.06	2518	35.92	101.48	181.02	2504
283	34.74	98.32	184.68	2554	35.11	99.36	183.64	2540	35.48	100.40	182.60	2525	35.84	101.44	181.56	2511
283.5	34.67	98.28	185.22	2562	35.03	99.32	184.18	2547	35.40	100.36	183.14	2533	35.77	101.40	182.10	2519
284	34.59	98.24	185.76	2569	34.96	99.28	184.72	2555	35.32	100.32	183.68	2540	35.69	101.35	182.65	2526
284.5	34.52	98.20	186.30	2577	34.88	99.24	185.26	2562	35.25	100.28	184.22	2548	35.61	101.31	183.19	2533
285	34.44	98.16	186.84	2584	34.81	99.20	185.80	2570	35.17	100.24	184.77	2555	35.53	101.27	183.73	2541
285.5	34.37	98.12	187.38	2591	34.73	99.16	186.34	2577	35.09	100.19	185.31	2563	35.46	101.23	184.27	2548
286	34.29	98.08	187.92	2599	34.66	99.12	186.88	2585	35.02	100.15	185.85	2570	35.38	101.19	184.81	2556
286.5	34.22	98.04	188.46	2606	34.58	99.07	187.43	2592	34.94	100.11	186.39	2578	35.31	101.15	185.35	2563
287	34.14	98.00	189.00	2614	34.51	99.03	187.97	2600	34.87	100.07	186.93	2585	35.23	101.11	185.89	2571
287.5	34.07	97.96	189.55	2621	34.43	98.99	188.51	2607	34.79	100.03	187.47	2593	35.15	101.07	186.43	2578
288	34.00	97.91	190.09	2629	34.36	98.95	189.05	2615	34.72	99.99	188.01	2600	35.08	101.03	186.97	2586
288.5	33.92	97.87	190.63	2636	34.28	98.91	189.59	2622	34.64	99.95	188.55	2608	35.00	100.99	187.51	2593
289	33.85	97.83	191.17	2644	34.21	98.87	190.13	2630	34.57	99.91	189.09	2615	34.93	100.94	188.06	2601
289.5	33.78	97.79	191.71	2651	34.14	98.83	190.67	2637	34.50	99.87	189.63	2623	34.85	100.90	188.60	2608
290	33.71	97.75	192.25	2659	34.06	98.79	191.21	2644	34.42	99.83	190.18	2630	34.78	100.86	189.14	2616
290.5	33.63	97.71	192.79	2666	33.99	98.75	191.75	2652	34.35	99.78	190.72	2638	34.71	100.82	189.68	2623
291	33.56	97.67	193.33	2674	33.92	98.71	192.29	2659	34.28	99.74	191.26	2645	34.63	100.78	190.22	2631
291.5	33.49	97.63	193.87	2681	33.85	98.66	192.84	2667	34.20	99.70	191.80	2653	34.56	100.74	190.76	2638
292	33.42	97.59	194.41	2689	33.78	98.62	193.38	2674	34.13	99.66	192.34	2660	34.49	100.70	191.30	2646
292.5	33.35	97.55	194.96	2696	33.70	98.58	193.92	2682	34.06	99.62	192.88	2668	34.41	100.66	191.84	2653
293	33.28	97.50	195.50	2704	33.63	98.54	194.46	2689	33.99	99.58	193.42	2675	34.34	100.62	192.38	2661
293.5	33.21	97.46	196.04	2711	33.56	98.50	195.00	2697	33.91	99.54	193.96	2682	34.27	100.58	192.92	2668
294	33.14	97.42	196.58	2719	33.49	98.46	195.54	2704	33.84	99.50	194.50	2690	34.20	100.53	193.47	2676
294.5	33.07	97.38	197.12	2726	33.42	98.42	196.08	2712	33.77	99.46	195.04	2697	34.12	100.49	194.01	2683
295	33.00	97.34	197.66	2734	33.35	98.38	196.62	2719	33.70	99.42	195.59	2705	34.05	100.45	194.55	2691
295.5	32.93	97.30	198.20	2741	33.28	98.34	197.16	2727	33.63	99.37	196.13	2712	33.98	100.41	195.09	2698
296	32.86	97.26	198.74	2749	33.21	98.30	197.70	2734	33.56	99.33	196.67	2720	33.91	100.37	195.63	2706
296.5	32.79	97.22	199.28	2756	33.14	98.25	198.25	2742	33.49	99.29	197.21	2727	33.84	100.33	196.17	2713
297	32.72	97.18	199.82	2764	33.07	98.21	198.79	2749	33.42	99.25	197.75	2735	33.77	100.29	196.71	2721
297.5	32.65	97.14	200.37	2771	33.00	98.17	199.33	2757	33.35	99.21	198.29	2742	33.70	100.25	197.25	2728
298	32.58	97.09	200.91	2779	32.93	98.13	199.87	2764	33.28	99.17	198.83	2750	33.63	100.21	197.79	2735
298.5	32.51	97.05	201.45	2786	32.86	98.09	200.41	2772	33.21	99.13	199.37	2757	33.56	100.17	198.33	2743
299	32.45	97.01	201.99	2793	32.79	98.05	200.95	2779	33.14	99.09	199.91	2765	33.49	100.12	198.88	2750
299.5	32.38	96.97	202.53	2801	32.72	98.01	201.49	2787	33.07	99.05	200.45	2772	33.42	100.08	199.42	2758
300	32.31	96.93	203.07	2808	32.66	97.97	202.03	2794	33.00	99.01	201.00	2780	33.35	100.04	199.96	2765
300.5	32.24	96.89	203.61	2816	32.59	97.93	202.57	2802	32.93	98.96	201.54	2787	33.28	100.00	200.50	2773
301	32.18	96.85	204.15	2823	32.52	97.89	203.11	2809	32.86	98.92	202.08	2795	33.21	99.96	201.04	2780
301.5	32.11	96.81	204.69	2831	32.45	97.84	203.66	2817	32.80	98.88	202.62	2802	33.14	99.92	201.58	2788
302	32.04	96.77	205.23	2838	32.39	97.80	204.20	2824	32.73	98.84	203.16	2810	33.07	99.88	202.12	2795
302.5	31.98	96.73	205.78	2846	32.32	97.76	204.74	2832	32.66	98.80	203.70	2817	33.00	99.84	202.66	2803
303	31.91	96.68	206.32	2853	32.25	97.72	205.28	2839	32.59	98.76	204.24	2825	32.94	99.80	203.20	2810
303.5	31.84	96.64	206.86	2861	32.18	97.68	205.82	2846	32.53	98.72	204.78	2832	32.87	99.76	203.74	2818
304	31.78	96.60	207.40	2868	32.12	97.64	206.36	2854	32.46	98.68	205.32	2840	32.80	99.71	204.29	2825
304.5	31.71	96.56	207.94	2876	32.05	97.60	206.90	2861	32.39	98.64	205.86	2847	32.73	99.67	204.83	2833
305	31.65	96.52	208.48	2883	31.99	97.56	207.44	2869	32.33	98.60	206.41	2855	32.67	99.63	205.37	2840
305.5	31.58	96.48	209.02	2891	31.92	97.52	207.98	2876	32.26	98.55	206.95	2862	32.60	99.59	205.91	2848
306	31.52	96.44	209.56	2898	31.85	97.48	208.52	2884	32.19	98.51	207.49	2870	32.53	99.55	206.45	2855
306.5	31.45	96.40	210.10	2906	31.79	97.43	209.07	2891	32.13	98.47	208.03	2877	32.47	99.51	206.99	2863
307	31.39	96.36	210.64	2913	31.72	97.39	209.61	2899	32.06	98.43	208.57	2885	32.40	99.47	207.53	2870
307.5	31.32	96.32	211.19	2921	31.66	97.35	210.15	2906	32.00	98.39	209.11	2892	32.33	99.43	208.07	2878
308	31.26	96.27	211.73	2928	31.59	97.31	210.69	2914	31.93	98.35	209.65	2899	32.27	99.39	208.61	2885
308.5	31.19	96.23	212.27	2936	31.53	97.27	211.23	2921	31.87	98.31	210.19	2907	32.20	99.35	209.15	2893
309	31.13	96.19	212.81	2943	31.47	97.23	211.77	2929	31.80	98.27	210.73	2914	32.14	99.30	209.70	2900
309.5	31.07	96.15	213.35	2951	31.40	97.19	212.31	2936	31.74	98.23	211.27	2922	32.07	99.26	210.24	2908
310	31.00	96.11	213.89	2958	31.34	97.15	212.85	2944	31.67	98.19	211.82	2929	32.01	99.22	210.78	2915
310.5	30.94	96.07	214.43	2966	31.27	97.11	213.39	2951	31.61	98.14	212.36	2937	31.94	99.18	211.32	2923
311	30.88	96.03	214.97	2973	31.21	97.07	213.93	2959	31.54	98.10	212.90	2944	31.88	99.14	211.86	2930
311.5	30.81	95.99	215.51	2981	31.15	97.02	214.48	2966	31.48	98.06	213.44	2952	31.81	99.10	212.40	2937

Body Composition   MALE   280-311.5 Lb.

Weight: Lb.	Waist: 54 inches				54.25 inches				54.5 inches				54.75 inches			
	Fat: %	Fat: Lb.	LBM: Lb.	RMR: Cal.	Fat: %	Fat: Lb.	LBM: Lb.	RMR: Cal.	Fat: %	Fat: Lb.	LBM: Lb.	RMR: Cal.	Fat: %	Fat: Lb.	LBM: Lb.	RMR: Cal.
280	36.69	102.72	177.28	2452	37.06	103.76	176.24	2437	37.43	104.80	175.21	2423	37.80	105.83	174.17	2409
280.5	36.61	102.68	177.82	2459	36.98	103.72	176.78	2445	37.35	104.75	175.75	2431	37.72	105.79	174.71	2416
281	36.53	102.64	178.36	2467	36.90	103.68	177.32	2452	37.26	104.71	176.29	2438	37.63	105.75	175.25	2424
281.5	36.45	102.60	178.90	2474	36.82	103.63	177.87	2460	37.18	104.67	176.83	2446	37.55	105.71	175.79	2431
282	36.37	102.56	179.44	2482	36.74	103.59	178.41	2467	37.10	104.63	177.37	2453	37.47	105.67	176.33	2439
282.5	36.29	102.52	179.99	2489	36.66	103.55	178.95	2475	37.02	104.59	177.91	2460	37.39	105.63	176.87	2446
283	36.21	102.47	180.53	2497	36.58	103.51	179.49	2482	36.94	104.55	178.45	2468	37.31	105.59	177.41	2454
283.5	36.13	102.43	181.07	2504	36.50	103.47	180.03	2490	36.86	104.51	178.99	2475	37.23	105.55	177.95	2461
284	36.05	102.39	181.61	2512	36.42	103.43	180.57	2497	36.78	104.47	179.53	2483	37.15	105.50	178.50	2469
284.5	35.98	102.35	182.15	2519	36.34	103.39	181.11	2505	36.71	104.43	180.07	2490	37.07	105.46	179.04	2476
285	35.90	102.31	182.69	2527	36.26	103.35	181.65	2512	36.63	104.39	180.62	2498	36.99	105.42	179.58	2484
285.5	35.82	102.27	183.23	2534	36.18	103.31	182.19	2520	36.55	104.34	181.16	2505	36.91	105.38	180.12	2491
286	35.74	102.23	183.77	2542	36.11	103.27	182.73	2527	36.47	104.30	181.70	2513	36.83	105.34	180.66	2499
286.5	35.67	102.19	184.31	2549	36.03	103.22	183.28	2535	36.39	104.26	182.24	2520	36.75	105.30	181.20	2506
287	35.59	102.15	184.85	2557	35.95	103.18	183.82	2542	36.31	104.22	182.78	2528	36.68	105.26	181.74	2513
287.5	35.51	102.11	185.40	2564	35.88	103.14	184.36	2550	36.24	104.18	183.32	2535	36.60	105.22	182.28	2521
288	35.44	102.06	185.94	2571	35.80	103.10	184.90	2557	36.16	104.14	183.86	2543	36.52	105.18	182.82	2528
288.5	35.36	102.02	186.48	2579	35.72	103.06	185.44	2565	36.08	104.10	184.40	2550	36.44	105.14	183.36	2536
289	35.29	101.98	187.02	2586	35.65	103.02	185.98	2572	36.01	104.06	184.94	2558	36.36	105.09	183.91	2543
289.5	35.21	101.94	187.56	2594	35.57	102.98	186.52	2580	35.93	104.02	185.48	2565	36.29	105.05	184.45	2551
290	35.14	101.90	188.10	2601	35.50	102.94	187.06	2587	35.85	103.98	186.03	2573	36.21	105.01	184.99	2558
290.5	35.06	101.86	188.64	2609	35.42	102.90	187.60	2595	35.78	103.93	186.57	2580	36.13	104.97	185.53	2566
291	34.99	101.82	189.18	2616	35.35	102.86	188.14	2602	35.70	103.89	187.11	2588	36.06	104.93	186.07	2573
291.5	34.91	101.78	189.72	2624	35.27	102.81	188.69	2610	35.63	103.85	187.65	2595	35.98	104.89	186.61	2581
292	34.84	101.74	190.26	2631	35.20	102.77	189.23	2617	35.55	103.81	188.19	2603	35.91	104.85	187.15	2588
292.5	34.77	101.70	190.81	2639	35.12	102.73	189.77	2624	35.48	103.77	188.73	2610	35.83	104.81	187.69	2596
293	34.69	101.65	191.35	2646	35.05	102.69	190.31	2632	35.40	103.73	189.27	2618	35.76	104.77	188.23	2603
293.5	34.62	101.61	191.89	2654	34.97	102.65	190.85	2639	35.33	103.69	189.81	2625	35.68	104.73	188.77	2611
294	34.55	101.57	192.43	2661	34.90	102.61	191.39	2647	35.25	103.65	190.35	2633	35.61	104.68	189.32	2618
294.5	34.48	101.53	192.97	2669	34.83	102.57	191.93	2654	35.18	103.61	190.89	2640	35.53	104.64	189.86	2626
295	34.40	101.49	193.51	2676	34.76	102.53	192.47	2662	35.11	103.57	191.44	2648	35.46	104.60	190.40	2633
295.5	34.33	101.45	194.05	2684	34.68	102.49	193.01	2669	35.03	103.52	191.98	2655	35.38	104.56	190.94	2641
296	34.26	101.41	194.59	2691	34.61	102.45	193.55	2677	34.96	103.48	192.52	2663	35.31	104.52	191.48	2648
296.5	34.19	101.37	195.13	2699	34.54	102.40	194.10	2684	34.89	103.44	193.06	2670	35.24	104.48	192.02	2656
297	34.12	101.33	195.67	2706	34.47	102.36	194.64	2692	34.82	103.40	193.60	2677	35.16	104.44	192.56	2663
297.5	34.05	101.29	196.22	2714	34.39	102.32	195.18	2699	34.74	103.36	194.14	2685	35.09	104.40	193.10	2671
298	33.97	101.24	196.76	2721	34.32	102.28	195.72	2707	34.67	103.32	194.68	2692	35.02	104.36	193.64	2678
298.5	33.90	101.20	197.30	2729	34.25	102.24	196.26	2714	34.60	103.28	195.22	2700	34.95	104.32	194.18	2686
299	33.83	101.16	197.84	2736	34.18	102.20	196.80	2722	34.53	103.24	195.76	2707	34.87	104.27	194.73	2693
299.5	33.76	101.12	198.38	2744	34.11	102.16	197.34	2729	34.46	103.20	196.30	2715	34.80	104.23	195.27	2701
300	33.69	101.08	198.92	2751	34.04	102.12	197.88	2737	34.39	103.16	196.85	2722	34.73	104.19	195.81	2708
300.5	33.62	101.04	199.46	2759	33.97	102.08	198.42	2744	34.31	103.11	197.39	2730	34.66	104.15	196.35	2715
301	33.55	101.00	200.00	2766	33.90	102.04	198.96	2752	34.24	103.07	197.93	2737	34.59	104.11	196.89	2723
301.5	33.48	100.96	200.54	2774	33.83	101.99	199.51	2759	34.17	103.03	198.47	2745	34.52	104.07	197.43	2730
302	33.42	100.92	201.08	2781	33.76	101.95	200.05	2767	34.10	102.99	199.01	2752	34.45	104.03	197.97	2738
302.5	33.35	100.88	201.63	2788	33.69	101.91	200.59	2774	34.03	102.95	199.55	2760	34.38	103.99	198.51	2745
303	33.28	100.83	202.17	2796	33.62	101.87	201.13	2782	33.96	102.91	200.09	2767	34.31	103.95	199.05	2753
303.5	33.21	100.79	202.71	2803	33.55	101.83	201.67	2789	33.89	102.87	200.63	2775	34.24	103.91	199.59	2760
304	33.14	100.75	203.25	2811	33.48	101.79	202.21	2797	33.82	102.83	201.17	2782	34.17	103.86	200.14	2768
304.5	33.07	100.71	203.79	2818	33.41	101.75	202.75	2804	33.76	102.79	201.71	2790	34.10	103.82	200.68	2775
305	33.01	100.67	204.33	2826	33.35	101.71	203.29	2812	33.69	102.75	202.26	2797	34.03	103.78	201.22	2783
305.5	32.94	100.63	204.87	2833	33.28	101.67	203.83	2819	33.62	102.70	202.80	2805	33.96	103.74	201.76	2790
306	32.87	100.59	205.41	2841	33.21	101.63	204.37	2826	33.55	102.66	203.34	2812	33.89	103.70	202.30	2798
306.5	32.80	100.55	205.95	2848	33.14	101.58	204.92	2834	33.48	102.62	203.88	2820	33.82	103.66	202.84	2805
307	32.74	100.51	206.49	2856	33.08	101.54	205.46	2841	33.41	102.58	204.42	2827	33.75	103.62	203.38	2813
307.5	32.67	100.47	207.04	2863	33.01	101.50	206.00	2849	33.35	102.54	204.96	2835	33.68	103.58	203.92	2820
308	32.61	100.42	207.58	2871	32.94	101.46	206.54	2856	33.28	102.50	205.50	2842	33.62	103.54	204.46	2828
308.5	32.54	100.38	208.12	2878	32.88	101.42	207.08	2864	33.21	102.46	206.04	2850	33.55	103.50	205.00	2835
309	32.47	100.34	208.66	2886	32.81	101.38	207.62	2871	33.14	102.42	206.58	2857	33.48	103.45	205.55	2843
309.5	32.41	100.30	209.20	2893	32.74	101.34	208.16	2879	33.08	102.38	207.12	2865	33.41	103.41	206.09	2850
310	32.34	100.26	209.74	2901	32.68	101.30	208.70	2886	33.01	102.34	207.67	2872	33.35	103.37	206.63	2858
310.5	32.28	100.22	210.28	2908	32.61	101.26	209.24	2894	32.94	102.29	208.21	2879	33.28	103.33	207.17	2865
311	32.21	100.18	210.82	2916	32.55	101.22	209.78	2901	32.88	102.25	208.75	2887	33.21	103.29	207.71	2873
311.5	32.15	100.14	211.36	2923	32.48	101.17	210.33	2909	32.81	102.21	209.29	2894	33.15	103.25	208.25	2880

Body Composition　MALE　280-311.5 Lb.

Weight: Lb.	Waist: 55 inches Fat: %	Fat: Lb.	LBM: Lb.	RMR: Cal.	55.25 inches Fat: %	Fat: Lb.	LBM: Lb.	RMR: Cal.	55.5 inches Fat: %	Fat: Lb.	LBM: Lb.	RMR: Cal.	55.75 inches Fat: %	Fat: Lb.	LBM: Lb.	RMR: Cal.
280	38.17	106.87	173.13	2394	38.54	107.91	172.09	2380	38.91	108.95	171.06	2366	39.28	109.98	170.02	2351
280.5	38.09	106.83	173.67	2402	38.46	107.87	172.63	2388	38.82	108.90	171.60	2373	39.19	109.94	170.56	2359
281	38.00	106.79	174.21	2409	38.37	107.83	173.17	2395	38.74	108.86	172.14	2381	39.11	109.90	171.10	2366
281.5	37.92	106.75	174.75	2417	38.29	107.78	173.72	2402	38.66	108.82	172.68	2388	39.03	109.86	171.64	2374
282	37.84	106.71	175.29	2424	38.21	107.74	174.26	2410	38.57	108.78	173.22	2396	38.94	109.82	172.18	2381
282.5	37.76	106.67	175.84	2432	38.12	107.70	174.80	2417	38.49	108.74	173.76	2403	38.86	109.78	172.72	2389
283	37.68	106.62	176.38	2439	38.04	107.66	175.34	2425	38.41	108.70	174.30	2411	38.78	109.74	173.26	2396
283.5	37.60	106.58	176.92	2447	37.96	107.62	175.88	2432	38.33	108.66	174.84	2418	38.69	109.70	173.80	2404
284	37.51	106.54	177.46	2454	37.88	107.58	176.42	2440	38.25	108.62	175.38	2426	38.61	109.65	174.35	2411
284.5	37.43	106.50	178.00	2462	37.80	107.54	176.96	2447	38.16	108.58	175.92	2433	38.53	109.61	174.89	2419
285	37.35	106.46	178.54	2469	37.72	107.50	177.50	2455	38.08	108.54	176.47	2441	38.45	109.57	175.43	2426
285.5	37.27	106.42	179.08	2477	37.64	107.46	178.04	2462	38.00	108.49	177.01	2448	38.36	109.53	175.97	2434
286	37.20	106.38	179.62	2484	37.56	107.42	178.58	2470	37.92	108.45	177.55	2455	38.28	109.49	176.51	2441
286.5	37.12	106.34	180.16	2492	37.48	107.37	179.13	2477	37.84	108.41	178.09	2463	38.20	109.45	177.05	2449
287	37.04	106.30	180.70	2499	37.40	107.33	179.67	2485	37.76	108.37	178.63	2470	38.12	109.41	177.59	2456
287.5	36.96	106.26	181.25	2507	37.32	107.29	180.21	2492	37.68	108.33	179.17	2478	38.04	109.37	178.13	2464
288	36.88	106.21	181.79	2514	37.24	107.25	180.75	2500	37.60	108.29	179.71	2485	37.96	109.33	178.67	2471
288.5	36.80	106.17	182.33	2522	37.16	107.21	181.29	2507	37.52	108.25	180.25	2493	37.88	109.29	179.21	2479
289	36.72	106.13	182.87	2529	37.08	107.17	181.83	2515	37.44	108.21	180.79	2500	37.80	109.24	179.76	2486
289.5	36.65	106.09	183.41	2537	37.00	107.13	182.37	2522	37.36	108.17	181.33	2508	37.72	109.20	180.30	2494
290	36.57	106.05	183.95	2544	36.93	107.09	182.91	2530	37.28	108.13	181.88	2515	37.64	109.16	180.84	2501
290.5	36.49	106.01	184.49	2552	36.85	107.05	183.45	2537	37.21	108.08	182.42	2523	37.56	109.12	181.38	2508
291	36.42	105.97	185.03	2559	36.77	107.01	183.99	2545	37.13	108.04	182.96	2530	37.48	109.08	181.92	2516
291.5	36.34	105.93	185.57	2566	36.69	106.96	184.54	2552	37.05	108.00	183.50	2538	37.41	109.04	182.46	2523
292	36.26	105.89	186.11	2574	36.62	106.92	185.08	2560	36.97	107.96	184.04	2545	37.33	109.00	183.00	2531
292.5	36.19	105.85	186.66	2581	36.54	106.88	185.62	2567	36.90	107.92	184.58	2553	37.25	108.96	183.54	2538
293	36.11	105.80	187.20	2589	36.46	106.84	186.16	2575	36.82	107.88	185.12	2560	37.17	108.92	184.08	2546
293.5	36.04	105.76	187.74	2596	36.39	106.80	186.70	2582	36.74	107.84	185.66	2568	37.10	108.88	184.62	2553
294	35.96	105.72	188.28	2604	36.31	106.76	187.24	2590	36.67	107.80	186.20	2575	37.02	108.83	185.17	2561
294.5	35.88	105.68	188.82	2611	36.24	106.72	187.78	2597	36.59	107.76	186.74	2583	36.94	108.79	185.71	2568
295	35.81	105.64	189.36	2619	36.16	106.68	188.32	2605	36.51	107.72	187.29	2590	36.87	108.75	186.25	2576
295.5	35.74	105.60	189.90	2626	36.09	106.64	188.86	2612	36.44	107.67	187.83	2598	36.79	108.71	186.79	2583
296	35.66	105.56	190.44	2634	36.01	106.60	189.40	2619	36.36	107.63	188.37	2605	36.71	108.67	187.33	2591
296.5	35.59	105.52	190.98	2641	35.94	106.55	189.95	2627	36.29	107.59	188.91	2613	36.64	108.63	187.87	2598
297	35.51	105.48	191.52	2649	35.86	106.51	190.49	2634	36.21	107.55	189.45	2620	36.56	108.59	188.41	2606
297.5	35.44	105.44	192.07	2656	35.79	106.47	191.03	2642	36.14	107.51	189.99	2628	36.49	108.55	188.95	2613
298	35.37	105.39	192.61	2664	35.72	106.43	191.57	2649	36.06	107.47	190.53	2635	36.41	108.51	189.49	2621
298.5	35.29	105.35	193.15	2671	35.64	106.39	192.11	2657	35.99	107.43	191.07	2643	36.34	108.47	190.03	2628
299	35.22	105.31	193.69	2679	35.57	106.35	192.65	2664	35.92	107.39	191.61	2650	36.26	108.42	190.58	2636
299.5	35.15	105.27	194.23	2686	35.50	106.31	193.19	2672	35.84	107.35	192.15	2657	36.19	108.38	191.12	2643
300	35.08	105.23	194.77	2694	35.42	106.27	193.73	2679	35.77	107.31	192.70	2665	36.11	108.34	191.66	2651
300.5	35.00	105.19	195.31	2701	35.35	106.23	194.27	2687	35.70	107.26	193.24	2672	36.04	108.30	192.20	2658
301	34.93	105.15	195.85	2709	35.28	106.19	194.81	2694	35.62	107.22	193.78	2680	35.97	108.26	192.74	2666
301.5	34.86	105.11	196.39	2716	35.21	106.14	195.36	2702	35.55	107.18	194.32	2687	35.89	108.22	193.28	2673
302	34.79	105.07	196.93	2724	35.13	106.10	195.90	2709	35.48	107.14	194.86	2695	35.82	108.18	193.82	2681
302.5	34.72	105.03	197.48	2731	35.06	106.06	196.44	2717	35.40	107.10	195.40	2702	35.75	108.14	194.36	2688
303	34.65	104.98	198.02	2739	34.99	106.02	196.98	2724	35.33	107.06	195.94	2710	35.68	108.10	194.90	2696
303.5	34.58	104.94	198.56	2746	34.92	105.98	197.52	2732	35.26	107.02	196.48	2717	35.60	108.06	195.44	2703
304	34.51	104.90	199.10	2754	34.85	105.94	198.06	2739	35.19	106.98	197.02	2725	35.53	108.01	195.99	2710
304.5	34.44	104.86	199.64	2761	34.78	105.90	198.60	2747	35.12	106.94	197.56	2732	35.46	107.97	196.53	2718
305	34.37	104.82	200.18	2768	34.71	105.86	199.14	2754	35.05	106.90	198.11	2740	35.39	107.93	197.07	2725
305.5	34.30	104.78	200.72	2776	34.64	105.82	199.68	2762	34.98	106.85	198.65	2747	35.32	107.89	197.61	2733
306	34.23	104.74	201.26	2783	34.57	105.78	200.22	2769	34.91	106.81	199.19	2755	35.25	107.85	198.15	2740
306.5	34.16	104.70	201.80	2791	34.50	105.73	200.77	2777	34.84	106.77	199.73	2762	35.17	107.81	198.69	2748
307	34.09	104.66	202.34	2798	34.43	105.69	201.31	2784	34.77	106.73	200.27	2770	35.10	107.77	199.23	2755
307.5	34.02	104.62	202.89	2806	34.36	105.65	201.85	2792	34.70	106.69	200.81	2777	35.03	107.73	199.77	2763
308	33.95	104.57	203.43	2813	34.29	105.61	202.39	2799	34.63	106.65	201.35	2785	34.96	107.69	200.31	2770
308.5	33.88	104.53	203.97	2821	34.22	105.57	202.93	2807	34.56	106.61	201.89	2792	34.89	107.65	200.85	2778
309	33.82	104.49	204.51	2828	34.15	105.53	203.47	2814	34.49	106.57	202.43	2800	34.82	107.60	201.40	2785
309.5	33.75	104.45	205.05	2836	34.08	105.49	204.01	2821	34.42	106.53	202.97	2807	34.75	107.56	201.94	2793
310	33.68	104.41	205.59	2843	34.02	105.45	204.55	2829	34.35	106.49	203.52	2815	34.68	107.52	202.48	2800
310.5	33.61	104.37	206.13	2851	33.95	105.41	205.09	2836	34.28	106.44	204.06	2822	34.62	107.48	203.02	2808
311	33.55	104.33	206.67	2858	33.88	105.37	205.63	2844	34.21	106.40	204.60	2830	34.55	107.44	203.56	2815
311.5	33.48	104.29	207.21	2866	33.81	105.32	206.18	2851	34.15	106.36	205.14	2837	34.48	107.40	204.10	2823

Body Composition   MALE   280-311.5 Lb.

Weight: Lb.	Waist: 56 inches				56.25 inches				56.5 inches				56.75 inches			
	Fat: %	Fat: Lb.	LBM: Lb.	RMR: Cal.	Fat: %	Fat: Lb.	LBM: Lb.	RMR: Cal.	Fat: %	Fat: Lb.	LBM: Lb.	RMR: Cal.	Fat: %	Fat: Lb.	LBM: Lb.	RMR: Cal.
280	39.65	111.02	168.98	2337	40.02	112.06	167.94	2323	40.39	113.10	166.91	2308	40.76	114.13	165.87	2294
280.5	39.56	110.98	169.52	2344	39.93	112.02	168.48	2330	40.30	113.05	167.45	2316	40.67	114.09	166.41	2301
281	39.48	110.94	170.06	2352	39.85	111.98	169.02	2338	40.22	113.01	167.99	2323	40.59	114.05	166.95	2309
281.5	39.40	110.90	170.60	2359	39.76	111.93	169.57	2345	40.13	112.97	168.53	2331	40.50	114.01	167.49	2316
282	39.31	110.86	171.14	2367	39.68	111.89	170.11	2353	40.05	112.93	169.07	2338	40.41	113.97	168.03	2324
282.5	39.23	110.82	171.69	2374	39.59	111.85	170.65	2360	39.96	112.89	169.61	2346	40.33	113.93	168.57	2331
283	39.14	110.77	172.23	2382	39.51	111.81	171.19	2368	39.88	112.85	170.15	2353	40.24	113.89	169.11	2339
283.5	39.06	110.73	172.77	2389	39.43	111.77	171.73	2375	39.79	112.81	170.69	2361	40.16	113.85	169.65	2346
284	38.98	110.69	173.31	2397	39.34	111.73	172.27	2383	39.71	112.77	171.23	2368	40.07	113.80	170.20	2354
284.5	38.89	110.65	173.85	2404	39.26	111.69	172.81	2390	39.62	112.73	171.77	2376	39.99	113.76	170.74	2361
285	38.81	110.61	174.39	2412	39.17	111.65	173.35	2397	39.54	112.69	172.32	2383	39.90	113.72	171.28	2369
285.5	38.73	110.57	174.93	2419	39.09	111.61	173.89	2405	39.45	112.64	172.86	2391	39.82	113.68	171.82	2376
286	38.65	110.53	175.47	2427	39.01	111.57	174.43	2412	39.37	112.60	173.40	2398	39.73	113.64	172.36	2384
286.5	38.56	110.49	176.01	2434	38.93	111.52	174.98	2420	39.29	112.56	173.94	2406	39.65	113.60	172.90	2391
287	38.48	110.45	176.55	2442	38.84	111.48	175.52	2427	39.21	112.52	174.48	2413	39.57	113.56	173.44	2399
287.5	38.40	110.41	177.10	2449	38.76	111.44	176.06	2435	39.12	112.48	175.02	2421	39.48	113.52	173.98	2406
288	38.32	110.36	177.64	2457	38.68	111.40	176.60	2442	39.04	112.44	175.56	2428	39.40	113.48	174.52	2414
288.5	38.24	110.32	178.18	2464	38.60	111.36	177.14	2450	38.96	112.40	176.10	2435	39.32	113.44	175.06	2421
289	38.16	110.28	178.72	2472	38.52	111.32	177.68	2457	38.88	112.36	176.64	2443	39.24	113.39	175.61	2429
289.5	38.08	110.24	179.26	2479	38.44	111.28	178.22	2465	38.80	112.32	177.18	2450	39.15	113.35	176.15	2436
290	38.00	110.20	179.80	2487	38.36	111.24	178.76	2472	38.72	112.28	177.73	2458	39.07	113.31	176.69	2444
290.5	37.92	110.16	180.34	2494	38.28	111.20	179.30	2480	38.63	112.23	178.27	2465	38.99	113.27	177.23	2451
291	37.84	110.12	180.88	2502	38.20	111.16	179.84	2487	38.55	112.19	178.81	2473	38.91	113.23	177.77	2459
291.5	37.76	110.08	181.42	2509	38.12	111.11	180.39	2495	38.47	112.15	179.35	2480	38.83	113.19	178.31	2466
292	37.68	110.04	181.96	2517	38.04	111.07	180.93	2502	38.39	112.11	179.89	2488	38.75	113.15	178.85	2474
292.5	37.61	110.00	182.51	2524	37.96	111.03	181.47	2510	38.31	112.07	180.43	2495	38.67	113.11	179.39	2481
293	37.53	109.95	183.05	2532	37.88	110.99	182.01	2517	38.24	112.03	180.97	2503	38.59	113.07	179.93	2488
293.5	37.45	109.91	183.59	2539	37.80	110.95	182.55	2525	38.16	111.99	181.51	2510	38.51	113.03	180.47	2496
294	37.37	109.87	184.13	2546	37.72	110.91	183.09	2532	38.08	111.95	182.05	2518	38.43	112.98	181.02	2503
294.5	37.29	109.83	184.67	2554	37.65	110.87	183.63	2540	38.00	111.91	182.59	2525	38.35	112.94	181.56	2511
295	37.22	109.79	185.21	2561	37.57	110.83	184.17	2547	37.92	111.87	183.14	2533	38.27	112.90	182.10	2518
295.5	37.14	109.75	185.75	2569	37.49	110.79	184.71	2555	37.84	111.82	183.68	2540	38.19	112.86	182.64	2526
296	37.06	109.71	186.29	2576	37.41	110.75	185.25	2562	37.76	111.78	184.22	2548	38.12	112.82	183.18	2533
296.5	36.99	109.67	186.83	2584	37.34	110.70	185.80	2570	37.69	111.74	184.76	2555	38.04	112.78	183.72	2541
297	36.91	109.63	187.37	2591	37.26	110.66	186.34	2577	37.61	111.70	185.30	2563	37.96	112.74	184.26	2548
297.5	36.84	109.59	187.92	2599	37.18	110.62	186.88	2585	37.53	111.66	185.84	2570	37.88	112.70	184.80	2556
298	36.76	109.54	188.46	2606	37.11	110.58	187.42	2592	37.46	111.62	186.38	2578	37.80	112.66	185.34	2563
298.5	36.68	109.50	189.00	2614	37.03	110.54	187.96	2599	37.38	111.58	186.92	2585	37.73	112.62	185.88	2571
299	36.61	109.46	189.54	2621	36.96	110.50	188.50	2607	37.30	111.54	187.46	2593	37.65	112.57	186.43	2578
299.5	36.53	109.42	190.08	2629	36.88	110.46	189.04	2614	37.23	111.50	188.00	2600	37.57	112.53	186.97	2586
300	36.46	109.38	190.62	2636	36.81	110.42	189.58	2622	37.15	111.46	188.55	2608	37.50	112.49	187.51	2593
300.5	36.39	109.34	191.16	2644	36.73	110.38	190.12	2629	37.08	111.41	189.09	2615	37.42	112.45	188.05	2601
301	36.31	109.30	191.70	2651	36.66	110.34	190.66	2637	37.00	111.37	189.63	2623	37.35	112.41	188.59	2608
301.5	36.24	109.26	192.24	2659	36.58	110.29	191.21	2644	36.93	111.33	190.17	2630	37.27	112.37	189.13	2616
302	36.16	109.22	192.78	2666	36.51	110.25	191.75	2652	36.85	111.29	190.71	2638	37.19	112.33	189.67	2623
302.5	36.09	109.18	193.33	2674	36.43	110.21	192.29	2659	36.78	111.25	191.25	2645	37.12	112.29	190.21	2631
303	36.02	109.13	193.87	2681	36.36	110.17	192.83	2667	36.70	111.21	191.79	2652	37.05	112.25	190.75	2638
303.5	35.94	109.09	194.41	2689	36.29	110.13	193.37	2674	36.63	111.17	192.33	2660	36.97	112.21	191.29	2646
304	35.87	109.05	194.95	2696	36.21	110.09	193.91	2682	36.55	111.13	192.87	2667	36.90	112.16	191.84	2653
304.5	35.80	109.01	195.49	2704	36.14	110.05	194.45	2689	36.48	111.09	193.41	2675	36.82	112.12	192.38	2661
305	35.73	108.97	196.03	2711	36.07	110.01	194.99	2697	36.41	111.05	193.96	2682	36.75	112.08	192.92	2668
305.5	35.66	108.93	196.57	2719	36.00	109.97	195.53	2704	36.34	111.00	194.50	2690	36.67	112.04	193.46	2676
306	35.58	108.89	197.11	2726	35.92	109.93	196.07	2712	36.26	110.96	195.04	2697	36.60	112.00	194.00	2683
306.5	35.51	108.85	197.65	2734	35.85	109.88	196.62	2719	36.19	110.92	195.58	2705	36.53	111.96	194.54	2690
307	35.44	108.81	198.19	2741	35.78	109.84	197.16	2727	36.12	110.88	196.12	2712	36.46	111.92	195.08	2698
307.5	35.37	108.77	198.74	2749	35.71	109.80	197.70	2734	36.05	110.84	196.66	2720	36.38	111.88	195.62	2705
308	35.30	108.72	199.28	2756	35.64	109.76	198.24	2742	35.97	110.80	197.20	2727	36.31	111.84	196.16	2713
308.5	35.23	108.68	199.82	2763	35.57	109.72	198.78	2749	35.90	110.76	197.74	2735	36.24	111.80	196.70	2720
309	35.16	108.64	200.36	2771	35.49	109.68	199.32	2757	35.83	110.72	198.28	2742	36.17	111.75	197.25	2728
309.5	35.09	108.60	200.90	2778	35.42	109.64	199.86	2764	35.76	110.68	198.82	2750	36.09	111.71	197.79	2735
310	35.02	108.56	201.44	2786	35.35	109.60	200.40	2772	35.69	110.64	199.37	2757	36.02	111.67	198.33	2743
310.5	34.95	108.52	201.98	2793	35.28	109.56	200.94	2779	35.62	110.59	199.91	2765	35.95	111.63	198.87	2750
311	34.88	108.48	202.52	2801	35.21	109.52	201.48	2787	35.55	110.55	200.45	2772	35.88	111.59	199.41	2758
311.5	34.81	108.44	203.06	2808	35.14	109.47	202.03	2794	35.48	110.51	200.99	2780	35.81	111.55	199.95	2765

Body Composition MALE 280-311.5 Lb.

Weight: Lb.	Waist: 57 inches Fat: %	Fat: Lb.	LBM: Lb.	RMR: Cal.	57.25 inches Fat: %	Fat: Lb.	LBM: Lb.	RMR: Cal.	57.5 inches Fat: %	Fat: Lb.	LBM: Lb.	RMR: Cal.	57.75 inches Fat: %	Fat: Lb.	LBM: Lb.	RMR: Cal.
280	41.13	115.17	164.83	2280	41.50	116.21	163.79	2265	41.87	117.25	162.76	2251	42.24	118.28	161.72	2237
280.5	41.04	115.13	165.37	2287	41.41	116.17	164.33	2273	41.78	117.20	163.30	2258	42.15	118.24	162.26	2244
281	40.96	115.09	165.91	2295	41.33	116.13	164.87	2280	41.70	117.16	163.84	2266	42.06	118.20	162.80	2252
281.5	40.87	115.05	166.45	2302	41.24	116.08	165.42	2288	41.61	117.12	164.38	2273	41.97	118.16	163.34	2259
282	40.78	115.01	166.99	2310	41.15	116.04	165.96	2295	41.52	117.08	164.92	2281	41.89	118.12	163.88	2266
282.5	40.70	114.97	167.54	2317	41.06	116.00	166.50	2303	41.43	117.04	165.46	2288	41.80	118.08	164.42	2274
283	40.61	114.92	168.08	2324	40.98	115.96	167.04	2310	41.34	117.00	166.00	2296	41.71	118.04	164.96	2281
283.5	40.52	114.88	168.62	2332	40.89	115.92	167.58	2318	41.26	116.96	166.54	2303	41.62	118.00	165.50	2289
284	40.44	114.84	169.16	2339	40.80	115.88	168.12	2325	41.17	116.92	167.08	2311	41.53	117.95	166.05	2296
284.5	40.35	114.80	169.70	2347	40.72	115.84	168.66	2333	41.08	116.88	167.62	2318	41.45	117.91	166.59	2304
285	40.27	114.76	170.24	2354	40.63	115.80	169.20	2340	40.99	116.84	168.17	2326	41.36	117.87	167.13	2311
285.5	40.18	114.72	170.78	2362	40.55	115.76	169.74	2348	40.91	116.79	168.71	2333	41.27	117.83	167.67	2319
286	40.10	114.68	171.32	2369	40.46	115.72	170.28	2355	40.82	116.75	169.25	2341	41.19	117.79	168.21	2326
286.5	40.01	114.64	171.86	2377	40.38	115.67	170.83	2363	40.74	116.71	169.79	2348	41.10	117.75	168.75	2334
287	39.93	114.60	172.40	2384	40.29	115.63	171.37	2370	40.65	116.67	170.33	2356	41.01	117.71	169.29	2341
287.5	39.85	114.56	172.95	2392	40.21	115.59	171.91	2377	40.57	116.63	170.87	2363	40.93	117.67	169.83	2349
288	39.76	114.51	173.49	2399	40.12	115.55	172.45	2385	40.48	116.59	171.41	2371	40.84	117.63	170.37	2356
288.5	39.68	114.47	174.03	2407	40.04	115.51	172.99	2392	40.40	116.55	171.95	2378	40.76	117.59	170.91	2364
289	39.60	114.43	174.57	2414	39.95	115.47	173.53	2400	40.31	116.51	172.49	2386	40.67	117.54	171.46	2371
289.5	39.51	114.39	175.11	2422	39.87	115.43	174.07	2407	40.23	116.47	173.03	2393	40.59	117.50	172.00	2379
290	39.43	114.35	175.65	2429	39.79	115.39	174.61	2415	40.15	116.43	173.58	2401	40.50	117.46	172.54	2386
290.5	39.35	114.31	176.19	2437	39.71	115.35	175.15	2422	40.06	116.38	174.12	2408	40.42	117.42	173.08	2394
291	39.27	114.27	176.73	2444	39.62	115.31	175.69	2430	39.98	116.34	174.66	2416	40.34	117.38	173.62	2401
291.5	39.19	114.23	177.27	2452	39.54	115.26	176.24	2437	39.90	116.30	175.20	2423	40.25	117.34	174.16	2409
292	39.10	114.19	177.81	2459	39.46	115.22	176.78	2445	39.82	116.26	175.74	2430	40.17	117.30	174.70	2416
292.5	39.02	114.15	178.36	2467	39.38	115.18	177.32	2452	39.73	116.22	176.28	2438	40.09	117.26	175.24	2424
293	38.94	114.10	178.90	2474	39.30	115.14	177.86	2460	39.65	116.18	176.82	2445	40.01	117.22	175.78	2431
293.5	38.86	114.06	179.44	2482	39.22	115.10	178.40	2467	39.57	116.14	177.36	2453	39.92	117.18	176.32	2439
294	38.78	114.02	179.98	2489	39.14	115.06	178.94	2475	39.49	116.10	177.90	2460	39.84	117.13	176.87	2446
294.5	38.70	113.98	180.52	2497	39.06	115.02	179.48	2482	39.41	116.06	178.44	2468	39.76	117.09	177.41	2454
295	38.62	113.94	181.06	2504	38.98	114.98	180.02	2490	39.33	116.02	178.99	2475	39.68	117.05	177.95	2461
295.5	38.54	113.90	181.60	2512	38.90	114.94	180.56	2497	39.25	115.97	179.53	2483	39.60	117.01	178.49	2468
296	38.47	113.86	182.14	2519	38.82	114.90	181.10	2505	39.17	115.93	180.07	2490	39.52	116.97	179.03	2476
296.5	38.39	113.82	182.68	2527	38.74	114.85	181.65	2512	39.09	115.89	180.61	2498	39.44	116.93	179.57	2483
297	38.31	113.78	183.22	2534	38.66	114.81	182.19	2520	39.01	115.85	181.15	2505	39.36	116.89	180.11	2491
297.5	38.23	113.74	183.77	2541	38.58	114.77	182.73	2527	38.93	115.81	181.69	2513	39.28	116.85	180.65	2498
298	38.15	113.69	184.31	2549	38.50	114.73	183.27	2535	38.85	115.77	182.23	2520	39.20	116.81	181.19	2506
298.5	38.07	113.65	184.85	2556	38.42	114.69	183.81	2542	38.77	115.73	182.77	2528	39.12	116.77	181.73	2513
299	38.00	113.61	185.39	2564	38.34	114.65	184.35	2550	38.69	115.69	183.31	2535	39.04	116.72	182.28	2521
299.5	37.92	113.57	185.93	2571	38.27	114.61	184.89	2557	38.61	115.65	183.85	2543	38.96	116.68	182.82	2528
300	37.84	113.53	186.47	2579	38.19	114.57	185.43	2565	38.54	115.61	184.40	2550	38.88	116.64	183.36	2536
300.5	37.77	113.49	187.01	2586	38.11	114.53	185.97	2572	38.46	115.56	184.94	2558	38.80	116.60	183.90	2543
301	37.69	113.45	187.55	2594	38.04	114.49	186.51	2579	38.38	115.52	185.48	2565	38.72	116.56	184.44	2551
301.5	37.61	113.41	188.09	2601	37.96	114.44	187.06	2587	38.30	115.48	186.02	2573	38.65	116.52	184.98	2558
302	37.54	113.37	188.63	2609	37.88	114.40	187.60	2594	38.23	115.44	186.56	2580	38.57	116.48	185.52	2566
302.5	37.46	113.33	189.18	2616	37.81	114.36	188.14	2602	38.15	115.40	187.10	2588	38.49	116.44	186.06	2573
303	37.39	113.28	189.72	2624	37.73	114.32	188.68	2609	38.07	115.36	187.64	2595	38.41	116.40	186.60	2581
303.5	37.31	113.24	190.26	2631	37.65	114.28	189.22	2617	38.00	115.32	188.18	2603	38.34	116.36	187.14	2588
304	37.24	113.20	190.80	2639	37.58	114.24	189.76	2624	37.92	115.28	188.72	2610	38.26	116.31	187.69	2596
304.5	37.16	113.16	191.34	2646	37.50	114.20	190.30	2632	37.84	115.24	189.26	2618	38.19	116.27	188.23	2603
305	37.09	113.12	191.88	2654	37.43	114.16	190.84	2639	37.77	115.20	189.81	2625	38.11	116.23	188.77	2611
305.5	37.01	113.08	192.42	2661	37.35	114.12	191.38	2647	37.69	115.15	190.35	2632	38.03	116.19	189.31	2618
306	36.94	113.04	192.96	2669	37.28	114.08	191.92	2654	37.62	115.11	190.89	2640	37.96	116.15	189.85	2626
306.5	36.87	113.00	193.50	2676	37.21	114.03	192.47	2662	37.54	115.07	191.43	2647	37.88	116.11	190.39	2633
307	36.79	112.96	194.04	2684	37.13	113.99	193.01	2669	37.47	115.03	191.97	2655	37.81	116.07	190.93	2641
307.5	36.72	112.92	194.59	2691	37.06	113.95	193.55	2677	37.40	114.99	192.51	2662	37.73	116.03	191.47	2648
308	36.65	112.87	195.13	2699	36.98	113.91	194.09	2684	37.32	114.95	193.05	2670	37.66	115.99	192.01	2656
308.5	36.57	112.83	195.67	2706	36.91	113.87	194.63	2692	37.25	114.91	193.59	2677	37.58	115.95	192.55	2663
309	36.50	112.79	196.21	2714	36.84	113.83	195.17	2699	37.17	114.87	194.13	2685	37.51	115.90	193.10	2671
309.5	36.43	112.75	196.75	2721	36.77	113.79	195.71	2707	37.10	114.83	194.67	2692	37.44	115.86	193.64	2678
310	36.36	112.71	197.29	2729	36.69	113.75	196.25	2714	37.03	114.79	195.22	2700	37.36	115.82	194.18	2685
310.5	36.29	112.67	197.83	2736	36.62	113.71	196.79	2722	36.95	114.74	195.76	2707	37.29	115.78	194.72	2693
311	36.21	112.63	198.37	2743	36.55	113.67	197.33	2729	36.88	114.70	196.30	2715	37.22	115.74	195.26	2700
311.5	36.14	112.59	198.91	2751	36.48	113.62	197.88	2737	36.81	114.66	196.84	2722	37.14	115.70	195.80	2708

Body Composition MALE 280-311.5 Lb.

Weight: Lb.	Waist: 58 inches				58.25 inches				58.5 inches				58.75 inches			
	Fat: %	Fat: Lb.	LBM: Lb.	RMR: Cal.	Fat: %	Fat: Lb.	LBM: Lb.	RMR: Cal.	Fat: %	Fat: Lb.	LBM: Lb.	RMR: Cal.	Fat: %	Fat: Lb.	LBM: Lb.	RMR: Cal.
280	42.61	119.32	160.68	2222	42.98	120.36	159.64	2208	43.36	121.40	158.61	2194	43.73	122.43	157.57	2179
280.5	42.52	119.28	161.22	2230	42.89	120.32	160.18	2215	43.26	121.35	159.15	2201	43.63	122.39	158.11	2187
281	42.43	119.24	161.76	2237	42.80	120.28	160.72	2223	43.17	121.31	159.69	2208	43.54	122.35	158.65	2194
281.5	42.34	119.20	162.30	2245	42.71	120.23	161.27	2230	43.08	121.27	160.23	2216	43.45	122.31	159.19	2202
282	42.25	119.16	162.84	2252	42.62	120.19	161.81	2238	42.99	121.23	160.77	2223	43.36	122.27	159.73	2209
282.5	42.16	119.12	163.39	2260	42.53	120.15	162.35	2245	42.90	121.19	161.31	2231	43.27	122.23	160.27	2217
283	42.08	119.07	163.93	2267	42.44	120.11	162.89	2253	42.81	121.15	161.85	2238	43.18	122.19	160.81	2224
283.5	41.99	119.03	164.47	2275	42.35	120.07	163.43	2260	42.72	121.11	162.39	2246	43.08	122.15	161.35	2232
284	41.90	118.99	165.01	2282	42.26	120.03	163.97	2268	42.63	121.07	162.93	2253	42.99	122.10	161.90	2239
284.5	41.81	118.95	165.55	2290	42.18	119.99	164.51	2275	42.54	121.03	163.47	2261	42.90	122.06	162.44	2246
285	41.72	118.91	166.09	2297	42.09	119.95	165.05	2283	42.45	120.99	164.02	2268	42.81	122.02	162.98	2254
285.5	41.64	118.87	166.63	2305	42.00	119.91	165.59	2290	42.36	120.94	164.56	2276	42.73	121.98	163.52	2261
286	41.55	118.83	167.17	2312	41.91	119.87	166.13	2298	42.27	120.90	165.10	2283	42.64	121.94	164.06	2269
286.5	41.46	118.79	167.71	2319	41.82	119.82	166.68	2305	42.19	120.86	165.64	2291	42.55	121.90	164.60	2276
287	41.37	118.75	168.25	2327	41.74	119.78	167.22	2313	42.10	120.82	166.18	2298	42.46	121.86	165.14	2284
287.5	41.29	118.71	168.80	2334	41.65	119.74	167.76	2320	42.01	120.78	166.72	2306	42.37	121.82	165.68	2291
288	41.20	118.66	169.34	2342	41.56	119.70	168.30	2328	41.92	120.74	167.26	2313	42.28	121.78	166.22	2299
288.5	41.12	118.62	169.88	2349	41.48	119.66	168.84	2335	41.84	120.70	167.80	2321	42.20	121.74	166.76	2306
289	41.03	118.58	170.42	2357	41.39	119.62	169.38	2343	41.75	120.66	168.34	2328	42.11	121.69	167.31	2314
289.5	40.95	118.54	170.96	2364	41.31	119.58	169.92	2350	41.66	120.62	168.88	2336	42.02	121.65	167.85	2321
290	40.86	118.50	171.50	2372	41.22	119.54	170.46	2357	41.58	120.58	169.43	2343	41.94	121.61	168.39	2329
290.5	40.78	118.46	172.04	2379	41.13	119.50	171.00	2365	41.49	120.53	169.97	2351	41.85	121.57	168.93	2336
291	40.69	118.42	172.58	2387	41.05	119.46	171.54	2372	41.41	120.49	170.51	2358	41.76	121.53	169.47	2344
291.5	40.61	118.38	173.12	2394	40.97	119.41	172.09	2380	41.32	120.45	171.05	2366	41.68	121.49	170.01	2351
292	40.53	118.34	173.66	2402	40.88	119.37	172.63	2387	41.24	120.41	171.59	2373	41.59	121.45	170.55	2359
292.5	40.44	118.30	174.21	2409	40.80	119.33	173.17	2395	41.15	120.37	172.13	2381	41.51	121.41	171.09	2366
293	40.36	118.25	174.75	2417	40.71	119.29	173.71	2402	41.07	120.33	172.67	2388	41.42	121.37	171.63	2374
293.5	40.28	118.21	175.29	2424	40.63	119.25	174.25	2410	40.98	120.29	173.21	2396	41.34	121.33	172.17	2381
294	40.19	118.17	175.83	2432	40.55	119.21	174.79	2417	40.90	120.25	173.75	2403	41.25	121.28	172.72	2389
294.5	40.11	118.13	176.37	2439	40.46	119.17	175.33	2425	40.82	120.21	174.29	2410	41.17	121.24	173.26	2396
295	40.03	118.09	176.91	2447	40.38	119.13	175.87	2432	40.73	120.17	174.84	2418	41.09	121.20	173.80	2404
295.5	39.95	118.05	177.45	2454	40.30	119.09	176.41	2440	40.65	120.12	175.38	2425	41.00	121.16	174.34	2411
296	39.87	118.01	177.99	2462	40.22	119.05	176.95	2447	40.57	120.08	175.92	2433	40.92	121.12	174.88	2419
296.5	39.79	117.97	178.53	2469	40.14	119.00	177.50	2455	40.49	120.04	176.46	2440	40.84	121.08	175.42	2426
297	39.71	117.93	179.07	2477	40.06	118.96	178.04	2462	40.40	120.00	177.00	2448	40.75	121.04	175.96	2434
297.5	39.63	117.89	179.62	2484	39.97	118.92	178.58	2470	40.32	119.96	177.54	2455	40.67	121.00	176.50	2441
298	39.54	117.84	180.16	2492	39.89	118.88	179.12	2477	40.24	119.92	178.08	2463	40.59	120.96	177.04	2449
298.5	39.46	117.80	180.70	2499	39.81	118.84	179.66	2485	40.16	119.88	178.62	2470	40.51	120.92	177.58	2456
299	39.39	117.76	181.24	2507	39.73	118.80	180.20	2492	40.08	119.84	179.16	2478	40.43	120.87	178.13	2463
299.5	39.31	117.72	181.78	2514	39.65	118.76	180.74	2500	40.00	119.80	179.70	2485	40.35	120.83	178.67	2471
300	39.23	117.68	182.32	2521	39.57	118.72	181.28	2507	39.92	119.76	180.25	2493	40.26	120.79	179.21	2478
300.5	39.15	117.64	182.86	2529	39.49	118.68	181.82	2515	39.84	119.71	180.79	2500	40.18	120.75	179.75	2486
301	39.07	117.60	183.40	2536	39.41	118.64	182.36	2522	39.76	119.67	181.33	2508	40.10	120.71	180.29	2493
301.5	38.99	117.56	183.94	2544	39.33	118.59	182.91	2530	39.68	119.63	181.87	2515	40.02	120.67	180.83	2501
302	38.91	117.52	184.48	2551	39.26	118.55	183.45	2537	39.60	119.59	182.41	2523	39.94	120.63	181.37	2508
302.5	38.83	117.48	185.03	2559	39.18	118.51	183.99	2545	39.52	119.55	182.95	2530	39.86	120.59	181.91	2516
303	38.76	117.43	185.57	2566	39.10	118.47	184.53	2552	39.44	119.51	183.49	2538	39.78	120.55	182.45	2523
303.5	38.68	117.39	186.11	2574	39.02	118.43	185.07	2560	39.36	119.47	184.03	2545	39.71	120.51	182.99	2531
304	38.60	117.35	186.65	2581	38.94	118.39	185.61	2567	39.29	119.43	184.57	2553	39.63	120.46	183.54	2538
304.5	38.53	117.31	187.19	2589	38.87	118.35	186.15	2574	39.21	119.39	185.11	2560	39.55	120.42	184.08	2546
305	38.45	117.27	187.73	2596	38.79	118.31	186.69	2582	39.13	119.35	185.66	2568	39.47	120.38	184.62	2553
305.5	38.37	117.23	188.27	2604	38.71	118.27	187.23	2589	39.05	119.30	186.20	2575	39.39	120.34	185.16	2561
306	38.30	117.19	188.81	2611	38.64	118.23	187.77	2597	38.97	119.26	186.74	2583	39.31	120.30	185.70	2568
306.5	38.22	117.15	189.35	2619	38.56	118.18	188.32	2604	38.90	119.22	187.28	2590	39.24	120.26	186.24	2576
307	38.15	117.11	189.89	2626	38.48	118.14	188.86	2612	38.82	119.18	187.82	2598	39.16	120.22	186.78	2583
307.5	38.07	117.07	190.44	2634	38.41	118.10	189.40	2619	38.74	119.14	188.36	2605	39.08	120.18	187.32	2591
308	37.99	117.02	190.98	2641	38.33	118.06	189.94	2627	38.67	119.10	188.90	2613	39.01	120.14	187.86	2598
308.5	37.92	116.98	191.52	2649	38.26	118.02	190.48	2634	38.59	119.06	189.44	2620	38.93	120.10	188.40	2606
309	37.85	116.94	192.06	2656	38.18	117.98	191.02	2642	38.52	119.02	189.98	2627	38.85	120.05	188.95	2613
309.5	37.77	116.90	192.60	2664	38.11	117.94	191.56	2649	38.44	118.98	190.52	2635	38.78	120.01	189.49	2621
310	37.70	116.86	193.14	2671	38.03	117.90	192.10	2657	38.37	118.94	191.07	2642	38.70	119.97	190.03	2628
310.5	37.62	116.82	193.68	2679	37.96	117.86	192.64	2664	38.29	118.89	191.61	2650	38.63	119.93	190.57	2636
311	37.55	116.78	194.22	2686	37.88	117.82	193.18	2672	38.22	118.85	192.15	2657	38.55	119.89	191.11	2643
311.5	37.48	116.74	194.76	2694	37.81	117.77	193.73	2679	38.14	118.81	192.69	2665	38.47	119.85	191.65	2651

Body Composition   MALE   280-311.5 Lb.

Weight: Lb.	Waist: 59 inches Fat: %	Fat: Lb.	LBM: Lb.	RMR: Cal.	59.25 inches Fat: %	Fat: Lb.	LBM: Lb.	RMR: Cal.	59.5 inches Fat: %	Fat: Lb.	LBM: Lb.	RMR: Cal.	59.75 inches Fat: %	Fat: Lb.	LBM: Lb.	RMR: Cal.
280	44.10	123.47	156.53	2165	44.47	124.51	155.49	2150	44.84	125.55	154.46	2136	45.21	126.58	153.42	2122
280.5	44.00	123.43	157.07	2172	44.37	124.47	156.03	2158	44.74	125.50	155.00	2144	45.11	126.54	153.96	2129
281	43.91	123.39	157.61	2180	44.28	124.43	156.57	2165	44.65	125.46	155.54	2151	45.02	126.50	154.50	2137
281.5	43.82	123.35	158.15	2187	44.19	124.38	157.12	2173	44.55	125.42	156.08	2159	44.92	126.46	155.04	2144
282	43.73	123.31	158.69	2195	44.09	124.34	157.66	2180	44.46	125.38	156.62	2166	44.83	126.42	155.58	2152
282.5	43.63	123.27	159.24	2202	44.00	124.30	158.20	2188	44.37	125.34	157.16	2174	44.74	126.38	156.12	2159
283	43.54	123.22	159.78	2210	43.91	124.26	158.74	2195	44.28	125.30	157.70	2181	44.64	126.34	156.66	2167
283.5	43.45	123.18	160.32	2217	43.82	124.22	159.28	2203	44.18	125.26	158.24	2188	44.55	126.30	157.20	2174
284	43.36	123.14	160.86	2225	43.73	124.18	159.82	2210	44.09	125.22	158.78	2196	44.46	126.25	157.75	2182
284.5	43.27	123.10	161.40	2232	43.63	124.14	160.36	2218	44.00	125.18	159.32	2203	44.36	126.21	158.29	2189
285	43.18	123.06	161.94	2240	43.54	124.10	160.90	2225	43.91	125.14	159.87	2211	44.27	126.17	158.83	2197
285.5	43.09	123.02	162.48	2247	43.45	124.06	161.44	2233	43.82	125.09	160.41	2218	44.18	126.13	159.37	2204
286	43.00	122.98	163.02	2255	43.36	124.02	161.98	2240	43.72	125.05	160.95	2226	44.09	126.09	159.91	2212
286.5	42.91	122.94	163.56	2262	43.27	123.97	162.53	2248	43.63	125.01	161.49	2233	44.00	126.05	160.45	2219
287	42.82	122.90	164.10	2270	43.18	123.93	163.07	2255	43.54	124.97	162.03	2241	43.91	126.01	160.99	2227
287.5	42.73	122.86	164.65	2277	43.09	123.89	163.61	2263	43.45	124.93	162.57	2248	43.81	125.97	161.53	2234
288	42.64	122.81	165.19	2285	43.00	123.85	164.15	2270	43.36	124.89	163.11	2256	43.72	125.93	162.07	2241
288.5	42.56	122.77	165.73	2292	42.92	123.81	164.69	2278	43.27	124.85	163.65	2263	43.63	125.89	162.61	2249
289	42.47	122.73	166.27	2299	42.83	123.77	165.23	2285	43.19	124.81	164.19	2271	43.54	125.84	163.16	2256
289.5	42.38	122.69	166.81	2307	42.74	123.73	165.77	2293	43.10	124.77	164.73	2278	43.46	125.80	163.70	2264
290	42.29	122.65	167.35	2314	42.65	123.69	166.31	2300	43.01	124.73	165.28	2286	43.37	125.76	164.24	2271
290.5	42.21	122.61	167.89	2322	42.56	123.65	166.85	2308	42.92	124.68	165.82	2293	43.28	125.72	164.78	2279
291	42.12	122.57	168.43	2329	42.48	123.61	167.39	2315	42.83	124.64	166.36	2301	43.19	125.68	165.32	2286
291.5	42.03	122.53	168.97	2337	42.39	123.56	167.94	2323	42.75	124.60	166.90	2308	43.10	125.64	165.86	2294
292	41.95	122.49	169.51	2344	42.30	123.52	168.48	2330	42.66	124.56	167.44	2316	43.01	125.60	166.40	2301
292.5	41.86	122.45	170.06	2352	42.22	123.48	169.02	2338	42.57	124.52	167.98	2323	42.93	125.56	166.94	2309
293	41.78	122.40	170.60	2359	42.13	123.44	169.56	2345	42.48	124.48	168.52	2331	42.84	125.52	167.48	2316
293.5	41.69	122.36	171.14	2367	42.04	123.40	170.10	2352	42.40	124.44	169.06	2338	42.75	125.48	168.02	2324
294	41.61	122.32	171.68	2374	41.96	123.36	170.64	2360	42.31	124.40	169.60	2346	42.66	125.43	168.57	2331
294.5	41.52	122.28	172.22	2382	41.87	123.32	171.18	2367	42.23	124.36	170.14	2353	42.58	125.39	169.11	2339
295	41.44	122.24	172.76	2389	41.79	123.28	171.72	2375	42.14	124.32	170.69	2361	42.49	125.35	169.65	2346
295.5	41.35	122.20	173.30	2397	41.70	123.24	172.26	2382	42.06	124.27	171.23	2368	42.41	125.31	170.19	2354
296	41.27	122.16	173.84	2404	41.62	123.20	172.80	2390	41.97	124.23	171.77	2376	42.32	125.27	170.73	2361
296.5	41.19	122.12	174.38	2412	41.54	123.15	173.35	2397	41.89	124.19	172.31	2383	42.24	125.23	171.27	2369
297	41.10	122.08	174.92	2419	41.45	123.11	173.89	2405	41.80	124.15	172.85	2391	42.15	125.19	171.81	2376
297.5	41.02	122.04	175.47	2427	41.37	123.07	174.43	2412	41.72	124.11	173.39	2398	42.07	125.15	172.35	2384
298	40.94	121.99	176.01	2434	41.29	123.03	174.97	2420	41.63	124.07	173.93	2405	41.98	125.11	172.89	2391
298.5	40.86	121.95	176.55	2442	41.20	122.99	175.51	2427	41.55	124.03	174.47	2413	41.90	125.07	173.43	2399
299	40.77	121.91	177.09	2449	41.12	122.95	176.05	2435	41.47	123.99	175.01	2420	41.81	125.02	173.98	2406
299.5	40.69	121.87	177.63	2457	41.04	122.91	176.59	2442	41.38	123.95	175.55	2428	41.73	124.98	174.52	2414
300	40.61	121.83	178.17	2464	40.96	122.87	177.13	2450	41.30	123.91	176.10	2435	41.65	124.94	175.06	2421
300.5	40.53	121.79	178.71	2472	40.87	122.83	177.67	2457	41.22	123.86	176.64	2443	41.56	124.90	175.60	2429
301	40.45	121.75	179.25	2479	40.79	122.79	178.21	2465	41.14	123.82	177.18	2450	41.48	124.86	176.14	2436
301.5	40.37	121.71	179.79	2487	40.71	122.74	178.76	2472	41.06	123.78	177.72	2458	41.40	124.82	176.68	2443
302	40.29	121.67	180.33	2494	40.63	122.70	179.30	2480	40.97	123.74	178.26	2465	41.32	124.78	177.22	2451
302.5	40.21	121.63	180.88	2502	40.55	122.66	179.84	2487	40.89	123.70	178.80	2473	41.24	124.74	177.76	2458
303	40.13	121.58	181.42	2509	40.47	122.62	180.38	2495	40.81	123.66	179.34	2480	41.15	124.70	178.30	2466
303.5	40.05	121.54	181.96	2516	40.39	122.58	180.92	2502	40.73	123.62	179.88	2488	41.07	124.66	178.84	2473
304	39.97	121.50	182.50	2524	40.31	122.54	181.46	2510	40.65	123.58	180.42	2495	40.99	124.61	179.39	2481
304.5	39.89	121.46	183.04	2531	40.23	122.50	182.00	2517	40.57	123.54	180.96	2503	40.91	124.57	179.93	2488
305	39.81	121.42	183.58	2539	40.15	122.46	182.54	2525	40.49	123.50	181.51	2510	40.83	124.53	180.47	2496
305.5	39.73	121.38	184.12	2546	40.07	122.42	183.08	2532	40.41	123.45	182.05	2518	40.75	124.49	181.01	2503
306	39.65	121.34	184.66	2554	39.99	122.38	183.62	2540	40.33	123.41	182.59	2525	40.67	124.45	181.55	2511
306.5	39.57	121.30	185.20	2561	39.91	122.33	184.17	2547	40.25	123.37	183.13	2533	40.59	124.41	182.09	2518
307	39.50	121.26	185.74	2569	39.84	122.29	184.71	2554	40.17	123.33	183.67	2540	40.51	124.37	182.63	2526
307.5	39.42	121.22	186.29	2576	39.76	122.25	185.25	2562	40.09	123.29	184.21	2548	40.43	124.33	183.17	2533
308	39.34	121.17	186.83	2584	39.68	122.21	185.79	2569	40.02	123.25	184.75	2555	40.35	124.29	183.71	2541
308.5	39.27	121.13	187.37	2591	39.60	122.17	186.33	2577	39.94	123.21	185.29	2563	40.27	124.25	184.25	2548
309	39.19	121.09	187.91	2599	39.52	122.13	186.87	2584	39.86	123.17	185.83	2570	40.20	124.20	184.80	2556
309.5	39.11	121.05	188.45	2606	39.45	122.09	187.41	2592	39.78	123.13	186.37	2578	40.12	124.16	185.34	2563
310	39.04	121.01	188.99	2614	39.37	122.05	187.95	2599	39.70	123.09	186.92	2585	40.04	124.12	185.88	2571
310.5	38.96	120.97	189.53	2621	39.29	122.01	188.49	2607	39.63	123.04	187.46	2593	39.96	124.08	186.42	2578
311	38.88	120.93	190.07	2629	39.22	121.97	189.03	2614	39.55	123.00	188.00	2600	39.88	124.04	186.96	2586
311.5	38.81	120.89	190.61	2636	39.14	121.92	189.58	2622	39.47	122.96	188.54	2607	39.81	124.00	187.50	2593

Body Composition MALE 280-311.5 Lb.

Weight: Lb.	Waist: 60 inches Fat: %	Fat: Lb.	LBM: Lb.	RMR: Cal.	60.25 inches Fat: %	Fat: Lb.	LBM: Lb.	RMR: Cal.	60.5 inches Fat: %	Fat: Lb.	LBM: Lb.	RMR: Cal.	60.75 inches Fat: %	Fat: Lb.	LBM: Lb.	RMR: Cal.
280	45.58	127.62	152.38	2107	45.95	128.66	151.34	2093	46.32	129.70	150.31	2079	46.69	130.73	149.27	2064
280.5	45.48	127.58	152.92	2115	45.85	128.62	151.88	2101	46.22	129.65	150.85	2086	46.59	130.69	149.81	2072
281	45.39	127.54	153.46	2122	45.76	128.58	152.42	2108	46.13	129.61	151.39	2094	46.49	130.65	150.35	2079
281.5	45.29	127.50	154.00	2130	45.66	128.53	152.97	2116	46.03	129.57	151.93	2101	46.40	130.61	150.89	2087
282	45.20	127.46	154.54	2137	45.57	128.49	153.51	2123	45.93	129.53	152.47	2109	46.30	130.57	151.43	2094
282.5	45.10	127.42	155.09	2145	45.47	128.45	154.05	2130	45.84	129.49	153.01	2116	46.20	130.53	151.97	2102
283	45.01	127.37	155.63	2152	45.38	128.41	154.59	2138	45.74	129.45	153.55	2124	46.11	130.49	152.51	2109
283.5	44.91	127.33	156.17	2160	45.28	128.37	155.13	2145	45.65	129.41	154.09	2131	46.01	130.45	153.05	2117
284	44.82	127.29	156.71	2167	45.19	128.33	155.67	2153	45.55	129.37	154.63	2139	45.92	130.40	153.60	2124
284.5	44.73	127.25	157.25	2175	45.09	128.29	156.21	2160	45.46	129.33	155.17	2146	45.82	130.36	154.14	2132
285	44.64	127.21	157.79	2182	45.00	128.25	156.75	2168	45.36	129.29	155.72	2154	45.73	130.32	154.68	2139
285.5	44.54	127.17	158.33	2190	44.91	128.21	157.29	2175	45.27	129.24	156.26	2161	45.63	130.28	155.22	2147
286	44.45	127.13	158.87	2197	44.81	128.17	157.83	2183	45.18	129.20	156.80	2169	45.54	130.24	155.76	2154
286.5	44.36	127.09	159.41	2205	44.72	128.12	158.38	2190	45.08	129.16	157.34	2176	45.44	130.20	156.30	2162
287	44.27	127.05	159.95	2212	44.63	128.08	158.92	2198	44.99	129.12	157.88	2183	45.35	130.16	156.84	2169
287.5	44.18	127.01	160.50	2220	44.54	128.04	159.46	2205	44.90	129.08	158.42	2191	45.26	130.12	157.38	2177
288	44.08	126.96	161.04	2227	44.44	128.00	160.00	2213	44.81	129.04	158.96	2198	45.17	130.08	157.92	2184
288.5	43.99	126.92	161.58	2235	44.35	127.96	160.54	2220	44.71	129.00	159.50	2206	45.07	130.04	158.46	2192
289	43.90	126.88	162.12	2242	44.26	127.92	161.08	2228	44.62	128.96	160.04	2213	44.98	129.99	159.01	2199
289.5	43.81	126.84	162.66	2250	44.17	127.88	161.62	2235	44.53	128.92	160.58	2221	44.89	129.95	159.55	2207
290	43.72	126.80	163.20	2257	44.08	127.84	162.16	2243	44.44	128.88	161.13	2228	44.80	129.91	160.09	2214
290.5	43.63	126.76	163.74	2265	43.99	127.80	162.70	2250	44.35	128.83	161.67	2236	44.71	129.87	160.63	2221
291	43.55	126.72	164.28	2272	43.90	127.76	163.24	2258	44.26	128.79	162.21	2243	44.62	129.83	161.17	2229
291.5	43.46	126.68	164.82	2280	43.81	127.71	163.79	2265	44.17	128.75	162.75	2251	44.52	129.79	161.71	2236
292	43.37	126.64	165.36	2287	43.72	127.67	164.33	2273	44.08	128.71	163.29	2258	44.43	129.75	162.25	2244
292.5	43.28	126.60	165.91	2294	43.64	127.63	164.87	2280	43.99	128.67	163.83	2266	44.34	129.71	162.79	2251
293	43.19	126.55	166.45	2302	43.55	127.59	165.41	2288	43.90	128.63	164.37	2273	44.25	129.67	163.33	2259
293.5	43.10	126.51	166.99	2309	43.46	127.55	165.95	2295	43.81	128.59	164.91	2281	44.17	129.63	163.87	2266
294	43.02	126.47	167.53	2317	43.37	127.51	166.49	2303	43.72	128.55	165.45	2288	44.08	129.58	164.42	2274
294.5	42.93	126.43	168.07	2324	43.28	127.47	167.03	2310	43.64	128.51	165.99	2296	43.99	129.54	164.96	2281
295	42.84	126.39	168.61	2332	43.20	127.43	167.57	2318	43.55	128.47	166.54	2303	43.90	129.50	165.50	2289
295.5	42.76	126.35	169.15	2339	43.11	127.39	168.11	2325	43.46	128.42	167.08	2311	43.81	129.46	166.04	2296
296	42.67	126.31	169.69	2347	43.02	127.35	168.65	2332	43.37	128.38	167.62	2318	43.72	129.42	166.58	2304
296.5	42.59	126.27	170.23	2354	42.94	127.30	169.20	2340	43.29	128.34	168.16	2326	43.64	129.38	167.12	2311
297	42.50	126.23	170.77	2362	42.85	127.26	169.74	2347	43.20	128.30	168.70	2333	43.55	129.34	167.66	2319
297.5	42.42	126.19	171.32	2369	42.76	127.22	170.28	2355	43.11	128.26	169.24	2341	43.46	129.30	168.20	2326
298	42.33	126.14	171.86	2377	42.68	127.18	170.82	2362	43.03	128.22	169.78	2348	43.37	129.26	168.74	2334
298.5	42.25	126.10	172.40	2384	42.59	127.14	171.36	2370	42.94	128.18	170.32	2356	43.29	129.22	169.28	2341
299	42.16	126.06	172.94	2392	42.51	127.10	171.90	2377	42.86	128.14	170.86	2363	43.20	129.17	169.83	2349
299.5	42.08	126.02	173.48	2399	42.42	127.06	172.44	2385	42.77	128.10	171.40	2371	43.12	129.13	170.37	2356
300	41.99	125.98	174.02	2407	42.34	127.02	172.98	2392	42.69	128.06	171.95	2378	43.03	129.09	170.91	2364
300.5	41.91	125.94	174.56	2414	42.26	126.98	173.52	2400	42.60	128.01	172.49	2385	42.95	129.05	171.45	2371
301	41.83	125.90	175.10	2422	42.17	126.94	174.06	2407	42.52	127.97	173.03	2393	42.86	129.01	171.99	2379
301.5	41.74	125.86	175.64	2429	42.09	126.89	174.61	2415	42.43	127.93	173.57	2400	42.78	128.97	172.53	2386
302	41.66	125.82	176.18	2437	42.00	126.85	175.15	2422	42.35	127.89	174.11	2408	42.69	128.93	173.07	2394
302.5	41.58	125.78	176.73	2444	41.92	126.81	175.69	2430	42.26	127.85	174.65	2415	42.61	128.89	173.61	2401
303	41.50	125.73	177.27	2452	41.84	126.77	176.23	2437	42.18	127.81	175.19	2423	42.52	128.85	174.15	2409
303.5	41.41	125.69	177.81	2459	41.76	126.73	176.77	2445	42.10	127.77	175.73	2430	42.44	128.81	174.69	2416
304	41.33	125.65	178.35	2467	41.67	126.69	177.31	2452	42.02	127.73	176.27	2438	42.36	128.76	175.24	2424
304.5	41.25	125.61	178.89	2474	41.59	126.65	177.85	2460	41.93	127.69	176.81	2445	42.27	128.72	175.78	2431
305	41.17	125.57	179.43	2482	41.51	126.61	178.39	2467	41.85	127.65	177.36	2453	42.19	128.68	176.32	2438
305.5	41.09	125.53	179.97	2489	41.43	126.57	178.93	2475	41.77	127.60	177.90	2460	42.11	128.64	176.86	2446
306	41.01	125.49	180.51	2496	41.35	126.53	179.47	2482	41.69	127.56	178.44	2468	42.03	128.60	177.40	2453
306.5	40.93	125.45	181.05	2504	41.27	126.48	180.02	2490	41.61	127.52	178.98	2475	41.94	128.56	177.94	2461
307	40.85	125.41	181.59	2511	41.19	126.44	180.56	2497	41.52	127.48	179.52	2483	41.86	128.52	178.48	2468
307.5	40.77	125.37	182.14	2519	41.11	126.40	181.10	2505	41.44	127.44	180.06	2490	41.78	128.48	179.02	2476
308	40.69	125.32	182.68	2526	41.03	126.36	181.64	2512	41.36	127.40	180.60	2498	41.70	128.44	179.56	2483
308.5	40.61	125.28	183.22	2534	40.95	126.32	182.18	2520	41.28	127.36	181.14	2505	41.62	128.40	180.10	2491
309	40.53	125.24	183.76	2541	40.87	126.28	182.72	2527	41.20	127.32	181.68	2513	41.54	128.35	180.65	2498
309.5	40.45	125.20	184.30	2549	40.79	126.24	183.26	2535	41.12	127.28	182.22	2520	41.46	128.31	181.19	2506
310	40.37	125.16	184.84	2556	40.71	126.20	183.80	2542	41.04	127.24	182.77	2528	41.38	128.27	181.73	2513
310.5	40.30	125.12	185.38	2564	40.63	126.16	184.34	2549	40.96	127.19	183.31	2535	41.30	128.23	182.27	2521
311	40.22	125.08	185.92	2571	40.55	126.12	184.88	2557	40.89	127.15	183.85	2543	41.22	128.19	182.81	2528
311.5	40.14	125.04	186.46	2579	40.47	126.07	185.43	2564	40.81	127.11	184.39	2550	41.14	128.15	183.35	2536

Body Composition MALE 280-311.5 Lb.

Weight: Lb.	Waist: 61 inches				61.25 inches				61.5 inches				61.75 inches			
	Fat: %	Fat: Lb.	LBM: Lb.	RMR: Cal.	Fat: %	Fat: Lb.	LBM: Lb.	RMR: Cal.	Fat: %	Fat: Lb.	LBM: Lb.	RMR: Cal.	Fat: %	Fat: Lb.	LBM: Lb.	RMR: Cal.
280	47.06	131.77	148.23	2050	47.43	132.81	147.19	2036	47.80	133.85	146.16	2021	48.17	134.88	145.12	2007
280.5	46.96	131.73	148.77	2058	47.33	132.77	147.73	2043	47.70	133.80	146.70	2029	48.07	134.84	145.66	2014
281	46.86	131.69	149.31	2065	47.23	132.73	148.27	2051	47.60	133.76	147.24	2036	47.97	134.80	146.20	2022
281.5	46.77	131.65	149.85	2072	47.13	132.68	148.82	2058	47.50	133.72	147.78	2044	47.87	134.76	146.74	2029
282	46.67	131.61	150.39	2080	47.04	132.64	149.36	2066	47.40	133.68	148.32	2051	47.77	134.72	147.28	2037
282.5	46.57	131.57	150.94	2087	46.94	132.60	149.90	2073	47.31	133.64	148.86	2059	47.67	134.68	147.82	2044
283	46.47	131.52	151.48	2095	46.84	132.56	150.44	2081	47.21	133.60	149.40	2066	47.57	134.64	148.36	2052
283.5	46.38	131.48	152.02	2102	46.74	132.52	150.98	2088	47.11	133.56	149.94	2074	47.48	134.60	148.90	2059
284	46.28	131.44	152.56	2110	46.65	132.48	151.52	2096	47.01	133.52	150.48	2081	47.38	134.55	149.45	2067
284.5	46.19	131.40	153.10	2117	46.55	132.44	152.06	2103	46.92	133.48	151.02	2089	47.28	134.51	149.99	2074
285	46.09	131.36	153.64	2125	46.46	132.40	152.60	2110	46.82	133.44	151.57	2096	47.18	134.47	150.53	2082
285.5	46.00	131.32	154.18	2132	46.36	132.36	153.14	2118	46.72	133.39	152.11	2104	47.09	134.43	151.07	2089
286	45.90	131.28	154.72	2140	46.26	132.32	153.68	2125	46.63	133.35	152.65	2111	46.99	134.39	151.61	2097
286.5	45.81	131.24	155.26	2147	46.17	132.27	154.23	2133	46.53	133.31	153.19	2119	46.89	134.35	152.15	2104
287	45.71	131.20	155.80	2155	46.07	132.23	154.77	2140	46.44	133.27	153.73	2126	46.80	134.31	152.69	2112
287.5	45.62	131.16	156.35	2162	45.98	132.19	155.31	2148	46.34	133.23	154.27	2134	46.70	134.27	153.23	2119
288	45.53	131.11	156.89	2170	45.89	132.15	155.85	2155	46.25	133.19	154.81	2141	46.61	134.23	153.77	2127
288.5	45.43	131.07	157.43	2177	45.79	132.11	156.39	2163	46.15	133.15	155.35	2149	46.51	134.19	154.31	2134
289	45.34	131.03	157.97	2185	45.70	132.07	156.93	2170	46.06	133.11	155.89	2156	46.42	134.14	154.86	2142
289.5	45.25	130.99	158.51	2192	45.61	132.03	157.47	2178	45.96	133.07	156.43	2163	46.32	134.10	155.40	2149
290	45.16	130.95	159.05	2200	45.51	131.99	158.01	2185	45.87	133.03	156.98	2171	46.23	134.06	155.94	2157
290.5	45.06	130.91	159.59	2207	45.42	131.95	158.55	2193	45.78	132.98	157.52	2178	46.13	134.02	156.48	2164
291	44.97	130.87	160.13	2215	45.33	131.91	159.09	2200	45.68	132.94	158.06	2186	46.04	133.98	157.02	2172
291.5	44.88	130.83	160.67	2222	45.24	131.86	159.64	2208	45.59	132.90	158.60	2193	45.95	133.94	157.56	2179
292	44.79	130.79	161.21	2230	45.15	131.82	160.18	2215	45.50	132.86	159.14	2201	45.86	133.90	158.10	2187
292.5	44.70	130.75	161.76	2237	45.05	131.78	160.72	2223	45.41	132.82	159.68	2208	45.76	133.86	158.64	2194
293	44.61	130.70	162.30	2245	44.96	131.74	161.26	2230	45.32	132.78	160.22	2216	45.67	133.82	159.18	2202
293.5	44.52	130.66	162.84	2252	44.87	131.70	161.80	2238	45.23	132.74	160.76	2223	45.58	133.78	159.72	2209
294	44.43	130.62	163.38	2260	44.78	131.66	162.34	2245	45.14	132.70	161.30	2231	45.49	133.73	160.27	2216
294.5	44.34	130.58	163.92	2267	44.69	131.62	162.88	2253	45.04	132.66	161.84	2238	45.40	133.69	160.81	2224
295	44.25	130.54	164.46	2274	44.60	131.58	163.42	2260	44.95	132.62	162.39	2246	45.31	133.65	161.35	2231
295.5	44.16	130.50	165.00	2282	44.51	131.54	163.96	2268	44.86	132.57	162.93	2253	45.22	133.61	161.89	2239
296	44.07	130.46	165.54	2289	44.42	131.50	164.50	2275	44.77	132.53	163.47	2261	45.13	133.57	162.43	2246
296.5	43.99	130.42	166.08	2297	44.34	131.45	165.05	2283	44.69	132.49	164.01	2268	45.04	133.53	162.97	2254
297	43.90	130.38	166.62	2304	44.25	131.41	165.59	2290	44.60	132.45	164.55	2276	44.95	133.49	163.51	2261
297.5	43.81	130.34	167.17	2312	44.16	131.37	166.13	2298	44.51	132.41	165.09	2283	44.86	133.45	164.05	2269
298	43.72	130.29	167.71	2319	44.07	131.33	166.67	2305	44.42	132.37	165.63	2291	44.77	133.41	164.59	2276
298.5	43.64	130.25	168.25	2327	43.98	131.29	167.21	2313	44.33	132.33	166.17	2298	44.68	133.37	165.13	2284
299	43.55	130.21	168.79	2334	43.90	131.25	167.75	2320	44.24	132.29	166.71	2306	44.59	133.32	165.68	2291
299.5	43.46	130.17	169.33	2342	43.81	131.21	168.29	2327	44.16	132.25	167.25	2313	44.50	133.28	166.22	2299
300	43.38	130.13	169.87	2349	43.72	131.17	168.83	2335	44.07	132.21	167.80	2321	44.41	133.24	166.76	2306
300.5	43.29	130.09	170.41	2357	43.64	131.13	169.37	2342	43.98	132.16	168.34	2328	44.33	133.20	167.30	2314
301	43.21	130.05	170.95	2364	43.55	131.09	169.91	2350	43.89	132.12	168.88	2336	44.24	133.16	167.84	2321
301.5	43.12	130.01	171.49	2372	43.46	131.04	170.46	2357	43.81	132.08	169.42	2343	44.15	133.12	168.38	2329
302	43.04	129.97	172.03	2379	43.38	131.00	171.00	2365	43.72	132.04	169.96	2351	44.07	133.08	168.92	2336
302.5	42.95	129.93	172.58	2387	43.29	130.96	171.54	2372	43.64	132.00	170.50	2358	43.98	133.04	169.46	2344
303	42.87	129.88	173.12	2394	43.21	130.92	172.08	2380	43.55	131.96	171.04	2365	43.89	133.00	170.00	2351
303.5	42.78	129.84	173.66	2402	43.12	130.88	172.62	2387	43.47	131.92	171.58	2373	43.81	132.96	170.54	2359
304	42.70	129.80	174.20	2409	43.04	130.84	173.16	2395	43.38	131.88	172.12	2380	43.72	132.91	171.09	2366
304.5	42.61	129.76	174.74	2417	42.96	130.80	173.70	2402	43.30	131.84	172.66	2388	43.64	132.87	171.63	2374
305	42.53	129.72	175.28	2424	42.87	130.76	174.24	2410	43.21	131.80	173.21	2395	43.55	132.83	172.17	2381
305.5	42.45	129.68	175.82	2432	42.79	130.72	174.78	2417	43.13	131.75	173.75	2403	43.47	132.79	172.71	2389
306	42.37	129.64	176.36	2439	42.70	130.68	175.32	2425	43.04	131.71	174.29	2410	43.38	132.75	173.25	2396
306.5	42.28	129.60	176.90	2447	42.62	130.63	175.87	2432	42.96	131.67	174.83	2418	43.30	132.71	173.79	2404
307	42.20	129.56	177.44	2454	42.54	130.59	176.41	2440	42.88	131.63	175.37	2425	43.21	132.67	174.33	2411
307.5	42.12	129.52	177.99	2462	42.46	130.55	176.95	2447	42.79	131.59	175.91	2433	43.13	132.63	174.87	2418
308	42.04	129.47	178.53	2469	42.37	130.51	177.49	2455	42.71	131.55	176.45	2440	43.05	132.59	175.41	2426
308.5	41.96	129.43	179.07	2476	42.29	130.47	178.03	2462	42.63	131.51	176.99	2448	42.96	132.55	175.95	2433
309	41.87	129.39	179.61	2484	42.21	130.43	178.57	2470	42.55	131.47	177.53	2455	42.88	132.50	176.50	2441
309.5	41.79	129.35	180.15	2491	42.13	130.39	179.11	2477	42.46	131.43	178.07	2463	42.80	132.46	177.04	2448
310	41.71	129.31	180.69	2499	42.05	130.35	179.65	2485	42.38	131.39	178.62	2470	42.72	132.42	177.58	2456
310.5	41.63	129.27	181.23	2506	41.97	130.31	180.19	2492	42.30	131.34	179.16	2478	42.63	132.38	178.12	2463
311	41.55	129.23	181.77	2514	41.89	130.27	180.73	2500	42.22	131.30	179.70	2485	42.55	132.34	178.66	2471
311.5	41.47	129.19	182.31	2521	41.81	130.22	181.28	2507	42.14	131.26	180.24	2493	42.47	132.30	179.20	2478

Body Composition MALE 280-311.5 Lb.

Weight: Lb.	Waist: 62 inches Fat: %	Fat: Lb.	LBM: Lb.	RMR: Cal.	62.25 inches Fat: %	Fat: Lb.	LBM: Lb.	RMR: Cal.	62.5 inches Fat: %	Fat: Lb.	LBM: Lb.	RMR: Cal.	62.75 inches Fat: %	Fat: Lb.	LBM: Lb.	RMR: Cal.
280	48.54	135.92	144.08	1993	48.91	136.96	143.04	1978	49.28	138.00	142.01	1964	49.65	139.03	140.97	1950
280.5	48.44	135.88	144.62	2000	48.81	136.92	143.58	1986	49.18	137.95	142.55	1971	49.55	138.99	141.51	1957
281	48.34	135.84	145.16	2008	48.71	136.88	144.12	1993	49.08	137.91	143.09	1979	49.45	138.95	142.05	1965
281.5	48.24	135.80	145.70	2015	48.61	136.83	144.67	2001	48.98	137.87	143.63	1986	49.35	138.91	142.59	1972
282	48.14	135.76	146.24	2023	48.51	136.79	145.21	2008	48.88	137.83	144.17	1994	49.24	138.87	143.13	1980
282.5	48.04	135.72	146.79	2030	48.41	136.75	145.75	2016	48.78	137.79	144.71	2001	49.14	138.83	143.67	1987
283	47.94	135.67	147.33	2038	48.31	136.71	146.29	2023	48.67	137.75	145.25	2009	49.04	138.79	144.21	1994
283.5	47.84	135.63	147.87	2045	48.21	136.67	146.83	2031	48.57	137.71	145.79	2016	48.94	138.75	144.75	2002
284	47.74	135.59	148.41	2052	48.11	136.63	147.37	2038	48.47	137.67	146.33	2024	48.84	138.70	145.30	2009
284.5	47.65	135.55	148.95	2060	48.01	136.59	147.91	2046	48.37	137.63	146.87	2031	48.74	138.66	145.84	2017
285	47.55	135.51	149.49	2067	47.91	136.55	148.45	2053	48.28	137.59	147.42	2039	48.64	138.62	146.38	2024
285.5	47.45	135.47	150.03	2075	47.81	136.51	148.99	2061	48.18	137.54	147.96	2046	48.54	138.58	146.92	2032
286	47.35	135.43	150.57	2082	47.72	136.47	149.53	2068	48.08	137.50	148.50	2054	48.44	138.54	147.46	2039
286.5	47.26	135.39	151.11	2090	47.62	136.42	150.08	2076	47.98	137.46	149.04	2061	48.34	138.50	148.00	2047
287	47.16	135.35	151.65	2097	47.52	136.38	150.62	2083	47.88	137.42	149.58	2069	48.24	138.46	148.54	2054
287.5	47.06	135.31	152.20	2105	47.42	136.34	151.16	2091	47.78	137.38	150.12	2076	48.15	138.42	149.08	2062
288	46.97	135.26	152.74	2112	47.33	136.30	151.70	2098	47.69	137.34	150.66	2084	48.05	138.38	149.62	2069
288.5	46.87	135.22	153.28	2120	47.23	136.26	152.24	2105	47.59	137.30	151.20	2091	47.95	138.34	150.16	2077
289	46.78	135.18	153.82	2127	47.13	136.22	152.78	2113	47.49	137.26	151.74	2099	47.85	138.29	150.71	2084
289.5	46.68	135.14	154.36	2135	47.04	136.18	153.32	2120	47.40	137.22	152.28	2106	47.76	138.25	151.25	2092
290	46.59	135.10	154.90	2142	46.94	136.14	153.86	2128	47.30	137.18	152.83	2114	47.66	138.21	151.79	2099
290.5	46.49	135.06	155.44	2150	46.85	136.10	154.40	2135	47.21	137.13	153.37	2121	47.56	138.17	152.33	2107
291	46.40	135.02	155.98	2157	46.75	136.06	154.94	2143	47.11	137.09	153.91	2129	47.47	138.13	152.87	2114
291.5	46.30	134.98	156.52	2165	46.66	136.01	155.49	2150	47.02	137.05	154.45	2136	47.37	138.09	153.41	2122
292	46.21	134.94	157.06	2172	46.57	135.97	156.03	2158	46.92	137.01	154.99	2143	47.28	138.05	153.95	2129
292.5	46.12	134.90	157.61	2180	46.47	135.93	156.57	2165	46.83	136.97	155.53	2151	47.18	138.01	154.49	2137
293	46.03	134.85	158.15	2187	46.38	135.89	157.11	2173	46.73	136.93	156.07	2158	47.09	137.97	155.03	2144
293.5	45.93	134.81	158.69	2195	46.29	135.85	157.65	2180	46.64	136.89	156.61	2166	46.99	137.93	155.57	2152
294	45.84	134.77	159.23	2202	46.19	135.81	158.19	2188	46.55	136.85	157.15	2173	46.90	137.88	156.12	2159
294.5	45.75	134.73	159.77	2210	46.10	135.77	158.73	2195	46.45	136.81	157.69	2181	46.81	137.84	156.66	2167
295	45.66	134.69	160.31	2217	46.01	135.73	159.27	2203	46.36	136.77	158.24	2188	46.71	137.80	157.20	2174
295.5	45.57	134.65	160.85	2225	45.92	135.69	159.81	2210	46.27	136.72	158.78	2196	46.62	137.76	157.74	2182
296	45.48	134.61	161.39	2232	45.83	135.65	160.35	2218	46.18	136.68	159.32	2203	46.53	137.72	158.28	2189
296.5	45.39	134.57	161.93	2240	45.74	135.60	160.90	2225	46.08	136.64	159.86	2211	46.43	137.68	158.82	2196
297	45.29	134.53	162.47	2247	45.64	135.56	161.44	2233	45.99	136.60	160.40	2218	46.34	137.64	159.36	2204
297.5	45.21	134.49	163.02	2254	45.55	135.52	161.98	2240	45.90	136.56	160.94	2226	46.25	137.60	159.90	2211
298	45.12	134.44	163.56	2262	45.46	135.48	162.52	2248	45.81	136.52	161.48	2233	46.16	137.56	160.44	2219
298.5	45.03	134.40	164.10	2269	45.37	135.44	163.06	2255	45.72	136.48	162.02	2241	46.07	137.52	160.98	2226
299	44.94	134.36	164.64	2277	45.28	135.40	163.60	2263	45.63	136.44	162.56	2248	45.98	137.47	161.53	2234
299.5	44.85	134.32	165.18	2284	45.19	135.36	164.14	2270	45.54	136.40	163.10	2256	45.89	137.43	162.07	2241
300	44.76	134.28	165.72	2292	45.11	135.32	164.68	2278	45.45	136.36	163.65	2263	45.80	137.39	162.61	2249
300.5	44.67	134.24	166.26	2299	45.02	135.28	165.22	2285	45.36	136.31	164.19	2271	45.71	137.35	163.15	2256
301	44.58	134.20	166.80	2307	44.93	135.24	165.76	2293	45.27	136.27	164.73	2278	45.62	137.31	163.69	2264
301.5	44.50	134.16	167.34	2314	44.84	135.19	166.31	2300	45.18	136.23	165.27	2286	45.53	137.27	164.23	2271
302	44.41	134.12	167.88	2322	44.75	135.15	166.85	2307	45.10	136.19	165.81	2293	45.44	137.23	164.77	2279
302.5	44.32	134.08	168.43	2329	44.67	135.11	167.39	2315	45.01	136.15	166.35	2301	45.35	137.19	165.31	2286
303	44.24	134.03	168.97	2337	44.58	135.07	167.93	2322	44.92	136.11	166.89	2308	45.26	137.15	165.85	2294
303.5	44.15	133.99	169.51	2344	44.49	135.03	168.47	2330	44.83	136.07	167.43	2316	45.17	137.11	166.39	2301
304	44.06	133.95	170.05	2352	44.40	134.99	169.01	2337	44.75	136.03	167.97	2323	45.09	137.06	166.94	2309
304.5	43.98	133.91	170.59	2359	44.32	134.95	169.55	2345	44.66	135.99	168.51	2331	45.00	137.02	167.48	2316
305	43.89	133.87	171.13	2367	44.23	134.91	170.09	2352	44.57	135.95	169.06	2338	44.91	136.98	168.02	2324
305.5	43.81	133.83	171.67	2374	44.15	134.87	170.63	2360	44.49	135.90	169.60	2346	44.83	136.94	168.56	2331
306	43.72	133.79	172.21	2382	44.06	134.83	171.17	2367	44.40	135.86	170.14	2353	44.74	136.90	169.10	2339
306.5	43.64	133.75	172.75	2389	43.98	134.78	171.72	2375	44.31	135.82	170.68	2360	44.65	136.86	169.64	2346
307	43.55	133.71	173.29	2397	43.89	134.74	172.26	2382	44.23	135.78	171.22	2368	44.57	136.82	170.18	2354
307.5	43.47	133.67	173.84	2404	43.81	134.70	172.80	2390	44.14	135.74	171.76	2375	44.48	136.78	170.72	2361
308	43.38	133.62	174.38	2412	43.72	134.66	173.34	2397	44.06	135.70	172.30	2383	44.39	136.74	171.26	2369
308.5	43.30	133.58	174.92	2419	43.64	134.62	173.88	2405	43.97	135.66	172.84	2390	44.31	136.70	171.80	2376
309	43.22	133.54	175.46	2427	43.55	134.58	174.42	2412	43.89	135.62	173.38	2398	44.22	136.65	172.35	2384
309.5	43.13	133.50	176.00	2434	43.47	134.54	174.96	2420	43.80	135.58	173.92	2405	44.14	136.61	172.89	2391
310	43.05	133.46	176.54	2442	43.39	134.50	175.50	2427	43.72	135.54	174.47	2413	44.06	136.57	173.43	2399
310.5	42.97	133.42	177.08	2449	43.30	134.46	176.04	2435	43.64	135.49	175.01	2420	43.97	136.53	173.97	2406
311	42.89	133.38	177.62	2457	43.22	134.42	176.58	2442	43.55	135.45	175.55	2428	43.89	136.49	174.51	2413
311.5	42.80	133.34	178.16	2464	43.14	134.37	177.13	2450	43.47	135.41	176.09	2435	43.80	136.45	175.05	2421

Body Composition MALE 280-311.5 Lb.

Weight: Lb.	Waist: 63 inches				63.25 inches				63.5 inches				63.75 inches			
	Fat: %	Fat: Lb.	LBM: Lb.	RMR: Cal.	Fat: %	Fat: Lb.	LBM: Lb.	RMR: Cal.	Fat: %	Fat: Lb.	LBM: Lb.	RMR: Cal.	Fat: %	Fat: Lb.	LBM: Lb.	RMR: Cal.
280	50.03	140.07	139.93	1935	50.40	141.11	138.89	1921	50.77	142.15	137.86	1907	51.14	143.18	136.82	1892
280.5	49.92	140.03	140.47	1943	50.29	141.07	139.43	1928	50.66	142.10	138.40	1914	51.03	143.14	137.36	1900
281	49.82	139.99	141.01	1950	50.19	141.03	139.97	1936	50.56	142.06	138.94	1921	50.93	143.10	137.90	1907
281.5	49.71	139.95	141.55	1958	50.08	140.98	140.52	1943	50.45	142.02	139.48	1929	50.82	143.06	138.44	1915
282	49.61	139.91	142.09	1965	49.98	140.94	141.06	1951	50.35	141.98	140.02	1936	50.72	143.02	138.98	1922
282.5	49.51	139.87	142.64	1973	49.88	140.90	141.60	1958	50.24	141.94	140.56	1944	50.61	142.98	139.52	1930
283	49.41	139.82	143.18	1980	49.77	140.86	142.14	1966	50.14	141.90	141.10	1951	50.51	142.94	140.06	1937
283.5	49.31	139.78	143.72	1988	49.67	140.82	142.68	1973	50.04	141.86	141.64	1959	50.40	142.90	140.60	1945
284	49.20	139.74	144.26	1995	49.57	140.78	143.22	1981	49.94	141.82	142.18	1966	50.30	142.85	141.15	1952
284.5	49.10	139.70	144.80	2003	49.47	140.74	143.76	1988	49.83	141.78	142.72	1974	50.20	142.81	141.69	1960
285	49.00	139.66	145.34	2010	49.37	140.70	144.30	1996	49.73	141.74	143.27	1981	50.10	142.77	142.23	1967
285.5	48.90	139.62	145.88	2018	49.27	140.66	144.84	2003	49.63	141.69	143.81	1989	49.99	142.73	142.77	1974
286	48.80	139.58	146.42	2025	49.17	140.62	145.38	2011	49.53	141.65	144.35	1996	49.89	142.69	143.31	1982
286.5	48.70	139.54	146.96	2032	49.07	140.57	145.93	2018	49.43	141.61	144.89	2004	49.79	142.65	143.85	1989
287	48.60	139.50	147.50	2040	48.97	140.53	146.47	2026	49.33	141.57	145.43	2011	49.69	142.61	144.39	1997
287.5	48.51	139.46	148.05	2047	48.87	140.49	147.01	2033	49.23	141.53	145.97	2019	49.59	142.57	144.93	2004
288	48.41	139.41	148.59	2055	48.77	140.45	147.55	2041	49.13	141.49	146.51	2026	49.49	142.53	145.47	2012
288.5	48.31	139.37	149.13	2062	48.67	140.41	148.09	2048	49.03	141.45	147.05	2034	49.39	142.49	146.01	2019
289	48.21	139.33	149.67	2070	48.57	140.37	148.63	2056	48.93	141.41	147.59	2041	49.29	142.44	146.56	2027
289.5	48.11	139.29	150.21	2077	48.47	140.33	149.17	2063	48.83	141.37	148.13	2049	49.19	142.40	147.10	2034
290	48.02	139.25	150.75	2085	48.38	140.29	149.71	2071	48.73	141.33	148.68	2056	49.09	142.36	147.64	2042
290.5	47.92	139.21	151.29	2092	48.28	140.25	150.25	2078	48.63	141.28	149.22	2064	48.99	142.32	148.18	2049
291	47.82	139.17	151.83	2100	48.18	140.21	150.79	2085	48.54	141.24	149.76	2071	48.89	142.28	148.72	2057
291.5	47.73	139.13	152.37	2107	48.08	140.16	151.34	2093	48.44	141.20	150.30	2079	48.80	142.24	149.26	2064
292	47.63	139.09	152.91	2115	47.99	140.12	151.88	2100	48.34	141.16	150.84	2086	48.70	142.20	149.80	2072
292.5	47.54	139.05	153.46	2122	47.89	140.08	152.42	2108	48.25	141.12	151.38	2094	48.60	142.16	150.34	2079
293	47.44	139.00	154.00	2130	47.80	140.04	152.96	2115	48.15	141.08	151.92	2101	48.50	142.12	150.88	2087
293.5	47.35	138.96	154.54	2137	47.70	140.00	153.50	2123	48.05	141.04	152.46	2109	48.41	142.08	151.42	2094
294	47.25	138.92	155.08	2145	47.61	139.96	154.04	2130	47.96	141.00	153.00	2116	48.31	142.03	151.97	2102
294.5	47.16	138.88	155.62	2152	47.51	139.92	154.58	2138	47.86	140.96	153.54	2124	48.22	141.99	152.51	2109
295	47.06	138.84	156.16	2160	47.42	139.88	155.12	2145	47.77	140.92	154.09	2131	48.12	141.95	153.05	2117
295.5	46.97	138.80	156.70	2167	47.32	139.84	155.66	2153	47.67	140.87	154.63	2138	48.02	141.91	153.59	2124
296	46.88	138.76	157.24	2175	47.23	139.80	156.20	2160	47.58	140.83	155.17	2146	47.93	141.87	154.13	2132
296.5	46.78	138.72	157.78	2182	47.13	139.75	156.75	2168	47.48	140.79	155.71	2153	47.83	141.83	154.67	2139
297	46.69	138.68	158.32	2190	47.04	139.71	157.29	2175	47.39	140.75	156.25	2161	47.74	141.79	155.21	2147
297.5	46.60	138.64	158.87	2197	46.95	139.67	157.83	2183	47.30	140.71	156.79	2168	47.65	141.75	155.75	2154
298	46.51	138.59	159.41	2205	46.86	139.63	158.37	2190	47.20	140.67	157.33	2176	47.55	141.71	156.29	2162
298.5	46.42	138.55	159.95	2212	46.76	139.59	158.91	2198	47.11	140.63	157.87	2183	47.46	141.67	156.83	2169
299	46.33	138.51	160.49	2220	46.67	139.55	159.45	2205	47.02	140.59	158.41	2191	47.37	141.62	157.38	2177
299.5	46.23	138.47	161.03	2227	46.58	139.51	159.99	2213	46.93	140.55	158.95	2198	47.27	141.58	157.92	2184
300	46.14	138.43	161.57	2235	46.49	139.47	160.53	2220	46.84	140.51	159.50	2206	47.18	141.54	158.46	2191
300.5	46.05	138.39	162.11	2242	46.40	139.43	161.07	2228	46.74	140.46	160.04	2213	47.09	141.50	159.00	2199
301	45.96	138.35	162.65	2249	46.31	139.39	161.61	2235	46.65	140.42	160.58	2221	47.00	141.46	159.54	2206
301.5	45.87	138.31	163.19	2257	46.22	139.34	162.16	2243	46.56	140.38	161.12	2228	46.91	141.42	160.08	2214
302	45.78	138.27	163.73	2264	46.13	139.30	162.70	2250	46.47	140.34	161.66	2236	46.81	141.38	160.62	2221
302.5	45.69	138.23	164.28	2272	46.04	139.26	163.24	2258	46.38	140.30	162.20	2243	46.72	141.34	161.16	2229
303	45.61	138.18	164.82	2279	45.95	139.22	163.78	2265	46.29	140.26	162.74	2251	46.63	141.30	161.70	2236
303.5	45.52	138.14	165.36	2287	45.86	139.18	164.32	2273	46.20	140.22	163.28	2258	46.54	141.26	162.24	2244
304	45.43	138.10	165.90	2294	45.77	139.14	164.86	2280	46.11	140.18	163.82	2266	46.45	141.21	162.79	2251
304.5	45.34	138.06	166.44	2302	45.68	139.10	165.40	2288	46.02	140.14	164.36	2273	46.36	141.17	163.33	2259
305	45.25	138.02	166.98	2309	45.59	139.06	165.94	2295	45.93	140.10	164.91	2281	46.27	141.13	163.87	2266
305.5	45.16	137.98	167.52	2317	45.50	139.02	166.48	2302	45.84	140.05	165.45	2288	46.18	141.09	164.41	2274
306	45.08	137.94	168.06	2324	45.42	138.98	167.02	2310	45.76	140.01	165.99	2296	46.09	141.05	164.95	2281
306.5	44.99	137.90	168.60	2332	45.33	138.93	167.57	2317	45.67	139.97	166.53	2303	46.01	141.01	165.49	2289
307	44.90	137.86	169.14	2339	45.24	138.89	168.11	2325	45.58	139.93	167.07	2311	45.92	140.97	166.03	2296
307.5	44.82	137.82	169.69	2347	45.16	138.85	168.65	2332	45.49	139.89	167.61	2318	45.83	140.93	166.57	2304
308	44.73	137.77	170.23	2354	45.07	138.81	169.19	2340	45.41	139.85	168.15	2326	45.74	140.89	167.11	2311
308.5	44.65	137.73	170.77	2362	44.98	138.77	169.73	2347	45.32	139.81	168.69	2333	45.65	140.85	167.65	2319
309	44.56	137.69	171.31	2369	44.90	138.73	170.27	2355	45.23	139.77	169.23	2340	45.57	140.80	168.20	2326
309.5	44.48	137.65	171.85	2377	44.81	138.69	170.81	2362	45.15	139.73	169.77	2348	45.48	140.76	168.74	2334
310	44.39	137.61	172.39	2384	44.73	138.65	171.35	2370	45.06	139.69	170.32	2355	45.39	140.72	169.28	2341
310.5	44.31	137.57	172.93	2392	44.64	138.61	171.89	2377	44.97	139.64	170.86	2363	45.31	140.68	169.82	2349
311	44.22	137.53	173.47	2399	44.55	138.57	172.43	2385	44.89	139.60	171.40	2370	45.22	140.64	170.36	2356
311.5	44.14	137.49	174.01	2407	44.47	138.52	172.98	2392	44.80	139.56	171.94	2378	45.14	140.60	170.90	2364

Body Composition   MALE   280-311.5 Lb.

Weight: Lb.	Waist: 64 inches				64.25 inches				64.5 inches				64.75 inches			
	Fat: %	Fat: Lb.	LBM: Lb.	RMR: Cal.	Fat: %	Fat: Lb.	LBM: Lb.	RMR: Cal.	Fat: %	Fat: Lb.	LBM: Lb.	RMR: Cal.	Fat: %	Fat: Lb.	LBM: Lb.	RMR: Cal.
280	51.51	144.22	135.78	1878	51.88	145.26	134.74	1863	52.25	146.30	133.71	1849	52.62	147.33	132.67	1835
280.5	51.40	144.18	136.32	1885	51.77	145.22	135.28	1871	52.14	146.25	134.25	1857	52.51	147.29	133.21	1842
281	51.29	144.14	136.86	1893	51.66	145.18	135.82	1878	52.03	146.21	134.79	1864	52.40	147.25	133.75	1850
281.5	51.19	144.10	137.40	1900	51.56	145.13	136.37	1886	51.93	146.17	135.33	1872	52.29	147.21	134.29	1857
282	51.08	144.06	137.94	1908	51.45	145.09	136.91	1893	51.82	146.13	135.87	1879	52.19	147.17	134.83	1865
282.5	50.98	144.02	138.49	1915	51.35	145.05	137.45	1901	51.71	146.09	136.41	1887	52.08	147.13	135.37	1872
283	50.87	143.97	139.03	1923	51.24	145.01	137.99	1908	51.61	146.05	136.95	1894	51.97	147.09	135.91	1880
283.5	50.77	143.93	139.57	1930	51.14	144.97	138.53	1916	51.50	146.01	137.49	1902	51.87	147.05	136.45	1887
284	50.67	143.89	140.11	1938	51.03	144.93	139.07	1923	51.40	145.97	138.03	1909	51.76	147.00	137.00	1895
284.5	50.56	143.85	140.65	1945	50.93	144.89	139.61	1931	51.29	145.93	138.57	1916	51.66	146.96	137.54	1902
285	50.46	143.81	141.19	1953	50.82	144.85	140.15	1938	51.19	145.89	139.12	1924	51.55	146.92	138.08	1910
285.5	50.36	143.77	141.73	1960	50.72	144.81	140.69	1946	51.08	145.84	139.66	1931	51.45	146.88	138.62	1917
286	50.25	143.73	142.27	1968	50.62	144.77	141.23	1953	50.98	145.80	140.20	1939	51.34	146.84	139.16	1925
286.5	50.15	143.69	142.81	1975	50.51	144.72	141.78	1961	50.88	145.76	140.74	1946	51.24	146.80	139.70	1932
287	50.05	143.65	143.35	1983	50.41	144.68	142.32	1968	50.77	145.72	141.28	1954	51.14	146.76	140.24	1940
287.5	49.95	143.61	143.90	1990	50.31	144.64	142.86	1976	50.67	145.68	141.82	1961	51.03	146.72	140.78	1947
288	49.85	143.56	144.44	1998	50.21	144.60	143.40	1983	50.57	145.64	142.36	1969	50.93	146.68	141.32	1955
288.5	49.75	143.52	144.98	2005	50.11	144.56	143.94	1991	50.47	145.60	142.90	1976	50.83	146.64	141.86	1962
289	49.65	143.48	145.52	2013	50.01	144.52	144.48	1998	50.37	145.56	143.44	1984	50.72	146.59	142.41	1969
289.5	49.55	143.44	146.06	2020	49.91	144.48	145.02	2006	50.26	145.52	143.98	1991	50.62	146.55	142.95	1977
290	49.45	143.40	146.60	2027	49.81	144.44	145.56	2013	50.16	145.48	144.53	1999	50.52	146.51	143.49	1984
290.5	49.35	143.36	147.14	2035	49.71	144.40	146.10	2021	50.06	145.43	145.07	2006	50.42	146.47	144.03	1992
291	49.25	143.32	147.68	2042	49.61	144.36	146.64	2028	49.96	145.39	145.61	2014	50.32	146.43	144.57	1999
291.5	49.15	143.28	148.22	2050	49.51	144.31	147.19	2036	49.86	145.35	146.15	2021	50.22	146.39	145.11	2007
292	49.05	143.24	148.76	2057	49.41	144.27	147.73	2043	49.76	145.31	146.69	2029	50.12	146.35	145.65	2014
292.5	48.96	143.20	149.31	2065	49.31	144.23	148.27	2051	49.66	145.27	147.23	2036	50.02	146.31	146.19	2022
293	48.86	143.15	149.85	2072	49.21	144.19	148.81	2058	49.57	145.23	147.77	2044	49.92	146.27	146.73	2029
293.5	48.76	143.11	150.39	2080	49.11	144.15	149.35	2066	49.47	145.19	148.31	2051	49.82	146.23	147.27	2037
294	48.66	143.07	150.93	2087	49.02	144.11	149.89	2073	49.37	145.15	148.85	2059	49.72	146.18	147.82	2044
294.5	48.57	143.03	151.47	2095	48.92	144.07	150.43	2080	49.27	145.11	149.39	2066	49.62	146.14	148.36	2052
295	48.47	142.99	152.01	2102	48.82	144.03	150.97	2088	49.17	145.07	149.94	2074	49.53	146.10	148.90	2059
295.5	48.38	142.95	152.55	2110	48.73	143.99	151.51	2095	49.08	145.02	150.48	2081	49.43	146.06	149.44	2067
296	48.28	142.91	153.09	2117	48.63	143.95	152.05	2103	48.98	144.98	151.02	2089	49.33	146.02	149.98	2074
296.5	48.18	142.87	153.63	2125	48.53	143.90	152.60	2110	48.88	144.94	151.56	2096	49.23	145.98	150.52	2082
297	48.09	142.83	154.17	2132	48.44	143.86	153.14	2118	48.79	144.90	152.10	2104	49.14	145.94	151.06	2089
297.5	47.99	142.79	154.72	2140	48.34	143.82	153.68	2125	48.69	144.86	152.64	2111	49.04	145.90	151.60	2097
298	47.90	142.74	155.26	2147	48.25	143.78	154.22	2133	48.60	144.82	153.18	2118	48.95	145.86	152.14	2104
298.5	47.81	142.70	155.80	2155	48.15	143.74	154.76	2140	48.50	144.78	153.72	2126	48.85	145.82	152.68	2112
299	47.71	142.66	156.34	2162	48.06	143.70	155.30	2148	48.41	144.74	154.26	2133	48.75	145.77	153.23	2119
299.5	47.62	142.62	156.88	2170	47.97	143.66	155.84	2155	48.31	144.70	154.80	2141	48.66	145.73	153.77	2127
300	47.53	142.58	157.42	2177	47.87	143.62	156.38	2163	48.22	144.66	155.35	2148	48.56	145.69	154.31	2134
300.5	47.43	142.54	157.96	2185	47.78	143.58	156.92	2170	48.12	144.61	155.89	2156	48.47	145.65	154.85	2142
301	47.34	142.50	158.50	2192	47.69	143.54	157.46	2178	48.03	144.57	156.43	2163	48.38	145.61	155.39	2149
301.5	47.25	142.46	159.04	2200	47.59	143.49	158.01	2185	47.94	144.53	156.97	2171	48.28	145.57	155.93	2157
302	47.16	142.42	159.58	2207	47.50	143.45	158.55	2193	47.84	144.49	157.51	2178	48.19	145.53	156.47	2164
302.5	47.07	142.38	160.13	2215	47.41	143.41	159.09	2200	47.75	144.45	158.05	2186	48.10	145.49	157.01	2171
303	46.97	142.33	160.67	2222	47.32	143.37	159.63	2208	47.66	144.41	158.59	2193	48.00	145.45	157.55	2179
303.5	46.88	142.29	161.21	2229	47.23	143.33	160.17	2215	47.57	144.37	159.13	2201	47.91	145.41	158.09	2186
304	46.79	142.25	161.75	2237	47.13	143.29	160.71	2223	47.48	144.33	159.67	2208	47.82	145.36	158.64	2194
304.5	46.70	142.21	162.29	2244	47.04	143.25	161.25	2230	47.38	144.29	160.21	2216	47.73	145.32	159.18	2201
305	46.61	142.17	162.83	2252	46.95	143.21	161.79	2238	47.29	144.25	160.76	2223	47.63	145.28	159.72	2209
305.5	46.52	142.13	163.37	2259	46.86	143.17	162.33	2245	47.20	144.20	161.30	2231	47.54	145.24	160.26	2216
306	46.43	142.09	163.91	2267	46.77	143.13	162.87	2253	47.11	144.16	161.84	2238	47.45	145.20	160.80	2224
306.5	46.34	142.05	164.45	2274	46.68	143.08	163.42	2260	47.02	144.12	162.38	2246	47.36	145.16	161.34	2231
307	46.26	142.01	164.99	2282	46.59	143.04	163.96	2268	46.93	144.08	162.92	2253	47.27	145.12	161.88	2239
307.5	46.17	141.97	165.54	2289	46.50	143.00	164.50	2275	46.84	144.04	163.46	2261	47.18	145.08	162.42	2246
308	46.08	141.92	166.08	2297	46.42	142.96	165.04	2282	46.75	144.00	164.00	2268	47.09	145.04	162.96	2254
308.5	45.99	141.88	166.62	2304	46.33	142.92	165.58	2290	46.66	143.96	164.54	2276	47.00	145.00	163.50	2261
309	45.90	141.84	167.16	2312	46.24	142.88	166.12	2297	46.58	143.92	165.08	2283	46.91	144.95	164.05	2269
309.5	45.82	141.80	167.70	2319	46.15	142.84	166.66	2305	46.49	143.88	165.62	2291	46.82	144.91	164.59	2276
310	45.73	141.76	168.24	2327	46.06	142.80	167.20	2312	46.40	143.84	166.17	2298	46.73	144.87	165.13	2284
310.5	45.64	141.72	168.78	2334	45.98	142.76	167.74	2320	46.31	143.79	166.71	2306	46.64	144.83	165.67	2291
311	45.56	141.68	169.32	2342	45.89	142.72	168.28	2327	46.22	143.75	167.25	2313	46.56	144.79	166.21	2299
311.5	45.47	141.64	169.86	2349	45.80	142.67	168.83	2335	46.14	143.71	167.79	2321	46.47	144.75	166.75	2306

Body Composition MALE 280-311.5 Lb.

Weight: Lb.	Waist: 65 inches				65.25 inches				65.5 inches				65.75 inches			
	Fat: %	Fat: Lb.	LBM: Lb.	RMR: Cal.	Fat: %	Fat: Lb.	LBM: Lb.	RMR: Cal.	Fat: %	Fat: Lb.	LBM: Lb.	RMR: Cal.	Fat: %	Fat: Lb.	LBM: Lb.	RMR: Cal.
280	52.99	148.37	131.63	1820	53.36	149.41	130.59	1806	53.73	150.45	129.56	1792	54.10	151.48	128.52	1777
280.5	52.88	148.33	132.17	1828	53.25	149.37	131.13	1814	53.62	150.40	130.10	1799	53.99	151.44	129.06	1785
281	52.77	148.29	132.71	1835	53.14	149.33	131.67	1821	53.51	150.36	130.64	1807	53.88	151.40	129.60	1792
281.5	52.66	148.25	133.25	1843	53.03	149.28	132.22	1829	53.40	150.32	131.18	1814	53.77	151.36	130.14	1800
282	52.56	148.21	133.79	1850	52.92	149.24	132.76	1836	53.29	150.28	131.72	1822	53.66	151.32	130.68	1807
282.5	52.45	148.17	134.34	1858	52.82	149.20	133.30	1844	53.18	150.24	132.26	1829	53.55	151.28	131.22	1815
283	52.34	148.12	134.88	1865	52.71	149.16	133.84	1851	53.07	150.20	132.80	1837	53.44	151.24	131.76	1822
283.5	52.23	148.08	135.42	1873	52.60	149.12	134.38	1858	52.97	150.16	133.34	1844	53.33	151.20	132.30	1830
284	52.13	148.04	135.96	1880	52.49	149.08	134.92	1866	52.86	150.12	133.88	1852	53.22	151.15	132.85	1837
284.5	52.02	148.00	136.50	1888	52.39	149.04	135.46	1873	52.75	150.08	134.42	1859	53.12	151.11	133.39	1845
285	51.92	147.96	137.04	1895	52.28	149.00	136.00	1881	52.64	150.04	134.97	1867	53.01	151.07	133.93	1852
285.5	51.81	147.92	137.58	1903	52.17	148.96	136.54	1888	52.54	149.99	135.51	1874	52.90	151.03	134.47	1860
286	51.71	147.88	138.12	1910	52.07	148.92	137.08	1896	52.43	149.95	136.05	1882	52.79	150.99	135.01	1867
286.5	51.60	147.84	138.66	1918	51.96	148.87	137.63	1903	52.33	149.91	136.59	1889	52.69	150.95	135.55	1875
287	51.50	147.80	139.20	1925	51.86	148.83	138.17	1911	52.22	149.87	137.13	1896	52.58	150.91	136.09	1882
287.5	51.39	147.76	139.75	1933	51.75	148.79	138.71	1918	52.11	149.83	137.67	1904	52.48	150.87	136.63	1890
288	51.29	147.71	140.29	1940	51.65	148.75	139.25	1926	52.01	149.79	138.21	1911	52.37	150.83	137.17	1897
288.5	51.19	147.67	140.83	1948	51.55	148.71	139.79	1933	51.91	149.75	138.75	1919	52.27	150.79	137.71	1905
289	51.08	147.63	141.37	1955	51.44	148.67	140.33	1941	51.80	149.71	139.29	1926	52.16	150.74	138.26	1912
289.5	50.98	147.59	141.91	1963	51.34	148.63	140.87	1948	51.70	149.67	139.83	1934	52.06	150.70	138.80	1920
290	50.88	147.55	142.45	1970	51.24	148.59	141.41	1956	51.59	149.63	140.38	1941	51.95	150.66	139.34	1927
290.5	50.78	147.51	142.99	1978	51.13	148.55	141.95	1963	51.49	149.58	140.92	1949	51.85	150.62	139.88	1935
291	50.68	147.47	143.53	1985	51.03	148.51	142.49	1971	51.39	149.54	141.46	1956	51.75	150.58	140.42	1942
291.5	50.58	147.43	144.07	1993	50.93	148.46	143.04	1978	51.29	149.50	142.00	1964	51.64	150.54	140.96	1949
292	50.47	147.39	144.61	2000	50.83	148.42	143.58	1986	51.19	149.46	142.54	1971	51.54	150.50	141.50	1957
292.5	50.37	147.35	145.16	2007	50.73	148.38	144.12	1993	51.08	149.42	143.08	1979	51.44	150.46	142.04	1964
293	50.27	147.30	145.70	2015	50.63	148.34	144.66	2001	50.98	149.38	143.62	1986	51.34	150.42	142.58	1972
293.5	50.17	147.26	146.24	2022	50.53	148.30	145.20	2008	50.88	149.34	144.16	1994	51.24	150.38	143.12	1979
294	50.08	147.22	146.78	2030	50.43	148.26	145.74	2016	50.78	149.30	144.70	2001	51.13	150.33	143.67	1987
294.5	49.98	147.18	147.32	2037	50.33	148.22	146.28	2023	50.68	149.26	145.24	2009	51.03	150.29	144.21	1994
295	49.88	147.14	147.86	2045	50.23	148.18	146.82	2031	50.58	149.22	145.79	2016	50.93	150.25	144.75	2002
295.5	49.78	147.10	148.40	2052	50.13	148.14	147.36	2038	50.48	149.17	146.33	2024	50.83	150.21	145.29	2009
296	49.68	147.06	148.94	2060	50.03	148.10	147.90	2046	50.38	149.13	146.87	2031	50.73	150.17	145.83	2017
296.5	49.58	147.02	149.48	2067	49.93	148.05	148.45	2053	50.28	149.09	147.41	2039	50.63	150.13	146.37	2024
297	49.49	146.98	150.02	2075	49.84	148.01	148.99	2060	50.19	149.05	147.95	2046	50.53	150.09	146.91	2032
297.5	49.39	146.94	150.57	2082	49.74	147.97	149.53	2068	50.09	149.01	148.49	2054	50.44	150.05	147.45	2039
298	49.29	146.89	151.11	2090	49.64	147.93	150.07	2075	49.99	148.97	149.03	2061	50.34	150.01	147.99	2047
298.5	49.20	146.85	151.65	2097	49.54	147.89	150.61	2083	49.89	148.93	149.57	2069	50.24	149.97	148.53	2054
299	49.10	146.81	152.19	2105	49.45	147.85	151.15	2090	49.79	148.89	150.11	2076	50.14	149.92	149.08	2062
299.5	49.01	146.77	152.73	2112	49.35	147.81	151.69	2098	49.70	148.85	150.65	2084	50.04	149.88	149.62	2069
300	48.91	146.73	153.27	2120	49.26	147.77	152.23	2105	49.60	148.81	151.20	2091	49.95	149.84	150.16	2077
300.5	48.81	146.69	153.81	2127	49.16	147.73	152.77	2113	49.51	148.76	151.74	2099	49.85	149.80	150.70	2084
301	48.72	146.65	154.35	2135	49.06	147.69	153.31	2120	49.41	148.72	152.28	2106	49.75	149.76	151.24	2092
301.5	48.63	146.61	154.89	2142	48.97	147.64	153.86	2128	49.31	148.68	152.82	2113	49.66	149.72	151.78	2099
302	48.53	146.57	155.43	2150	48.88	147.60	154.40	2135	49.22	148.64	153.36	2121	49.56	149.68	152.32	2107
302.5	48.44	146.53	155.98	2157	48.78	147.56	154.94	2143	49.12	148.60	153.90	2128	49.47	149.64	152.86	2114
303	48.34	146.48	156.52	2165	48.69	147.52	155.48	2150	49.03	148.56	154.44	2136	49.37	149.60	153.40	2122
303.5	48.25	146.44	157.06	2172	48.59	147.48	156.02	2158	48.94	148.52	154.98	2143	49.28	149.56	153.94	2129
304	48.16	146.40	157.60	2180	48.50	147.44	156.56	2165	48.84	148.48	155.52	2151	49.18	149.51	154.49	2137
304.5	48.07	146.36	158.14	2187	48.41	147.40	157.10	2173	48.75	148.44	156.06	2158	49.09	149.47	155.03	2144
305	47.97	146.32	158.68	2195	48.31	147.36	157.64	2180	48.65	148.40	156.61	2166	48.99	149.43	155.57	2151
305.5	47.88	146.28	159.22	2202	48.22	147.32	158.18	2188	48.56	148.35	157.15	2173	48.90	149.39	156.11	2159
306	47.79	146.24	159.76	2210	48.13	147.28	158.72	2195	48.47	148.31	157.69	2181	48.81	149.35	156.65	2166
306.5	47.70	146.20	160.30	2217	48.04	147.23	159.27	2203	48.38	148.27	158.23	2188	48.71	149.31	157.19	2174
307	47.61	146.16	160.84	2224	47.95	147.19	159.81	2210	48.28	148.23	158.77	2196	48.62	149.27	157.73	2181
307.5	47.52	146.12	161.39	2232	47.85	147.15	160.35	2218	48.19	148.19	159.31	2203	48.53	149.23	158.27	2189
308	47.43	146.07	161.93	2239	47.76	147.11	160.89	2225	48.10	148.15	159.85	2211	48.44	149.19	158.81	2196
308.5	47.34	146.03	162.47	2247	47.67	147.07	161.43	2233	48.01	148.11	160.39	2218	48.35	149.15	159.35	2204
309	47.25	145.99	163.01	2254	47.58	147.03	161.97	2240	47.92	148.07	160.93	2226	48.25	149.10	159.90	2211
309.5	47.16	145.95	163.55	2262	47.49	146.99	162.51	2248	47.83	148.03	161.47	2233	48.16	149.06	160.44	2219
310	47.07	145.91	164.09	2269	47.40	146.95	163.05	2255	47.74	147.99	162.02	2241	48.07	149.02	160.98	2226
310.5	46.98	145.87	164.63	2277	47.31	146.91	163.59	2262	47.65	147.94	162.56	2248	47.98	148.98	161.52	2234
311	46.89	145.83	165.17	2284	47.22	146.87	164.13	2270	47.56	147.90	163.10	2256	47.89	148.94	162.06	2241
311.5	46.80	145.79	165.71	2292	47.13	146.82	164.68	2277	47.47	147.86	163.64	2263	47.80	148.90	162.60	2249

Body Composition MALE 280-311.5 Lb.

Weight: Lb.	Waist: 66 inches Fat: %	Fat: Lb.	LBM: Lb.	RMR: Cal.	66.25 inches Fat: %	Fat: Lb.	LBM: Lb.	RMR: Cal.	66.5 inches Fat: %	Fat: Lb.	LBM: Lb.	RMR: Cal.	66.75 inches Fat: %	Fat: Lb.	LBM: Lb.	RMR: Cal.
280	54.47	152.52	127.48	1763	54.84	153.56	126.44	1749	55.21	154.60	125.41	1734	55.58	155.63	124.37	1720
280.5	54.36	152.48	128.02	1771	54.73	153.52	126.98	1756	55.10	154.55	125.95	1742	55.47	155.59	124.91	1727
281	54.25	152.44	128.56	1778	54.62	153.48	127.52	1764	54.99	154.51	126.49	1749	55.36	155.55	125.45	1735
281.5	54.14	152.40	129.10	1785	54.51	153.43	128.07	1771	54.87	154.47	127.03	1757	55.24	155.51	125.99	1742
282	54.03	152.36	129.64	1793	54.39	153.39	128.61	1779	54.76	154.43	127.57	1764	55.13	155.47	126.53	1750
282.5	53.92	152.32	130.19	1800	54.28	153.35	129.15	1786	54.65	154.39	128.11	1772	55.02	155.43	127.07	1757
283	53.81	152.27	130.73	1808	54.17	153.31	129.69	1794	54.54	154.35	128.65	1779	54.91	155.39	127.61	1765
283.5	53.70	152.23	131.27	1815	54.06	153.27	130.23	1801	54.43	154.31	129.19	1787	54.80	155.35	128.15	1772
284	53.59	152.19	131.81	1823	53.95	153.23	130.77	1809	54.32	154.27	129.73	1794	54.68	155.30	128.70	1780
284.5	53.48	152.15	132.35	1830	53.84	153.19	131.31	1816	54.21	154.23	130.27	1802	54.57	155.26	129.24	1787
285	53.37	152.11	132.89	1838	53.74	153.15	131.85	1824	54.10	154.19	130.82	1809	54.46	155.22	129.78	1795
285.5	53.26	152.07	133.43	1845	53.63	153.11	132.39	1831	53.99	154.14	131.36	1817	54.35	155.18	130.32	1802
286	53.16	152.03	133.97	1853	53.52	153.07	132.93	1838	53.88	154.10	131.90	1824	54.24	155.14	130.86	1810
286.5	53.05	151.99	134.51	1860	53.41	153.02	133.48	1846	53.77	154.06	132.44	1832	54.14	155.10	131.40	1817
287	52.94	151.95	135.05	1868	53.30	152.98	134.02	1853	53.67	154.02	132.98	1839	54.03	155.06	131.94	1825
287.5	52.84	151.91	135.60	1875	53.20	152.94	134.56	1861	53.56	153.98	133.52	1847	53.92	155.02	132.48	1832
288	52.73	151.86	136.14	1883	53.09	152.90	135.10	1868	53.45	153.94	134.06	1854	53.81	154.98	133.02	1840
288.5	52.62	151.82	136.68	1890	52.98	152.86	135.64	1876	53.34	153.90	134.60	1862	53.70	154.94	133.56	1847
289	52.52	151.78	137.22	1898	52.88	152.82	136.18	1883	53.24	153.86	135.14	1869	53.60	154.89	134.11	1855
289.5	52.41	151.74	137.76	1905	52.77	152.78	136.72	1891	53.13	153.82	135.68	1877	53.49	154.85	134.65	1862
290	52.31	151.70	138.30	1913	52.67	152.74	137.26	1898	53.03	153.78	136.23	1884	53.38	154.81	135.19	1870
290.5	52.21	151.66	138.84	1920	52.56	152.70	137.80	1906	52.92	153.73	136.77	1891	53.28	154.77	135.73	1877
291	52.10	151.62	139.38	1928	52.46	152.66	138.34	1913	52.82	153.69	137.31	1899	53.17	154.73	136.27	1885
291.5	52.00	151.58	139.92	1935	52.35	152.61	138.89	1921	52.71	153.65	137.85	1906	53.07	154.69	136.81	1892
292	51.90	151.54	140.46	1943	52.25	152.57	139.43	1928	52.61	153.61	138.39	1914	52.96	154.65	137.35	1900
292.5	51.79	151.50	141.01	1950	52.15	152.53	139.97	1936	52.50	153.57	138.93	1921	52.86	154.61	137.89	1907
293	51.69	151.45	141.55	1958	52.04	152.49	140.51	1943	52.40	153.53	139.47	1929	52.75	154.57	138.43	1915
293.5	51.59	151.41	142.09	1965	51.94	152.45	141.05	1951	52.30	153.49	140.01	1936	52.65	154.53	138.97	1922
294	51.49	151.37	142.63	1973	51.84	152.41	141.59	1958	52.19	153.45	140.55	1944	52.55	154.48	139.52	1929
294.5	51.39	151.33	143.17	1980	51.74	152.37	142.13	1966	52.09	153.41	141.09	1951	52.44	154.44	140.06	1937
295	51.28	151.29	143.71	1988	51.64	152.33	142.67	1973	51.99	153.37	141.64	1959	52.34	154.40	140.60	1944
295.5	51.18	151.25	144.25	1995	51.54	152.29	143.21	1981	51.89	153.32	142.18	1966	52.24	154.36	141.14	1952
296	51.08	151.21	144.79	2002	51.43	152.25	143.75	1988	51.78	153.28	142.72	1974	52.14	154.32	141.68	1959
296.5	50.98	151.17	145.33	2010	51.33	152.20	144.30	1996	51.68	153.24	143.26	1981	52.03	154.28	142.22	1967
297	50.88	151.13	145.87	2017	51.23	152.16	144.84	2003	51.58	153.20	143.80	1989	51.93	154.24	142.76	1974
297.5	50.78	151.09	146.42	2025	51.13	152.12	145.38	2011	51.48	153.16	144.34	1996	51.83	154.20	143.30	1982
298	50.69	151.04	146.96	2032	51.03	152.08	145.92	2018	51.38	153.12	144.88	2004	51.73	154.16	143.84	1989
298.5	50.59	151.00	147.50	2040	50.93	152.04	146.46	2026	51.28	153.08	145.42	2011	51.63	154.12	144.38	1997
299	50.49	150.96	148.04	2047	50.84	152.00	147.00	2033	51.18	153.04	145.96	2019	51.53	154.07	144.93	2004
299.5	50.39	150.92	148.58	2055	50.74	151.96	147.54	2040	51.08	153.00	146.50	2026	51.43	154.03	145.47	2012
300	50.29	150.88	149.12	2062	50.64	151.92	148.08	2048	50.99	152.96	147.05	2034	51.33	153.99	146.01	2019
300.5	50.20	150.84	149.66	2070	50.54	151.88	148.62	2055	50.89	152.91	147.59	2041	51.23	153.95	146.55	2027
301	50.10	150.80	150.20	2077	50.44	151.84	149.16	2063	50.79	152.87	148.13	2049	51.13	153.91	147.09	2034
301.5	50.00	150.76	150.74	2085	50.35	151.79	149.71	2070	50.69	152.83	148.67	2056	51.03	153.87	147.63	2042
302	49.91	150.72	151.28	2092	50.25	151.75	150.25	2078	50.59	152.79	149.21	2064	50.94	153.83	148.17	2049
302.5	49.81	150.68	151.83	2100	50.15	151.71	150.79	2085	50.50	152.75	149.75	2071	50.84	153.79	148.71	2057
303	49.71	150.63	152.37	2107	50.06	151.67	151.33	2093	50.40	152.71	150.29	2079	50.74	153.75	149.25	2064
303.5	49.62	150.59	152.91	2115	49.96	151.63	151.87	2100	50.30	152.67	150.83	2086	50.64	153.71	149.79	2072
304	49.52	150.55	153.45	2122	49.86	151.59	152.41	2108	50.21	152.63	151.37	2093	50.55	153.66	150.34	2079
304.5	49.43	150.51	153.99	2130	49.77	151.55	152.95	2115	50.11	152.59	151.91	2101	50.45	153.62	150.88	2087
305	49.33	150.47	154.53	2137	49.67	151.51	153.49	2123	50.01	152.55	152.46	2108	50.35	153.58	151.42	2094
305.5	49.24	150.43	155.07	2145	49.58	151.47	154.03	2130	49.92	152.50	153.00	2116	50.26	153.54	151.96	2102
306	49.15	150.39	155.61	2152	49.49	151.43	154.57	2138	49.82	152.46	153.54	2123	50.16	153.50	152.50	2109
306.5	49.05	150.35	156.15	2160	49.39	151.38	155.12	2145	49.73	152.42	154.08	2131	50.07	153.46	153.04	2117
307	48.96	150.31	156.69	2167	49.30	151.34	155.66	2153	49.64	152.38	154.62	2138	49.97	153.42	153.58	2124
307.5	48.87	150.27	157.24	2175	49.20	151.30	156.20	2160	49.54	152.34	155.16	2146	49.88	153.38	154.12	2132
308	48.77	150.22	157.78	2182	49.11	151.26	156.74	2168	49.45	152.30	155.70	2153	49.78	153.34	154.66	2139
308.5	48.68	150.18	158.32	2190	49.02	151.22	157.28	2175	49.35	152.26	156.24	2161	49.69	153.30	155.20	2146
309	48.59	150.14	158.86	2197	48.93	151.18	157.82	2183	49.26	152.22	156.78	2168	49.60	153.25	155.75	2154
309.5	48.50	150.10	159.40	2204	48.83	151.14	158.36	2190	49.17	152.18	157.32	2176	49.50	153.21	156.29	2161
310	48.41	150.06	159.94	2212	48.74	151.10	158.90	2198	49.08	152.14	157.87	2183	49.41	153.17	156.83	2169
310.5	48.32	150.02	160.48	2219	48.65	151.06	159.44	2205	48.98	152.09	158.41	2191	49.32	153.13	157.37	2176
311	48.22	149.98	161.02	2227	48.56	151.02	159.98	2213	48.89	152.05	158.95	2198	49.23	153.09	157.91	2184
311.5	48.13	149.94	161.56	2234	48.47	150.97	160.53	2220	48.80	152.01	159.49	2206	49.13	153.05	158.45	2191

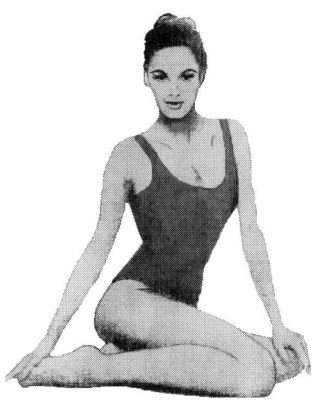

Special Weight Class—Male and Female

IF YOU are an adult, and if Body Composition Tables are not available for your weight and/or waist size, use the following sequence of formulas to calculate your:

1. Pounds of Lean Body Mass (LBM)
2. Pounds of Body Fat
3. Percentage Body Fat
4. Resting Metabolic Rate (RMR)

Pounds of Lean Body Mass (LBM):

(A) = Your Waist Size (Inches)
       Multiplied by 4.15
(B) = Your Body Weight (Pounds)
       Multiplied by 1.082
(B) − (A) = (C)
(C) + 98.42 (Male) = Pounds of LBM
(C) + 76.76 (Female) =   "   " LBM

example:
   30 inches x 4.15 = 124.5 (A)
   154 pounds x 1.082 = 166.628 (B)
   166.628 (B) − 124.5 (A) = 42.128 (C)
   42.128 (C) + 98.42 (Male) = 140.548*
                       pounds

Pounds of Body Fat:

Your Total Body Weight Minus Your Pounds of LBM.

example:
   154 − 140.548 = 13.452* pounds

Percentage Body Fat:

Divide Your Pounds of Body Fat by Your Total Body Weight and Multiply by 100.

example:
   (13.452 ÷ 154) x 100 = 8.735%*

Resting Metabolic Rate (RMR):

Multiply Your Pounds of LBM by 13.83 Calories.

example:
   140.548 x 13.83 = 1943.778** calories

---

* On the Body Composition Tables, this figure is rounded off to two decimal places.

** On the Body Composition Tables, this figure is rounded off to the nearest whole calorie.

Energy Balance Chart

MEASUREMENTS			BODY COMPOSITION			ENERGY OUTPUT				CALORIE INTAKE	
Date	Weight	Waist	Fat	Fat	LBM	RMR	+ Activity Calories		= Total	Diet	Net
Month/Day	Lb.	Inches	%	Lb.	Lb.	Calories	Aerobic	Anaerobic	Calories	Calories	+/-

MEASUREMENTS			BODY COMPOSITION			ENERGY OUTPUT				CALORIE INTAKE	
Date	Weight	Waist	Fat	Fat	LBM	RMR	+ Activity Calories		= Total	Diet	Net
Month/Day	Lb.	Inches	%	Lb.	Lb.	Calories	Aerobic	Anaerobic	Calories	Calories	+/-

<u>**Activity Intensity Levels:**</u>

Sedentary/Light .... **200–300 calories** *per day* (**dressing, eating, washing, etc.**)

Moderate .... **200 calories** *per hour* (**housework, slow walking, standing while using arms**)

Vigorous .... **300 calories** *per hour* (**brisk walking, 3.5 mph, 5.6 km/h**) *

Strenuous .... **400–500+ calories** *per hour* (**stop-and-go type sporting activities**)

                8 calories *per minute* (**weight lifting**)

Very Strenuous .... **600–1000+ calories** *per hour* (**cross country skiing, fast running**)

* **Calories** *per hour* **at 3.5 mph**
   = **2 x body weight**

Calories *per mile* **on foot**
(**walking, jogging, running**)
= **2 x body weight** ·/· **3.5**
   (·/· **5.6** *per kilometer*)

Energy Balance Chart

MEASUREMENTS			BODY COMPOSITION			ENERGY OUTPUT				CALORIE INTAKE	
Date	Weight	Waist	Fat	Fat	LBM	RMR	+ Activity Calories		= Total	Diet	Net
Month/Day	Lb.	Inches	%	Lb.	Lb.	Calories	Aerobic	Anaerobic	Calories	Calories	+/-

MEASUREMENTS			BODY COMPOSITION			ENERGY OUTPUT				CALORIE INTAKE	
Date	Weight	Waist	Fat	Fat	LBM	RMR	+ Activity Calories		= Total	Diet	Net
Month/Day	Lb.	Inches	%	Lb.	Lb.	Calories	Aerobic	Anaerobic	Calories	Calories	+/-

Activity Intensity Levels:
Sedentary/Light .... 200–300 calories *per day* (dressing, eating, washing, etc.)
Moderate .... 200 calories *per hour* (housework, slow walking, standing while using arms)
Vigorous .... 300 calories *per hour* (brisk walking, 3.5 mph, 5.6 km/h) *
Strenuous .... 400–500+ calories *per hour* (stop-and-go type sporting activities)
         8 calories *per minute* (weight lifting)
Very Strenuous .... 600–1000+ calories *per hour* (cross country skiing, fast running)

* Calories *per hour* at 3.5 mph
= 2 x body weight

Calories *per mile* on foot
(walking, jogging, running)
= 2 x body weight ·/· 3.5
(·/· 5.6 *per kilometer*)

Electronic Energy Balance Chart

IMAGINE: YOU stroll over to your personal computer, enter in your weight and waist size, and *presto*—your body composition information is automatically calculated. The monitor screen displays your:

Percentage Body Fat
Pounds of Body Fat
Pounds of Lean Body Mass
Resting Metabolic Rate

Enter in the number of calories from your daily activities, and your total Energy Output appears on the screen. Enter in the number of calories from your diet, and your Net Calorie Intake appears on the screen.

All you need to create your own Electronic Energy Balance Chart is a simple spreadsheet program and a personal computer. Lay out your chart on a spreadsheet as shown in the diagram below. Males require separate charts from females. Follow the instructions in your spreadsheet program manual and enter the following formulas onto your spreadsheet (round off your cell entries to 2 decimal places):

$F5 = (B5 * 1.082) - (C5 * 4.15) + 98.42$
 for males or $+ 76.76$ for females

$E5 = B5 - F5$

$D5 = (E5 / B5) * 100$

$G5 = F5 * 13.83$

$J5 = G5 + H5 + I(5)$

$L5 = K5 - J5$

NOTE: Numbers or error messages may appear in some columns after you enter these formulas, but this should not affect the accuracy of the spreadsheet.

OPTIONAL: Break down your energy output into requirements for grams of fat, protein and carbohydrates. For a diet containing 30% fat, 15% protein, and 55% carbohydrates, add 3 more columns, each with one of the following formulas:

Grams of fat $= J5 * (.3 / 9)$
Grams of protein $= J5 * (.15 / 4)$
Grams of carbohydrates $= J5 * (.55 / 4)$

To automatically convert distance covered on foot into calories: Add a column to enter distance (miles or kilometers). Add another column with the following formula to convert distance into calories:

Calories $=$ distance cell $* (B5 +$ pounds of clothing) $*$ $(2 / 3.5$ for miles or $2 / 5.6$ for kilometers.)

Add these calories to your energy output, J5.

	A	B	C	D	E	F	G	H	I	J	K	L
1	*ENERGY BALANCE CHART MALE*											
2	MEASUREMENTS			BODY COMPOSITION			ENERGY OUTPUT				CALORIE INTAKE	
3	Date	Weight	Waist	Fat	Fat	LBM	RMR	+ Activity Calories		= Total	Diet	Net
4	Month/Day	Lb.	Inches	%	Lb.	Lb.	Calories	Aerobic	Anaerobic	Calories	Calories	+/-
5												
6												
7												
8												
9												
10												
11												

(Values are approximate for edible portions.) *Food CalorieTable* Based on U.S. Dept. of Agriculture's Home and Garden Bulletin, No. 72: Nutritive Value of Foods.

Fruit		Cal.
Apple	2^{3}/$_{4}$" diameter	80
Apple juice	1 cup	115
Applesauce	1 cup unsweetened	105
Apricot	3 medium	50
Avocado	1 medium	305
Banana	1	105
Blueberries	1 cup	80
Cantaloupe	^{1}/$_{2}$ of 5" diameter	95
Cherries	1 cup	90
Dates	10	230
Grapefruit	^{1}/$_{2}$	40
Grapes, green	1 cup	90
Honeydew	6^{1}/$_{2}$" wedge	45
Kiwi	1	45
Mango	4 ounces	75
Nectarine	1	75
Orange	1 medium	70
Orange juice	1 cup	105
Papaya	4 ounces	45
Peach	1 medium	50
Pear	1	100
Pineapple	8 ounces	60
Pineapple juice	4 ounces	60
Plum	1	30
Prunes	2 ounces	130
Raisins	^{1}/$_{4}$ cup	120
Raspberries	1 cup	70
Strawberries	1 cup	55
Tangerine	1 medium	37
Watermelon	4" x 8"	155

Vegetables		Cal.
Artichoke	1 medium	50
Asparagus	4 ounces	20
Beets	4 ounces	35
Beet greens	1 cup	25
Broccoli	4 ounces	30
Brussel sprouts	1 cup	50
Cabbage, raw	1 cup	25
Carrot	1	30
Cauliflower, raw	1 cup	30
Celery	1 stalk	5
Collard greens	1 cup	25
Corn, on cob	1 ear	85
Corn, kernels	1 cup	165
Cucumber	8"	15
Dandelion	4 ounces	50

Vegetables		Cal.
Eggplant	1 cup	25
Endive/Escarole	1 cup	10
Green beans	4 ounces	40
Kale, raw	1 cup	40
Leeks	^{1}/$_{2}$ cup	16
Lettuce, head	1 cup	15
Lettuce, romaine	4 ounces	25
Mushrooms	^{1}/$_{2}$ cup	9
Okra	1 cup	50
Onions, green	6 small	25
Onions, white, raw	4 ounces	40
Parsnips	1 cup	95
Peas	1 cup	125
Pepper, sweet green	1 medium	20
Pepper, sweet red	1 medium	25
Potato, baked	4 ounces	125
Potato chips	10	105
Potato, French fried	6	100
Potato, mashed	^{1}/$_{2}$ cup	90
Potato salad	1 cup	360
Potato, sweet	5 ounces	200
Pumpkin	1 cup	50
Radishes	4 small	8
Sauerkraut	1 cup	45
Spinach	1 cup	10
Squash, summer	^{1}/$_{2}$ cup	55
Squash, winter	^{1}/$_{2}$ cup	45
Squash, zucchini	1 cup	40
Tomato	1 medium	20
Turnips	1 cup	55
Turnip greens	1 cup	45
Watercress	4 ounces	25

Legumes, Nuts		Cal.
Almonds, shelled	1 cup	795
Beans, lima	1 cup	260
Beans, navy	1 cup	225
Beans, kidney	1 cup	230
Brazil nut, shelled	1 ounce	185
Cashews, raw	^{1}/$_{4}$ cup	196
Chestnuts, shelled	1 cup	350
Chickpeas	1 cup	270
Coconut, shelled	2" x 2" x ^{1}/$_{2}$"	160
Coconut, dried	1 cup	410
Filberts, shelled	1 ounce	180
Lentils	1 cup	215
Macadamias	1 ounce	196

(Values are approximate for edible portions.)

Legumes, Nuts		Cal.
Peanuts, shelled	1 ounce	160
Peanut butter	1 tablespoon	95
Peas, raw	1/2 cup	58
Pecans, halves	1 ounce	190
Pine nuts	1 ounce	160
Pistachios, shelled	1 ounce	165
Pumpkin seeds	1 ounce	155
Sesame seeds, hulled	1 tablespoon	45
Sesame butter	1 tablespoon	95
Soybeans	1 cup	235
Sprouts, mung	4 ounces	36
Sprouts, soybean	4 ounces	40
Sprouts, alfalfa	4 ounces	32
Sunflower seeds	1 ounce	160
Tofu, raw	1/2 cup	94
Walnut pieces	1 ounce	180

Cereals, Grains		Cal.
Bagel	1 medium	165
Barley	4 ounces	390
Biscuit	1 medium	90
Bran flakes	1 cup	105
Bread crumbs	1 cup	340
Bread, French	1 slice	70
Bread, Italian	1 slice	70
Bread, pita	1	80
Bread, pumpernickel	1 slice	70
Bread, rye	1 slice	50
Bread, whole wheat	1 slice	60
Bread, white	1 slice	70
Corn flakes	1 cup	100
Corn grits	1 cup	125
Croutons	6	35
Farina	1 cup	100
French toast	1 slice	130
Granola	1 cup	225
Melba toast	1 slice	30
Muffin, bran	1 medium	150
Muffin, corn	1 medium	130
Muffin, English	1	150
Oatmeal, cooked	1 cup	150
Pancake	4"	60
Pasta, cooked	1 cup	190
Popcorn	1 cup	55
Rice cake	1	35
Rice, white, cooked	1/2 cup	100
Rice, brown	1/2 cup	110

Cereals, Grains		Cal.
Rice, wild	1/2 cup	85
Roll, hamburger	1	120
Roll, hot dog	1	160
Roll, onion	1	130
Wheat, cream of	1/2 cup	65
Wheat germ	1/2 cup	220

Fats, Dressings		
Butter, regular	1 tablespoon	102
Butter, whipped	1 tablespoon	65
Catsup	1 tablespoon	15
Dressing, 1000 Island	1 tablespoon	80
Dressing, French	1 tablespoon	65
Dressing, Italian	1 tablespoon	50
Dressing, low-calorie	1 tablespoon	15
Hollandaise sauce	1 cup	240
Margarine, regular	1 tablespoon	102
Margarine, whipped	1 tablespoon	68
Mayonnaise	1 tablespoon	100
Mustard	1 teaspoon	5
Vegetable shortening	1 tablespoon	110
Vegetable oil	1 tablespoon	120

Mixed Dishes		
Beef chop suey	1 cup	300
Chesseburger	1 med.	300
Cheeseburger, 1/4 lb.	1	525
Chili con carne	1 cup	340
Egg muffin sandwich	1 medium	280
Fish filet sandwich	1 medium	370
Hamburger	1 medium	245
Hamburger, 1/4 lb.	1	445
Pasta & meatballs	1 cup	330
Pizza, cheese	1/8 of 15" pie	290
Quiche Lorraine	1/8 of 8" dish	600
Roast beef sandwich	1 medium	345
Soup, chicken noodle	1 cup	75
Soup, clam chowder	1 cup	165
Soup, cream of tomato	1 cup	160
Soup, vegetable beef	1 cup	80
Taco	1 medium	183

Sweets, Desserts		
Cake, angel food	1/12	140
Cake, cheese	1/8	250
Cake, chocolate	1/8	270
Cake, strawberry short	1/14	270

(Values are approximate for edible portions.)

Sweets, Desserts

		Cal.
Candy, chocolate	1 ounce	145
Cookie, chocolate chip	1	60
Donut, plain	1	190
Ice cream, vanilla	1/2 cup	150
Ice milk	1/2 cup	95
Frozen yogurt	1/2 cup	105
Jam	1 tablespoon	55
Pie, fruit-filled	1/8 regular	300
Pie, lemon meringue	1/8 regular	275
Pie, pecan	1/8 regular	430
Pudding, chocolate	1/2 cup	200
Pudding, custard	1 cup	305
Sugar	1 tablespoon	45
Syrup, chocolate	1 tablespoon	47
Syrup, corn/maple	1 tablespoon	60

Beverages

Beer	12 ounces	160
Cola	12 ounces	144
Cocoa	8 ounces	250
Coffee, black	6 ounces	4
Ginger ale	12 ounces	115
Tea, black	8 ounces	1
Tomato juice	6 ounces	35
Wine, dry	4 ounces	100
Wine, sweet	4 ounces	160

Meat, Poultry, Fish

Bacon	3 strips	100
Bacon, Canadian	2 ounces	155
Bluefish	4 ounces	130
Bologna	2 ounces	165
Chicken breast	3 ounce fillet	140
Chicken breast, battered	4.9 ounces	365
Chicken leg	1.6 ounces meat	75
Chicken leg, battered	2.5 ounces	195
Chicken liver	4 ounces	185
Chicken pot pie	4 ounces	350
Chicken salad	1.9 ounces	90
Clams	6	100
Cod fish cakes	4 ounces	185
Corned beef	4 ounces	250
Crab meat	4 ounces	100
Duck, roast	4 ounces	190
Filet mignon	4 ounces	250
Frankurter	1 regular	180
Ground beef	4 ounces	320

Meat, Poultry, Fish

		Cal.
Ham, Virginia	4 ounces	300
Lamb chop	1	385
Leg of lamb	4 ounces	217
Liver, broiled	4 ounces	290
Lobster meat	4 ounces	111
Pork chop	1	275
Pork sausage	1 ounce	130
Roast beef	4 ounces	198
Salami	1 ounce	120
Salmon, baked	3 ounces	140
Salmon, smoked	3 ounces	150
Scallops	4 ounces	140
Shrimp	3 ounces	100
Sirloin steak	4 ounces	229
Spareribs	6	505
Tuna, in oil	3 ounces	165
Tuna, in water	3 ounces	135
Tuna salad	1.9 ounces	80
Turkey, dark meat	4 ounces	320
Turkey, white meat	4 ounces	200
Veal chop	1	260

Dairy, Eggs

Cheese, cheddar	1 ounce	120
Cheese, cottage	4 ounces	110
Cheese, cottage, skim	4 ounces	90
Cheese, cream	1 ounce	100
Cheese, feta	1 ounce	75
Cheese, process	1 ounce	100
Cheese, ricotta	1 cup	430
Cheese, ricotta, skim	1 cup	340
Cheese, Swiss	1 ounce	105
Cream, coffee	1 tablespoon	29
Cream, half & half	1 tablespoon	20
Cream, heavywhip	1 tablespoon	26
Cream, lightwhip	1 tablespoon	22
Cream, sour	1 tablespoon	25
Egg	1 large	80
Egg white	1 large	15
Egg yolk	1 large	65
Milk, buttermilk	1 cup	100
Milk, skim	1 cup	85
Milk, whole	1 cup	150
Omelet, cheese	2 eggs	260
Yogurt, fruit-flavor	1 cup	230
Yogurt, low-fat	1 cup	127
Yogurt, whole	1 cup	140

Activity Calorie Table

ACTIVITY	CALORIES per hour (Approximate for 150 lb. person)
Automobile driving	140
Bicycling (slow, 6 mph)	300
Bicycling (medium, 8 mph)	400
Bicycling (fast)	600
Bowling	250
Calisthenics	350
Golf (no cart)	360
Housework (moderate)	200
Ice/Roller Skating	420
Jogging (5 mph)*	430
Rowing (slow)	400
Running (6 mph)*	515
Skiing (downhill)	450
Skiing (cross country)	1200
Squash	550
Swimming (medium)	400
Tennis (singles)	450
Tennis (doubles)	350
Walking (slow, 2 mph)*	170
Walking (medium, 3 mph)*	260
Walking (fast, 5 mph)*	430
Weight Lifting	480

See page 302 for metric conversion

Activity Intensity Levels:
Sedentary/Light .... 200–300 calories *per day* (dressing, eating, washing, etc.)
Moderate .... 200 calories *per hour* (housework, slow walking, standing while using arms)
Vigorous .... 300 calories *per hour* (brisk walking, 3.5 mph, 5.6 km/h) **
Strenuous .... 400–500+ calories *per hour* (stop-and-go type sporting activities)
　　　　　　　　　 8 calories *per minute* (weight lifting)
Very Strenuous .... 600–1000+ calories *per hour* (cross country skiing, fast running)

* Calories *per mile* on foot (walking, jogging, running) = 2 x body weight ·/· 3.5 (·/· 5.6 *per kilometer*)

** Calories *per hour* at 3.5 mph = 2 x body weight

Standard Measurement Table
North American

MASS
1 ounce = 28.35 grams
1 pound = 16 ounces = 453.59 grams
1 kilogram = 2.2 pounds = 35.27 ounces = 1000 grams

VOLUME (Dry)
1 tablespoon = 3 teaspoons
1 cup = 16 tablespoons
1 pint = 2 cups = 32 tablespoons

VOLUME (Water)
1 fluid ounce = 2 tablespoons = 30 milliliters
1 cup = 8 fluid ounces = 16 tablespoons = 240 milliliters
1 pint = 16 fluid ounces
1 quart = 2 pints = 32 fluid ounces = .946 liters
1 gallon (8 pounds) = 4 quarts = 128 fluid ounces = 3.785 liters
1 liter = 1000 milliliters

LINEAR
1 inch = 2.54 centimeters
1 metre = 39.37 inches
1 mile = 1.6 kilometers

Glossary

Activity intensity levels   sedentary, light, moderate, vigorous, strenuous.

Adipose tissue   body tissue that stores fat.

Adult-onset diabetes   later-life disturbance in the utilization of blood glucose.

Adrenal glands   secrete hormones, including fight-or-flight hormones and cortisol.

Aerobic activity   activity that uses oxygen to burn fat for energy.

Amino acids   building blocks of protein.

Anaphylaxis   allergic blood-hypersensitivity.

Anaerobic activity   activity that burns glycogen for energy without using oxygen.

Anorexia nervosa   eating disorder based on the obsession to be thin.

Anthropometry   the science of measuring the human body.

Arthritis   bone joint disease.

Atherosclerosis   hardening of the arteries.

Bioelectrical impedance   test for body fat using electric current.

Biosynthesis   the creation of new tissue in the body.

Body composition   combination of body fat and lean body mass.

Body fat   fat stored in the body's tissues.

Body Mass Index   health tables based on weight and height.

Body weight   total combined weight of body fat and lean body mass.

Bodybuilding   training to increase muscular development.

Buffalo torso   body fat redistributed into upper back, neck and abdomen.

Bulimia   eating disorder based on purging.

Caffeine   habituating drug in coffee, cola, chocolate (theobromine) and tea (theine).

Calorie intake   amount of calories in the food eaten.

Calorie   unit of heat used to measure energy.

Carbohydrate   starch or sugar food that supplies energy to the body.

Carnivore   meat-eating organism.

Cellulite   puckering layer of body fat.

Chlorophyll   green pigment in plants that helps build blood.

Cholesterol   steroid lipid in blood—level indicates risk of circulatory disease.

Comparative anatomy   human anatomy compared to animals.

Coronary occlusion   obstruction of artery to the heart.

Cortisol   adrenal hormone that regulates mobilization of body fat.

Crash diet   sacrificing muscle to lose weight quickly—quick fix diet.

Crunch   abdominal exercise—sit-up with knees bent.

Cushing's syndrome   changed body appearance due to excessive cortisol secretion.

Deadlift   exercise for lower back, legs, hips and buttocks.

Dietary fat   fat found in food.

Dietary fiber found in unrefined foods—regulates digestion.

Distilled water pure, uncontaminated water.

Ectomorph narrow and thin body type.

Endomorph soft and wide body type.

Energy balance balance between energy output and calorie intake.

Energy output total amount of calories burned from activity plus RMR.

Essential body fat permanent fat in cell membranes, nerves and around organs.

Essential dietary fat type of fat that must be obtained from food.

Fasting no intake of food—just water.

Fight-or-flight hormones prepares your body for defensive action.

Fluid retention excess liquid held in body tissues.

Food addiction uncontrollable urge to eat food.

Freehand exercise resistance exercise that does not require equipment.

Fructose sugar found in fruit.

Frugivore fruit-eating organism.

Galactose natural sugar found in milk.

Gastrointestinal tract the stomach, small intestines and large intestines.

Glucose sugar found in carbohydrates—also in the blood.

Gluconeogenesis body tissue used as source of glucose.

Glucostat monitors blood glucose.

Glutes gluteal muscles—buttocks.

Glycogen starch stored in muscle—fuel for anaerobic activity.

HDL high-density lipoprotein—transports cholesterol out of circulation.

Hormones secreted by glands to regulate the body.

Hydrogenation saturating fat with hydrogen molecules. Creates trans—fatty-acids.

Hydrostatic weighing water-immersion body fat test

Hyperglycemia elevated blood sugar.

Hypertension high blood pressure.

Intramuscular within the muscle.

Isometric muscle contraction without limb motion.

Labile protein protein easily broken down and replaced by the body.

LBM lean body mass.

LDL low-density lipoprotein—transports cholesterol into circulation.

Lean body mass includes muscle, bone, blood, organs.

Mediterranean diet low animal-protein diet of southern Europe.

Mesomorph muscular and strong body type.

Metabolism all the processes that build up the body and remove waste.

Metabolic acids waste products of metabolism.

Midriff area of abdomen above waist.

Minerals food substances that build and regulate the body.

Monosaccharides simple sugars in food—also from digested starch.

Monounsaturated fat in peanuts, olives, avocados and nuts.

Moon face body fat redistributed into face.

Negative calorie balance energy output is greater than calorie intake.

Net calorie intake — the difference in calories (+ or −) between calorie intake and energy output.

Neutral calorie balance — calorie intake equals energy output.

Nicotine — addictive drug in tobacco.

Obesity — 20% over ideal body weight.

Osteoarthritis — worn away bone cartilage.

Overcompensation — extra replenishment following exercise—new growth.

Perceived rate of exertion — judging the intensity of activity by "feel."

Percentage body fat — percent of total body weight that is fat.

Pernicious anemia — caused by disturbance of vitamin B_{12} usage.

pH — the acid/alkaline balance of the body's fluids.

Polyunsaturated fat — found mainly in plant foods.

Positive calorie balance — calorie intake is greater than energy output.

Premenstrual syndrome — bloating, cramping and other symptoms in menstrual cycle.

Protein — main nutrient that builds the body.

Recovery — replenishment of body nutrients after activity.

Resistance — force applied against muscle in exercise.

Resistance (organic) — the power of the body to overcome damaging agents.

Resting metabolic rate — calories burned by lean body mass at rest.

RMR — resting metabolic rate.

Salt — sodium chloride—causes water retention.

Saturated fat — found mainly in animal foods and processed foods.

Serotonin — brain neurotransmitter.

Skeletal frame — large-, medium-, or small-boned.

Skeletal muscle — muscle attached to bone.

Skin-fold calipers — a device to measure body fat in a fold of skin.

Spot reducing — exercise to shrink body part—burns muscle, not body fat.

Squat — lower-body exercise—deep knee-bend.

Steroids — drugs that increase intramuscular weight.

Strain-gage scale — computerized electronic scale.

Structural proteins — proteins that are permanent part of body structure.

Subcutaneous body fat — body fat stored under skin.

Suppression — reducing symptoms by weakening the body's resistance.

Taste buds — sensory nerve receptors in the mouth.

Testosterone — male sex hormone.

Thromboembolic disease — blood vessel blocked by detached blood clot—causes heart attack or stroke.

Toleration — accommodation of damaging agents within the body.

Toning — shaping and firming muscle.

Vacuum — exercise for internal abdomen.

Vegan — strict vegetarian diet with no animal foods.

Vitamins — food substances that regulate nutrition.

Waistline — located at level of navel.

Waist-to-hip ratio — waist size divided by hip size—above .80 is health risk.

Weigh-in — scheduled time to weigh and measure the body.

Bibliography

"Adults Still Too Fat." Associated Press. February 6, 1996.

Altman, Nathaniel. *Eating For Life, A Book About Vegetarianism.* Wheaton, Illinois: The Theosophical Publishing House, 1973.

Bailey, Covert. *The New Fit Or Fat.* Boston, Massachusetts: Houghton Mifflin, 1991.

———————— *Smart Exercise.* Boston, Massachusetts: Houghton Mifflin, 1994 .

Barnard, Neal D. *"T. Colin Campbell, Ph.D."* Health Science. January/February 1995, p.8.

Bass, Clarence. *Ripped, The Sensible Way To Achieve Ultimate Muscularity.* Albuquerque, New Mexico: Clarence Bass' Ripped Enterprises, 1980.

Clarke, David H. *Exercise Physiology.* Englewood Cliffs, New Jersey: Prentice-Hall Inc., 1975.

Darden, Ellington, Ph.D. *Big: Bulkbuilding Instructional Guide.* New York, New York: Perigee Books, 1990.

"Diet and Disease: The China Study." Health Science. September/October 1992, p.6.

Edgren, Gretchen. *The Playmate Book: Five Decades Of Centerfolds.* Los Angeles, California: General Publishing Group, 1996

Everson, Cory, et al. *Cory Everson's Fat-Free & Fit.* New York, New York: Perigee Books, 1994.

"Factors You Can Control That Affect Cholesterol Levels." Health Science. July/August 1991, p.8.

"Find Your % Body Fat." Muscle And Health. Spring 1993, p.28.

Fry, T.C. *Program For Dynamic Health.* Chicago, Illinois: Natural Hygiene Press, 1974.

Grunwald, Lisa. *"Do I Look Fat To You?"* Life. February 1995, p.58.

Haney, Lee, et al. *Lee Haney's Ultimate Bodybuilding.* New York, New York: St. Martin's Press, 1993.

Heritage, Ford, BS., M.E. *Composition And Facts About Food.* Mokelumne Hill, California: Health Research, 1971.

"Inflammation May Be Major Factor In Heart Disease, Strokes." Washington Post. April, 1997.

Jordan., et al. *Eating Is Okay, The Behavioral Control Diet.* New York, New York: Signet, 1976.

Kapit, Wynn, et al. *The Physiology Coloring Book.* New York, New York: Harper & Row, 1987.

Kenton, Leslie, et al. *Raw Energy.* London, England: Arrow Books, 1987.

Kreutler, Patricia A., Ph.D. *Nutrition In Perspective.* Englewood Cliffs, New Jersey: Prentice-Hall, 1980.

Kumer, Vinay, et al. *Basic Pathology.* Philadelphia, Pennsylvania: W. B. Saunders Company, 1992.

Kurzweil, Raymond. *The 10% Solution For A Healthy Life.* New York, New York: Crown Publishers, 1993.

Lorey, Nicole Garris. *"Lipo: Permanent Fat Loss Or Quick Fix?"* Vie. May 1996.

Lüllmann, Heinz, et al. *Color Atlas Of Pharmacology.* New York, New York: Theime Medical Publishers, 1993.

Myers, Clayton R. *The Official YMCA Physical Fitness Handbook.* New York: Popular Library, 1975.

Kraus, Barbara. *Calorie Guide To Brand Names And Basic Foods.* New York, New York: Signet, 1996.

Olinekova, Gayle. *Go For It.* New York, New York: Fireside/ Simon And Schuster, 1982.

Ornish, Dean, M.D. *Dr. Dean Ornish's Program For Reversing Heart Disease.* New York, New York: Ballantine Books, 1990.

Parrillio, John. *The Parrillo Performance BodyStat Manual.* Cincinnati, Ohio: Parrillo Performance, 1989-90.

Peele, Stanton. *Love And Addiction.* New York, New York: Signet, 1976.

"Red Meat, All Alcohol Make Cancer Group's Hit List." Associated Press. September, 1996.

Schiffer, Claudia. *Memories.* London, England: Mandarin Hardback, 1995.

Schwarzenegger, Arnold. *Encyclopedia Of Modern Bodybuilding.* New York, New York: Fireside/Simon And Schuster, 1985.

———————— *Arnold's Bodybuilding For Men.* New York, New York: Simon And Schuster, 1981.

Shelton, Herbert M. *Exercise!* Chicaco, Illinois: Natural Hygiene Press, 1971.

——————— *Health For The Millions.* Chicago, Illinois: Natural Hygiene Press, 1969.

——————— *Human Beauty: Its Culture And Hygiene.* San Antonio, Texas: Dr. Shelton's Health School, 1958.

——————— *The Hygienic System, Vol. 2, Orthotrophy.* San Antonio, Texas: Dr. Shelton's Health School, 1975.

——————— *The Science And Fine Art Of Fasting; The Hygienic System, Vol. 3.* Tampa, Florida: Natural Hygiene Press, 1993.

Taber, Clarence Wilbur. *Taber's Cyclopedic Medical Dictionary.* Philadelphia, Pennsylvania: F. A. Davis Company, 1989.

Tant, Lisa. *"The Runway Vs. Reality."* Southham Newspapers. August 22, 1996.

Van De Graaff, Kent M. *Human Anatomy.* Dubuque, Iowa: Wm. C. Brown Publishers, 1992.

Vander, Arthur J., M.D., et al. *Human Physiology.* New York, New York: McGraw-Hill Publishing Company, 1990.

Vetrano, Virginia. *"The Vitamin B_{12} Hoax."* Dr. Shelton's Hygienic Review. August 1979, p. 353.

Viccellio, Peter, M.D. *Handbook Of Medical Toxicology.* Boston/ Toronto/ London: Little, Brown And Company, 1993.

Young, Frank Rudolph, D.C. *Yoga For Men Only.* West Nyack, New York: Parker Publishing Company, Inc., 1969.

Zane, Frank and Christine. *The Zane Way To A Beautiful Body.* New York, New York: Simon And Schuster, 1979.

Suggested Reading

In addition to the books listed in the Bibliography, the following are recommended:

- A catalogue of books, audiotapes and videotapes on health topics, such as natural foods, food combining, fasting, exercise, and vegetarianism, may be ordered from:

  The American Natural Hygiene Society
  P.O. Box 30630
  Tampa, Florida, USA 33630
  Phone (813) 855-6607

To analyze your diet on your computer:

- Expert Software carries a *Diet Expert* program. Contact:
  N-Squared Computing
  3040 Commercial St. SE
  Suite 240
  Salem, OR, USA 97302
  Phone (503) 364-9118

- Cory Everson has a multimedia CD called *Body, Mind and Soul* that contains a full diet and exercise guide. Contact:
  Philips Media Inc. and
  Primal Media Corporation
  10960 Wilshire Blvd.
  Los Angeles, CA, USA 90024
  Catalog No: 31069 1069–2 BK01

Calorie books include:
- Barbara Kraus.
  Calorie Guide To Brand Names & Basic Foods. Contact:
  Penguin USA
  P.O. Box 999—Dept. #17109
  Bergenfield, New Jersey, USA 07621

- Corinne T. Netzer.
  The Corinne T. Netzer Calorie Counter. Contact:
  Dell Readers Service
  Box DR
  1540 Broadway
  New York, NY, USA 10036

Index

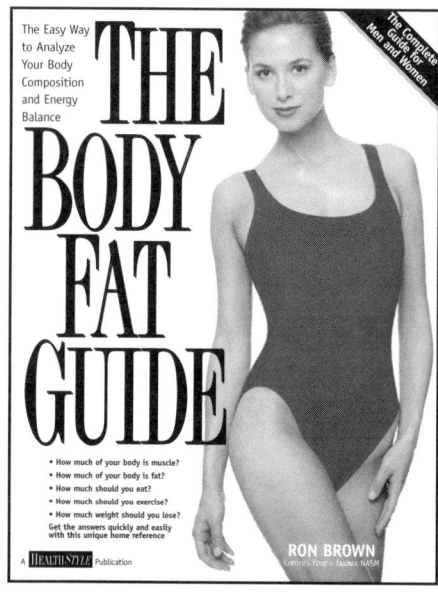 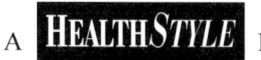